Mental Health Nursing

A Holistic Approach

Mental Health Nursing

A Holistic Approach

ELAINE ANNE PASQUALI, R.N., Ph.D.

Professor, Adelphi University
Garden City, New York
Anthropologist; Volunteer Therapist in a community mental
health day treatment program; Consultant; Humor Therapist

HELEN MARGARET ARNOLD, R.N., Ph.D., C.S.

Professor, Adelphi University
Garden City, New York
Holder of postdoctoral certificate in psychoanalysis and
psychotherapy; Derner Institute of Advanced Psychological
Studies

NANCY DeBASIO, R.N., Ph.D.

Associate Dean for Academic Affairs
and Associate Professor
Research College of Nursing—Rockhurst College
Kansas City, Missouri

THIRD EDITION

The C. V. Mosby Company

ST. LOUIS · BALTIMORE · TORONTO   1989

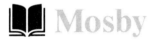

Editor: Linda L. Duncan
Assistant editor: Joanna May
Project editor: Teri Merchant
Cover and book design: Gail Morey Hudson
Editing and production: Cracom Corporation

THIRD EDITION

Copyright © 1989 by The C.V. Mosby Company

Previous editions copyrighted 1981, 1985

Printed in the United States of America

The C.V. Mosby Company
11830 Westline Industrial Drive, St. Louis, Missouri 63146

Library of Congress Cataloging in Publication Data

Pasquali, Elaine Anne
    Mental health nursing.

    Rev. ed. of: Mental health nursing / Elaine Anne Pasquali . . . [et al.]. end ed. 1985.
    Includes bibliographies and index.
    1. Psychiatric nursing.   I. Arnold, Helen Margaret.
II. DeBasio, Nancy.   III. Title. [DNLM: 1. Psychiatric Nursing. WY 160 P284m]
RC440.P362   1989   610.73'68   88-31403
ISBN 0-8016-3578-0

TS/VH/VH   9 8 7 6 5 4 3 2

To our families with love, affection, and appreciation.

Elaine Anne Pasquali
Helen Margaret Arnold
Nancy DeBasio

Preface

What is mental health? What is mental illness? When is a person ill enough to require treatment? These questions have long concerned society in general and mental health practitioners in particular. Of all mental health workers, nurses are in the best position to become actively involved in a broad range of mental health care activities. In primary prevention roles, nurses provide health education and perform health promotion activities. In secondary prevention roles, nurses play an important and integral part in identifying health care needs and providing therapeutic care. In tertiary prevention roles, nurses help reduce the severity and limitations of disabilities and are actively involved in rehabilitation.

The concepts and skills of mental health nursing are not limited to any particular practice setting. Staff nurses, nurse practitioners, community health nurses, industrial nurses, and nurse educators may all actively participate in the promotion of mental health. The health education and emotional support that nurses offer to persons facing maturational and situational stress help these persons mobilize resources, resolve crises, and maintain emotional stability. When mental illness does develop, it is often these same nurses who recognize the early signs of maladaptive behavior or emotional distress and help the involved individuals obtain early treatment. At this point, these clients may come into contact with psychiatric nurses, who may then assume a vital role in all aspects of treatment. Later, community mental health nurses may help the clients reestablish family and social networks and reassume social roles. Regardless of whether nurses function in psychiatric settings or other health care settings, they may be engaged in a variety of activities that serve to promote and restore mental health.

PHILOSOPHICAL APPROACH

This book advocates an eclectic and holistic systems approach to mental health nursing. It is our belief that no one theory or model can provide a complete basis for understanding all aspects of human functioning or the complexities of human behavior. We believe further that anyone practicing mental health nursing must acknowledge, identify, and explore the many interrelationships among biological, psychological, intellectual, spiritual, and sociocultural dimensions of behavior.

Although many nurses conceptually agree with this approach, most textbooks and many nurses in practice tend to emphasize a particular dimension to the minimization or exclusion of others. To fail to recognize all the dimensions of behavior and their interrelationships, however, is to fail to address the primary objectives of mental health nursing

1. Promotion of mental health
2. Intervention in mental illness
3. Restoration of mental health

Drawing on a variety of theories and concepts from a number of sources, this book develops a theoretical framework that examines and integrates concepts and skills involving all the dimensions of behavior.

Rather than emphasizing only theory, however, this holistic systems approach focuses on *people* and on the myriad interrelated factors that both affect and are affected by them. Nursing should not be hospital oriented or community oriented but *people oriented*. Because people—their behavior and the reasons for their behavior—are the focus of mental health nursing, nurses must learn to view and understand the ways in which people interrelate within a wide social field. By using the nursing process, nurses can endeavor to promote healthy behavior, sustain people during stress-producing situations, intervene during maladaptive behavior, and restore adaptive behavior.

The major objectives of this book are to provide a theoretical background for the understanding of human coping with stress and crisis and to present a basis for therapeutic intervention designed to promote, maintain, or restore mental health. In keeping with the holistic, humanistic philosophy of nursing and the belief that mental health nursing is an integral part of all nursing as well as a specialized area of professional practice, this book emphasizes nursing interventions both for persons who are coping with physical illness and injury and for individuals with psychiatric disorders. Attention is also given to the functions of the nurse as a collaborative member of the mental health team and to the social forces of power and politics as they relate to mental health nursing.

ORGANIZATION AND COVERAGE

Building on the strengths of the first and second editions, this book has been logically and cohesively organized to provide

1. A theoretical framework for understanding human behavior
2. A historical perspective on mental health nursing
3. An understanding of political and other forms of power inherent in the health care system and the nursing profession
4. A theoretical foundation for understanding and practicing psychiatric nursing
5. An understanding of how people cope with stress
6. A framework and methods for the implementation of the nursing process in primary, secondary, and tertiary prevention

An introduction and three new chapters have been added to expand the book's coverage and provide for a more in-depth exploration of pertinent issues and topics in mental health nursing. The following

is a brief description of the organization, the new chapters, and other expanded coverage.

Introduction: The Student Experience, new to this edition, has been added in an effort to acknowledge and allay students' fears as they begin their mental health experience. Unit 1, The Domain of Mental Health Nursing, consists of three chapters that provide the reader with an orientation to mental health nursing. Chapter 1, Framework for Mental Health Nursing Practice, defines mental health, mental illness, and mental health nursing and presents the holistic and eclectic theoretical framework used and further developed throughout the book. Selected nursing theories with a systems focus and their application to mental health nursing are explored. The concepts of primary, secondary, and tertiary prevention are also presented—as part of a systems-theory approach—along with a discussion of how these concepts can be used as an organizing framework for nursing intervention. Discussion of the biological basis for mental illness has been expanded, reflecting the most current research and focus in both psychiatry and mental health nursing. Chapter 2, Historical Overview of Psychiatric Nursing, examines historical aspects of psychiatry and psychiatric nursing and considers their influence on contemporary nursing practice. Focusing on contemporary nursing practice, Chapter 3, Power, Politics, and Psychiatric Nursing, provides both a theoretical and a practical basis for understanding the political forces that are inherent in any situation in which groups of people work together. Describing strategies for utilizing power and political action to promote mental health, this chapter also discusses the roles of the nurse as client advocate and change agent.

Unit 2, Concepts Basic to Understanding Behavior and to Nursing Intervention, explores in depth the fundamental concepts of mental health nursing. Because the ways in which people perceive and respond to stress and to health problems are culturally influenced, Chapter 4, The Sociocultural Context of Behavior, introduces theories that provide a foundation for understanding enculturation and acculturation. Sociocultural influences related to stress and coping are explored, as are theories that provide approaches to understanding and assessing ethnic or cultural factors in relation to health care.

The discrepancies that may exist between the cultural values of a client and those of a health care provider are also discussed. A section on attitude clarification explores how a professional nurse's own cultural and ethnic values may affect the nurse-client relationship. This section also explores the influence of the nurse's self-awareness and self-understanding on the therapeutic interpersonal process between nurse and client.

Chapter 5, The Family, investigates the many factors that influence the composition, form, and dynamics of the family. The family is viewed as a social system whose effective functioning depends not only on internal variables but also on the family's relationship with the social, cultural, emotional, and physical environment.

Experiences early in life have a major influence on the ways in which each of us perceives and copes with the stress caused by anxiety, fear, frustration, loss, and other threats to emotional and mental well-being. Chapter 6, Human Development, discusses the processes of human development from biological, psychological, and sociocultural perspectives. A variety of theories are presented and integrated to provide a comprehensive understanding of this important topic, which continues as a conceptual strand throughout the book. This chapter provides the theoretical basis for nursing interventions for clients at all stages of the life cycle and aids in understanding behavioral responses that may have their origins in early developmental experiences. New to this edition, Chapter 7, Human Sexuality, explores human sexual response patterns, alternative lifestyles, and sexual dysfunction and treatment, acknowledging how this aspect of the client affects mental health and illness.

Because dealing with stress is an ongoing process throughout life, it is a theme that recurs throughout the book. However, this theme serves as the focus for Chapter 8, Stress and Anxiety. Concepts such as biological, psychological, spiritual, intellectual, and sociocultural stressors are explored. Responses to stress are discussed in relation to mechanisms for adaptation in mental health and mental illness. In Chapter 9, Commonly Encountered Stressors, such stressors as pain, threats to body image, loss, and immobilization are described and explored. Primary, secondary, and tertiary prevention in

cases involving these threats to mental health are discussed in terms of the nurse-client interpersonal process as a tool of nursing practice.

The therapeutic interpersonal process is fundamental to all areas of practice in mental health nursing. A knowledge of communication theory and the ability to use therapeutic communication processes with individuals and groups are at the heart of psychiatric nursing. Chapter 10, Basic Concepts of Communication, provides a theoretical basis for understanding communication. Theories of verbal, kinesic, and proxemic communication are discussed. Communication theory and the relationships among different levels of communication are discussed to promote an understanding of the use of the therapeutic interpersonal process with clients from various ethnic backgrounds. Chapter 11, Therapeutic Communication and the Nursing Process, specifically addresses the nurse-client relationship and the application of the nursing process to mental health nursing.

Unit 3, Therapeutic Settings and Modalities, focuses on the application of theory and explores a variety of treatment settings and the more common forms of treatment in conjunction with the many roles of the psychiatric nurse. The material in this unit, much of which is new to this edition, provides the reader with an opportunity to examine and explore new and expanding roles and responsibilities in mental health nursing. Chapter 12, The Therapeutic Milieu, introduces a wide range of therapeutic modalities and the concepts and realities of the therapeutic milieu. The client is considered an integral part of the health care team. The role of the nurse is emphasized.

Chapters 13, 14, and 15 focus on nursing functions in relation to group therapy, crisis intervention, and family therapy. Chapter 13, Group Therapy, has been strengthened, exploring group processes and dynamics along with a variety of approaches to group therapy. Chapter 14, Family Dysfunction and Family Therapy, discusses the stressors that may contribute to family dysfunction and their impact on the dynamics of the family and the role of the nurse. Chapter 15, Crisis Intervention, defines and describes both maturational and situational crises and examines the role of the nurse in this important short-term form of therapy.

Chapter 16, Community Mental Health, focuses on mental health services that are oriented toward defined communities or catchment areas. Characteristics of the community mental health movement are described, as are the scope of mental health problems and the current status of community mental health services. The organization of community mental health services is considered in terms of primary, secondary, and tertiary prevention, and in relation to the roles and functions of community mental health nurses.

Unit 4, Client Behavior and Nursing Practice, identifies and discusses major psychogenic and psychiatric conditions of children, adolescents, and adults. Although most of these chapters consider the development and implications of particular disorders throughout the life cycle, Chapter 17, Patterns of Conflict and Stress in Childhood and Adolescence, explores in depth and within a family context selected disorders specific to children or adolescents. An important new addition to this text is Chapter 18. Patterns of Conflict and Stress in the Elderly . The elderly represent the fastest growing segment of the population, and they have special needs that must be met by health care professionals. Psychiatric nurses are in a unique position to meet these needs and therefore must be knowledgeable about developmental tasks, biopsychosocial influences, and specific problems afflicting this group.

In Chapters 19 through 26, patterns of coping with stress are discussed. The earlier chapters concern conditions that involve relatively little interference with psychosocial functioning, such as the psychophysiological and neurotic disorders. The later chapters concern conditions, such as schizophrenia, affective disorders, and organic brain disorders, in which there may be great interference with psychosocial functioning. A new chapter, Patterns of Human Abuse, has been added to address domestic and criminal violence. The chapter on substance and practice abuse, virtually all of which is new to this edition, examines these widespread problems in today's society. Chapter 24, Patterns of Emotional Turbulence and Primitive Defenses, explores disruptive, borderline personality disorders and the role of the nurse in helping affected clients maintain psychological equilibrium.

A new appendix, Selected Psychotropic Drugs, discusses common psychotropic drugs, their indications and side effects, and implications for the nurse's role in administration.

PEDAGOGY

To facilitate the teaching-learning process, we have included a number of pedagogical aids. Each unit opens with a brief introduction, with an overview of chapters within that unit. Each chapter begins with an outline of its contents and a brief statement of chapter focus. These tools should help orient the reader to the logical progression in subject matter as well as the purposes and coverages of individual chapters.

Throughout the text, many new case studies have been added to help the reader understand and apply the theoretical concepts to practical situations. Sample interaction boxes have also been included throughout, providing realistic communication examples to help students better interact with clients.

The five-step nursing process has been used in the secondary prevention sections of chapters, and care plans have been added that reflect the latest 8th NANDA approved diagnoses with corresponding DSM-III-R classification codes.

Many new summary tables and boxes have been created to synthesize important information in an easy-to-use format and to aid student learning. A new section at the end of each chapter, Self-Directed Learning, features sensitivity awareness exercises that help students better understand themselves so that they may intervene effectively with clients. Also included in this section are Questions to Consider, featuring multiple-choice and matching questions that help students review concepts presented in the chapter.

As in the first edition, references, annotated suggested readings, and further readings are included for all chapters to provide the reader with a basis for further exploration of the topics presented.

Package

To enable nurse educators and students to benefit optimally from use of this text, we have provided an instructor's manual, which includes learning objectives, lists of terms and concepts introduced in each chapter, topical lecture outlines, suggested course syllabi, classroom discussion/questions, and lists of audiovisual aids. At the end of this manual, instructors will find a testbank consisting of over 200 multiple-choice questions from which they can construct examinations.

Also for use by instructors or students are two interactive CAI software disks covering crisis intervention and psychiatric assessment. The menu for both disks includes a pretest, review of concepts, clinical simulations, and posttest. Software is available for Apple II+, Apple IIe, and IBM-PC microcomputers.

• • •

We believe that people should be actively involved in their own health care. Since the term *client* denotes such a participatory role, this term is used predominantly in this book. However, there are times in the delivery of health care when people are (or have historically been) acted upon, when they are forced by illness or other circumstances to assume a submissive, dependent role—the role of patient. Thus, in appropriate instances we have used the term *patient* instead.

The terminology in many of the chapter titles in Unit 4 reflects patterns of coping with stress rather than psychiatric diagnostic categories. Psychiatric terminology is used in the text, however, when it is appropriate to learning objectives and when it facilitates communication.

We would like to take this opportunity to thank a number of people who have contributed in various ways to the development of this book. We are indebted to the hundreds of students who have taken our courses. Their learning needs have motivated us to write the book, and their learning experiences have formed the basis for much that appears in it.

We would also like to acknowledge the original contributions of the late Eleanore Alesi. We remember Eleanore with love, affection, and admiration.

Finally we want to thank our friends and families, who have patiently lived with the development of the book and who have offered constant encouragement. Without their support this book might never have been written.

Elaine Anne Pasquali
Helen Margaret Arnold
Nancy DeBasio

Introduction: the student experience

Any new clinical experience generates a certain amount of anxiety, concern for one's own skills, and lack of confidence in the ability to meet client needs effectively. The psychiatric nursing experience, however, is most often looked upon with much trepidation—preconceived ideas and past negative experiences of other students influence students' perceptions. Often students consider the psychiatric experience to be "just talking" with the implication that goals cannot be set; thus, nothing can be achieved with the client. Unrealistic expectations of what can be accomplished may be deterministic in the perceived value of the experience as well. The goals of the psychiatric clinical experience may also be framed differently from other clinical experiences. Goals that reflect an increased awareness of self as a therapeutic tool may initially be threatening. Students are accustomed to performing specific skills, which can then be measured by direct observation. The therapeutic use of self may befuddle students who generally come to the bedside with all types of equipment.

Fears and concerns about the ability to function competently in the psychiatric clinical area are normal. The purpose of this introduction is to reduce the sense of "pluralistic ignorance," better known as "I must be the only student who has felt this way—I must be a terrible person!" Through our shared experiences as faculty working with these students, we can hope to minimize those fears as well as enhance students' ability to function effectively and to experience satisfaction in the psychiatric clinical setting. Students must be encouraged to utilize their listening and communicating skills—those same skills they have utilized with friends and family. Respect, honesty, and a genu-ine commitment to listen and to care for another human being are critical variables in the development of therapeutic relationships. Satisfaction for the student may be gained by enabling a client to express himself to a willing listener or by returning again and again to a client who does not believe he is capable of another individual's caring. Students may lose sight of the fact that psychiatric clients are human beings—the fear of "who" they are and "what" they might do may preclude this important premise. Validation of feelings experienced in the psychiatric clinical area is vital. Concurrently, developing an understanding of one's self within the context of the therapeutic relationship as having an affect on and being affected by another individual is also necessary.

Common fears and issues arise in the psychiatric experience. The following discussion will explore these issues and possible reasons for these feelings.

Will I be hurt?

Students have perceptions that crazy people are kept behind locked bars waiting to harm others. Such films as "One Flew over the Cuckoo's Nest" reaffirm the belief that psychiatric clients have no control over their behavior. In fact, clients in some cases do not have control over their behavior and require control from health care providers. Students feel vulnerable in the sense that they may not have the skills to provide necessary controls, thus leading to the fear of clients either physically or psychologically harming them. One student stated that she was told by the staff that she could no longer see her client because she had been transferred to a maximum security unit, which would not be safe for her to visit. Another student shared that his client kept pacing back and forth and glaring at him. He felt that if he approached the client, the client would "haul off and whack" him. A group of students described their first day on a locked unit. A common thread of apprehension and dread was voiced upon being "left" on the unit without keys. Each identified a fear that they would be left with the clients and be unable to "get out."

Will I become crazy?

Students describe a fear of "catching" mental illness or becoming like their clients. One student shared in post-conference that he felt as though he was analyzing his own mood swings rather than viewing them as a normal part of his life. Another student stated that during the psychiatric rotation her roommate noticed that each day after clinical, the student would go back to her room and pull the cover over her head until dinner. Students in a private psychiatric hospital noted that "many of the clients looked just like them." There was a concern as to what actually separated "us" from "them." The use of street clothes in the psychiatric setting prevents separation by generally accepted symbols of authority: the uniform, the scissors, the stethescope. Students have described the need to find some symbol—a name pin, a lab coat—which will reduce the perceived dissonance and role blurring. Although the fear of mental illness is a real one, the issue can be utilized to demonstrate to students that clients are not "crazy" in all areas of their lives. Mentally ill individuals may utilize the same defense mechanisms healthy individuals do, but the degree and frequency of usage is different. This perspective often assists students to reframe their perceptions of the mentally ill.

What can I do to help clients?

Most students express an overwhelming sense of helplessness on initial entry into the psychiatric setting. Comments such as "I don't have anything to do," "The client is in activities all day; what does he need me for?" "I feel like an appendage; all I do is follow my client around," "How does talking help

when someone is really depressed or delusional?" Each of these comments deserves merit, yet students are unaware of what they can potentially bring to the client's situation. Just as they learned skills to effect outcomes in other clinical settings so too can they develop effective use of their communication skills to develop a relationship with a client who is mentally ill. The reaffirmation that students' feelings are valid is most important, particularly in the early stages of the psychiatric clinical experience.

Will I hurt the client?

In conjunction with the above concern, students express a fear that they might say the wrong thing. For example, one student who was working with a suicidal client feared that he might say something that would "send the client over the edge." In this same situation, the student also feared that he might not pick up clues that would be indicative of impending suicidal activity. Students working with depressed clients shared the belief that they might make the client feel worse by saying the wrong thing. There is also a fear that clients might lose control and act out, precipitated by something the student said. Two factors must be identified in relation to this issue. First, clients have much more strength than we attribute to them. They are able to tolerate in many cases the clumsy attempts of students to intervene therapeutically. Secondly, there seems to be an inherent belief that students have the power or influence to cause clients to discuss subjects or behave in certain ways. This can be described as analogous to the discussion of suicide or birth control—students do not put thoughts into clients' heads but rather provide an environment where thoughts and feelings are accepted and encouraged.

Will I be rejected?

The fear of being rejected by the client is valid and quite commonly experienced among students. Students' feelings of incompetence lead them to believe they have little to offer; thus, why should a client want to establish a relationship with them? During a pre-conference, a student stated that his client was described as withdrawn and noncommunicative, having not developed relationships with many people on the unit. The student had already determined that he would be rejected—prior to even entering the unit. Another student described an experience with a client she had been seeing for two weeks. The client was sitting in the dayroom when the student arrived for pre-conference. The student acknowledged the client with a brief wave and went with her peers to conference. At the scheduled time of their meeting, the client did not appear and was found in the recreation room with another staff member. She ignored the student. The student assumed the responsibility for the client's actions. It must have been something she did or did not do. Through processing the event in post-conference, the student became aware that the client's past experiences may have caused this specific response. It was known through the client's history that she had had little success with relationships. The student then utilized this experience to enable the client to explore her own feelings of rejection and to develop strategies to engage in successful relationships—initiated by a successful relationship with the student. In some instances, clients feel the need to have more space or distance between themselves and health care providers. The reasons for this may be unknown to the client on a conscious level and are acted out behaviorally. Clients may also reject students because a particular student may interact with a client similarly to a significant other with whom the client has had negative experiences. For example, an elderly depressed woman refused to engage in an initial interview with a young student. When evaluating this behavior in the supervisory relationship, the faculty member suggested that the student might remind the client of a significant person in her life with whom she has some conflictual feelings. The student was able to determine from staff input that the woman's granddaughter, a woman similar in age to the student, had recently committed suicide. The woman had not spoken to her granddaughter in several years because the grandmother had disapproved of her lifestyle. Clients often feel a low sense of self-worth, which generates feelings of "Why would anyone want to be with me?" which in turn leads to rejecting behavior on the part of the

client. Other clients may use the rationale that they "talk" to too many other health professionals or that they "don't have time to talk to the student." In many cases, the client often fears rejection by the student so in turn rejects the student before he or she can reject the client. Through the exploration of this issue, students are able to understand the dynamics of rejection from the client's perspective. Students are also encouraged to give up the notion that they are personally responsible for the rejecting behavior of the client.

Am I using the client?

Often students feel that they are using clients as guinea pigs—attempting to get information from a client to write process recordings or a nursing care plan. Students have shared that they have nothing to offer clients or can't make them better as they can in other clinical settings. This feeling may be reaffirmed by psychiatric clients who may accuse students of doing just that in order to intimidate new students and empower themselves as important people. One student stated that his client shouted at him, "You don't like me; you just want to see what all the nuts look like!" Students need to be encouraged to be honest with clients, that is, to reiterate their desire to genuinely be involved with this person because of that person—not his or her information. Nonverbal messages are critical in conveying commitment to the individual. Clients are often astute enough to realize the student's lack of concern for them. Students may share their feelings of ineptness in this new situation yet convey a genuine sense of caring, of making a conscious choice to be with this individual in a therapeutic relationship.

Can I have feelings too?

Students are often not clear whether they should have feelings about their clients, and if they do, what do they do with them? One student explained after listening to a group of borderline clients who were trying to "one up" the other in their descriptions of their suicide attempts that she was so angry and frustrated that she had to leave the unit. She felt guilty for feeling angry. Later that day her interaction with her client was described by the student as "disastrous." During post-conference, several students concurred that they weren't sure if they could be angry, frustrated, or disappointed. Sharing positive feelings was much easier. The process of the supervisory relationship between student and faculty member can facilitate the student's understanding of his or her feelings and how they can be utilized in a positive sense within the context of the student-client interaction. Once trust has been established between student and client, the client can learn more adaptive methods of coping with anger, frustration, and disappointment through the student's expression of how he or she copes with those same feelings.

What do I need to know before I see the client for the first time?

There are differing schools of thought as to whether students should have information prior to making the initial contact with the client. Generally in other clinical areas, students have access to charts and often preplan care the day before the clinical experience. Students share their concern that they feel little clinical competence; not having information prior to the initial contact is anxiety provoking and frustrating. On the other hand, some students feel that they would like to go in "cold" so as not to form preconceived ideas about their clients. It seems that there is no right or wrong answer but rather a consideration for the individual student and the individual client as to how their mutual needs are best met.

• • •

In conclusion, several issues and fears that are common to the initial psychiatric clinical experience have been explored. Role dissonance in the psychiatric setting is expected. Validation by faculty and professional staff are critical in the facilitation of a positive psychiatric clinical experience. Students *do* bring something with them into this clinical arena: honesty, caring, respect, and the ability to listen. Small but significant goals such as the client's ability to sit with the student for ten minutes longer each session are viewed as equally important to changing a dressing or making a bed. The process of the therapeutic interaction between student and client is a mutual one where each influences and is influenced by the other. The analysis of this relationship through group conference or individual supervision provides a learning experience through which clients can learn more adaptive measures of coping. Students are encouraged to gain insight into their own behaviors as they relate to their clients, peers, and instructor. In some cases, the psychiatric clinical experience may elicit unresolved conflictual issues for students. The student may then choose to examine these issues further in a therapeutic relationship outside of the clinical setting.

Contents

Mental Health Nursing

A Holistic Approach

The domain of mental health nursing

Mental health nursing concepts and principles are an integral part of professional nursing practice today. By nature, nursing is a people-oriented profession, and every contact or interaction provides an opportunity for the nurse to observe and intervene on behalf of people who have emotional needs. To enhance such interactions, it is important to understand the various ways to view behavior, the evolution of those theories and approaches, and their implications for contemporary nursing practice. This unit provides such an orientation to the practice and profession of psychiatric nursing.

Chapter 1 defines mental health nursing and describes a number of the more influential and dominant theories of behavior. A holistic systems approach is explored and endorsed as the theoretical framework used throughout this book. The three levels of prevention—primary, secondary, and tertiary—are defined as an organizing structure for nursing intervention. The five-step nursing process is described in relationship to the three levels of prevention.

To know where we are and where we are going, it is important to understand where we have been. Chapter 2 provides a historical overview of psychiatric nursing and briefly discusses how events in the past have had an impact on contemporary nursing practice.

Focusing on contemporary issues, Chapter 3 describes strategies for utilizing power and political action to promote mental health and to meet such professional objectives as client advocacy and improvement of mental health facilities and services.

CHAPTER 1

Framework for mental health nursing practice

CHAPTER FOCUS

Professional nursing is essentially an interpersonal process. Professional nursing acknowledges the complexities of human nature and promotes a holistic view—the person as a system composed of biological, psychological, intellectual, spiritual, and sociocultural subsystems. Mental health, or psychiatric, nursing is that aspect of professional nursing which is concerned with people's emotional responses to stress and crisis and with the interplay of the many health factors that enhance and/or inhibit the ability to cope with stress. Psychiatric nursing is both an integral part of all professional nursing and a specialized area of nursing practice. There are two levels of preparation for psychiatric nursing—the generalist and the psychiatric nursing specialist.

The concepts of wellness and holistic health stress an evolving rather than an absolute state of mental health. Wellness is a process of ongoing growth toward self-actualization. Stress disrupts this process. People participate in the process of becoming mentally ill, and they should also participate in the process of getting well and staying well. Thus, crisis can be an opportunity to grow toward one's fullest potential. In their roles as counselors, teachers, and advocates, mental health nurses help clients to make life-style changes directed toward high-level wellness. Because a systems-theory approach explores how a myriad of factors interrelate and contribute to human behavior, systems theory can be effectively applied to wellness and holistic health and to nursing intervention. Since it incorporates the concepts of stress, coping, and levels of prevention that are set forth in this book, Neuman's systems-theory model is most compatible with the

3

orientation of this book. Systems models developed by other nursing theorists are used, when appropriate, to discuss behavior and to provide a frame of reference for professional nursing practice.

Nursing intervention is based on the nursing process and is organized according to the concepts of primary, secondary, and tertiary prevention. These concepts offer a framework for providing holistic mental health care to clients.

PHILOSOPHY OF PROFESSIONAL NURSING

The activities of the health professionals are predicated upon certain beliefs about the nature of human beings, the nature of society, and the role of the professions within that society. These fundamental beliefs provide a philosophical foundation for the attitudes, ideals, and theoretical concepts underlying professional education and practice. Professional philosophy also recognizes the dynamic nature of society and of the health professions and incorporates the ideals toward which the professions strive.

Professional nursing is essentially an *interpersonal process*, and psychiatric nursing is an integral part of that process (Travelbee, 1971). The primary concern and central focus of nursing is people coping with present and potential health problems. People and the interactions between them are a central component of the nursing process (Peplau, 1952).

Nursing is a *humanistic* profession. It shares with other health professions the responsibility for meeting the health needs of society. These needs include the maintenance and promotion of health, the prevention and treatment of health problems, and the rehabilitation of clients after treatment. Inherent in the concept of humanism is a belief in the worth, dignity, and human rights of every individual. Among the rights of concern to the nursing profession are the right to an optimum level of health and the right to comprehensive health services. The protection of human rights and civil rights, including the right to privacy and the right

to participate in health care processes, has a high priority in professional nursing practice.

Professional nursing acknowledges the complexities of human nature and promotes a *holistic* view—the person as a biological, psychological, intellectual, spiritual, and sociocultural being. Knowledge and understanding of the complex interactions and interrelationships between these dimensions of behavior, as each individual continually adapts and adjusts to his or her internal and external environments, are essential to the practice of nursing. Inherent in the holistic concept is an awareness that many aspects of human nature are universal and that others are unique to the individual. Sullivan's statement (1953) that "we are all more simply human than otherwise" expresses the common humanity that each of us shares with all other people on our planet. The uniqueness can be observed in so basic a biological phenomenon as fingerprints, which are so individual that they are used to distinguish one person from every other. Each personality is even more complex and unique. Each individual is more than a biopsychosocial being. Each has needs and aspirations as a part of the self, which may be referred to as spiritual being. Recognition of the uniqueness of each personality and of the cultural and ethnic variations in our society is a basic precept of professional nursing practice.

Because nursing is a profession, nurses are responsible for the quality of practice and accountable to the public. A professional level of practice is maintained through a continuing process of formal and informal study. Formal education for professional nursing is a blend of liberal arts and professional education.

Definition of mental health nursing

Mental health, or psychiatric,* nursing is that aspect of professional nursing which is concerned with a person's emotional responses to stress and crisis and with the interplay of the many factors that

---

*We use the terms *mental health nursing* and *psychiatric nursing* interchangeably throughout this book, since both terms describe the same area of nursing practice.

enhance and/or inhibit the ability to cope with stress. The therapeutic interpersonal process is central to the practice of mental health nursing. Nursing intervention emphasizes interpersonal interactions with individuals and groups coping with present or potential mental health problems. The objectives of nursing intervention are as follows: maintenance and promotion of mental health (primary prevention), early identification and intervention in maladaptive disorders (secondary prevention), and rehabilitation in chronic disorders (tertiary prevention). Psychiatric nursing practice extends across the spectrum of human behavior, from the most adaptive to the least adaptive levels of coping with stress, and involves persons of all stages of the life cycle.

To meet their objectives, psychiatric nursing professionals collaborate with other health professionals and community groups in social, political, and educational activities that promote the mental health of individuals, families, and communities. Psychiatric nursing is both an integral part of all professional nursing and a specialized area of nursing practice (Travelbee, 1971).

As in all other areas of professional nursing, the level of psychiatric nursing practice varies with the educational preparation and clinical expertise of the practitioners. There are two levels of preparation for psychiatric nursing. The *generalist* has educational preparation at the undergraduate level and has demonstrated clinical ability in psychiatric nursing. The *psychiatric nursing specialist* has educational preparation at the master's or doctoral level, has supervised clinical experience, and has evidenced in-depth knowledge, ability, and skill in psychiatric nursing (American Nurses' Association, 1982).

Clinical expertise is assessed through a formal review process. Professional nurses who meet the criteria for either of the levels of preparation are prepared to function as members of mental health teams in any clinical setting that provides mental health services. The psychiatric nursing specialist must, in addition, be prepared in research, teaching, clinical supervision, and independent practice. The term *psychiatric nurse* is applied to persons working at either of the two levels of practice.

Relevance of psychiatric nursing to all areas of professional nursing practice

The professional nurse practitioner with basic preparation in nursing, including biopsychosocial theory and therapeutic interpersonal skills, views the psychiatric nursing component as an integral part of nursing practice to meet the comprehensive health needs of clients.

There is general consensus in the profession that the theories of human behavior and interpersonal skills encompassed in psychiatric nursing are essential aspects of basic nursing education and professional practice. In 1950, the National League for Nursing, the organization responsible for accrediting nursing education programs, required that psychiatric nursing be included in all nursing curricula. Sometime thereafter, the federal government, through the National Institute for Mental Health, provided grant funds for faculty in baccalaureate programs in nursing for the purpose of integrating psychiatric nursing concepts and skills into curricula.

The practice of mental health nursing is not limited to any particular health care setting or to any age group of clients. Rather, it is an integral part of nursing in all areas of professional practice and for clients throughout the life span. The nursing profession has long been committed to the concepts of health maintenance and prevention of physical and psychological disorders. Providing emotional support to adults and children who are coping with physical illness and injury has long been part of nursing practice in hospitals, clinics, and the home. Health teaching, supervision, and anticipatory guidance practiced by parent-child nurses are forms of primary prevention in physical and mental health that are accepted aspects of professional practice. Nurses working in community health programs, schools, and industry engage in a variety of activities that promote mental and physical health.

Recent developments in health care have placed increased emphasis upon the need for the integration of mental health concepts. Among these developments are the public criticism of the health care delivery system for failure to meet the health needs of many segments of society, particularly the elderly, the poor, and ethnic groups in inner-city ghettos. The demand for comprehensive health care and the focus upon physical and mental health maintenance—in addition to treatment and rehabilitation—place a responsibility upon professional nursing and other health professions for meeting these needs.

THE MENTAL HEALTH TEAM

Professional nurses work with other health professionals in the delivery of comprehensive mental health care. The nurse and the other health professionals are collectively referred to as the mental health team. The roles, educational preparation, and some of the professional backgrounds of the members of the mental health team are discussed below.

The nurse

Nursing actions are many and varied. According to the American Nurses' Association's "Statement on Psychiatric and Mental Health Nursing Practice," the functions of a psychiatric nurse include the following:

1. Responsibility for maintaining a therapeutic milieu
2. Working with clients to help resolve some of their problems in living
3. Acceptance of the surrogate parent role
4. Supervision of the physical aspects of the client's health needs, including responses to medications and treatments
5. Health education, particularly in the area of emotional health
6. Helping to improve the client's recreational, occupational, and social competence
7. Providing supervision and clinical assistance to other health workers, including other nurses
8. Psychotherapy
9. Involvement in social action related to the mental health of the community

Psychiatric mental health nurses carry out these functions in such varied settings as hospitals, hospices, other institutional facilities, and community agencies. (The nurse's roles and functions will be discussed in more depth in Chapters 12 and 16.)

The social worker

Social workers function in many settings—for example, medical services, public welfare programs, family and adoption agencies, prisons, community health clinics, and psychiatric facilities. While the largest portion of social workers work in psychiatric settings, the term *psychiatric social worker* is considered obsolete. Most professional social workers are prepared at the master's level (M.S.W.); a smaller number are graduates of baccalaureate programs with a major in social welfare. Some social workers have doctorates in social work (D.S.W. or Ph.D.) or in related fields. Some states have licensing or certification laws for social workers (C.S.W.). The national professional organization is the National Association of Social Workers (N.A.S.W.). A social worker who has a master's degree, who has completed 2 years of supervised practice, and who has passed a qualifying examination administered by the N.A.S.W. may be admitted to the Academy of Certified Social Workers. The worker is then entitled to use the designation A.C.S.W.

At the master's level, social workers are trained in individual, group, and family treatment. At this level there seems to be a good deal of overlapping with the functions of the master's-educated clinical specialist in psychiatric nursing. Social workers and clinical specialists work cooperatively in many settings. Some social workers and clinical specialists are enrolled in postdoctoral programs that provide training in psychoanalysis.

The clinical psychologist

The clinical psychologist is educated at the Ph.D. level. Four to five years of graduate school and one year of clinical internship are usually required. Clinical psychologists are trained in individual, group, and family psychotherapy. In several states they are licensed through qualifying examinations and other criteria. Some psychologists also receive several years of postdoctoral training in psychoanalysis. The professional organization is the

American Psychological Association, which maintains standards and sponsors various professional activities.

The psychiatrist

The psychiatrist is a medical doctor who has specialized in psychiatry. Some psychiatrists are *board certified*, a designation that involves meeting clinical requirements and passing written examinations administered by the American Board of Psychiatry and Neurology. Like psychologists, some psychiatrists seek additional training as psychoanalysts. The professional organization for psychiatrists is the American Psychiatric Association.

The physician

The client is a biopsychosocial organism, a *whole person*. Too often in psychiatric settings, however, there is a tendency to focus only on the psychosocial aspects of a client and to neglect the physical aspects. Most general hospital psychiatric units therefore include a medical internist or general practitioner as an active team member. Another important role that such a physician plays is in the area of referral. Indeed, many referrals of clients to psychiatric care originate with family doctors.

The occupational therapist

Occupational therapists have been educated and trained to promote the recovery and rehabilitation of clients through manual, creative, and self-help activities. There are two entry levels for the occupational therapist—the B.A. degree and the M.S. degree. Certification is granted by the Occupational Therapist Association, which is the professional organization for occupational therapists.

The recreational therapist

Most recreational and occupational therapists have majored in the specialty in college, and some have advanced degrees (M.A. or Ph.D.). In addition to their specialty, they are educated in counseling and other social sciences. Recreational therapists often utilize volunteer services to maintain

the necessary link between client and community. They also plan and supervise trips from the agencies to such places as shopping centers, theaters, beaches, and cultural and sports events. Registration for recreational therapists is, at present, on a voluntary basis and is administered by the National Recreation and Parks Association (N.R.P.A.). Within the N.R.P.A., the Division of Therapeutic Recreation provides the professional organization for recreational therapists.

The psychiatric aide or clinical assistant

The preparation of psychiatric aides varies greatly. Many are high school graduates, but an increasing number of people with additional education—including persons who have master's degrees in psychology and are either working toward a doctoral degree or awaiting admission to a doctoral program—are functioning as psychiatric aides to increase their clinical experience and competence.

In many psychiatric facilities these people are referred to as psychiatric technicians; they are given more responsibility and greater remuneration than the less-educated aide, but there is little upward mobility.

● ● ●

Since mental health services are provided through a system of cooperating health, welfare, and social systems in a geographically defined community, the mental health team may function in any of a variety of settings. The therapeutic services offered in any setting depend upon whether the major focus is primary, secondary, or tertiary prevention, although some treatment modalities may be utilized in all three levels of prevention. Table 1-1 outlines some unique roles and functions of mental health team members.

DEFINITIONS OF MENTAL HEALTH AND MENTAL ILLNESS

The terms *mental health* and *mental illness* are used in a very broad, general sense to imply some optimum level of psychosocial functioning or some

TABLE 1-1 Health team members

Team member	Unique roles and functions
Nurse	Works with client health needs and problems in living; coordinates client therapies; supervises and provides clinical assistance to other health workers
Social worker	Works with client social problems and with clients' families, social networks, and communities; initiates appropriate referrals
Clinical psychologist	Administers and interprets psychological tests that aid in diagnosis, treatment, and research
Psychiatrist	Diagnoses psychiatric disorders; admits and discharges clients; prescribes and supervises medications and other somatic therapies
Physician	Supervises physical health of psychiatric clients; refers emotionally disturbed clients for psychiatric care
Occupational therapist	Assesses client needs for and prescribes manual, creative, and self-help activities that promote learning of job skills and mastery of activities of daily living
Recreational therapist	Assesses client needs in areas of sports, recreation, and cultural enrichment and plans programs to meet those needs
Psychiatric aide	Provides much direct client care under the supervision of a nurse

level of deviation from such a state. Although these terms are widely used in the literature, they have not been clearly defined.

Peplau (1952), one of the outstanding leaders in psychiatric nursing, has written: "Health has not been clearly defined; it is a word symbol that implies forward movement of personality and other ongoing processes in the direction of creative, constructive, productive personal and community living." Doona (1979) observes: "The problem in defining mental health (and health in general) derives from the fact that health is not a scientific term." Science is concerned with particular, or specific and discrete, aspects that can be clearly defined and measured, while concepts such as "health" and "illness" relate to very general, nonspecific characteristics of an individual or a group or a segment of a population.

Problems arise when one attempts to apply concepts of health and illness to human behavior—to the complex ways in which people think, feel, and behave in relation to the joys and troubles of life. Each culture sanctions some types of defensive behavior that provide culturally acceptable means of coping with stress, anxiety, and other noxious feelings. Definitions of mental health and illness tend to be based upon particular cultural or ethnic orientations, a situation that may lead to subjective or judgmental attitudes and values being used to assess mental health status. Helman (1984, 141–142) points out that culture not only defines normal and abnormal behavior in a particular society but may also contribute to the development of psychiatric disorders, influence their clinical manifestations and distributions, and determine how mental illness is "recognized, labelled, explained and treated." Thus, society and culture interact in the construction and maintenance of mental health–mental illness.

Kendell (1975) observes that diagnoses of mental health–mental illness tend to reflect the particular orientation or values of the examining psychiatrist, who often models his or her diagnostic behavior after influential teachers and therapy trends. The psychiatrist's experience, methods of data collection and decision making, social class, ethnicity, and religious and political orientations also influence the nature of psychiatric diagnoses (Kendell 1975; Helman 1984).

Mental health

Despite the difficulties involved in finding a satisfactory definition of mental health, there remains a need for some objective standard based on a general concept of mental health or psychological maturity. Cox (1974) has identified "trends or themes of a mature person" that she believes are "most nearly universal and timeless." These include a firm grasp of reality, a value system, a sense of self, and the ability to care for others, to work productively, and to cope with stress. Travelbee (Doona, 1979) views mental health not as something one has but as "something one is." She incorporates themes similar to those listed above into "the ability to love," which includes the love of self, "the ability to face reality," and "the ability to find meaning." Concepts of mental health will be discussed further in Chapter 6.

Mental illness

Mental illness may be defined as psychosocial responses to stress that interfere with or inhibit a person's ability to comfortably or effectively meet human needs and function within a culture. It may be viewed more simply as problems in living precipitated by stress.

Medical terms such as *illness* or *pathology* suggest the presence of a disease process, which cannot be substantiated in the majority of psychiatric conditions, although recent research indicates biological components in many psychological disorders. Of even greater concern is the use of diagnostic categories inherent in the medical model. Diagnostic labeling can have "some very unfortunate effects" (Baron, Byrne, and Kantowitz, 1978). One such effect is that it tends to assign the person to a dependent status. Once the label "mentally ill" is assigned to a person, cultural cues instruct the person about the enactment of the social role of sick person or dependent patient. Only society-at-large can then release the person from the sick role through a process of "de-labeling" (Waxler, 1977).

In addition, labeling clients by means of psychiatric nomenclature subjects them to public and professional attitudes toward mental illness in general and toward certain diagnostic categories in particular. For example, labeling a person "schizophrenic" in childhood or adolescence may have a profound and lasting impact upon the person's life, especially if the label becomes known to school systems, employers, law enforcement agents, and the like.

Questions have also been raised about attempts to fit people of various ethnic backgrounds, and with innumerable behavioral responses to stress, into specific diagnostic categories. Such an effort may focus upon the diagnostic category rather than upon the person who is suffering.

Although psychological suffering is found in all societies, the "language of distress" that expresses this suffering and its definition, explanation, and treatment vary from culture to culture. The expressions and manifestations of psychological distress usually reflect the symbols, imagery, and motifs of a particular cultural context. Syndromes or clusters of symptoms unique to a particular culture or geographic area are referred to as *culture-bound disorders* (Helman, 1984). (Specific culture-bound disorders will be discussed in Unit IV.) Mindful of the influence of culture, we can best understand abnormal or maladaptive behavior if we think of it as a way of coping with stress (Baron, Byrne, and Kantowitz, 1978).

Psychosocial threat and stress are inherent in the human condition. Threats or stressors may include any perceived threat to the physical or psychosocial self, any loss or threat of loss, and so on. Coping processes are strategies for dealing with stress. These strategies may be instrumental (attempting to problem solve or modify the environment) or palliative (attempting to regulate emotions) (Lazarus and Launier, 1978). Coping processes serve the purpose of psychological equilibrium. Behavioral responses to psychosocial stress may be expressed through the emotions, through motor behavior, and through thought processes, including language.

Responses to stress become maladaptive (we prefer "least adaptive") when coping processes are unable to control noxious feelings or when the coping mechanisms themselves result in symptoms. For example, in an acute anxiety attack, the defensive or coping mechanisms have failed to contain or master the emotion of anxiety. In obsessive-compulsive behavior, the coping processes result in the behavior. However, all coping processes, regardless of whether they are socially acceptable, are adaptive in the sense that they help a person maintain some level of psychological equilibrium. An individual's ability to cope effectively with stress is influenced by a combination of factors, which include the degree of stress perceived, the current psychosocial situation, and the individual's holistic health status.

THEORETICAL FRAMEWORK
Wellness–holistic health orientation

A holistic orientation toward health encompasses the relationship of microcosm to macrocosm and the concept of complementarity. As with any system, change in one part changes the whole. Balance with the natural world is essential to wellness and holistic health (Scheper-Hughes and Lock, 1987).

We believe that the practice of mental health nursing requires knowledge of the biological, psychological, intellectual, spiritual, and sociocultural subsystems of a person and that these subsystems are interrelated in human responses to stress. In this book we have therefore adopted a wellness–holistic health orientation to human behavior and mental health. However, in the discussions of human behavior and mental health, we have often synthesized these concepts into a three-faceted approach, in which the intellectual subsystem is considered part of the psychological subsystem and the spiritual subsystem is considered part of the sociocultural subsystem.

The concepts of wellness and holistic health stress an evolving process rather than an absolute state of mental health. A state of wellness or well-being evolves from the integration of the five subsystems of a person. Wellness is therefore a process of ongoing growth toward self-actualization. One's goals become not merely the avoidance of disorders and premature death but progress toward self-actualization and the optimum enjoyment of life.

A wellness–holistic health orientation toward human behavior rests on the following premises (Flynn, 1980; Goldwag, 1979; Tulloch and Healy, 1982):

1. Wellness evolves out of the integration and balance of a person's five subsystems—biological, psychological, intellectual, spiritual, and sociocultural.

2. Stress disrupts a person's inner balance or wellness.
3. Unhealthy life-styles (for example, value conflicts, acculturative pressures, substance abuse, noise pollution, compulsive working) produce stress. People respond to stress with biochemical, physiological, and psychological changes. Prolonged or multiple stressors may precipitate psychophysiological or psychopathological disorders (see Chapters 8, 9, and 19).
4. Once a psychophysiological or psychopathological disorder develops, a person needs assistance to relieve symptoms and to prevent a relapse or recurrence.
5. A person participates in (contributes to) the process of becoming mentally ill and should also participate in the processes of getting well and staying well.
6. All therapies are temporary expedients until a person can be helped to understand how life-style influences mental health.
7. A crisis can be an opportunity to grow toward one's fullest potential.

People should actively participate in the changes that are necessary to achieve high-level wellness. By increasing self-awareness and by clarifying values and establishing realistic and attainable goals, people can begin to develop positive approaches to their lives. Self-esteem then begins to improve, and feelings of hopelessness and helplessness (a victim orientation) begin to diminish. The locus of decision making for achieving high-level wellness rests ideally with the client. Clients who agree to changes or who make decisions to please the nurse or other care givers usually do not integrate these changes into their life-styles. Such changes are usually short-lived. Clients should be encouraged to explore and to utilize both traditional and nontraditional approaches that support the life-style changes toward high-level wellness that they desire.

The roles of nurses and other care givers in facilitating change* toward high-level wellness consist primarily in (1) counseling (viewing and accepting

*Refer to Chapter 3 for discussions of the process of change and client advocacy.

clients as whole people, assessing their health statuses, supporting them, and guiding them toward high-level wellness), (2) teaching (educating clients about the processes of problem solving and change so that they can increase their self-awareness and learn to appreciate and integrate the five dimensions of the self), and (3) advocacy (ensuring clients' rights and the quality of care) (Goldwag, 1979; Flynn, 1980; Tulloch and Healy, 1982).

Wellness–holistic health assessment guide

The following assessment guide has been developed to assist clients in assessing their levels of wellness and to enable students to assess their own levels of wellness. The five major areas of assessment correspond to the five interrelated subsystems of a "whole" person. Assessments should be made within the context of a person's family, social networks, and community, since it is within this context that a person's ideology, values, and behavior are developed and reinforced.

I. Biological subsystem
  A. Physical activity
    1. Frequency, duration, and types of planned exercise (for example, brisk walking, jogging, aerobics)
    2. Frequency and types of activity required by social roles (for example, sedentary versus physically active job)
  B. Health habits
    1. Personal habits (for example, smoking versus nonsmoking; number of hours of sleep required versus number obtained)
    2. Personal and family history of physical illness and/or organ weakness
  C. Nutritional status
    1. Daily food intake (for example, amount of fiber in diet; consumption of foods from four basic food groups)
    2. Types of food preparation: broiled, boiled, fried, baked, etc.
    3. Frequency and types of food additives (for example, preservatives, sugars, salt), processed foods, and "empty calo-

rie" foods (for example, soda, candy, alcoholic beverages) ingested
    4. Adherence to special dietary practices: cultural, religious, or social (for example, fad diets, fast foods)
    5. Frequency and types of dietary supplements consumed (for example, vitamins, lecithin)
    6. Frequency of snacking and types of foods eaten (for example, candy versus fruit)
  D. Environmental input
    1. Frequency and types of sensory stimulation, sensory deprivation, and/or perceptual monotony (for example, noise level, intensity of lights)
    2. Degree of exposure to atmospheric pollutants (for example, smog, smoke, vinyl chloride)
    3. Types of territorial imperatives*
      a. Built territories (for example, rooms that afford much or little privacy; architecture that facilitates accessibility [ramps, elevators] or impedes accessibility [stairs, curbs])
      b. Personal spacing (for example, clearly defined and acknowledged claims to space versus ambiguous or disputed claims; adequate space versus overcrowding)
    4. Frequency and degree of exposure to pathogens (for example, exposure to bacteria and viruses; level of immunity)
    5. Degree of relatedness to nature (exhibited through nature walks, gardening, ecological activities, and so on)
II. Intellectual subsystem
  A. Formal idea stimulation
    1. Frequency and types of activity (for example, formal schooling, seminars, adult education courses)
    2. Valuation of and commitment to education
  B. Informal idea stimulation
    1. Frequency and types of activity (for ex-

---

*See Chapter 10 for a discussion of territoriality.

ample, reading, educational television programs, discussion groups)
2. Frequency and effectiveness of use of a problem-solving approach to life situations and difficulties

III. Sociocultural subsystem
A. Support systems
1. Types of help offered (for example, emotional, economic)
2. Constituents of support system (for example, family, friends, colleagues)
3. Degree of availability of support systems (for example, available in crisis; must be asked for help; volunteer help)
B. Sensitivity to others
1. Degree of ability to listen to and empathize with others
2. Degree of ability to reach out to help others
3. Degree of ability to ask for help from others
C. Cultural orientation (see Chapter 4 for a cultural orientation assessment guide)
1. Nature of the family (for example, members composing family unit; sense of obligation among family members)
2. Nature of role relationships (for example, rigid versus flexible sex-defined roles; egalitarian male-female relationships versus unequal statuses; long-established versus disrupted role relationships)
3. Verbal, kinesic, and proxemic communication patterns
4. Relationship to time (for example, past oriented, present oriented, or future oriented)

IV. Psychological subsystem (see Chapter 11 for a mental health assessment guide)
A. Personal insight
1. Degree of awareness of own attitudes, feelings, beliefs, goals, and plans
2. Degree of awareness of sources of and/or influences on own attitudes, feelings, beliefs, goals, and plans
3. Nature of self-concept (for example, perception of own strengths and weak-

nesses, modes of interaction with the social and physical environment, and personal appearance)
4. Degree of awareness of own locus of control (for example, autonomous, fatalistic, victim oriented)
5. Frequency, types, and outcomes of own risk-taking behaviors
B. Concept of happiness or well-being
1. Description of happiness or well-being (for example, characteristics; how it is obtained; who deserves it)
2. Degree to which attainment of happiness or well-being depends on oneself; degree to which it depends on others
C. Behavior patterns
1. Nature of thought patterns (for example, delusions, flight of ideas, confusion)
2. Nature of sensory processes (for example, degree of sensory functioning, type of disorder, type of hallucination)
3. Nature of speech patterns (for example, mutism, confabulation, irrelevancy)
4. Nature of affect (for example, elation, depression, anxiety, anger)
D. Stressors*
1. Identification of perceived positive stressors (for example, challenges, excitements) and of perceived negative stressors (for example, threats, problems) and of their sources
2. Perception of probable durations of stressors (for example, short-lived, long-term, chronic)
3. Identification of types of coping behavior that are adaptive (for example, sublimation, verbalization, problem solving) and those that are maladaptive (for example, substance abuse, compulsive eating, hypochondriasis)
4. Personal and family history of maladaptive coping behavior

V. Spiritual subsystem
A. Ideology

---

*See Chapters 8 and 9 for a discussion of stress.

1. Nature of belief in a supernatural being and/or supernormal energy
2. Nature of belief in communion between a supernatural being or supernormal energy and people alive and dead
3. Conceptualizations about good, evil, and forgiveness
4. Conceptualizations about the quality of life and the quality of death
5. Nature of belief about life after death
6. Effectiveness or ineffectiveness of ideology as a coping mechanism

B. Inner life
  1. Frequency and type of inner-life activity (for example, meditation, yoga, prayer)
  2. Interrelationship between one's spiritual life and the other parts of one's life (for example, meditate when under stress; pray when in trouble)
  3. Effectiveness or ineffectiveness of inner-life activity as a coping mechanism

After they have assessed their levels of wellness, clients and/or students should decide whether they want to make changes in their lifestyles and in what areas they want to make these changes. Tulloch and Healy (1982) suggest that only one behavior be modified at a time; that a concrete, measurable, and attainable goal be set; and that a time frame be established for achieving the goal. Support systems, such as self-help groups, families, and friends, may be helpful to clients or students who are attempting to make changes toward high-level wellness.

Locus of decision making

Since we are basing the nurse-client relationship on a wellness–holistic health model of care, the *locus of decision making* ideally rests with clients. These are clients who are able to assume responsibility for meeting their own mental health needs and who require nursing assistance for health education and health promotion and for guidance in establishing an environment that will support high-level wellness. Some clients, however, may be only partially able to assume responsibility for meeting their mental health needs, and they may require a therapeutic regimen to meet those needs. In these situations, the locus of decision making is shared by the client and the nurse. Other clients may have such severely impaired reality-testing ability or such severe emotional problems that therapeutic intervention is necessary to improve their mental health before they can assume self-responsibility. In these situations, the locus of decision making rests primarily with the nurse (National Council of State Boards of Nursing, Inc., 1980).

Dorothy Orem's (1971) self-care model is pertinent to any discussion of the locus of decision making. According to Orem, self-care actions or systems of self-care can be considered therapeutic when they contribute to the following outcomes:

1. Maintenance and promotion of life processes and functioning
2. Promotion of normal growth and development, both physical and social
3. Prevention, treatment, or cure of disease conditions and injuries
4. Prevention of disability or rehabilitation after a disabling injury or disease

The first two outcomes are pertinent to everyone, while the last two are pertinent only to people who are at risk for, or who are suffering from, disease or injury.

Because self-care is goal- or outcome-seeking activity, it may be characterized as deliberate action. A client appraises a situation, weighs the anticipated results of alternative courses of action, determines which result he or she desires, makes a thoughtful and deliberate choice of one appropriate course of action, and then follows through on the selected course of action. Therefore, according to Orem, deliberate action is a process that is "self-initiated, self-directed, controlled," and based on informed judgment.

To have informed judgment, a client needs to be (1) knowledgeable about the demands of self-care, the actions necessary to accomplish self-care, and factors in the environment (such as social values and rules and availability of resources) that may facilitate or impede self-care and (2) skillful in performing tasks, making judgments, and validating judgments. Any deficiencies in these areas of knowledge or skill may limit a client's ability to assume responsibility for self-care and may shift the locus of decision making partially or totally from the client to the nurse.

Because the locus of decision making is not always centered in clients, in this book both long- and short-term goals are stated without reference to a locus of control. Goals can then be modified to reflect a client's status. For example, the goal "select activities that provide an outlet for angry feelings" can be modified as follows:

Locus of decision making	Goal
Client	Client will select activities that provide an outlet for angry feelings.
Client and nurse	With assistance from the nurse, client will select activities that provide an outlet for angry feelings.
Nurse	Nurse will select activities that provide an outlet for client's angry feelings.

In a situation in which the locus of decision making is not centered in the client, changing this situation should be the objective toward which the client and the nurse work.

Since we believe that people should be actively involved in their health care and that the term *client* denotes such a participatory role, this term is predominantly used in this book. We recognize however, that there are times when, in the delivery of health care, people are (or have historically been) acted upon, when they are placed in a submissive, dependent role—the role of patient. Therefore, in appropriate instances, we depart from the term *client* and use the term *patient*.

Major theories

The complex nature of human mental functioning, the large quantity of ongoing research, and the extensive literature available in relation to human behavior make it impossible for a single book to cover the field fully. The mental health practitioner is responsible for continued study to keep abreast

of developments. Selected theories are introduced in this section to provide a historical perspective and some background for the discussions in the various chapters of this book.

BIOLOGICAL THEORIES

A report of the National Institute of Mental Health task force on research observed that "more has been learned about the brain and behavior in the last quarter-century than in all previous history" (Segal and Boomer, 1975). Research in neurophysiology has increased our knowledge of the complex processes through which messages or impulses are transmitted in the brain and the central nervous system. This has led to theories about alterations in neurochemical processes that may contribute to such mental disorders as schizophrenia and the depressions. Table 1-2 summarizes these theories.

▶ Psychoneuroimmunological theories

a new field of biology, psychoneuroimmunology (PNI), utilizes the techniques of psychology, neurobiology, and immunology and explores how the brain, emotions, and the body's immune system interact. Recent PNI studies indicate that the brain and the immune system form a closed circuit. Chemicals from the brain govern immune defenses, and the immune system, functioning much as a sensory organ functions, is capable of sending chemical communications to the brain about microorganisms and tumors invading the body. PNI researchers suggest that when an infection is present in the body, the immune system not only fights invading microorganisms but also influences such brain-regulated functions as heart rate, sleep, and body temperature. The possibility that chemical messages from the immune system may also be sent to the emotional and rational areas of the brain may explain why such symptoms as irritability and compromised mental functioning often are associated with reduced resistance to infection. In addition, studies by National Institute of Health neuropharmacologist Candace Pert and immunologist Michael Ruff not only indicate that neuropeptides may be the biochemical units of emotion, each linked to a particular emotional state, but also suggest that, because neuropeptides are capable of

TABLE 1-2 Biological theories

Biological orientation	Biological focus	Example of application in psychiatric nursing practice
Psychoneuroimmunological	Interaction of brain, emotions, and immune system	Nurses deliver holistic health care to clients
Genetic	Genes, genetic transmission, and genetic aberrations	Nurses refer clients with family histories of Huntington's disease for genetic counseling
Neurophysiological	Neural transmission of impulses	Nurses administer medications whose actions affect neuraltransmission of impulses, aiding in the treatment of psychoses and depressions
Developmental	Adequate nutrition and environmental stimulation for brain cell development	Nurses teach parents about the importance of adequate prenatal and infant nutrition for optimal biopsychosocial child development

linking onto macrophages, emotions can influence the way that macrophages combat disease. PNI studies are in their infancy, but such research holds hope for discovering the mechanisms that underlie the holistic health approach (Wechsler, 1987).

▶ **Genetic theories**

Research in genetics, particularly the discovery by Watson and Crick of chromosomal structure, and developments in research methodology, such as the electron microscope, have increased the ability to identify genetic abnormalities responsible for some forms of mental retardation and other hereditary disorders.

At present, no single gene aberration has been found that can be cited as a factor in the etiology of schizophrenia (Kety, 1978) or in other functional mental disorders. Huntington's disease, however, is genetically transmitted. If one parent has the disease, there is a 50% chance that each offspring has inherited it. Huntington's disease destroys brain cells, primarily those in the caudate nuclei. In 1983, a test was designed to screen for Huntington's gene. The test is 96% accurate in identifying if a person has the gene for Huntington's disease and

makes genetic counseling possible (Brady, 1987) (see Chapter 26 for further discussion).

The observation that such psychiatric disorders as the schizophrenias and the depressions tend to run in families has led naturally to an assumption that these disorders may be hereditary. Research studies of the incidence of schizophrenia in children of schizophrenic parents, and particularly the study of monozygotic and dizygotic twins of schizophrenic parents, have provided statistical evidence to support this theory. Many studies have found that there is a higher incidence of schizophrenia in the children of schizophrenic parents than in children whose parents are not schizophrenic and an even higher incidence among monozygotic twins of schizophrenic parents. (Studies involving twins will be discussed further in Chapter 25.) To avoid the psychological and sociocultural influences that can result from growing up in a family in which the parents are schizophrenic, studies of children and twins raised by adoptive parents who were not schizophrenic have also been conducted. These studies, too, have found the incidence of schizophrenia higher in children of schizophrenic parents than in children whose biological parents are not schizophrenic.

▶ Neurophysiological theories

Neurophysiological research has been going on for more than a quarter of a century, during which time many theories about the biological nature of mental disorders have been studied. For example, research studies have identified changes in the neurons of the cerebral cortex in victims of Alzheimer's disease. The results of the neuronal changes in Alzheimer's disease are of two types: neurofibrillary tangles and senile plaques. Further research may provide an understanding of the etiology, treatment, and prevention of Alzheimer's disease.

Fairly recent developments in neurophysiological research have contributed to our knowledge of the complex processes by which messages, or impulses, are transmitted from one nerve cell, or neuron, to another. Several chemicals called neurotransmitters have been identified, among them dopamine, norepinephrine, and serotonin. Because of their chemical structure, neurotransmitters are also referred to as biogenic amines and as monoamines. In the transmission of messages or impulses from the axon, or nerve ending, of one neuron to a receptor site in an adjacent neuron, a chemical neurotransmitter, dopamine, for example, is released into the synaptic space between the neurons. Following transmission, the neurotransmitter in the synaptic space is either taken back into the axon of the transmitter neuron through the cell membrane (re-uptake) or metabolized by enzymes or other chemical substances. An enzyme, monoamine oxidase, is believed to be essential to the neutralization of the neurotransmitter and possibly to the re-uptake process (Schildkraut, 1978). Nerve cells are highly specialized in the neurotransmitters that they produce and respond to and in their locations and functions in relation to other neurons (Segal and Boomer, 1975).

Research in neurochemistry has been stimulated and influenced by study of the action and side effects of the psychopharmaceuticals that are effective in the treatment of psychoses and depressions. The dopamine hypothesis, for example, which posits some disturbance in the neurotransmitter dopamine, was stimulated by the observation that parkinsonism was a prominent side effect of treatment with the phenothiazines and other antipsychotic drugs. Since it was known that in Parkinson's disease there is a deficiency of dopamine or a disturbance in dopamine transmission, the assumption was made that the antipsychotic drugs acted by blocking dopamine receptors (see Chapter 25). Other studies have focused upon the group of antidepressant drugs that are monoamine oxidase inhibitors. Such drugs are effective in treating certain forms of depression (see Chapter 22).

▶ Developmental theories

The relationship between experience and psychological development, particularly in the early years of life and personality development, has been a major concern in psychological theories since the works of Freud early in this century. Biological research in recent years has focused upon the importance of adequate nutrition and environmental stimulation to brain cell development. Nutritional deficiencies during the prenatal period and during infancy, when the brain is undergoing the most rapid development, have been found to have a direct impact upon brain cell development. Studies in mice have demonstrated that malnutrition during these critical periods "permanently reduces the number of neurons in the brains of mice" (Segal and Boomer, 1975). Lack of environmental stimulation during the early developmental years also has a negative impact upon brain cell development and function (Segal and Boomer, 1975). (See Chapter 6.)

PSYCHOLOGICAL THEORIES

A variety of psychological theories or schools of psychological thought have developed during the last century. Two major schools of psychological theory began at about the same time with the works of Freud in Austria and Pavlov in Russia. Freud introduced the psychodynamic, or intrapsychic, theory, which has led to a variety of additional theories of intrapsychic functioning. In his studies of animals, Pavlov introduced behavior theory, which has also been expanded upon and applied to human behavior.

Some of the basic concepts of each of these and other schools of thought will be presented here. Table 1-3 summarizes these theories. Additional

TABLE 1-3 Psychological theories

Psychiatric orientation	Psychiatric focus	Example of application in psychiatric nursing practice
Psychodynamic	Unconscious processes motivate behavior; id, ego, and superego are interacting structures of the personality; symptoms are symbolic representation of intrapsychic conflicts	Nurses help clients develop insight into their feelings and the way those feelings influence their behavior so they may modify their behavior
Interpersonal	Interpersonal interactions, including the impact of social forces on the individual, influence the origin and perpetuation of behavior; the nature of interpersonal relationships is important to an individual's mental health	Nursing is an interpersonal process; by experiencing a satisfying relationship with the nurse, clients can learn to form satisfying relationships with others
Behavioral	Behavior, rather than thoughts or feelings, is paramount; all behavior, including psychiatric symptoms, is learned through conditioning (either operant or respondent)	Nurses use praise or "token" rewards (operant conditioning) to teach and/or reinforce clients' adaptive behaviors, while giving demerits for maladaptive behavior

theoretical formulations will be discussed in the chapters in which they are relevant.

▶ **Psychodynamic theory**

Psychodynamic, or intrapsychic, theory, upon which psychoanalysis is based, is a conceptual framework pioneered by Freud that aids in the understanding of the complex forces and functions related to human behavior and personality. Several aspects of this theory will be discussed.

Levels of awareness or consciousness. The concept of levels of consciousness, often referred to as the topographical theory, is important in psychodynamic theory. According to this concept, there are three levels of awareness, or consciousness, which influence behavior—the conscious level, the preconscious level, and the unconscious level.

The conscious level is that part of experience which is in awareness. This level encompasses the broad range of intellectual, emotional, and interpersonal aspects of behavior, among others, over which we have conscious control. The preconscious level includes those areas of mental functioning that, although not in immediate awareness, can be recalled with some effort. Anyone who has had

some difficulty recalling information necessary to answer a question on an examination, even when the information has been reviewed the night before, has had experience with this level of awareness. The preconscious level serves an important function in screening out extraneous data and incoming stimuli when one is trying to concentrate on a particular matter.

The unconscious level is characterized by mental functioning that is out of awareness and that cannot be recalled. Inherent in Freud's view of the unconscious is the idea that the level of mental functioning in early life, prior to the development of language and logical thought processes, still exists within the psyche and must be maintained on the unconscious level to protect one's ability to function as a mature adult. This is accomplished, after the ability for logical thought has developed, through the process of repression. Repression is one of the counterforces or ego-defense mechanisms that maintain a hypothetical boundary between conscious and unconscious levels of functioning. Thoughts, wishes, ideas, and so on that are in conflict with one's internalized standards and ideals are also maintained in the unconscious level through repression and other counterforces.

An important aspect of the unconscious level of functioning is that such forces as drives and wishes that are kept out of awareness are dynamic forces that seek expression, even in a disguised form—hence the need for counterforces. Therefore, in topographical theory the unconscious level of functioning is viewed as one of the motivating forces of behavior. Some of the forms through which unconscious forces may be expressed are dreams, slips of the tongue, and impulsive acts. Expression may also be seen in disturbances in thinking and behavior that appear in symptoms of psychoses and neuroses.

The idea of a dynamic unconscious process as one of the motivating forces of human behavior—the idea of unconscious motivation—is one of the Freudian views that aroused controversy. The idea that all of our thinking, feeling, and acting is not under fully conscious control is threatening to our view of ourselves as fully rational people. This concept has, however, become a part of our language and can be useful in understanding otherwise inexplicable behavior, such as that often displayed in symptoms of mental disorder.

Personality structure. The id is the part of the personality with which one is born and from which the ego and the superego, the more mature parts of the personality, develop as the individual progresses through the stages of psychosexual development from infancy to adulthood (see Chapter 6). The infant is born with the potential for such development and with innate or inborn drives for the survival of the self and the survival of the species. Survival of the self requires that such basic biological needs as those for food, sleep, and shelter be met; since the infant is helpless, these needs must be met by the mother or by others in the environment. The sexual and aggressive drives are also viewed as inborn tendencies or instincts present in the id. The id is therefore often referred to as the seat of the passions.

Freud introduced the term *pleasure principle* to describe one aspect of functioning at the id level of personality. The pleasure principle means that internal needs, experienced by the infant as tension, demand immediate gratification, that is, relief of tension. This principle is in accord with Cannon's theory of homeostasis, which holds that an organism always seeks a return to a steady state. There is no ability to discriminate, at this early level of development, between an object that will satisfy a need and one that will not. Any available vehicle will be utilized to reduce tension. For example, to reduce hunger tension, the young infant will suck upon anything near the mouth. In later life, similar indiscriminate behavior can often be observed as psychiatric symptoms. Compulsive hand washing, for example, may be utilized to reduce the tension of anxiety and conflict.

Primary process thinking is another aspect of the id level of functioning that can be helpful in understanding behavior. Primary process thinking is a form of mental functioning that precedes the ability to use logical thought processes. It is the form of thought believed to occur in early life, before the development of language. Dreams are one example of primary process thinking, and it is, perhaps, through dreams that this level of mental functioning can best be understood. One feature of dreams is their incomprehensibility. Dreams are highly symbolic, and much of the symbolism is of the earlier or more primitive level of mental functioning. One symbol may represent more than one unconscious wish, thought, emotion, or object. Put another way, many forces that are seeking expression may be condensed into a single symbolic expression. Another aspect of dreams is the lack of logic. Contradictory or mutually exclusive wishes, thoughts, and so on can occur together.

Dreams serve an important function in mental life in that they provide expression, in a disguised form, of some of the unconscious forces of the personality and thus help to maintain mental health. Primary process thinking can also be seen in some of the behavioral symptoms in mental disorders. For example, the compulsive hand washing mentioned earlier makes no sense from the logical point of view. But in relation to the symbolism of primary process, this symptom becomes more comprehensible when it is viewed as a means of reducing the tension of anxiety, conflict, and guilt.

The ego is the part of the personality that interacts with both the external environment and the somatic and psychic aspects of the individual's internal environment. The ego is a highly complex system of functions that is sometimes referred to as the executive part of the personality and the site of reason. The ego develops over time as an individual matures physically, psychologically, and socially. Since the ego is involved with learning, reason, and creativity, ego development continues over a lifetime. Ego functions encompass all of the intellectual and social abilities that we think of as being particularly human. Imagination, creativity, and the ability to use spoken and written language, logic, and abstract thought are but a few of these complex human functions. The ego is also the system that experiences emotions, which range from joy to fear, anxiety, and depression. Another major function of the ego that is of special importance to mental health is that of maintaining the integrity of the personality when it is coping with stress. The noxious feelings often aroused by internal and external stress threaten the integrity of the personality by upsetting the balance between unconscious forces seeking expression and counterforces preventing a breakthrough of the unconscious forces into awareness. The ego maintains the delicate balance between the conscious and unconscious aspects of the personality through such mental mechanisms as repression, denial, and projection. Stress and the anxiety that accompanies it can bring about the need for additional, often more primitive, mental mechanisms, or ego-defense mechanisms, to cope with it. When stress is severe, such mechanisms may result in symptoms of mental illness. (Ego-defense mechanisms and concepts of anxiety will be discussed further in Chapters 6 and 8.)

The superego represents the internalization of the ethical precepts, standards, prohibitions, and taboos of parents and other authority figures responsible for the enculturation of the child. This complex system develops in childhood through a process of rewards and punishments, approval and disapproval, and through identification with parents, peers, and others in one's culture. The superego provides an individual with a system of internal controls over thoughts, feelings, and actions that is essential to independent, adult functioning in the culture. The ego ideal, a part of the superego system, is an internalized ideal image of the self toward which the ego strives and against which ego functioning is measured. Striving to realize the ide-

alized image provides some of the motivation for achievement of a person's higher aspirations. When the idealized image is too far removed from the real self, however, the struggle to achieve unrealistic ideals can lead to frustration and feelings of hopelessness.

The conscience is another aspect of the complex superego system. The conscience monitors thoughts, feelings, and actions and measures them against internalized values and standards. When one's internalized values are not adhered to in a particular sphere of behavior, feelings of guilt and shame are aroused. A person who has a strict, inflexible superego is highly susceptible to experiencing guilt and other painful emotions. Since portions of ego and superego functioning are unconscious, the person who is unduly susceptible to experiencing guilt is often unaware that the feeling arises from within the self. In such instances, the feeling is perceived as coming from a punitive environment. In contrast, people in whom the superego is weak or nonexistent do not experience feelings of guilt or shame, even when behavior grossly violates cultural norms. Such individuals lack the internal controls needed to function responsibly in society.

Personality development. One of Freud's major contributions to the understanding of human behavior was the introduction of the theory of personality development, or psychosexual development, as he termed it. Although Freud's ideas about infantile sexuality remain controversial, the concept that there are predictable developmental stages has been generally accepted. The importance of personality development to mental health is implicit in all schools of psychoanalytic thought. Since theories of personality development will be the focus of Chapter 6, they will not be discussed here. It is important to note, however, that the degree to which one masters the sequential, developmental tasks of one stage can have an impact upon mastery of the tasks of succeeding stages. For example, difficulty in developing trust in self and others can inhibit the ability to develop autonomy.

The theoretical formulations of Freud have been expanded and given new focus by many theorists during the years following his work. Anna Freud, for example, further developed the concept of the ego and the mental mechanisms utilized in coping with stress. Erik Erikson expanded Freud's theory of personality development to cover the entire life span. Erikson also refocused developmental theory to incorporate social science concepts concerning the interaction of the individual with the environment. Others have advanced different aspects of Freudian theory.

▶ Interpersonal theories

The interpersonal theorists, sometimes referred to as neo-Freudians, placed emphasis upon the interaction between the individual and society in relation to mental health and mental illness. Karen Horney, Harry Stack Sullivan, and Erich Fromm utilized modern concepts from such disciplines as sociology and anthropology to a greater extent than Freud had in developing their theories.

Horney's theory of neurosis emphasizes the importance of interpersonal interactions in the origin and perpetuation of neurotic behavior. Sullivan also views the individual as primarily a socially interacting organism. Sullivan developed a comprehensive theory to explain human behavior in mental health and mental illness. His theory of personality development and functioning is often considered to be couched more in operational terms than in concepts. Sullivan's terms are often utilized by nurses and other health professionals. Fromm's theory has focused more broadly upon social forces and their impact upon the individual. (The interpersonal theories will be discussed more fully in later chapters.)

▶ Behavior theory

Behavior theory, which was developed in the laboratory through experimental research with animals, had its origins in the work of Ivan Pavlov in Russia. Interest in this field has steadily expanded, and it is now one of the major branches of psychology in Europe and America. The best known contemporary American in this field is B.F. Skinner, whose *Beyond Freedom and Dignity* (1971) applies some of the behavioral concepts to aspects of society. More recent research in behavior, or learning, theory has also focused upon human, rather than animal, behavior, and advances have been made in the study of human motivation and biological rhythms.

One basic premise of behavior is that all behavior is learned—that is, conditioned by events in the development of the organism that arouse the behavior or perpetuate it. From this point of view, psychiatric symptoms are also learned, or, to use the behavioral term, conditioned. Learning occurs in one of two ways, either by respondent conditioning or by operant conditioning.

Wolpe (1974) and others have applied behavior, or learning, theory to the treatment of some symptoms of mental disorders. Many neurotic and psychotic symptoms are regarded by behaviorists as learned but unadaptive behavioral patterns that are maintained by their consequences, that is, by their reinforcements. Behavior therapy, sometimes referred to as behavior modification, focuses upon the overt behavior or symptom that is unadaptive rather than upon the underlying dynamics or subjective experience, which is the focus of the intrapsychic therapists.

The methods employed in behavior therapy for humans include the operant conditioning techniques of positive and negative reinforcement, extinction, and aversive control. Behavior is positively reinforced by the provision of attention, approval, praise, or other forms of reward by people in the environment. Behavior is negatively reinforced by avoidance of an aversive reinforcer. For example, client A leaves the day room when clients B and C try to involve him in their argument and he thereby avoids a confrontation. Client A will be likely in the future to leave the room whenever clients B and C begin to argue. Extinction is accomplished when reinforcing stimuli (both negative or positive) are omitted. The "token economy," in which tokens can be exchanged for candy, cigarettes, and so on as a reward for desired behavior, is often used in the treatment of chronically ill clients in mental hospitals (see Chapter 25). Aversive control is achieved through some form of aversive stimulus when clearly identified undesirable behavior occurs. Negative reinforcement and aversive control are quite often used in adolescent treatment centers, the former by the ignoring of unacceptable behavior that has been identified as attention seeking and the latter through a system of demerits for undesirable behavior.

Other forms of behavior therapy include desensitization techniques (which are combined with forms of deep muscle relaxation to enable the individual to cope with anxiety and other noxious feelings), assertiveness training, persuasion, and advice giving. Desensitization techniques have been used extensively in the treatment of phobias. In such a method, the phobic person is repeatedly exposed in a limited way to the stimulus that induces anxiety. The therapy is combined with deep muscle relaxation. When the client is completely relaxed, the suggestion is made by the therapist that the person imagine being in the situation that produces the phobic response. An elevator or a bus, for example, may be the object of the abnormal fear. The treatment may be repeated several times until the anxiety response is reduced. Then another step is taken—for example, the client walks toward the elevator with the therapist. This gradual approach is continued until the client is able to overcome the phobia.

Any behavior therapy should be designed and carried out, or directed, by a skilled behavioral therapist or by a person who has extensive knowledge of theory and techniques. Prior to any attempt to institute behavior therapy, the particular behavior to be modified must be clearly identified. The contingencies, or events that reinforce the behavior, must also be understood. Then a program can be developed that can be followed consistently by everyone who will participate in the therapy. The client who is the object of the behavior modification techniques should be included in decisions about the behavior to be modified and the techniques to be used and should agree to participate in the program.

SOCIOCULTURAL THEORIES

A sociocultural perspective on mental health focuses on the influence of social definitions, social norms, and social values on human behavior. Sociocultural theory explores social processes in an attempt to better understand mental illnesses and to promote mental health. The sociocultural theories

used in this book may be divided into three categories: functionalism model, psychocultural model, and communication model. Table 1-4 summarizes these theories.

▶ Functionalism model

The functionalism model holds that society is an organismic whole. The various parts of society (that is, institutions and groups) articulate smoothly with one another and thereby maintain equilibrium. New ideas and practices that maintain the existing social order are readily accepted by members of society. Ideas and practices that seriously disrupt the existing social order tend to be resisted. Disjunctions in society may produce social strain.

Functionalists like Durkheim, Merton, Srole, and Parsons use social strain theory to explain social deviance and psychopathology. Society stresses certain values, roles, and standards, but the social structure may make it difficult to act in accordance with them. There may be a disjunction between socially sanctioned goals and access to legitimized ways of achieving those goals, or the social system may make the rules contradictory and meaningless. Sociocultural disjunctions may result in inadequate socialization of children. Family patterns, kinship obligations, child-rearing practices, and economic activities may be disrupted. Value systems and role relationships may become confused, fragmented, or conflicting. Children may fail to learn socially sanctioned values, standards, and roles. The resultant frustration, alienation, and tension may produce socially deviant or maladaptive behavior.

▶ Psychocultural model

The psychocultural model focuses upon the relationship between the individual psyche and the social field. Society is viewed as having a profound impact upon the development of an individual's personality. Society provides an individual with opportunities for role development, independence, and socially acceptable emotional expression.

Children are born into a family unit. The family unit becomes the first socializing agent. Later in life, children encounter other socializing agents,

TABLE 1-4 Sociocultural theories

Sociocultural orientation	Sociocultural focus	Example of application in psychiatric nursing practice
Functionalism	Society is an organismic whole; social disjunctions may produce social strain; frustration and alienation associated with social strain may produce socially deviant or maladaptive behavior	Nurses identify social disjunctions such as disorganized families or a high incidence of social deviance in a community and intervene by counseling disorganized families and pressing for social changes that will modify the sociocultural environment
Psychocultural	Socializing agents teach children socially acceptable norms, standards, and values; mentally healthy individuals use socially approved ways of coping with stress; others use stress-reduction behaviors society defines as socially deviant or mentally ill	Nurses help clients develop socially acceptable ways of coping with anxiety, frustration, anger, low self-esteem, etc.
Communication	Verbal and nonverbal communication are interrelated; the form and meaning of communication are influenced by sociocultural context; all behavior, including deviant or pathologic behavior, is communication; behavior that is socially approved in one culture may be labeled deviant or pathological in another culture; impaired communication may disrupt role relationships and contribute to mental illness	Nurses assess the meaning and effectiveness of client communication within the sociocultural context in which it occurs; nurses give clients feedback about congruence between verbal and nonverbal communication; nurses act as role models in teaching clients socially acceptable communication behaviors

such as teachers, clergymen, and peers. A socializing agent serves as a cultural ideal. Children identify with socializing agents, emulate their behavior, and thereby inculcate the norms, standards, and values of society. Through the process of socialization, individuals eventually want to act the way society demands and desire what society needs.

Since family units are never identical, what a child learns at home may later come into conflict with what is learned from other socializing agents. The manner of resolving such conflict, as well as the inherent conflict between the desires of the individual and the demands of society, varies from one society to another. While every society defines what is acceptable and unacceptable behavior, each society offers a range of acceptable alternatives from which an individual may choose.

Social scientists like Fromm, Wallace, Whiting,

and Child look at the sociocultural context in which individuals develop and at the mechanisms individuals use to adjust to society. While the majority of a society's members are usually able to use socially sanctioned techniques for keeping stress within tolerable limits, some persons may find socially sanctioned stress-reduction behavior ineffective and may try alternative techniques. Some of these alternative types of behavior may be defined by society as social deviance or mental illness.

► **Communication model**

The communication model focuses upon the cultural specificity of communication. Communication is a process of regulating relationships and exchanging ideas, information, values, and feelings with others. Communication occurs on both verbal and nonverbal levels. Verbal communication is the use of spoken language. Nonverbal communication embraces kinesics (the way people use body parts to communicate) and proxemics (the way people use space to communicate). These different types of communication are systematically interrelated to reinforce, supplement, or contradict one another.

Communication specialists like Birdwhistle, Hall, Scheflen, and Ashcraft maintain that kinesic and proxemic communication are as culturally specific as verbal communication. The form and meaning of linguistic, kinesic, and proxemic behavior are dependent upon the sociocultural context in which they occur. Ethnicity, age, sex, social class, institutional membership, and geographic locale are only a few of the factors that influence the form and meaning of verbal and nonverbal communication.

When people from different cultural backgrounds interact, using dissimilar linguistic, kinesic, or proxemic cues and having different assumptions and orientations, communication is impaired and role relationships may be disrupted. A sense of nonrelatedness to persons with a different cultural heritage may develop. In addition, culturally determined and culturally acceptable behavior that is foreign to members of a dominant culture may be misinterpreted and labeled as deviant or pathological. (Sociocultural theories will be discussed further in Chapter 4 and in other chapters in which they are relevant.)

GENERAL SYSTEMS THEORY

The current state of systems theory is built on the classic works of such people as Bertalanffy, Bateson, Buckley, Fuller, Miller and Hall, and Fagan.

General systems theory is founded on assumptions inherent in the holistic paradigm. This paradigm holds a monistic view of the universe as one grand, interconnected system. According to the holistic paradigm, truth and knowledge are obtained through the interaction of inner experience and external verification, and this interaction accounts for both the subjective and objective aspects of knowledge. Stability and change within a system are accounted for by transformation. While form is maintained through the permanent transformation matrix (or structure) of a system, change occurs when the system is transformed as a result of infor-

mation-processing feedback loops (Battista, 1977; Harman, 1974; Laszlo, 1972; Lifton, 1975; Sutherland, 1973).

Any particular system can be described by both its concrete and abstract aspects. The objects or parts that make up a system are known as the concrete aspect of the system. These parts, which take on different attributes or characteristics over time, are referred to as system variables. When a system is examined at a particular moment in time, the interaction between system variables accounts for the form of that system; the way that the total system is characterized is referred to as the state of the system. The abstract aspect, or the pattern of organizational rules and functions that interconnect the variables of a system, reflects the organizational framework of the system and is referred to as the structure of the system (Battista, 1977).

Whether a system is defined as a complex of elements in interaction (Bertalanffy, 1955) or as "a set of objects together with the relationships between the objects and between their attributes," any system is composed of subsystems (smaller systems within the system), which can be further broken down into sub-sub-systems, components, elements, units, or parts that are tied together by their interdependence into a total system (Hall and Fagan, 1968, 81–84). Systems exist as a synthesis of their parts so that "the whole is greater than the sum of its parts." Outside any particular system is a suprasystem or larger system of which the given system is an integral part (Miller 1965, 218). According to Fuller (1969), by focusing on any given system, you are simultaneously identifying what is included (its "insideness") and what is excluded (its "outsideness"). The basic notion of a system is that dynamic relationships or interrelatedness unite its parts ("insideness") and its suprasystem (environment or "outsideness") into a meaningful whole. Figure 1-1 shows how a system is hierarchically organized into a more inclusive suprasystem as well as being a synthesis of component subsystems or parts.

Systems are characterized by such properties as wholeness, hierarchical organization, interdependence, activity, self-maintenance, and self-transformation. The properties of wholeness, hierarchical organization, and interdependence have already

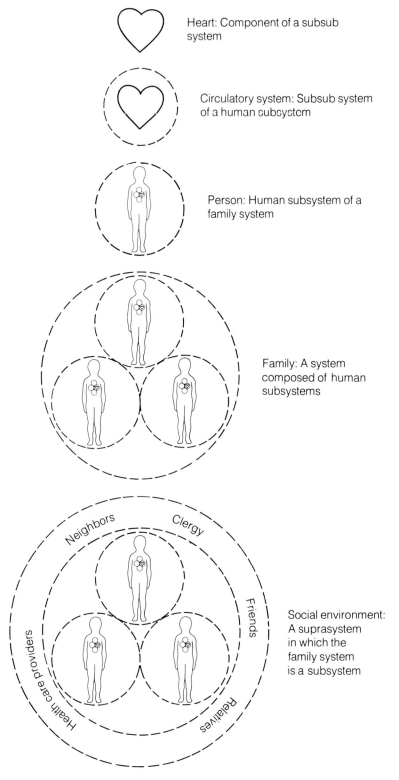

Heart: Component of a subsub system

Circulatory system: Subsub system of a human subsystem

Person: Human subsystem of a family system

Family: A system composed of human subsystems

Social environment: A suprasystem in which the family system is a subsystem

Fig. 1-1 System organization: synthesis of component parts hierarchically organized. System within suprasystem is composed of interacting subsystems and subsubsystems.

been discussed. Because of the properties of wholeness, hierarchical organization, and interdependence, alteration in any particular variable may affect a transformation of all system variables and partially affect the condition of every other variable within a particular hierarchical level of the system. For example, through a process of mutual interaction, psychological counseling of a husband-father may affect not only his relationships with significant others (both within and outside the family system) but also the ways that family members relate with him, with each other, and with people outside the family (suprasystem). Ultimately, these interaction changes may circle back and affect the husband-father. Bateson (1958, 176-177) explains that "We have to consider not only A's reaction to B's behavior but we must go on to consider how these affect B's later behavior and the effect of this on A." An unending feedback loop is created that keeps the system in a continuous process of transformation. This is referred to as the property of activity or the dynamic state of systems. Positive feedback facilitates change within a system, while negative feedback promotes system stability. Feedback thus has a regulatory function. It serves to monitor, reinforce, and correct the structure and conditions of a system.

Flow of information is utilized for feedback. Buckley (1967) holds that any system must be able to incorporate a "full flow" of three types of information to sustain effective functioning of the system. These three categories of information are: (1) external information (data concerning conditions outside the system, such as the nature of socioeconomic conditions or the quality of support systems), (2) historical information (data of a historical nature that affects the system, such as a person's past experiences with psychotherapy or past state of health) and (3) internal information (data concerning conditions within the system, such as a person's values or thought patterns).

Self-maintenance refers to the ability of a system to keep its form and properties not only over time but also under varying environmental conditions. For example, despite the biopsychosociocultural changes inherent in immigrating from a tropical country to a temperate zone country and the fact that, over time, every cell in the human body is replaced by another, a person is able to maintain his or her body shape over a period of time. On the other hand, the ability of a system to alter its structure and properties is known as self-transformation. Self-transformation on a particular level is exemplified by learning and adaptation, while evolution is an example of self-transformation that generates hierarchical reordering (Bateson, 1972; Battista, 1977).

General systems theory is an approach to conceptualizing and analyzing relationships between interacting units. It allows us to explore problems beyond the level of the individual person and to see how myriad relationships—biological, physiological, social, economic, and psychological—are involved.

Social scientists such as Moynihan, Janchill, and Hazzard describe systems as being either open or closed. An open system has a permeable boundary, and it is characterized by active interaction with the outside environment. An example of an open system is a family that has many social relationships; that utilizes such social institutions as church, school, and health facilities; and that buys consumer goods from both local and nonlocal merchants. A closed system is self-contained; it has a definite boundary, and interaction with the outside environment is nonexistent. Few families represent such a system, but we may find families whose networks are restricted or limited. For example, an elderly couple living in a depressed urban area may have lost contact with relatives and may be hesitant to make new friends and afraid to venture outside an apartment. The man and the woman in such a couple rely upon each other for support and may have little social interaction with others. However, even such a seemingly closed system has some avenues of interaction with the outside environment. Food must be purchased at the market. Health problems require the services of physicians or nurses. A clergyman may attend to religious needs. Nevertheless, such a family is very vulnerable during crisis periods because of the large expenditure of energy needed to defend its boundaries and the paucity of support resources.

In contrast, a family that is an open system has more access to outside resources and social networks that can provide support and assistance when they are needed. In addition, more energy is available for problem solving and life pursuits, since it is not being expended on maintaining boundaries.

Nurses and nursing focus on many different types of human systems. Individuals, themselves a synthesis of such subsystems as cardiovascular, neurological, digestive, etc., are at the same time hierarchically organized into more inclusive supra-systems such as family, small group, and community. This set of human systems and subsystems is the focus of nursing practice. For example, when dealing with an individual, nurses might focus on alteration in mood or impaired nutrition; when dealing with a small group or family, on family or group process; when dealing with a community, on underutilization of services or populations at risk.

Systems therapy takes into consideration all factors that may contribute to a problem. The illness of one member of a family often indicates that a pervasive, stress-producing problem may exist within the family unit. Treatment may involve all members of the family and may even include other relatives, as well as friends. During a period of hospitalization, other clients may also be included in this social network. Through the inclusion of many vital linkages in a social system, there is increased opportunity for feedback and exploration of alternative avenues of problem solving. Change in any one of the component linkages in a system ultimately affects, and is affected by, the other linkages in the system.

A nurse can become a linkage in the social system of an emotionally ill person. The nurse thus can focus on the person's relationships with other people and with the environment. The actions of either the nurse or the client may affect the entire system. Concentrating on making the system open and adaptable facilitates the evaluation of health care stratagems, the development of a holistic approach to health care, and an understanding of mentally disturbed individuals and their place in society. To work on improving people's feelings of self-worth, only to discharge them back into families that scapegoat and derogate them and into communities that are fearful of them and reluctant to employ them, is self-defeating. The hospital, the family, and the community are component linkages in the emotionally disturbed person's social field. Negative feedback from one will undermine the efforts of other linkages.

NURSING THEORIES: SYSTEMS MODELS

Nursing theories or conceptual models, which are often based on theories and concepts from other disciplines, help to clarify the domain of nursing activity. Nursing theories provide a framework for professional nursing practice. Depending on the nursing theory/concept used, the focus of nursing practice will vary. Stanton (1985) points out that Florence Nightingale, the first nursing theorist, by focusing on environmental manipulation and the prevention and alleviation of unnecessary suffering laid a foundation on which nurses could later build their theories. In this section we will explore how some nursing theorists focus on human systems and how their theories assist in the implementation of nursing practice.

King's (1981) *theory of goal attainment* identifies the individual as the central focus of nursing. Individuals are personal systems. Groups are interpersonal systems. Society is a social system. The functional concept for individuals is perception, for groups it is interaction, for society it is organization. King examines the impact of *perception, interaction,* and *organization* on individuals. King defines perception as each person's impression or image of reality. People are reacting, time-oriented, social beings. As such, they interact with other people in existential moments to accomplish a purpose or goal. Goal attainment is achieved through transactions (energy and information exchanges among interacting individuals). Social interaction and learning occur through the avenues of communication and exchange of ideas and opinions.

King states that both clients and nurses are affected by perceptual influences on judgment and decision making. The focus of nursing is on people and their environments. Nursing practice involves assisting people to attain, maintain, and restore health (defined as a biopsychosocial state where people are able to carry out their social roles). This orientation views nursing practice as a process of action, reaction, interaction, and transaction that helps people to meet daily needs, perform activities of daily living, and cope with health and illness.

Johnson's (1980) *behavioral system model* views human beings as behavioral systems that exist in particular cultural settings. These behavioral systems are composed of *seven universal subsystems:* attachment (or affiliative), dependency, ingestive, eliminative, sexual, aggressive, and achievement. Each subsystem has structural components (drive, set, choice, and behavior) that interrelate with one another, thereby engendering the overall function of the system. *Drive* refers to stimulation toward a desired goal; *set* refers to predisposition for particular ways of acting; *choice* refers to selecting a particular action from a repertoire of alternatives that will best accomplish the sought-after goal; and *behavior* refers to response competency and effectiveness in goal attainment. Although behavior is an integrated response to external or internal stimuli, environmental factors are capable of modifying it. Therefore, a behavioral system is manifested by complex, overt, functional, and purposeful responses to a multiplicity of environmental stimuli. Biological, sociocultural, and psychological systems regulate behavioral responses through such factors as genetics, values, roles, self-concept, and problem-solving ability and sometimes mask the universal nature of human behavior.

According to Johnson, because a behavioral system aims to produce an integrated response to the environment that will enable relatively stable balance, it adjusts to ever-changing internal and external environmental demands. This process of adjusting is referred to as *behavioral adaptation*. When a behavioral system is threatened by the loss of order and predictability, a person experiences illness. The goal of nursing, an external regulator force, is to preserve or effect system stability. This is accomplished by using a five-step nursing process that includes assessment (data collection about biopsychosociocultural factors, environmental factors, and general regulator factors), analysis (examination of subsystems for functional and structural stress by identifying drive, set, choice, and behavior), diagnosis (delineating conditions of insufficiency, discrepancy, incompatibility, or dominance), intervention (carrying out nursing actions), and evaluation (determining the effectiveness of intervention strategies and their consequences, both intended and unintended).

Roy's (1970, 1976, 1980) *adaptation model* views an individual as an open system capable of adapting to an ever-changing environment. Every individual is a biopsychosocial being with distinctive ways of responding to environmental changes. *Modes of adaptation* include physiological needs, role function, interdependence, and self-concept, and problems of adaptation can occur in any of these four modes. Adaptive mechanisms are of two major types: a *regulator mechanism* that operates through the autonomic nervous system and prepares a person for such coping responses as approach, fight, or flight and a *cognator mechanism* that operates by identifying, amassing, and relating stimuli, thereby permitting the formation of symbolic responses. Individual adaptation levels are influenced by such factors as focal stimuli (those stimuli presently facing a person), residual stimuli (consisting of attitudes, beliefs, experiences, or traits), and contextual stimuli (all other stimuli).

Roy applies such an adaptation approach to health. Individual adaptation is a function of a person's position along a health-illness continuum (the polarities being peak wellness and death). The focus of nursing practice, to promote adaptation, is therapeutic because it conserves client energy. The nursing process is used to facilitate client adaptation. Nurses assess client behavior in each of the four adaptive modes by locating the client on the health-illness continuum and by noting influential focal, contextual, and residual factors. Nursing diagnosis is accomplished by identifying problems related not only to adaptive and maladaptive behavior but also to major focal, contextual, and residual stimuli. Goals are then established that will alter maladaptive behavior and strengthen adaptive behavior. Goal implementation includes managing or controlling focal, contextual, and residual stimuli, and evaluation consists of determining the effectiveness of interventions. It is evident that throughout Roy's adaptation model, the concepts of biological, psychological, and social integrity are prominent.

Orem's (1971) *self-care theory* focuses on the individual and the need for self-care. Self-care refers to consistent, purposeful, controlled, and effective care actions carried out by a mature person for him or her self. Self-care is divided into three types: *universal self-care* (activities that meet such basic human needs as air, food, excretion, and social intercourse), *developmental self-care* (activities that meet developmental needs throughout the life span) and *health deviation self-care* (activities that meet needs that develop as a result of illness, injury, or disability). Regardless of the type of self-care activity, it is learned, involves some degree of decision making, and is influenced by one's social position and roles, culture, and state of health.

Orem states that self-care at any level is therapeutic because it helps to support life processes and normal functioning, fosters normal growth and development, and prevents, limits, compensates for, or cures illness, injury, or disability. This theory of self-care is based on the premise that human beings are differentiated from other living creatures by their ability to manage themselves and their environments. They are capable of reflection and symbolic thinking and are able to apply these functions to communication and actions that are beneficial to self and others.

According to Orem, individuals and their environments are integrated into functional wholes (systems). Awareness of the nature of individual-environmental interaction is essential if change elements are to be introduced that will alter the balance of a system. This concept is important for nurses who provide or assist clients with self-care. Nurses plan, manage, and maintain *systems of self-care* for clients who have some degree of self-care deficit. These self-care systems may be either completely compensatory, partially compensatory, or supportive educative, but they are all designed to govern the need for therapeutic self-care and to promote clients' own self-care abilities. The framework for implementing these self-care systems, the nursing process, consists of identifying clients' self-care needs, planning nursing assistance or actions that will meet these self-care needs, and providing or managing nursing actions. Nursing assistance should be based on one or a combination of the three basic self-care systems. Nursing assistance should be implemented according to the plan of care and should keep in mind not only the desired goal but also goal-pertinent environmental, technological, and human factors. Altered conditions and progress toward goal attainment should be considered whenever contemplating revision of a plan for nursing assistance.

Rogers's (1980, 1983) *theory of the nature of unitary human beings* focuses on the wholeness of people and their interaction with the environment. Unitary human beings are open systems that are characterized by *four dimensionality* (a synthesis of the three space coordinates and time). Underlying this four dimensionality are certain basic premises concerning the integral relationship between human and environmental fields: (1) noncausality, (2) nonspatiality, (3) nontemporality, (4) nonlineality, (5) rhythmical, nonrepetitive patterning, and (6) irreducibility to parts. Change, since it is rhythmical, nonrepetitive, and nonlineal, is delineated as an irregular spiral rather than as a cycle. Unitary human beings exhibit qualities that are both different from the parts and not predictable from knowledge of the parts. They are negentropic energy fields containing pattern, organization, unity, and arbitrary boundaries. The pattern and organization describing a field are engendered by motion, interaction, rhythmicity, and change. Pattern persists throughout this mutual process and provides both continuity and change. Other properties of unitary human beings can be described by the principle of *complementarity* (refers to the ongoing, mutual interaction between human and environmental fields), the principle of *helicy* (refers to the nature of human and environmental change, which is a continuous developmental process that is evolutionary, creatively complex, diverse, differentiated, probabilistic, and goal-directed) and the principle of *resonancy* (refers to the tendency of human and environmental fields to function according to patterns that can be identified and studied).

Rogers explains nursing by relying on principles that explain human beings, and human beings are explained by referring to principles that Rogers believes describe the universe. Rogers views the focus of nursing as the movement of human beings toward maximum health. The principles of complementarity, resonancy, and helicy are holistic ways of viewing human beings and should be used by nurses to deliver holistic health care that considers biopsychosocial aspects and problems of clients. The framework for nursing practice is a conceptual system that includes empirical observation, identification of meaningful relationships between knowledges, and verification or evaluation of concepts and knowledge. The amassing of data from empirical evidence and "unexpected relationships" arising from empirical evidence are used to "support hypotheses" or to generate additional questions for study. Rogers believes that the science of nursing is the science of unitary human beings.

Neuman's *systems-theory model* (1982) incorporates the concepts of stress, coping, and levels of prevention. Neuman's model is based upon a person's dynamic relationship to stress. Neuman views systems theory as "a unifying force for scientific exploration," one that can provide nurses a fresh perspective for understanding and intervening in people's responses to stress.

Neuman defines a system as a set of component parts in dynamic interaction. The "pervasive order" of the system is maintained through regulatory mechanisms that evolve from the dynamics of the open system.

Neuman applies such a systems approach to health. People, whether they are well or ill, are dynamic systems having four component parts— physiological, psychological, developmental, and sociocultural. Wellness exists when all component parts or subparts are "in harmony with the whole of man." Disharmony thus contributes to various degrees of nonwellness. *Environment* (both internal and external) affects and is affected by human needs, drives, perceptions, and goals. People are open systems, constantly interacting with their environments, and this interaction contributes to their states of wellness or illness.

Any system strives for a dynamic state of balance. Forces (harmful or beneficial) that tend to disrupt this state of balance, or *normal line of defense*, Neuman labels *stressors*. Stressors are characterized by their nature, timing, duration, and intensity, and they can affect more than one human component part. In addition, not only do stressors influence people's behavior but they are also influenced by people's responses to them.

A *flexible line of defense*, consisting of coping mechanisms that can be mobilized to deal with stressors, acts as a buffer between a person's normal line of defense and the stressors in the environment. When the flexible line of defense is ineffective in protecting a person from stressors, the stressors penetrate the normal line of defense, and the person experiences a state of disequilibrium. Such a state of imbalance is accompanied by a "violent energy flow," as the person tries to cope with the stressors and the resultant disorganization. At this point, the person's internal resistance factors, or *lines of resistance*, try to stem the disorganization and to reinstate the normal line of defense (a state of homeodynamics).

If the lines of resistance are effective in stabilizing the system, the energy flow is arrested and the person may begin to move toward a state of wellness (negentropy). If the lines of resistance are ineffective in stabilizing the system, large amounts of energy continue to be expended. As more energy is expended than is stored or produced, illness (entropy) and, eventually, death may occur.

According to Neuman, the function of nursing is to help clients conserve energy. The framework for nursing practice is a three-phase nursing process that incorporates client perspective into each phase. The nursing diagnosis phase encompasses both assessment and diagnosis. A holistic assessment includes data about the four aspects of the client system (psychological, physiological, developmental, and sociocultural), potential and actual stressors that threaten the stability of the client system, characteristics of lines of defense and resistance, condition of energy resources, nature of client-environment interaction, and variations in wellness. Client and nurse perceptions concerning wellness variations are compared for differences that might interfere with client attainment of a maximum level of wellness. In the nursing goals phase, an integral part of the preparation of a nursing care plan includes negotiating with the client about desired outcomes and interventions. Interventions are planned to implement goals of retention, attainment, and/or maintenance of client system stability. The nursing outcome phase focuses on goal implementation and evaluation. Nursing care is delivered through primary, secondary, and tertiary preventive intervention. Evaluation of outcome goals following nursing intervention either indicates goal attainment or serves as a basis for revision of the care plan. Client expectations are an integral part of goal evaluation and revision of care plans.

Applying this systems approach, Neuman looks

at the three levels of preventive intervention—primary, secondary, and tertiary.

1. Primary prevention. Stressors are primarily covert, and nursing actions are designed to *promote* or *retain* system stability by strengthening the flexible line of defense. Nursing actions include the identification and modification of risk factors associated with stressors, through education, desensitization, and the strengthening of coping behaviors.

2. Secondary prevention. Stressors are primarily overt, and nursing actions are designed to *reinstate* system stability. Such nursing actions as early case finding, establishing intervention priorities, and instituting appropriate treatment are aimed at decreasing the severity of reactions to stressors.

3. Tertiary prevention. Stressors are primarily overt or residual, and nursing actions are designed to *attain* or *maintain* system stability. Such nursing measures as progressive goal setting, reeducation, and optimum utilization of health services support internal and external resources for reconstitution.

Neuman's systems-theory model, incorporating the concepts of stress, coping, and levels of prevention, is consistent with the orientation set forth in this book. No one nursing model or theory, however, can comprehensively encompass the emerging parameters of professional psychiatric–mental health nursing. In keeping with the eclectic nature of this book, other major nursing theories discussed in this section will also be utilized at appropriate times to discuss behavior and to provide a frame of reference for professional nursing practice. Table 1-5 summarizes these theories and indicates areas of similarities and differences in emphasis and orientation.

As we apply systems theory in this book, we will take a holistic and multifactor approach to the etiology of mental disorders, one that looks at the interrelationship of the factors and feedback loops. Within this systems model, the role of the nurse is to assist a client to remain in a state of system stability. This is accomplished by assessing the whole person and the person's interrelationship with the environment. The collection of data includes analysis of each system (biological, psychological, intellectual, spiritual, and sociocultural) and identification of patterns of relationships or behavior. Goal setting and goal implementation aim at repatterning or manipulating maladaptive patterns, thereby contributing to increased system stability and high-level wellness. At each step in this process, locus of decision making ideally rests with the client.*

ORGANIZATION OF NURSING INTERVENTION

Health maintenance and prevention of disease have long been basic goals of professional nursing. Thus psychiatric nursing, as a part of the nursing profession, has a commitment to mental health promotion and maintenance, as well as to treatment of the mentally ill. In addition, the public and many health professionals have been encouraging the health professions to place more emphasis upon maintenance and promotion of health. The chapters on maladaptive disorders therefore include discussion of the nurse's role in primary, secondary, and tertiary prevention in each mental health problem.

Preventive psychiatry is a term coined by Caplan (1964) to describe a body of theoretical and practical knowledge that can be used to plan and implement programs whose goals are the improvement of the mental health of the community and its residents. Prevention, as defined by Caplan, consists of primary, secondary, and tertiary levels. Primary prevention seeks to reduce the incidence of mental illness in a community, secondary prevention attempts to reduce the duration of mental illness and to prevent sequelae, and tertiary prevention seeks to reduce residual effects of mental disorders through rehabilitation. This concept of prevention has been widely utilized in the community mental health movement in planning and implementing treatment and prevention programs to serve the mental health needs of individuals and communities with a variety of sociocultural characteristics.

We have found the concept of preventive psychiatry an effective approach in professional nursing. It is an approach that can be used in any area of

---

*Refer to the earlier section in this chapter for a discussion of locus of decision making.

TABLE 1-5 Nursing theories

Nurse theorist	System focus	Nursing focus	Framework for nursing practice
King	Personal system of a reacting, time-oriented, social being	People and their environments	Process of mutuality between client and nurse that includes action, reaction, interaction, and transaction to attain, maintain, and restore health
Johnson	Behavioral system composed of 7 universal subsystems	Preservation of or effecting of system stability	Process of assessing biopsychosocial factors, environmental factors, and general regulator factors; analysis of subsystems for functional and structural stress; diagnosis of insufficiency, discrepancy, incompatibility, or dominance; intervention and evaluation
Roy	Person as an open system capable of adapting to a changing environment	Promotion of adaptation	Process of assessing 4 adaptive modes, diagnosing problems related to adaptive and maladaptive stimuli and focal, contextual, and residual stimuli; goal setting; goal implemention and evaluation
Orem	Person and environment as a functional whole	Design, management and maintenance of systems of therapeutic self-care that meet universal needs, developmental requisites, and health deviation requisites	Process of identifying client self-care needs, planning nursing actions to meet client self-care needs, implementing nursing assistance, and revising care plan as needed
Rogers	Unitary human being interacting with the environment	Movement of unitary human beings toward maximum health	Conceptual process of empirical observation, identification of knowledge relationships, utilization of data to support or generate hypotheses, and validation of concepts and knowledge
Neuman	Person as an open system interacting with the environment	Conservation of client energy	Process consisting of nursing diagnosis phase (assess/diagnose 4 parts of the human system), nursing goals phase (care plan stating expected outcomes/interventions), and nursing outcome phase (nursing care delivered through primary, secondary, and tertiary preventive intervention; evaluation of outcome goals; revision of care plan)

professional practice to meet the comprehensive health needs of clients. Applying the concepts of primary, secondary, and tertiary prevention to the nursing process, on the basis of a holistic philosophy of the nature of human beings, offers a theoretical framework for meeting a client's health needs in the biological, psychological, spiritual, intellectual, and sociocultural subsystems. The level of prevention and the priority of needs in each subsystem vary from one individual to another and depend on the nature of the health problem and other factors related to it.

Primary prevention

Primary prevention is oriented toward limiting or reducing the incidence of psychiatric disorders in a community. This type of prevention involves an epidemiological, public health approach, which has achieved marked success in eliminating communicable diseases. It places emphasis on the community as well as on the individual or family coping with stress. The focus is upon diminishing or removing sources of stress in the community and upon early identification of, and intervention for, persons in crisis situations, with the goal being to prevent the development of psychiatric disorders. Primary prevention of mental health problems is an aspect of many health and social welfare activities that involve cooperation with community groups in the planning and implementation of preventive services. These services include providing consultation and education programs to increase understanding of psychiatric problems, identifying potential threats to mental health, and providing assistance to community groups and residents who may be at risk for developing psychiatric disorders. Preventive measures may also include efforts to strengthen or increase support systems for groups who may be isolated or alienated and participation in social and political action to reduce such sources of stress as poverty, joblessness, and poor or inadequate housing.

Secondary prevention

Secondary prevention is oriented toward reducing the duration of psychiatric disturbances in a community through early identification and effective treatment. The underlying theory is that, in many disorders, early and effective treatment will reduce the duration of illness. Measures to accomplish secondary prevention include screening programs in schools, golden age centers, and other places where groups of residents gather, case finding by public and community health workers, and education programs oriented toward members of the population who may be at risk. Inherent in the

TABLE 1-6 Levels of preventive nursing intervention

Level of prevention	Prevention focus	Examples of psychiatric nursing activities
Primary	Decreasing or removing sources of stress to prevent psychiatric disorders	Identification of people at risk for mental illness; identification of potential stressors; development of programs that remove sources of stress or modify risk factors through education, desensitization, and strengthening of coping behaviors
Secondary	Decreasing the impact of stressors to reduce the duration of psychiatric disorders	Case finding and intake screening; provision of crisis intervention, psychotherapy, and a therapeutic milieu; supervision of clients receiving medication
Tertiary	Decreasing the impact of stressors to prevent or decrease long-term impairment from psychiatric disorders	Progressive goal setting; reeducation; resocialization; utilization of appropriate health and social services; referral to psychiatric aftercare programs

concept of secondary prevention is the availability in the community of referral resources for diagnosis and treatment.

Therapeutic modalities utilized in secondary prevention may include any of those used in the treatment of psychiatric disorders. Individual therapy, group and family therapy, brief hospitalization, and chemotherapy may be employed, depending upon the nature of the mental health problem. Brief psychotherapy, crisis intervention, and short-term hospitalization in a psychiatric unit of a general hospital are often employed in secondary intervention.

Tertiary prevention

Tertiary prevention is concerned with preventing or reducing the long-term disability that is often a residual effect of such major psychiatric disorders as schizophrenia, organic brain dysfunction, and some of the psychiatric disorders of childhood. The treatment and rehabilitative objectives are to restore the person to an optimum level of functioning.

Treatment in tertiary prevention depends upon the particular psychiatric disorder. Treatment may include any of the somatic therapies, the individual and group psychotherapies, and other measures employed to ameliorate psychological distress and maladaptive coping processes. In addition, rehabilitative measures, which are designed to prevent or to shorten the period of long-term disability, are important aspects of tertiary prevention. Table 1-6 summarizes the levels of preventive intervention.

The nursing process

The nursing process* is the framework for nursing intervention. Although the nursing process is used in primary, secondary, and tertiary prevention of mental illness, in this book we have delineated the nursing process only for the secondary level of preventive intervention.

The nursing process is a form of the scientific method. Although the steps in the nursing process

---

*Refer to Chapter 11 for an in-depth discussion of the nursing process.

have been described in various ways, in this book we are using a five-step process: assessment, analysis, planning, implementation, and evaluation. *Assessment* refers to collecting and verifying data about clients, whether they be individuals, aggregates, or communities. The aims of assessment are to systematically gather information, to confirm it through consensual validation or additional information, and to communicate it to other health team members, verbally and through charting. *Analysis* refers to the making of inferences based on the collected data. The aim of this step of the nursing process is to understand the meaning of a client's behavior patterns. During the analysis phase a *nursing diagnosis* of the client's actual or potential behavior problem is made. Step three of the nursing process, *planning*, refers to establishing goals and developing intervention for client care. The aims of planning are twofold: (1) to develop a plan of action for initiating change or for enabling a client to better cope with an existing situation and (2) to design and modify a client care plan that is based on psychiatric nursing principles, psychiatric literature, and nurses' own experiences with effective approaches to specific behavior problems. *Implementation*, step four of the nursing process, refers to instituting and completing nursing actions that are necessary for the achievement of established goals and the facilitation of growth-promoting behavior. The aims of implementation are to counsel a client and to provide care that will facilitate the accomplishment of therapeutic goals. The last step of the nursing process, *evaluation*, refers to determining the degree of goal achievement. One aim of this step is to have the client participate in the estimation of his or her progress toward the attainment of goals.

In this book, we use the nursing diagnoses of the North American Nursing Diagnosis Association (NANDA) whenever possible, suffixing to the diagnosis the related or associated condition or situation. Because the NANDA nursing diagnosis system is still evolving, there are times when the NANDA system does not have appropriate diagnoses for particular client behaviors, and, in those instances, the authors have developed their own nursing diagnoses. In addition, after each nursing diagnosis, the DSM-III-R category and code associated with the specific maladaptive behavior pattern is given.

DSM-III-R categories and codes* are used by physicians when they make diagnoses and by nurses when they compile statistics and complete insurance forms. *The Diagnostic and Statistical Manual of Mental Disorders* (1987), published by the American Psychiatric Association, lists the following reasons for developing these categories and codes: (1) facilitates arriving at treatment and management decisions in different clinical settings, (2) provides reliability of diagnostic categories, (3) is accepted by clinicians and researchers with different and varied theoretical backgrounds (4) is helpful in educating health professionals, (5) fosters compatibility with ICD-9-CM categories (an international classification system for such dysfunctions as diseases, morbid conditions, and mental disorders. It is primarily for the purpose of statistical information concerning diseases, morbidity, and mortality but it is also used as a nomenclature for medical records.), (6) avoids using nontraditional terminology and concepts except when obviously necessary, (7) provides a means of developing consensus on the meaning of new and inconsistently used diagnostic terms and of discouraging the use of outdated terms, (8) provides consistency with research information concerning the validity of diagnostic categories, (9) is useful in characterizing research subjects, and (10) addresses the critiques of researchers and clinicians.

Currently, some nurses are suggesting the prioritization of nursing diagnoses along an axial system similar to the five axes of DSM-III-R. They believe such prioritizing would eliminate intuition and feelings as a basis for prioritizing and would standardize nursing diagnoses. Axis 1 would encompass nursing diagnoses that need immediate intervention; Axis 2 would list nursing diagnoses that are essential to accomplishment of long-range goals; Axis 3 would include medical and physical diagnoses; Axis 4 would designate currently experienced client stress levels; Axis 5 would evaluate client functional status in the year prior to "help-seeking

---

*Refer to Appendix A for DSM-III-R classifications and codes and for further discussion.

behavior" (Coler and Vincent, 1987). This approach for standardizing nursing diagnoses, while creative, interesting, and challenging, is new and needs further study.

Some nurses question whether the nursing process is too reductionistic a method to use with a holistic systems approach. Barnum (1987) argues that the concept of holism, which is based on integrity and inseparableness of components, is incompatible with a nursing process that reduces material to discrete parts or linkages between parts. She points out that the steps in the nursing process lead nurses to focus on discrete components and to view clients as constellations of nursing diagnoses rather than as whole, indivisible beings. Henderson (1987) criticizes the nursing process for being substantively too closely aligned to the process of medicine and for emphasizing the science of nursing to the exclusion of the art of nursing. She sees the nursing process as oriented toward the "biomedical and science-based practice of the physician" rather than toward a psychosocial nursing approach. In addition, Henderson cautions that the nursing process supports independent rather than collaborative practice by health care givers.

Other nurses believe that nursing process can be effectively utilized with a holistic, systems approach. For example, Neuman's (1982) systems model of holistic care utilizes a three-step nursing process. The North American Nursing Diagnoses Association's (NANDA) health assessment framework is based on Rogers's concept of unitary person-environment interaction patterns and points the way for nurses to use the nursing process for pattern recognition. Pattern is one characteristic of people's wholeness, and identification of sequential patterns of person-environment interaction is one way of getting in touch with the whole (Newman 1987). Donnelly (1987) points out that, although the nursing process has been criticized for being a linear, scientific approach, the term *process* indicates ongoing, dynamic interaction with the environment and active involvement rather than passive reaction. The nursing process allows nurses to creatively utilize science, art, humanity, and skills in the practice of nursing.

Although the nursing process is most often used in secondary and tertiary prevention, its usefulness in primary prevention is being explored. The delphi survey of 104 nurses showed favorable support but not total support for positive nursing diagnoses that would be directed at healthy populations not at risk, at health promotion and health care rather than illness care, and at nursing interventions that would not only ensure continued health but that would also encourage clients to continue their present health care actions (Frenn et al., 1987).

Thus, the nursing process provides a framework for nursing intervention, guiding nurses as they assess and analyze client behavior, develop plans for client care, implement those care plans, and evaluate the outcomes.

CHAPTER SUMMARY

Professional nursing acknowledges and promotes the view that people are multidimensional beings. Mental health nursing is the aspect of professional nursing that deals with human responses to stress and crisis and with the relationships between the many factors that influence a person's ability to cope with stress.

A wellness–holistic health approach to mental health and mental illness stresses an evolving rather than an absolute state of mental health. Wellness, a process of ongoing growth toward self-actualization, can be disrupted by stress. Mental health nurses, in their roles as change facilitators, help clients to make life-style changes toward high-level wellness. Therefore, a crisis may provide a client with an opportunity to grow to his or her fullest potential. Because a systems-theory approach facilitates the exploration of how various interrelated factors contribute to human behavior, systems theory can effectively be applied to nursing intervention. Neuman's systems-theory model, which incorporates the concepts of stress, coping, and levels of prevention, is most compatible with the orientation of this book. Other nursing theories are used when appropriate to discuss behavior and to provide a frame of reference for professional nursing practice.

Nursing intervention is based on the nursing process. The concepts of primary, secondary, and tertiary prevention provide a framework for organizing nursing intervention and for providing holistic mental health care to clients.

SELF-DIRECTED LEARNING

Sensitivity-Awareness Exercises

The purposes of the following exercises are to:
- Develop awareness of the many different ways that behavior can be explained
- Develop awareness of the way in which mental health team members are perceived by society and depicted by the media
- Develop awareness of the way that mental health and mental illness are perceived by society and the media

1. Select a character from a novel, a movie, or a television program. How many different types of theories (e.g. genetic, interpersonal, communication) can you use to explain the character's behavior?

2. Watch a movie or a television program that depicts all or some members of the mental health team.
   a. What are the roles and functions that are enacted by the mental health team members?
   b. How do those roles and functions compare with the roles and functions discussed in the chapter?
3. Read the comic strips in your local newspaper for one month. Cut out those comic strips that relate to mental health and mental illness.
   a. What are the messages that the comic strips convey about mental health or mental illness?

Continued.

SELF-DIRECTED LEARNING — cont'd

Sensitivity-Awareness Exercises — cont'd

    b. How are mentally healthy comic strip characters depicted?

    c. How are comic strip characters who are experiencing stress or emotional problems depicted?

    d. Do the comic strips stereotype or stigmatize mental illness? If so, how is it done?

Questions to Consider

1. Administering and interpreting psychological tests is done by the
   a. Nurse
   b. Social worker
   c. Clinical psychologist
   d. Psychiatrist
2. The interrelationship between culture and mental illness includes
   a. Defining abnormal behavior
   b. Contributing to the development of psychiatric disorders
   c. Determining how mental illness is explained and treated
   d. All of the above
3. A wellness–holistic health orientation toward human behavior rests on all *but* which of the following premises?
   a. A person has little input into the process of becoming mentally ill
   b. Stress disrupts a person's inner balance
   c. Crisis can be an opportunity for growth
   d. Therapies are only temporary expedients until a person can understand how life-style influences mental health
4. A psychiatric nursing activity associated with secondary prevention of mental illness is
   a. Identification of potential stressors
   b. Referal to psychiatric aftercare programs
   c. Intake screening
   d. Modification of risk factors

5. After assessing a client, the psychiatric nurse decides that a partially compensatory self-care system is indicated. Which of the following goals is consistent with a partially compensatory self-care system?
   a. The client will select activities that provide an outlet for anxiety
   b. With assistance from the nurse, the client will select activities that provide an outlet for anxiety
   c. The nurse will select activities that provide an outlet for anxiety

Match each of the following terms with the statement that is associated with it:

6. Psychodynamic theory	a. Behavioral system composed of seven universal subsystems
7. Nursing assessment	b. Unconscious processes motivate behavior
8. Psychoneuroimmunology	c. Collecting and verifying data about clients
9. Rogers	d. Interaction of brain, emotions, and immune system
10. Johnson	e. Unitary human being interacting with the environment

Answer key

1. c	6. b
2. d	7. c
3. a	8. d
4. c	9. e
5. b	10. a

REFERENCES

American Nurses' Association Division on Psychiatric–Mental Health Nursing Practices: Standards of psychiatric and mental health nursing practice, Kansas City, Mo, 1982, ANA Publications.

Barnum BJ: Holistic nursing and nursing process, Holistic Nurs Prac 1(3):27-35, 1987.

Baron R, Byrne D, and Kantowitz B: Psychology: understanding behavior, Philadelphia, 1978, W.B. Saunders Co.

Bateson G: Naven. Stanford, Cal, 1958, Stanford University Press.

Bateson G: Steps to an ecology of mind, New York, 1972, Ballantine.

Battista JR: The holistic paradigm and general system theory, Gen Sys 22:65-71, 1977.

Bertalanffy L von: General system theory, Main Curr Mod Thought 2:75-83, 1955.

Brady D: The ticking of a time bomb in the genes, Discover 8(6):26-39, 1987.

Buckley W: Sociology and modern system theory, Englewood Cliffs, NJ, 1967, Prentice-Hall.

Caplan G: Principles of preventive psychiatry, New York, 1964, Basic Books, Inc., Publishers.

Coler MS and Vincent KG: Coded nursing diagnoses on axes: a prioritized, computer-ready diagnostic system for psychiatric/mental health nurses, Arch Psychiatr Nurs 1(2):125-131, 1987.

Cox RD: The concept of psychological maturity. In Arieti S, editor: American handbook of psychiatry, ed 2, vol 1, New York, 1974, Basic Books, Inc., Publishers.

Diagnostic and Statistical Manual of Mental Disorders/DSM-111-R, ed 3, rev, Washington, DC, 1987, American Psychiatric Association.

Donnelly GF: The promise of nursing practice: an evaluation, Holistic Nurs Prac 1(3):1-6, 1987.

Doona ME: Travelbee's intervention in psychiatric nursing, ed 2, Philadelphia, 1979, F.A. Davis Co.

Flynn P: Holistic health: the art and science of care, Bowie, Md, 1980, Robert J. Brady Co.

Frenn MD, Jacobs CA, Lee HA, Sanger MT, and Strong KA: Delphi survey to gain consensus on wellness and health promotion nursing diagnoses. In McLane AM, editor: Classification of nursing diagnosis: proceedings of the seventh conference, St. Louis, 1987, C.V. Mosby Co.

Fuller RB: Operating manual for spaceship earth, New York, 1969, Clarion.

Goldwag EM, editor: Inner balance: the power of holistic healing. Englewood Cliffs, NJ, 1979, Prentice-Hall, Inc.

Hall AD and Fagan RE: Definition of a system. In Modern systems research for the behavioral scientist: A sourcebook, Chicago, 1968, Aldine.

Harman W: The new Copernician revolution. In Muses C and Young A, editors: Consciousness and reality, New York, 1974, Discus.

Helman C: Culture, health and illness: an introduction for health professionals, Bristol, Great Britain, 1984, John Wright & Sons Ltd.

Henderson V: Nursing process—a critique, Holistic Nurs Prac 1(3):7-18, 1987.

Johnson DE: The behavioral system model for nursing. In Riehl JP and Roy C, editors: Conceptual models for nursing practice, ed 2, New York, 1980, Appleton-Century-Crofts.

Kendell RE: The role of diagnosis in psychiatry, Oxford, 1975, Blackwell Scientific Publications.

Kety SS: Genetic and biochemical aspects of schizophrenia. In Nicholi, AM Jr, editor: The Harvard guide to modern psychiatry, Cambridge, Mass, 1978, The Belknap Press of Harvard University Press.

King IM: A theory for nursing: Systems, concepts and process, New York, 1981, John Wiley & Sons, Inc.

Lazarus RS and Launier R: Stress-related transactions between person and environment. In Pervin LA and Lewis M, editors: Perspectives in interactional psychology, New York, 1978, Plenum Press.

Lazlo E: The systems view of the world, New York, 1972, George Braziller.

Lifton R: From analysis to form: Towards a shift in psychological paradigm, Salmagundi 28:43-78, 1975.

Miller J: Living systems: Basic concepts, Behav Sci 10:93-237, 1965.

National Council of State Boards of Nursing, Inc: Test plan for the National Council Licensure Examination for registered nurses, Chicago, 1980, The Council.

National Institutes of Health: Alzheimer's disease, Department of Health, Education and Welfare Publication No. 79-6146. Washington, DC, 1979, U.S. Government Printing Office.

Neuman B: The Neuman systems model, New York, 1982, Appleton-Century-Crofts.

Newman MA: Nursing's emerging paradigm: the diagnosis of pattern. In McLane AM, editor: Classification of nursing diagnoses: proceedings of the seventh conference. St. Louis, 1987, C.V. Mosby Co.

Offer D and Sabshin M: The concept of normality. In Arieti S, editor: The American handbook of psychiatry, ed 2, vol 1, New York, 1974, Basic Books, Inc.

Orem DE: Nursing: concepts of practice. New York, 1971, McGraw-Hill Book Co.

Peplau H: Interpersonal relations in nursing, New York, 1952, G.P. Putnam's Sons.

Portnoy I: The school of Karen Horney. In Arieti S, editor: The American handbook of psychiatry, ed 2, vol 1, New York, 1974, Basic Books, Inc., Publishers.

Portnoy I: Report to the President of the President's Commission on Mental Health. Washington, DC, 1978, US Government Printing Office.

Rickelman B: Brain bio-amines and schizophrenia: a summary of research findings and implications for nursing, Psychiatr Nurs Mental Health Serv 17:9, 1979.

Riehl JB and Callista R: Conceptual models for nursing practice, ed 2, New York, 1980, Appleton-Century-Crofts.

Rogers M: A science of unitary man. In Reihl J and Roy C, editors: Conceptual models for nursing practice, ed 2, New York, 1980, Wiley & Sons.

Rogers M: Science of unitary human beings: a paradigm for nursing. In Clements IW and Roberts FB, editors: Family health: a theoretical approach to nursing care, New York, 1983, Wiley & Sons.

Roy C: Adaptation: a conceptual framework for nursing. Nurs Outlook 18(3):42-45, 1970.

Roy C: Introduction to nursing: an adaptation model, Englewood Cliffs, NJ: 1976, Prentice-Hall, Inc.

Roy C: The Roy adaptation model. In Riehl JP and Roy C, editors: Conceptual models for nursing practice, ed 2, New York, 1980, Appleton-Century Crofts.

Scheper-Hughes N and Lock MM: The mindful body: a prolegomenon to future work in medical anthropology. Med Anthropol Q 1(1):6-31, 1987.

Schildkraut JJ: Depressions and biogenic amines. In Hamburg D and Brodie KH, editors: The American handbook of psychiatry, ed 2, vol 6, New York, 1974, Basic Books, Inc. Publishers.

Schildkraut, JJ: The biochemistry of affective disorders. In Nicholi AM Jr, editor: The Harvard guide to modern psychiatry, Cambridge, Mass, 1978, The Belknap Press of Harvard University Press.

Segal J and Boomer D, editors: Research in the service of mental health: summary report of the research task force of the National Institute of Mental Health. Department of Health, Education and Welfare Pub No (ADM) 75-237, Washington, DC, 1975, US Government Printing Office.

Seltzer B and Frazier SH: Organic mental disorders. In Nicholi AM, Jr, editor: The American handbook guide to modern psychiatry, Cambridge, Mass, 1978, The Belknap Press of Harvard University Press.

Seltzer B and Sherwin I: Organic brain syndromes: an empirical study and critical review, Am J Psychiatr 135:1, 1978.

Skinner BF: Beyond freedom and dignity, New York, 1971, Alfred A. Knopf, Inc.

Spector RE: Cultural diversity in health and illness, New York, 1979, Appleton-Century-Crofts.

Stanton M: Nursing Theories: the base for nursing process. In George JB, editor: Nursing theories: the base for professional nursing practice, Englewood Cliffs, NJ, 1985, Prentice-Hall, Inc.

Sullivan HS: Conceptions of modern psychiatry, New York, 1953, W.W. Norton & Co., Inc.

Sullivan HS: Ideology and insanity, New York, 1970, Doubleday & Co., Inc.

Sutherland J: A general systems philosophy for the social and behavioral sciences, New York, 1973, Braziller.

Szaz T: The myth of mental illness, New York, 1961, Harper & Row, Publishers, Inc.

Travelbee J: Interpersonal aspects of nursing, ed 2, Philadelphia, 1971, F.A. Davis Co., Inc.

Tulloch J and Healy C: Changing lifestyles: a wellness approach, Occup Health Nurs, 45:13-21, 1982.

Waxler N: Is mental illness cured in traditional societies? a theoretical analysis, Cultural Med Psychiatr 1:233-253, 1977.

Wechsler R: A new prescription: mind over malady. Discover 8(2):51-61, 1987.

Wells CE: Chronic brain disease: an overview, Am J Psychiatr 135:1, 1978.

Werner HD: New understandings of human behavior: non-Freud readings from professional journals, 1960-1968, New York, 1970, Associated Press.

Wittkower ED and Prince R: A review of transcultural psychiatry. In Caplan G, editor: The American handbook of psychiatry, ed 2, vol 2, New York, 1974, Basic Books, Inc., Publishers.

Wolpe J: The practice of behavior therapy, ed 2, New York, 1973, Pergamon Press, Inc.

Wolpe J: The behavior therapy approach. In Arieti S, editor: The American handbook of psychiatry, ed 2, vol 1, New York, 1974, Basic Books, Inc., Publishers.

ANNOTATED SUGGESTED READINGS

Riehl JP and Roy C, editors: Conceptual models for nursing practice, ed 2, New York, 1980, Appleton-Century-Crofts.
This is a book of readings. Selected theorists, such as Rogers, Neuman, Roy, Orem, and Johnson, set forth their theories of nursing with implications for nursing education, nursing practice, and/or nursing research.

Tulloch J and Healy C: Changing lifestyles: a wellness approach, Occupational Health Nurs, 45, 13-21, 1982.
The authors discuss the concept of a wellness approach to health and set forth areas to be included in a wellness assessment. Tulloch and Healy then discuss factors that influence change toward high-level wellness and the role of the nurse as a change facilitator.

Wechsler R: A new prescription: mind over malady. Discover 8(2):51-61, 1987.
This article cites the holistic health approaches of such practitioners as Stephanie and Carl Simonton at the Cancer Counseling and Research Center in Dallas, Texas, and explains some of the psychoneuroimmunology (PNI) research currently being conducted in support of a holistic health orientation. PNI researchers are exploring the interrelationship among brain, emotions, and immune system and seem to be discovering mechanisms that underlie a holistic approach to health.

FURTHER READINGS

Baer C, editor: Nursing diagnosis, Topics in Clin Nurs 5(4):1-96, 1984.

Donnelly GF: Nursing theory: evolution of a sacred cow. Holistic Nurs Practice 1(1):1-7, 1986.

Lundh U, Soder M, and Waerness K: Nursing theories: a critical review, Image 20(1)36-40, 1988.

Silva MC and Rothbart D: An analysis of changing trends in philosophies of science on nursing theory development and testing, Adv Nurs Science 6(2):1-13, 1984.

Williams K: The facilitation of wholeness, Holistic Nurs Prac 2(3):1-8, 1988.

CHAPTER 2

Historical overview of psychiatric nursing

CHAPTER FOCUS

This chapter explores some of the important developments in mental health care in general, and psychiatric nursing in particular, during several eras. The effects of scientific and clinical discoveries in the medical and behavioral fields, as well as the profound influences of social and political change, are noted.

HISTORICAL ASPECTS OF MENTAL HEALTH CARE

Mental disorders are believed to have been a part of human experience throughout history. The *Nei Ching* (also known as the *Yellow Emperor's Classic of Internal Medicine*), written in China as early as the twenty-seventh century BC, states:

When the minds of the people are closed and wisdom is locked out they remain tied to disease. Yet their feelings and desires should be investigated and made known, their wishes and ideas should be followed; and then it becomes apparent that those who have attained spirit and energy are flourishing. . . . (Veith, 1965)

Insanity was mentioned by Homer in the *Iliad*. Plato distinguished between "divine madness," the madness given by the gods, and "natural madness." Hippocrates, a Greek physician who lived from 460 to 370 BC, described depressed states. Claudius Galen, a Roman physician who lived from 138 to 250 AD, wrote a treatise on melancholia that remained an important work on the subject for many centuries (Manfreda and Krampitz, 1977). Justinian, an emperor of the Eastern or Byzantine Empire in the sixth century AD, established many charitable institutions, including some for the care of the mentally ill (Ellenberger, 1974).

As early as the thirteenth century, the people of Gheel, in what is now Belgium, had pioneered in community psychiatry to meet the needs of the mentally ill, many of whom made pilgrimages to the Shrine of St. Dymphna, the patron saint of the mentally ill. Some of the pilgrims to St. Dymphna's shrine stayed on in Gheel, and a practice of foster family care evolved that has continued to the present time.

Attitudes toward mental illness and the treatment of people regarded as being mentally ill have not always been so enlightened. During the Middle Ages, a theory of demonology, or possession by the devil or evil spirits, was prevalent in some areas of Western Europe. Such views persisted at least into the seventeenth century—for example, in the town of Salem, Massachusetts. In some cases, people who may have been mentally ill were regarded as witches and, at times, burned at the stake. In other instances, rites of exorcism were practiced as a means of driving out evil spirits.

Developments in mental health care have always been influenced by cultural attitudes, the level of knowledge available, and the religious beliefs and sociopolitical events of particular eras. Johan Weier (1515–1588) a Dutch physician and humanist, was moved by the plight of the many women who were being tortured and executed as witches. Weier believed that these women were mentally ill—melancholic and prone to believing that their fantasies were true. He spoke out for treatment rather than torture and did so at no small peril to himself (Swales, 1982).

Phillipe Pinel, who has been credited with liberating mental patients from their chains in Salpetrière hospital in France in 1795, was also influenced by the problems of his time. His work received public support as a result of the spirit of "libertè, ègalitè, and fraternitè" that prevailed in France around the period of the French Revolution. The spirit of humanism and concern for humane treatment of the mentally ill was greatly influenced by Pinel's philosophy that mental illness was caused by an individual's experiences in life rather than by some lesion in the brain or by demons or devils. The humanistic philosophy and the enlightened treatment of the mentally ill embraced by Pinel could also be found in the work of Vincenzo Chiarugi in Italy and William and Samuel Tuke in England.

Benjamin Rush (1745–1813), an American physician who is sometimes described as the "father of American psychiatry," provided humane treatment for the mentally ill in the late eighteenth and early nineteenth centuries (Greenblatt, 1977; Manfreda and Krampitz, 1977). During this time the people of the United States were fairly homogeneous in cultural background, and they often were highly dependent upon one another for survival because they lived predominantly in small, largely agricultural communities. The shared sense of responsibility was reinforced by the Christian ethic. These factors influenced Rush and others to provide humanistic treatment and care for the mentally ill. The humanistic movement lasted until about the middle of the nineteenth century (Greenblatt, 1977).

In the latter half of the nineteenth century there was a decline in public interest in mentally ill persons in the United States and a concurrent decline in the number and quality of facilities available for their care. This change in public attitude was related to the wave of poor immigrants from Europe. Many of the immigrants suffered from poverty and culture shock, which increased the incidence of mental disorders and the need for mental health services but also taxed the nation's ability to provide humanistic care. In addition, the nation's growing preoccupation with the Industrial Revolution tended to reduce the importance placed on the individual.

Dorothea Lynde Dix (1802–1887), a retired Boston schoolteacher, became alarmed by the condition of the mentally ill and the prevailing practice of incarcerating mentally ill persons in filthy almshouses and jails. She traveled thousands of miles in the United States and abroad, urging state legislatures and other governmental agencies to assume responsibility and to establish hospitals for the care of mental patients. Miss Dix's reform effort was successful in that the individual states assumed responsibility for mental health care and built state hospitals to care for persons with emotional disorders. The state hospitals, often large, understaffed, and built in locations remote from population centers, served primarily to provide custodial care. These hospitals were a major mental health resource until the community mental health movement of the 1960s.

In 1903, a book by Clifford Beers entitled *The Mind That Found Itself*, in which he described his experiences in a custodial institution, attracted the attention of several prominent people. Among them were William James, the great American psychologist, Adolph Meyer, a leading American psychiatrist, and William Welch, the father of American pathology. They joined with Beers and others to form the National Committee for Mental Hygiene. Under the leadership of Adolph Meyer, the movement took a preventive approach to mental illness similar to that of the community mental health movement of the 1960s. The movement failed, however, to attract public and governmental support.

The work of Freud, in the late nineteenth and early twentieth centuries, and that of his contemporaries and of the neo-Freudians who followed, dominated psychiatric thought in the first half of the twentieth century. Although Freud's work markedly increased our knowledge of human behavior, it had a limited effect upon the treatment of patients in the large state hospitals, where canvas restraints and locked doors often replaced the chains of Salpetrière.

World War II, which brought universal conscription of young men for military service in the United States, focused national attention upon the extent of the nation's mental health problems. Levenson (1974) notes that "approximately 40% of the 5,000,000 men rejected for military service for medical reasons, during this time, were rejected because of some neuro-psychiatric defect." Levenson also notes that such disturbances were responsible for the greatest number of medical discharges from the armed services during the war. In addition, the success of military psychiatry in returning soldiers to active duty following brief crisis-intervention treatment near the front lines served to alert the nation to the possibility of more effective treatment of mental disorders.

World War II focused attention upon the scope of the nation's mental health problems, but it was not until the 1950s that several important developments in the therapeutic measures available for treating the mentally ill occurred. These developments improved the quality of health care and changed the attitudes of both the general public and health professionals about psychiatric disorders. Among the developments were group therapy, which was adaptable to meeting a variety of treatment goals; crisis intervention; the therapeutic community concept, developed by Maxwell Jones in England; and chemotherapy, which was in wide use by the mid-1950s. In addition to improving the treatment of people with psychiatric disorders, these advances spurred research into etiology and treatment modalities for such disorders.

The 1960s and 1970s saw the growth and development of the community mental health movement (see Chapter 16), which focused on the delivery of health care to the mentally ill population and made a strong effort in the direction of prevention of mental illness. The emergence of advocacy roles for clients and their families was also taking place during this time.

THE DEVELOPMENT OF MODERN PSYCHIATRIC NURSING

The roots of nursing care of the mentally ill can, of course, be traced back to very early times. The ancient Greeks cared for their emotionally ill citizens in the enlightened and humanistic way described in the following quotation from an ancient writing found in the temple of Aesculapius:

As often as they had phrenetic patients or such as were unhinged they did make use of nothing so much for the cure and restoration of their health as symphony, sweet harmony and concert voices. (Manfreda and Krampitz, 1977).

The power of suggestion, human kindness, music and dance, and something called "temple sleep" were all incorporated into the nursing care or milieu therapy of the time (Ducey and Simon, 1975; Howells and Osborn, 1975). The Greek Pythagoras traveled to Egypt to observe the treatment modalities commonly practiced in nursing the mentally ill back to health. He found that cold baths, amusements, and reading were all in vogue (Manfreda and Krampitz, 1977).

Even earlier—roughly 1400 BC—an ancient Hindu writing contained in the Ayur-Veda classified mental illnesses, while another of the Vedas set down functions and qualifications for nurses who cared for the mentally disturbed. Such a nurse was instructed to be

Cool headed, pleasant, kind-spoken, strong and attentive to the needs of the sick and indefatigable in following the physician's orders. (Manfreda and Krampitz, 1977)

Certainly psychiatric nursing has grown in complexity since these early descriptions were written (see Appendix C, "ANA Standards of Psychiatric and Mental Health Nursing Practice"), but one can definitely see the beginnings of *interpersonal relationship* and *management of the milieu* as tools for psychiatric nursing.

1882 to 1930

Psychiatric nursing in the United States is a little over 100 years old. It had its beginning in 1882, at McLean Hospital in Belmont, Massachusetts. This private facility (known then as the McLean Asylum) was the setting for the first training school for psychiatric nurses in this country. *Linda Richards*, famous as America's "first trained nurse," was instrumental in the establishment of the school.

Linda Richards had graduated in 1873 from the New England Hospital for Women and Children in Boston. She was profoundly influenced by the work of *Florence Nightingale*, who had established her own St. Thomas School of Nursing in 1860. In England, before the work of Nightingale, the care of patients in hospitals was carried out by family members, servants, religious orders, and sometimes even by convicts from the local prisons. After her graduation in 1873, Linda Richards traveled to England to meet with Florence Nightingale.

When she returned to this country, Richards was able to establish several hospitals for the mentally ill and also to help establish the school at McLean. The value of this school was quickly appreciated, and within the short period of 10 years there were 19 American institutions providing training programs for psychiatric nurses.

In 1886, four years after it opened, the training school at the McLean Asylum pioneered in nursing

education by becoming affiliated with the Massachusetts General Hospital. Nurses-in-training from Massachusetts General could complete the senior year at McLean. As early as 1906, nurse educators began to work toward establishing similar affiliations for *all* students enrolled in general hospital schools of nursing. By 1935, one half of the existing schools of nursing offered a single course in psychiatric nursing. The goal of incorporating psychiatric nursing theory and practice into the curriculum of all professional nursing programs in the country was not reached until the 1950s, when completion of a course in psychiatric nursing became a requirement for eligibility for state license as a registered nurse.

As stated earlier, nursing care of the mentally ill in ancient times had much in common with some of the modern trends in psychiatric nursing. But there is a dramatic contrast between psychiatric nursing as it is practiced today and the roles and functions of psychiatric nurses during the period of 1882 to approximately 1930. Santos and Stainbrook, in their article "A History of Psychiatric Nursing in the Nineteenth Century" (1949), describe the functions of the psychiatric nurse as follows:

Her duties included carrying out or assisting the physician with the psychiatric procedures of the day; administering such as whiskey, chloroform, and paraldehyde; and therapeutic measures such as hot and cold douches, showers, continuous baths and wet sheet packs. Various methods of inducing patients to take food also played an important part in the therapeutic measures practiced by physicians and nurses. However, the nineteenth century psychiatric nurse had very few psychological nursing skills at her command.

Custodial care was the main focus, and "habit training" was part of the required course content in psychiatric nursing. Habit training was aimed at assisting patients toward greater conformity or "acceptable" behavior (Peplau, 1981). Hildegarde Peplau notes that many of the routine nursing activities, such as "sharp counts," "bed counts," "belt counts," and periodic "body counts," were effective in reinforcing an atmosphere of mistrust between patients and their nurses (Peplau, 1981). In the years from 1882 to 1930, this custodial role for psychiatric nurses did not change greatly. Substantial changes did not occur until the 1950s, when the importance of the therapeutic nurse-patient relationship was finally realized (Lego, 1980). In 1920, one psychiatric nursing text had been published—*Nursing Mental Diseases*, by Harriet Bailey—but psychiatric nursing in the period was mainly concentrated on providing for the patients' physical needs and safety through *control* of the patients. Hydrotherapy, tube feedings, and restraint procedures were part of the usual nursing measures. Some psychological interventions on the part of nurses existed, but they consisted primarily in the expectation that nurses should be kind and tolerant toward their patients. Few psychodynamic techniques were available to nurses, and they were often discouraged by the prevalent view in psychiatry that almost all mental illness was incurable—all that could be done was to "classify" the various conditions and provide custodial care. In addition, there was the stress associated with caring for very large numbers of patients. Individualized care was all but impossible. Peplau has pointed out that psychiatric nursing from the 1890s to the 1950s was not a particularly attractive field in which to work. In spite of this, the number of registered nurses employed in psychiatric settings grew from 471 in 1891 to 12,000 in 1951 (Peplau, 1981).

1930 to the 1950s

As descriptive, Kraepelinian psychiatry was gradually replaced by the new psychodynamic concepts, roles of psychiatric nurses also began to change. In private psychiatric facilities such as the well-known Chestnut Lodge in Maryland, nurses were actively involved in the treatment of mentally ill patients. Through their experiences in these settings, they became more aware of the value of healing relationships and therapeutic communication techniques. An effort was made to incorporate these concepts into the body of knowledge for education and clinical practice.

In the 1930s and 1940s, the somatic treatments for mental illness became prevalent, and the participation of nurses was crucial. Deep sleep therapy, psychosurgery, and insulin and Metrazol shock therapy all had their eras. The rapid growth in the use of these modalities contributed to the development of psychiatric nursing. These therapies all involved intensive nursing care, and Florence Nightingale had long since shown, through her hospital mortality statistics, the necessity of skilled nursing services in carrying out any somatic therapy.

The somatic therapies added another element to the evolution of psychiatric nursing. Patients were helped by these therapies and thus became more amenable to psychological intervention. This increased the demand for mental health workers, including psychiatric nurses, who could use their skills and knowledge of psychodynamic concepts to interact therapeutically with their patients. The psychodynamic concepts that had the greatest impact on psychiatric nursing were psychoanalytic theory, interpersonal theory, communication theory, and systems theory.

World War II was also an important influence. Since 43% of all army discharges were attributed to psychiatric disorder, the country became aware that mental illness was a major health problem (Kalkman and Davis, 1974). The *National Mental Health Act* (passed in 1946) authorized, among other things, a program for training professional psychiatric personnel. Psychiatric nursing was one of the four specific professions included in this training program, and this stimulated the growth and development of several undergraduate and graduate programs in colleges throughout the country. In 1950, a study by the National League for Nursing concluded that special training was required for psychiatric nurses. Psychologists, psychiatric residents, social workers, and psychiatric nurses (the four groups singled out for National Institute of Mental Health [N.I.M.H.] training) often took classes together during this period, and nurses began to work on a collegial basis with their fellow team members. The graduate-level programs in psychiatric nursing served to produce qualified teachers in psychiatric nursing for programs at all levels—practical nursing, diploma schools, and associate degree, baccalaureate, and graduate programs. Funds from the N.I.M.H. and the Bolton Act (the first federal program to subsidize nursing education for school and student) continued to support psychiatric nursing from 1946 until approximately 1979, when most of the funds were used up.

Also in the 1950s, psychiatric nursing began to focus on the importance of the nurse's "therapeutic use of self" in the nurse-patient relationship. Hildegarde Peplau's *Interpersonal Relations in Nursing,* published in 1952, helped to revolutionize the teaching and practice of psychiatric nursing by providing the theoretical basis for the therapeutic role that is practiced today. Another important event that occurred during this period, and one that greatly affected the care of the mentally ill population, was the discovery of the antipsychotic drugs. By alleviating acute symptoms, these drugs enabled the patient to participate actively in psychological treatments of all kinds, including psychiatric nursing therapy and milieu therapy.

In the 1950s, just prior to the widespread use of these medications, a typical listing of psychiatric nursing procedures might include the following:

1. Nursing care of the lobotomized patient.
2. Supervision of the admission of a patient, with a cataloguing of all clothing and belongings (Since most patients came into the hospital to stay for a long time, there were numerous belongings to store and keep track of.).
3. Safe transportation of large groups of patients from one building to another.
4. Proper procedure for conducting utensil counts after every meal.
5. Intensive nursing care of the patient undergoing insulin coma therapy.
6. Correct procedure for continuous tub baths, wet sheet packs, showers, and other forms of hydrotherapy.
7. Surveillance and supervision of patients at dances and religious services.
8. Tube feeding or intravenous feeding and complete bed care for withdrawn, chronically schizophrenic patients, who lay in the dormitories of the "back wards." These patients were often ankylosed into fetal positions after many years of withdrawal and inadequate nursing care.
9. Preparation of patients for "shock therapy." This procedure was quite different from the electroconvulsive therapy procedure that is

presently practiced; nursing care often involved joining a "posse" that searched for a frightened patient who was hiding to avoid the treatment.

10. The correct and safe way to enter and leave a seclusion room. There was not just one "quiet room," as is the custom in today's psychiatric facilities. Each ward had several seclusion rooms, and patients did not go into them for a few hours of therapeutically reduced stimuli but spent months or even years living in them.

1960s and 1970s

The 1960s and the 1970s constituted a golden age for psychiatric nursing. Graduate education expanded, and the incorporation of psychiatric nursing principles into the undergraduate curriculum was well established. The community mental health movement flourished, and progressive psychiatric inpatient units were opened in several general hospitals. A liaison role for psychiatric nurses evolved—clinical specialists became consultants to nurses in other areas of the hospital. Maternity, pediatric, and medical and surgical units all sought the expertise of the psychiatric clinical nurse specialist to help them deal with nursing care problems. Maxwell Jones's therapeutic community concept influenced the nurse's role in milieu therapy. The prestigious psychiatric nursing journal *Perspectives in Psychiatric Care* began to be published in 1963. Psychiatric nurses published clinically focused articles in *Perspectives* and in several other professional journals. Many excellent textbooks became available. In the 1970s an increasing number of psychiatric nurses began to be involved in their own private practices.

The role of the psychiatric nurse was becoming increasingly interesting and challenging. Group dynamics, family therapy, and systems theory were some of the concepts that were added to the graduate-level curriculum and, later, to the undergraduate level. Clinical specialists, prepared at the master's level, became proficient in the treatment modalities of group therapy, couples therapy, and family therapy. Some clinical nurses specialists focused their education and practice on the field of child psychiatry. The number of psychiatric nurses with earned doctorates increased dramatically in this period—from approximately 200 in the 1960s to over 2,000 in 1983.*

The role of the clinical specialist in psychiatric nursing became more clearly defined. Standards and functions were described by the American Nurses' Association for both the professional nurse working in a psychiatric setting and for the master's-level clinical specialist.

Another important development occurred in the middle to late 1970s—a certification process became available. Psychiatric nurses who wished to achieve certification could do so, either on a generalist level or as a clinical specialist, through the American Nurses' Association. The two levels have different educational standards and requirements; both involve written examinations, documented experience, and supervised practice. The ANA publishes a directory of all nurses who have been certified through this process.

In 1972, the ANA's *Division on Psychiatric–Mental Health Nursing Practice* established the *Council of Advanced Practitioners in Psychiatric Mental Health Nursing.*

The 1980's

In 1979 the council's name was changed to the *Council of Specialists in Psychiatric–Mental Health Nursing.* In 1981 the council defined practice for such nurses as follows:

Psychiatric and mental health nursing is a specialized area of nursing practice directed toward prevention, treatment, and rehabilitative aspects of mental health care. Nursing treatments are based on assessment of need, diagnosis and evaluation of progress. They include individual and group psychotherapy, family therapy, screening and evaluation, making house calls, conducting health teaching activities, providing support and medication surveillance and responding to clients' needs through community action, if appropriate." (American Nurses' Association, 1981)

The council also noted that specialists work in a variety of settings, such as acute care and long-term

*Figures from the research departments of the American Nurses' Association and the National League for Nursing.

care institutions, outpatient clinics, community mental health centers, offices, schools, courts, and industrial surroundings. In 1983, 675 nurses were listed as members of the council, and in 1984, the council merged with the *Division on Psychiatric and Mental Health Nursing Practice* to become the *Council on Psychiatric and Mental Health Nursing.* (Pacesetter, 1984)

What are some of the current issues in psychiatric nursing? In Chapter 3, "Power, Politics, and Psychiatric Nursing," current issues are discussed in depth. One important issue of the late 1980s was the liability insurance coverage problem. Psychiatric–mental health nurses in independent practice were excluded from certain insurance programs in 1985 and faced substantial rate increases in other programs in 1986. In 1987, the problem reached crisis proportions (American Nurses' Association, September 1987). In November 1987, *The American Nurse* reported that liability coverage to self-employed psychiatric–mental health practitioners was now available (American Nurses' Association, November 1987). The following brief list indicates some of the possible future directions for psychiatric nursing:

1. The problems associated with applying the primary nursing model to psychiatric nursing practice need to be resolved. There is some conflict between the principles of milieu therapy and those of primary nursing. (For further discussion of this topic, see Ronoff and Kane, 1982.)
2. Nursing research must continue to develop. The number of nurses with earned doctorates is still relatively small, but it is increasing. An example of an appropriate and timely topic for research in psychiatric nursing is the effectiveness of therapy provided by psychiatric clinical nurse specialists (Smoyak, 1982). Other examples would be mental health problems of older women; depression in women; the interrelationships among body image, eating disorders, exercise, nutrition, and self-esteem; the interrelationships among role conflict, stress, social support and coping in families (McBride, 1987). The publication of the DSM-III-R has prompted the ANA to encourage nursing research into the contro-

versial new diagnoses listed in the appendix (Late Luteal Phase Dysphoric Disorder, Self-Defeating Personality Disorder, and Sadistic Personality Disorder). Concerned that these diagnoses are based on an inadequacy of scientific data and that there may be a tendency to apply them inconsistently and mostly to a female population were the inspiration for a June 1987 House of Delegate's communication to the American Psychiatric Association (Pacesetter, 1987).

3. Third-party payments for psychiatric nurses is an important issue. In December 1981, a third-party reimbursement plan was approved by one large health insurance plan, CHAMPUS (Civilian Health and Medical Programs for Uniformed Services). After an experimental program providing for such reimbursement was authorized and carried out in fiscal 1980, the Defense Appropriations Conference Committee of the U.S. Senate adopted a proposal to make the program permanent. It provided that state-licensed nurse practitioners and certified psychiatric clinical nurse specialists be considered regular CHAMPUS authorized providers. The sponsor of the amendment was Senator Daniel Inouye of Hawaii (American Nurses' Association, 1982). This was an encouraging start toward promoting the autonomy of psychiatric nurse practitioners.

4. Networking, as a support system and as a communication facilitator for the psychiatric nurse practitioner, is becoming an important reality (Pacesetter, 1982).

5. Patricia Pothier (1987), chairperson of the *Council on Psychiatric and Mental Health Nursing*, outlined the council's goals for 1987–88.
   They sound appropriate for the 1990s, too:
   a. To improve psychiatric and mental health nursing practice
   b. To provide mechanisms for communication among psychiatric and mental health nurses, with ANA organizational units and outside groups
   c. To provide for the professional development of council affiliates
   d. To increase the understanding of the collegial role of psychiatric and mental health nurses among the mental health professions and administrators
   e. To increase the number and authority of qualified psychiatric and mental health nurses in government, education, and the health care delivery system
   f. To influence federal and state political and legislative processes

CHAPTER SUMMARY

The roots of mental health can be traced to ancient times. Modern American psychiatric nursing, however, is considered to have begun in 1882, when the first training school for psychiatric nurses was established. From that time to the 1950s, the role of the psychiatric nurse did not change very much; it consisted primarily of "custodial care giver." The impetus for change in the profession came from outside forces: the widespread acceptance of psychodynamic concepts, World War II, the National Health Act, the development of psychotropic drugs, the community mental health movement. At present the profession continues to grow—to increase its body of theoretical knowledge, to improve its scope of clinical experience, and to develop network systems for mutual support and exchange of information. Psychiatric nursing is coming of age in that the stimulation for growth is coming from within the profession itself.

SELF-DIRECTED LEARNING

Sensitivity-Awareness Exercises

The purpose of these exercises is to:
- Develop an awareness of some of the past procedures, concerns, issues, and trends of psychiatric nursing
- Develop an awareness of the possible future issues and trends for psychiatric nursing in this country

1. Read some early issues of nursing journals and psychiatric nursing journals. Choose from several decades and make some notes about the differences in topics, procedures described, and level of scientific knowledge demonstrated.
2. Read one of the older textbooks in psychiatric nursing (e.g., *Nursing Mental Diseases* by Harriet Bailey or *A Guide to Psychiatric Nursing* by Charmichael and Chapman or *Interpersonal Relations in Nursing* by Hildegard Peplau). Or survey all of them at once and note differences in approach. Compare them with your textbooks.
3. Read Florence Nightingale's *Notes on Nursing: What It Is and What It Is Not*. What are her principles of psychosocial nursing?
4. Interview two clinical specialists in psychiatric–mental health nursing. For each interview, focus on his or her views of the future of psychiatric nursing. Write down your own reaction to each interview.

Questions to Consider

Match each of the following:

1. Dorothea Dix   4
2. Phillipe Pinel   3
3. Linda Richards   5
4. Hildegard Peplau   2
5. Benjamin Rush   6
6. Clifford Beers   1
7. Johan Weier   7

a. *Interpersonal Relations in Nursing* (a text).
b. Helped establish the first training school for psychiatric nurses
c. The "father of American psychiatry"
d. Liberated mental patients from being chained
e. *The Mind That Found Itself:* A pioneering book for mental health.
f. A retired schoolteacher and champion of the mentally ill in the nineteenth century
g. Spoke out for the women who were accused of witchcraft and cruelly tortured in the sixteenth century

Answer key

1. f   5. c
2. d   6. e
3. b   7. g
4. a

REFERENCES

American Nurses' Association: Fact Sheet of Division on Psychiatric–Mental Health Nursing Practice, Council of Specialists in Psychiatric–Mental Health Nursing. Kansas City, Mo, 1981, The Association.

American Nurses' Association: Am Nurse 14(2):19, 1982.

American Nurses' Association: ANA arranges for study of nursing liability claims, Am Nurse, pp 3 and 6, September 1987.

American Nurses' Association: Liability plan is extensive, unique. Am Nurse, pp 3 and 22, November 1987.

Ducey C and Simon B: Ancient Greece and Rome. In Howells JG, editor: World history of psychiatry. New York, 1975, Brunner/Mazel, Inc.

Ellenberger HF: Psychiatry from ancient to modern times. In Arieti S, editor: American handbook of psychiatry, ed 2, vol 1, New York, 1974, Basic Books, Inc.

Greenblatt M: Introduction to psychiatry and the third revolution, Psychiatr Ann 7(10):7-9, 1977.

Howells JG and Osborn ML: Great Britain. In Howells JG, editor: World history of psychiatry, New York, 1975, Brunner/Mazel, Inc.

Kalkman ME and Davis AJ: New dimensions in mental health–psychiatric nursing, ed 4, New York, 1974, McGraw-Hill Book Co.

Lego SM: The one-to-one nurse-patient relationship, Persp Psychiatr Care 18(2):67-89, 1980.

Levenson AI: A review of the federal community mental health centers programs. In Caplan G, editor: American handbook of psychiatry, ed 2, vol 2, New York, 1974, Basic Books, Inc.

Manfreda M and Krampitz SD: Psychiatric nursing, ed 10, Philadelphia, 1977, F.A. Davis Co.

McBride A: Developing a women's mental health research agenda, Image: J Nurs Scholarship, 19(1):4-8, 1987.

Pacesetter: Newsletter of the American Nurses' Association Council of Specialists in Psychiatric–Mental Health Nursing, 7(1):2 and 5, 1982.

Pacesetter: New council formed. Newsletter of the American Nurses' Association, Council on Psychiatric–Mental Health Nursing, 11(3):1, 1984.

Pacesetter: APA response to ANA. Concerns regarding potential DSM-III-R diagnoses. Newsletter of the American Nurses' Association Council on Psychiatric–Mental Health Nursing, 14(6):1, 1987.

Peplau H: Reflections on earlier days in psychiatric nursing. Paper presented at the Elizabeth Palmieri Memorial Lecture, Adelphi University, Oct. 12, 1981.

Pothier P: Report from the chairperson—Pacesetter. Councils' Annual Report Newsletter, June 1987. American Nurses' Association Division of Constituent Affairs—Nursing Practice Programs and Council Services, pp. 22 and 23.

Ronoff V and Kane I: Primary nursing in psychiatry: an effective and functional model, Persp Psychiatr Care 20(2): 73-78, 1982.

Santos E and Stainbrook E: A history of psychiatric nursing in the nineteenth century. J Hist Med Allied Sci Winter, pp. 40-74, 1949.

Smoyak S: Psychiatric/mental-health nursing research: what difference does a psychiatric nurse make? Pacesetter 7 (1):4-5, 1982.

Swales PJ: A fascination with witches. The Sciences 22(8):21-23, 1982.

Veith I, translator: The yellow emperor's classic of internal medicine, Berkeley, 1965, University of California Press.

ANNOTATED SUGGESTED READINGS

Church O: Emergence of training programs for asylum nursing at the turn of the century, Adv Nurs Sc (Nursing History), 7(2):35-46, 1985.
This describes the transition of psychiatric nursing from its identification as custodial caretaking to an accepted and unique part of the nursing profession as a whole. During this period "attendants" become "nurses," and "inmates" become "patients." Some of the issues, politics, and problems of the time are reviewed. The pioneering efforts of early nurses in the areas of nursing practice and nursing education are discussed.

Doona M: At least as well cared for . . . Linda Richards and the mentally ill. Image: J Nurs Scholarship, 16(2):51-56, 1984.
This article is a chronicle of Linda Richards's activities on behalf of the mentally ill and the nurses who cared for them. Time covered is from the time of her efforts toward nursing reform at the Massachusetts State Hospitals in 1899 to the end of her career when she was Superintendent Emerita at Taunton Hospital (1911). Personal characteristics of Linda Richards as viewed by others of the time are included, and the article gives us an interesting picture of this remarkable woman and her times.

Osborne O: Intellectual traditions in psychiatric mental health nursing, J Psychosoc Nurs, 22(11):27-32, 1984.
A historical review of some of the psychiatric textbooks through the ages, the article also acts as a concise overview of the development of modern psychiatric nursing in America. The author's view is that earlier texts were more vigorous in developing statements unique to psychiatric nursing and that the conceptual strength of psychiatric nursing has not been evident in recent texts.

Power, politics, and psychiatric nursing

CHAPTER FOCUS

Power is a dynamic of interpersonal relationships. Power arises from many sources, has many forms, and comprises many strategies. To influence the nature and direction of mental health care and professional nursing, nurses must understand the interrelationship between power, politics, gender bias, and planned change. Institutions, consumers, and nurses are major components of the contemporary mental health care delivery system. Within this system, power strategies and power struggles sometimes arise around such issues as quality of care, client rights, ethical dilemmas, and allocation of resources. Trends in mental health often portend the issues around which future power strategies and power struggles may revolve. In the United States today some major trends in mental health are consumerism, a questioning of the insanity defense, decreased funding for mental health research, prioritizing research needs, and independent nursing practice.

Power is the ability to act, to do, and/or to control others. Everyone needs to experience some form of power. In her classic investigation of themes in nursing, Peplau (1953) stated that the need for power enters into every nursing situation. Whether a nursing situation involves clients, families of clients, health team members, or agency administrators, interacting participants are usually striving for, relinquishing, exerting, or submitting to power. Certain basic assumptions underlie this concept of power:

1. Power is a resource. It is neither innately

good nor innately evil. Power may be used constructively to solve social problems or destructively for corrupt and selfish purposes.

2. Power is an essential dynamic of human interaction. For power to operate in an interaction, it must be acknowledged through "empowering responses."
3. Power is dynamic. Its supply is constantly being increased, decreased, and redistributed (Votaw, 1979).
4. Power may be exerted covertly or overtly. People may be subtly influenced (covert power) or coerced (overt power) into complying with the wishes of others (Ashley, 1975; Leininger, 1978, 1979).

Power is wielded in three predominant ways, which are often referred to as instruments of power. Instruments of power include *condign, compensatory,* and *conditioned* power (Galbraith, 1983). Table 3-1 illustrates these different instruments of power.

Power arises from various sources. Three major sources are leadership, property, and organization. Leadership refers to one's ability to utilize physical, mental, moral, or personality traits to gain access to power. Leadership is usually associated with conditioned power. Property (or wealth), because it bestows an aspect of authority, also provides access to power. Because having property or wealth provides

the means to purchase submission, it is associated with compensatory power. In contemporary society, organization (the unity of people or groups around a central purpose or work) is the most important source of power. Although it is most often associated with conditioned power, organization also uses condign and compensatory power.

Institutions are characterized by hierarchies of organization, and power plays and power struggles often occur among the groups of people within those hierarchies. In such instances, internal power (manifested by commitment to and submission to the aims of one hierarchical group) often becomes the basis for that group's external power (power imposed on other hierarchical groups). For example,

---

The contract for nurses working in a psychiatric hospital had expired. The nurses had identified the following two issues as vital: an end to mandatory overtime and a salary increase above the annual rise in the cost of living. The nurses saw these issues as vital not only to their own well-being but also to the well-being of the clients in their care. Without competitive salaries, the hospital could not attract qualified nurses. The fatigue factor inherent in compulsory overtime not only compromised quality of client care, but compulsory overtime also discouraged many qualified nurses from applying for staff nurse positions. The nurses felt very

TABLE 3-1 Instruments of power

Type	Explanation	Example
Condign	Imposes unpleasant consequence for not submitting to the wishes of authority figures	*Nurse*: rebuke by nursing supervisor for not following dress code *Client*: being labeled a "bad patient" and avoided by the nursing staff
Compensatory	Offers rewards for submitting to the wishes of authority figures	*Nurse*: merit raise for complying with mandatory overtime *Client*: being labeled a "good patient" and getting extra attention from the nursing staff
Conditioned	Changes beliefs through persuasion, education, or social commitment (since belief change results in selecting the preferred course of action, the person does not generally feel that he or she is submitting to the wishes of authority figures)	*Nurse*: identifies with the purposes of a day treatment program and implements its goals *Client*: after receiving health teaching about reasons lithium is being prescribed, complies with medication regimen

strongly about the importance of achieving these changes in salary and working conditions and were unified in their determination to strike if necessary to obtain these benefits. A one-day strike did occur, and 90% of the nurses participated. The solidarity of the nurses as a collective-bargaining group communicated their unity of purpose to the hospital administrators. The nurses obtained a contract that included an acceptable salary increase and an end to compulsory overtime.

The solidarity of the nurses as a collective-bargaining organization reflects the high degree of internal submission to the goals of their group. Galbraith (1983) points out that when internal submission is high, then power is effectively exercised and the likelihood of winning the submission of the employer to collective-bargaining demands is good. If internal submission is weak, as evidenced by reluctance to follow the strategies of the collective-bargaining organization, then the likelihood of winning the submission of the employer is poor. Therefore, internal power becomes the basis for external power.

Other expressions of internal and external power are evident in health care institutions. For example, when health team members present a "unified front" to clients, the likelihood of clients' submitting to the power of the health team and complying with treatment plans and institutional rules and regulations is greater than if health team members criticize each other's competence. The external exercise of power is dependent on submission to internal rules of conduct. In health care settings as in any other setting, teamwork involves conditioned submission to the power of the group.

The right to use power to command behavior, enforce rules, and make decisions is referred to as *authority* (Leininger, 1979; McFarland and Shiflett, 1979). Authority is often based on rank or position in a social hierarchy. Authority may be either of two types—line authority or staff authority. Line authority is based on job status. People with line authority have a position of power that enables them to hire, fire, and command. Overt use of power tends to predominate. Staff authority is based on interpersonal relationships. People with staff authority do not have the power to hire, fire,

or command. A relatively nonthreatening environment is created, and the covert use of power tends to predominate.

Power may be used either constructively or destructively (Ashley, 1975; Leininger, 1978, 1979). The constructive use of power facilitates the functioning of those subject to it. For instance, a nursing care coordinator may use power to enable nurses to work toward specific goals of nursing care or to achieve desired results of nursing actions. The destructive use of power inhibits the functioning of those who must submit to it. For example, a director of nurses may decide, in collaboration with a medical director, that only psychiatrists, psychologists, and social workers should hold therapy groups. Nurses prepared in group therapy would not be permitted to function as group therapists. Such destructive use of power may be repressive, suppressive, and demoralizing.

POWER, GENDER BIAS, AND MENTAL HEALTH CARE

Lengermann and Wallace (1985;118-120) assert that "our traditional gender system is founded on an assumption of inequality" between men and women and that women have traditionally experienced institutionalized powerlessness. People's gender identities center on the age and sex norms, values, and expectations of the society in which they are reared. Gender identity is central not only to individual self-identity but also to the organization of society. Gender identity is operative on intrapersonal, interpersonal, and societal levels (refer to Chapters 6 and 7 for further discussion of gender identity).

During periods of extreme sociocultural change, people often find that responsibilities and commitments that have previously given meaning and direction to life, what Bardwick (1979) calls "existential anchors," are lost. Gender roles, a source of gender identity, serve as existential anchors or sources of stable identity.

The decade of the 1970s brought enormous changes in American values and attitudes about gender roles. For women to gain power in the public sphere, however, men must give up some power. Similarly, for men to share roles and responsibilities in the domestic sphere, women must relinquish some control. These changes generate feelings of confusion, fear, and anger that are often manifested as resistance. Resistance to gender-role change may be found among men, women, and children. Many men feel threatened by the feminist movement because they perceive a trend toward sharing with women what has traditionally been masculine power and privilege. Conservative men tend to idealize traditional feminine roles, while cynical men tend to devalue women who take on the challenges of nontraditional gender roles. Women who have been socialized into traditional gender roles and are ambivalent about assuming nontraditional roles also evidence resistance to gender-role changes. On a conscious level some women may be angry at having missed opportunities, but on an unconscious level they may be fearful about their ability to fulfill nontraditional roles. In addition, many women perceive traditionally female roles as creative and meaningful and resist help with such activities as child care, thereby limiting their commitment to their careers at a time when male age-mates are most fully career oriented. Possibly because of their own gender-related developmental issues as well as selective reward and punishment for traditional gender appropriate-inappropriate behaviors and role models, children also tend to resist changing concepts of male-female roles and try to reinforce sex-role stereotypes (Bardwick, 1979).

Female and male liberation movements are attempting to facilitate some gender-role changes. The ideal for many feminists is represented by gender-role equality in both public and domestic spheres. Such equality involves egalitarian families, absence of sexist stereotypes, and women and men with equal access to opportunities in education, occupation, and the law. The primary orientation of the male liberation movement is the reduction of stress and other health problems associated with traditional male roles and establishment of more meaningful interpersonal relationships with men and women. The secondary orientation of the male liberation movement is political. It involves changing the occupational structure by introducing flextime, child care, job sharing, etc., thereby making the occupational structure more compatible with family living, as well as ending male discrimination in such areas as child custody laws and alimony (Lengermann and Wallace, 1985).

Even with the societal changes that are occurring, boys tend to have fewer parental and institutional restrictions imposed upon them than do girls. These differential restrictions serve to shelter girls not only from opportunities but also from the consequences of seeking out socially disallowed choices. In adulthood, most women continue to have fewer opportunities for decision making and power than do men, and this situation affords them relatively little control over the environment. For example, discrimination and limited opportunities often result in women working in less satisfying jobs or receiving less money for the same jobs as men. Moreover, the roles and responsibilities of work outside the home are often superimposed on those of being a wife-mother, producing role overload and overburdening. Because the role expectations of women tend to be more ambiguous than the role expectations of men, they may contribute to confused female identity and negative female self-concept (Grove and Tudor 1973; Litman 1978). Lengermann and Wallace (1985) suggest that those people who deviate from society's gender expectations often experience legal, economic, and mental health sanctions.

Legal sanctions are illustrated by discrimination in the areas of child custody, alimony, and the handling of family violence.* When a couple divorces, unless she is proven to be "unfit," the courts usually award custody of the children to the mother. Afterward, more than half of the mothers who are awarded child custody experience legal impasses in getting their ex-husbands to comply with child support payments. In the case of family violence, although 46 of the states have some type of law against spouse abuse, loopholes often make the laws difficult to enforce.

Economic sanctions are manifested by economic discrimination in salaries and occupational positions. On average, male salaries are higher than female salaries in all occupational groups. Men dominate all occupational categories except service and household workers. Women are underrepre-

---

*Refer to Chapter 21 for a discussion of family violence.

sented in professional/technical occupations and, when they do have professional/technical jobs, they are usually either nurses or teachers below the college level.

The mental health profession is also dominated by men. The President's Commission on Mental Health (1978) reported that women are the major consumers of a health care delivery system that is predominantly controlled by men. An issue that has generated considerable discussion is gender bias in mental health care. A classic study by Broverman et al. (1970) found that gender is very influential in determining standards for mental health. Professional clinicians were asked to characterize (1) a mentally healthy person, (2) a mentally healthy man, and (3) a mentally healthy woman. Descriptive terminology for a mentally healthy person and for a mentally healthy man were almost identical. In contrast, a mentally healthy woman was described as being overly emotional and easily excitable; more vain, submissive, and dependent than a man; and less risk taking, aggressive, competitive, and objective than a man.

Another issue of gender bias in mental health care involves DSM-III categories and codes. Kaplan (1983) criticizes DSM-III for classifying as symptomatic those aspects of dependency which are typified by the female stereotype while ignoring male dependency. The Council on Psychiatric and Mental Health Nursing (1987), in reviewing changes made by the American Psychiatric Association in DSM-III-R, is similarly concerned about gender bias. The introduction of Late Luteal Phase Disorder establishes a mental diagnosis restricted to women. Council members note that this diagnosis reinforces the rationalization that women may be periodically impaired in their ability to function on the job. As a result, this category can be used detrimentally against women in the marketplace. The council believes that if a woman suffers from premenstrual dysphoria, she can be treated either under the ICD-9 gynecological diagnostic category or under a depressive disorder category.

The council also criticizes the DSM-III-R diagnosis of Self-Defeating Personality Disorder because: (1) It can reflect gender bias. As a result, women could be inappropriately and disproportionately labeled with this disorder. (2) It can

reflect ethnocentricity. As a result, sociocultural factors that may account for similar behaviors that are unassociated with any personality disorder may be discounted. (3) The behaviors identified may be a response to abuse and victimization and not a personality disorder. (4) It is a psychoanalytically oriented diagnosis. Therefore it is antithetical to the atheoretical norm of DSM-III-R. The council suggests that Post Abuse Syndrome would be a more appropriate and useful diagnosis.

Research in the 1980s indicates that sexual bias may be becoming less prevalent, especially among female clinicians. Increased knowledge about the problems of women and sensitivity to discriminatory attitudes, ideas, and practices may also be contributing to a decrease in sexual stereotyping and bias against women (Brodsky and Hare-Mustin 1980a, 1980b). There continues to be differential treatment of male and female clients by psychotherapists, however. For example, when severity of symptoms is controlled for, women are given more medication (more than 70% of psychotropic medications prescribed are prescribed for women), receive more potent medication, and are subjected to more therapy sessions than are men (Stein, Del Gaudio, and Ansley, 1976; Stephenson and Walker, 1979; Fidell, 1980). In addition, women are sometimes viewed and used as sex objects by their therapists. Approximately 6 to 10% of psychiatrists admit to seducing their clients (Gartrell et al., 1986). In a national survey of 1,423 psychiatrists, 65% had treated clients who had been sexually active with previous therapists (88% of the clients were women). Although it was acknowledged that sexual involvement between therapist and client had been harmful to the client in 87% of the cases, only 8% of the incidents were reported to ethics committees, licensing boards, or legal authorities (Gartrell et al., 1987). Bouhoutsos and others (1983) found that 11% of clients who had been sexually involved with their therapists were hospitalized as a consequence of that seduction and that 1% of them committed suicide.

Power is a complex concept; it has many sources and forms. There are various types of power strategies and various ways in which power can be used. To influence the nature and direction of mental health care and professional nursing, nurses need to understand that power, politics, and planned change are interrelated. We will explore this interrelationship.

POWER, POLITICS, AND THE PROCESS OF PLANNED CHANGE

Politics is the process of achieving and using power for the purpose of influencing decisions and resolving disputes between factions. A political system is a network of ideas and interpersonal relationships that effectively influences the thoughts, decisions, and behavior of people within formal, organized institutions (Ashley, 1975; Leininger, 1978). Each political system contains ideologies, goals, loyalties, interests, norms and rules that foster cohesion within the political system and differentiate it from other political systems (Scheflen and Scheflen, 1972). For example, a neighborhood drug rehabilitation program will have a political system that is different from that of a neighborhood crisis center. The political system of a federal psychiatric hospital will differ from that of a state psychiatric hospital. An agency operated by a board of directors composed of community residents will have a political system that is different from that of an agency operated by a board of directors composed of mental health professionals.

To apply knowledge about power processes and strategies and to influence the nature and direction of mental health care and professional nursing, nurses must understand the process of planned change. Planned change involves the formulation of a program or scheme for altering the status quo. There are three basic types of planned change—collaborative, coercive, and emulative. Collaborative change involves mutual goal setting and planning. Interactions are characterized by the covert use of power. In contrast, coercive change involves the overt use of power to impose goals and plans on others. Emulative change is characterized by people identifying with an authority figure and adopting the goals and plans of the authority figure. The authority figure usually uses power covertly and serves as a role model.

Planned change is characterized by four phases: motivation, establishing a change relationship,

TABLE 3-2 Phases of planned change

Phase	Accomplishment
Motivation	1. Development of a need for change 2. Identification of a need for change
Establishing a change relationship	1. Clarification of problems and situations requiring change 2. Examination of alternative procedures
Changing	1. Establishment of goals and a plan of action 2. Transformation of the plan of action into actual change efforts 3. Incorporation of change efforts into the system
Assimilating and stabilizing	1. Achievement of the desired goal 2. Positive feedback from significant people that reinforce the change efforts 3. Establishment of a state of equilibrium

Sources consulted include Lewin (1974), Miller (1979), and Gerrard, Boniface, and Love (1980).

changing, and assimilating and stabilizing. Table 3-2 describes these phases of planned change.

Essential to the success or failure of planned change are motivational and resistive factors. *Motivational factors* include desire for alleviation of an intolerable situation, disparity between a hoped-for situation and an actual situation, external demands for change, and internal demands for change. *Resistive factors* include reluctance to accept any change, refusal to accept a particular change, satisfaction with the status quo, conflict in the relationship between an agent for change and a health care delivery system, and transformation of initially obscure factors into major obstacles to change (Gerrard et al., 1980).

When planned change is contemplated, it is essential that the people who will be affected by the change be involved in all aspects of the process of change. Whenever responsibility is given for effecting change, it is necessary that the authority to implement change also be delegated. Otherwise the persons trying to effect change will be powerless, and their efforts will be frustrated.

In an understaffed unit where there were many chronically ill clients who had been hospitalized for more than 12 months, a clinical nurse specialist was given the responsibility of instituting milieu therapy (see Chapter 12 for a discussion of milieu therapy). However, he was not empowered to fire staff members who were committed to a custodial care approach or to hire new staff members who would implement milieu therapy. In addition, he was not empowered to spend money for renovating the unit or for purchasing supplies.

Although the clinical nurse specialist was initially enthusiastic about establishing a therapeutic milieu on the unit, his lack of power thwarted all his efforts to implement change. After 6 months in this situation, he became so frustrated that he resigned from his position.

When faced with a need for change, a person can adapt to a situation, leave a situation, or change a situation. If either of the first two options is selected, the status quo is maintained. If the last option is selected, change occurs. People who try to influence the making and implementing of decisions in a way that fosters change are referred to as change agents.

Change agents act as resource people, as catalysts for change, and as educators in techniques of planned change. To fulfill these roles, change agents need to be skilled in the following areas:

1. Identifying and helping others recognize a need for change
2. Assessing factors that may facilitate or impede change
3. Helping people view themselves as a group that can effect change
4. Helping a group explore its mode of interaction and correct disruptive interaction patterns
5. Helping a group establish goals for change
6. Selecting appropriate roles and techniques to assist a group in achieving goals
7. Helping a group develop methods for achieving goals
8. Supporting and guiding a group through the phases of change

9. Maintaining channels of communication within the health delivery system
10. Helping a group evaluate change efforts and results (Gerrard et al., 1980)

Gerrard et al. (1980) believe that people who are committed to effecting change need to possess high degrees of candor and trust, a sound knowledge base, be willing to take risks, and be able to tolerate ambiguity in the system. These personal attributes are especially important when change requires the adoption of deviant behavior (for example, promoting a policy that differs markedly from previous agency policy) or self-corrective behavior (self-evaluation or self-improvement), the changing of present behavior, or a high degree of interdependence among participants in a group or situation.

Whenever nurses are involved in planned change, they need to examine the ethical issues inherent in the change situation. Nurses should ask themselves the following questions: (1) What values do the goals of the planned change maximize? (2) What values do the goals of the planned change minimize? (3) What is the target population (e.g., clients, staff, environment)? (4) Whose interests is the planned change satisfying? For instance, are the needs of the target client population being met or those of the mental health team proposing the change? (5) Is the power of one group (e.g., clients) being eroded to strengthen the power of another group (e.g., the mental health team)? The ethical dimension needs to be included whenever planned change is being considered (Warwick and Kelman, 1973; Aroskar, 1982).

Power, politics, and planned change are complex and interrelated processes. We will now look at the utilization of these processes in mental health care.

POWER, POLITICS, PLANNED CHANGE, AND PSYCHIATRIC CARE
Institutions

Institutions* are organizations that fulfill normative functions and purposes in society. An institution is a subsystem of a larger system (Blase, 1973).

---

*Refer to Chapter 4 for a discussion of institutions and culture shock.

Federal, state, and local psychiatric hospitals and community mental health agencies are examples of institutions.

An institution usually officially communicates its philosophy of health care in verbal and written statements. An institution's unofficial philosophy may, however, be reflected in symbols (for example, use or nonuse of uniforms, locked or unlocked psychiatric units). Institutions also officially and unofficially state expectations about members' performance. These expectations define acceptable behavior for all members (both staff members and clients). Members are then evaluated on the basis of their desire and ability to fulfill these expectations. Staff members who satisfy these expectations may be promoted or given salary increases. Clients who fulfill the expectations may be judged mentally healthy and discharged from the institution. Scheflen and Scheflen (1972) emphasize that kinesic monitors*, especially those which convey negative feedback, are very effective in evaluating and controlling behavior.

A clinical nurse specialist thought that the wearing of uniforms in a psychiatric setting conveyed messages of control and authority, reinforced the passive client role, and contributed to an interaction theme of dominance (nurse)–submission (client). When she discussed this issue with the director of nurses, the director took a deep breath and rolled her eyes upward toward the ceiling. The director's kinesic monitor conveyed the message: "Here we go again. I've heard this before. I don't approve of the idea." The clinical nurse specialist felt intimidated and did not pursue the idea any further.

Because staff members and clients, to differing degrees, depend on an institution for gratification of security needs, negative kinesic monitors tend to be very effective in controlling behavior.

Often there is incongruity between the verbal and kinesic levels of institutional communication. For instance, an administrator's verbal philosophy of care may emphasize client participation in the

*Refer to Chapter 10 for a discussion of nonverbal communication.

setting of treatment goals, while his kinesic behavior may severely restrict client input into the treatment program. Such inconsistency between verbal and kinesic messages tends to confuse staff members and to render them powerless to change the system. Kinesic monitors derive much of their power from the incongruity produced in the communication system (Scheflen and Scheflen, 1972).

A system of reinforcement that includes both kinesic monitors and negative and positive sanctions helps regulate the behavior of an institution's members. For instance, staff members who display institutionally approved behavior may be rewarded with job security, job advancement, and salary increments. This is an example of the use of compensatory power. Staff members who deviate markedly from institutionally approved behavior may be threatened with demotion, firing, and negative references for future jobs, or they may actually be demoted or fired (use of condign power).

Members of an institution may be, to varying degrees, indoctrinated into institutional *ideology*. An ideology projects an institution's ideas and purpose for existing outward onto its social environment. Indoctrination into institutional ideology promotes cohesion and commitment among members and is an example of the use of conditioned power. The more controversial an institution's programs and services, the greater the importance of ideology in defending and supporting its activities (Zentner, 1973; Galbraith, 1983).

Members who are fully indoctrinated into institutional ideology tend to believe and think along institutional lines—to engage in "institutional think." When institutional think occurs, members are apt not to recognize discrepancies, problems, or alternatives. At this point, members may so closely identify with the institution that an attack on it becomes an attack on them (Scheflen and Scheflen, 1972).

Some nursing students felt overwhelmed by course requirements. In addition, they felt that there was a degree of overlap and redundancy in such course requirements as process recordings, supervisory conferences, log entries, and sharing of clinical experiences in seminar. When the students complained to the faculty and asked that the assignments be reeval-

uated and streamlined, the faculty became very defensive. Not only had the faculty required these assignments for a number of years, but particular faculty members had also designed particular assignments. The rationale for the assignments reflected the philosophy of the program. The faculty's identification with the program and the assignments made the faculty members resistant to any suggestions for change. They were unable to hear the students' complaints or to see any value in the students' suggestions for change. The faculty members were victims of "institutional think."

Any discussion of planned change in institutions must include three elements—institutional variables, networks, and transactions.

Institutional variables include leadership, ideology, programs, resources, and internal structure. Leadership must be displayed by the people who are actively involved in making policies and decisions and in directing institutional operations. Ideology consists of an institution's stated philosophy and its purpose for existing. Programs are methods for translating institutional ideology into actions and for allocating resources for accomplishing those actions. Resources include money, materials, labor, and political support, all of which may be necessary for implementation of programs. Internal structure, the organizing and channeling of power, authority, and decision making within an institution, may be either lateral or hierarchical* (Perrow, 1970; Argyris, 1972; Bumgardner et al., 1972; Blase, 1973; Zaltman, Duncan, and Holbeck, 1973).

Networks are interrelationships between an institution and its social environment that influence and maintain the institution and provide it with a capacity for change. Table 3-3 describes several types of networks.

Transactions are the actual interactions between an institution and the component linkages in its network, which both influence and are influenced by the institution. Transactions involve planning and strategy decisions. These plans and strategies comprise the matrix of planned change in institutions (Bumgardner et al., 1972; Scheflen and Scheflen, 1972; Blase, 1973).

Institutional variables, networks, and transactions can interrelate to produce planned change

---

*Lateral structure involves a dispersed locus of authority, with all members presumably enjoying equal power and authority. Hierarchical structure involves a centralized locus of authority and a chain of command.

TABLE 3-3 Types of networks

Type	Composition	Example
Enabling	Organizations that give an institution both legal authority and resources for its existence	Community Mental Health Centers Act of 1963 authorized establishment of community mental health centers and Title 11 provided funds for their establishment
Normative	Interrelationships between an institution and an organized body of people who determine norms and standards for the operation of an institution	Community Mental Health Centers Act amendments of 1975 established standards and guidelines for the operation of community mental health centers
Diffuse	Interrelationships between an institution and the public	National Association of Mental Health and organized consumer groups may work toward the same goals
Functional	Interrelationships between an institution and a body of people who provide the institution with such resources as clients and professional staff	Mental health professionals may refer clients to an institution; an institution may agree to provide clinical experience for students in exchange for tuition remission for nonprofessional staff who want to pursue professional education

within an institution. When institutional ideology is not viable, impetus for change tends to develop from forces outside the institution (from component linkages in the institution's networks). The internal structure of the institution will then either respond to or resist pressure for change. If institutional structure is of a lateral type, all members will presumably be equally involved in the process of change and will respond to pressure for change. If institutional structure is of a hierarchical type, however, pressure from outside the institution for change will usually be met by resistance (Perrow, 1970; Argyris, 1972; Bumgardner et al., 1972; Blase, 1973).

When institutional ideology is variable, impetus for planned change tends to develop from forces within the institution. For instance, professional staff may realize that mental health services do not meet the needs of the catchment population. If commitment to institutional ideology is weak, then a hierarchical structure will be most effective in mandating and effecting planned change. If commitment to institutional ideology is strong, a lateral structure will be most effective in initiating and implementing planned change (Bumgardner et al., 1972; Blase, 1973).

Consumers

A consumer is an individual, a group, or a community that utilizes a product or service. In the area of mental health, consumerism refers to the utilization of all levels of mental health services (services designed for primary, secondary, and tertiary prevention of mental illness).

The ability to impose power on others through the use of authority supposes a relationship of domination-submission. Those who are powerless in most aspects of their lives are vulnerable to the wills of others.

In the relationship between power and vulnerability, Janeway (1980) sees the "ordered power to disbelieve" as basic to refuting the definition of self that is advanced by the powerful. By disbelieving and questioning the opinions, perceptions, rules, codes, and norms of people in power, powerless people may find that there are other ways of perceiving and coping with events than the people in

power prescribe. The power to disbelieve, however, has to have validation through shared experience with others in similar circumstances. This can be accomplished by forming consumer groups that create a bond of trust, a sense of community, and a belief that their purposes are important enough to work for. Groups such as the Mental Patients Liberation Movement (composed of people who have been treated for mental illness) and the Federation of Parents' Organization (composed of parents and other relatives of the mentally ill) accomplish just such aims (see the section on consumers in this chapter for further discussion).

Gonzalez (1976) points out that consumer groups have been organized on all levels—local, state, national, and international. These groups, which may operate either independently or corporately, often grow out of special interest movements in schools, health agencies, government, and industry.

Consumers, individually and organized as groups, serve two functions—to monitor and to regulate. In their function as monitors, consumers ascertain the need for and the accessibility, availability, and effectiveness of health care services; check into the cost effectiveness of health care activities; and watch for unethical behavior on the part of mental health professionals. In their function as regulators, consumers are concerned with the credentials and competence of mental health professionals and with standards of professional practice (Gonzalez, 1976).

To carry out these functions, consumers assume roles as planners, advisors, and educators. Consumers are actively involved in the following areas:

1. Lobbying for legislation that will upgrade mental health care
2. Lobbying for adequate funding of mental health programs
3. Reordering of local, state, and national priorities
4. Utilizing community resources for the planning and implementation of programs that will meet the mental health needs of the community
5. Contributing to the preparation of mental health workers by acquainting them with the

needs, values, and goals of the community that the workers are servicing (Health Task Force of the Urban Coalition, 1970; National Association for Mental Health, 1974)

Consumers, individually or in groups, tend to have certain basic concerns. Fundamental to these concerns is the idea that mental health professionals have too much power over clients. Consumer groups point out that the courts usually accept a psychiatrist's observations or predictions of dangerous behavior over a client's request for discharge from a psychiatric institution. Consumer groups also express concern that, once a person is labeled mentally ill, the focus of mental health professionals is on abnormal rather than normal behavior. In addition, consumer groups are concerned that some psychiatric institutions do not provide adequate treatment and that transitional and aftercare facilities are insufficient.

Consumers of mental health services do not have the vested interest in protecting a mental health agency or program that mental health professionals may have. Moreover, consumers are the people who experience the health care delivery system. For these reasons, it is often easier for consumers to identify areas where change is needed than it is for mental health professionals. Some mental health professionals may become accustomed to the status quo and may not be aware of a need to change practices. Other mental health professionals may fear the effect change will have on their role status and functioning and may therefore deny a need for change.

Consumers often have a better understanding of their mental health needs or of the mental health needs of their community than do mental health professionals. Epstein (1974) observes that the social class and life-style of mental health professionals often differ from those of their clients. Epstein suggests that even mental health professionals who originally came from backgrounds similar to those of the majority of their clients usually drastically alter their life-styles once they achieve the position of mental health professional. It becomes the function of indigenous workers, who still share the same life-styles as the clients, to serve as liaisons between clients and professionals. Indigenous workers may help professionals view clients within the

sociocultural context of the community, facilitate communication between clients and practitioners, and articulate needs for change from the perspective of the client (Ruiz and Behrens, 1973; Epstein, 1974).

If change is to occur in the mental health care delivery system, consumers must be involved in the decision-making process. To effectively participate in decision making, consumer groups are demanding information about mental health care. They want to know about the efficacy of various therapeutic approaches, the comparative costs of therapies, and the anticipated therapeutic results and side effects of various treatment modalities (Gonzalez, 1976).

Comprehensive health care programs operated by boards of directors composed of consumers have demonstrated that consumers are able to

1. Make decisions and policies based on an intimate knowledge of a community's health needs
2. Identify areas that require professional expertise and seek consultation in those areas
3. Evaluate services and staff behavior from the perspective of the client
4. Identify areas that need change and effectively use power to achieve change in a mental health program (Ruiz and Behrens, 1973; Epstein, 1974)

The consumer movement has successfully used power to effect changes in the field of mental health that range from research to delivery of care. For example, in one year, consumers

1. Initiated a lawsuit that resulted in release of $126 million for research, alcoholism, and manpower programs
2. Influenced the amending of a health maintenance organization bill to include basic mental health coverage
3. Helped amend a rehabilitation act so that affirmative action in hiring would include the "mentally handicapped"
4. Succeeded in getting the United States Civil Service Commission to remove a question about previous treatment for mental illness from employment applications
5. Instituted and awarded National Association for Mental Health Research Fellowships

6. Successfully lobbied so that the Federal Education Act would allocate funds to states for the establishment of programs for mentally ill children
7. Sponsored a conference, under the auspices of the National Association for Mental Health, on critical issues related to mental health research (National Association for Mental Health, 1974)

Nurses

Nurses are important members of the interdisciplinary mental health team. Many nurses work in psychiatric agencies. Some clinical specialists work independently or in group practice situations. Chapters 1 and 12 emphasize the role and functions of nurses as care providers in an interdisciplinary mental health setting. Later in this chapter we will define the various levels of practice in psychiatric nursing. In this section, we will focus on the nursing role of client advocacy.

NURSES AS CLIENT ADVOCATES

Because nurse-advocates have to be able to offer information objectively to clients and to support clients in their decisions, even when those decisions may not be the ones the nurses would have chosen, it is essential for nurse-advocates to be open minded. Kohnke (1982) suggests that to develop the open-mindedness essential to the advocate rule, nurses should be able to inform and support clients, analyze systems, utilize ethics, identify the effects of social issues on advocacy, understand the role of the medical-industrial complex, and recognize the impact of laws on advocacy. The advocate self-assessment guide on p. 61 is based on these abilities.

As nurses develop the aforementioned abilities, they will be better able to carry out their responsibilities as advocates. As client advocates, nurses are responsible for the following functions:

1. Ensuring ethical practice. Nurses need to be committed to basic human rights, able to assess possible consequences of actions, and sensitive to situations that may influence the application of principles pertinent to accountable nursing practice (Nations, 1973; Annas and Healey, 1974; Curtin, 1978a, 1978b).

2. Ensuring client rights. Nurses assist clients to learn about, protect, and assert their rights. Nurses may explain civil rights, retention status, and institutional procedures to clients and may help them to obtain legal counsel. In addition, nurses act as monitors to ensure that client rights are not violated.
3. Acting as liaisons. Nurses help clients and staff members develop effective interpersonal relationships, investigate clients' complaints, and assist clients in using institutional resources for problem solving (refer to Chapter 12).
4. Ensuring high-quality care. Nurses participate in and cooperate with quality assurance programs. Data are collected, analyzed, and utilized for planning, assessing, and improving the quality of mental health care.

POWER, POLITICS, AND ETHICAL PRACTICE

Nursing is a "moral art." Nursing combines a concern for people's well-being with the technical skills needed to achieve that end. The interconnectedness of individuals and society means that the well-being of the individual must be balanced with the well-being of society. Such balancing requires interaction between ethics and the use of power.

An ethical caring relationship involves two participants: the one who is doing the caring ("one-caring") and the one who is receiving the caring ("one-cared-for"). When the one-caring is open to another person, a feeling mode is entered. This feeling mode is not necessarily an emotional mode, but it is a receptive-intuitive mode where the other person is accepted without evaluation or judgement. What Buber (1970) describes as an I-Thou relationship is established. The one-caring "sees" from both his or her perspective and from the perspective of the one-cared-for. This relationship is characterized by interdependence. For example, in the nurse-client relationship, if the one-cared-for is overly demanding or complaining, the one-caring may become overwhelmed, resentful, and/or angry and may cease caring. When the one-cared-for responds with authenticity or personal growth, then there is genuine reciprocity in the I-Thou

Advocate self-assessment guide

ABILITY TO INFORM AND SUPPORT A CLIENT

1. Do I have the facts necessary to thoroughly inform the client?
2. If I do not have the necessary facts, do I know where to get the information?
3. Do I believe the client should have this information?
4. Do I present this information to the client in a meaningful manner and in an appropriate context?
5. What people (other staff members, family) might object to the client having this information? How can I cope with these objections?
6. Do I allow the client to make a decision, or do I try to influence the client's decision? Do I play the role of rescuer when the decision does not work out?

ABILITY TO ANALYZE A SYSTEM

1. What is an institution's official philosophy? What is its unofficial philosophy?
2. What are the stated and unstated expectations of myself and others?
3. What factors in a system, including vested interests of participants, constitute risks to informing and supporting clients? For example, an institution's official philosophy may be to encourage client participation in treatment planning, but the vested interests of staff members may operate to ensure their own power and status within the institution. A hierarchy is thereby created, with the client at the bottom. This situation might present a problem to a nurse-advocate who is supporting a client's right to accept or refuse a course of treatment.
4. What strategies might I utilize for dealing with these risks?

ABILITY TO USE ETHICS* TO ANALYZE A SITUATION

1. Am I familiar with the ethics that should guide the conduct of psychiatric nurses?
2. How do these ethical positions guide my conduct and affect the decisions that I make?
3. How might differing ethical positions of the client and others (family, staff members) affect my ability to inform and support the client?

ABILITY TO IDENTIFY THE EFFECTS OF SOCIAL ISSUES ON ADVOCACY

1. What issues (racism, sexism, ageism) are operative in a situation?
2. What risks do these issues present for client advocacy? For example, if mental health professionals believe that Hispanics are volatile, emotional people, the staff may try to withhold information from an Hispanic client so as not to "upset" the client and cause the client to become "irrational" or to "overreact." This prejudicial attitude of staff members may present a problem to a nurse-advocate who is trying to ensure the right of Hispanic clients to information about their psychiatric conditions and treatment plans.
3. What strategies are needed for dealing with these risks?

ABILITY TO UNDERSTAND THE ROLE OF THE MEDICAL-INDUSTRIAL COMPLEX

1. What vested interest groups (pharmaceutical companies, mental health boards, consumer groups) might affect client care?
2. How might these groups affect my advocate role? For example, an agency's concern about liability suits may interfere with a nurse-advocate's responsibility to ensure that a client has the least restrictive conditions that will meet the aims of retention.

ABILITY TO RECOGNIZE HOW LAWS AFFECT ADVOCACY

1. How do laws affect the care of mentally ill clients?
2. How do these laws affect my advocate role? For example, the right of clients to confidentiality affects the information about the therapeutic relationship that a nurse can and cannot give the parents of an emotionally ill child.
3. What are the risks that might be encountered when, as an advocate, I ensure a client's rights? For example, if a nurse, in the advocacy role, gives a client information about the right to refuse treatment, will the client's family or the staff retaliate? Who will they retaliate against— the client? the advocate? the system?

*Ethics is discussed in more depth in subsequent pages of this chapter.

TABLE 3-4 Relationship among ethics, health behavior, and advocacy

Ethical philosophy	Health behavior	Advocacy
Kantian: People should have freedom of decision making and action (or inaction)	Client undergoes treatment because he or she wants to recover from an emotional disorder	Nurse focuses on client advocacy: supports a client's right to accept or reject treatment
Natural law: People have personal autonomy, but they also have obligations and responsibilities for the common good	Client undergoes treatment because he or she feels an obligation to the family to recover from an emotional disorder and resume social roles	Nurse focuses on social advocacy: supports human rights in general and obligations and responsibilities to society

Sources consulted include Becker (1986), Francoeur (1983), Ramsey (1970), and Burckhardt (1986).

relationship and the relationship is nurtured (Noddings, 1984).

One's ethical self develops out of a fundamental awareness of relatedness of self-to-others and of self-to-self. It is an active relationship between a person's actual and ideal selves that acknowledges not only that one cares for others but also that one is cared for by others. Noddings (1984,49) states, "As I care for others and am cared for by them, I become able to care for myself."

A difficult area in nursing involves conflicting responsibilities to individuals and society. The need to balance ethical and political dimensions is paramount. For example, Burkhardt (1986) discusses the moral-ethical dilemmas surrounding the issue of client compliance. Most nurses support the concept of individual autonomy over one's own body. But individual autonomy has two aspects: personal freedom and social responsibility. If a nurse has a Kantian philosophy, then the nurse holds that personal autonomy and freedom are paramount to all other considerations. Clients with a Kantian philosophy, in deciding to act or not to act, consider what is best for themselves at that time. On the other hand, if a nurse has a natural law philosophy, then the nurse holds that one's responsibilities and obligations to the common good are of paramount importance. Clients with a natural law philosophy, in deciding to act or not to act, consider the ramifications of their actions on others. Nurses who have a Kantian orientation tend to focus on client advocacy, while those who have a natural law orientation tend to focus on social advocacy. Table

3-4 illustrates the relationship among ethics, health behavior, and advocacy.*

Basic ethical dilemmas encountered by nurses center around two major areas: (1) institutional policies and/or physicians' orders that affect quality of client care and (2) the appropriation of nurses' legitimate authority to make decisions about nursing care (Curtin, 1978a, 1978b). Rouslin (1976) states that mental health nurses should be guided by two rules: (1) optimal behavior concerning client welfare and (2) optimal professional conduct.

Nurses should use a *code of ethics* to direct their professional conduct. These codes emphasize that the primary responsibilities of nurses are the preservation of life, the relief of suffering, and the promotion and maintenance of health. These codes also stress the responsibilities that nurses have as citizens to follow laws, to carry out the duties of citizenship, and to work with other citizens to improve and preserve the health of communities on local, state, national, and international levels.

Some nurses' associations have adopted *codes of ethics for psychiatric nurses.* Such codes of ethics usually include the following provisions:

1. The promotion of mental health is a primary responsibility of psychiatric nursing.
2. Through continuing education, psychiatric nurses must increase their professional knowledge and competencies.
3. Maintenance and utilization of professional

*Advocacy will be discussed in more depth later in this chapter.

competencies are essential to the provision of optimal mental health care.

4. Regardless of the color, race, religion, or gender of clients, clients should be respected as individuals and should be the focus of nursing concern both during and after therapy.
5. Client-nurse interaction should be confidential except when there is a possibility of harm to self or others.
6. Psychiatric nurses are accountable for their own psychiatric nursing decisions and actions.
7. Psychiatric nurses work with and sustain confidence in other health professionals.
8. Psychiatric nurses should report incompetence or unethical conduct of health team members to appropriate authorities.
9. Psychiatric nurses assume responsibility as concerned citizens for promoting efforts to meet the mental health needs of a community.
10. Psychiatric nurses collaborate with other health professionals in informing clients of treatment plans and of the anticipated outcomes and side effects of treatment procedures.
11. Psychiatric nurses follow laws that relate to the practice of mental health nursing.
12. Psychiatric nurses should not engage in a nursing practice that violates the code of ethics (Psychiatric Nurses Association of Canada, 1977; American Nurses' Association, 1982).

Codes of professional ethics try to assist nurses to deal with ethical dilemmas in nursing by establishing guidelines for professional behavior. Codes of professional ethics cannot by themselves, however, resolve all ethical dilemmas in psychiatric nursing. What is often necessary is for nurses to systematically analyze complex ethical issues and to understand how they arrive at ethical decisions. Kohlberg's (1973) theory of moral development, which has been utilized and expanded upon by Lande and Slade (1979), is useful for this purpose. The theory of moral development has six stages. Table 3-5 identifies the stages and the characteristics of each stage.

The following situation shows how the stages of moral development can be applied to the analysis of ethical dilemmas in psychiatric nursing:

Thirteen months ago, Chad Johnston, a twenty-six-year-old high school teacher, was diagnosed as having AIDS. At first Chad denied the diagnosis, asserting that the result of the blood test was in error. When a second blood test confirmed the AIDS diagnosis, Chad began to accept his diagnosis. He became alternately angry at the "unfairness of life" and hopeful that a cure would be found. However, as Chad's physical condition deteriorated, his mood also changed to one of hopelessness and depression. Chad discussed with his family his plan to commit suicide before he became "an invalid living a life of pain." His family supported Chad in this decision.

Two days ago, one of Chad's friends discovered Chad unconscious from an overdose of barbiturates. Chad's friend called the paramedics, and Chad was brought to the hospital emergency room where he was successfully resuscitated. Chad is angry that he was resuscitated and is refusing all treatment. He states that he is still determined to commit suicide.

Some of the nurses on Chad's unit feel that, because of Chad's physical condition and prognosis, it was wrong to resuscitate Chad. Other nurses feel that suicide is wrong no matter what the circumstances and that they have a professional and moral obligation to prevent suicide.

The above example shows the responses that psychiatric nurses may have concerning an ethical-moral dilemma such as a person's right to commit suicide. The question also arises, "If a client has a right to commit suicide, should nurses respect that right?" The positions that psychiatric nurses take on ethical issues such as suicide are usually based on one or more of the following ethical-moral arguments:

1. People have the right to live and die as they choose, even to the extent of committing suicide. This argument is indicative of Stage 2 reasoning: People may do whatever they wish with their own bodies and belongings. There is no reason to sacrifice one's self (e.g., through suffering) unless you can expect some benefit or gain in return.

TABLE 3-5 Stages of moral development

Stage	Characteristics
One	This is the stage of obedience or punishment. There is no internal sense of right or wrong. Actions are labeled good or bad according to the judgment of others (people who have power to reward or punish behavior). Following rules is all-important. Concern is with consequences of rule following (reward or punishment) for one's self. Stage One is primarily operative with children.
Two	This is the stage of the "morality of the marketplace." Concern is primarily with one's own well-being, but there is a rudimentary idea of sharing reflected in the reciprocity of doing a favor and expecting a favor in return. Sacrificing for another is done with the expectation of reciprocation. Rules are usually followed. If rules are broken, it is for personal gain. Values are relative and viewed in terms of materialistic or social usefulness.
Three	This is the stage of conformity to peer group standards and ideals concerning behavior. Group solidarity is of paramount importance, and favors are done for members of one's peer group to please them and gain their approval.
Four	This is the stage of law and order. Concern is no longer just for one's peer group but for society in general. Society is viewed as a network of complimentary roles, obligations, rules, and authority. Mutual trust, honesty, dependability, and moral conformity are expected of everyone (both leaders and followers). Values, laws, and customs (the status quo) are not questioned, and they are staunchly (and sometimes emotionally) upheld.
Five	This is the stage of the social contract. One's moral conduct is based on principles that have been self-chosen. Concern is for protecting the rights of others and for meeting one's social and legal responsibilities. Rules must ensure the rights of everyone. The rights of individuals assume the same importance as the well-being of society. It is held that society should protect the rights of all individuals. Human life is valued more than property. Rules may be broken to ensure justice and fairness.
Six	This is the stage of universal human rights. Judgments are predicated on universal moral principles, the most inviolate being the value of human life. The needs of others and self are viewed as equally important. Behavior is based on a concern for human dignity. One has a moral responsibility to uphold just laws and to break unjust laws. Even though disobeying unjust laws may be an attempt to raise the consciousness of society, one must be ready to accept the consequences of law breaking. Stage Six individuals may be viewed as heroes, as revolutionaries, or as rabble-rousers.

2. The dilemma arises because the health team, who is trying to keep a client alive, and the client's family, who may support the decision to commit suicide, all have the client's best interest at heart. This argument is indicative of Stage 3 reasoning: People act out of concern for the well-being and happiness of others.

3. The dilemma concerns the client's right to commit suicide versus the health team's obligation to sustain life. This argument is indicative of Stage 4 reasoning: People's legal rights should not be violated, and moral judgments should uphold rules, laws, and authority.

4. The risks associated with treatment (such as chemotherapy) and the emotional trauma of living with a terminal illness must be weighed against the possibility of the client going into remission or recovering. This argument is indicative of Stage 5 reasoning: The welfare of the individual is as important as the welfare of society, and society must protect the interests of the individual. Conflict often occurs when the interests of society (or a subsystem of society, such as the health care delivery system) clash with the wishes or beliefs of an individual.

5. The rules or laws against taking one's own life are unjust and should be openly disobeyed. This is indicative of Stage 6 reasoning: People's actions must be based on a concern for human dignity. People have a moral obligation to disobey unjust rules, but they must

TABLE 3-6 Ethical analysis

Step	Actions
Obtain a data base of relevant information	Gather information pertaining to the situation, circumstances, and factors that directly influence the situation.
Identify ethical constituents	Sort out ethical from nonethical issues. Ethical issues may include alleviation of aggressive behavior vs. loss of ability to generate and express ideas (as with psychosurgery) and freedom vs. restriction of rights (as in the treatment of mental illness).
Identify ethical agents and their roles in the situation	Identify those people who are engaged in or will engage in or be affected by a decision. Clients, families, clergy, court judges, and health team members are examples of ethical agents. Explore the rights, duties, and responsibilities of ethical agents, as well as factors that may facilitate or impede their freedom to make and carry out a decision.
Explore alternative actions	Consider the possible consequences of each action. Instances in which duty or responsibility conflicts with consequences of an action may be especially difficult to resolve. For example, a nurse may be confronted with the dilemma: "If I intervene to prevent a client from committing suicide (responsibilty as a nurse), I am denying the client's right to self-determination (the right to take one's own life).
Develop an approach based on ethical principles	Identify the ethical principles (e.g., ideas about the nature of human beings and self-determination, the manner of ethical thinking and decision making). For example, nurses who rely on the authority of the Scriptures may hold that the taking of life is always wrong. On the other hand, nurses who hold that actions that deny human freedom are wrong may view suicide as an act of self-determination and therefore a rightful act.
Resolve the dilemma	Make a decision based on the above process of obtaining pertinent information, identifying ethical agents and their roles, exploring alternative courses of action, and developing an approach based on ethical principles. The decision arrived at may involve only the nurse or it may involve assisting a client or a client's family to decide on a course of action.

also be willing to accept the penalties for their actions.

In making ethical decisions, psychiatric nurses must learn to critically analyze situations. Curtin (1978a, 1978b) has developed a model for critical ethical analysis. Using Curtin's model, we can extrapolate the steps illustrated in Table 3-6.

Ensuring client rights

Ensuring client rights is a primary responsibility of nurses. To fulfill this responsibility, nurses should be knowledgeable about the legal aspects of mental health nursing practice. Nurses need to be aware of retention procedures, client rights, and client advocacy services.

There are three reasons for retaining a person in an institution: danger to self, danger to others, and need for psychiatric treatment. Each state in the

United States has its own statues or mental health code on which retention procedures are based. The purpose of legally defined retention procedures is to protect against retention abuses. A person may be retained in a psychiatric hospital or in a psychiatric unit of a general hospital. Retention procedures generally involve three steps. (1) application, (2) assessment and evaluation, and (3) commitment to an institution. Most states recognize four types of retention: informal, voluntary, emergency, and involuntary.

To be informally retained, a person verbally requests admission to an institution for psychiatric treatment. In most states, a person who is being informally retained may leave the institution simply by notifying the director of the institution (through the professional mental health staff) of a plan to leave. If the mental health professionals think a client needs to remain in the institution, then application must be made to convert the client's status from informal to involuntary.

Voluntary retention has two components: a written request for admission to an institution and a voluntary seeking of psychiatric treatment. People who are voluntarily retained usually do not relinquish their civil rights and may vote, manage property, and conduct business. If a client wants to leave the institution before he or she has been discharged, the client must make a written request to the director of the institution. The director must either honor the client's request or get a court order authorizing involuntary retention. Each state specifies the length of time a voluntary client may be retained after requesting discharge. For example, in New York and Pennsylvania, the director of an institution has 72 hours to either honor a client's request for discharge or obtain a court order converting the client's status to involuntary.

A person who is acutely mentally ill may be admitted to an institution on an emergency status. This type of admission is time limited. For example, in New York (see Fig. 3.1), emergency retention is valid for 15 days. If at the end of the time period it is felt that a client is not ready to be discharged, the client can agree to voluntary retention or the director of the institution can petition the court to convert the client's status to involuntary.

There are two avenues to involuntary retention:

1. Medical certification. A specified number of physicians certify that a person is mentally ill and *potentially dangerous to self or others*. The number of physicians required for certification is established by state statue and varies from state to state. In many states the assessment of two physicians is necessary for certification. The director of the institution then presents this assessment to the court and requests a court order for involuntary retention.
2. Status conversion. By court order, retention status is converted from informal, voluntary, or emergency to involuntary.

A court order for involuntary retention is time limited. The time period may vary from state to state. If at the expiration of the first court order it is felt that a client still needs to be retained in the insti-

tution, the director of the institution can petition the court for an extension of the involuntary retention order. Each time the order for involuntary retention is extended the time period may be increased. For example, in New York the first court order is valid for 60 days, the second for 6 months, and the third for 1 year. In many states, when the court is considering a retention order of 1 year or more, the client must be physically present in court. At any time, by using a habeas corpus procedure, a client or a client's family can petition the court for repeal of the retention order and discharge from the institution.

Ensuring client rights encompasses more than knowledge about retention procedures. A person with mental illness is the only "patient" who has to be granted, by state statutes, rights previously guaranteed to him or her as a citizen. These rights include the right to vote (by absentee ballot, if necessary), the right to personal freedom unless convicted of a crime, the right to a court hearing (in cases of involuntary retention), and the right of appeal and review by a higher court (Ennis and Siegel, 1978; Offir, 1974). Even persons certified as insane retain the civil rights of citizenship. In addition, no institutional regulation may deprive mentally ill clients of rights guaranteed them by state mental health statutes or codes. Although state statutes vary, most state mental hygiene codes guarantee certain rights of mentally ill adults. Table 3-7 illustrates the rights of the mentally ill and nursing actions that facilitate those rights.

Recent legal developments have further extended the rights of the mentally ill to control their own lives. The concepts of self-determination, self-actualization, and protectable interest as they apply to people who have psychiatric disorders center around the following three basic issues: (1) the cultural relativity of "normal" and "abnormal" behavior, (2) the function of psychiatry as an agent of social control (identifying and treating behavior that deviates from sociocultural norms), and (3) the presumption of personhood, of an actualized self. This last issue poses questions concerning the type of or extent of limits that society can place on people's expression of their individuality and individual self-expression versus the rights of others and the common good (Tancredi, 1983; Feather, 1985).

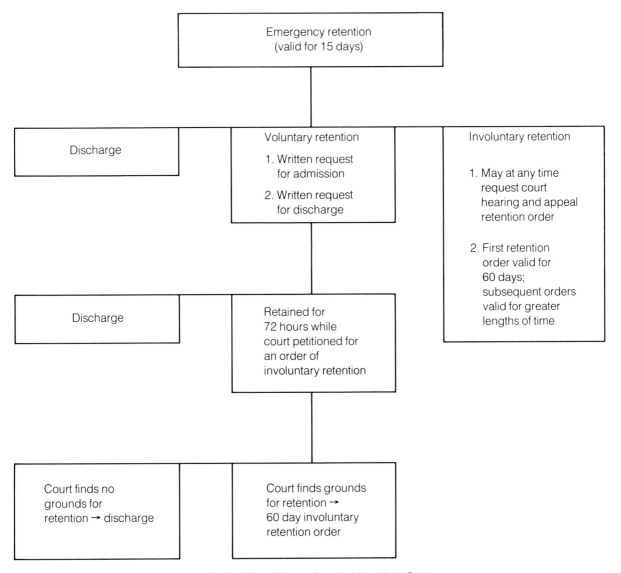

Fig. 3-1 Retention options in New York State.

Explicitly stated rights represent the strides that have been made in guaranteeing the civil rights of mentally ill clients. Yet, as Shindul and Snyder (1981) point out, such advances in the civil rights of clients may also pose dilemmas for mental health professionals. For example, courts have ruled that competent adults have the right to refuse treatment. The procedure for an informed refusal of treatment is similar to that for an informed consent.

In Lane vs. Candura (1978), it was ruled that a competent adult must be advised of the nature of the diagnosis, the expected action of the treatment, possible risks and side effects associated with the treatment, alternative treatments (if available), and the risks and consequences associated with refusing treatment.

Later court cases determined that the right to refuse treatment is contingent on the circum-

TABLE 3-7   Rights of mentally ill adults

Guaranteed right	Facilitating nursing action
To know one's retention status	Notify a client-advocate or a representative of the Mental Health Information Service (who may be a lawyer) of client's admission to the unit so that the client can be officially notified of retention status and rights.
To the least restrictive retention	Talk with an agitated client. Use chemical or physical restraints as last resorts and never as punishment.
To periodic review of one's mental health status if one is involuntarily retained	Ensure that procedural process of review is followed by periodically reviewing client's mental health status with health team members.
To an explanation of one's psychiatric condition and treatment plan and of untoward reactions that may occur as a result of treatment	Routinely review with client progress made and areas to work on. Whenever possible, include client in setting, implementing, and evaluating goals. Explain actions and side effects of somatic therapies and chemotherapy and determine client's understanding of the explanations.
To treatment	Establish an individualized treatment plan within a specified period after admission (e.g., 5 days). Develop a discharge plan and, when appropriate, provide for transitional care. Contact a physician whenever a client appears physically ill or expresses physical complaints. Do not assume that clients' physical complaints are manifestations of hypochondriasis or somatic delusions. Such measures will facilitate prompt and adequate treatment of physical illness.
To refuse or accept treatment	Explain purpose of treatment and ramifications of accepting or refusing treatment. Unless client behavior is dangerous to self or others, abide by client wishes. Do not threaten client (e.g., if you do not take this oral medication, you will receive an injection) or use punitive actions toward client (e.g., avoiding client).
To judicious use of medication	Check that medications are prescribed in writing, have a maximum termination date, and are reviewed periodically. Do not administer medications as a form of punishment, for staff convenience, or in dosages that conflict with a treatment program.
To judicious use of physical restraints and seclusion	Use physical restraints and seclusion only in a situation in which a client is deemed dangerous to self or others. Physical restraints and seclusion can only be ordered by a physician who has personally seen the client. Check that the order is in writing and that it specifies a time period—for example, 24 hours. Do not exceed the specified time period. Monitor and record the client's physical and psychiatric status—for example, every hour. Bathroom privileges must be allowed, and the client must be bathed regularly—for example, every 12 hours.
To privacy and to be treated with dignity	Respect client's territorial boundaries. Unless contraindicated by the treatment plan, allow a client privacy when dressing, bathing, and toileting. Do not intrude when client has visitors or eavesdrop on client's conversations and telephone calls.

Sources consulted include Shapiro (1974), Miller, Dawson, and Parnas (1976), Stone (1979), and Feather (1985).

TABLE 3-7 Rights of mentally ill adults—cont'd

Guaranteed right	Facilitating nursing action
To communicate with people outside the institution	Allow clients access to telephones and visitors. Mentally ill clients have the same right of access to telephones and visitors as clients in general hospitals. This right can be denied only by written order from a qualified mental health professional who is responsible for a client's therapeutic regimen. Check that such an order is reviewed at regular intervals. Be sure that visits from lawyers, private physicians, and other health professionals are not denied. Allow clients to receive sealed mail from attorneys, health professionals, courts, and government officials. Be sure that a client's right to receive mail is only restricted or denied by written order from a qualified mental health professional responsible for the client's treatment.
To informed consent	Determine that a client has been informed about the purposes, untoward effects, and risks associated with potentially dangerous treatments. Be sure that the client has given consent or has legal counsel prior to administration of such potentially dangerous treatment modalities as electroconvulsive therapy, psychosurgery, and aversion therapy or prior to experimental research. Research must be reviewed and approved by a human subjects committee. If a client is incompetent to consent, a judge or lawyer may become a proxy consenter.
To confidentiality	Do not discuss a client's diagnosis, type of treatment, or the fact that the client is receiving treatment with people who are not part of the client's treatment team. If information needs to be shared outside the treatment team, obtain the client's written consent. "Privileged communication" is a legal term referring to a client's right not to have information gained through psychiatric therapy divulged in court. A client may waive, in writing, the right of privileged communication.
To be adequately clothed	Allow clients to wear their own clothes and keep personal belongings unless such a right is denied or restricted in writing by a qualified mental health professional. If clients do not have adequate clothing, they have the right to be clothed by the institution.
To regular physical exercise	Allow clients to go out of doors on a regular basis, unless they are physically ill. The institution must supply facilities and equipment for exercising.
To be paid the minimum wage for any work that contributes to operation and maintenance of the institution	Check that clients are receiving the minimum wage for such operational or maintenance services as working in the institution's laundry room, working in the institution's kitchen and bussing tables in the institution's dining areas.
To engage in religious worship	Allow clients to attend religious services of their own denominations. Upon client request, contact the clergy of the client's choice. Unless contraindicated in writing by a qualified mental health professional, respect a client's privacy when praying or conversing with the clergy.

stances of each individual case (Rennie vs. Klein, 1981). Among the circumstances that qualify the right to refuse treatment are:

1. Emergency situations where treatment is necessary to protect the safety of the client, staff, or other clients.

2. Involuntary commitment situations where treatment is needed to prevent deterioration of the client's condition or to prevent injury. The treatment must be the least intrusive and restrictive available that will accomplish the desired effects.

3. Voluntary commitment situations where the client's refusal of treatment poses a threat to the safety of the client or others. Then involuntary commitment procedures should be considered.

4. Incompetency situations where the client has been declared incompetent by the courts. In this circumstance, a court-appointed guardian must consent to treatment. Should the legal guardian and the client disagree about treatment, then a judicial review may be ordered before treatment is forced on a client.

Doris Peters had been voluntarily admitted to a psychiatric unit following a suicide attempt. She was severely depressed and she was experiencing self-accusatory delusions and suicidal ideation. When the client's depression was not helped by antidepressants, the psychiatrist decided to try electroconvulsive therapy. The client consented. As electroconvulsive therapy progressed, the client showed some mood elevation. Then, midway through the treatments, the client decided she did not wish to continue with electroconvulsive therapy.

As the above vignette illustrates, the rights of clients can sometimes pose dilemmas for mental health professionals:

1. Does Doris have the right to refuse treatment?

2. Does the staff have the right to force Doris to accept treatment?

3. Does Doris's behavior pose a danger to herself or others?

4. Does Doris's commitment status have any

bearing on the way in which this situation should be handled?

5. Does this situation qualify as a psychiatric emergency?

As a voluntary client, Doris has the right to refuse treatment unless the lethality of her suicidal ideation is assessed as a threat to her own safety. What also needs to be considered is whether discontinuing electroconvulsive therapy would contribute to deterioration of Doris's condition. Complicating this determination is the fact that Doris's depression had not responded to antidepressive medications. Since Doris has a voluntary commitment status, if the staff believes that there is a need for forced treatment, then they will have to initiate involuntary commitment procedures.

In addition to the legal recourse that mental health professionals have when clients refuse treatment, some lawyers, clients, and their advocates state that subtle pressures are used to make clients comply with treatment regimens. For example, privileges may be withheld or honor cards may be withdrawn from a noncompliant client (Talan, 1987).

Another area that may pose a dilemma for mental health professionals centers around the issue of when a client is ready for discharge. A client's right to the least restrictive mode of treatment may sometimes conflict with the social responsibility to protect clients and others from potential harm. Recent court decisions have identified "duties" that mental health professionals owe clients and the public. These duties include the duty to warn, the duty to protect, and the duty to predict. In the event that a recently discharged client harms self or others, mental health professionals must be able to substantiate that these duties were fulfilled in order to avoid the charge of negligent release. Risk-management strategies that can be used to establish that release decisions were appropriate and met reasonable standards of professional care include:

1. Peer review. Release procedures should be developed and subjected to a peer review panel of five to ten mental health experts recruited nationwide. Peer reviewers should also submit written critiques of the standards for release that include statements about whether the release procedures are in accord with national standards of care.

2. Independent case consultation. An independent clinician should review all high-risk management discharges, for example, the discharge of a client with a history of violent behavior, to determine whether all release procedures were followed and carefully implemented (Poythress, 1987).

Nurses also are responsible for ensuring the *rights of mentally ill children and adolescents*. Although these rights vary from state to state, most state mental health statutes guarantee the following:

1. Right to free educational services
2. Right to be free from involuntary sterilization (Parents cannot authorize the sterilization of their child.)
3. Right to have legal counsel for any retention procedures
4. Right to the least restrictive conditions that will meet the aims of retention
5. Right to treatment (A child or an adolescent has the right to an individualized treatment plan that considers the developmental stage of the child or adolescent and to treatment by a qualified mental health professional who is a specialist in child or adolescent mental health. There should be interaction between mental health personnel and the child or adolescent's family. When parents deny treatment for a child or an adolescent, the court may act as an advocate and make a decision on the child's or adolescent's behalf.)
6. Right to informed consent (Whenever possible, informed consent should be obtained from a child or an adolescent.)
7. Right to confidentiality (A child of any age has the right not to have detailed information derived from therapeutic relationships disclosed to parents. An adolescent over 16 years of age usually can decide what information he or she wants disclosed. When a child is unable to give consent, because of age or for other reasons, parents have the right to know the type of treatment their child is receiving and their child's progress in treatment and the right to decide about releasing information to a third party [Burgdorf, 1979].)

Nurses can function as formal or informal child advocates. Formal advocacy involves appearing in court as a witness or being primary initiator of a lawsuit on a child's behalf. Informal advocacy involves educating parents, administrators, and health team members about the rights of mentally ill children and adolescents and guaranteeing these rights.

State statutes usually provide a client advocacy service that is under the jurisdiction of the state courts. The purpose of a client advocacy service is to safeguard the rights of child and adult clients. For example, in New York State, the Mental Health Information Service informs clients of their retention status and rights, including their right to counsel from the service. It reviews annually the status of involuntarily retained clients. If there is any doubt about the need for retention, the Mental Health Information Service must request a court hearing to resolve the issue.

Nurses are responsible for guaranteeing client rights, for educating others about the rights of mentally ill individuals, and for acting as liaisons between clients and a state-established client advocacy service. Nurses may be directly or indirectly involved in safeguarding client rights. For instance, when a nurse performs a nursing procedure (for example, administers a medication), he or she must explain the purpose, anticipated results, and possible side effects of the procedure to the client. If the client then allows the nurse to perform the procedure, the client is implicitly giving consent. If the client refuses the procedure, the nurse should comply with the client's refusal and should then inform the psychiatrist. For nonnursing procedures (such as aversion therapy), nurses are responsible for ascertaining that clients are giving informed and voluntary consent. Occasionally, nurses are asked to ensure that a client's consent is voluntary and informed. This entails detailed recording of the discussion with the client. The questions and responses of both nurse and client and the client's mental status should be included. These are instances of direct involvement of nurses in the safeguarding of client rights (Creighton, 1970; Willeg, 1970).

Sometimes nurses are indirectly involved in the protection of client rights. Education of nonprofessional staff about the rights of clients is an example of indirect protection of client rights. If a staff member does not believe in a particular right, he or she probably will not be vigilant in guaranteeing it. In a study of psychiatric aides, Daugherty (1978) found that aides supported rights that concerned abstract concepts or basic human needs (for example, adequate nutrition and treatment of medical problems) but had reservations about rights that might affect ward management or give increased responsibility to clients (for example, the right to be paid for work necessary to the operation of a psychiatric center and the right to judicious use of physical restraints and medications).

Nurses, as client advocates, are responsible for ensuring client rights. To fulfill this responsibility, they should be aware of retention procedures, the nature of client rights, client advocacy services, and the attitudes of the mental health staff members with whom they work.

Ensuring high-quality care

As client advocates, nurses should be concerned with the quality of care provided, and they should be active participants in quality assurance programs. *Quality assurance* refers to activities designed to indicate the quality of health care and efforts aimed at improving the quality of health care (Towery and Windle, 1978; ANA Standards of Psychiatric and Mental Health Nursing Practice, 1982).

In 1975, the Community Mental Health Centers Amendment (Public Law 94-63) made three stipulations concerning quality assurance in community mental health centers:

1. Development of national standards for community mental health centers
2. Development of quality assurance programs
3. Collection of data for the evaluation of quality assurance programs including operating costs and patterns of service utilization (acceptability of services, accessibility of services, and responsiveness of services to the needs of the catchment population)

A minimum of 2% of the previous year's operating expenses of a center must be allocated and used for implementation and evaluation of quality assurance programs (Towery and Windle, 1978).

Depending on the level of program development, either a formative or a summative evaluation may be used. A formative evaluation involves the collection of empirical data for the purpose of developing a program. To date, designs for formative evaluation have not been well developed. A summative evaluation involves the collection of data for the purpose of assessing the effectiveness of an already existing program. A summative evaluation may be conducted internally by the personnel responsible for the program, or it may be conducted externally by individuals or groups outside the program. Whether a summative evaluation is internal or external, it has the following objectives:

1. To establish outcome criteria for specific populations of clients. Comparing results of health care with outcome criteria gives an indication of the effectiveness of services.
2. To determine the least number of cost-effective activities and resources required to accomplish outcome criteria. Relating the expense incurred for required activities and resources to outcomes services gives a measure of efficiency.
3. To ascertain the degree to which a health delivery program meets the needs of the catchment population. Identifying factors that facilitate or inhibit the use of program services provides a measurement of accessibility of services (Zimmer, 1974; Towery and Windle, 1978).

Nurses may participate in formative and summative evaluation of mental health programs. The collection and analysis of data for the purpose of planning, assessing, and improving the quality of mental health care is a vital component of client advocacy.

NURSES AND PLANNED CHANGE

The effectiveness of nurses as client advocates is often hampered by inadequate knowledge about the process of change and the use of power. Nursing education may not adequately prepare nurses to understand change and provides them with limited experience with power strategies.

Within an agency or institution, the power structure usually comprises three groups: administrative personnel, medical personnel, and nursing personnel. Power tends to shift continuously, through negotiation, among these three groups and among the individuals within these groups. It is not unusual for a given person (for example, a director of nurses) to belong to more than one group. The intergroup power system creates a balance of power. To participate effectively within this balance of power, nurses, especially nurse-leaders, should learn to negotiate for power. When power is controlled by one group or when one group has little power, there may be diminished morale, ineffective functioning of the group having little power, or abuse of power by the group controlling power (McFarland and Shiflett, 1979).

Conflicts in the vested interests of the individuals and groups that make up the health delivery system may result in a *power struggle.* A power struggle often occurs between nurses and other professionals within the health delivery system. In mental health settings, power struggles often are related to such advocacy functions as ensuring ethical practice and quality care. Struggles may be centered around issues such as the following:

1. Agency or institutional philosophy and delivery of mental health care
2. Negotiation for limited strategic resources (human and material)
3. Autonomy in mental health nursing practice
4. Roles and functions of nurses within the mental health care delivery system

In a broader social context, power struggles sometimes exist between nurses, special interest groups, and legislators, on local, state, or federal levels. Such power struggles often center around client advocacy issues such as the following:

1. Allocation of money for mental health research and preventive intervention
2. Legislation concerning client rights and affirmative action programs for children and adults with a history of mental illness
3. Legislation forbidding discrimination against children and adults because of a history of mental illness
4. Insurance coverage for the treatment of mental illness (including third-party payment)

Political nursing is the use of knowledge about power processes and strategies to influence the nature and direction of health care and professional nursing (Ashley, 1975; Leininger, 1978). To be effective client advocates, nurses need to learn how to use power for planned change. The goals of political nursing are the same as the goals of the mental health care system: the availability, quality, accessibility, and funding of mental health care (Brown, Gebbie, and Moore, 1978; McFarland and Shiflett, 1979). The constituency of political nursing is clients: communities, groups, and individuals—both identified and potential.

Through political nursing, nurses attempt to provide input into power systems and to establish power strategies that can be used to regulate information and influence people in power. Methods for regulating information include rapid acquisition and distribution of accurate information by organizations to members; verification of information so that people do not have to act on the basis of rumor; and dissemination of knowledge about who to contact, how to initiate contact, and methods for conveying ideas to people in power. Involvement in local government, participation in public hearings, and lobbying are ways of influencing people in power (Ver Steeg, 1979).

Knowing how to regulate information and influence people in power is important in effecting change. Nurses can be instrumental in effecting change in their own mental health agencies or in the broader social contexts of community, state, and nation. To effect change, nurses should utilize the steps for expanding their bases of power and authority shown in Table 3-8.

Because of the risks to personal security (for example, job security), nurses are sometimes hesitant to initiate change in their own agencies or institutions. However, these risks can be minimized. Epstein (1974) suggests that nurses minimize risks to personal security by identifying with like-minded colleagues, by expanding their power bases, and, whenever possible, by utilizing supportive agency policy. Identification with people who view the need for change in a similar way creates a network of support and action. Within this network, nurses can develop power strategies, evaluate progress, revise plans for change, and support one another in both success and failure. By talking with other members of the mental health team and with administrators, nurses can broaden their support bases both quantitatively and qualitatively. In addition, if an agency has a clearly and concisely written policy that supports a proposed change, nurses should use the policy in effecting change. If the

TABLE 3-8   Steps in expanding bases of power and authority

Step	Purpose
Increase nursing knowlege and clinical expertise	Develops a base for expert power
Develop strong, creative, and knowlegeable nursing leadership	Serves as a source for role models, gives novices an opportunity to develop power strategies and to be socialized into leadership roles, and provides a foundation for assertive and effective action
Identify sources of one's own power and learn to use power strategies effectively	Recognizes that power is a component of interpersonal relationships
Develop alliances that will increase support and power	Serves to diminish power struggles and to increase associative power
Identify people who can serve as intermediaries in expediting change	Serves to understand the channels of communication

Sources consulted include Leininger (1979), McFarland and Shiflett (1970), and Gerrard, Boniface, and Love (1980).

policy is violated, violators may be confronted with the written policy. Whenever possible, such confrontation should be done by a group of people who are committed to the change. Confrontation by a group reduces the risk of retaliation against an individual.

Effecting change in the broader social contexts of community, state, and nation involves the use of many of the same strategies that are used in effecting change in an individual mental health agency. Burke (1979) suggests that nurses apply the interpersonal skills utilized in nurse-client relationships to relationships with community leaders and legislators. She suggests that a nurse should first establish a working relationship and then should identify appropriate contact people. Often local community leaders and their staffs can act as liaisons with other people and agencies. Maintaining an ongoing relationship is important. Even when a nurse is not lobbying for change, he or she should keep in touch with community leaders and legislative staff. Nurses must be knowledgeable: They should learn the names and functions of leaders who are involved with health issues, and they should be well informed about those issues. They should support lobbies and special interest groups that share their concerns. A nurse should provide community leaders and legislators with the local perspective—the way people in the community feel about an issue. Community leaders and legislators tend to be polit-

ically sensitive to this type of feedback (Burke, 1979; Donley, 1979).

Through political nursing, nurses use power processes and strategies to influence the nature and direction of health care and professional nursing. Political nursing is an essential element in client advocacy. McFarland and Shiflett (1979) caution nurses to consider the ethical implications of power strategies, not to use power solely for self-serving ends, and to be mindful of the responsibilities and obligations associated with the use of power.

Institutions, consumers, and nurses are the major components of the contemporary mental health care delivery system. Within this delivery system, power strategies and power struggles sometimes arise around such issues as quality of care, client rights, affirmative action, and allocation of resources. We will now examine some major issues and trends in mental health that may indicate the areas in which future power strategies and struggles will occur.

ISSUES AND TRENDS IN MENTAL HEALTH

Issues* and trends in mental health develop within a social context and need to be examined

---

*Other mental health issues, such as family violence and abuse (Chapter 21) are discussed elsewhere in this book.

within that social context. Consumerism, questioning of the insanity defense, decreases in funding for mental health research, and independent nursing practice are trends that affect and are affected by such social factors as inflation, political activism, and community attitudes. As these trends evolve and ramify, implications for the future are suggested.

Consumerism
CONSUMER POWER

A philosophy is emerging that encourages equal participation in decision making between consumers and providers of mental health care. The trend toward increased involvement of and power for consumers is moving ahead on two levels—individual and community.

On the first level, individuals are being given knowledge that will make them educated consumers of and effective participants in the therapeutic process. Clients have a right to, and are being given, explanations about their psychiatric conditions, treatment plans, alternative types of treatment and their costs, and any untoward reactions that might occur as a consequence of treatment. Within the therapeutic relationship, mutuality between clients and nurses (or other mental health professionals) is also being encouraged. Stone (1979) notes that the introduction of mutuality between client and therapist restructures the therapeutic relationship from a status relationship (a relationship based on hierarchical positions) to a contract relationship (a relationship based on voluntary individual arrangements). Clients have an opportunity for more autonomy in contractual than in status relationships (Stone, 1979).

Many clients are turning for assistance to self-help groups composed of people who have recovered from specific psychosocial problems. Alcoholics Anonymous, Gamblers Anonymous, and Overeaters Anonymous are examples of such groups. In many instances, these self-help groups constitute the major treatment modality. In other instances, self-help groups are used in conjunction with other therapies or to prevent the development of psychosocial problems (for example, Compassionate Friends is a support group for bereaved parents).

Client decisions to utilize the therapeutic properties of self-help groups and the assumption of care-provider roles by some recovered clients exemplify the increasing autonomy of consumers in the mental health care delivery system.

Recently, a national organization of people who are currently or were formerly mentally ill was formed. The primary goals of this organization, the National Mental Health Consumers' Association, is to remove the stigma from mental illness, to improve the quality of life for people with psychiatric problems, and to empower the mentally ill to fight for their rights. Among the rights that the National Mental Health Consumers' Association is fighting for are (1) representation on decision-making bodies that have input into the mental health care delivery system, to increase the responsiveness and accountability of the mental health care delivery system to the needs of the mentally ill; (2) to increase the development of self-help groups throughout the United States, linked by a national clearinghouse; (3) to stop discrimination against the mentally ill in housing and employment; (4) to lobby for increased public benefits; and (5) to work with the media and communities to remove the stigma from mental illness (Rogers, 1986).

The second level of the trend in consumerism is characterized by collaboration between the community and nurses and other professionals in community mental health centers. Increasingly, community representatives are sitting on the boards of community mental health centers. Community mental health boards thereby become a point of articulation between community residents and care providers. Such collaboration between community representatives and mental health professionals is a potentially educational experience. Community representatives may learn firsthand about the community mental health movement—its philosophy, goals, and problems. This educational process helps to demystify mental health and mental illness, to teach consumers (and potential consumers) about treatment modalities and the roles and functions of members of the mental health team, and to sensitize residents to the mental health problems in their community.

Community residents may become aware of the influence their involvement and support can have on a community mental health program. Community representatives may develop an increased understanding of their sources of power and of how power relationships affect budgeting, service priorities, and programming.*

Nurses and other mental health professionals can better view clients within the sociocultural context of the community. The values, ideologies, and traditions of subgroups (such as ethnic groups and classes) within the community may be better identified and understood. Nurses and other mental health professionals can also increase their awareness of the perceptions that subgroups within the community have about the definition, cause, and treatment of mental illness (Borus, 1976; Ruiz and Behrens, 1973; Borus and Klerman, 1976; Landsberg and Hammer, 1978).

IMPLICATIONS FOR THE FUTURE

The role of consumers (actual and potential) in the mental health delivery system will probably continue to expand. Presently, people who have recovered from specific psychosocial problems (such as alcoholism, drug abuse, and compulsive overeating) are effectively intervening in the treatment of people who have not yet recovered. Gonzalez (1976) suggests that this trend may grow to include other psychosocial problems (for example, depression, phobias, and compulsive working).

In addition, consumers are becoming more vocal about their perceptions of effective treatment for mental illness, and nurses and other mental health professionals are becoming more responsive to the ideas of consumers. Gonzalez (1976) and Warner (1977) note that many consumers rely on the native healers and folk medicines of their cultures. Client belief in folk medicine and confidence in native healers need not rule out treatment by nurses and other mental health professionals. Torrey (1973) explains that both native healers and mental health professionals function as therapists in the treatment of mental illness and that both achieve therapeutic results. Native healers are important mental health resources and should be actively integrated into mental health programs.

---

*Chapter 16 discusses the effect of recent governmental budget cutbacks on community mental health centers.

Questioning of the insanity defense
CURRENT ATTITUDES

An increase of violence in the United States, underscored by the history of violent acts against public figures, has precipitated an outcry against the verdict "not guilty by reason of insanity." Although the insanity defense has recently become the focus of much attention, it should be noted that most violent people are not mentally ill and most mentally ill people are not violent. People with a history of mental illness who commit violent acts usually have a history of criminal activity that predates their mental illness (Babich, 1981; Schell-King and Finneran, 1982; Steadman, 1982).

Forensic psychiatry is that specialty in psychiatry that deals with the legal facets of mental illness (Sadoff, 1975). People accused of crimes can be found incompetent to stand trial because of a mental condition, or they can plead not guilty on the basis of insanity and be so found by a jury.

A determination that a person is incompetent to stand trial is based upon his or her inability to understand the charges and to participate with a lawyer in his or her own defense because of mental disorder (Stone, 1975).

Many of our laws and legal procedures have developed from English common law. This is true of one of the most frequently invoked rules in cases involving the insanity plea—the *McNaughton Rule*. This rule, which was handed down in England in 1843, holds that a person is not guilty of a crime if the person did not understand the nature and quality of the act or did not know that the act was wrong (Stone, 1975). Although the McNaughton Rule has been criticized by legal scholars and members of the psychiatric profession, it has remained an important aspect of the insanity defense in many jurisdictions in the United States.

Another defense that is valid in some states is the *Irresistible Impulse Test*, which was introduced in Alabama in 1887 and has since been adopted by many states. The Irresistible Impulse Test expanded upon the McNaughton Rule by adding criteria for determining people's ability to control their behavior (Stone, 1975).

Both the McNaughton Rule and the Irresistible Impulse Test have been criticized by legal scholars and members of the psychiatric profession because of their moralistic quality and because they do not reflect current knowledge of human psychology. A recent attempt to develop a test or rule governing responsibility for criminal acts in relation to mental disorders resulted in the *American Law Institute Test*. According to this test, a person is not responsible for criminal behavior if at the time of committing a crime the person lacked substantial capacity either to appreciate the criminality of the act or to control his or her behavior so that it conformed to the law (Stone, 1975; Bower, 1984).

Those who would retain the insanity defense argue as follows:

1. If the insanity defense were eliminated, both the criminal law and the public conscience would no longer distinguish between mental illness and evil.
2. People who are charged with crimes should have defense choices available to them.
3. The decision to convict and punish or detain and treat should be arrived at democratically by a jury rather than by a panel of experts in forensic psychiatry.
4. The public's perception that people who benefit from the insanity defense are murderers and rapists is very inaccurate (Steadman, 1982; Schell-King and Finneran, 1982).

Those who would abolish the insanity defense argue as follows:

1. The questions asked of psychiatrists and psychologists by the law are beyond their scope of knowledge.
2. In practice, the insanity defense is a wealthy person's defense.
3. The ambiguous and confusing wording of the various insanity tests results in intuitive moral judgments rather than in objective determinations.
4. Insanity acquitees usually are incarcerated in correctional institutions for periods of time comparable to periods for criminals, but insanity acquitees detained in mental health facilities usually serve approximately six months less time than do comparable felons.
5. The legal system should not function in one manner for a "normal" defendant and in another manner for an "abnormal" defendant

(Steadman, 1982; Schell-King and Finneran, 1982; Bower 1984).

IMPLICATIONS FOR THE FUTURE

Central to any discussion of the insanity defense is concern about the lack of criteria for assessing—and, in effect, predicting—whether individuals will be dangerous to themselves or others because of mental disease or disorder. In many, if not in most, instances, a prediction of violence* is very difficult to make. Although such situational and environmental factors as poorly functioning family, peer, or occupational support systems seem to contribute to violent behavior, the common denominator among people who are violent appears to be simply a history of violent behavior (Babich, 1981).

Among others, Clarke (1982) wonders why the American public becomes outraged when someone who commits a violent act is found not guilty by reason of insanity but similar outrage is not expressed at the failure of psychiatry to more accurately predict violent behavior and to institute preventive therapy. Shindul and Snyder (1981) stress the fact that research into the predictability of violent behavior is necessary for preventive intervention. This is an area in which nurses and other mental health professionals should develop proposals, write grants, and otherwise engage in research.

Status of mental health research
CURRENT STATUS

National trends have been toward decreased National Institute of Mental Health (NIMH) research training monies, elimination of NIMH support for clinical training, and decreased numbers of clinical researchers applying for and receiving federal or private research funding (Fagin, 1986).

Because trained researchers are having difficulty obtaining research grants, many researchers are entering other fields of mental health, such as practice or teaching. Brown (1976) predicts that not only will the scarcity of research grants affect the

---

*Refer to Chapter 21 for an in-depth discussion of violence.

current level of mental health research, but, because young scientists have limited research opportunities, there will also be a dearth of prepared researchers for the next 10 or 20 years.

There is also a trend in American society toward evaluating the worth of a program in terms of its cost effectiveness. Mental health researchers have difficulty translating their results into a dollar amount. While dollar savings can be attached to decreases in the number of people hospitalized for mental illness, similar cost effectiveness cannot as readily be demonstrated for such improvements in human functioning as increased sense of well-being or more effective coping behavior. The difficulty of translating research results into cost-effectiveness formulae plus the stigma that much of the general public still attaches to mental illness result in a lack of public support for mental health research (Brown, 1976).

IMPLICATIONS FOR THE FUTURE

Nurses and other mental health professionals will need to become more politically active and politically effective in educating legislators and the general public about the importance of mental health research. Brown (1976) suggests that such an educational program should encompass the crisis in mental health research, as well as the process, purpose, and importance of mental health research. Public support will be essential if mental health professionals are to successfully compete for scarce research resources. The National Association for Mental Health, a consumer citizen group that in the past used its political influence to engender support for mental health services, is beginning to use its political influence to engender support for mental health research.

Nurses and other mental health professionals are becoming politically active. They will need to direct some of their political activity toward influencing legislation concerning mental health research. Such political activity should involve more than lobbying and contacting legislators. Ver Steeg (1979) believes that mental health professionals who are experts in their fields and who are also politically active are more apt to be asked to serve on advisory committees. Serving on advisory committees may increase the opportunities for mental health professionals to influence legislation concerning research in mental health.

In examining mental health research priorities for the coming decade, Fagin (1986) points to findings of the Institute of Medicine that speak to six areas of research need. These areas are

1. Childhood and adolescent disorders. Although 2 million children have severe mental disorders necessitating immediate care and 8 to 10 million children have mental disorders requiring less immediate care, only 500,000 children are receiving treatment. Developmental disorders of infants, hyperkinetic behavioral and attention deficit disorders, psychotic disorders, depression, drug abuse, eating disorders, and child abuse are among the many childhood and adolescent problems needing to be researched.
2. Family systems. Both functional and dysfunctional family systems need to be studied. The influence of family systems on the development of childhood trust, self-acceptance, achievement, and responsibility needs to be researched. In addition, ways of increasing childhood resistance to the disruptive effects of family members' mental illness or substance abuse need to be explored.
3. Chronic mental illness. The problems of the chronically mentally ill as well as biological, psychosocial, psychopharmacological, and ecological approaches to chronic mental illness need to be studied. The research effort expended on chronic mental illness is far less than the effort expended on chronic physical illness. For example, for every person undergoing cancer treatment, more that $300 is spent on research, while for every person with schizophrenia, only $7 is spent on research.
4. Efficacy and cost effectiveness of treatment. Controlled studies and outcome evaluations are needed to assess various psychotherapies and the disorders for which they are effective. Prospective payment and Diagnosis Related Groups (DRGs) are being considered for psychiatric disorders. Clinical research on the possible impact of prospective payment and DRGs on cost effectiveness and efficacy of psychiatric treatment is essential.

5. Assessment of clinical programs and clinical practice. Rigorous research methodology and replication is needed to evaluate the effectiveness of traditional psychiatric interventions as well as newer innovative interventions. Studies need to look at both short-term improvements and long-term progress of clients.

6. Mental disorders of the elderly. Research is needed to increase knowledge about the mental health and mental disorders of the elderly so that preventive and treatment interventions may be developed. Research should also focus on family and group process as it applies to the elderly and to problems of caring for the elderly. A Women's Mental Health Research Agenda, developed for NIMH, emphasized the need to understand the experience of older women and the impact of poverty, human abuse and role conflict/overload on their mental health (McBride, 1986).

Psychotherapy is derived from a science of behavior. The psychotherapist nurse needs to become involved in clinical research. Such research generates theory that guides psychiatric nurses in selecting effective therapeutic nursing actions. Then the theoretical principles underlying psychiatric nursing practice can be systematically taught using both didactic and supervisory teaching techniques (Jones, 1987).

The American Nurses' Association, in its Standards of Psychiatric and Mental Health Nursing Practice (1982), states that nurses have a responsibility to engage in research so that knowledge in the field of mental health will be advanced. To help nurses achieve this aim, the ANA has enumerated the following process criteria:

1. Nurses should maintain inquisitiveness and open-mindedness in their practice of nursing.
2. They should apply the research findings of others to their own nursing practice.
3. They should participate in the development, implementation, and evaluation of research projects appropriate to their levels of education.
4. They should use responsible investigative standards whenever engaging in research.

5. They should ensure that the rights of human subjects are protected.
6. They should consult with and/or seek the supervision of experts whenever necessary.

Independent nursing practice
CURRENT STATUS

In the past few decades, mental health nursing has expanded both its clinical base and its range of clinical practice.* Recently, nurses have departed from the medical model and have developed a model that embraces the nursing process. Nurses are now making nursing diagnoses, writing nursing orders, treating human responses to illness, and evaluating outcome effectiveness. Enough of this terminology has been legislated into nurse practice acts to enable some psychiatric nurses to expand their role from that of dependent practitioner to that of independent practitioner.

The psychiatric nurse practitioner demonstrates *clinical ability* and has achieved educational preparation beyond a baccalaureate degree with a major in nursing. This additional education may be accomplished through continuing education courses. The clinical nurse specialist has a minimum of a master's degree in psychiatric and mental health nursing, demonstrates *clinical expertise* in psychiatric nursing, and is prepared in research, teaching, clinical supervision, and/or independent practice. Psychiatric clinical nurse specialists are employed in a variety of settings that include, but are not limited to, acute and long-term institutions, outpatient clinics, community mental health agencies, schools, and industry. Psychiatric and mental health clinical nurse specialists who evidence high-level proficiency with interpersonal skills, nursing process, and psychiatric treatment modalities and who have a minimum of two years of supervised direct client contact (8 hours a week) may take a written certification examination to qualify as a Certified Specialist (C.S.).

The expanded role of the nurse has provided an opportunity for many psychiatric nurses to become direct providers of mental health care. Along with this change in employee role a problem has arisen about payment for service. Although psychiatric

---

*Refer to Chapter 2 for a history of psychiatric nursing.

nurses in private practice bill clients directly for services provided, these nurses have usually been unable to receive payment from clients' insurance companies or from such social programs as Medicare and Medicaid. This means that clients are not reimbursed for care provided by psychiatric nurses, although similar care provided by licensed social workers, psychologists, and psychiatrists will be reimbursed. In essence, clients are being financially penalized by third-party carriers for seeking mental health care from psychiatric nurses.

A survey prepared for the Council of Specialists in Psychiatric and Mental Health Nursing showed that psychiatric and mental health clinical nurse specialists should be eligible for third-party reimbursement because:

1. Psychiatric and mental health clinical nurse specialists are fulfilling the recommendation of the President's Commission on Mental Health to "serve the underserved" by devoting part of their practice to serving poor people, minority group members, the elderly, and children.
2. Since their services are not directly reimbursed by many insurance companies, it causes financial hardships for agencies and clinics to hire psychiatric and mental health clinical nurse specialists.
3. Of the clinical nurse specialists who participated in the survey, 67% provided direct client services, but less than 3% received third-party reimbursement for their services.
4. The policy of insurance carriers to require a nurse who receives third-party reimbursement to practice under the supervision of a physician limits the rendering of services in rural and other areas.
5. Since psychiatric and mental health clinical nurse specialists who are not eligible for third-party reimbursement must be employed in salaried positions, which are usually found in populated areas, it prevents many

clinical nurse specialists from providing services to people in rural areas (American Nurses' Association Division on Psychiatric and Mental Health Nursing Practice, 1980).

IMPLICATIONS FOR THE FUTURE

Third-party reimbursement for state-licensed nurse-practitioners and for certified psychiatric nurses is beginning to occur. In December 1981, the U.S. Defense Department's Civilian Health and Medical Programs for Uniformed Services (CHAMPUS) approved the reimbursement of state-licensed nurse-practitioners and certified psychiatric nurses as CHAMPUS-authorized care providers ("Nurse Reimbursement Plan Approved for CHAMPUS," 1982).

More recently, the Colorado Society for Clinical Specialists in Psychiatric Nursing (CSCSPN) successfully negotiated with Colorado Blue Cross/Blue Shield for third-party payment. Blue Cross/Blue Shield now holds that, as long as the supervision process set forth by the Colorado Insurance Statute (that psychotherapy done by psychiatric clinical nurse-specialists be supervised by a licensed physician or psychologist) is followed, claims will be paid. However, a letter from the clinical nurse-specialist's supervisor verifying the supervisory requirements must accompany every claim ("Third-Party Reimbursement," 1982).

Obviously, some progress is being made in recognizing nurse-practitioners and psychiatric clinical nurse-specialists as autonomous providers of mental health care. Yet much work still needs to be done to promote the autonomy and credibility of psychiatric nurses engaged in independent practice. As nurses become more politically active, as they establish networks of support, and as they advocate third-party payment for nurses, the autonomy and credibility of nurses engaged in independent practice will be advanced (Chaisson, 1982).

CHAPTER SUMMARY

Power, which is a dynamic of all interpersonal relationships, has many sources and forms, and it is the basis of many strategies. To have input into power systems that affect the direction of mental health care and professional nursing, nurses need to understand the interrelationship between power, politics, gender bias, and planned change. Institutions, consumers, and nurses are major elements of the contemporary mental health care delivery system. Within this system, issues related to quality of care, client rights, ethical dilemmas, and allocation of resources often lead to power strategies and power struggles. Trends in mental health can indicate the issues around which future power struggles will revolve. Currently, some major mental health trends are consumerism, a questioning of the insanity defense, decreased funding for mental health research, prioritizing research needs, and independent nursing practice.

SELF-DIRECTED LEARNING

Sensitivity-Awareness Exercises

The purposes of these exercises are to:
- Develop insight into the operation of power and politics in your own life
- Develop awareness of your own reactions to change
- Develop an understanding of how you can influence issues and trends in mental health

1. Think about a situation in which you have experienced planned change. The change may have occurred in your personal or professional life. Identify and describe:
   a. The factors that facilitated change
   b. The factors that impeded change
   c. The agent(s) of change
   d. The channels of communication among the people involved in the change situation
   e. Your reaction to the proposed change
2. Analyze and describe the following in regard to an institution (for instance, a health care agency, hospital, school) with which you are associated:
   a. The stated philosophy vs. the operational philosophy
   b. The regulation of behavior (expectations concerning acceptable and unacceptable behavior; negative and positive sanctions on behavior; achievement of upward mobility)
   c. The institutional variables (type of leadership, ideology, programs, resources)
   d. The type(s) of networks that exist between the institution and its social environment
   e. Instances in which you or others were victims of "institutional think"

3. Peruse your local newspaper for 1 month. Collect newspaper articles that relate to such issues or trends in mental health as consumerism, mental health research, the insanity defense, and independent nursing practice. On the basis of the articles you have collected, how would you describe the current state of each issue? What do you foresee happening with regard to each issue in the future? What emerging trends might influence the practice of psychiatric nursing on local, state, national, and international levels? What input can you have into future developments?

Questions to Consider

1. For women to gain power in the public sphere, gender-role changes must occur. Role change often generates confusion, fear, anger, and resistance. Nurses who are working with clients who are experiencing such role change need to know that resistance to gender-role change may be manifested by
   a. relaxing sex-role stereotypes
   b. questioning sex-linked roles
   c. assuming nontraditional gender roles
   d. resisting help with housework and childcare
2. When roles and responsibilities associated with work outside the home are superimposed on those of wife-mother, women may evidence all *but* which of the following?
   a. role overload and overburdening
   b. role security
   c. confused self-identity
   d. negative self-concept
3. A clinical nurse specialist was working with a group of nurses who wanted to start nurse-led

Continued.

SELF-DIRECTED LEARNING — cont'd

Questions to Consider — cont'd

group therapy. The nurses had set goals and developed a plan of action. The nurses are in which phase of planned change?
a. motivation
b. establishing a change relationship
c. changing
d. assimilating and stabilizing

4. Community mental health nurses were in disagreement about the right of homeless ex-psychiatric patients to live on the street. Some of the nurses (group "A") felt that they should be allowed to live the way they wanted, as long as they did not harm others. The other nurses (group "B") disagreed and felt that they should be made to submit to psychiatric treatment. The positions held by group "B" nurses are indicative of which of the following stages of moral development?
a. stage one: following rules is all-important
b. stage two: people may do whatever they wish with their own bodies and belongings
c. stage three: people act out of concern for the well-being of others
d. stage four: people's legal rights should not be violated
e. stage five: the welfare of the individual is as important as the welfare of society
f. stage six: actions must be based on a concern for human dignity

5. When a nurse talks with an agitated client and uses physical or chemical restraints only as a last resort, the nurse is facilitating the client's right to
a. the least restrictive retention
b. treatment
c. informed consent
d. be treated with dignity

Match each of the following terms with the statement that is associated with it:

6. Psychiatric clinical nurse specialist
7. Condign power
8. Psychiatric nurse practitioner
9. Compensatory power
10. Politics

a. imposes unpleasant consequences for not submitting to authority
b. demonstrates clinical ability
c. offers rewards for submitting to authority
d. demonstrates clinical expertise
e. process of achieving and using power

Answer key

1. d	6. d
2. b	7. a
3. c	8. b
4. c	9. c
5. a	10. e

REFERENCES

American Nurses' Association Division on Psychiatric and Mental Health Nursing Practice: Council of Specialists in Psychiatric and Mental Health Nursing FACT SHEET on Clinical Specialist in Psychiatric and Mental Health Nursing, Kansas City, Mo, 1980, ANA Publications.

American Nurses' Association Division on Psychiatric and Mental Health Nursing Practice: Standards of psychiatric and mental health nursing practice, Kansas City, Mo, 1982, The Association.

Annas G and Healey J: The patient's rights advocate. Vanderbilt Law Review 27:243-269, 1974.

Archer R and Lloyd B: Sex and gender, London, 1985, Cambridge University Press.

Argyris C: The applicability of organizational sociology, Cambridge, 1972, Cambridge University Press.

Aroskar MA: Ethical issues in community health nursing. In Spradley BW, editor: Readings in community health nursing, Boston, 1982, Little, Brown & Co.

Ashley JA: Power, freedom and professional practice in nursing, Supervisor Nurse 1:12-29, 1975.

Babich KS: Useful research findings on violence: a summary. In Babich KS, editor: In assessing patient violence in the health care setting, Boulder, Colo, 1981, Western Interstate Commission for Higher Education.

Bardwick JM: In transition: how feminism, sexual liberation, and the search for self-fulfillment have altered our lives, New York, 1979, Holt, Rinehart & Winston.

Becker PH: Advocacy in nursing: perils and possibilities, Holistic Nurs Practice 1(1):54-63, 1986.

Biegel A: The politics of mental health funding: two views. Hosp Commun Psychiatr 28(3):194-195, 1977.

Blase MG, editor: Institution-building, a source book. Washington, D.C., 1973, US Government Printing Office (U.S. Dept. of State).

Borus JF: Neighborhood health centers as providers of primary mental health care. N Engl J Med 295(3):140-145, 1976.

Borus JF and Klerman GL: Consumer-professional collaboration for evaluation in neighborhood mental health programs. Hosp Commun Psychiatr 27(6):401-404, 1976.

Bouhoutsos J et al: Sexual intimacy between psychotherapists and patients. Profess Psychol 14(2):185-196, 1983.

Bower B: Not popular by reason of insanity. Sci News 126:218-219, 1984.

Brodsky AM and Hare-Mustin RT: Psychotherapy and women: priorities for research. In Brodsky AM and Hare-Mustin RT, editors: Women and psychotherapy: an assessment of research and practice, New York, 1980a, Guilford Press.

Brodsky AM and Hare-Mustin RT: Women and psychotherapy: An assessment of research and practice, New York, 1980b, Guilford Press.

Broverman IK et al: Sex role stereotypes and clinical judgements of mental health, J Consult Clin Psychol 34:1-7, 1970.

Brown BJ, Gebbie K, and Moore JF: Affecting nursing goals in health care. Nurs Admin Q 2(3):17-31, 1978.

Brown BS: The crisis in mental health research. Address presented at the 1976 Annual Meeting of the American Psychiatric Association, 1976.

Buber M: I and thou, New York, 1970, Charles Scribner's Sons (Translated by W Kaufman).

Bumgardner HL et al: Institution building: basic concepts and implementation, Chapel Hill, 1972, University of North Carolina (mimeographed).

Burckhardt CS: Ethical issues in compliance, Topics Clin Nurs 7(4):9-16, 1986.

Burgdorf MP: Legal rights of children: implications for nurses, Nurs Clin North Am 14(3):405-416, 1979.

Burke S: What the Washington professionals expect. Am J Nurs 79(10):1949, 1979.

Chaisson MG: Candidate's statement. Am Nurse 14(3):20, 1982.

Chesler P and Goodman EJ: Women, money and power, New York, 1976, William Morrow & Co., Inc.

Clarke AR: Editorial comment. Persp Psychiatr Care 20(2):64, 1982.

Connolly PM: Psychiatric and mental health nursing research, Pacesetter 7(3):3, 1982.

Council on Psychiatric and Mental Health Nursing: DSM-III-R Criteria, Pacesetter 14(1):1, 1987.

Creighton H: Law every nurse should know, Philadelphia, 1970, W. B. Saunders Co.

Curtin LL: Nursing ethics: theories and pragmatics, Nurs Forum 17(1):4-11, 1978a.

Curtin LL: A proposed model for critical ethical analysis, Nurs Forum 17(1):12-17, 1978b.

Daugherty LB: Assessing the attitudes of psychiatric aides toward patients' rights, Hosp Commun Psychiatr 29(4):225-229, 1978.

Donley R: An inside view of the Washington health scene, Am J Nurs 79(10):1946-1949, 1979.

Ennis BJ and Siegel L: The rights of mental patients: the basic ACLU guide to a mental patient's rights, New York, 1978, Richard W. Baron Publishing Co., Inc.

Epstein C: Effective interaction in contemporary nursing, Englewood Cliffs, NJ, 1974, Prentice-Hall, Inc.

Fagin CM: The research agenda, Am J Orthopsychiatr 56(3):340-346, 1986.

Feather RB: The institutionalized mental health patient's right to refuse psychotropic medication, Persp Psychiatr Care 23(2):45-68, 1985.

Fidell LS: Sex role stereotypes and the American physician, Psychol Women Q 4:313-330, 1980.

Francoeur RT: Biomedical ethics: a guide in decision making, New York, 1983, Wiley & Sons.

Galbraith JK: The anatomy of power, Boston, 1983, Houghton Mifflin Co.

Garfield SL: Psychotherapy: a 40 year appraisal. Am Psychol 36:174-183, 1981.

Gartrell N et al: Psychiatrist-patient sexual contact: results of a national survey, Am J Psychiatr 143(9):1126-1131, 1986.

Gartrell N et al: Reporting practices of psychiatrists who knew of sexual misconduct by colleagues, Am J Orthospsychiatr 57(2):287-295, 1987.

Gerrard BA, Boniface WJ, and Love BH: Interpersonal skills for health professionals, Reston, Va, 1980, Reston Publishing Co., Inc.

Gonzalez HH: The consumer movement: the implications for psychiatric care, Persp Psychiatr Care 14(4):186-190, 1976.

Grove W and Tudor J: Adult sex roles and mental illness, Am J Sociol 77:812-835, 1973.

Hare-Mustin RT: An appraisal of the relationship between women and psychotherapy, Am Psychol 38(5):593-601, 1983.

Health Task Force of the Urban Coalition: Rx. for Action. Washington, D.C., 1970, US Government Printing Office (The Urban Coalition).

Janeway E: Powers of the weak, New York, 1980, Alfred A. Knopf.

Jones SL: The psychotherapist nurse as clinical researcher, Arch Psychiatr Nurs 1(4):217-218, 1987.

Kaplan M: The issue of sex bias in DSM-III: comments on the articles by Spitzer, Williams, and Kass, Am Psychol 38:802-803, 1983.

Kohnke MF: Advocacy: risk and reality. St. Louis, 1982, The CV Mosby Co.

Kohlberg L: Stages and aging in moral development, Gerontologist 13(4):497-502, 1973.

Lande N and Slade A: Stages: understanding how you make your moral decisions, New York, 1979, Harper & Row.

Landsberg G and Hammer R: Involving community representatives in CMHC evaluation and research, Hosp Commun Psychiatr 29(4):245-247, 1978.

Lane vs. Candura. Massachusetts Apellate Court. 376 N.E. 2d 1232, 1978.

Leininger M: Political nursing: essential for health service and education systems of tomorrow, Nurs Admin Q 2(3):1-16, 1978.

Leininger M: Territoriality, power, and creative leadership in administrative nursing contexts, Nurs Dimensions: Power in Nurs 7(2)33-42, 1979.

Lengermann PM and Wallace RA: Gender in America: social control and social change, Englewood Cliffs, NJ, 1985, Prentice-Hall, Inc.

Lewin K: Frontiers in group dynamics. Human Relations 7:15-41, 1974.

Litman GK: Clinical aspects of sex-role stereotyping. In Chetwynd J and Hartnett O, editors: The sex role system: psychological and sociological perspectives, London, 1978, Routledge & Kegan Paul.

McBride AB: Developing a women's mental health agenda. Image 19(1):4-8, 1986.

McFarland DE, and Shiflett N: The role of power in the nursing profession. Nurs Dimensions: Power in Nurs 7(2):1-14, 1979.

Miller M: The nurse as change agent, Nurs Clin N Am 14(2):347-356, 1979.

Miller W, Dawson RO, and Parnas RI: The mental health process, New York, 1976, New York Foundation Press.

National Association for Mental Health: Citizens making a difference, Mental Health 58(4):16-17, 1974.

National Commission on Community Health Services: Health is a community affair, Cambridge, Mass, 1966, Harvard University Press.

Nations W: Nurse lawyer is patient advocate. Am J Nurs 73:1039-1041, 1973.

Noddings N: Caring: a feminine approach to ethics and moral education, Berkeley, 1984, University of California Press.

Nurse reimbursement plan approved for CHAMPUS, Am Nurse 14(2):19, 1982.

Offir CW: Civil rights and the mentally ill: revolution in Bedlam, Psychol Today 8(5):60-62, 1974.

Peck C: Current legislative issues. Psychiatry 38:303-317, 1975.

Peplau HE: Themes in nursing situations. Am J Nurs 53:1221-1223, 1953.

Perrow C: Organizational analysis: a sociological view, Belmont, Calif, 1970, Wadsworth, Inc.

Poythress, NG: Avoiding negligent release: a risk-management strategy, Hosp Commun Psychiatr 38(10):1051-1052, 1987.

President's Commission on Mental Health: Report to the President, Washington, DC, 1978, US Government Printing Office.

Psychiatric Nurses Association of Canada: Code of ethics, Can J Psychiatr Nurs 18(6):8, 1977.

Ramsey P: The patient as person. New Haven, Conn, 1970, Yale University Press.

Rennie vs. Klein. 462 F. Supp. 1131; 653 F. 2d 836; vacated, 102 S. Ct. 3506 (1982), 1981.

Rogers S: First national mental patients organization is formed. Tie Lines 3(3):5, 1986.

Rouslin S: Commentary on professional ethics. Persp Psychiatr Care 14(1):12-13, 1976.

Ruiz P and Behrens M: Community control in mental health: how far can it go? Psychiatr Q 47(3):317-324, 1973.

Sadoff R: Forensic psychiatry. Springfield, Ill, 1975, Charles C Thomas, Publisher.

Scheflen AE and Scheflen A: Body language and social order, Englewood Cliffs, NJ, 1972, Prentice-Hall, Inc.

Schell-King M and Finneran MR: The role of forensic psychiatry and the insanity defense, Persp Psychiatr Care 20(2):55-64, 1982.

Shapiro M: Legislating the control of behavior control; autonomy and coercive use of organic therapies, Southern California Law Rev 47:237-56, 1974.

Shindul JA and Snyder ME: Legal restraints on restraint, Am J Nurs 81(2):393-394, 1981.

Steadman HJ: Insanity defense: some questions answered, This Month in Mental Health (September):6, 1982.

Stein LS, Del Gaudio AC, and Ansley MY: A comparison of female and male neurotic depressives, J Clin Psychol 32:19-21, 1976.

Stephenson PS and Walker GA: The psychiatrist-woman patient relationship, Can J Psychiatr 24:5-16, 1979.

Stone AA: The right to treatment. Am J Psychiatr 132:1125-1134, 1975.

Stone AA: Informed consent: special problems for psychiatry. Hosp Commun Psychiatr 30(5):321-326, 1979.

Talan J: When mental patients say no. Newsday, Part III, Discovery, October 20, 1987, pp 1, 3.

Tancredi LR: Psychiatry and social control. In Romanucci-Ross L, Moerman DE, and Tancredi LR, editors: The anthropology of medicine: from culture to method, South Hadley, Mass, 1983, Bergin & Garvey Publishers, Inc.

Third-party reimbursement, Pacesetter 7(3):5-6, 1982.

Torrey EF: cited in Tending the spirit, Wall Street Journal, pp 1 and 17, March 26, 1973.

Towery OB and Windle C: Quality assurance for community mental health centers: impact of P.L. 94-63, Hosp Commun Psychiatr 29(5):316-319, 1978.

Ver Steeg DF: The political process; or, the power and the glory, Nurs Dimensions: Power in Nurs 7(2):50-63, 1979.

Warner R: Witchcraft and soul loss: implications for community psychiatry, Hosp Commun Psychiatr 28(9):686-690, 1977.

Warwick DP and Kelman HC: Ethical issues in social intervention. In Process and phenomena of social change, New York, 1973, Wiley.

Willeg SH: The nurses' guide to the law, New York, 1970, McGraw-Hill Book Co.

Zentner MJ: Organizational ideology: some functions and problems, Int Rev His Poli Sci 10(2):75-84, 1973.

ANNOTATED SUGGESTED READINGS

Kohnke MF: Advocacy: risk and reality, St Louis, 1982, CV Mosby Co.
The author deals with the many aspects of advocacy. Among these aspects are the functions of advocacy, the importance of open-mindedness, and the levels of advocacy (self-advocacy, client advocacy, community advocacy).

Noddings N: Caring: a feminine approach to ethics and moral education, Berkeley, 1984, University of California Press.

In taking a classical feminine approach to ethics, the author deals with the importance of receptivity, relatedness, and responsiveness. This approach is not to negate the role of logic or to imply that women are incapable of logical thinking. Instead, the author sets out to provide readers with an alternative approach based on caring and being cared for—an approach that is very applicable to nursing.

Schell-King M and Finneran MR: The role of forensic psychiatry and the insanity defense, Persp Psychiatr Care 20(2):54-64, 1982.

The authors examine the relationship between the criminal justice and mental health systems within a historical framework. Several approaches to the problems of forensic psychiatry are explored: the traditional, the reform, and the rethinking. Special attention is given to the issues defining mental illness, the expert witness, and the insanity defense.

FURTHER READINGS

Bandman EL: The nurse as advocate in everyday ethics, J N.Y.S.N.A. 18(1):19-28, 1987.

Chaska N, editor: The nursing profession: a time to speak, New York, 1983, McGraw-Hill Book Co.

DelBueno DJ: How well do you use power? Am J Nurs 87:1495-1498, 1987.

McBride AB: Mental health effects of women's multiple roles, Image 20(1):41-47, 1988.

Pincus HA, West J, and Goldman H: DRGs and clinical research in psychiatry, Arch Gen Psychiatr 42:627-633, 1985.

Simon RI: Clinical psychiatry and the law, Washington, DC, 1986, American Psychiatric Press, Inc.

Concepts basic to understanding behavior and to nursing intervention

In this unit concepts that are vital to the understanding and practice of mental health nursing are presented. The first chapter in this unit discusses the sociocultural aspects of mental health nursing in a theoretical, as well as practical, sense. The cultural diversity of our society is examined, and discussions are included on how the nurse's cultural background may influence interactions with clients.

Chapter 5 looks at sociocultural factors that influence the composition, form, and dynamics of the family. Viewing the family as a social system, this chapter explores interrelationships and interactions. The stages of human development are the focus of Chapter 6. The theoretical basis for nursing intervention for clients at all stages of the life cycle is provided. Chapter 7 discusses human sexuality (normal sexual response, sexual dysfunctions, and alternative sexual life styles) and its relationship to mental health, including implications for nursing practice. Chapters 8 and 9 present the concepts of stress, anxiety, and commonly encountered stressors. Discussions are centered on biological, psychological, and sociocultural factors and their relationship to stress and anxiety in mental health and mental illness.

Thoughts, emotions, needs, and ideas are communicated in various ways. Chapter 10 describes the process of communication and develops a theoretical basis for understanding communication in relation to culture and mental processes. The therapeutic use of communication skills and techniques is discussed in Chapter 11. Application of the nursing process to the establishment of a nurse-client relationship is the focal point of this chapter.

The sociocultural context of behavior

CHAPTER FOCUS

Society is one type of social system, and ethnic groups are subsystems within the total system. The population of the United States is composed of people from many different ethnic groups, each of which has its own culture. Through the process of enculturation, people learn the conceptual and behavioral systems of their culture. Enculturation is an essential mechanism for cultural continuity. When persons of differing ethnic backgrounds interact, some degree of another process, acculturation, usually occurs. Acculturation refers to the reciprocal retentions, losses, and adaptations that occur when members of two or more ethnic groups interact.

Because each culture codifies reality in its own way, members of different ethnic groups act upon different premises in behaving and evaluating behavior. When members of one ethnic group come into contact with the culturally coded orientations of another ethnic group, cognitive dissonance and culture shock may develop. Moving to a foreign country, moving to another neighborhood, or even entering a hospital may precipitate cognitive dissonance and culture shock, which engender stress and make people more vulnerable to mental illness.

Awareness of ethnic differences and their significance enables nurses to understand the cultural dimension of mental health and mental illness. In addition, a nurse's awareness of his or her own attitudes and the influence of ethnic heritage on them are essential to therapeutic nursing intervention. For nurses to engage in the therapeutic use of self, they must have a high degree of self-awareness and self-understanding. Attitude clarification helps them develop insight into many factors that influence their behavior.

SOCIETY AS A SOCIAL SYSTEM

Society is a social system—an organic whole that persists as long as total system needs are met. These needs generate institutions and patterns of interrelated activities that foster system stability and predictability. System stability is promoted by a dynamic equilibrium of reciprocally interlocking institutions and patterns. Other characteristics of a social system include complementarity, boundary maintenance, mutuality of role expectations, and pattern consistency of norms and values. Through the process of enculturation these values and norms are transmitted to society's members. Once values and norms become internalized, they serve as motivators for maintaining the social system.

Society comprises subsystems that mutually interact with each other and with systems external to the social system (e.g., ecological system, other social systems). Ethnic groups, as subsystems of society, not only have all the characteristics of a system but also engage in reciprocal boundary exchanges with the rest of the social system. In some instances boundary interchange is limited, and there is only minimal intergroup interaction and sharing of values and norms. In other instances, boundary exchange is greater, and, through the reciprocal processes of acculturation and assimilation, ethnic group members, over time and to different extents, fit into mainstream society. Conflict, however, manifested by interethnic strife, resistance to acculturation, etc., may be present in varying degrees. Social integration sometimes is maintained through conflict, while at other times conflict provides the mechanism for attainment of a new level of social integration (Smith, 1970; Teske and Nelson, 1974; Schermerhorn, 1978).

With this systems orientation in mind, we will now look at the United States as a multiethnic society.

THE UNITED STATES AS A MULTIETHNIC SOCIETY

The population of the United States is composed of many ethnic groups. An *ethnic group* is a collectivity of people organized around an assumption of common origin. The members of an ethnic group hold basically similar value and ideological systems and share systems of communication, social interaction, and world view. In addition, an ethnic group sees itself and is seen by others as a distinct category.

Novak (1973) describes several aspects of America's "New Ethnicity" movement: The movement acknowledges the United States as a multiethnic society, dispels the melting pot myth, and discourages cultural homogenization. Advantages of ethnic differences are emphasized, and ethnic consciousness raising is encouraged. Awareness of ethnic traditions and practice of ethnic customs are stressed. Involvement in the social and political needs of one's ethnic group is encouraged.

Kluchkhohn and Strodtbeck (1961) have identified basic aspects of any ethnic group's world view. Their classic theory of variation in cultural value orientations identifies complex patterns that grow out of the interaction of cognitive, affective, and directive domain and that provide order and direction to human behavior (both thoughts and actions). That these value orientations help to form certain aspects of any cultural group's world view has been supported and expanded by others (e.g., Spiegel, 1982). Central to any group's world view are the aspects of human nature, activity, time, interpersonal relationships, and person-nature (or environment) relationships. Table 4-1 outlines these aspects. These value orientations, however, are not mutually exclusive. While members of a cultural group may have a preference for one orientation, they may utilize alternative orientations as second- or third-order choices. For example, while mainstream Americans emphasize the future in their time orientation, they do spend part of their lives living in the present and acknowledging the past (e.g., reminiscing or feeling nostalgic).

The British-American middle class is often referred to as mainstream America or as dominant American society. Table 4-2 compares preferred

TABLE 4-1   Aspects of world view

Value orientation	Description
Human nature	Human nature may be viewed as basically good, evil, or a blank slate
Activity	Three activity alternatives: *doing* (tangible accomplishments, goal-directed behavior, competitiveness, and autonomy); *being* (spontaneous expression of inner feelings or self); *being-in-becoming* (process of developing different aspects of the self as an integrated whole)
Time	Having a past, present, or future orientation
Relational	Three alternative relationship patterns within the primary group: *individual* (individualistic, egalitarian, autonomous preference; emphasis on goals and well-being of the individual); *collateral* (define self in relation to one's laterally extended primary group; emphasis on goals and well-being of the laterally extended primary group; sense of responsibility to and for the primary group); *lineal* (hierarchical pattern of authority and status within the primary group; emphasis on the continuity of the primary group over time and the order of succession in the primary group)
Person-to-nature (or environment)	Three alternatives: *control-over-nature* (stresses importance of problem solving; assumes that most problems can be mastered by technology and money); *harmony-with-nature* (stresses importance of balance between people and nature; views imbalance as the source of problems); *subjugated-to-nature* stresses submissiveness to a god or natural forces and endurance of suffering; sense of fatalism and powerlessness over problems)

TABLE 4-2   Comparison of world views

	Mainstream American	Italian	Irish
Human nature	Neutral	Mixed	Evil
Activity	Doing	Being	Being
Time	Future	Present	Present
Relational	Individual	Collateral	Lineal
Person to nature or environment	Control over	Subject to	Subject to

	Native American	Chinese	Afro-American
Human nature	Good	Mixed	Mixed
Activity	Being-in-becoming	Being-in-becoming	Being-in-becoming
Time	Present	Past	Present
Relational	Collateral	Collateral	Collateral
Person to nature or environment	Harmony with	Harmony with	Harmony with

Sources consulted include M'biti (1969), Hsu (1970), McGoldrick (1982), Spiegel (1982), Attneave (1982), Hines and Boyd-Franklin (1982), Pinderhughes (1982), Lee (1982).

world view orientations of mainstream Americans with *traditional* world views of five ethnic groups.

It is important to realize that even when two cultural groups appear to share similar aspects of world view, there may be subtle differences. For example, although Table 4-2 indicates that traditional Italians and traditional Chinese tend to view human nature as mixed, the Italian "mixed" refers solely to a capacity for both good and evil, while the Chinese "mixed" refers to a capacity for good and evil that is predestined in accordance with deeds performed in one's own previous life or in the lives of one's ancestors.

Dominquez (1975) holds that many minority ethnic group members consider assimilation into mainstream American society either impossible or undesirable. The Glazer-Moynihan study (1970) found that many people prefer to live in ethnic enclaves. An *ethnic enclave* is a geographic area in a city, town, or village that is populated by a minority ethnic group.

It has been suggested that it is the interaction of cultural heritage with immigration and postimmigration experiences that produces American ethnic group culture (Greeley and McReady, 1975). Greeley (1974) stresses that in the study of ethnicity it is important to differentiate among the concepts of ethnic identification, ethnic heritage, and ethnic culture.

Ethnic identification refers to where people place themselves on the "ethnic chart." For example, do people identify themselves as Hispanic-Americans? Afro-Americans? Sino-Americans? Some studies have indicated that the higher the educational, occupational, and income levels of immigrants, the more rapidly they identify themselves as Americans and become integrated into mainstream America (Rogg, 1974; James, 1977).

Ethnic heritage refers to the cultural history of people, and it may be perpetuated by ethnic schools, ethnic churches, and ethnic folk festivals. For example, *El Día de la Raza* (The Day of the Race), an Hispanic folk festival, is a time when various Hispanic ethnic groups come together to celebrate and to share with each other their distinctive folk dances, music, and foods.

Ethnic culture refers to attitudinal, value, and

behavioral patterns associated with an ethnic group. For example, North Americans and Latin Americans perceive time differently. In the United States, time is perceived as something fixed that can be divided into discrete segments. Time is valued for the pursuit of achievement and success. Promptness and adherence to schedules are highly valued, and efficiency is associated with doing one thing at a time. However, in Latin American societies, time is perceived as a relative and flexible phenomenon. Latin Americans tend not to adhere strictly to schedules, and they frequently function in a context where several things are going on simultaneously. These different orientations toward time can sometimes present problems in health care settings. For example,

A mental health after-care clinic operated on an appointment basis. If clients were more than 15 minutes late for their appointments, they were not seen and had to reschedule their appointments. Clients who were habitually late for appointments were labeled "uncooperative," "unmotivated toward health," or "resistive to treatment."

Although the clinic's catchment area included a large Hispanic population, Hispanic clients were underrepresented on the clinic's roster. The nurse-anthropologist employed by the clinic was aware of the different conceptualizations of time held by North Americans and Latin Americans. She spoke with Hispanic clients who attended the clinic and with those who had been referred to the clinic but who did not attend. Both groups of clients cited the clinic staff's "rigidity" concerning promptness and appointment schedules as a reason why Hispanics did not attend the clinic.

The nurse-anthropologist discussed this situation with other staff members, and she explained to them the different orientations toward time held by Latin Americans and North Americans. The staff decided to develop a pilot program whereby on Monday, Wednesday, and Friday evenings clients could be seen without an appointment. The number of Hispanic clients attending the clinic increased measurably.

A fourth concept in the study of ethnicity is *ethnic interaction*. Ethnic interaction refers to the degree to which people's interpersonal relationships are based on ethnic affiliation. For example,

Pasquali (1982) found that first-generation Long Island Cubans who had immigrated as adults were more likely to base friendships and marriage on shared ethnicity and that they were less likely to be integrated into American social networks than were first-generation Cubans who had immigrated as youths.

Equally important to the definition of an ethnic group is the way people outside an ethnic group perceive the ethnic group (Isajiw, 1974). For example, Caucasian Americans may lump anyone who is oriental into the social interaction category "Chinese," regardless of the person's ethnicity.

If such an ascribed category of social interaction is accepted both by the individuals who are being categorized and by others, then the category becomes established. If either party rejects the category, then alternatives may be proposed and compromises arrived at. For example,

---

At a neighborhood health center, the Caucasian staff tended to view all black clients as having similar cultural backgrounds. However, the black clients rejected the category "black American," and they educated the staff about the cultural differences among black people from the southern United States, from the Caribbean, and from Africa.

Eventually, categories of social interaction become accepted by the media, the public, and by the minority group members themselves. When minority group members accept this "other definition" as Irish, Italian, or Chinese and stop thinking of themselves by their village or regional identities, immigrants have become ethnics (Horowitz, 1975).

Immigrants may accept the broad category of identity assigned by outsiders and identify themselves on a national rather than a regional or village level as a defense against the prejudice and hostility of society at large. Ethnic organizations may be formed and symbols may be created by immigrants who are unifying in national groups. Symbols may serve as representation of and stimulation for ethnic unity and ethnic consciousness (Sarna, 1978).

ENCULTURATION

Every ethnic group has its unique culture. *Enculturation* is the process of learning the conceptual and behavioral systems of one's culture. The goal of enculturation is to transform a person from a predominantly biogenic being (motivated by physiological states) into a predominantly sociogenic being (motivated by social values, sanctions, and constraints). To achieve this end, a culture must teach youngsters survival skills that provide for the biosocial continuity of society and standards and rules that govern behavior and the distribution of social and material assets (Hamburg, 1975). Through this process members of an ethnic group learn how their ethnic group is distinguished from all others.

Sense of self

It is probable that all people, regardless of their culture, are aware of their own mind-body integration, of their own internal body image, and of their spatial separateness from other people. Scheper-Hughes and Lock (1987), in their literature review, point out that the concept of body-self is believed to be universal and a precultural given. In some societies the body-self may consist of multiple selves, with each self related to a specific body area. This is the case with the Cuna Indians of Panama whose personality is determined by which part of the body dominates (e.g., domination by the head results in an intellectual person, while domination by the heart results in a romantic person).

Universal body-self awareness should not be confused with the Western social sense of "I" as an individual with legal rights and moral responsibilities. For example, in some societies the body-self consists of many selves that mirror one's interpersonal relationships. This is true for the Bororo, whose identity comprise multiple selves (e.g., the perception of one's self held by one's parents, by one's kinspeople, by one's enemies). In other societies, such as Japan, Java, and Bali, one's body-self and social self are fused and one's identity is established through structured social roles and one's obligations to and dependency on the family. This is very different from the concept of individuation from family that many Western mental health professionals hold as a "normal" stage in growth and development.

The relationship between body-self and social self is evident in the concept of basic group identity. Basic group identity, which evolves from membership in an ethnic group, results from shared social characteristics, such as world view, language, values, and beliefs. Isaacs (1975) points out that two concepts figure predominantly in the development of basic group identity: body and name.

The body is the most fundamental feature of basic group identity. Partly because exogamy (marriage outside the ethnic group) threatens the physical similarity of an ethnic group, many ethnic groups have taboos and constraints surrounding exogamy. Many ethnic groups have also created ways of physically distinguishing their members from all others (for example, through tattooing, scarification, or molding the shape of head, nose, or lips).

Some people try to "pass" from their own ethnic group to an ethnic group of perceived higher status. Whether passing is achieved through intermarriage or other means, the degree of social mobility possible is closely associated with the degree of physical similarity to the ethnic group of higher status.

The name, or names, associated with an ethnic group carries much meaning. Names that ethnic groups give to themselves and others tell much about inter-ethnic relations. Both names and meaning may change over time (for example, "colored," "negro," "black").

Individual surnames may serve as badges of ethnic group identity and current ethnic orientation. For example, "Americanizing" a surname may indicate a desire to be assimilated into mainstream United States society.

Agents of enculturation
FAMILY

The earliest and generally most effective enculturating agent is the family.* The family experience is essential to the development of basic group identity. Ethnically specific (unique to an ethnic group)

---

*See Chapter 5 for an in-depth discussion of the family.

norms, values, role relationships, communication patterns, and world views are taught within the family context.

There are many different family forms, some of which are associated with specific ethnic groups. Two major types of family organization may be distinguished: extended and nuclear. Table 4-3 compares some aspects of these two major forms of family organization.

Whether the ethnic family is extended or nuclear, it often gives its members conflicting messages: Succeed in mainstream America, but do not become part of it. Participate in society, but retain strong bonds with your ethnic group. At the same time, the ethnic family may try to protect children from discrimination by other ethnic groups. This protectiveness may deprive children of opportunities for full participation in mainstream American life and thereby prevent them from successfully competing in society (Gambino, 1974).

Ethnicity also influences the duration of life-cycle stages and the emphasis placed on life-cycle transitions. For example, among Mexican Americans, the stages of early and middle childhood are longer and adolescence is shorter than are the comparable mainstream American stages, while Mexican American middle age extends into what most mainstream Americans consider old age. Italians focus on marriage and the wedding as a most important life-cycle transition, the Irish emphasize death and the wake, Jews celebrate the transition to communal adult status with a *bar* or *bat mitzvah*, and Cubans mark a girl's social transition to womanhood with a *fiesta de quince años* (Falicov, 1980; Herz and Rosen, 1982; McGoldrick, 1982; Pasquali, 1982).

NEIGHBORHOOD

The concept of ethnicity centers around group identity. An ethnic group residing in an enclave feels a strong sense of belonging and community. Gans's (1962) classic study of "urban villages" and Fried's (1974) more recent study show that members of ethnic enclaves have a strong sense of "neighborhood." Neighborhood constitutes a protective social milieu. It encompasses shops with familiar wares, social clubs, a church, often a school, and a supportive social network composed of reliable neighbors.

TABLE 4-3 Comparison of family functioning

Family form	Function	Description
Extended (encompasses three or more generations of kinsmen)	Provides family members with security and dignity	Aged members have a place to live; aged members hold positions of authority and respect; adult family members share in child rearing and serve as role models; potentially large labor force; many opportunities for division of labor; *disadvantages:* young family members may live out much of their lives under the supervision of elders; security may be gained at the expense of personal growth and individualism
Nuclear (parent(s) and their children)	Facilitates the individual growth of young family members	Family members are encouraged to develop as individuals; children are encouraged to assume responsibilities appropriate to their ages; children are allowed input into age-appropriate decision making; *disadvantages:* non family relationships and occupational demands may compete with and weaken family ties and relations with other relatives; during periods of crisis, sources of support may be inadequate; personal growth may be gained at the expense of security

Sources consulted include Scheflen and Scheflen (1972) and McGoldrick (1982).

Neighborhood groups, such as peer groups and ethnic associations, contribute to enculturation by helping their members cope with conflicts and tensions that may be engendered when the values and customs of the ethnic group clash with those of mainstream America. Table 4-4 outlines the functions and characteristics of these two types of neighborhood groups.

It is important to note that, while ethnic neighborhoods help to strengthen traditional cultural values, norms and behaviors, they also may impede the assimilation and acculturation of immigrants into mainstream American society (Gelfand and Fandetti, 1986).

The ethnic association is another type of neighborhood group that contributes to enculturation. Ethnic associations form as a response to immigration to America. In America, the immigrant family often cannot provide for all areas of family well-being without some outside assistance. Historically, local, state, and federal governments were not forthcoming with such assistance, so ethnic fraternal and community self-help groups formed and offered members burial services, illness insurance, unemployment insurance, etc.

In a multiethnic society like the United States, ethnic associations help reinforce ethnic identity and ethnic consciousness. Symbols may be created that serve as representations of and stimulation for ethnic unity. Ethnic associations also provide social and cultural activities for people who speak the same native language and eat the same ethnic foods. The multiplicity of services provided by ethnic associations enhances neighborhood life. In addition, these associations often become focal points of ethnic and neighborhood power and leadership and the foundations for ethnic political machines. Associations such as La Orden Cabellero de la Luz (for Cubans), the Sons of Italy, and the India Association establish new bonds of fellowship to replace those severed by migration and develop the rudiments of an ethnopolitical consciousness.

RELIGION

Religion plays an important role in the lives of many Americans. Religion serves as an institutional mechanism for explaining, justifying, and supporting particular values, and it addresses such core human concerns as the meanings of life, suffering,

TABLE 4-4 Neighborhood groups

Group	Function	Characteristics
Peer group	Provides support and a sense of belonging; structures relationships in the neighborhood and with outside communities; helps members cope with acculturative tensions	Members are bound together by age and/or gender in addition to ethnicity; same peer group may be influential throughout a person's life; within the peer group, there is usually consensus about norms and role relationships and peer pressure to conform to them
Ethnic association	Helps reinforce ethnic identity, ethnic unity, and ethnic consciousness; provides social and cultural activities; may serve as focal points of ethnic and neighborhood power and leadership; may serve as basis for ethnopolitical machines and ethnopolitical consciousness; develops bonds to replace those severed by migration; provides mutual aid	Forms as a response to immigration; symbols may be created to represent and stimulate ethnic unity; social and cultural center for people who speak the same native language and eat the same ethnic foods; historically offered members burial services, illness insurance, and unemployment insurance; multiplicity of services provided enhances neighborhood life; by serving as a reference group, it keeps ethnic culture alive with ethnic Americans; examples of ethnic associations are La Orden Cabellero de la Luz (for Cubans), Sons of Italy, and the India Association

Sources consulted include Krickus (1976), Sarna (1978), Pasquali (1982).

and death. Positively correlated with conventional religions is an ideological system that supports prevailing social institutions and that may reflect such traditional values as opposition to divorce, birth control, abortion on demand, and premarital sex (Larson, 1978).

Not all religious movements, however, espouse and reinforce the values and institutions of society. During periods of societal unrest and revolution, religious groups often arise that vigorously oppose the prevailing social order and serve as a "counterculture." Such sects are usually under the leadership of a charismatic person or "prophet." These countercultural religious movements may oppose the existing social order in one of the following ways: (1) repudiate the present by attempting either to revitalize the past or to build a utopian future, (2) repudiate moderation by emphasizing asceticism or lack of moral restraint, or (3) repudiate cooperation and negotiation by interfacing with established society passively or violently. Examples of contemporary countercultural religious movements are Sun Myung Moon's Unification Church,

Hare Krishna movement, Meher Baba movement, and Maharaj Ji's Divine Light Mission (Yinger, 1982).

According to Burnett (1979), religion is such an essential part of many people's lives that understanding a person's religion is an interal part of understanding the person. O. F. Larson (1978) suggests that rural populations tend to be more religiously oriented than urban populations, to view themselves as "fairly" or "very" religious, to read the Bible frequently, and to believe that religion holds the answer to all or most of their problems. Because fewer religious sects may exist in rural areas than in urban areas, the values and attitudes of rural communities may be based on the religious orientations of community residents (Oates, 1977). In such instances, religious attitudes may affect a community's way of life, influencing ideas about such seemingly nonreligious issues as governmental reform and desegregation (Swanson, Swanson, and Cohen, 1979).

Bergin (1980) observes that the effects of religion tend to be diverse. For example, in rural areas where evangelical or fundamentalist beliefs tend to be strong, fundamentalist Christians tend to view men as dominant over women. Conflict may be engendered as the media focuses on women's rights, as economics necessitates women's working outside the home, and as new opportunities arise for women that give them alternatives to farm life and offer them some degree of financial independence (Kuczynski, 1981). J. A. Larson (1978, 261) believes that in situations that engender family conflict, the families that seek professional help are usually those which are religiously divided. Families characterized by shared religious outlook tend to be able to work out their difficulties within the family. For those religious families which seek professional help, Larson contends that the best therapeutic approach is one that works within the family's "religious value and belief system and that efforts to alter values and beliefs are counterproductive."

There is also a historical association between ethnic groups and religious denominations. In addition to inculcating and reinforcing ethnic values, norms, and behavior, religious groups may act as political reference groups, militating for changes that will advance an ethnic group's aims. For example, Afro-American churches have been influential in the social and political lives of American blacks from the antebellum period to contemporary times. Such was the case when black religious sects in the southern United States spearheaded the civil rights movement for desegregation and justice for Afro-Americans. Religious groups often try to advance ethnic goals by appealing to an abstract and idealistic moral order (Staples, 1976; Holt, 1980).

SCHOOL

When children reach school age, teachers join the ranks of significant others who are instrumental in enculturation. A teacher may be the first significant other with whom a child relates outside the family and the neighborhood. Especially to young children, teachers may represent the end product of the process of enculturation. Neighborhood schools in ethnic enclaves are sometimes staffed with teachers of similar ethnicity or with teachers who are knowledgeable about and supportive of the ethnic group's culture. However, when children of one ethnic group attend school with children of other ethnic minorities or with children from mainstream America, there may be little articulation between values taught at home and those taught at school (Dickerman, 1973).

Ethnic children may quickly realize that there are two value systems: one that reflects the values of their ethnic group and one that reflects the values of mainstream America. For example, Hsu (1970) points out that American values of equality before the law, of relying on lawyers to settle disputes on the basis of absolute concepts of legal right and wrong, and of personal growth and individual responsibility for becoming successful contrast sharply with Chinese values of deference to age, of a middleman or peacemaker settling disputes on the basis of situational or relative concepts of right and wrong, and of responsibility to one's extended family even at the expense of personal growth and individuation. Hsu also notes that while some Chinese-Americans may become anglicized, those who prefer to live in an enclave still hold much of the Chinese value system.

Ethnic children are usually not helped to view the two value systems as complementary. The school may try to socialize ethnic children into the culture of mainstream America by undermining and discouraging any manifestation of ethnicity (Krickus, 1976). Behavior and customs taught and practiced at home may be derogated or forbidden in school.

Maria was a first-generation Italian-American. When she began kindergarten she was very outgoing and talkative. Her speech was accompanied by gesturing. The teacher was British-American and used little gesturing. The teacher frequently admonished Maria to "calm down" and "not to talk with your hands." Occasionally while Maria was talking the teacher would gently hold Maria's hands.

At the middle of the school year the teacher noticed that Maria had become very quiet. She spoke only when spoken to and then made only brief responses. The teacher consulted the school nurse.

The school nurse spent some time in the classroom observing Maria's behavior. The nurse, who was also Italian, noticed that Maria appeared very tense when speaking and that she used very little gesturing. The nurse shared this observation with the teacher. The teacher then disclosed that she had tried to help Maria learn to speak without gesturing. The nurse explained that this was an ethnic communication pattern and suggested that interference with it might be related to Maria's noncommunicative behavior. The nurse also referred the teacher to studies on ethnicity and communication.

The teacher decided she had been wrong to try to control Maria's gesturing and explained this to Maria. Maria gradually became more comfortable in the teacher's presence and more communicative. *

Thus criticism of ethnic children by teachers may be aimed at the core of the children's identity. Ethnic customs and values may be derogated or discouraged in the schoolroom, and ethnic literature, art, music, and heroes may be absent. This atmosphere may undermine ethnic identity and make it difficult for ethnic minority students to relate to the aims of formal education. Covello (1972) maintains that such students often find the experience of schooling an experience of cultural criticism.

In school, ethnic children become acquainted with ideas and behavior that are new and different and that may be held up as superior. The culture of mainstream America is attractive because it is the dominant, "superior" culture. The world of ethnic culture is attractive because it is familiar and secure. Thus conflict often occurs. Children may try to resolve this conflict through accommodation, which usually requires the maintenance of a dichotomy between public and private behavior. In public, ethnic children may reject ethnic behavior and try to use the behavior of mainstream America. In the private world of home and enclave, they may use ethnic behavior. For example, when they are at school, Chinese-American children may speak English and eat the "American" food that is served in the school cafeteria. When they are at home, the children may speak Chinese and eat such Chinese foods as rice, bean curd, snow peas, and water chestnuts. The degree of rejection of ethnic behavior depends largely on the ethnic composition of the school population (both students and teachers)

*See Chapter 10 for a discussion of ethnicity and communication.

and the ethnic homogeneity of the community. When a large percentage of the school population is composed of members of the child's ethnic group and when the child comes from an ethnically homogeneous neighborhood, the probability of culture conflict is smaller than it is when school and neighborhood populations are ethnically heterogeneous (Covello, 1972; Gambino, 1974; Krickus, 1976).

POVERTY

Poverty may be defined as the lack of the necessary resources to participate in a life-style that society commonly deems acceptable. Table 4-5 outlines some characteristics associated with poverty. The anthropologist Oscar Lewis (1966) was the first to clearly identify and describe what he referred to as the "culture of poverty." Lewis stressed that poverty involves more than being poor or experiencing the negative consequences of being poor. He delineated a descriptive model of poverty—a subculture of Western society composed of structure, rationale, and ways of dealing with life—a life-style perpetuated "from generation to generation along family lines."

Such a model fails to look at the context in which poverty occurs. Because of the interrelationship between scarcity and abundance, poverty is interrelated with affluence. The United States experienced tremendous economic growth after World War II. Although most sectors of the economy expanded, housing and automobiles led the growth pattern. In the 1960s, 8 million youths attended college, and suburbs, primarily zoned for single-family houses, sprang up. Numerically, suburbanites started to outnumber urbanites. During this period of economic growth, however, there were still too few jobs for all who wanted to work, and unemployment and underemployment did exist. High schools that served middle-class areas usually provided programs that enabled students to attend college. Students were prepared for jobs that required skills essential to white collar and professional careers, and most were able to find employment in growth industries. In lower-class areas, high school programs tended to prepare students for unskilled or semiskilled jobs, jobs that would either become obsolete or would pay a salary inadequate to the rising cost of living. In addition, rac-

TABLE 4-5 Characteristics of poverty

Characteristic	Description
Deprivation	Lack of money, loss of human dignity, inability to engage in such activities as eating in a restaurant or taking a vacation, lack of ready access to and choice of legal and medical services, scarcity of employment and educational opportunities, lack of political power
Helplessness	Sense of powerlessness, low self-esteem, hopelessness about ability to alter one's own socioeconomic conditions
Present orientation	Desire for immediate gain, short-term goals, education often not a priority
Loss of self-determination	Dependency on agencies to meet one's socioeconomic and health needs, bureaucratic structure of agencies may strip one of decision-making responsibility; hostility, apathy, low self-esteem, hopelessness and failure to achieve may be associated with the loss of self-determination

Sources consulted include Shrewbridge (1972) and Meltzer (1986).

ism contributed to the poverty of many black Americans who were not prepared to avail themselves of skilled job opportunities. A gap between the affluent and the poor developed, and it has steadily grown. Poor neighborhoods tend to be characterized by high-density population and scarce resources. Goods and services that are available in impoverished neighborhoods are often high in price and poor in quality (Ashcraft and Scheflen, 1976; Meltzer, 1986).

Allocation of social service resources is often inadequate. For example, money may not be allocated for carfare and suitable clothing, definitely handicapping people who have the potential to work, be self-supportive, and break out of the cycle of poverty. Because they may have to wait several weeks before financial assistance begins, the work-

ing poor may be thrown into crisis when the breadwinner loses his or her job. Living from paycheck to paycheck leaves no financial cushion to fall back on and little if any money for job hunting (e.g., carfare for job interviews, money to purchase newspapers for employment possibilities) (Shewbridge, 1972).

Avenues out of poverty may also be blocked. For example, people who attend vocational training or university extension courses may find that their support payments have stopped. Financially impoverished children may have difficulty achieving academically. Teachers and social workers often blame this lack of achievement on poor parental motivation and involvement. Little attention may be paid to the roles of overcrowding, lack of privacy, frequent distractions, poor nutrition, inadequate clothing, and such recurring crises as nonreceipt of welfare checks, utility shut-offs because of nonpayment of bills, and frequent moving with associated change of school. In addition, there may be little or no money allocated for school supplies (Shewbridge, 1972).

The elderly in our society who are also poor have other problems. Many aged people—because they have outlived their friends, are geographically or emotionally distant from relatives, and/or have physical disabilities or emotional problems— become socially isolated. If the aged person is also poor, then life may be very bleak. Residency may be in a single-room-occupancy dwelling. This building is often a walk-up with inadequate heat in the winter and excessive heat and inadequate ventilation in the summer. Organizations that provide socializing opportunities for the elderly often try to avoid accepting the aged poor. Many of the aged poor "are trapped in a wall of loneliness and isolation" (Shewbridge, 1972, 92).

For people who are without family or friends, release from a psychiatric hospital or a prison often is a prelude to vagrancy or homelessness. All the homeless are not mentally ill or ex-convicts, however. Homelessness is an absolute form of poverty. Either because they cannot be accommodated at a public shelter or because they are fearful of being assaulted in one, they often live in skid rows or in train or bus terminals and beg for money to subsist on (Shewbridge, 1972; Meltzer, 1986). Bahr (1973) observes that the primary problems of these people are not their homelessness, advanced age, or physical or emotional problems. It is the stigma that society attaches to them. They are stereotyped as derelicts, drunks, and degenerates, and their struggle to maintain adequate self-esteem to support life is ongoing. (See Chapter 16 for further discussion of homelessness.)

Cross-cutting social class, race, ethnicity, and age is gender, and women tend to be poorer than the men in these categories. Scott (1984) notes that since poverty is concerned with access to economic and political resources and power, women, because they have the least access to these assets, are the most likely to be poor. "Woman's work" has traditionally taken place outside the economic sphere and therefore is economically devalued.

The "feminization of poverty" refers to a multiplicity of factors that keep women in a more economically vulnerable position than men while at the same time increasing their economic responsibilities. Although woman-headed households account for only 15% of all households in the United States, approximately 50% of poverty-level households are woman-headed. These woman-headed households often come about through the desertion, death, or divorce of husbands. Many divorced women are not receiving child support or alimony. In addition, many of these women never held a job, having devoted themselves to their role as wife-mother. They often have no skills and end up as "displaced homemakers" who are responsible for the sole support of their children. Lack of day-care services and job-training programs militate against these women becoming self-supportive (Oakley, 1981; Sawhill, 1980; Scott, 1984).

Since many women have traditionally found employment in labor-intensive light industries and in office work, the automation of industry and the computerization of clerical jobs has adversely affected job opportunities for women. Scott (1984) notes that women are less likely than men to make the transition to data processing, programming, and systems analysis jobs because (1) fewer women than men have these high-level technical skills, (2) men have staked these jobs out as their territory and they do not want to share this niche with women, (3) women are less apt than men to have access to job retraining programs, and (4) women

tend not to participate in all levels of union organization, and this renders them powerless to fight discrimination.

Historically the poor have been stereotyped and stigmatized, along with the mentally ill and the disabled, as moral inferiors and disaffiliated from society. Poor families tend to be uninvolved in community or social organizations and church groups. This pattern of borderline affiliation to societal organizations is perpetuated from generation to generation. The social networks of the poor tend to shrink. This is often a consequence of deteriorating transportation systems and communication systems in impoverished neighborhoods coupled with attempts by surrounding neighborhoods to close their borders to the residents of these impoverished neighborhoods. Poor people may risk physical harm by crossing into neighborhoods that have closed their borders, just as others may fear entering deteriorated, impoverished areas. As a result, not only is social intercourse between the poor and the nonpoor curtailed, but the passage of goods and services into impoverished neighborhoods is also curtailed (Ashcraft and Scheflen, 1976; Bahr, 1973; Meltzer, 1986).

Ethnicity is inculcated through the process of enculturation. For many people, enculturation occurs within a context of poverty. For most people, family, neighborhood, church, and school serve as agents of enculturation. Kin, peers, clergymen, and teachers are profoundly influential in the transmission of norms, values, role relationships, communication patterns, and world view.

Sociocultural context and mental health behaviors

Mental health behaviors are greatly influenced by sociocultural factors.* For example, Westermeyer, Vang, and Neider (1983), in a study of Hmong refugees, found that change of residence is associated with increased psychiatric symptoms. Those Hmong who had not moved evidenced the

---

*Refer to Chapter 16 for further discussion of sociocultural factors and mental health–mental illness and to Chapters 5 and 14 for discussion of family influences on mental health–mental illness.

least psychopathology. Those Hmong who had moved but were in close proximity to other Hmong evidenced an intermediate rate of psychopathology. Those Hmong who had moved and were not in close proximity to other Hmong evidenced the highest rate of psychopathology. Gelfand and Fandetti (1986) note that when people of the same ethnic background live in an ethnic community, traditional life-style, including ways of problem solving, may be reinforced and that family networks, rather than professional practitioners, may be sought to assist with crises.

Although religion can be a source of psychosocial conflict, for religiously-oriented people religion also offers many sources of assistance. While it does not seem to be as effective as relaxation training in reducing tension, prayer has been found to significantly lower tension (Anchor, Elkias, and Sandler, 1979). In addition, religious congregations serve as sources of group support, providing a sense of acceptance and personal value, offering hope, and counteracting loneliness and isolation. Religion may also help people cope with acculturative pressures. This is especially true of religious groups that organize around a specific ethnic group (Gelfand and Fandetti, 1986).

Poor people and poorly educated people (especially women) are vulnerable to depression. Seligman (1975) views poverty and school failure in terms of learned helplessness. Both poverty and poor education contribute to a sense of having little control over one's life, decrease one's opportunities to learn effective coping behaviors, and increase one's vulnerability to depression. Since childhood poverty and poor education are often associated with low-status, poor-paying jobs or unemployment as an adult, the cycle of depression continues. Seligman concludes that not only are poor people predisposed to depression by their past experiences but also that their present experiences expose them to more depression-precipitating factors.

The Report of Consensus Conferences on Access to Prenatal Care and Low Birthweight (1987) identified stressors that can be generalized to most impoverished people. Stressors include

1. Inadequacies of food, shelter, and employment

2. Living with chronic or recurring crises
3. Concerns about being unmarried, alone, or unsupported
4. Employment conditions
5. Everyday life changes such as moving, family illness, or change of employment

The Report of Consensus Conferences also identified values that interfere with poor people obtaining adequate health care. Primary among these is the attitude that health care is earned by one's ability to be self-supporting. A ramification of this attitude is that people are poor because they do not work hard enough. Concomitantly, there is a stigmatizing of poor people, especially poor women, and an erection of obstacles to obtaining health care. Ruffin (1979) summarizes the conclusions of several sociological studies related to poverty and health as follows: (1) the effects of poverty contribute to a higher incidence of and more serious types of morbidity and (2) poverty hinders health maintenance (e.g., preventive health care) and health restitution (e.g., early casefinding and treatment).

Bullough and Bullough (1972) conclude that ethnic minority status added to poverty status hampers attaining high-level wellness and complicates acquiring health care. In a study of Mexican-American migrant farmworkers, O'Brien (1982) found that pragmatic survivalism influences perception and experience of illness, health-seeking behaviors, and treatment response. Table 4-6 outlines the interrelationship between pragmatic survivalism and health.

Clara Montoya, a Mexican living in the United States, worked as a factory pieceworker. If she did not work, she did not get paid. Because she was an illegal alien, she was not a member of a union and had no health benefits.

Clara began complaining of headaches, loss of appetite, listlessness, and fatigue. She did not seek medical care until she felt so ill that she was unable to get out of bed each morning and go to work. At this point she sought the assistance of a curandero *(a folk healer) and, at the insistence of her daughter, also went to see a medical doctor. The* curandero *determined that Clara was suffering from* susto *(a condition of soul loss which is precipitated by severe, sudden fright) and performed a* limpia *ceremony to reclaim her soul. The physician diagnosed Clara as depressed, prescribed an antidepressant medication, and referred her to the local mental health clinic. The physician was unaware of the cultural stigma many Mexicans attach to mental illness and mental health facilities. Neither was the physician aware that Clara was simultaneously being treated by a* curandero.

Clara took the antidepressant medication until she began feeling better. She paid little attention to the food and beverage restrictions that the physician had told her must be followed while taking the antidepressant medication. She did not go to the mental health clinic. Whenever she began feeling a recurrence of her earlier symptoms, she would take a few of the antidepressants and visit the curandero.

The implications of pragmatic survivalism for psychiatric nursing are evident in the preceding vignette. Chronic psychosocial disorders that have periods of remission or disorders whose symptoms are controlled by medication may be ignored by disadvantaged clients unless the nurse is able to educate clients about their psychosocial disorders and the importance of continuing follow-up care. Disadvantaged clients who seek help from the mental health care system may simultaneously be utilizing a folk health care system, and communication between the practitioners of the two systems is advisable. It is also important to determine client perception of the disorder and treatment and any stigma that may be attached to the disorder. Disadvantaged clients who have chronic psychosocial disorders need much support to follow through with plans for long-term care, and the support and help of family members should be enlisted.

ACCULTURATION

During the process of enculturation members of an ethnic group learn the conceptual and behavioral systems of their culture. However, in a culturally plural society like the United States, members of different ethnic groups come into contact and interact with one another. The reciprocal retentions, losses, or adaptations of cultural patterns that result when members of two or more ethnic groups interact constitute the process referred to as acculturation. Acculturation is sometimes also referred to as

TABLE 4-6 Pragmatic survivalism and health

Characteristic	Influence on health
Role-constrained perception of illness	The more a condition interferes with role performance, the more likely it is that a person will view it as an illness
Parochial-restricted health behavior	Disadvantaged minorities tend to use indigenous health care systems more often than they use the professional-scientific system
Reality-accommodated treatment response	The less a course of treatment interferes with role performance, the more disadvantaged minorities will comply with the treatment plan

behavioral assimilation (Spindler, 1977; Luhman and Gilman, 1980).

The degree of rigidity of ethnic group boundaries and the quality of inter-ethnic relationships influence the response of ethnic group members to acculturative pressures.

Ethnic boundaries

Every ethnic group has a unique culture. Ethnic groups function as systems and have the properties of systems. The properties of interacting ethnic groups influence the process of acculturation of ethnic group members.

Ethnic groups are bounded. Boundaries maintain the distinctiveness of an ethnic group. *Boundary maintenance mechanisms* are practices and types of behavior that exclude outsiders from the customs and values of a particular ethnic group. Such mechanisms protect the group from foreign influence and create a "we-they" orientation. Some examples of boundary maintenance mechanisms are ritual initiations, secret societies, fear of outsiders, social controls (such as gossip and rumor), racism, and ethnocentrism (Greeley, 1974; Spindler, 1977).

The degree to which an ethnic group uses boundary maintenance mechanisms largely determines how closed (resistant) or open (susceptible) the group is to acculturation pressures.

A community health nurse had recently been transferred from one district to another. The nurse had observed that the former district had been composed of third- and fourth-generation Americans of many ethnic backgrounds. Neighbors shared recipes for the preparation of ethnic foods. Teachers discussed the ethnic traditions of many countries. It was common for children and adults to have close friends with ethnic backgrounds different from theirs. Ethnicity did not seem to play a role in the selection of a physician.

The community health nurse's new district was different in many respects from the old one. The new district was composed largely of members of a single ethnic group. The residents were primarily immigrants or second-generation Americans. Local grocery stores sold traditional ethnic goods. While teachers in the school came from various ethnic backgrounds, the students were ethnically homogeneous. It was rare for children or adults to have friends from a different ethnic group. Ethnicity played a large role in the selection of a physician. People felt more comfortable with a physician who spoke their language and shared their customs. Residents were reserved in the presence of "outsiders" and seemed to mistrust them. The community health nurse was of an ethnic background different from that of the people in the district and initially had difficulty establishing rapport. Only after many months of attending local activities and events, shopping at local stores, talking with local merchants and residents, and otherwise demonstrating interest in and respect for their culture was the nurse accepted by the people in the district.

The residents of the first district described here exhibit open ethnic boundaries; there is much inter-ethnic exchange. The people in the second district exhibit closed ethnic boundaries. There is a very strong "we-they" orientation. Ethnocentrism and suspicion of outsiders operate to maintain ethnic boundaries, and acculturation is resisted.

Interethnic relationships

Triandis (1977) defines stereotyping as the assigning of a "set of characteristics" by one group of people to themselves (autostereotyping) or to others (heterostereotyping). The function of both types of stereotyping is to simplify, by categorizing traits, complicated information. Stereotyping arises from an attributional process. The attribution of qualities or traits is based on behavioral differences that are observed during interactions and the stereotyping that ensues serves to explain those differences. According to Jaspars and Hewstone (1982, 153), "Ethnic stereotypes or, in general, evaluative judgements of in-and-out group members, should be seen as the outcome of an attribution process and not simply as distorted perceptions."

In-group–out-group relationships among ethnic groups influence the process of acculturation. Unique socio-politico-economic relationships may exist among the members of an ethnic group and differentiate that group from all other ethnic groups. Relationships within a group are characterized by camaraderie, order, rules, and industry. Relationships between groups are characterized by hostility and conflict. Each ethnic group tends to view its own folkways as superior and right and those of other groups as inferior and wrong. Each ethnic group uses its culture as a standard for judging all other cultures (ethnocentrism).

A student nurse had been assigned to a pediatric unit to gain clinical experience. One client that the student cared for was a 4-year-old child who was recovering from meningitis. When the child was discharged from the hospital, the student decided to make a follow-up home visit. During the visit, the student observed the child eating a lunch of beans, rice, hearts of palm, and plantain. The student concluded that this meatless lunch was not very nutritious and that the family's eating habits were poor.

The family had recently emigrated from the Caribbean, where beans, rice, heart of palm, and plantain are traditional foods. The student nurse was unfamiliar with these foods and therefore viewed them as inferior. The student's judgment was influenced by ethnocentrism, a common in-group theme that contributes to in-group–out-group polarization (Kelley, 1972, 1973; Tajfel 1974, 1978).

Under certain acculturative conditions, an out-group may become a source of positive rather than negative reference. People may wish to belong to, feel loyalty toward, or emulate the behavior of an out-group and to reject the behavior of their own group. Emulation of out-group behavior tends to be in the direction of the technologically superior culture (Horowitz, 1975; Spindler, 1977). Horowitz (1975) suggests that the more dominant and prestigious an ethnic group is, the more successful it will be in recruiting and in making itself appealing as a reference group.

When members of different ethnic groups interact, role relationships are established that usually reflect interethnic status, power, values, and needs. These relationships provide culturally patterned ways for people of differing ethnic groups to interact (Barnett et al., 1954; McGoldrick, 1982).

The Hsu family followed a very strong Chinese tradition when in their ethnic enclave. The family members spoke Chinese, wore traditional Chinese dress, ate Chinese foods, consulted a herbalist, and followed a Chinese value system. However, whenever they attended a family-practice clinic, they wore Western-style clothes, spoke English, and accepted prescriptions for Western medicines.

Interethnic role relationships thus may produce private and public spheres of interaction, each with its appropriate behavior. By enclosing ethnic differences in a sphere of intraethnic articulation (private sphere), members of an ethnic group may maintain ethnic identity and still engage in a sphere of interethnic articulation (public sphere).

The maintenance of dichotomous spheres of behavior is not the only option open to members of minority ethnic groups who wish to participate in mainstream America. Instead, they may try to "pass" and become assimilated into dominant mainstream society, or they may exaggerate their ethnic characteristics and use them to achieve status and desired socioeconomic rewards. Social scientists have been unable to determine the variables that influence the selection of an option or to speculate on the degree of success that any one option will

provide minority group members who attempt to participate in mainstream society.

Indices of acculturation

Barnett et al. (1954) and Gordon (1964) have conducted some of the classic research on acculturation. The process of acculturation has two stages. In the first stage, cultural acculturation, members of a minority ethnic group accept and use the dominant ethnic group's language, customs, dress, and foods. Members of the minority group may be reluctant to alter their value system. Isolated ideas and values are altered more readily than those that are integral parts of the minority group's culture. In the second stage, structural acculturation, members of the minority ethnic group are incorporated into the dominant ethnic group's social networks (for example, play and peer groups, country clubs, and neighborhoods). This stage of acculturation necessitates acceptance by members of the dominant ethnic group and occurs more slowly than cultural acculturation.

In trying to measure degree of acculturation, anthropologists have considered the type and extent of interethnic contact and the degree to which such contact results in identification with another ethnic group. Chance (1965) and Shannon (1968) were among the first to develop criteria for determining degree of interethnic contact:

1. Knowledge and use of the other culture's language
2. Residential mobility
3. Occupational mobility
4. Access to mass media
5. National Guard or military service

Chance and Shannon have also developed the following indices for measuring identification with the culture of another ethnic group:

1. Preference for activities of another culture over those of one's own culture
2. Preference for foods of another culture when foods from both cultures are equally available
3. Preference for the clothing, hair styles, and cosmetic styles of another culture over one's own culture

4. Use of another culture's language
5. Acceptance of another culture's world view

Cultural assessment guide

Indices of acculturation can be used to develop a tool for assessing cultural orientation. Fong (1985) strongly recommends that nurses assess their own cultural orientations and note similarities and differences with the cultural orientations of clients. Since people's cultural orientations and ethnic identities have strong influences on their values and behavior, nurses need to incorporate cultural assessment into overall assessment strategies. Information from the following areas should be included in such an assessment*:

1. Demographics. Client's name. Proper pronunciation of client's name. Client's age. If client is an immigrant, length of time in the United States and age at time of immigration. Place of current residence (for example, interethnic neighborhood or ethnic enclave).
2. Family organization. Type of family. Generations represented. Members composing the family unit. Members vested with family authority. Members involved in child rearing. Sense of obligation to family members. Members residing in the same household or in different households. Interaction of family with society. Family values.
3. Sex-defined roles. Stereotyped male and female roles. Amount of independence permitted men and women. Degree of intimacy permitted between married men and women and degree of intimacy permitted between unmarried men and women.
4. Communication patterns. Languages spoken at home and outside home. Use of eye contact, touching, and gesturing. Interpersonal spacing. Use of humor. Use of proverbs.
5. Type of dress. Traditional ethnic dress or Western-style dress?

6. Type of food. Ethnic food or "American" food? Types of food preparation (for example, broiled, fried, baked; seasonings used). Food taboos. Use of food for health maintenance and/or treatment.
7. View of human nature. Good, evil, mixed, or neutral?
8. Activity mode. Doing, being, or being-in-becoming?
9. Relationship to people. Individual, collateral or lineal? Egalitarian or authoritative?
10. Relationship to time. Past-, present-, or future-oriented?
11. Relationship to nature. Control-over-nature, harmony-with-nature, or subjugated-to-nature?
12. Health care patterns. Definition of health and illness. Ideas concerning causes of illness (for example, germs, evil spirits, punishment for sins). Ideas concerning treatment of illness. Coping behaviors. Acculturative pressures. Minority status stressors. People consulted when ill (for example, family member, native healing specialist, physician, pharmacist) and order in which they are consulted.
13. Religious practices. Beliefs and rituals concerning birth, illness, suffering, and death. Nature of belief in a supernatural being or supernormal energy. Conceptualizations about the quality of life and the quality of death. Conceptualizations about good, evil, and forgiveness.

CULTURE, COGNITION, AND CULTURE SHOCK
Codification of reality and behavior

Over a span of many years, people acquire and store information in their nervous systems. *Cognition* is the processing of information by the nervous system. This processing structures reality and gives meaning to human experience. Cognitive activity includes the focusing of attention, comprehension, problem solving, and information storage and retrieval (memory) (Estes, 1975; Fiske and Taylor, 1984).

One of the most important aspects of cognition is

---

*Sources consulted in the preparation of this cultural assessment tool include Kluckhohn and Strodtbeck (1961), Spradley and Phillip (1972), and Mosley and Clift (1977).

coding, the process of categorizing information. Information is sorted and then stored by means of various types of memory codes: iconic codes (visual images), echoic codes (auditory images), motor codes (motor skills), and symbolic codes (representative images) (Hunt and Lansman, 1975). Although culture influences all types of cognitive coding, symbolic codes are especially influenced by culture. For example, communication systems, one type of symbolic coding, vary from culture to culture. Even a sound such as hissing may communicate either approval (in Japan) or disapproval (in the United States).

All cultures provide a cultural code for perceiving, interpreting, and synthesizing reality. This culturally structured codification of reality is referred to as world view. *Culture* may be defined as an ordered system of shared and socially transmitted symbols and meanings that structures world view and guides behavior (Geertz, 1957), or it may be defined as a "system of social institutions, ideologies, and values—that are systematically transmitted to succeeding generations" (Hamburg, 1975, 387). Members of an ethnic group, by virtue of their shared cultural background, usually have a common world view and similar values, ideologies, and standards of behavior. Although these thought and behavior patterns are similar among members of an ethnic group, they are not identical. Members of a group usually operate within the boundaries of established custom, but there may be a wide range of individual variation.

Because each culture codifies reality in its own way, members of dominant mainstream America may act upon premises for behaving and evaluating behavior that are different from those of members of minority ethnic groups. In the process of interethnic contact and acculturation, change may occur in the culturally structured cognitive order of individual members of an ethnic group. Any such change involves learning new values, beliefs, and attitudes.

Individual members of an ethnic group, mindful of alternatives, make choices—usually between a traditional practice, value, or idea and a new one. Ogionwo (1975) analyzed how networks of information and influence are involved in the decision to adopt a new idea. He found that personal communication is more effective than mass media and that when mass media are used, broadcast media (radio and television) are more effective than print media (magazines and newspapers). Ogionwo also found that the flow of information is not simply from the source to the individual. Group interaction is also important. Family, friends, and social norms may all exert pressure on a person either to adopt or to resist a new idea.

A community mental health nurse identified a need for child care education for new parents. Counseling on a one-to-one basis proved unsuccessful. The nurse evaluated the program and realized that it had not considered the ethnic background of the clients.

The people in the community were immigrants and second-generation Hispanic Americans. In traditional Hispanic culture, child care is the sole responsibility of women. In addition, the extended family is central to Hispanic family life.

The nurse considered these cultural factors when revising the child care education program. The revised program was designed for the new mother and the female relatives in her extended family. This approach to child care education proved effective.

This vignette illustrates how important it is for nurses to recognize that informational flow is not simply from the nurse to the individual client. Group interaction is also important. The composition of the group and the influence of the group on the individual vary from culture to culture.

Cultural change and cognitive dissonance

When, through interethnic contact and acculturation, change occurs in people's culturally structured cognitive orders, *cognitive dissonance* may develop. Cognitive dissonance refers to a state of inconsistent cognitions that generates discomfit (an aversive state of arousal). There is then a drive to lessen the discomfit, and this drive often precipitates cognitive change. People may try to avoid cognitive dissonance through

1. Selective exposure: seeking new information

that will be consistent with current cognitions

2. Selective attention: focusing on consistent information and denying the existence of discrepant information
3. Selective interpretation: comprehending ambiguous information as consistent (Wallace, 1970; Kleinhesselink and Edwards, 1975; Abelson, 1983).

Fiske and Taylor's (1984) evaluation of research about selective perception shows that, while data supporting selective exposure are ambiguous, findings supporting selective attention and selective interpretation are indisputable. They conclude that from the outset people's tendency toward selective attention and selective interpretation leads them to information that strengthens their original beliefs.

Cognitive dissonance and culture shock

Culture shock, which results from a drastic change in the cultural environment, is both precipitated by and a response to cognitive dissonance. Culture shock is engendered by unfamiliar cues of social interaction. When ethnic groups use dissimilar cues during interaction with each other, conflicts in communication and role relationships may result. Brink and Saunders (1976) have identified the following factors in social interaction as the ones that most frequently create cognitive dissonance and engender culture shock:

1. Different systems of communication
2. Unfamiliar physical environment
3. Isolation from family and friends
4. Foreign customs
5. Different or new role relationships

Any alteration in people's verbal or nonverbal systems of *communication* creates a barrier in the giving and receiving of behavioral cues. Even if people are familiar with the language of another ethnic group, they may have difficulty with nuances of meaning, styles of humor, and colloquialisms.

Alterations in the *physical environment* may also prove difficult. If people have recently immigrated to a country, utilities formerly taken for granted, such as electricity and telephone, may operate dif-

ferently or be absent. House styles, clothes, shopping facilities, and food may also seem strange. It takes time and energy to learn to manipulate the mechanical environment. Fatigue and frustration may develop.

In addition, patterns of customary behavior and *role relationships* may be disrupted. People may have to become accustomed to new and different sex-linked roles, rules of etiquette, and status and kinship systems. Value and belief systems may also be challenged. Since people's ideological systems are usually implicit rather than explicit, they may not be aware of their own values and beliefs until they are questioned. They may realize only then that their standards and ideologies are different from those of their neighbors. These changes in life-style may create cognitive dissonance and result in culture shock.

Cognitive dissonance acts as a stressor and requires adaptive responses. The greater the number of changes required by the new cultural environment, the more difficult the cultural readjustment. Cultural readjustment is part of the process of acculturation. Having to unlearn old cognitive patterns may often prove more stressful than learning new cognitive patterns.

Oberg (1954) was one of the first to observe and describe the phases of adaptation to culture shock: excitement, disenchantment, and resolution. During the excitement phase, people begin to learn about their new country or neighborhood. They become acquainted with new customs, taste unfamiliar foods, sightsee, and begin to establish new work and social roles. As people begin to "settle in," they enter the disenchantment phase. Changes in life-style that earlier had seemed exciting now seem frustrating. Ethnocentrism surfaces as people tend to view the customs, values, and communications systems of other ethnic groups as inferior and infuriating. Feelings of inadequacy, loneliness, anger, and nostalgia predominate. If people remain in a new country or neighborhood and begin to learn the behavioral and communication systems of other ethnic groups, resolution of culture shock is under way. During this phase, new friendships are formed and feelings of inadequacy, isolation, and loneliness dissipate. With the termination of this phase, culture shock is successfully resolved.

Responses to culture shock are not always adaptive, however. Spradley and Phillip (1972) have found that when people's usual coping responses prove ineffective and opportunity to learn new coping responses is unavailable, people may respond to culture shock with psychosis, depression, suicide, or homicide.

The following operational definition of culture shock describes the dynamic interrelationship between enculturation, cognitive dissonance, and culture shock:

1. People, through interaction with significant others, learn the skills necessary for participating in a particular ethnic group in a particular society.

2. When these people, through choice or force, interact with members of another ethnic group, the skills that were effective in their own culture may prove ineffective in varying degrees.

3. The people perceive the situation as stressful. Old role relationships, values, expectations, and types of behavior are either less effective or not effective. Culturally coded meanings for objects and events are not shared by members of the other ethnic group with whom they have to interact.

4. This drastic change in the cultural environment produces cognitive dissonance, which acts as a stressor and requires accommodation or readjustment of life-style and behavior. This situation is known as *culture shock.*

5. The people develop stress responses to the culture shock. During the process of cultural readjustment involved in resolving culture shock, they either (a) accommodate themselves to the other ethnic group by learning new behavioral, communication, and ideological systems and thus become acculturated or (b) are unable to learn the skills required for cultural readjustment and become aggressive, depressed, or withdrawn. Mental illness may develop in the latter situation.

Culture shock and mental illness

Social scientists have found a relationship between culture shock and mental illness. Frost (1938) was among the first to study the incidence of mental illness in American immigrants. He found that the first 18 months in a new country is the period when they are most vulnerable. Dayton (1940) found that, for all age groups, the admission rate to psychiatric hospitals in the United States is significantly higher for foreign-born persons than for persons born in this country. A later study by Tyhurst (1955) corroborated the findings of Frost and Dayton by describing some of the maladaptive effects of migration. During the first 2 months in the host country, an immigrant usually experiences a general sense of well-being, with an associated increase in psychomotor activity. This hyperactivity serves to relieve tension. As the immigrant settles into the new country and encounters social difficulties engendered by unfamiliar language, customs, and values, culture conflict and emotional strain develop and gradually heighten. Flights into nostalgia often help an immigrant cope with the realities of culture shock. Approximately 6 months after having arrived in the new country, the immigrant may begin to evidence high anxiety, suspiciousness, depression, psychosomatic disorders, or any combination of these characteristics.

The incidence of psychiatric disorders in immigrants seems to be higher among women than among men. Chesler (1972) observed that during periods of rapid sociocultural change, disjunctions often occur more acutely and more pervasively in the roles of women than in the roles of men. Such disjunctions contribute to greater role conflict among women than among men. For example, Pasquali (1982) found that among Cubans living on Long Island, the post-immigration role adjustment for women was tremendous. In Cuba, their role primarily had been one of supervisor of household help. After immigration, almost all of these women had to take jobs outside the home. In addition, their domestic role changed from supervising servants to doing housework and child care. These Cuban women suddenly had to juggle work roles with domestic roles, and this often contributed to overburdening, role conflict, and role stress. Similar observations of role conflict and role stress have been made for Cuban women in other parts of the United States (Szapocznik and Kurtiness, 1980). Pasquali (1982) cautions that although Cuban men have not admitted to psychoneurotic or affective symptoms, it should not be concluded that they are not experiencing role conflict. It may be that the concept of *machismo* keeps Cuban men from admitting to feelings of stress and depression. Generally, when men cope maladaptively with stress, they develop what Chesler (1972) terms "male diseases." Such socially deviant behavior* as alcoholism, gambling, and aggressive acts have been termed male diseases by Chesler because they constitute an exaggerated stereotype of the male role.

Several hypotheses might explain the high rate of mental illness among immigrants. These are the selection hypothesis (that individuals who have a history of mental illness may view emigration as a way to deal with their problems), the stress hypothesis (that immigration, with its culture shock and socioeconomic deprivation, generates stress levels high enough to precipitate mental illness in vulnerable people), and the prejudice hypothesis (that the higher admission rates of immigrants into psychiatric facilities reflects moral and political prejudice as well as misinterpretation as psychopathology certain cultural beliefs and culturally acceptable behaviors) (Cox, 1977; Littlewood and Lipsedge, 1982; Helman, 1984).

The rate of mental illness among immigrants varies by ethnic group. For instance, in Britain factors such as dissatisfaction with food and climate, sexual deprivation, language difficulties, discrimination, legal and economic problems, and fear of grant termination in the event of academic failure account for some of the hardships predisposing West African students to mental illness. Also, political refugees who are forced to emigrate to Britain and who cannot return to their homelands have a high rate of mental illness. In contrast, Chinese, Italians, and Asian Indians who decide to emigrate to Britain for economic gain, who are "entrepreneurial," make little attempt to assimilate and intend to return to their homelands have the lowest rate of mental illness of all ethnic groups (Littlewood and Lipsedge, 1982). Among Hmong refugees in the United States, Westermyer and others (1983) found that

*Refer to Chapters 20 and 21 for a discussion of socially deviant behavior.

TABLE 4-7   Relationship between immigration and mental illness

Factor	Description
Reason for immigrating	Includes forced immigration (as with political refugees who cannot return to their homelands) and immigration by choice (as with people who immigrate for economic gain and who are able to visit their homelands or who intend return to their homelands)
Hardships endured in the host country	Includes dissatisfaction with climate and other conditions generating cognitive dissonance and culture shock
Social conditions in the host country	Includes institutionalized racism, discrimination, and politicoeconomic conditions
Culturogenic stressors	Includes rigid sex role stereotyping, social isolation of women, and religious and/or cultural taboos and prescriptions of one's own culture

Sources consulted include Cox (1977), Littlewood and Lipsedge (1982), Helman (1984).

while remaining in one residence and maintaining contact with a sponsor are associated with a low rate of mental illness, employment is associated with depression, obsessive-compulsive behavior, and high anxiety. The researchers suggest that the realization of their low-status jobs and limited opportunities for socioeconomic upward mobility precipitate emotional distress and advise that the refugees receive "social and emotional support" to assist them in adjusting to the social realities of their lives in the United States. Although the explanation is complex, Table 4-7 outlines some factors that seem to contribute to differential rates of mental illness among ethnic groups.

The stress of culture shock is not limited to immigrants. Second- and even third-generation Americans may experience stress engendered by conflict between ethnic ideology and the ideology of mainstream America. Ethnic identity is formed early in life through interaction with family, peers, and significant others. Therefore, social networks are often composed of members of similar ethnic heritage. However, as Dickerman (1973) points out, to succeed in the United States and become assimilated into mainstream American society, members of minority ethnic groups must often deny much of their ethnic heritage. Ethnically oriented customs, behaviors, beliefs, and values must often be unlearned and replaced by those of mainstream America. Such denial of ethnicity often requires people to disavow affiliation with family and other significant members of their ethnic groups. Dickerman maintains that disavowal of ethnic identity is demanded of all Americans who wish to participate in mainstream society but have not been born into it.

Culture shock and hospitalization

The transition from person to patient* may be marked by culture shock. Goffman's (1961) classic study of total institutions describes this transition. In a total institution, such as a hospital, a significant number of persons are isolated from society, and their lives are organized according to the rules and regulations of a bureaucracy. People in total institutions fall into one of two categories: a large group of supervised inmates or a small group of supervisory staff. Social intercourse and mobility between the two groups are severely limited and usually formally prescribed. Through the bureaucratic management of blocks of people, total institutions try to provide for at least minimal gratification of human needs. A consequence of this enclosed, bureaucratically administered life is the molding of people's personalities and behavior. To change people into inmates (or patients), a total institution must use certain techniques, based on the principles of role loss and humiliation, that are built into its structure. These maneuvers are part of a "stripping process" that breaks down people's self-concepts and

life-styles so that they will more readily fit into the institutional mold.

The stripping process may be facilitated in a number of ways. Such procedures as issuing hospital gowns, history taking, and confiscating personal belongings all succeed in undermining patients' self-images. Most people view wearing an open-in-the-back gown, even for a short time, as humiliating. Many people feel dehumanized when aides, technicians, nurses, and doctors do not know their names and have to check name tags to be certain they are talking with the right person. Being known by one's name is very important to one's self-image.

In addition, dependency is fostered by such common practices as being confined in bed, being served meals only at specified times, and having to ask for permission or assistance to get out of bed.

The abrupt transition from a familiar social system to an unfamiliar one is fundamental to the culture shock of hospitalization.* The following factors that are inherent in hospitalization may create cognitive dissonance and engender culture shock.

COMMUNICATION

A new language, "hospitalese," must be learned. People are asked if they have "voided." It is explained to patients that they will receive IMs, IVs, or ECT. Even previously familiar expressions may suddenly have different meanings. For example, instead of being an expletive, "S.O.B." stands for "short of breath." In addition, in psychiatric units nurses may or may not wear uniforms, and they may be addressed by their first or their last names. Such informal practices as nurses wearing street clothes and being called by their first names may facilitate nurse-patient communication. However, such informality may confuse some patients about the nurse's role and impede nurse-patient communication.

MECHANICAL ENVIRONMENT

People must become familiar with new mechanical devices and forms of transportation. In a general hospital, patients often must learn to use bedpans and call buttons and must allow themselves,

---

*The term *patient* is used here instead of *client* to denote a passive, acted-upon role.

*Brink and Saunders (1976) have also discussed this transition.

even when ambulatory, to be transported to various parts of the hospital in wheelchairs or on stretchers. Although patients in a psychiatric hospital usually encounter fewer mechanical devices, they may encounter physical restraints. They may also have to become accustomed to various types of surveillance systems, such as grating on windows, locked units, and suicide or escape precautions.

CUSTOMS

To fit into hospital routine, all patients must learn a new life-style. General hospital patients are expected to wear pajamas day and night. Patients in psychiatric hospitals often are not permitted to have access to such sharp objects as razors and mirrors. When to awaken, when to go to sleep, when to visit with family and friends, and when and what to eat are no longer matters of personal choice. While staff members may intrude into patient's domains—their rooms—patients are usually not permitted to enter the staff's domain—the nurse's station.

ISOLATION

Another characteristic of hospitals is the isolation of patients from their families and communities. Visiting hours are often brief (several hours twice a day) and may be scheduled at times when many people are at work. Children often are not allowed in hospital units. In some hospitals, patients do not have private telephones and may only have access to a telephone in the hall. Such a situation not only makes it difficult to place and receive calls but also violates a person's privacy. One's nearest human contact often is a hospital roommate. Roommates may or may not be compatible, and they may be from different social classes or ethnic groups. Thus a patient who views the mixing of socioeconomic and ethnic backgrounds as an invasion of privacy may be even further isolated from social interaction. Newspapers, television, or radio may become the major contacts with the outside world.

ROLE RELATIONSHIPS

Patients have to learn a new role, and it is a socially undesirable one. Our society values assertiveness and independence, but the role of patient is often characterized by dependence and subordination. Doctors, nurses, and aides often assume authority roles. Orders are passed from physicians and nurses to aides and finally to the patient. While staff members may both give and receive orders, the patient often can do only the latter. In addition, during the time that a person is assuming the role of patient, other role relationships—those of parent, spouse, employee, or student—may be temporarily interrupted. Occasionally, role reversals occur. For example, a self-supporting independent father may suddenly have to be cared for by his children.

• • •

An altered communication system, an unfamiliar mechanical environment, different customs, a sense of isolation, and new role relationships are inherent in the experience of hospitalization. These dramatic changes in life-style may create cognitive dissonance and result in culture shock.

During the first days of hospitalization, patients usually ask many questions and inquire into hospital routines. This period corresponds to Oberg's first phase of adaptation to culture shock. In phase two, the disenchantment phase, patients become frustrated with hospitalization and respond with depression, anger, or withdrawal. When they learn the communication system and routines of the hospital, become friendly with staff and other patients, and demonstrate a sense of humor, they are beginning to resolve the culture shock of hospitalization. However, if patients stay in the hospital long enough to resolve culture shock completely, problems may develop. Unless they are in a long-term facility or a nursing home, such an adjustment is counterproductive. They feel "at home"; they can function comfortably and easily within the framework of the hospital. They thus have become dependent and institutionalized. They are fearful of discharge and unwilling to face the resumption of life outside the hospital.

Culture, cognition, and the practice of nursing
NURSES AND CLIENTS AS MEMBERS OF ETHNIC GROUPS

Each person is born into a culture, and his or her enculturation includes assuming the cognitive system of that culture. It is important to remember that culture is persistent. Through the process of immigration, cultural patterns are transplanted from the country of origin to the new country, and then from the immigrant generation to succeeding generations. Even when a person from one ethnic group has extensive contact with people from other ethnic backgrounds, many of the thought and behavior patterns acquired during childhood persist.

Therefore, in the United States, both nurses and clients are usually influenced not only by the American cultural system but also by the cultural systems of their respective ethnic groups, of which British-Americans, Italian-Americans, German-Americans, Afro-Americans, and Sino-Americans are only a few. As a result of interethnic marriage, some people have a mixture of ethnic heritages.

Ethnic heritage can be very influential.

James and Tony were nursing students. Although both young men had been born in the United States, their grandparents had been born in Europe. James was British-American, and Tony was Italian-American.

During a seminar discussion entitled "The Crying Client," James and Tony evidenced very different reactions. While both young men felt uncomfortable when people cried, James believed it was "unnatural and unmanly" for a man to cry. Tony did not see anything wrong with men crying.

James and Tony were influenced by different ethnic backgrounds. Each young man's ethnically specific values, beliefs, and standards of behavior were reflected in his attitude about crying. James' British heritage sanctioned stoicism as a reaction to stress. Tony's Italian heritage sanctioned crying both for men and women as a response to stress.

There are several reasons why nurses need to be sensitive to cultural diversity and aware of the influences of culture on health care. First, nurses often tend to be ethnocentric about their own health-oriented values, norms, and behaviors. It is not uncommon for nurses to feel that their own culturally influenced beliefs and practices are superior to those of clients who are influenced by other cultural orientations. Awareness of culturally diverse beliefs and practices that have effectively helped people from other cultures maintain health and cope with illness may keep nurses from imposing their cultural beliefs and practices on clients and may assist nurses to be less ethnocentric. Second, when nurses learn about other cultures it helps them to develop more insight into their own cultural orientations. The Society for Intercultural Education, Training, and Research (SIETAR) states that as a people increase their understanding about their own values, identity, and needs, there is an increased ability to let go of old behaviors surrounding core identity and to learn new behaviors. Learning about the life-styles of different cultural groups helps nurses to be more culturally sensitive. Cultural sensitivity enables nurses to recognize and respect the culturally specific health beliefs and practices of clients, to incorporate many of those practices into nursing care, and to act as client advocates for ethnic clients who are being deprived of quality health care. Third, awareness of cultural diversity among clients and incorporation of culturally specific care into treatment plans promotes client satisfaction with health care and lessens the possibility of noncompliance (Fong, 1985).

ATTITUDES AND ATTITUDE CLARIFICATION

An *attitude* is a verbal or nonverbal stance that reflects innermost convictions about what is good or bad, right or wrong, desirable or undesirable. People's attitudes, which are largely unconscious, are based on value systems that are influenced by their enculturation and on life experiences that are interpreted in terms of that enculturation. Nurses who regard their values, standards, beliefs, and perceptions of reality as absolutes may experience cognitive dissonance when they are confronted with other cultural systems.

After vacationing in the Caribbean, Jeanette decided to move there. Up to that time, she had lived in the northeastern United States. Initially, she was very happy with the move. She rented a house, did a good deal of sight-seeing, and went to the beach every day.

After a few months of becoming acquainted with her new environment, Jeanette began working as a nurse in a local hospital. The hospital was not air condi-

tioned, and Jeanette found the heat oppressive. She could not understand how people could be expected to recuperate under such adverse conditions, and she became impatient with the staff, who thought that the heat was not an adversity. Jeanette also began to realize that her conception of time was different from that of the native population. While the natives viewed time as something flexible and relative and they did not strictly adhere to schedules, Jeanette highly valued adherence to schedules and punctuality. She became increasingly annoyed about "people's inability to be on time," and she began to view the native population as "irresponsible" and "unmotivated."

In addition, Jeanette was unable to reconcile folk healing practices with her belief in the efficacy of modern medicine. She felt that folk medicine was "ridiculous and dangerous."

Jeanette's interaction with a foreign culture resulted in cognitive dissonance and culture shock. The differences in value judgments between her and the native population served as stressors.

Opposing value judgments may also lead to value conflict. In the example of Jeanette, the following incompatible value judgments could constitute value conflict:

1. Jeanette's value judgments
   a. Absence of air conditioning during hot weather is an *unacceptable* situation for the recuperation of clients.
   b. Punctuality is *important*.
   c. Folk medicine is *bad*.
   d. Blending of modern medicine with folk medicine is *undesirable*.
2. Natives' value judgments
   a. Absence of air conditioning during hot weather is an *acceptable* situation for the recuperation of clients.
   b. Punctuality is *unimportant*.
   c. Folk medicine is *good*.
   d. Blending of modern medicine with folk medicine is *desirable*.

The differences between Jeanette's value judgments and those of the native population are what Meux (1980) terms the direct source of value conflict. Factors such as prejudice, concrete thinking, and stress, which may affect the perceptions and understanding of people about the degree of value

judgment incompatibility operating in a particular situation, Meux considers direct sources of value conflict. People's value judgments are reflected in their attitudes about what is right or wrong, desirable or undesirable, important or unimportant.

The practice of nursing involves three levels of exploration: the factual, the comprehensive, and the attitudinal. For example, on the factual level a nurse may learn the definitions of defense mechanisms. On the comprehension level, he or she may consider the function of defense mechanisms and may differentiate between the adaptive and maladaptive use of defense mechanisms. On the attitudinal level, a nurse may explore questions such as the following: What do I consider healthy use of defense mechanisms? What do I consider unhealthy use of defense mechanisms? What defense mechanisms do I use? When do I use them? How often do I use them?

It is important that nurses become aware of their own attitudes. They need to understand how ethnic heritage influences attitudes—especially their attitudes about mental health and mental illness. Attitude clarification is one way that nurses may become more aware of their own attitudes. Because attitudes are often unconscious, a nurse may need to work with a colleague or supervisor who can provide objective information about behavior that reflects attitudes and who will assist in the clarification process. Attitude clarification can help nurses develop insight into some of the factors influencing their behavior.

The process of attitude clarification involves exploring alternatives and setting personal priorities. Using the work of Smith (1977) and Uustal (1977), we can identify the following six steps in this process:

1. An attitude should be the nurse's own attitude and not one that the nurse thinks is expected. For example, a nurse may believe that a person has a right to self-determination, even when suicide is a possibility. It is this attitude that needs to be acknowledged and explored, not an attitude that the nurse may believe is more acceptable to colleagues.
2. Alternative attitudes should be identified. If we again use the example of the permissibility of suicide, the following attitudes may be con-

sidered: nurses have a moral and/or professional obligation to prevent suicide; a person contemplating suicide is irrational and cannot be allowed to make such an important decision; suicide is sinful.

3. The consequences and significance of an attitude should be explored. What are the legal ramifications of ignoring a communication that indicates the possibility of suicide? What are the personal ramifications? What are the professional ramifications?

4. Personal priorities should be established. For example, does the nurse believe that being self-sufficient makes life worth living and that it is better to be dead than to be disabled, despondent, or dependent? Does the nurse believe that a person has a right to decide when to die?

5. An attitude should be affirmed. An attitude may be communicated to relatives, friends, or colleagues. For example, a nurse might say, "Mr. Jones is terminally ill. He is despondent. If I learned that he was saving pills to use to commit suicide, I would not try to stop him."

6. An attitude should be incorporated into a person's behavioral system. This is the point at which an attitude is acted upon. When the nurse who believes that a person has a right to decide when to die intentionally ignores clues to suicide, (mindful of the ethical and legal consequences of that professional decision) the nurse's attitude has been incorporated into his or her behavioral system.

Attitude clarification is an essential component of the practice of mental health nursing. In order for nurses to engage in the therapeutic use of self, they must have a high degree of self-awareness and self-understanding.* Attitude clarification helps nurses develop insight into many factors that influence their behavior.

Very often nurses and their clients have different and somewhat conflicting attitudes. When these attitudes are radically different, frustration and misunderstandings may result. How often has a

---

*See Chapter 11 for further discussion of the importance of self-awareness for therapeutic communication.

nurse tried to refer a client for psychotherapy, only to have the client hold tenaciously to the belief that "shrink therapy" is useless? How often has a nurse been taken aback at the stigma that is still attached to mental illness? The community health nurse who tries to help discharged psychiatric clients make places for themselves in the community is only too well aware of the prejudice that family, friends, neighbors, and employers still have about mental illness. How often has a nurse shaken his or her head in bewilderment over the number of people who spend a small fortune on over-the-counter drugs while condemning drug abuse?

Attitudes among health professionals frequently differ also. How often has a nurse shivered over incidents involving the too readily prescribed tranquilizer? How often has a nurse been astounded to hear colleagues refer disparagingly to persons with psychosomatic or psychoneurotic symptoms as malingerers and complainers? How often has a nurse encountered sexual bias?

Attitudes are deeply ingrained and are influenced by systems of cultural cognition and codification. Attitudes reflect beliefs, values, and standards of behavior. Attitudes are operative in all aspects of life. Thus it is unrealistic to think that nurses can be attitude free and totally objective. Through attitude clarification, however, they can become increasingly aware of their own behavior and less judgmental about others' behavior. Attitude clarification is essential to therapeutic nursing practice.

CHAPTER SUMMARY

The people of the United States come from various ethnic backgrounds. Each ethnic group has its own cultural system. Through the process of enculturation, people learn the conceptual and behavioral systems of their culture. When people from different ethnic backgrounds interact, some degree of acculturation usually occurs.

Because each culture codifies reality in its own way, members of different ethnic groups act upon different premises in behaving and evaluating behavior. Dissimilar culturally coded orientation often engender cognitive dissonance and culture shock. Moving to a foreign country, moving to another neighborhood, or even entering a hospital may precipitate cognitive dissonance and culture shock. Persons experiencing cognitive dissonance and culture shock are vulnerable to mental illness.

Awareness of ethnic differences and their significance enables nurses to understand the cultural dimension of mental health and mental illness. In addition, a nurse's awareness of his or her own attitudes and the influence of ethnic heritage on those attitudes is essential to therapeutic nursing intervention.

SELF-DIRECTED LEARNING

Sensitivity-Awareness Exercises

The purposes of the following exercises are to:
- Develop awareness that your way of structuring reality is not the only way
- Develop insight into some of your own behaviors and customs
- Develop awareness of the behaviors and customs of others
- Develop sensitivity to differences in behaviors and customs that contribute to culture shock in immigrants and culture conflict in ethnic Americans
- Develop awareness of the impact of culture on the nurse-client relationship

1. Visit an ethnic grocery store and acquaint yourself with its wares.
   a. Plan one well-balanced meal using ethnic foods. To do this, you will have to talk with the shopkeeper or with customers about the nature of the foods and their methods of preparation.
   b. Identify how you felt entering and shopping in the store. What were your reactions to the sights, sounds, and smells of the store? In what ways was the grocery store similar or different from the one in which you or your family shop? What were your feelings when conversing with the shopkeeper and/or customers? What were their reactions to you?
2. Visit an ethnic grocery store and purchase at least one ethnic food with which you are unfamiliar.
   a. Find out from the shopkeeper or from customers how to prepare the food.
   b. Prepare the food. How does it smell, look, and feel during its preparation?
   c. Prepare to eat the food. How does it smell, look, and feel? How do you anticipate it will taste?
   d. Eat the food. How does it taste? How does its taste compare with what you had anticipated?
   e. What were your feelings during this exercise?
3. With a friend or classmate, role play that, while visiting a foreign country, you become ill and go to a hospital. You are not familiar with the language or customs of the country. Try to make your symptoms and discomfit known to the "nurse" (your friend or classmate) without using verbal language. Remember, your life may depend on your ability to make yourself understood. At the end of 15 minutes, discuss with your friend or classmate
   a. Your feelings during the exercise
   b. The behavior you demonstrated
   c. The behavior and reactions of the "nurse"
   d. The feelings of the "nurse" during the exercise

Now reverse roles and reenact the exercise.
4. Using Kluckholn's and Strodtbeck's value orientations toward human nature, activity, time, relationships, and person to nature/environment as a guide
   a. Identify the world view that you hold
   b. Identify the world view that a friend or classmate with an ethnic heritage that is different from yours holds
   c. Compare the similarities and difference in world view held by you and your friend or classmate

Continued.

SELF-DIRECTED LEARNING—cont'd

Questions to Consider

1. A community health nurse worked in a neighborhood where the majority of the residents had incomes at or below the poverty level. In working with these residents, the nurse should recognize that poor people are at risk for stress because they may encounter all *but* which of the following stressors
   a. A sense of powerlessness over their lives
   b. Impoverished social networks
   c. Inadequate food, shelter, and employment
   d. Overinvolvement in community or church groups
2. A psychiatric nurse noticed that many of the clients on the psychiatric unit were immigrants. A hypothesis that may explain the high rate of mental illness among immigrants is the
   a. Inattention hypothesis
   b. Selective exposure hypothesis
   c. Prejudice hypothesis
   d. Dissatisfaction hypothesis
3. Culture shock for clients who are admitted to a hospital may be generated by which of the following conditions
   a. Familiarity with hospital routines
   b. Altered role relationships
   c. Wearing their own clothes
   d. Liberal visiting hours
4. Cultural sensitivity enables nurses to
   a. Strengthen their own ethnocentric values
   b. Impose their own cultural practices on clients
   c. Incorporate culturally specific health practices of clients into nursing care
   d. Encourage clients to adopt the culturally specific health practices of the health team

Match the following terms:

5. Ethnic identification   a. Process of learning the conceptual and behavioral system of one's own culture

6. Enculturation   b. Assigning a set of characteristics by one group of people to themselves or others

7. Acculturation   c. Where people place themselves on the ethnic chart

8. Stereotyping   d. Process of reciprocal retentions, losses, or adaptations of cultural patterns occurring when members of different ethnic groups interact

9. Culture shock   f. Process of exploring one's convictions, looking at alternatives, and setting personal priorities

10. Attitude clarification   e. Response to a drastic change in the cultural environment

Answer key

1. d   6. a
2. c   7. d
3. b   8. b
4. c   9. e
5. c   10. f

REFERENCES

Abelson RP: Whatever became of consistency theory? Personality Soc Psychol Bull 9:37-54, 1983.

Anchor K, Elkias D, and Sandler H: Relaxation training and prayer behavior as tension reduction techniques. Behavioral Engineering 5:81-87, 1979.

Ashcraft N and Scheflen AE: People space: the making and breaking of human boundaries, Garden City, NY, 1976, Anchor Press/Doubleday.

Attneave C: American Indians and Alaska native families: emigrants in their own homeland. In McGoldrick M, Pearce JK, and Giordano J, editors: Ethnicity and family therapy, New York, 1982, The Guilford Press.

Bahr HM: Skid row: an introduction to disaffiliation, New York, 1973, Oxford University Press.

Barnett H et al: Acculturation: an explanatory formulation, Am Anthropol 56:973-1002, 1954.

Bergin AE: Psychotherapy and religious values. J Consult Clin Psychol 48:95-105, 1980.

Brink PJ and Saunders JM: Cultural shock: theoretical and applied. In Brink PJ, editor: Transcultural nursing: a book of readings, Englewood Cliffs, NJ, 1976, Prentice-Hall, Inc.

Bullough B and Bullough VL: Poverty, ethnic identity, and health care, New York, 1972, Appleton-Century-Crofts.

Burnett DW: Religion, personality and clinical assessment, J Religion Health 18:308-312, 1979.

Chance NA: Acculturation, self-identification and personality adjustment, Am Anthropol 67:372-393, 1965.

Chesler P: Women and madness, New York, 1972, Doubleday & Co., Inc.

Covello L: The social background of the Italian-American school child, Totowa, NJ, 1972, Rowman & Littlefield.

Cox JL: Aspects of transcultural psychiatry. Br J Psychiatr 130:211-221, 1977.

Dayton NA: New facts on mental disorders, Springfield, Ill, 1940, Charles C Thomas, Publisher.

Dickerman M: Teaching cultural pluralism. In Banks JA, editor: Teaching ethnic studies: concepts and strategies, Washington, DC, 1973, National Council for the Social Studies.

Dominquez VR: From neighbor to stranger: the dilemma of Caribbean peoples in the United States, Antilles Research Program, New Haven, Conn, 1975, Yale University Press.

Estes WK: The state of the field: general problems and issues of theory and metatheory. In Estes WK, editor: Handbook of learning and cognitive processes. Hillsdale, NJ, 1975, Lawrence Erbaum Associates, Inc.

Falicov C: Cultural variations in the family life cycle. In Carter EA and McGoldrick M, editors: The family life cycle: a framework for family therapy. New York, 1980, Gardner Press.

Fiske ST and Taylor SE: Social cognition, Reading, Mass, 1984, Addison-Wesley.

Fong CM: Ethnicity and nursing practice, Topics in Clini Nurs 7(3):1-10, 1985.

Fried M: The world of the urban working class. Cambridge, 1974, Harvard University Press.

Frost I: Sickness and immigrant psychoses: Australian and German domestic servants and basis of study. J Mental Sci 84:801, 1938.

Gambino R: Blood of my blood: the dilemma of Italian Americans, New York, 1974, Doubleday & Co., Inc.

Gans H: The urban villagers, Glencoe, NY, 1962, The Free Press.

Gelfand DE and Fandetti DV: The emergent nature of ethnicity: dilemmas in assessment, Social Casework 67(9):542-550, 1986.

Geertz C: Ritual and social change: a Javanesse example. Am Anthropol 59:32-54, 1957.

Glazer N and Moynihan DP: Beyond the melting pot. Cambridge, Mass, 1970, The MIT Press.

Goffman E: Asylums: essays on the social situation of mental patients and other inmates, New York, 1961, Doubleday & Co., Inc.

Greeley AW: Ethnicity in the United States: a preliminary reconnaissance, New York, 1974, John Wiley & Sons, Inc.

Greeley AW and McCready WC: The transmission of cultural heritages: the case of the Irish and the Italians. In Glazer N and Moynihan DP, editors: Ethnicity—theory and experience, Cambridge, Mass, 1975, Harvard University Press.

Hamburg BA: Social change and the problems of youth. In Arieti S, editor: American handbook of psychiatry, ed 2, New York, 1975, Basic Books.

Helman C: Culture, health and illness, Bristol, England, 1984, John Wright & Sons, Ltd.

Herz RM and Rosen EJ: Jewish families. In McGoldrick M, Pearce JK, and Giordano J, editors: Ethnicity and family therapy, New York, 1982, The Guilford Press.

Hines PM and Boyd-Franklin N: Black families. In McGoldrick M, Pearce JK, and Giordano J, editors: Ethnicity and family therapy. New York, 1982, The Guilford Press.

Holt TC: Afro-Americans. In Ternstrom S, editor: Harvard encyclopedia of American ethnic groups, Cambridge, 1980, Harvard University Press.

Horowitz DL: Ethnic identity. In Glazer N and Moynihan DP, editors: Ethnicity—theory and experience, Cambridge, Mass, 1975, Harvard University Press.

Hsu FLK: Americans and Chinese: reflections on two cultures and their people, Garden City, NY, 1970, Doubleday Natural History Press.

Hsu FLK: Americans and Chinese. New York, 1970, Doubleday Natural History Press.

Hunt E and Lansman M: Cognitive theory applied to individual difference. In Estes WK, editor: Handbook of learning and cognitive process, Hillsdale, NJ, 1975, Lawrence Erbaum Associates, Inc.

Isaacs HR: Idols of the tribe: group identity and political change, New York, 1975, Harper & Row, Publishers, Inc.

Isajiw WW: Definitions of ethnicity. Ethnicity 1:111-124, 1974.

James A: Economic adaptations of a Cuban community. Ann NY Acad Sci 293:194-205, 1977.

Jaspars J and Hewstone M: Cross-cultural interaction, social attribution and inter-group relations. In Bochner S, editor: Cultures in contact: studies in cross-cultural interaction, New York, 1982, Pergamon Press.

Kelley HH: Causal schemata and the attribution process, New York, 1972, General Learning Press.

Kelley HH: The process of causal attribution. Am Psychol 28:107-128,1973.

Kleinhesselink RR and Edwards RE: Seeking and avoiding belief-discrepant information as a function of its perceived refutability, J Personal Soc Psychol 31:787-790, 1975.

Kluckhohn F and Strodbeck F: Variations in value orientations, Evanston, IL, 1961, Row, Peterson & Co.

Krickus R: Pursuing the American dream: white ethnics and the new populism. Bloomington, 1976, Indiana University Press.

Kuczynski K: New tensions in rural communities, Hum Serv Rural Environment 6:50-55, 1981.

Larson JA: Dysfunction in the evangelical family: treatment considerations, Family Coordinator 27:261+, 1978.

Larson OF: Values and beliefs of rural people. In Ford T, editor: Rural U.S.A., Iowa City, 1978, Iowa State University Press.

Lee E: A social systems approach to assessment and treatment for Chinese American families, In McGoldrick M, Pearce JK, and Giordano J, editors: Ethnicity and family therapy, New York, 1982, The Guilford Press.

Lewis O: The culture of poverty, Sci Am 215(16):19-25, 1966.

Littlewood R and Lipsedge M: Aliens and alienists, Harmondworth, England, 1982, Penguin.

Luhman R and Gilman S: Race and ethnic relations: the social and political experience of minority groups, Belmont, Calif, 1980, Wadsworth Publishing Co.

M'biti JS: African religions and philosophy, New York, 1969, Frederick A. Praeger, Inc.

McGoldrick M: Ethnicity and family therapy: an overview. In McGoldrick M, Pearce JK, and Giordano J, editors: Ethnicity and family therapy, New York, 1982, The Guilford Press.

Meltzer M: Poverty in America, New York, 1986, William Morrow & Co.

Meux M: Resolving interpersonal value conflicts, Adv Nurs Sci 2(4):41-69, 1980.

Mosley HJ and Clift VA: The evaluation of cultural dimensions in the curriculum. In Cultural dimensions in the baccalaureate nursing curriculum, New York, 1977, National League for Nursing.

Myers JK and Roberts BH: Family and class dynamics in mental illness, New York, 1959, John Wiley.

Novak M: The rise of the unmeltable ethnics: politics and culture in the seventies, New York, 1973, Macmillan Publishing Co., Inc.

Oakley A: Subject women, New York, 1981, Pantheon.

Oates J: A systems' approach to rural communities, Hum Serv Rural Environment 3:67-75, 1977.

O'Brien ME: Pragmatic survivalism: behavior patterns affecting low-level wellness among minority group members, Adv Nurs Sci 4(3):13-21, 1982.

Ogionwo WW: The adoption of technological innovations in Nigeria: a study of factors associated with adoption of farm practices. Ph.D. thesis, University of Leeds, Cited in Goldthorp JE, editor: The sociology of the third world: disparity and involvement, New York, 1975, Cambridge University Press.

Oberg K: Culture shock, Indianapolis, 1954, The Bobbs-Merrill Co, Inc.

Pasquali E: Assimilation and acculturation of Cubans on Long Island, Ph.D. dissertation, State University of New York at Stony Brook, 1982.

Peterson JH: Assimilation, separation and out-migration in an American Indian group, Am Anthropol 74:1286-1295, 1972.

Pinderhughes E: Afro-American families and the victim system, In McGoldrick M, Pearce JK, and Giordano J, editors: Ethnicity and family therapy, New York, 1982, The Guilford Press.

Report of Consensus Conferences: Access to prenatal care: key to preventing low birthweight, Kansas City, Mo, 1987, American Nurses Association.

Rogg EM: The assimilation of Cuban exiles: the role of community and class, New York, 1974, Aberdeen Press.

Ruffin JE: Changing perspectives on ethnicity and health, In A strategy for change, Kansas City, Mo, 1979, American Nurses' Association.

Sarna J: From immigrants to ethnics: toward a theory of 'ethnicization', Ethnicity 5:370-378, 1978.

Sawhill I: Discrimination and poverty among women who head families, In Blaxall M and Regan B, editors: Women and the workplace, Chicago, 1980, University of Chicago Press.

Scheflen A and Scheflen A: Body language and social order, Englewood Cliffs, NJ, 1972, Prentice-Hall, Inc.

Scheper-Hughes N and Lock MM: The mindful body: a prolegomenon to future work in medical anthropology, Med Anthropol Q 1(1): 6-33, 1987.

Schermerhorn RA: Comparative ethnic relations: a framework for theory and research, Chicago, 1978, The University of Chicago Press.

Schneider L and Lysgaard S: The deferred gratification pattern: a preliminary study, Am Sociol Rev 18:142-149, 1953.

Scott H: Working your way to the bottom: the feminization of poverty, London, 1984, Pandora Press.

Seligman MEP: Helplessness: on depression, development, and death, San Francisco, 1975, W.H. Freeman.

Shannon LW: The study of migrants as members of social systems. In Helm J, editor: Spanish speaking people of the United States, Seattle, 1968, University of Washington Press.

Shewbridge EA: Portraits of poverty, New York, 1972, WW Norton & Company, Inc.

Smith M: A practical guide to value clarification, La Jolla, Calif, 1977, University Associates, Inc.

Smith MG: Afro-American research: a critique. In Comitas L and Lowenthal D, editors: Work and family life: West Indian perspectives, New York, 1973, Doubleday & Co., Inc.

Smith RT: Social stratification in the Caribbean, In Plotnicov L and Tuden A, editors: Essays in comparative social stratification, Pittsburgh, 1970, University of Pittsburg Press.

Spiegel J: An ecological model of ethnic families. In McGoldrick M, Pearce JK, and Giordano J, editors: Ethnicity and family therapy, New York, 1982, The Guilford Press.

Spindler L: Culture change and modernization: mini-models and case studies, New York, 1977, Holt, Rinehart & Winston.

Spradley JP and Phillip M: Culture and stress: a quantitative analysis, Am Anthropol 4:518-529, 1972.

Staples R: Introduction to black sociology, New York, 1976, McGraw-Hill, Inc.

Swanson B, Swanson E, and Cohen R: Small towns and small towners: a framework for survival and growth, Beverly Hills, Calif, 1979, Sage.

Szapocznik J and Kurtiness W: Acculturation, biculturalism and adjustment among Cuban Americans, In Padilla AM, editor: Acculturation, theory, models and some new findings, Boulder, Colo, 1980, Westview Press, Inc.

Tajfel H: Social identity and intergroup behavior, Soc Sci Information 13:65-93, 1974.

Tajfel H: Differentiation between social groups: studies in inter-group behavior, London, 1978, Academic Press.

Teske RHC and Nelson BH: Acculturation and assimilation: a clarification, Am Ethnol 1:351-367, 1974.

Triandis HC: Interpersonal behavior, Monterey, Calif, 1977, Brooks/Cole.

Tyhurst L: Psychosomatic and allied disorders. In Murphy

HBM editor: Flight and resettlement, Paris, 1955, UNESCO.

Uustal D: The use of values clarification in nursing practice. J Continuing Ed Nurs 8:8-13, 1977.

Wallace AFC: Culture and personality, New York, 1970, Random House, Inc.

Westermyer J, Vang TF, and Neider J: Migration and mental health among refugees: association of pre- and post-migration factors with self-rating scales, J Nervous Mental Dis 17(2):92-96, 1983.

Yinger JM: Countercultures: the promise and the peril of a world turned upside down, New York, 1982, The Free Press.

ANNOTATED SUGGESTED READINGS

Brink PJ and Saunders JM: Cultural shock: theoretical and applied. In Transcultural nursing: a book of readings, Englewood Cliffs, NJ, 1976, Prentice-Hall, Inc., pp 126-138.
This essay explores culture shock as a stress syndrome and the implications for nursing care. The authors discuss such categories as stressors, phases of culture shock, coping behavior, and hospitalization as culture shock.

Dunham HW: Society, culture and mental disorder, Arch Gen Psychiatr 33(2):147-156, 1976.
Dunham critically examines theories and hypotheses relating societal and cultural factors to the etiology or precipitation of specific emotional disorders. The author identifies many unresolved methodological difficulties involved in such research. The article concludes with a summary of definitive results that relates sociocultural factors to specific mental illness.

Helman C: Culture and illness: an introduction for health professionals, Bristol, England, 1984, John Wright & Sons, Ltd.
The author applies basic ideas and research in medical anthropology to health care and preventive medicine. Chapters commence with a theoretical framework and then utilize case studies to illustrate sociocultural dimensions of health and illness as well as implications for clinical practice. Each chapter concludes with recommended readings that relate to the topic under discussion.

Oberg K: Culture shock, Indianapolis, 1954, The Bobbs-Merrill Co, Inc.
In this classic discussion of culture shock the author explores the nature and phases of culture shock and briefly suggests ways of coping with it.

FURTHER READINGS

Abernethy V: Cultural perspective on the impact of women's changing roles on psychiatry, Am J Psychiatr 133:657-666, 1976.

Fabega H: Disease and social behavior, Cambridge, Mass, 1974, The MIT Press.

Guttentag M, Salasin S, and Belle D, editors: The mental health of women, New York, 1980, Academic Press.

Merta RJ, Stringham EM, and Ponterotto JG: Simulating culture shock in counselor trainees: an experiential exercise for cross-cultural training, J Couns Dev 66(5):242-245, 1988.

Pasquali E: East meets west: a transcultural aspect of the nurse-patient relationship, J Psychiatr Nurs Mental Health Serv 12:20-22, 1974.

Sizemore BA: Shattering the melting pot myth, In Banks JE, editor: Teaching ethnic studies: concepts and strategies, Washington, DC, 1973, National Council for the Social Studies, pp 73-101.

Staples R and Mirande A: Racial and cultural variations among American families: a decennial review of the literature on minority families, J Marriage Family 42:887-903, 1980.

Westemeyer J: Anthropology and mental health, Chicago, 1976, Aldine Publishing Co.

Wittkower ED and Prince R: A review of transcultural psychiatry, In Caplan G and Arieti S, editors: American handbook of psychiatry, ed 2, vol 2, New York, 1974, Basic Books, Inc.

CHAPTER 5

The family

CHAPTER FOCUS

Sociocultural factors have great influence on the composition, form, and dynamics of the family. The concept of "family" may vary depending on the stage of the developmental cycle that the family occupies and on the interactions, relationships, and organizational patterns among family members.

The family is a system and has the properties of any social system. There is an interrelationship between the family system and the context (physical, social, cultural, and emotional) in which it functions. This interrelationship is one of reciprocal influence.

THE NATURE OF THE FAMILY

The earliest and generally the most effective enculturating agent is the family.* Fundamental to any discussion of the family is a definition of the term *family*. Does it refer only to parent(s) and children? Does it include married children and their spouses? Does it encompass grandparents? Aunts and uncles? Cousins? Family friends or significant others?

Definition of the family

Any definition of the family must first shed the assumption that the nuclear family (parents and their children) is the basic or universal family form. Rather, when the family is viewed cross culturally, the fundamental relational components seem to be

*Refer to Chapter 4 for a discussion of the family as an agent of enculturation.

dyadic. Two dyadic relationships, because of their biological correlates, are essential to the formation of the nuclear family and to other family forms. These two relationships are the sexual dyad, which is the reproductive unit of society, and the maternal dyad, which is the temporal linkage between generations. The nuclear family is only one way of combining these two basic dyads. If other kin and other dyads are added to these two basic dyadic relationships, other family forms become recognizable. For example, if grandparents are added to the sexual and maternal dyads, a three-generation extended family is formed.

An *extended family* encompasses at least three generations of kin. The stem family of Japan (composed of eldest son, his wife and children, and his parents) is an example of an extended family. The extended family has a potentially larger labor force and more options for the division of labor than either the nuclear family or the single-parent family. The extended family may be further characterized as follows:

1. Many adult members to share in child rearing and with whom children may identify
2. Provision of security to aged family members
3. Restricted opportunities for the personal growth of young adult family members because of the authority vested in elders
4. Extended kin support systems during situational and maturational crises (Scheflen and Scheflen, 1972)

In West Indian and Hispanic extended families the bond between mother and child may be very strong, and it may be considered primary to all other relationships. Daughters often consider their mothers "best friends" and confide in them about problems and conflicts (Gilmore, 1980; Pasquali, 1982).

An 18-year-old unmarried Hispanic woman became pregnant. When she confided this to her mother, her mother offered to help her raise the child. During an antepartum examination, the nurse asked the young woman, who was accompanied by her mother, what plans she had made for the baby. When the young woman said her mother was going to help raise the baby, the nurse began to explain that there were other options available, such as placing the baby for adoption. The young woman's mother became very upset and interrupted the nurse by saying, "If you don't love your baby, who do you love? Not yourself. Not your mother. Nobody. Any man who comes to you is gonna say, 'If you don't love your children, you don't love me.' So the men will come and use you and say 'goodbye.' "

The nurse, who was not Hispanic, did not understand the primacy that many Hispanics give to the mother-child relationship. The nurse viewed the mother's behavior as "interfering, domineering, and rude." The nurse became defensive. The young woman rallied to her mother's aid and said to the nurse, "My mother is my best friend. She always has my best interest at heart." The counseling session ended abruptly.

Thus, the importance attached by some ethnic groups to the mother-child bond may not be understood by people with a different orientation to the family unit.

Another family form, at variance with the extended family, is the *nuclear family*. The nuclear family, long regarded by mainstream America as the "normal" family form, emerged as an adaptation to the Industrial Revolution. As farms became mechanized and people began working in factories and moving to cities, extended families were no longer an economic necessity. A nuclear family consists of a man, a woman, and their children. The nuclear family may be characterized as follows:

1. Many opportunities for the personal growth of children and young adults
2. Few adults who share in child rearing and with whom children can identify
3. Nonkin support systems during times of crisis
4. Inadequate extended family support systems during periods of situational or maturational crisis (Scheflen and Scheflen, 1972)

Another increasingly common family form is the *single-parent* family. In the single-parent family, the sexual dyad that produced the children was temporary in nature either because it was not sanctioned by marriage or because the marriage was terminated by death or divorce. Sometimes the sexual dyad may be unrelated to the parent, as when a single woman or man adopts a child. The single-parent family, while offering many opportunities for the personal growth of children, may present some of the following difficulties:

1. The parent may look to the child for emotional support.
2. The child may manipulate separated parents, playing one against the other.
3. The child may become the pawn of separated parents.
4. The child may have to deal with evidences of the parent's sexuality (for example, affairs, live-in relationships).
5. The child may form positive relationships with parental lovers and then have to deal with feelings of loss when the lovers leave (Meagher, 1980; Critchley, 1981).

On the opposite end of the continuum from the single-parent family is the omnigenous (or "blended") family. The term *omnigenous family* refers to the family formed when parents divorce and remarry. Since many people divorce and remarry more than once, a complex kinship system of relatives and steprelatives may develop. An array of alliances and interpersonal relationships of differing meaning and intensity may also evolve. The strengths and weaknesses of an omnigenous family are not very different from those of the extended family (Tiger, 1978; Jordheim, 1980; Johnson, Klee, and Schmidt, 1988).

The basic forms of family organization differ in their potential for meeting the needs of their members. The extended family and the omnigenous family provide members with security. Children benefit from the collective presence of many adults, who help to rear them and who serve as role models. However, since age usually carries respect and the exercise of family authority, younger members may live out much of their lives under the supervision of elders. Therefore, in extended and omnigenous families, security is sometimes gained at the expense of personal growth. Nuclear and single-parent families usually encourage and facilitate the individual development of their young members. However, nonfamily relationships and occupational bonding tend to compete with and weaken family ties. Relationships with extended kin are often inadequate. Consequently, during periods of

maturational or situational crisis, family members may not receive necessary support or security. For instance, during a divorce, parents may be distraught and unable to offer their children adequate emotional support. At the same time, the children may be physically and affectionally estranged from relatives who could serve as a support system. Aunts and uncles might live many miles away and grandparents may be isolated in a nursing home. Therefore, in the nuclear or single-parent family, opportunity for personal development is sometimes gained at the expense of security.

Just as the definition of the family should not be restricted to the nuclear family but should be flexible enough to include kin that people regard as "family," the word "kin" does not refer only to people related by consanguinal or affinal bonds but also to fictive kin. *Fictive kin* are usually regarded as "just like family." For example,

---

A Cuban client told a nurse: "This woman is not really my mother, but I call her Mamá Jolie. She and my mother were close friends all of their lives. They were always together, and this woman became like a mother to me. On Mother's Day, I always visit my mother and Mamá Jolie. Now that Mamá Jolie is ill and her children live in Cuba, I am the only daughter she has. I will help care for her when she leaves the hospital."

Fictive kinship is usually established through co-parentage (godparentage) of a child or by longtime and close friendship with the entire family. Fictive kinship binds people together in ties of affection and concern as well as in a sense of obligation, responsibility, and expectation concerning loyalty and exchanges of goods and services. Fictive kinship thus establishes a sense of relatedness among people unrelated by ties of consanguinity or affinity, and it helps people to adapt to their environmental conditions and changes (Gubrium and Buckholdt, 1982; Pasquali, 1982). For example, among the acquaintances of the elderly, there is often a sense of relatedness that enables them to establish confidant relationships and that serves as a support network or quasi-family. This quasi-family functions as a buffer against problems that the

TABLE 5-1 Phases of the domestic cycle

Phase	Characteristics
Expansion	Begins with marriage and continues until completion of the natal family; may be physiologically limited by a woman's period of fertility; may be extended beyond a woman's fertility period by absorbing children into the family system (e.g., through adoption, foster care, raising grandchildren)
Fission	Begins when the first child marries or leaves home; lasts until all children are married or leave home; sometimes referred to as the "empty nest" stage; because of economic problems, divorce, or other factors, adult children may return to the parental home after having left (often referred to as the "refilled nest")
Replacement	Begins when the first child establishes a family; continues as each succeeding child establishes a family; ends with the death of the ancestral parents

elderly may experience concerning aging and institutionalization (Butler and Lewis, 1982).

In addition to discussing the various forms that the family may take and the members that it may encompass, when defining the family we also need to consider what stage of the domestic cycle the family occupies. Fortes (1958) was one of the first to describe three phases in the domestic cycle: expansion, fission, and replacement (see Table 5-1). These stages are progressive, and they often overlap.

Family versus household

Residents of a household may or may not be united by bonds of kinship. Also, members of a family may reside in different households. For example, after parents are divorced, children and their mother often live in one household while the children's father lives in another household.

A household is a group of people bound together by common residence, economic cooperation, and the task of child rearing. A household is *not* concerned with the function of procreation. This is a function of the family. In those instances when family and household do not coincide, the household needs to be viewed as a separate but extremely influential adjunct or alternative to the family.

One type of household is a *commune.* Communal living is not new. The nineteenth century saw the rise of more than 200 communes in the United States. Many of these early Americans were participating in a life-style that violated the norm of monogamous family life. However, while a few communes, notably those of the Shakers, insisted on celibacy, most other religious communes have sanctioned monogamy. In both religious and secular communes, labor and money are usually shared among members. Communes are one way to collectively raise children. Commune participants share the bonding that sometimes becomes burdensome in nuclear and single-parent families (Jordheim, 1980).

Another type of household may be formed by cohabiting heterosexual couples. Cohabiting couples usually share household tasks and expenses. Many cohabiting couples view themselves and their mates as being like spouses. They share bonds of affection and concern, and they have a sense of obligation, responsibility, and expectation concerning loyalty and exchange of goods and services. In these instances, cohabiting couples may be regarded as fictive kin rather than as unrelated people (Sedgwick, 1981).

Still another type of household may be formed by homosexuals. Some homosexual households include children. Often two gay partners live together with their children from a heterosexual relationship.

A homosexual orientation does not mean that people cannot be dependable, nurturing parents or that children raised by homosexual parents will become homosexual. The incidence of children living with their homosexual parent and their parent's partner seems to be greater among lesbian mothers than among gay fathers. Gay fathers seem to more frequently remain in their marriages while engaging in homosexual relationships than do lesbian mothers (Jordheim, 1980). A primary parenting concern of gay fathers is the decision about disclosure of their homosexuality. Gay fathers fear that self-disclosure will mean rejection by or decreased respect from their children. However, nondisclosure entails monitoring all aspects of their lives that might reveal their homosexuality. Research indicates that although there is a wide range of response (from complete rejection to total acceptance) by children to paternal self-disclosure of gay identity, in the majority of cases, the increased understanding that children gain about parental marital problems decreases family tensions and the liklihood of children blaming themselves for domestic conflicts (Miller, 1979; Maddox, 1982; Bozett, 1984).

Thus, the definition of the family and the difference between the family and the household need to be considered when the nature of the family is examined. Social organization is flexible enough to permit different forms of the family to coexist in different parts of the world and even in different subsystems of the same society. Each of these different family forms may serve different functions and fill different needs of individuals and society. It is important for nurses working with families to include all the people that the client-family regards as family and to be aware of the cultural relativity of family form.

Functions of the family

A family system is more than a collection of actual or fictive kin. The concept of "family" includes interactions, relationships, and functional and organizational patterns that strive to effectively meet the needs of family members and the expectations of society. Family functions refer to what the family does; these functions include economic cooperation, procreation, child rearing (including socialization and enculturation), and the growth and development of family members. The family is further involved in information gathering, decision making, conflict resolution, and the promotion of acceptance, authenticity, trust, and cooperation among family members. The emphasis given to family functions and the way that family functions are implemented will vary from culture to culture. The mental health status of individual family members is believed to reflect the level of family functioning.

It is important to view the *context* in which a family functions—in other words, the family's physical, social, cultural, and emotional environments. Context includes the nation, the state, and the neighborhood in which the family lives, the social institutions (for example, schools, churches, and organizations) with which it interacts, the social networks with which it relates, and the cultural, racial, and socioeconomic orientations of the family. The interaction between family and context is characterized by reciprocal influence: the context influences the family and the family influences the context. The degree of a family's involvement with or isolation from its context affects the family's ability to exert as much influence on its *total* environment as the environment exerts on the family. The environment may be especially influential in such areas of family functioning as exchange of ideas; incorporation of norms, expectations, and attitudes; effectiveness of support systems; and direction of goals (Sedgwick, 1981). For example,

---

Five years ago, families A and B both moved from Korea to the United States. Family A moved into a Korean enclave. They share an apartment with already settled extended family members. All the adults in Family A work at two jobs. They do not socialize with their neighbors. Because there are no adults at home when the children return from school, the children are told to stay in the apartment, to do their homework, and to complete household chores. They are not permitted to go out to play or to invite other children into the apartment. The members of Family A have few friends in the neighborhood, have much difficulty speaking English, and have learned little about American norms and attitudes.

In contrast, Family B moved into an integrated Korean-American neighborhood. Although all the adults in Family B work at two jobs, they have arranged their days off so that an adult is always home when the children return from school. The children in Family B play with both Korean and American children, and the adults in Family B have made friends with many of the parents of these children. The members of *Family B are conversant in English, and they have learned enough about American norms and attitudes to decide which are compatible with their life-style and which are not.*

Thus, family functioning and social context are integrally related, and for nurses to assess family functioning, they must be cognizant of the social context in which the family lives (see Fig. 5-1 for an example of a family and its social context).

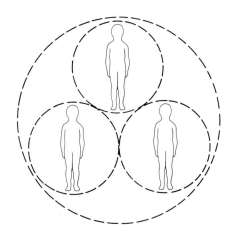

Family: A system composed of interacting members

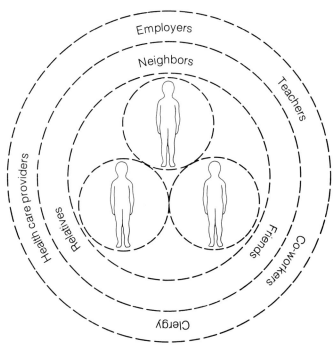

Family and its social environment: Suprasystem in which family is a subsystem

Fig. 5-1 Family and its social context.

Two interrelated issues that affect family functioning are *working parents* (either dual-earner families or single-parent families) and *child care* for children of working parents. Any one or a combination of factors may influence the decision to have a dual-earner family. These factors include economic (e.g., inadequate finances, desire for a higher standard of living), societal (e.g., changing sex roles, changing occupational roles), and personal (e.g., need for fulfillment unrelated to domestic roles, desire to utilize educational or vocational training).

Many working parents, especially women, experience conflict as they try to balance work-related assignments with family demands. Working parents may also experience guilt about such unavoidable situations as accidents or illnesses that befall their children or about placement of children in child care. The nature of supportive relationships is crucial to the functioning of families with dual-earner parents or employed single-parents. Spouses (in dual-earner families), children, friends, and relatives may serve as support systems. However, research on dual-earner families indicates that the majority of husbands do not substantially share domestic roles with their working wives (Smith and Reid, 1986). This often creates role conflict and overburdening for women. For example,

---

Both Jean and Harold Jones work full-time. They have three children, ages 4, 7, and 11. Jean is a kindergarten teacher, and Harold manages a local supermarket. Jean leaves for school at 7:30 in the morning; Harold leaves for work at 8. Although Harold puts the two school-age children on the school bus, it is Jean who supervises their dressing, prepares breakfasts (including Harold's), and brings the preschooler to day care.

On her way home from work, Jean picks the youngest child up from day care. The two school-age children stay with a neighbor until Jean gets home. Once Jean gets in the house, she prepares a snack for the children, gets them started on their homework, and then prepares supper. When Harold gets home, he checks the children's homework. Then the family eats supper. After supper, Harold reads to the children while Jean washes the supper dishes and prepares the children's school lunches. On the weekends, Jean

does the housework and Harold does the family's food shopping. When the children are too ill to go to school or day care, Jean stays home with them.

The patterns illustrated in the above vignette often exist as much because of women's reluctance to share domestic roles with men as because of men's reluctance to participate in housework and child care. For instance, sharing child care may pose a threat to the identity of some women, while other women may feel their children will be neglected.

Working parenthood also impacts on power and control in the family. For example, parents in dual-career families may have to decide whether one career will be given priority and for how long. Another issue surrounding power in the family includes the partial relinquishing of nurturing and control over children to nonparental caretakers. These nonparental caretakers may include relatives, friends, or child care personnel. In some neighborhoods, child care is a cottage industry. Mothers who are not employed outside the home care for the children of working parents. Although some child care services may be funded by voluntary or community organizations, overall, affordable child care programs greatly fall short of demand. There is also inadequate government support for families that require child care services (Kutzner and Toussie-Weingarten, 1984; Googins and Burden, 1987). Inadequacy of child care facilities contributes to an increasing population of latchkey children. The growing national awareness about latchkey children has resulted in Project Home Safe, an outreach program that plans to establish a hot line for latchkey children and to develop standards for school-age child care programs (Short Takes, 1987).

Thus, the effective functioning of the family is dependent on the relationship between the family and its context.

FAMILY PROCESS
Family theory

The models that family theorists use to study the operation of the family can be categorized as follows: (1) structural-functional analysis, (2) interactional analysis, (3) developmental analysis (Jones and Dimond, 1982).

The *structural-functional model* views the family as an open social system and explores the relationships between the family and other social institutions. For example, the contribution of status-role functions of family members to the maintenance of the family system may be examined. Individual family members are seen as reactive, rather than as action-initiating; they behave according to the demands or constraints of the family system. In turn, the family system is viewed as a passive adaptor, rather than as a change-initiating agent, that functions to maintain the broader social system (Spindler, 1977; Adams, 1980).

In contrast to the structural-functional model, which looks at the functions of individual family members in family system maintenance, the *interactional model* focuses on the interacting personalities and interaction patterns of individual family members. The structural-functional model approaches the family as an open system and examines the relationships between the family and other social institutions, while the interactional model views the family as a self-contained unit. In the interactional model, the family system is analyzed by looking at the internal functioning of the family, such as its processes of communication, conflict resolution, and decision making (Van Servellen, 1984).

Like the two previous models, the *developmental model* focuses on individual family members. The family is viewed as an open social system. Within the context of the family, individual members are seen as holding dyadic positions (for example, wife-mother, daughter-sister). Norms prescribe acceptable role behavior, and changes in role behavior are studied over time. According to the developmental model, the needs and tasks of the family vary according to the phase of the developmental cycle it is in. The role behavior of family members fulfilling these needs and tasks is the focus of study. This analysis of family role behavior is conducted on three levels.

1. Alterations in the developmental tasks and role expectations of *children*
2. Alterations in the developmental tasks and role expectations of *parents*
3. Alterations in the developmental tasks of the *family unit* in response to cultural influences at various phases of the developmental cycle of the family (Jones and Dimond, 1982)

Each of the three family theory models focuses on the *health* of family systems. Nurses involved in primary prevention of family dysfunction need to be knowledgeable about family theory to accurately assess family dynamics and to promote optimal family functioning (Jones and Dimond, 1982). (See Table 5-2.)

Application of family theory to family process

The family is a dynamic system of interrelated parts that form a whole. As was previously pointed out, the family system includes members and their relationships with one another and with their physical, social, cultural, and emotional environments.

TABLE 5-2 Comparison of family theory models

Family theory model	Boundaries of the family system	Unit of analysis	Focus of analysis
Structural-functional	Open	Individual family members	Relationships between the family and other social institutions
Interactional	Closed	Individual family members	Internal functioning of the family
Developmental	Open	Individual family members	Role behavior of family members over time

THE FAMILY SYSTEM

To understand the family as a system, one must have an understanding of general systems theory.*

▶ Properties of systems

Central to all systems are the properties of *interrelatedness, flow of information,* and *feedback.* Any system, including a family system, must be able to interrelate and incorporate information. Information sought and used by families is of two types: information that reinforces what the family already knows or believes (negative feedback) and information that questions or disagrees with the family's ideas, values, and behaviors (positive feedback) (Sedgwick, 1981). Positive feedback facilitates change within the family system, while negative feedback promotes family system stability. For example,

1. Information of an expected nature, gathered from relatives or friends, is fed back into the family system and reinforces the family system's stability or balance (an example of negative feedback).
2. Information that challenges or offers alternatives to the family's way of life, sought from the media, friends with ideas different from the family's, etc., is used to alter the structure of the family system (an example of positive feedback).

Feedback thus has a regulatory function. It serves to monitor, reinforce, and correct the structure and conditions of the system. Because of feedback, change in any part of the family system affects the entire family. For example, when a family seeks counseling for one member (the identified client), positive feedback of two types, *learning* and *self-awareness,* is used not only to alter the behavior of the identified client but also to alter the structure and functioning of the family system.

Another property of any system, including a family system, is *homeostasis.* Homeostasis refers to the maintenance of equilibrium or to a steady state of balance. Many social scientists hold that because of the many forces of dysfunction and change that affect social systems, social systems are continuously in a state of flux and can only be in relative balance. This state of flux and relative balance is referred to as *homeodynamics.*

Like other social systems, a family system continuously strives for homeostasis. Often the balance within a family system incorporates the pathological conditions of its members. Jackson (1957) was one of the first to recognize that when the behavior or condition of an identified client improves, it is not uncommon for another family member to experience an emotional or psychophysiological problem. This seesawing of members evidencing dysfunction helps to maintain family equilibrium.

When a family directs most of its energy into the maintenance of family equilibrium, there is little residual energy to channel into personal or family development. For example, in a family system that does not permit dissension, much energy is directed toward maintaining harmony among family members and hiding instances of family dissension from people outside the family.

The Anderson family almost always presented a united, harmonious appearance. The parents never disagreed with each other in front of the children, and they rarely disagreed in private. Neither the children nor the parents ever raised their voices to each other. If the children began to misbehave, a stern look from the mother would curtail the misbehavior. On the rare occasions that dissension in the family did occur, the Andersons pretended it did not exist.

One such instance of dissension happened when Mrs. Anderson's brother, who had lived with the Andersons, died. Mr. Anderson had long resented the close relationship between Mrs. Anderson and her brother, a relationship that made Mr. Anderson feel "like an outsider in my own home." Thus, when Mrs. Anderson's brother died, Mr. Anderson did not attend the funeral. At the funeral, both Mrs. Anderson and the Anderson children acted as if nothing were amiss. Relatives noticed that Mr. Anderson was not at the funeral, and they wondered why, but no one, including Mrs. Anderson's sister, inquired for fear of "upsetting" Mrs. Anderson.

Obviously, the Anderson family used much energy to maintain an appearance of harmony and to mask

---

*Refer to Chapter 1 for a discussion of general systems theory.

dissension. Relatives facilitated and participated in this masking.

▶ Boundaries and boundary maintenance

Every system, including the family system, has boundaries. These boundaries may be distinct or ambiguous, flexible or rigid. In a social system, boundaries identify differences between social groups and maintain the distinctiveness of groups. Various forces may function as boundary-maintaining mechanisms. Family secrets and family suspiciousness of people outside the family are examples of boundary maintenance mechanisms in a family system. The degree of boundary flexibility and boundary maintenance affects the way that a family system interacts with other social systems (see Fig. 5-1):

1. It defines who is entitled to family membership and who must remain outsiders
2. It determines the degree of differentiation permitted between family members and outsiders and the amount of emotional involvement that family members should invest in the family
3. It defines the frequency and types of extrafamilial experiences available to family members and the criteria that should be used to evaluate extrafamilial experiences (Van Servellen, 1984; McGoldrick, 1982)

The degree of openness (characterized by flexible boundaries and little boundary maintenance) or closedness (characterized by rigid boundaries and much boundary maintenance) also regulates the adaptability of the family system to its environment. Table 5-3 summarizes the characteristics that influence the environmental adaptability of open and closed family systems.

Self-corrective mechanisms enable a social system to alter its functioning and to adapt internally. These adjustive mechanisms permit social systems, like the family, to counteract disruptive tendencies in society and to maintain equilibrium. Self-corrective mechanisms include such institutionalized measures of social control as enculturation techniques* and socially sanctioned opportunities to relax restrictive rules (for example, socially ap-

*Refer to Chapter 4 for a discussion of enculturation.

TABLE 5-3 Adaptability of family systems

Type of family system	Characteristics
Open	Flexibly interacts with other social systems; uses imput from sources outside the family; seeks information that questions or challenges family's ideas, values, and behaviors; broad scope of adaptability
Closed	Rigidly interacts with other social systems; ignores or misinterprets imput from outside the family; seeks information that supports family's ideas, values, and behaviors; restricted scope of adaptability

proved occasions for role turn-about or for the display of competition between family members). Self-corrective mechanisms act to resolve conflict and to stabilize a social system.

The aforementioned Anderson family used most of its energy to maintain family equilibrium. The family interacted with the social environment predominantly as a unit. Family members had a few acquaintances but no friends, and the family rarely socialized with relatives. Mr. and Mrs. Anderson discouraged their children from having friends because "the behavior of other children is a bad influence. When they (our children) come home from playing with other children, we have to brainwash them into the right way to behave." Relatives were only permitted to talk to the Anderson children about activities and things, never about ideas, feelings, or relationships. Mr. and Mrs. Anderson feared that relatives might express opinions that were different from theirs and thereby influence the children in a direction other than the one set by the parents.

When the oldest Anderson daughter turned 16, she convinced her parents to let her have a party at home. She invited many of her classmates. Some of these classmates smuggled beer into the party and smoked cigarettes. Mr. and Mrs. Anderson were very upset by the behavior of these few teenagers. The Anderson parents used the incident to justify to themselves and to their daughter that to have friends would expose her to "bad influences."

Authoritarian parental controls, prescribed activities and behavior patterns, and such self-corrective mechanisms as the socialization of the Anderson children to view people outside the nuclear family as bad influences created within the Anderson family a rigid family structure that counteracted social influences inconsistent with the family's approach to life. Although equilibrium in the Anderson family was maintained through the use of self-corrective mechanisms, the types of self-corrective mechanisms that the family used restricted the family's ability to adapt to their social environment.

It should be noted that there are no completely open or completely closed family systems. Even the rigidly bound Anderson family interacted with outsiders when its members attended school, shopped for groceries, went to work, and so on.

▶ Family structure and role relationships

As with any social system, a family system operates according to rules and statuses. These rules and statuses usually, but not always, influence people to behave in a predictable fashion. It is on the basis of rules and statuses that roles are assigned. For example, because parents usually have dominant status over young children, parents usually assume the roles of authority figures in the family. Family energy is directed toward helping members fulfill the roles that are essential for effective functioning of the family. Yet within any particular family, role assignments tend to be flexible and to change to reflect the stage of the developmental cycle that the family occupies.

Factors such as illness or unemployment may interfere with family members' desire or ability to fulfill allocated roles. In such instances, role conflict and family disequilibrium may develop. Parental roles usually reflect the male-female division of labor in society (Fife, 1985). However, in contemporary American society, many men and women are renegotiating these traditional roles. During the period of renegotiation, role conflict and family disequilibrium may occur.

Role conflict may also be found in other areas of family life. Role reversal may occur, and this role reversal may produce role conflict. For example, aged and infirm parents, who are no longer physically or economically able to care for themselves,

may have to rely on their children's assistance. In such situations, the roles of nurturer and provider, which are usually carried out by parents, are assumed by the children. Role reversal may also occur in times of social change, as when people immigrate to a new country.

When the Montaño family immigrated to the United States from Cuba, the family constellation consisted of Mr. and Mrs. Montaño, their 6-year-old son, their 5-year-old son, and Mrs. Montaño's parents. At the time of immigration, no one in the family spoke English. The adult Montaños had difficulty learning English. However, their sons, who attended school with Americans, not only learned English but also learned many American customs. The children served as agents of acculturation and as translators for their parents and grandparents. At the age of 7, one son acted as a translator during such major family transactions as the purchase of a car and the signing of a business lease. Mrs. Montaño told a neighbor, "They (the children) know that we need them, not they need us."

Except for instances of role reversal, parents and other significant adults usually serve as role models for children.

▶ Power in the family

Power refers to the ability to act, to do, and to control others, while *authority* refers to the right to use power to command behavior, enforce rules, and make decisions.* In a family, authority is often based on the rank or position of members in the family hierarchy. For example, the mother and the father usually exercise absolute authority over young children, but, in the parents' absence, adolescent children may be "left in charge" of their younger siblings. Authority is thus delegated by the parents to the next in family rank.

At various stages of the developmental cycle of the domestic group, power in the family may need to be redistributed and diffused among family members to avoid a power struggle. For example, when children grow into adolescence, they usually

---

*Refer to Chapter 3 for a discussion of power.

want to assume some of the power held by their parents. Later in the developmental cycle, if adult children remain in or move back to the family home or if grandparents move in with the family, power and authority may again need to be redistributed. There may be times, however, when family members give ambiguous messages about the redistribution of power. For example,

---

When their children were young, Mr. and Mrs. Johnson held all the power in the family, and they exercised it authoritatively. As their children approached adolescence, the parents encouraged their children to call them by their first names and to express opinions openly. Mr. and Mrs. Johnson told the children that they were the equals of adults and should not acquiesce to the opinions of adults simply because they were adults. Yet the Johnsons continued to unilaterally set curfews for their children and to have the final say about whom the children could date and when and where the children could go on dates.

When power is unambiguously redistributed, it provides opportunity for the personal growth of family members. Failure to redistribute power or the ambiguous redistribution of power may engender power struggles, limit the opportunities for personal growth of family members denied a share of family power, and otherwise act as a stressor in the family system. Unless the family finds another level on which to operate, family relationships may be endangered (Van Servellen, 1984).

Although power is a dynamic in all families, different orientations toward power may be evidenced by different families and even among different members of the same family. McClelland (1975) has categorized power orientations, ranking them from stage I to stage IV. Stage IV behavior is indicative of more social and emotional maturity than is stage I behavior. However, extremism in any stage may be pathological. Table 5-4 describes the characteristics of each stage of power orientation.

These categories of power orientation can be applied to power in the family. For example, the powerful person in stage I may be an authoritative parent on whom other family members totally de-

TABLE 5-4   Power orientations

Stage	Characteristics
I	"I am strengthened by others." Individuals rely on others for strength. If association with a perceived powerful person is terminated, the individual may experience a loss of control and become hysterical or become dependent on food, drugs, or religion.
II	"I can strengthen myself." Individuals gain a sense of power by exerting control over their bodies (e.g., involved in exercise programs) or by amassing material possessions. Extremism may be exhibited through obsessive-compulsive behavior.
III	"I can control others." Individuals obtain a sense of power by competing with, manipulating, or outsmarting others. The object is to dominate others. Extremism may be exhibited by engaging in crime, personal violence, or smother love to gain control over others.
IV	"I am influenced by others to carry out my obligations." Individuals may subordinate their desires and views to those of a higher authority. Extremism may be exhibited by an inability to differentiate one's own desires and views from those of a higher authority. Such behavior is known as "messianism."

pend. In stage IV, the higher authority on which decisions are based may be the "good of the family" or "the good of the children."

Sometimes a family member who nominally holds power is not the actual power holder. For example, the members of a family might say that the father is the authority figure, but a family therapist might observe that the mother is the family disciplinarian and decision maker. In this instance, the father *nominally* holds power but the mother *actually* holds power. In another family, the parents might consider themselves family authority figures when, in actuality, the children wield power by manipulating their parents.

CULTURAL INFLUENCES ON FAMILY PROCESS

The United States is a culturally plural society; it consists of people from various ethnic and religious groups. Culture influences the values, ideology, behavior, and life-style not only of immigrants but also of second-, third-, and fourth-generation ethnic Americans (McGoldrick, 1982).

In the United States, the mass media, especially television, are extremely influential in the formation of people's impressions and attitudes about the world around them. Seal (1983), who has investigated the effects of television on children, believes that television is an important socializing agent, often rivaling parents and the school. An average child watches 4 to 6 hours of television a day. The effects of television are different for children than for adults. While most adults can differentiate between the playacting world of television and the real world, children often cannot. Young children have difficulty distinguishing between the fantasy that is depicted in many children's programs and reality. As an example, Seal (1983) tells about a youngster who was asked if *Sesame Street*'s Big Bird is real. The child answered, "No, that's a costume. Under the costume is a real bird."

Adolescents also are influenced by television viewing. According to Seal (1983), they watch, almost exclusively, adult programs and believe that these programs depict reality. Two factors contribute to the credibility that adolescents give to television programs: (1) adolescents have limited life experience with which to compare the world depicted by television, and (2) television programming has the sanction of adults (the parents who allow and often encourage them to watch television and the adults who develop the shows).

Through television viewing, children and adolescents learn to accept ethnic stereotypes. They incorporate into their self-systems stereotypes about the beliefs, customs, rituals, occupations, behaviors, and family forms of various ethnic groups. These ethnic stereotypes are usually disparaging, demeaning, and based on erroneous information (Seal, 1983). For example, the family ethics of Italian-Americans includes the importance of hard work, saving, self-sacrifice, and investing in real estate (including ownership of one's own home).

Yet the stereotype often presented by the media is that Italian-American men are uneducated manual laborers who engage in domestic violence against their wives and children and that Italian-American women are uneducated domestic "slaves" to their families (Gambino, 1983).

Studies have shown that, in addition to stereotyping ethnic groups, television rarely presents positive images of them. Also, in the decade of 1971 to 1981, blacks and Hispanics experienced a decline in their representation in television programming, while the representation of white Anglo-Saxon types increased. This situation contributes to (1) a homogenization that ignores the diversity in values, attitudes, and beliefs of different ethnic groups in the United States; (2) a decrease in the exposure of the viewing public to the language patterns, dress, foods, family forms, and other behaviors of ethnics, and (3) a paucity of ethnic role models. As a result, the nuclear family is usually depicted on television as the "normal" family form, and ethnic family role models are missing, misrepresented, or disparaging (Seggar, Haffen, and Hannonen-Gladden, 1981; Seal, 1983; Gambino, 1983).

Because many health professionals, including nursing students and nurses, have incorporated ethnic stereotyping into their self-systems, it is important to become aware of these stereotypes and to understand the way in which culture influences family life, family behavior, and family process.

The way in which a person conceives of his or her environment (the person's system of cognition*) may be thought of as a map. People from different cultures have different cultural maps. This fact offers an explanation for differences in cultural behavior and for differences in conceptualizations of the family. The degree of agreement or disagreement between different cultural groups about the images, meaning, and priority given to the family is sometimes used as an index of the psychocultural distance between groups. For example, Szalay and Maday (1983) found that there is greater similarity, and thus less psychocultural distance, in the perceptions that black and white Americans have

---

*See Chapter 4 for a discussion of culture and cognition.

about the family than there is between whites and Hispanic-Americans or between blacks and Hispanic-Americans. Therefore, it should not be assumed that all minority groups have similar orientations toward the family. For example, black Americans include a broad network of relatives and friends-like-family in their definition of the family (Kennedy, 1980). Chinese-Americans extend their definition of the family to include ancestors and all their descendants, and these descendants may be very influential in child rearing (Hsu, 1970; McGoldrick, 1982). For example,

---

A Chinese-American client explained to a community health nurse that when the American young couples in her neighborhood become ill, the grandparents often come to help out with the children. However, the grandparents are supposed to follow the rules of the house and not undermine the way in which the young couples have been raising their children. "With Chinese it is different. When grandparents visit, they can do anything they want with their grandchildren, even if it means going against the rules laid down by the parents. If Chinese parents should object to the overindulgence of the grandparents, they would be ridiculed, not sympathized with, by others. The same thing is true for the way that Chinese aunts and uncles care for their nephews and nieces."

Italian-Americans achieve identity as individuals through their roles, rights, and responsibilities in the family. The Italian-American family therefore provides its members not only with a sense of security but also with a sense of identity (Gambino, 1983).

Culture also influences the definition of life-cycle phases of individual family members. For instance, among Mexican-Americans, early and middle childhood usually encompasses a more protracted period of time than is customary among mainstream Americans. Mexican-American adolescence tends to cover a shorter period of time than does mainstream American adolescence. Moreover, among Mexican-Americans, middle age covers a larger block of time, permeating into what mainstream Americans define as old age.

Life-cycle rites of passage are also subject to cul-

tural influence. For instance, among Cuban-Americans, a girl's fifteenth birthday signifies her social transition from girlhood to womanhood. The occasion is marked by a *fiesta de quince años* (fifteenth birthday party), at which the *quince años* girl is presented to that segment of society that constitutes the family's meaningful social relationships (Pasquali, 1982). Likewise, among Jewish-Americans, when a child turns 13, a bar (bas) mitzvah marks the social and religious transition from childhood to adulthood. Among Irish-Americans, death is seen as one of the most significant life-cycle transitions, and they therefore stress wakes, while among Italian-Americans, marriage is an extremely important life-cycle transition, and they emphasize weddings (McGoldrick, 1982).

Cultural differences also influence the boundaries between families and the community. Hispanic-American families tend to have flexible boundaries. This boundary flexibility may be evidenced in child lending among Puerto Ricans (McGoldrick, 1982) or in preparing enough food so that unexpected guests may be invited to dinner among Cubans (Pasquali, 1982). For example, a Cuban woman told a nurse, "The difference between Cubans and Americans is, if my child is in an American home at dinnertime, they send her home. If their child is in my house at dinnertime, I ask her to stay for dinner." In contrast to the flexible family boundaries of Hispanic-Americans, Italian-American and Greek-American families tend to have rigid boundaries. Although Italians may incorporate friends of long and close association into the family, the boundary between the family and "outsiders" is usually rigid. The rigid family boundaries among Greeks partially reflect Greek emphasis on the "blood line" and tend to discourage the adoption of children (McGoldrick, 1982).

All of the aforementioned differences in orientation toward the family demonstrate the significant role played by culture. Middlefort (1980) explains that it is not unusual for a subsystem in a family to assume dominance. When the cultural subsystem dominates family life, there may be a lack of individuation and an emphasis on one's relationship to and responsibility for the family. When the psychological subsystem dominates family life, the individual is stressed and the influence of the family on the individual is weakened. The individual's independence from the natal family may then be viewed as a goal and as an indication of emotional maturity. Middlefort believes that most psychotherapists view the psychological subsystem as the dominant subsystem in the family and ignore the cultural subsystem. Psychotherapists therefore espouse the importance of individuals achieving independence from the family hierarchy and especially from their parents. This approach may not be appropriate for families in which the dominant family subsystem is the cultural.

GENOGRAMS

Construction of a genogram is one way for nurses to tap into the process of the family system over time. A genogram is an outgrowth of the genealogies that anthropologists have long used to learn about family relationships. Genograms depict family relationships over at least three successive generations.

Social scientists have developed guidelines for the construction of genograms. These guidelines provide some consensus about the type of information that should be gathered and how this information should be recorded. Male family members are represented by squares, females by circles. Birth dates, death dates, marriage dates, separation and divorce dates, educational levels, occupations, and nature of relationships (for example, conflicts among members; with whom family alliances are formed) could be indicated alongside each symbol on the genogram. In addition, to present a more holistic picture, nurses might also indicate place of residence, ethnicity, major illnesses, religious affiliation (or absence of one), frequency and types of contact among family members (for example, visits, letters, telephone calls), fictive kin relationships, and immigration dates (where appropriate). This additional information can help nurses to begin to identify cultural orientations, extrafamilial relationships, and the physical and social distance that exists among family members. For example, family members may live in geographic proximity to each other but only infrequently interact with one another, or they may live at great geographic distance from one another but maintain frequent contact through visits, letters, and telephone calls. Possibly

decisions are not made without the input of these geographically distant but socially close relatives. Fig. 5-2 shows a genogram that includes much of this information.

Genograms can be useful in two ways: (1) they can help clients gain better understanding of their own family systems, and (2) they can assist nurses to assess the dynamics of client-families and to identify family orientations and process patterns that have been perpetuated over generations.

CHAPTER SUMMARY

Family dynamics, family form, and who is defined as family are very much influenced by sociocultural factors. In addition to the various forms that a family may take and the members that it may encompass, nurses also need to consider what stage of the developmental cycle a family is experiencing. The concept of "family" also includes the interactions, relationships, and organizational patterns among members that serve to effectively meet the needs of family members and the expectations of society.

The family is a dynamic system and has the properties of any social system. The effective functioning of the family system is dependent on the interrelationship between the family and its context (physical, emotional, cultural, and social).

REFERENCES

Adams B: The family: a sociological interpretation, Chicago, 1980, Rand McNally & Con.

Bozett FW: Parenting concerns of gay fathers, Topics Clin Nurs 6(3):60-71, 1984.

Butler RN and Lewis MI: Aging and mental health: positive psychosocial and biomedical approaches, ed 3, St. Louis, 1982, The C.V. Mosby Co.

Critchley DL: The child as patient: assessing the effects of family stress and disruption on the mental health of the child, Persp Psychiatr Care 5(5 and 6):144-155, 1981.

Fife BL: A model for predicting the adaptation of families to medical crisis, Image 17(4):108-112, 1985.

Fortes M: Introduction, In Goody J, editor: The developmental cycle in domestic groups, London, 1958, The Syndics of the Cambridge University Press.

Gambino R: Plenary session presentation at the National Conference on Ethnicity and the Media, Italian-Americans and the media: building a positive image, New York, April 9, 1983.

Gilmore DD: The people of the plain: class and community in lower Andalusia, New York, 1980, Columbia University Press.

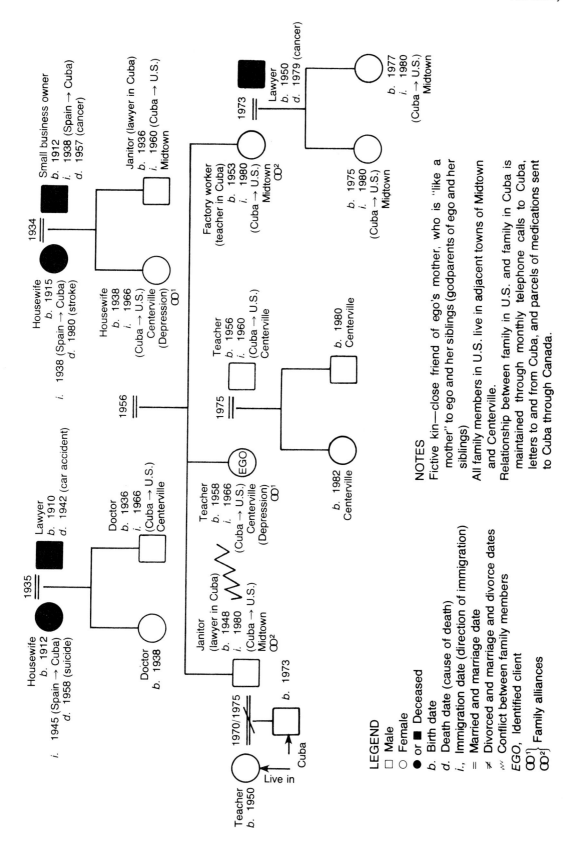

NOTES

Fictive kin—close friend of ego's mother, who is "like a mother" to ego and her siblings (godparents of ego and her siblings)

All family members in U.S. live in adjacent towns of Midtown and Centerville.

Relationship between family in U.S. and family in Cuba is maintained through monthly telephone calls to Cuba, letters to and from Cuba, and parcels of medications sent to Cuba through Canada.

Fig. 5-2 Genogram.

LEGEND

□ Male
○ Female
● or ■ Deceased
b. Birth date
d. Death date (cause of death)
i., Immigration date (direction of immigration)
= Married and marriage date
≠ Divorced and marriage and divorce dates
〰 Conflict between family members
EGO, Identified client
CO¹ }
CO² } Family alliances

SELF-DIRECTED LEARNING

Sensitivity-Awareness Exercises

The purposes of these exercises are to:

- Develop awareness about the dynamics, strengths, and limitations of your own family system and the family systems of clients
- Develop awareness about family orientations and process patterns that have been perpetuated over generations in your own family and in client families
- Develop awareness about the interrelationship between families and their context (physical, emotional, cultural, and social)

1. Construct a genogram of your family system. Be sure to include birth dates, death dates, marriage dates, separation and divorce dates, and immigration dates for family members. In addition, indicate educational levels, occupations, nature of relationships (for example, conflict among family members; alliances among family members), places of residence, ethnicity, major illnesses, religious affiliations (or nonaffiliation), frequency and types of contact among family members, and fictive kin relationships. On the basis of this genogram, how would you describe the dynamics in your family system? The physical and social distance among family members? The sociocultural orientation of family members? Next, construct a genogram for a client family and answer the aforementioned questions.

2. Use one or more of the following techniques to describe your family's dynamics: reviewing the family photograph album, writing a family history, drawing a family picture, or role playing.

3. Using a tape recorder or taking notes, prepare a life history of a grandparent, great-grandparent, or a sibling of such a family member (for example, a great aunt). This life history should contain the major people, relationships, and events in the person's life. You might start out by saying, "Tell me about your life when you were a child." This question might lead you to ask, "What was your life like when you were my age?" or "How was life the same (or different) then and now?" A life history will help you to better understand the beliefs, conceptualizations, and perceptions of past events of this family member.

Questions to Consider

1. The stage of the domestic cycle that may include both the "empty nest" and the "refilled nest" is

   a. expansion
   b. fission
   c. replacement

2. An increasing population of latchkey children may be traced to
   a. precocious school-age growth and development
   b. decreased number of women in the work force
   c. inadequate child care services
   d. family conflict about child care

3. The focus of analysis for the structural-functional family theory model is on
   a. relationships between the family and other social institutions
   b. internal functioning of the family
   c. role behavior of family members over time

4. According to McClelland, extremism in Stage III power orientation ("I can control others") may be exhibited by
   a. hysterical behavior
   b. obsessive-compulsive behavior
   c. violent behavior
   d. messianic behavior

5. Stereotyping and underrepresentation of ethnic groups in the media contributes to all *but* which of the following
   a. decreased exposure to the life-style of ethnics
   b. paucity of ethnic role models
   c. homogenization of values, attitudes, and beliefs
   d. exposure to ethnic diversity

Match the following terms:

6. Omnigenous family
7. Working parents
8. Extended family
9. Replacement
10. Concern of gay fathers

a. Encompasses at least three generations of kin
b. Stage of the domestic cycle
c. Self-disclosure to children
d. Blended family
e. Issue of child care

Answer key

1. b	6. d
2. c	7. e
3. a	8. a
4. c	9. b
5. d	10. c

Googins B and Burden D: Vulnerability of working parents: balancing work and home roles, Social Work 32(4):295-305, 1987.

Gubrium JF and Buckholdt DR: Describing care: image and practice in rehabilitation, Cambridge, Mass, 1982, Oelgeschlager, Gunn & Hain.

Hsu FLK: Americans and Chinese: reflections on two cultures and their people, New York, 1970, Doubleday & Co., Inc.

Jackson DD: The question of family homeostasis, Psychiatr Qu Suppl 1:79-90, 1957.

Johnson CL, Klee L, and Schmidt C: Conceptions of parentage and kinship among children of divorce, Am Anthropol 90(1):136-144, 1988.

Jones SL and Dimond M: Family theory and family therapy models: comparative review with implications for nursing practice, J Psychiatr Nurs Mental Health Serv 20(10):12-19, 1982.

Jordheim AE: Alternate life-styles and the family, In Reinhardt AM and Quinn, MD, editors: Family-centered community nursing: a sociocultural framework, vol 2, St. Louis, 1980, The C.V. Mosby Co.

Kennedy TR: You gotta deal with it: black family relations in a southern community, New York, 1980, Oxford University Press.

Kutzner SK and Toussie-Weingarten C: Working parents: the dilemma of child rearing and career, Topics Clin Nurs 6(3):30-37, 1984.

Maddox B: Married and gay, New York, 1982, Harcourt/Brace/Javanovich.

McClelland D: Power: the inner experience, New York, 1975, Irvington Publishers, Inc.

McGoldrick M: Ethnicity and family therapy, Fam Therapy Networker 6:22-26, 1982.

Meagher MAK: Separation, divorce, and subsequent coping problems of single-parent families, In Reinhardt AM and Quinn MD, editors: Family-centered community nursing: a sociocultural framework, vol 2, St. Louis, 1980, The C.V. Mosby Co.

Middlefort CF: Ethnic and religious factors in family illnesses, Bull Am Assoc Soc Psychiatr 1(3):16-21, 1980.

Miller B: Gay fathers and their children, Fam Coordinator 28:544-552, 1979.

Pasquali EA: Assimilation and acculturation of Cubans on Long Island, Ph.D. dissertation, State University of New York at Stony Brook, 1982.

Scheflen AE and Scheflen A: Body language and social order, Englewood Cliffs, NJ, 1972, Prentice-Hall, Inc.

Seal C: Television entertainment. Paper presented at the National Conference on Ethnicity and the Media, Italian-Americans and the media: building a positive image, New York, April 9, 1983.

Sedgwick R: Family mental health: theory and practice, St. Louis, 1981, The C.V. Mosby Co.

Seggar JF, Haffen JK, and Hannonen-Gladden H: Television's portrayals of minorities and women in drama and comedy drama, 1971-1981, Broadcasting 25:277-288, 1981.

Short Takes Part II: Newsday, November 30, p 2, 1987.

Smith AD and Reid WJ: Role expectations and attitudes in dual-earner families, Soc Casework 67(7):394-402, 1986.

Spindler LS: Culture change and modernization: mini-models and case studies, New York, 1977, Holt, Rinehart & Winston.

Szalay LB and Maday BC: Implicit culture and psychocultural distance, Am Anthropol 85:110-118, 1983.

Tiger L: Omnigamy: the new kinship system, Psychol Today 12:14, 1978.

Van Servellen GM: Group and family therapy: a model for psychotherapeutic nursing practice, St. Louis, 1984, The C.V. Mosby Co.

ANNOTATED SUGGESTED READINGS

Kutzner SK and Toussie-Weingarten C: Working parents: the dilemma of child and career topics, Clin Nurs 6(3):30-37, 1984.
The authors examine the parenting dilemmas of working couples. The authors then give suggestions of how nurses can help working parents as well as each other cope with the stressors engendered by the demands of job and family.

Googins B and Burden D: Vulnerability of working parents: balancing work and home roles, Soc Work 32(4):295-300, 1987.
This study explores the impact of working women on traditional family roles and responsibilities. Groups that are vulnerable to decreased physical and emotional well-being as a consequence of family role strain are identified.

Johnson CL, Klee L, and Schmidt C: Conceptualizations of parentage and kinship among children of divorce, Am Anthropol 90(1):136-144, 1988.
The authors examine the profound changes occurring in family form as a result of divorce. The research report focuses on children's perceptions of kinship systems in omnigenous families and the effect of gender differences on children's conceptualization of kinship after parental divorce and remarriage.

FURTHER READINGS

Adams B: The family: a sociological interpretation, Chicago, 1980, Rand McNally & Co.

Brazelton TB: Issues for working parents, Am J Orthopsychiatr 56(1):14-25, 1986.

Levant R: Sociological and clinical models of the family: an attempt to identify paradigms, Am J Fam Ther 8:5-20, 1980.

McBride AB: Mental health effects of women's multiple roles, Image 20(1):41-47, 1988.

Human development

CHAPTER FOCUS

A nurse must understand that the process of human development is crucial to the accurate assessment of clients. There is a variety of perspectives on how and why a person develops in the manner he or she does. Cognitive, cultural, economic, physiological, and psychological factors are thought to influence the development of each personality in various ways, making it unique. In this chapter, an eclectic view of the operation of these factors will be presented. The role of culture and its impact on the socialization of a human being will be identified as one of the major factors in the process called "development."

Personality can be described as progressing along a chronological schema. The philosophies of human development of four major theorists—Freud, Sullivan, Erikson, and Piaget—will be discussed. Incorporated within this discussion will be the concept of vulnerability and its subsequent impact on healthy adaptation. Mental health and mental illness will be presented as reflecting a dynamic continuum on which types of human behavior can be placed. Such a continuum reflects the fact that health is a dynamic state, constantly interacting with external and internal forces.

Knowledge of the needs and tasks associated with a particular stage of development, and of the tools required to accomplish those tasks, is significant to nurses in making accurate assessments regarding recurrent behavior patterns and their implications. Data from such assessments can then be used to determine areas in which further learning is necessary for a client to develop appropriate skills to meet developmental tasks. A brief discussion of Maslow's hierarchy of needs will be presented, along with its implications for personality development. This portion of the chapter will present each developmental era—infancy, childhood, and so on—as an interrelationship of the many factors that influence the development of a person's unique personality. The concept of dying and death as the final phase of life will be discussed, and strategies of nursing assessment and intervention will be presented.

UNDERLYING DYNAMICS
Socialization and personality

The process of personality development is a complex one that is often misunderstood or misinterpreted because individuals who study personality do so according to their own inclinations. For example, a social-learning theorist might disagree strongly with a cultural anthropologist or a traditional psychoanalyst on the interpretation of a particular incident. Different strategies of intervention result. The question, however, is not which intervention is correct but rather which intervention is most effective in terms of client response and positive directional change. A therapist who refuses to see that an approach is, in fact, ineffective is not helping the client. Nurses therefore must be aware of the varying psychological, sociocultural, and biological factors present. They must have a basic understanding of each factor and its implications. Culture is the first of these variables that will be presented.

We assume that one function of a culture is to inculcate the young with prescribed conceptual, moral, ethical, and behavioral standards. The continuation of the society is thus ensured, and socialized beings are produced. Our focus as nurses, however, is the *individual* and his or her unique responses. We will be aware of shared personality characteristics, yet the critical emphasis will be on individuals and their socialization into roles within the culture as a whole.

A human being is not a closed system ruled or governed by a given nature; a human being is an open system. He or she creates and imposes order of an acquired nature. An individual exists within the framework of culture and society as a being whose needs, attitudes, values, and behavior are defined and made meaningful in the social and cultural milieu. A variety of social types, diversified in time and space, results. Individuals can be viewed as having a common structure of probabilities that can only be realized in a cultural context. By first realizing that personality always comes into being in a cultural context, we can then consider how common cultural materials are utilized by individuals, rendering them unique beings. Although there are similarities in the composition of different personalities, individuals retain differences because of the unique ways they respond to and integrate various cultural patterns and traits. We can say that before their encounters with others, human beings are nothing substantial. They require the presence of others to stimulate the development of cognition, emotion, and, ultimately, sense of self.

Needs, as an aspect of personality, are noncognitive in origin. They can be divided into two categories: biological needs—such as thirst, hunger, and the need to eliminate—and needs acquired through interaction with society—such as the needs for affiliation and sense of self-worth. We need to bear in mind, however, that biological needs are themselves influenced by culture. For example, the need to eliminate is panhuman; however, each society has its own attitudes toward this need. What is considered modesty in one society might be considered inhibition in another. Nurses need to be aware that societal expectations are reflected in behavior clients use to meet needs.

Attitudes, as well as needs, reflect cultural orientation. Like needs, attitudes are major integrative forces in the development of personality; they give a sense of consistency to an individual's behavior. Attitudes are cognitive in origin. They are formed through interactions with the social environment. Attitudes serve to direct an individual's attention to his or her particular commitments and responsibilities. In a sense, they act as guidelines for the individual's present existence and help shape the future for the individual and for his or her progeny. An individual soon learns to attend to particular aspects of his or her environment on the basis of an attitudinal system. Ideas, social situations, and other people are grouped according to a person's "frame of reference," his or her own personal guidelines. Although overall cultural norms are reflected in an individual's tightly knit attitudinal system, they are integrated differently in each personality.

We have been placing various components of the individual into separate categories. Thompson (1975) states that the construction of these parts into some semblance of a being within a cultural context requires an entity that acts as coordinator. That entity is the concept of self—a basic requirement for the sound psychological functioning of the human animal.

Self-concept is a major variable in the development of healthy patterns of behavior. A person's self-concept is the person's view of his or her own strengths and weaknesses; it is the person's perception of self based on reflected appraisals from the environment. Self-concept, then, is an accumulation of what others think of a person as well as the person's own exploratory activities that assist the person in understanding his or her world.

One of the most salient features of the self-concept is its ability to grow, to become more sophisticated in acquiring and applying knowledge and experience. In early infancy, the self-concept is virtually nonexistent. However, as infants begin to experience themselves as being different from their environment, their motor activity increases. As children develop the tool of language, they become more capable of differentiating themselves from other objects and persons in the environment. Accomplishments bring positive reinforcement from significant persons, which serves to strengthen self-concept.

The mores of a culture are internalized and become such an integral part of a person that self-concept cannot be understood without cultural considerations. Internal needs and societal expectations are meshed to permit the individual as a social being to achieve a measure of consistency between the inner and outer selves.

The development of a positive self-concept allows an individual to experience a wide range of activities without feeling threatened. A perception of the world emerges that is unique to each person. As positive experiences accumulate, an individual's

self-concept is further enhanced. The individual who repeatedly encounters failure develops a poor self-concept, which is perpetuated through a phenomenon that amounts to a self-fulfilling prophecy. A person with a poor self-concept might continue to perceive his or her world in the most restricted sense unless the person can begin to perceive himself or herself as competent according to societal norms and values. A poor self-concept eventually results in maladaptive coping measures. One of our primary concerns as nurses is assisting such an individual to effect change that will potentiate a positive self-concept. This nursing function will be discussed further in this chapter, in the discussions of self-concept in relation to parent-child interactions and self-esteem.

It is evident that an individual can inherit biological characteristics, such as body size, weight, eye color, and hair color. However, the qualities that identify an individual as a human being are those which may not be genetically transmitted— thought patterns, emotions, and behavior responses, although some theorists indicate that certain types of behavior are in fact genetically transmitted. Those characteristics identified as congenital are passed on during the gestation period. However, our cultural heritage is acquired through our relationships with others. Even characteristics that seem to be predominantly biological can be related to cultural experience. For example, positive living conditions might be characteristic of a particular civilization because they are valued entities. The same factors might not be in evidence in another civilization, perhaps because they are not valued. A society might limit the availability of affection, physical warmth, and light. In such a case, an individual's physical growth as well as his or her emotional development might be retarded. Body size and weight might tend to be less than in a culture that placed a premium on factors that enhance these characteristics.

Locke and Rousseau were the first to oppose the view that the infant entered this world with a built-in set of responses—a mini-adult who had already been programmed for eternity. Locke introduced the concept of the *tabularasa*—that the newborn infant resembles a blank slate. The infant learns from the environment how, when, and eventually why he or she should respond. Itard, in his famous work with the Wild Boy of Aveyron, expanded this concept. This young child of about 11 or 12 had the characteristic behavior of a wild animal, posturing himself on all fours, scratching and biting those who came near him. He had no awareness of social restrictions on behavior. He operated on an immediate-gratification principle. It was apparent that there was little instinctive basis for rules of socialization. The young boy had adapted to his environment as would any animal in similar circumstances. When the Wild Boy was found by Frenchmen in 1799, he was compared to persons living in a European cultural environment. By European standards he was a freak, a subhuman. Although this case is an extreme example, it serves to point out the individual differences that result from the socialization process.

It is of little importance to identify one specific factor—biological, psychological, social, cultural—as having more impact on development than another. Behavior and development have a multifactorial base.

However, recognizing the role of culture is particularly relevant in nursing. By recognizing the impact of culture on behavioral responses, the nurse makes available a broadened scope of assessment and intervention strategies. Let us consider some examples of what might have previously been identified as having a strictly biological base. The sensory nerve endings respond to heat and cold. However, this response can be culturally as well as biologically induced. A certain element of learned response develops as children are repeatedly warned not to touch something because it is hot. Parents are continually requiring children to put their coats on when the temperature falls to a certain point. Thus a child might not have been biologically triggered, yet he or she puts on a sweater. In addition, culturally determined dietary preferences affect nutrition, and culturally determined mating preferences affect genetic pools.

Biological factors can be subject to environmental modification. A child who has been locked in a closet for the first 2 years of life will probably be retarded in motor development. Culture provides a milieu in which an individual can exercise his various options. A person may be biologically ready for

a higher-level task yet not have learned from his or her culture what the level means or how to reach it. The tools may be missing. We can look at a variety of situations in which a child may be identified as slow or backward based on the fact that he or she is biologically ready for a task but not performing it. For example, the sphincter of the bladder may be developed and functional, yet the child continues to have wet pants. Perhaps the child has not been socialized into a realization that this behavior is viewed negatively by the culture. A child's legs and arms may be coordinated sufficiently to propel him or her over to someone else; however, the question arises of what to do then. Is the answer to that question part of the process of socialization into a particular role by the culture? Socialization into roles continues into adulthood, and each individual may be socialized into a variety of roles. One of the prime examples of the socialization process is learning the roles of receiver of health care and health care provider.

In summary, we view the individual as emerging from a cultural context. A human being is born with the biological readiness to perform many functions; however, culture provides the basic materials for personality development, such as value systems, a knowledge base, and fundamental beliefs. Each individual then combines biological and cultural equipment in a unique way to emerge as a personality different from all others. The culture in turn is molded by the individual in a sort of circular pattern. It is necessary to state at this point that, although individuals share personality traits, a true group personality never exists. As we pointed out in Chapter 4, we use the concept of "basic group identity" to refer to shared traits rather than to a single personality type characteristic of an entire culture.

Factors influencing personality development

It seems appropriate to the discussion of personality development that we provide an overview of some of the many "panphasic" factors, or factors that span all the developmental epochs. We suggest that these influences be called to mind as one assesses an individual in relationship to his or her developmental status. Too often human beings are simply categorized into eras, task groups, or age groups for diagnostic purposes without considering such factors as parent-child relationships, intelligence, self-concept, genetic transmission, age, sex, and child-rearing practices. We have identified three general categories for the purpose of discussion: psychological, biological, and sociocultural.

PSYCHOLOGICAL FACTORS

The parent-child relationship has been the center of attention during the past decade or so, particularly since the studies of Bowlby and Spitz. The primary concern of theorists has been the impact of the parent, initially the mother, on the early development of the child. Bowlby (1973) found that the infant develops a strong sense of attachment to the mothering figure and quite vigorously protests her (or his) leaving. The implication is that the persistent attitudes and styles of the parental figure are imprinted on the child at a very early age and that the resulting value system pervades the developmental span until some point in young adulthood, when the individual is able to strike out alone.

▶ Family relationships

The nature of the family relationships that develop is crucial to each family member. It is within the family system that identification occurs, a major factor in personality development. We note that identification is particularly relevant to the oedipal phase but that it does, in fact, occur throughout the developmental cycle. Shifts in identification result from positive interpersonal relationships with others in the social system.

An infant who is isolated cannot develop into a mature, well-integrated individual. Indeed, physical growth itself must be facilitated by a system that nurtures, educates, and enculturates. The family unit is the chief molder of personality. It is a system that provides an atmosphere for the testing of unfamiliar techniques of adaptation. Within the family, one can become familiar with roles and institutions. There is a sense of stability and integration, a home base to which one may always return. The enculturating capacities of parents impinge upon children during whatever phase they may be in; they transcend all phases. Enculturation is a generational process. Each parent brings a value system and

characteristics of personality into a mating relationship. Offspring are produced, and the values and personality characteristics of the parents influence the development of those offspring.

It is important to note the deleterious influences that parents can have upon the personality development of children. The parent who feels little self-esteem and who has a poor image of himself or herself has difficulty responding to a child in a manner that promotes a positive self-concept in the child. For example, 7-year-old Jamie brings home his first homework assignment. After completing it, he asks his mother to check it for him. She repeatedly makes comments such as, "Are you sure this is the way you were supposed to do it?" and "Did the teacher tell you this was alright?" These comments reflect the parent's inability to accept the child's actions as being correct and indicate the parent's dependence on an authority figure. She is uncomfortable with accepting the responsibility for her own actions, and this message is transmitted to her child. The child thus is led to question his own abilities, a situation that results in a distorted estimation of them.

The effect of parental influence may be quite positive during one phase of development and quite negative during another. A mother may develop a sound relationship with her infant, based on the comfort she experiences in being depended upon. However, if the mother is unable to relinquish this relationship, the child may suffer the consequences in later periods of personality development.

Self-concept evolves out of the parent-child interaction and functions as a mediator of development. Parents and children interact with one another; in this process a self-concept is continually evolving for each family member, as was discussed earlier. Each self-concept reflects the appraisals of significant others in the environment. Thus family life nurtures each child, providing strong affectional and relational bonds. As Satir (1975) points out in *Peoplemaking*, parents have the tremendous responsibility of facilitating the development of a positive self-concept and a sound sense of self-esteem.

It is necessary to identify the meaning of self-esteem as it relates to self-concept. An individual with a healthy self-concept is able to integrate the appraisals reflected from his or her environment and to accept personal strengths and weaknesses. Self-esteem grows out of this positive self-concept; individuals with high self-esteem feel they are worthwhile in spite of mistakes or defeats. They feel capable of achieving realistically determined goals and accept responsibility for their actions. They do not have to be right all the time; when they fail, they reassess their coping skills and develop another plan. They perceive failure not as total defeat but rather as an opportunity to develop an alternative plan of action.

Parents with high senses of self-esteem are able to provide an atmosphere in which children feel comfortable with their self-concepts and their emerging identities. There are no obligations attached to behavior and no conditions for reward. Unmet parental needs do not become a burden to the next generation. Each child is free to "be." Conditions within the family system are such that trust, a secure identity, and a sense of autonomy are valued. In appropriate situations, children are permitted to explore the decision-making process and to experience independence. They are not forced to play out a symbiotic relationship to meet the needs of their parents.

Parents who are unsure of themselves or their own worth often unconsciously set up circumstances very much like ones they themselves experienced as children. Feelings of "bad me," guilt, and shame, which produce low self-esteem, are evoked in their own children just as they were evoked in themselves many years before. Unreasonable punishment and, ultimately, withdrawal of expression of love cause children of such parents to feel that their behavior must be unworthy if it has caused these responses from the persons they consider significant—their parents. They believe that they must truly be "bad." A pattern has been established that continues from generation to generation.

One needs to feel positive about one's self—aware of both limitations and strengths—before one can invest actively and positively in another human being. Such is the case in the parent-child relationship. If parents have experienced smooth developmental courses and if they are aware of

their own needs, they will be more able to share a sound, nurturing relationship with their children.

▶ Self-concept

A positive self-concept, initiated in the toddler period and nurtured throughout the developmental span, enables an individual to meet each challenge as it comes and to deal with it appropriately. Problems are viewed not as insurmountable obstacles but as potential learning situations. It would be unrealistic to say that each possible impediment is viewed with gleeful delight. A person with a strong sense of self recognizes that he or she has a wide range of capabilities, yet also acknowledges limitations. Such a person realizes that it is acceptable to work within the framework of those limitations. At each developmental level, the parameters of those limitations are altered. The individual with a healthy sense of self is able to adapt to those alterations.

Self-concept correlates with many factors, some of which will be discussed at greater length later in this chapter. A person whose self-evaluations are negative tends to experience consistently high levels of anxiety, which in turn lead to less positive interactions with peers. An individual with a poor self-concept feels a sense of powerlessness to change roles, thus perpetuating a cycle of feeling victimized. This sense of inability to bring about change can be connected with the perception of an external locus of control—the feeling that one has no real opportunity to actively effect change, that it is in the hands of fate. In contrast, a person with a positive self-concept has a sense of active participation in the environment and feels able to determine realistic life goals. These patterns serve to reinforce the notion that the self is the organizing factor in the personality.

Although each individual is unique, everyone is affected by interactions with the environment, and the process by which interactions affect a person is roughly the same for everyone. All aspects of human development interact, responding continuously to experiential and constitutional factors.

An individual's personality is a reflection of his or her input into the process of personality development. How one speaks to another person or how one puts thoughts into actions determines the response one receives from the environment. Environmental responses, in turn, determine behavior. Reciprocity exists in that the behavior of one individual has an impact on that of another, and vice versa. There is a continuous exchange of communication (both verbal and nonverbal) between persons (see Chapter 10). Future behavioral patterns are influenced by those interactions.

▶ Intelligence

One individual characteristic that is very relevant to personality development is intelligence. Intelligence is the aptitude or capacity for learning and includes problem-solving ability. Intelligence is biologically determined by virtue of the fact that a person inherits a nervous system. However, experiences provided by the environment may retard or facilitate the development of cognitive skills.

Differences in intelligence appear as early as infancy and gradually become more apparent during the childhood and adolescent years. The ability to reason through complex situations has many implications for personality development. Intelligence has a profound impact on many areas of development and behavior, such as talking, memory, understanding and applying new concepts, and creativity. It seems that children who learn rapidly and who can apply their knowledge develop a more positive self-concept—as a result of praise received from parents and teachers—than children who are poor achievers. They assume positions of leadership more frequently, recognize their limitations more readily, and are able to look at themselves and laugh when appropriate.

Intelligence was once considered completely hereditary. However, published studies have demonstrated that heredity is not the only factor. The effect of environment can no longer be negated. Children who were born to parents with low IQs who were then adopted by parents of average or high IQs have been shown to be able to reach the educational levels of their adoptive parents (McCandless and Evans, 1973)

Educational experiences play a definitive role in the development of intelligence, particularly during infancy and the preschool and adolescent periods. Thus parents need to provide an atmosphere that facilitates learning during these critical periods. Personality development will be enhanced, and a positive self-concept will be promoted.

▶ Loss

Object loss is discussed at length in the chapter on aggression against oneself (Chapter 22). However, it is relevant here to note the impact that loss has on personality development. Bowlby (1973) compares loss to separation from the mother figure. The manner in which loss is resolved, if in fact it is resolved, is crucial to the development of a positive sense of self and the ability to invest in trusting relationships. Although the interrelationship between positive self-concept and personality development has been emphasized several times in this book, we believe that it bears repetition. The sense of security one has in dealing with loss will be reflected in personality development over and over again. Since life is characterized by a series of losses, it is in this arena that nurses must focus to develop primary preventive strategies.

▶ Coping skills

The ability to cope with a variety of situations reflects an awareness of one's strengths and limitations and indicates a capacity to tap one's resources as necessary. Of great importance to personality development is the type of coping mechanism utilized as well as the degree and frequency to which it is called into play. For example, an individual may learn a coping skill such as the internalization of stress and its expression through a physiological route. This mechanism of reducing tension, learned in early interactions with significant persons in the environment, is then carried on throughout the life cycle. The nature of such early coping experiences and parental responses to them have a profound influence on future personality development. Coping skills that include an honest, open sharing of feelings provide the setting for the development of a sound sense of self. Coping skills that are rooted in, or fixated at, early levels of psychosexual development color the emerging personality. The terms *oral personality* and *anal personality* indicate levels of development in which individuals can be rooted. For example, the anal personality is characterized by a coping repertoire that includes retentive kinds of behavior with little sharing of feelings. An individual with this type of personality is stingy on a material level as well as an emotional level.

The nursing profession, by definition, had historically directed much of its effort toward secondary prevention. However, primary prevention efforts have awakened the awareness of parents on behalf of their children to facilitate the development of healthy coping skills during early childhood periods.

BIOLOGICAL FACTORS

The relationship of neurochemistry to the development of personality is a striking one. Two key hormones, androgen and estrogen, affect not only the biological sexual orientation but also the psychological assumption of sex roles. Aggression and maternalism are two types of behavior that are affected by these hormones. Androgen levels correlate positively with aggressive tendencies, and estrogen levels correlate positively with maternalistic tendencies. The neurochemical effect of hormones also has an impact on growth rates, weight, and bone ossification. Everyone grows at a different rate, a fact that is apparent if we look at a class of first-graders. There may be differences in height of as much as 8 inches. Size definitely affects the kinds of activities a child engages in and how he or she is perceived by peers. A boy who is considerably smaller than his classmates is often called a "runt" and may not be asked to participate in physical activities such as football or basketball. He may then assume a passive role among his peerage. Because of a biological "hand of fate," his personality development will have taken a particular course; the course might have been different if he had been larger. Thus a simple biological fact of life such as growth rate can have a wide-ranging effect on overall personality development. Again, the interrelatedness of biological and cultural factors is apparent.

The biological factors involved in personality development cannot be discussed without reference to the concept of maturation. Maturation is the process of developmental changes, a process that is controlled by genetic factors.

► Genetics

What is the significance of genetics to personality development? Various personal characteristics, such as physical appearance, motor activity, emotional reactivity, and energy level, are strongly related to genetic composition. Intellectual characteristics—and, to some degree, social characteristics—are shaped by heredity. As an individual matures, he or she experiences certain expected developmental changes. The timetable that controls these changes is laid down by genes yet may be vastly altered by environmental variables. Even under similar environmental conditions, it is quite possible that two male siblings will reach adolescence at very different times.

The task of nursing involves recognition of two basic facts: (1) each individual occupies his or her own given space on the developmental continuum, and (2) variables such as health care, stress, cultural expectations, and chronic illness affect an individual's rate of maturation irrespective of a genetic timetable. With these facts in mind, nurses can devise primary preventive strategies that promote optimum conditions for the development of each individual's unique personality.

► Age

Chronological age is probably one of the most common criteria used to categorize human development. Certain observable types of behavior have been identified for each particular age group. Within each age level, these common characteristics are studied in respect to frequency, variety, complexity, and organization. Mental age as well as chronological age need to be considered; individuals in the same chronological age group may have very different mental ages.

Obviously, there are significant limitations to the discussion of personality development in terms of chronological age. When age is considered alone, the very factors that we have just been discussing—genetic timetables and environmental influences—are negated. To say that a child is older is simply not sufficient to account for increased reading ability, for example. Many experiential factors need to be studied. Since environment plays such a great role in development, we need to identify

ate an atmosphere in which discussions about relationships (one vs. several), intimacy, feelings, lovemaking (when to and when not to), child bearing, and alternative forms of sexual expression (such as homosexuality or bisexuality) can occur. Development of a sense of responsibility in regard to one's "right" to be sexual and to exercise choices in sexual expression comes out of respect for others as well as respect for self. An environment that encourages discussion of sexual issues and their ramifications can only reinforce that concept of respect. Affirmation of one's sexual being, which cannot be separated from one's physical, emotional, intellectual, sociocultural, and spiritual dimensions, enables one to strive for high-level wellness.

No single determinant can be said to account for sexual behavior. It results from the interaction of biological, psychological, and sociocultural factors.

Biological determinants of sexual behavior have historically been rooted in the concept of instinct. Sex, in one sense, is the innate drive to mate and to reproduce. Yet in lower animals there is no awareness that coitus leads to pregnancy—a fact that leads one to believe that humans as well as lower animals engage in sexual activity for pleasurable reasons. Sex appears to involve a psychological drive that is correlated with feelings of pleasure, which can be traced back to the "pleasure centers"—the thalamus, the hypothalamus, and the mesencephalon. When these centers are electrically stimulated, animals experience pleasurable feelings of varying intensities.

One's sexuality is reflected in the complex interaction of the hypothalamus, the pituitary gland, and the gonads. This system is responsible for the stimulation and regulation of the hormones necessary for sexual development and activity. During intrauterine life the fetus seems to be under the direct influence of hormones, a situation that reflects a greater degree of genetic determination of sex roles and behaviors than is the case during the ensuing years of development. It appears that as an individual approaches adulthood, sexual roles and behaviors reflect the impact of cultural influences. Indirect data suggest that there is a prenatal influence, by fetal hormones, on the hypothalamus. This influence is exerted in a subtle manner

throughout the life cycle. However, there needs to be an awareness of the interaction of these innate, biological factors and the environmental factors that facilitate the expression of those factors.

Thus it is inaccurate to view sexuality from the singular perspective of biological determination. Psychological factors may be considered expressions of underlying biological sexual instincts. For example, Freud believed that libido (sex drive) was the psychological representation of a biological sexual instinct. Psychological determinants may exist in the form of learned patterns of behavior. Motivation may be mediated through the brain yet have at its base such learned patterns. Sexual behavior, its expression and purpose, may be learned through psychological and sociocultural mechanisms.

Sexuality can be viewed as an interpersonal process in which one individual chooses to share with and relate to a significant other. The process involves the experiencing of interrelated emotional, psychological, and physiological changes that are pleasurable to each partner. Each person enables the other to realize the potential for sexual fulfillment while recognizing the partner's as well as his or her own strengths and limitations. (See Chapter 7.)

SOCIOCULTURAL FACTORS

Child-rearing practices, as a major component of the cultural context, had been relatively ignored by social scientists until the 1950s. Concepts such as Freud's Oedipus complex and the family romance were applied universally with little regard for cultural variations. This is not to say that these psychoanalytic constructs should be negated; instead, their usefulness should be expanded. This can be accomplished most readily if they are linked to the cultural environment in which people and their symbols live. For example, Malinowski's (1927) study of the Trobriand Islanders, a society with a matrilineal and avunculocal psychological defense system, found that a male child developed a hatred of his mother's brother rather than his own father. Thus the Freudian concept has limitations. The primary point to draw from this study is that although the family romance exists, it differs from culture to culture. Thus we could say that Freud's work, although substantially valid, is not necessarily completely valid for every culture.

Whiting (1953) conducted a great deal of research in the area of cultural expectations, child-rearing practices, and individual development. They noted that excessive deprivation of affection during childhood could be correlated with pathological responses in later life and with related cultural beliefs.

As has been stated throughout this book, the impact of cultural context on personality development cannot be minimized. The interaction of biological, psychological, and cultural factors in the lifelong process called personality development cannot be ignored.

▶ Socioeconomic status

Socioeconomic status, social class, and social status are virtually synonymous. The educational level one's parents attained, the occupations they pursue, and the income they receive all contribute to one's social status. It is important to look at these functional correlates of an individual's particular class. What does being a part of an identifiable class mean? How do these correlates affect personality development?

Families of the middle class, whose members are often well-educated and have certain advantages, have been compared with families of the lower class, whose members are often poorly educated and have few community resources. There is a marked difference in family stability between the two groups, with a concurrent effect on parent-child relationships. It is within the realm of these relationships that the effects of socioeconomic status on personality development can be noted. The middle class tends to raise children to be high achievers, to control their emotions, and to share thoughts and ideas with their parents. The environment is one in which cultural, physical, and intellectual opportunities are available and encouraged. Value is placed on the appreciation of music and art. Advantaged families may be more liberal than disadvantaged families in child-rearing practices, possibly because, as Zigler (1970) suggests, they have more time and the vocabulary to devote to democracy. Physical punishment is less likely to be used in advantaged families. In contrast, the frus-

trations of little money, time, and energy may cause the less advantaged family to release pent-up tension through excessive physical punishment or child abuse. Children from less advantaged families tend not to do well on standardized tests (possibly because of cultural variations) or to learn as quickly in school (perhaps because of a self-fulfilling prophecy on the part of teachers). Children from disadvantaged families also tend to feel less secure about their own self-concepts, a situation that has significant effects on personality development.

We do not mean to imply that a person from a lower-class family is always doomed to failure or that a person from a middle-class family always achieves his or her optimal level of being. The task of nurses is to recognize that the developmental rate can be seriously impeded by conditions of poverty. These conditions need not be restricted to less advantaged families as defined by socioeconomic criteria. As is seen more and more often, children from "good" families can experience difficulty in adjusting to life situations and can have poor self-concepts. A socioemotional poverty can exist in a setting in which material goods are provided but little else. Parents who are caught up in enhancing their own status may show little concern for the emotional needs of their children.

Such data can be useful in the area of primary prevention. By being aware that certain conditions promote positive personality development while others do not, parents can make efforts to provide situations in which learning and growth are facilitated.

▶ Religion

Religion is a factor that affects personality development in general and child-rearing practices, family stability, and self-concept in particular. Child-rearing practices may be heavily influenced by religious beliefs. For example, the Protestant ethic ("good, hard work will accomplish all") may be transmitted to a child through a no-nonsense approach on the part of the parent. In such a family, the expression of feelings may be viewed as frivolous and unacceptable. In a family of another religious orientation, discipline may not be considered as important.

Knowledge, attitudes, and problem-solving

methods may be influenced by religious affiliation. A child pursuing a parochial school education may develop attitudes and values somewhat different from those developed by a child in public school. Differences in motivational levels may be accounted for, in part, by differences in religious background. Even if religion does not play a particularly important role in a family's child-rearing practices, it still can have a profound influence on the development of moral and ethical standards.

▶ **Education**

Education, although the last factor to be discussed here, is one of the most influential in personality development. Differences in problem-solving capacity, initiative, creativity, and self-concept have been noted among children who have attended different schools. Our goal is not to trace these differences to their respective sources but rather to recognize their implications for the developing personality. Hoy and Applebury (1970) suggest that the most important aspects of the school experience are peer relationships and student-teacher relationships. Students generally see teachers as role models and agents for change. Unfortunately, however, some teachers are instrumental in giving students negative attitudes about themselves. If a teacher considers a student primarily in terms of the student's race, social class, or ethnicity rather than in humanistic terms, a self-defeating cycle can be produced.

It has been shown by various studies that schools are direct reflections of the communities in which they exist. Therefore, it is logical to assume that they meet the needs of their students. However, this is not always the case, particularly in school districts composed of large groups of minorities but administered primarily by members of the middle class (see Chapter 4 for further discussion). For individual development to be enhanced, the values of the school must be consonant with those of the community. Each group must be working toward the same end. For example, if a school supports the notion of a college education for all its students, but the community views its members as blue-collar workers with little need for a college education, the student is caught in the middle. In such a situation, the effectiveness of the school is impaired and the

student is left with unmet needs and a feeling of frustration. Once the values and goals of community, teachers, and students are in consonance, the impact on personality development will be in a more positive, growth-promoting direction (McCandless and Evans, 1973).

• • •

Although a wide range of variables has been considered in terms of their impact on personality development, the most important concept is the interrelatedness of these factors. Biological factors are subject to environmental modification. A child raised in a vacuum, unable to learn from his or her environment, will be severely retarded in perceptual and motor development. Cognitive processes will also be affected. An individual's self-concept is greatly influenced by constitutional factors such as body height and weight. Genes determine the developmental timetable, but the timetable responds to environmental modifications.

Nurses are not as much concerned with determining the degree each component plays in the development of the individual personality as they are with recognizing that this interaction occurs and understanding its implications for the emerging personality.

Effect of early experiences on personality development

We have discussed in previous sections the impact of early life experiences on personality development. Adaptive mechanisms in early life may be quite primitive, yet they act as prototypes for future reactions to stress.

Freudian theory has emphasized the fact that a "foundation for pathology" is laid in the early years. This concept may be taken a step further, away from strict psychoanalytic concepts, if we view early sociocultural or environmental experiences as being significant to the development of personality disturbances later in life. It can be said that, regardless of whether psychosexual development is maturational, the response of a child's caretaker and the environment in which the child exists at the time of each stage serve to influence personality development.

The energy that is invested in the tasks of each stage, the tension that arises in stressful circumstances, and the coping skills that emerge result in patterns that serve as models for future adjustment to the same circumstances. Freud (1916) states that as a consequence of each stage, a certain amount of libidinal energy is fixated at that stage, building certain defenses and expectations into the personality. Major psychopathology occurs when too much libido or energy is fixated at an early stage, because the coping patterns developed at those early stages are not applicable to problem solving in adult life. In such an instance, the adult tends to use coping mechanisms that are not effective and that are not appropriate to his or her level of intelligence.

Probably the very first anxiety experience is that engendered by the birth process. The fetus moves quite rapidly from the warm, dark, quiet, and relatively safe environment of the womb into a bright, almost tumultuous environment. How does the infant respond to this barrage of stimuli? The adaptive mechanisms he or she develops become models for future adaptations.

The infant devises a number of methods of dealing with incoming stimuli. He or she selectively attends to stimuli, filtering out those he or she cannot or does not want to attend to. This cannot be done on a voluntary basis; however, the infant can focus on a specific activity that effectively blocks out other stimuli. He or she also becomes accustomed to a stimulus after it has been occurring for a long period of time. Anxiety then is no longer aroused.

What consequences do these experiences have in terms of personality development? Escalona and Leitch (1953) suggest that infants differ in responsiveness and in the speed at which they respond. It has been shown that there are infants who react more readily to stimuli—that is, startle more easily. A history of increased sensitivity to stimulation has been identified in children with pathology. Behavior patterns of the schizophrenic child may be maladaptive responses to this sensitivity. Such early mechanisms may serve to reduce anxiety initially, but they are ineffective in the long run.

Sleep is an effective method of reducing anxiety during infancy, and it is frequently utilized and reinforced. Can you recall instances when circumstances around you were overwhelming? It was quite comfortable to retreat to the bedroom, curl up in bed, and pull the covers over your head. Sleep relieves a person of the need to deal with anxiety. The development of this adaptive mechanism need not result purely from experiences during infancy. In adult life, one is told to "go to bed" or to "get some rest" to alleviate the anxiety of a tension-packed day. Sleep allows an individual the luxury of putting off dealing with a situation causing anxiety while realizing that it will be necessary to face the anxiety at some point. Sleep is but one mechanism of adaptation in the early phases of development.

Psychoanalytically oriented theorists believe that certain experiences may be perceived as being comforting because of their similarity to the birth process. A child, when anxious, may seek refuge in a warm, dark place—a place that is similar to the mother's womb. Although this view may stretch one's imagination, it is important to note that early experiences do set the stage for the use of certain adaptive mechanisms in later phases of life.

Factors such as self-concept, interactions with parents and significant others, socioeconomic background, and schooling experiences collectively and individually affect the development of adaptive mechanisms in later life. For example, individuals who feel comfortable with their self-concepts are able to relate successfully to others. They are more likely to perceive themselves as integral parts of their surroundings and to provide themselves with sources of continuous information about those surroundings. Maladaptive mechanisms tend to occur when people perceive their environments as threatening. If, in the early phases of life, they encounter continuous negative reinforcement from parents and other significant people, they develop mechanisms to protect their already suffering self-concepts. Withdrawal from reality, submission, and psychophysiological responses are utilized to deal with tension. These patterns continue to develop throughout the early periods of life until they become entrenched in the adult personality.

Thus the early periods of life are fertile territory for the development of adaptive (or maladaptive) mechanisms. Nurses need to be cognizant of the many factors that affect personality development. As Freud first pointed out, we need to recognize the implications of early childhood experiences and response patterns to understand adult adaptive mechanisms.

THEORIES OF DEVELOPMENT

A wide range of published material is related to the development of personality. We will present the concepts proposed by four major theorists: Freud, Erikson, Sullivan, and Piaget. We believe that these theories present a broad base of knowledge from which students can develop their understanding of the dynamics of personality.

Freud

Freud introduced the principle of epigenetics—the view that development follows a logical, sequential pattern. The critical tasks of each phase in the sequence must be completed to successfully move on to the next phase. If there is an interference in development at one of the stages, maladaptive behavior may result. However, since Freud's time it has been found that compensations are possible, to a certain degree. Deficiencies may be converted into strengths if they are recognized at an early stage.

In essence, Freud was arguing that sexual energy or libido is the prime motivator of human behavior. He viewed personality development in terms of libidinal investment, or cathexis, in the oral, anal, and phallic zones. He then correlated the process of physical maturation with the progression of the aforementioned zones.

Before Freud's view of psychosexual development is discussed further, his concept of the partitions of the mind—the id, the ego, and the superego—should be explained. The id represents the instinctual portion of the mind, controlled only by the blind strivings of Eros, the instinct of life, and Thanatos, the instinct of death. Thus the id is the origin of an individual's drives and motives. Normally, the actual forces of the id remain in the unconscious. Their effects are felt, however, as conscious perceptions of thoughts, desires, and feelings. The influence of the id is constantly and subtly felt by the ego, which is the rational reality-based component. The ego results from interaction with the environment; this interaction forms a boundary for the mind. The ego is the portion of the psyche that others "see" first. It serves a decision-making function in that it determines what kinds and amounts of stimuli are allowed into the mind as well as what is permitted to leave. What we say and do, how we perceive situations—these functions are dictated by the ego. The ego acts as a mediator between the id and the superego, which is the conscience, the dictator of moral and ethical standards. The superego is a differentiation of the ego, as the ego is a differentiation of the id. Both differentiations are a result of the interaction of id and environment and concurrent cognitive development. However, the development of the superego results primarily from interactions with specific parts of the environment, such as parents.

At birth the infant is predominantly operating under the pleasure principle, seeking immediate gratification for all needs and having little concern for the needs of others. He or she is all-encompassing, a concept that is supported by the orality or literally "eating alive" quality of the infant's responses to the mother. At the interfaces of the pleasure-driven id and reality there arise the beginnings of ego—the reality-oriented component of the mind. It is important to note that the thinking mechanisms associated with the initial, id-driven behavior can be connected to the dreams and fantasies of adults. This "primary process thinking" is frequently found in adaptive behavior of a regressive nature, such as in various types of psychosis. "Secondary process thinking" is related to reality situations.

Psychosexual development involves the concept of motivation. Freud believed that motivations remain constant throughout life but that the zones through which id gratification is sought vary. Much of motivation remains unconscious; however, in the course of the development of the ego, a person receives a limited insight into his motives. Knowledge that may not be conscious at the moment but that can be recalled at any time is said to exist in the "preconscious." Material that has never been permitted into conscious awareness, as well as repressed material, is said to exist in the "unconscious." The utilization of defense mechanisms to control anxiety points out the fact that individuals often do things for reasons they are unclear about or may even deny (see further discussion of defense mechanisms later in this chapter).

The oral stage of infancy encompasses approximately the first 15 months of life, in which children are unable to meet their most basic needs on their own. They depend upon others for that nurturance.

The channel of gratification is the mouth and lips, which are particularly sensitive. The stimulation of the mouth and lips sets off the sucking reflex. Libidinal energy is invested, or cathected, in the relevant channel of gratification, which in this psychosexual stage is the mouth. The gratifying objects are the mother's breast, a bottle, a pacifier, or the thumb. Energies of the infant are directed toward nursing, with the accompanying relationship to the parenting figure. The infant is unable to distinguish satisfying objects as being separate from his or her own body. They may, in fact, hold more attention than actual parts of the infant's own body. However, by approximately 9 months of age, the infant is able to discern the difference between self and the object of gratification.

Under favorable circumstances, the needs of an infant are met on a consistent basis. The way in which needs are met (or not met), particularly the responses of the parenting figure, has a great influence on an adult's ability to relate to another—to develop a sense of trust. If needs are met on a continuous basis by a warm, loving figure, a feeling of trust develops. We will discuss trust further when we consider the theories of Erikson.

It is interesting to note the paradox of infancy. It would seem that infants are totally helpless, dependent. However, their needs are met repeatedly without their actual recognition and identification of wanted objects. In a sense, then, there is an omnipotence inherent in the infant's personality. Parents of infants, who are often given to discussion of their problems, have frequently expressed the feeling that a mother's or father's life revolves around the infant. Activities must be planned around the infant's feeding and sleeping schedule. A person cannot simply get in the car and go shopping; such an operation requires very careful consideration of the hours of wakefulness and the "irritable" periods. This feeling of not having one's own life sometimes reaches extreme proportions. In such circumstances a parent may use maladaptive forms of behavior to adjust.

Orality means more than just gratification through the mouth and lips. The infant actually "takes in" various kinds of stimuli in his or her environment, a process that lays the groundwork for future cognitive and emotional processes. Lest we focus primarily on feeding as the representation of the oral phase, we must be aware that the infant is particularly sensitive to tactile stimulation. This sensation is most highly developed in the oral, or infancy, period. The relationship to the mother's body is very important in this phase; it is an intrinsic component of orality.

Defense mechanisms to reduce tension develop in the phase of infancy or orality. Sublimation, introjection, projection, and denial act as initial tension-alleviating mechanisms in this period. (See Table 6-1.)

It must be pointed out that defense mechanisms do not operate on a conscious level. Even in adulthood they operate below the awareness levels. The results of these mechanisms, however, are apparent.

The degree of libidinal energy invested during the oral phase is reflected in later activities such as gum chewing, nail biting, excessive eating and drinking, and smoking. All these activities are said to satisfy oral needs. Problems that develop during the oral phase may prohibit the release of energy for utilization during later stages, thereby causing a fixation in that stage. In such a situation, the individual's physical development progresses according to schedule, while psychosexual objectives remain the same as they were during that early period.

The toddler period is the stage in which the child begins to move throughout his or her environment, to exercise control, to be free to some degree. There is a shift of libidinal energy from the mouth as a channel of gratification to the anus. This area becomes highly sensitive and responds to stimulation. Baldwin (1967) suggests that the shift is not maturational but rather follows the attention that is directed toward the anus by the toilet-training pro-

TABLE 6-1 Defense mechanisms of oral stage

Defense	Example	Activity
Sublimation—directing of unacceptable libidinal energies into more socially acceptable channels	A young woman collects recipes while on a diet	Protection from those behaviors that are irrational
Introjection—incorporation of qualities or values of others into one's own personality	A 16-year-old boy tells his 13-year-old sister not to be late on her first date Healthy resolution of the grieving process	Critical in the development of the superego
Projection—attributing one's own unacceptable thoughts, wishes, fears to others	A 3-year-old boy tells his mother that his teddy bear is afraid of the dark A young man who has been fired blames it on the fact that the boss never liked him	Protection of self—may become pathological; extreme form of projection is paranoia
Denial—rejection or disavowal of elements of reality that may be unpleasant or painful	Postponement of diagnostic testing; refusal to confront diagnosis A newly diagnosed diabetic fails to take her insulin on a regular basis The father of a premature infant asks if there is hope after being told of the imminent death of the newborn	Protection of self from traumatic insult of an event; a determination of the nature of denial is critical to the assessment of and intervention in these situations

cess. The focus of the anal period is toilet training. Here the child finds himself or herself in a bind. The child wants to please the parents by having a bowel movement in the right place at the right time, yet this intention impinges upon his or her developing sense of autonomy. The child also desires the immediate gratification of the pleasurable feeling of the act of defecating. The question becomes one of either delaying gratification to receive parental approval or risking disapproval for immediate pleasure. There is a sense of ambivalence, a combination of positive and negative feelings directed toward the same object or situation.

According to Freud, various features of the anal period are crucial to later development. The retention of feces and "giving" them to the parents increases the significance attached to possessions. The person fixated at the anal stage of development is often characterized as parsimonious and unable

to tolerate ambiguity or confusion. The anal personality considers love objects as possessions and acts to control them rather than to permit them to act independently. This tendency may be reflected in the marital situation, with each partner "belonging" to the other.

The mechanism of sublimation is carried over into the anal phase, as are other mechanisms. Small children find pleasure in playing with feces, yet this is unacceptable to parents. Such activities as playing with mud, finger paints, sand, and modeling clay satisfy this instinctual drive in a socially acceptable fashion. See Table 6-2 for anal-stage defense mechanisms.

The phallic stage, or self-centered sexual stage, revolves around the concept of the Oedipus complex (or in the female, the Electra complex). There is a shift of libidinal energies from the anal region to the genitals. The male child directs his energies

TABLE 6-2 Defense mechanisms of anal stage

Defense	Example	Activity
Reaction formation—shift in feelings or attitudes from one point on the continuum to the extreme opposite point	A young man resents the fact that his best friend has been promoted but takes him out to dinner and is effusive in his support	Presents socially acceptable behavior; acts to support repression
Repression—a major defense whereby unpleasant thoughts, feelings, impulses are involuntarily excluded from conscious awareness	A young mother is unable to recall abusive experiences in her own childhood	Cornerstone of defenses which acts to preserve ego boundaries; other defenses reinforce repression
Regression—return to an earlier stage of development where modes of gratification were more satisfying and needs were met	A 4-year-old begins to wet the bed after the arrival of a new baby sister A young man is hospitalized for a myocardial infarction and is reliant upon others to make decisions	Provides opportunity to return to stage of development where needs are met; ego is acted upon

toward the mother, in direct competition with his father. He alternately loves and hates the father (ambivalence). The preschooler's ideas of sexual relations are often vague. The child sometimes places his hands all over the mother's body, particularly on the breasts. He imitates the way his father transmits affection to the mother. The mother tends to feel uncomfortable, particularly if she is unaware of her son's internal struggles at this time. The child, in any case, is not permitted to live out his fantasy. His feelings are condemned by both parents, yet those same feelings are accepted *between* the parents. The young boy fears the retaliation of his father in the form of castration. The subsequent aspect of this phase is the relinquishing of the sexual wishes because of fear of castration. Rather than be a rival of his father, the boy identifies with him. Hostility is repressed, as are sexual desires for the mother. In this way, the young boy begins to acquire masculine desires and values.

The Electra complex has not been as well defined as its male counterpart. Similar components exist: sexual desires are repressed, rivalry with the mother cannot be tolerated, so identification occurs, and acceptance of femininity results. The concept of castration anxiety is quite different for the female, since there is no penis. The resolution of

this part of the complex lies in the fact that women can reproduce and men cannot.

The beginning of the resolution of the Oedipus complex occurs in the phallic stage, as does the beginning of the development of the superego. As we will see, this resolution is carried over into the latency period. To present a clear picture of the development of the superego, we will discuss the mechanisms of introjection and identification. The child takes on aspects of the personality of the parent of the same sex. This process, termed *introjection*, was discussed previously. As a result of this internal process, identification comes about. The child introjects the values, attitudes, and goals of his or her parents—a ready-made conscience—into his or her ego structure (see Table 6-3). This process concurs with the child's concrete cognitive level of development. Introjection serves as the basis of the superego, yet it can be carried to an extreme. In such a situation, an individual may replace his or her entire ego structure with the characteristics of the significant other, losing his or her own identity in the process. As a person matures, the superego becomes more reality based and less harsh and demanding. The development of the superego relieves the child's castration anxiety or penis envy.

TABLE 6-3 Defense mechanisms of the phallic stage

Defense	Example	Activity
Identification—the process whereby the child imitates the desired behaviors of a significant other	An adolescent takes on qualities of a teacher she admires A newly graduated nurse models her behavior after her head nurse whom she admires for her caring attitude toward clients	Acts in concert with introjection; in extreme cases, one may replace the entire ego structure, incurring loss of identity of self

Faulty resolution of the Oedipus complex has far-reaching effects on later personality development. It can be said that at the base of almost all neurotic difficulties lies an inadequate resolution of the Oedipus complex. The adult who is fixated at this phase of development is characterized by poor sexual identity and difficulty with authority figures.

The period corresponding to the grade school years is referred to as the latency period. As we noted, there is a tremendous flow of energy in the phallic stage. Then there is a quieting of that energy in the latency period, perhaps a "calm before the storm" type of effect. It is the valley between the two peak periods—the phallic and the genital phases. A great deal of energy is devoted to intellectual pursuits. Sexual achievement and curiosity are replaced by a quest for knowledge and the motivation to achieve in school. Through sublimation, sexual drives are channeled into the socially accepted activity of the pursuit of education. The latency period is a time when culturally determined skills and values are acquired. The child moves out of the family system and is subjected to the values and attitudes of others. Throughout this period, the superego matures and becomes more organized, integrating the viewpoints of a variety of significant people in the environment.

The latency period, ranging from ages 6 to 12, is characterized by increasing sex-role development, which is facilitated by identification with the parent of the same sex. Testing of new sex roles can be seen in the development of sex-segregated gangs and cliques, which are quite common during this phase. Aggressive behavior, valued in males, takes the form of rebellion against authority. Reaction formation is in operation when the male child rejects not only sexuality but the whole opposite sex. This phenomenon can be noted in the attitude of boys toward girls in this age bracket. A 9-year-old boy would not be caught dead having a conversation with a girl! Adults fixated at this stage of development are often characterized by a lack of motivation and by an inability to appraise situations and solve problems creatively.

Freud did not actually include adolescence as a stage of personality development. It was his feeling that the personality is established by the beginning of adolescence. The genital stage differs from the phallic stage in that the genital stage is characterized by an overwhelming supply of sexual drives. But there is now a concern for others' feelings. The primary goal of this stage is the development of satisfactory relationships with persons of the opposite sex. The manner in which the Oedipus complex is resolved may have a definitive effect on an individual's choice of a partner. A girl often seeks out a boyfriend whose expectations in regard to her behavior are similar to her father's expectations about her mother. A man will often marry a girl who is quite similar to his own mother.

As a result of the Oedipus complex, the male identifies with the father. In the genital phase, repressed sexual feelings are allowed into consciousness, and acceptance of these feelings begins. It is at this point that libidinal energies are directed toward a relationship with the opposite sex.

Another major component of the adolescent phase is the development of a sense of self-worth. Inherent in this development is the defining of one's role in society. Up until this point, the adolescent had occupied a fairly secure role—knew where he or she belonged and who his or her

TABLE 6-4 Miscellaneous defense mechanisms

Defense	Example	Activity
Isolation—ego allows actual facts of experience, either past or present, to remain in consciousness, but breaks the linkage between facts and the emotions that belong with them	Nursing student giving postmortem care walls off emotions usually elicited by dead human bodies	Allows person to function without being overwhelmed by emotions that accompany activities of life
Displacement—certain strivings or feelings are unconsciously transferred from one object, activity, or situation to another	A husband is angry at his boss; upon arriving home, he criticizes his wife for not having dinner ready	Feelings are placed on objects that are considered safer
Rationalization—plausible reasons for one's behavior, feelings, and attitudes are constructed	An executive cheats on his income tax by saying "everyone else does it"	Permits person to cope with inability to meet certain societal and individual goals
Intellectualization—emotional responses to life situations that are painful are avoided by removing any personal significance	A young woman's failure to get the job she desired was explained by her statement that she really wasn't ready to go back to work anyway	Protects self-esteem in painful situations
Undoing—specific action or verbal statements that negate previous actions or statements that were of an oppositional nature	An employer reprimands a young, newly hired employee; the next day she invites the person to lunch	Provides a means to reduce the guilt associated with certain activities
Compensation—perceived deficits are made up for by emphasizing other more desirable characteristics	A young woman with little athletic ability stars on the chess team	Reinforces sense of self-worth
Substitution—replacement of an unavailable, highly valued object or person by a less valued object or person	A young man begins to date a woman who is very much like his recently deceased mother	Reduces impact of trauma or disappointment

friends were. But during this phase of life the adolescent must move out of this comfortable niche and find a place in society. This process can encompass a wide range of possibilities, such as further education, a vocation, and marriage. Finding one's place in society is, at best, a difficult task.

An adult who is fixated at the genital phase of development is characterized by an inability to enter into an intimate relationship with another individual and by a tendency to "float" from one occupation or educational setting to another.

In addition to the defense mechanisms already presented, several others are commonly utilized. They are summarized in Table 6-4.

In summary, according to Freud two series of changes take place concurrently in the development of the personality (see Table 6-5). The first is the maturation of the ego, with the attending recognition of reality and development of defense mechanisms. The final product of this series is an interpersonally oriented being. Second, cognitive processes develop that permit an individual to assess and interpret his or her environment, to give meaning and rationality to what is perceived. This

TABLE 6-5 Freudian stages

Developmental stage	Time period	Critical behaviors
Oral	Birth to 15 months	Mouth and lips are channels of gratification and means by which environment is explored
Anal	15 months to 3 years	Libidinal energy shifts to anal area; focus is on toilet training and muscle control
Phallic (oedipal)	3 to 6 years	Libidinal energy shifts to genital area; introjection and identification initiate development of superego
Latency	6 to 12 years	Focus of energy is on intellectual development, maturation of superego continues; child moves out of family system (through school) and is subjected to others' values
Genital	12 years to early adulthood	Overwhelming supply of sexual drives; primary goal is developing satisfactory relationships with persons of the opposite sex

framework leads to the discussion of the view of development of another psychoanalyst—Erik Erikson.

Erikson

Erikson added a new dimension to Freud's psychosexual stages: psychosocial development. He viewed society as having a profound impact on the emerging personality. Erikson identified critical tasks for each phase of development. These graduated tasks must be met for a person to move successfully on to the next phase. Society assures the proper socialization of the child by providing him or her with opportunities for (1) role development, (2) attainment of independence, and (3) healthy expression of emotions. The accomplishment of these tasks occurs differently in each culture.

Development, according to Erikson, is a gradual process. The ultimate goal is an individual who not only feels comfortable with his or her own identity but also is sensitive to the needs of others in the environment: a *social* animal. Like Freud, Erikson believed that the success or lack of success of adaptation in one phase influences an individual's ability to master the critical tasks of the next period. It is not a question of a child selecting the tasks that he or she would like to master. Tasks occur on a dynamic continuum, each leading to the next, with an ever-increasing repertoire of coping abilities being made available on a regular basis. (See Table 6-6.)

The *sensory* phase lasts from birth to approximately 18 months. The most crucial task to be dealt with is the development of a sense of being able to rely on others, to establish a sense of trust. During this period infants are totally dependent upon others in their environment. As their needs are consistently met, they begin to attain a basic sense of trust. The significant relationships that occur during this phase set the tone for all future relationships. Infants who are able to trust others, to be confident that their needs will be met, are more likely to achieve a feeling of confidence in themselves. This feeling of trust in others and the increasing sense of self-confidence permit them to feel secure in the knowledge that their needs will be met should they find themselves in a helpless, dependent position in later life. Adults who have not experienced trusting relationships in early life will be more pessimistic in their expectations of others. Their relationships with others are frequently doomed to failure. Their lack of self-esteem is often projected onto others in the form of the attitude, "He doesn't like me." This attitude elicits responses that reinforce it. The cycle then comes full circle. Individuals who do not have a basic sense of self are prevented from investing in open, two-way interactions with others.

The *muscular*, or toddler, phase approximates the period of ages 1 to 3 years. The critical task of this phase is the achievement of a sense of autonomy, as opposed to arousal of feelings of self-doubt.

TABLE 6-6   Erikson's stages

Developmental stage	Time periods	Critical behaviors (tasks*)
Sensory	Birth to 18 months	Trust vs. mistrust; development of significant trusting relationships
Muscular	1 to 3 years	Autonomy vs. shame and doubt; child learns to function autonomously within the context of the environment
Locomotor	3 to 6 years	Initiative vs. guilt; increasing awareness of own identity and relationship to multiple other systems; increasing awareness of influence on others
Latency	6 to 12 years	Industry vs. inferiority; energies are directed toward creative activities and the pursuit of learning
Adolescent	12 to 20 years	Identity vs. role diffusion; transition from childhood to adulthood; achievement of integration of values, beliefs, attitudes acquired up to this point
Young adulthood	18 to 25 years	Intimacy vs. isolation; ability to extend self into intimate relationships with others
Adulthood	21 to 45 years	Generativity vs. stagnation; logical extension of young adulthood; relationships reflect successful achievement of intimacy and the ultimate goal of developing a family
Maturity	45 years to death	Ego integrity vs. despair; perception of life as a culmination of both positive and negative events; acceptance of one's own life as it is; ultimately a positive sense of self remains intact

*Term specifically used by Erikson.

Lidz (1968) suggests that this cannot truly occur until the child achieves a sense of initiative, the critical task of the next developmental phase.

Perhaps the crucial concept here is the interrelationship of phases. Young children become independent of their parents as the parents provide opportunities to do so. They feel comfortable in seeking out new experiences in the environment because there has been the initial development of basic trust. They soon realize that they can take the initiative to explore their world, knowing full well that mother or father will be there if the need should arise. In this way children begin to feel independent, autonomous. They begin to be aware of the effects their bodies have on the environment around them.

Parents greatly influence the degree to which children attempt to master their environment. When constant barriers, both physical and verbal, are placed in the path of the development of autonomy, there is little room for growth of initiative. Children feel they are "bad" for not conforming to rules and regulations. Parents who lack confidence in their own abilities often project their inadequacies onto their children. In such a case, the child does not feel capable of extending his or her horizons further into the environment. Again, a basic lack of trust in oneself prevents the development of a satisfying relationship.

The critical task of the next stage, the *locomotor* phase, is the achievement of a sense of initiative. During the period from ages 3 to 6 years, the developing child seeks to balance initiative and guilt. Erikson (1950) suggests the child achieves this balance by identifying with the parent of the same sex, thereby reducing the guilt produced by the rivalry between the child and that parent. As a result of this phase, the child develops a conscience that serves to regulate primary id impulses.

The locomotor phase is characterized by a greater organization of personality. The child gains an appreciation of his own sense of identity, his own place as a system in relation to many other systems. He becomes increasingly aware of his influence on others as well as of his limitations. In a later section, we will discuss the impact of the broadening range of cognitive processes on the child's personality organization and development.

The *latency* period, ages 6 to 12, is concerned with the task of industry versus inferiority. The child utilizes energies in creative activities or in the pursuit of learning. The child seeks to become part of a group; a sense of belonging is crucial to this phase. The child begins to internalize the values and attitudes of others. There are new environments to become familiar with. The child finds a place among peers. The child gains feelings of self-worth as a result of appraisals from other persons in the environment—adults, playmates, and schoolmates. Recognition that some people like him or her and value his or her word while others do not is critical to the development of a capability for a healthy self-evaluation. The quality of leadership is one that becomes apparent in this period. The child learns to lead or sees himself or herself primarily as a follower. Or the child may see himself or herself as never being a part of the group and thus become habitually rebellious or alienated. In such a situation, the child often feels a sense of inferiority, which causes the child to act out in defiance against others—a protective shell made necessary by a lack of self-worth.

The *adolescent* phase, encompassing ages 12 to 20, is the transitional phase between childhood and adulthood. It is characterized by turmoil and change. There are individual variations in the rate of sexual maturation, as well as in the pace of emotional, intellectual, and social development. The adolescent is expected to integrate all experiences up to that point into a coherent sense of self and to emerge as an adult.

The achievement of an integrated self requires the successful accomplishment of the tasks of previous phases. The child comes equipped with a basic sense of trust, an ability to make some decisions regarding his or her life, and an ability to relate to others individually and in groups. These factors enable the personality to gel into a workable, integrated whole.

During the transitional period the individual can prepare for independence, yet still be under the protective umbrella of the parents. This situation may have a negative influence on successive development if parents do not permit children to exer-

cise some of their options. If an adolescent remains in a children's world within the family but is confronted with adult expectations in the total society, a sense of role confusion results.

Erikson (1950) stresses the significance of the next phase—*young adulthood* or late adolescence, which lasts from ages 18 to 25. The crucial task of this phase is the achievement of intimacy as opposed to isolation. The young person must gain an ego identity that reflects an individual who is a human being in his or her own right. The person is no longer considered someone's daughter or son. Once a firm sense of self has been established, the young adult is able to engage in an intimate relationship with another individual. Interdependence—the sharing with another of all that one values without fear of loss of self—is the crux of this period. (It seems that an inability to achieve a true sense of intimacy in our current society is being reflected in a rising divorce rate, although the divorce rate is influenced by many other factors as well.)

The phase of *adulthood*, ages 21 to 45, is concerned with the task of generativity as opposed to stagnation. As young adults move through the life cycle, they begin to identify life goals, including occupational and marital choices. The period of adulthood thus is a logical extension of the period of young adulthood, during which the capacity for a sharing relationship develops. The adult's choices reflect the successful achievement of a sense of self-worth and belonging, and the transition from operating under parental values and attitudes to operating under one's own.

During this period, a dyad is often transformed into a triad with the addition of a child. The partners who feel comfortable with themselves and who have had their needs met are able to direct their love and energy into the development of a new human being. We have come full circle; the phases of development begin again—with another life.

The final phase of development according to Erikson, is *maturity*, in which the task is to accomplish ego integrity as opposed to despair. Individuals review their life experiences, considering those objectives they have successfully completed and those they have not. Persons who can accept their lives for what they have achieved undergo a renewed sense of ego integrity. Life has meaning for them, in both its positive and negative events. They do not despair for what might have been. The end of life is perceived as a culmination of their many experiences rather than as something to be feared. The older person has thought a good deal about death and has usually had many experiences with it. Death is a phase of development that one must pass through, with the ultimate goal being achievement of a positive sense of self in this final stage.

Sullivan

Harry Stack Sullivan believed that individuals need to be socialized in their environments. His theory was based on the premise that each individual seeks to avoid anxiety. Inherent in this theory is the view that coping mechanisms are developed to reduce anxiety. Sullivan differed from Freud and Erikson in that he viewed biological changes as the stimuli for emerging needs and growth trends.

As an individual grows, there are changes in the inherent ability to relate to objects and persons in the environment. Abilities and body parts are considered an individual's *tools*. The goal of each developmental phase is considered the *task*. For example, the task of the infancy stage is to receive fulfillment of needs from others in the environment. To accomplish this goal, the infant utilizes

the mouth, the ability to cry. The mouth and the ability to cry are considered tools. As the child moves through the stages of development, the tasks becomes more sophisticated, as do the tools. During late adolescence, the individual utilizes the genital organs and the process of experimentation (tools) to develop an intimate, loving relationship with another (task). Like Freud, Sullivan described the individual who successfully completed the tasks of each developmental phase as being interdependent, capable of forming a lasting relationship, and comfortable with his or her concept of self. (See Table 6-7.)

To facilitate the understanding of Sullivanian theory, we will discuss some of its dynamic concepts. Reality orientation is referred to in terms of "mode." The prototaxic mode, occurring in infancy, is characterized by a lack of differentiation between self and the environment. Thus Sullivan's and Freud's concepts of self and its relationship to the environment are similar.

The parataxic mode is characterized by the breaking up of the undifferentiated whole. The resulting parts are illogical and disjointed and occur inconsistently. This mode is in operation primarily during childhood, but it also extends into the juvenile period. It is necessary for the child to separate the parts of the whole into discrete units so as to better understand their individuation and subsequent relatedness to the physical and social environment.

TABLE 6-7 Sullivan's stages

Developmental stage	Time period	Critical behaviors
Infancy	Birth to 18 months	Gratification of needs results in beginning level of trust
Childhood	18 months to 6 years	Learning to delay gratification to achieve longer-term rewards (i.e., parental approval)
Juvenile	6 to 9 years	Development of sense of belonging to one's peer group; "chum" relationships
Preadolescence	9 to 12 years	Primary relationships are with those of the same sex; switch of loyalty from family to peers
Early adolescence	12 to 14 years	Attempts to be independent while at the same time desiring dependence; primary goal is development of satisfactory relationships with members of opposite sex
Late adolescence	14 to 21 years	Achievement of an intimate love relationship without the fear of loss of self

The ability to perceive whole, logical, coherent pictures as they occur in reality characterizes the syntaxic mode. The syntaxic mode is used as a means of understanding the environment and relating to others. To gain assurance that perceptions are real, adults seek consensual validation. They are then able to identify areas that need development as well as those which do not.

Sullivan refers to the organization of experiences that defend against anxiety as the "self-system." To make an accurate assessment of an individual's feelings of worth, it is important to understand the concepts of "good-me," "bad-me," and "not-me." The child, based on his or her interpersonal experiences, assumes one of the above postures. Behavior that is regarded as valued by the parents is then learned and incorporated by the child as good-me. Behavior that does not receive parental approval is identified as bad-me. The child perceives from verbal and nonverbal cues that such behavior is not acceptable. For example, he or she may hear a parent talk about the unacceptability of tardiness. Behavior that generates large amounts of anxiety is denied and identified as not-me. A parallel can be drawn between the Freudian mechanism of reaction formation and the concept of not-me. Each involves an unacceptable feeling being denied, the opposing feeling being verbalized, and anxiety being reduced for the moment. For example, a person who is experiencing feelings of hostility may say, "I love everyone as a brother," saying, in effect, that the hostility is "not-me."

The focus of Sullivanian strategies is to develop appropriate, healthy responses as components of the syntaxic mode. Reduction of anxiety caused by developmental deficits is also a primary goal. One of the purposes of the nurse-client interaction is to permit the client to identify these deficits and to correct them. (See Chapter 9 for discussion of nurse-client interaction.)

Sullivan identified six basic phases of development, which are similar to those of Freud and Erikson. In *infancy,* the period from birth to approximately 1½ years, the primary task is the development of a basic sense of trust in others. The gratification of needs ensues as a result of the foundation of trust. The mouth, the ability to cry, the satisfaction response, empathic observation, autistic in-

vention (see Chapter 25), exploration, and emergency responses such as rage and anxiety are the developmental tools—the means by which the child accomplishes the task.

As individuals move through the developmental phases, they increase their repertoire of coping mechanisms as each task becomes more complex. The focus of the *childhood* period, 1½ years to about 6 years, is learning to delay gratification to receive long-term reward—for example, parental approval. Through the use of mouth, anus, autistic invention, experimentation, manipulation, identification, and emergency responses such as anxiety, guilt, shame, doubt, and anger, children begin to develop a more realistic sense of their own influence on the environment, which leads to a greater sense of independence and self-worth.

The *juvenile* period, ages 6 to approximately 9, is characterized by the development of a sense of belonging within one's peer group. It is especially important for a child in this period to form satisfying relationships with children of his or her own age group. Sullivan refers to these as the "chum" relationships. Often the child will place the family second to meet the needs of peers. The tools available to the child in this period include competition, compromise, cooperation, experimentation, manipulation, and exploration.

Following the juvenile period is *preadolescence,* which includes ages 9 to 12. During this time there is a marked switch of loyalty from family to peers. A friend of the same sex is the primary relationship. Exploration, manipulation, and experimentation, coupled with the capacity to love, consensual validation, and collaboration, are the primary tools of the period.

Early adolescence, ages 12 to 14, reflects the child's beginning attempts to be independent of parents and their set of values, attitudes, and beliefs. There is a sense of rebelliousness. It seems as though the child longs to be both independent and dependent at the same time, and anger arises from this seemingly impossible situation. The task at hand is learning to develop satisfactory relationships with members of the opposite sex. Another primary goal is the achievement of a sense of identity concurrently with a delineation of life goals. Lust, experimentation, exploration, manipulation, and anxiety are the tools most commonly utilized during this phase of development.

The last phase, *late adolescence*, encompasses ages 14 to approximately 21. The major task of this phase is similar to that of Erikson's late adolescent or young adulthood phase—achievement of an intimate, love relationship without the fear of loss of self. This is a culmination of the previous phases in that a sound sense of identity has developed, along with the ability to form trusting relationships with others. The appropriate tools of this period include genital organs, exploration, manipulation, and experimentation.

Sullivan believed that after completing the tasks of late adolescence, an individual would be capable of functioning interdependently in society. He thought it unnecessary to continue the discussion of personality development farther than this point, since the most crucial developmental tasks would already have been accomplished.

Piaget

Piaget describes personality development as a progression of cognitive processes. Initially the child is quite egocentric: he or she believes that all others in the environment share his or her feelings, thoughts, and beliefs. As children mature, they become aware of others' viewpoints and develop an ability to integrate those concepts into their own framework.

Like the other theorists discussed, Piaget views development as a series of stages. When a stage has been completed successfully, the child moves on to a more complex one. For Piaget, mature, intelligent behavior is the ability to critically assess and problem solve in virtually any situation. Thought processes progress from a concrete level to "formal operations," or abstract, logical thinking.

Four factors concurrently influence the development of cognition: biological maturation, experience with the physical world, social experience, and equilibration. Equilibration is the balancing and integrating of new experiences with those of the past as an individual progresses along the developmental course.

Two behavioral factors inherent in equilibration are *assimilation* and *accommodation*. Through the interaction of these two components, the child (and eventually, the adult) is able to reconcile and integrate any new behavior.

Assimilation is the ability to comprehend experiences. An individual is constantly being bombarded with new situations that require responses. What an individual learns as a result of new interactions with the environment needs to be incorporated into an already existing body of experiences. Thus new interactions are given meaning in terms of the experiences an individual has had up to that time. In other words, assimilation occurs.

When new concepts are introduced, a certain degree of upset or disequilibrium ensues, depending on the nature of the concept and its perceived effect. An individual directs energies toward identifying and eliminating the cause of the disequilibrium. As the disequilibrium decreases, the perception of the event becomes more accurate. The process is termed *accommodation*. For example, the infant views the mothering figure as an extension of self. Through the process of development, the infant begins to differentiate self from environment. New experiences impinge upon the infant. The meanings of these experiences need to be integrated with the meanings of past experiences. The infant must change the manner in which the mothering figure is perceived in order to develop a differentiated self. Thus the process of differentiation occurs as a result of assimilation and accommodation, in that order.

In summary, assimilation is the mechanism whereby the comprehension of a new experience occurs, up to the point where previous experience left off. Therefore, assimilation frequently results in incorrect plugging in (because of lack of experience). Accommodation occurs to rectify the inaccurate plugging in. This leads to restoration of equilibrium at a higher level of functioning. A parallel can be drawn between disequilibrium and anxiety; the ultimate goals of an individual are the reduction of anxiety and the incorporation of experiences—and thus higher-level functioning—cognitive, emotional, psychological, and biological.

Piaget divides his cognitively based developmental schema into four periods (see Table 6-8). The first is the *sensorimotor* period, which lasts from birth to 2 years of age. This period is charac-

TABLE 6-8 Piaget's stages of cognitive development

Developmental period	Time period	Critical behaviors
Sensorimotor	Birth to 2 years	Manipulation of environment through goal-directed behavior; child learns concepts of object permanence
Preoperational thought		Growing ability to utilize language as a tool; egocentrism,
Preoperational phase	2 to 4 years	or the belief that one's viewpoint is the only one, is a primary characteristic
Intuitive phase	4 to 7 years	Integration of concepts based on more than one dimension; increasing ability to comprehend rules and to recognize relationships
Concrete operations	7 to 11 years	Beginning use of logic and objectivity; reasoning is related to concrete or real events
Formal operations	11 to 15 years	Abstract thinking is reached during this period; emergence of self as well as recognition and validation of identity; development of relationships with others

terized by the infant's moving around in the environment. Meaning is attached to objects by way of manipulation. Young children begin to differentiate themselves from their environment through goal-directed behavior. One of the primary concepts children learn in this period is the permanence of objects, a concept that is basic to logical thought. Objects continue to exist, whether they are seen or not. Another concept that is basic to logical thought is that objects retain their identity even though the context in which they appear changes. Children in this period learn that grandma is the same person with her glasses off as she is with them on.

The second major period is that of *preoperational thought*. To describe the progression of cognition more clearly, Piaget divided this period into two phases—preoperational and intuitive.

The preoperational phase, ages 2 to 4 years, reflects the child's growing ability to use language as a tool to meet his or her needs. The seedlings of thought begin to appear as the child becomes more aware of the representation of objects by words. For example, a table is an object; we do not eat at the word "table" but at the actual object. The ability to make this distinction prepares the child for symbolic mental activity.

Children in this phase cannot categorize objects in more than one dimension—for example, an object cannot be both yellow and rectangular. They are capable of attending to only one primary char-

acteristic at a time. They are also unable to classify a group of similar objects in terms of their multifactorial similarity.

Another general feature of thinking of the preoperational period is egocentrism. The child believes that his or her viewpoint is the only one—it is difficult for the child to understand thoughts, perceptions, and ideas as being different from one's own. The child cannot understand why an event does not occur as he or she had thought it would. The child cannot allow for factors other than his or her own. When a parent admonishes the child, saying, "Don't do that—you wouldn't like it if someone did that to you," the child does not understand because he or she is unable to place himself or herself in the position of another.

As children become older, they are able to conceive of groups or classes as having relationships. In the intuitive phase, ages 4 to 7, they comprehend basic rules and are able to integrate concepts based on more than one dimension. The number of objects in a group no longer changes as the context of presentation changes—another cornerstone of logical thought. For example, children are able to discern that one set of dots is equal in number to another set of dots even though the presentation is different (see Fig. 6-1). By the end of the preoperational period, children see that each block contains six dots.

In the period of *concrete operations*, ages 7 to 11, children begin to use logic and objectivity. Reason-

Fig. 6-1   Integration of multiple concepts.

ing is related to concrete or real events—for example, all apples are fruit; then this apple is fruit. As a result of this phase, children can organize objects into hierarchies as well as reduce a whole into its component parts and combine it differently without causing a change in the whole.

The final step—abstract thinking—is reached during the period of *formal operations*, ages 11 to 15. By age 11, children are able to conceptualize a plan based on hypothetical events, consider more than one variable, and identify appropriate strategies of action. Potential relationships among objects can be visualized. As in the adolescent phases of Freud, Erickson, and Sullivan, there is emergence of self, recognition and validation of one's own identity, and then the development of relationships with others in the environment. The individual is able to reflect, review his or her experiences to that point, and evaluate their influence on self-appraisals.

Thus an individual's interaction with his or her environment is a fundamental premise of the Piagetian philosophy of personality development. The child moves from simple cognitive processes, such as understanding object permanence, to formal, abstract thought processes.

MASLOW'S HIERARCHY OF NEEDS

The previous section dealt primarily with the phases of development a child must complete to reach maturity. Parallels among four theorists discussed were drawn when appropriate; the tasks or crises of corresponding phases often seemed to be similar. It is important to understand the implications of this statement. Nurses must not assess clients on the basis of only one developmental theory; they must correlate the relevant aspects of many theories.

Maslow (1954) views individuals from a perspective that is somewhat different from those of the four theorists discussed—but one that is equally

important for health care providers to understand and apply. Maslow suggests that there is a priority or "hierarchy" of needs, that a person seeks to satisfy basic needs before moving on to complex ones.

The individual must be motivated to meet challenges, to satisfy needs. Motivation, a concept crucial to the understanding of human behavior, has been discussed in a variety of formats. It can be defined as the rationale or logical thought behind an individual's actions, plans, or ideas. A rationale operates on three levels—conscious, preconscious, and unconscious. Most of what motivates individuals operates on an unconscious level. This fact is of critical importance not only in a nurse's assessment of a client's behavioral responses but also in the nurse's understanding of his or her own reciprocal responses. Maslow proposed a list of five basic needs, each of which reflects a higher-level priority than the preceding one. The needs are as follows: (1) physiological, (2) safety, (3) love and belonging, (4) self-esteem, and (5) self-actualization. What meaning do these needs hold for the development of nursing care strategies? Nurse and client could be operating on two different levels. Imagine, for example, that a community health nurse enters a woman's home to discuss her feelings about becoming a mother for the first time but that the woman does not seem interested. Observations of the surrounding environment reveal leaky ceilings, no food in the refrigerator, little furniture, tattered clothing. What are this woman's priorities of needs? Obviously the nurse is concerned about a higher-level need (love and belonging) than the client. The client is concerned about physiological necessities and safety. Initially, lower-level needs must be satisfied. The client may then be more able to share her feelings about being a new mother. Nursing strategies must take into account the fact that lower-level needs must be satisfied to a greater extent than higher-level needs.

When the first three needs are, for the most part,

satisfied, a person seeks out appraisals and assurance from significant others in the environment. He or she needs to feel a sense of self-respect and self-confidence. Individuals value the appreciation and recognition received from their peers; however, the last two of the five needs are rarely satisfied completely. Self-fulfillment needs and the recognition of one's potential for continued self-development tend to remain below the level of consciousness. These two needs thus tend to be unconscious motivators of behavior (Maslow, 1954). This fact should alert nurses to be critically aware of verbal and nonverbal behavior that may be motivated by a client's desire for self-respect, autonomy, and self-development.

Maslow's levels of need overlap, just as the phases of development of the various theorists overlap. Higher-level needs emerge before lower-level needs are totally satisfied. Most people tend to be partially satisfied in each area and partially unsatisfied.

DYNAMIC CONTINUUM OF MENTAL HEALTH–MENTAL ILLNESS

We have noted that developmental "lags," fixations at early levels of development, or unsuccessful accomplishment of developmental tasks set the stage for mental illness. However, we must point out the fact that mental health, or mental illness, is not a static state. Behavior varies from minute to minute, day to day, month to month. Mental health can be likened to a series of peaks and valleys with plateaus interspersed periodically. Many factors interact, resulting in behavior. In addition, as we will note in succeeding chapters, culture influences the identification of mental illness. Sapir (1963) points out the role of culture as an etiological factor in mental illness—through child-rearing practices and stressful roles, for example—and as a symptom-molder, as in the case of syndromes peculiar to one culture. For example, in the United States, value is placed on rational, logical thought processes. Persons unable to behave in a rational manner are labeled "ill." The same behavior in another culture might be perceived as normal. Thus the criteria used to define and identify mental illness are linked to cultural heritage. It is necessary for

nurses to appreciate the arbitrary, culture-bound bases of what is viewed as "normal." Oddities of behavior in another culture are easily identifiable as culture bound. However, the identification of psychiatric disorders within one's own society as being culture bound is not readily accepted.

Jahoda (1953) describes six characteristics developed in infancy and childhood that reflect positive mental health. The first of these indicators is a positive attitude toward oneself. A person who understands his or her strengths and accepts his or her limitations possesses a strong sense of identity and is relatively secure in the environment.

Appropriate growth and development, as well as achievement of self-actualizing ability, constitute the second positive indicator. Erikson's eight stages of man can be used to measure this particular criterion. The individual who is unable to successfully complete developmental tasks may become maladapted. Positive reinforcement of self-concept is of great importance in enabling an individual to achieve his or her maximum level of functioning.

The third indicator of positive mental health is the ability to integrate and synthesize life events in such a way as to maintain equilibrium and to reduce anxiety or make it tolerable. Each person develops a philosophy of life that reflects an assessment of the environment and his or her relatedness to, or isolation from, that environment.

Autonomy is the ability to make appropriate decisions and to be self-directed, with specific goals and objectives in mind. A parallel can be drawn between this fourth indicator of positive mental health and Erikson's second phase of development—autonomy versus shame and doubt. Can a person separate self from the environment and its social influences? Is he or she able to make decisions on his or her own and willing to accept the consequences of his or her actions, whatever they may be? Throughout the life span, vast amounts of energy are directed toward achievement of independence, which is an important indicator of mental health.

The fifth indicator of positive mental health is the ability to perceive reality without distortion. A person's perceptions of the "real" world as opposed to what is fantasized are influenced by cul-

Text continued on p. 174.

TABLE 6-9   Overview of developmental stages

Stage of development	Play/social activities	Health promotion	Language/cognitive development
Infancy	Playing with self Understanding environment through movement Infant needs colorful, mobile, cuddly toys	Immunizations essential during this period Safety precautions relate to falls, burns, oral ingestion of foreign objects and poisons, drowning	Sensorimotor period—ability to recognize change and to adjust accordingly Vocalization begins about 4 months of age—relates to recognition of people and definition of needs; language in this phase is autistic; communication is goal-oriented by the end of the period
Toddler	Play is primary mode through which child organizes world, releases tension, improves muscular coordination, and develops spaciotemporal perception Stage characterized by solitary or parallel activities	Primary concerns are respiratory infections and accidents; parents "childproof" the home by removing scatter rugs and sharp or breakable objects and putting poisons out of reach	Preoperational/parataxic period—learning through imitation; lack of understanding of cause and effect relationships Child communicates in an understandable manner yet may not use words with meaning Syncretic speech—one word represents a certain object; emotions, objects, actions are fused to have one meaning Speech is autistic, vocabulary enlarges

Body image	Emotional development	Developmental tasks (From Duvall, 1971)
Diffuse feelings of hunger, pain, comfort, but no real body image; self not differentiated from environment; basis for positive perception of body image laid in early mother-child relationships By end of first year, internalization of sensory experiences into body image occurs Ego development and body image development occur simultaneously	Developmental task: trust versus mistrust Parent-child bonding crucial foundation for basic sense of trust and patterns of future relationships; essential that primary needs are gratified promptly	Achieve physiological equilibrium following birth Establish self as dependent person but separate from others Become aware of alive versus inanimate and familiar versus unfamiliar and develop rudimentary social interaction Develop feeling of and desire for affection and response from others Adjust somewhat to the expectations of others Manage the changing body; learn new motor skills; begin eye-hand coordination Learn to understand and control the world through exploration Develop beginning symbol system, preverbal communication Direct emotional expression to indicate needs and wishes
Body image gradually evolves as a component of self-concept Child becomes more aware of his or her body as having physical and emotional components Child not fully aware of the interaction of his or her body with the environment—i.e., the impact each has on the other Body products—e.g., feces—are not perceived as separate from self Self-concept develops from reflected appraisals of significant others; concept of "good-me" develops as a result of positive responses from others; critical period for development of positive self-concept	Developmental task: autonomy versus shame and doubt—"Me do it!" Child relies greatly on parental responses and support; need for attention and approval acts as primary motivator for socialization process Toilet training is major developmental accomplishment	Settle into healthy routines Master good eating habits Master the basics of toilet training Develop physical skills appropriate to stage of motor development Become a family member Learn to communicate effectively with others

Continued.

TABLE 6-9 Overview of developmental stages—cont'd

Stage of development	Play/social activities	Health promotion	Language/cognitive development
Preschool	Pre-gang stage; peers assume a new importance; child progresses from solitary play to cooperating with others in group; learns to follow rules, to compare self to others, and to be concerned about others; appraisals begin to come from persons other than parents—provides for reality testing and allows expression of emotion and creativity	Accident prevention—e.g., motor vehicles, burns, falling, drowning, child needs clear-cut safety rules explained consistently, simply; adult supervision is also warranted Immunization boosters Dental and medical checkups important on a regular basis	Concept formation begins—child moves from lack of differentiation to awareness of objects as concrete and separate from the environment Inability to differentiate own feelings from external events—everything is important on an equal basis Language is used to get attention, to maintain interpersonal relationships, and to gather information Reading becomes significant factor in language development
School age	Peer groups provide a broader circle of friends outside home environment Six- or seven-year-old enjoys assuming roles—e.g., fireman, mailman, teacher, doctor, nurse Older school-age children enjoy table games of a simple nature, riding bikes, swimming Later in this period, creativity appears in the areas of music, art, dance, drama Predominant partner is "chum"—of same sex and age, actually is an extension of child's self; sharing of very special thoughts and feelings occurs	Illness occurs for first time as child enters school; upper respiratory infections are common Immunization boosters are important Safety precautions in relation to motor vehicle accidents and drownings	Stage of concrete operations—reasoning through real or imagined situations Child progresses to greater understanding of meanings and feelings Child uses language to establish relationships and to increase knowledge base Syntaxic communication is utilized—cause and effect relationships are beginning to be recognized Child learns to express feelings and thoughts in a way that is meaningful to others

Body image	Emotional development	Developmental tasks (From Duvall, 1971)
Ego boundaries become more differentiated, as do physical body boundaries; in part because of an increase in sexual awareness, an increase in motor coordination, more mature play experiences, and positive parental relationships Fear of mutilation is quite common in this period	Child learns social roles and responsibilities and behaves more like adult counterparts Continuation of mastery of self and environment Developmental task—initiative versus guilt Child uses imagination and creativeness to greater degree Increasing awareness of feelings of love, hate, anger, tension—child learns modes of coping to reduce anxiety	Settle into healthy daily routine of adequate eating, resting, and playing Master skills of gross- and fine-motor coordination Become a participating family member Conform to others' expectations Express emotions healthily and for a wide variety of experiences Learn to communicate effectively with others Learn to use initiative tempered by a conscience Develop ability to handle potentially dangerous situations Lay foundations for understanding the meaning of life, self, the world, and ethical, religious, and philosophical ideas
School experience reinforces or weakens child's perceptions of body and self Fluidity of body image/self-concept, due to rapid physical, emotional, and social changes	Developmental task—industry versus inferiority Child progresses from self-centered to more other-directed behavior Child evidences concern for others—particularly "chum" in latter part of period More self-direction—continued imitation of adults Child still unaware of effects of self on others, yet becoming more tolerant of others' behavior	Decrease dependence on family and gain satisfaction from peers and adults Increase neuromuscular skills to participate in games and work with others Learn adult concepts, as well as concepts related to problem solving Learn to communicate with others realistically Become active family member Give affection to, and receive affection from, family and friends without expecting immediate return Learn socially acceptable ways of handling and saving money Learn to deal with strong feelings Adjust to changing body image and come to terms with sex roles Discover healthy ways to become an acceptable person Develop positive attitude toward own and other social, racial, and economic groups

Continued.

TABLE 6-9 Overview of developmental stages—cont'd

Stage of development	Play/social activities	Health promotion	Language/cognitive development
Adolescence	Peer groups most important; status and recognition derived from the group; behavior defined by group members Sense of identity results from appraisals by others in the social setting	Mood swings quite common in this period Accidents involving motor vehicles of some sort are leading cause of death Obesity, excessive loss of weight (anorexia nervosa), acne, venereal disease, suicide, and pregnancy are current health issues Drug and alcohol abuse are, historically, very characteristic of period	Period of greatest ability to acquire and use knowledge; adolescent is able to perform active problem solving to reach realistic solutions; considers alternatives to problems; is highly imaginative—this can be a very creative time
Young adulthood	Review of life options to decide what focus of life will be—e.g., marriage, work, family Person continues to have close circle of friends, usually based on similar interests, values, occupations Chooses social and recreational activities as pleasure-promoting as well as outlets for energy	Accidents—especially motor vehicle, industrial, drowning—are the leading cause of death	Full mental capacity has been attained, although knowledge may be increased in college or trade schools Person assumes more responsibility for own learning rather than expecting it to be handed to him or her Is able to make contributions to society of a social or intellectual nature

Body image	Emotional development	Developmental tasks (From Duvall, 1971)
Body image and self-concept closely tied to identity formation; experiences of a positive nature enable development of positive body image; adolescent is sensitive to rapid change in physical characteristics; may be overly aware of a defect, resulting in undervaluation of self Body is the channel through which rejection or acceptance occurs	Developmental task—identity versus role diffusion completion of task rests on successful completion of previous tasks—leads to secure sense of self Values, attitudes, beliefs of parents are internalized Adolescent feels a sense of wholeness—recognizes uniqueness of self	Accept changing body size, shape, and function Learn a variety of physical skills Achieve a satisfying and socially acceptable sex role Find the self as a member of one or more peer groups; develop interpersonal skills Achieve independence from parents and other adults yet maintain interdependence Select a satisfying occupation in line with interests and abilities Prepare to settle into a close relationship with another individual based on love rather than infatuation Develop intellectual and work skills and sensitivity to others Develop workable philosophy of life, mature values, and worthy ideals
Body continues to be channel of connection to the world; disturbances of the body influence self-concept If body undergoes changes, person must explore those changes and incorporate them into existing picture Body type and size influence personality development Illness causes changes in body image/self-concept that need to be integrated	Developmental task—intimacy versus isolation Inadequate resolution of identity crisis may lead to disturbances in sex-role identity Stress reactions, including physiological changes, may occur as a result of intolerable levels of anxiety Suicide is third leading cause of death Alcoholism and drug abuse are two other chronic problems	Accept self and stabilize self-concept and body image Establish independence from parental home and financial aid Become established in a vocation or profession that provides satisfaction and financial recompense Learn to appraise and express love responsibly through more than sexual contacts Establish an intimate bond with another Manage a residence Decide whether to have a family Find congenial social group Formulate a meaningful philosophy of life Become involved as a citizen in the community

Continued.

TABLE 6-9 Overview of developmental stages—cont'd

Stage of development	Play/social activities	Health promotion	Language/cognitive development
Middle age	Leisure time becomes a concern; as individual progresses toward retirement, assessment of leisure time is important; person needs to feel that it is acceptable to put aside time for leisure Recognition of the era in which one was raised and subsequent values developed Relationship with spouse is especially important—provides security and stability in a period of much change	Menopause—both male and female—occurs, with concurrent physiological changes Consideration of safety factors to prevent falls, burns Coronary artery disease is leading cause of death in men Other health problems include cancer, pulmonary disease, diabetes, depression, alcoholism	Learning enhanced by individual's resource of life experiences Motivation to learn is greater—increasing numbers of individuals in this age bracket are continuing their education Ability to integrate cognitive function with experiential factors, resulting in more meaningful interpretation of life experiences
Older adulthood	Older individual often surrounds himself or herself with his or her few special friends; period characterized by great sense of loss—loss of close friends, loss of function/independence, and eventual loss of self Person is comfortable with daily routines and same people Needs to maintain contact with outside world to preserve reality orientation and to prevent loneliness Retirement affects number and type of relationships—person may feel cut off from meaningful people	Safety factors are of prime consideration; impaired sensory input hampers the accurate perception of environment; falls, burns, forgetfulness in regard to the taking of medications are examples of potentially dangerous situations Alterations in all major systems begin; regular physicals and early detection of illness help to reduce ensuing problems	Many factors affect learning: reduced motivation, sensory impairment, educational level, deliberate caution; capacity to learn continues—logical associations between words and events are easily recalled Apprehension in new learning situations Slowness in reaction time

Body image	Emotional development	Developmental tasks (From Duvall, 1971)
Additional physical changes occur—graying hair, wrinkled skin, decreasing sensory functions Need to accept body changes as part and parcel of maturation process Need to recognize positive aspects of self, body, and other persons in age group	Developmental task—generativity versus stagnation Reassessment and evaluation of one's life are critical Acceptance of goals that were accomplished as well as those that were not Enjoyment of watching children carry on traditional values and beliefs Orientation toward needs and goals of others—willingness to extend self	Rediscover and develop new satisfactions as a mate Assist growing children to become more responsible Create pleasant, comfortable home, appropriate to own values Find pleasure in generativity and recognition in work Adjust to role reversal with aging parents Assume mature social and civic responsibilities Develop and maintain active organization membership Accept and adjust to physical changes Make an art of friendship Use leisure time with satisfaction Continue to form a philosophy of life
Physical changes cause alterations in function and appearance and thus in body image; sensory deficits cause individual to believe that he or she is weak and less worthy; feels the loss of independence; perceives prostheses, hearing aids, glasses, etc., as threats to wholeness	Developmental task—ego integrity versus despair; person defends his or her beliefs and life-style—because they hold meaning for the person; views life as worthwhile, productive rather than futile, and too short; individual who has had an intact ego throughout the life cycle is better equipped to deal with aging—feels completeness and satisfaction with his or her life; death then is not feared but accepted as part of life	Decide where and how to live out remaining years; find satisfactory home and living arrangements Continue a warm, supportive relationship with significant other Adjust living standards to a retirement income Maintain maximum level of health Maintain contact with children, grandchildren Maintain interest in people outside family Pursue new interests and maintain former activities Find meaning in life after retirement Work out significant philosophy of life Adjust to loss of loved one

tural values and mores. Through consensual validation, a Sullivanian concept, a person receives support from others in perceiving the environment validly. Similarly, we consider an individual to be mentally healthy, if he or she is sensitive to another human being's wants and needs—that is, if the individual is empathic. One of the most significant indicators of mental disorder is the inability to grasp reality. However, this factor must be assessed in relationship to the predominant culture, as well as to family constellation and significant others.

The sixth indicator of positive mental health is the ability to love others and to be loved. The ability to love others and be loved includes all aspects of interpersonal relationships, such as work and play. Environmental mastery is the crux of this criterion. The ability to adapt—to meet situations head-on, assess them appropriately, draw relevant conclusions, identify goals, and plan strategies—is a complex component of environmental mastery. The individual is no longer a slave of the environment; the individual is aware of his or her *impact* on other people, that he or she does have input. Environmental mastery begins shortly after birth and continues through senescence. At each level, different tasks serve to increase an individual's ability to problem solve in new and varied settings. Energy is directed toward mastering the tasks at hand. A paralyzed young adult devotes energies toward mastering an environment that functions on the concept of mobility. A perceptually or visually impaired person seeks to master his or her environment. Each individual assesses his or her environment to discover what meaning it holds at the time and devotes energy toward the accomplishment of tasks that will reinforce environmental mastery.

Thus far in this chapter, some of the major aspects of personality development have been presented. Assessment of clients must be based on an overview of psychosexual, biological, cognitive, interpersonal, and social characteristics, as well as on other factors that combine to form an integrated, whole being. Table 6-9 illustrates such an integration of the concepts we consider significant to the understanding of the unique personality of each client.

DEATH AS PUBLIC POLICY

What is the definition of death? When do socially appropriate behaviors that accompany death begin? Veatch (1988) notes that there has been a shift in the moral, social, and political position on the determination of death since the 1960s. Historically, there has been a controversy over various philosophical and theological positions yet little concern as to what it meant to be dead in a public policy sense. What does being labeled "dead" actually mean? Death-related behaviors such as the initiation of mourning as well as other social and cultural changes occur once an individual has been labeled as dead. Spouses assume the role of widow or widower. Organs may be donated. The processes of disposal of remains and the reading of the will are initiated. However, the point at which death occurs has become unclear and the cause for much debate. The precision of definition of death and the initiation of ensuing death behaviors assumes a role of greater significance in this age of increasing technology. Veatch indicates that two critical factors have influenced death as a public issue. First, technology has extended the capacity to prolong the dying process, thus increasing the number of potential indicators of what should be considered as death. Second, organ donation requires a precise definition of death to facilitate the removal and transplantation of viable tissue. Death then becomes a process rather than a finite point in time. This concept holds implications for death behaviors. Morally we may find that the body continues to live, yet the person no longer exists as a result of the consideration of dying as a series of events rather then one finite point. Veatch suggests, for the purpose of public policy definition, that death be considered as death of the whole human organism rather than some particular part. However, the notion of "brain death" as the determinant of the indicator of death has emerged. This term itself is shrouded in ambiguity. Several standards have been developed to measure brain death: the Harvard criteria, the President's Commission, and other groups'. Each has set different lengths of time and types of tests that should be utilized to determine brain death. In each case, if tests are applied for too short or too long a period of time, the determination of death will assume a different definition. Further is the consideration of the brain as the sole organ utilized to determine death. The standard of death then is basically what society considers the essential nature of man. Thus, the definition of death—how and when to treat individuals who are dead—is a matter of public policy and has implications for the nursing profession. The question of extraordinary life-support measures—withholding of nutritional support in terminal situations and removing individuals from life-support measures—rely in part on philosophical perspectives and also on the public domain's consideration of when death occurs.

Critical issues remain to be resolved in the issue of the determination of death. Veatch identifies them as follows: the problem of irreversibility; is the critical loss relative to death one of function or structure; is the critical loss at the cellular level or at the structural level; which functions and/or structures are essential for determining death; and can there be a difference of definition in the public domain since there is such a great deal of variation in the definition of death. Nurses, in their attempts to deal holistically with clients and their families, need to be cognizant of their own philosophical beliefs regarding death as well as the issue of death within the public domain. Forty-one states have adopted some form of criteria relative to brain death as the measure of cessation of life, yet no state has adopted a definition of death based on higher brain function. Perhaps this is due to the lack of specific measurements relative to higher brain function. In any case, the issue of the public definition of death and the care of those who are considered alive remains a crucial one for the health care profession.

Stages of the dying process

Although each person who faces death experiences the situation uniquely, six stages are commonly associated with the process of dying. These stages, identified by Elizabeth Kübler-Ross as a result of her extensive work with the dying, were incorporated into her book *On Death and Dying* (1969). See the box on this page.

Stages of dying

STAGE I—SHOCK AND DENIAL

"No, not me—it can't be true." Denial is healthy and acts as a buffer so that client can mobilize resources. Dependent upon client's previous experiences with loss; amount of time to prepare for death; and how the information of impending death was given to the client.

STAGE II—ANGER AND RAGE

"Why me?" Client directs anger at family and health professionals. Feels loss of control and frustration. May have difficulty sifting out and sharing emotions. Needs to assume as much of the decision making regarding care as is possible.

STAGE III—BARGAINING

"If I could just live to see my son be married this fall." Energies are directed towards bargaining for more time. After each goal is completed, another may be set. This mechanism permits the client to deal with dying a piece at a time.

STAGE IV—DEPRESSION

The impact of future as well as present and past losses becomes apparent. Changes in role imply changes in financial status, sense of identity as a productive person, and loss of self as one who has a future. Guilt and shame may also accompany depression.

STAGE V—PREPARATORY DEPRESSION

Period in which the client attempts to assimilate the losses facing him and to prepare for his impending death.

STAGE VI—ACCEPTANCE

This is not a sense of hopelessness but rather an understanding of the finality of one's life. There is little sense of struggle; energies are directed toward the living process of dying. The client may prefer to be with one significant person rather than with many during this time.

Although Elizabeth Kübler-Ross has identified the stages of the dying process, it is important to remember that individuals face dying in their own unique manner. Rando (1984) notes that specific variables influence the responses of dying clients. These variables may be classified into groups. The first of these is personal characteristics: personality; sex; age; coping style and abilities; religion and philosophy of life; social, cultural, and ethnic background; previous experiences with loss and death; maturity; intelligence; mental health; fulfillment in life; life-style; and perceived timeliness of impending death. The second group includes quality and quantity of the client's relationships, degree of support provided by relationships, degree of openness and communication between client and significant others, and social milieu of the client. The third group of variables include those relative to socioeconomic and environmental factors such as financial resources, economic status, degree of access to quality medical treatment, education, employment status, social class, and physical environment. The last group of variables relate specifically to the illness of the client. This group includes type of illness, the personal meaning of the illness and its location, presence and amount of pain, effects of mental and physical deterioration, effects of treatment regimen, rate of loss of control, rate of progression toward death. Research suggests that certain patterns of variables predict how well clients will cope with their illness. Weisman and Worden (1975) found that longer survivals were associated with those clients who had positive relationships with others; who asked for and received medical and emotional support; who accepted the seriousness of their illness but not the inevitability of their death; who expressed anger but did not alienate their support systems; and who refused to let others pull away from them. Those with shorter survival rates had poor social and intimate relationships from early life on; had considered suicide; tended to become depressed and pessimistic about progress; and described wanting to die. Other studies confirm these hypotheses. Rando synthesized the research by stating that clients who communicate openly about their feelings and needs; who express their anger directly and appropriately; and who have strong supportive relationships tend to cope better and live longer. To facilitate the coping process, nurses need to acknowledge the client who is more vocal, who expresses anger assertively, and who chooses to participate actively in the process of his own dying. The function of denial must be understood more clearly by nurses who have the misconception that denial is unhealthy. Weisman (1972) distinguishes between first-, second-, and third-order denial. First-order denial is the unequivocal denial of the primary facts of the illness. For example, a woman is diagnosed with Hodgkins disease yet refuses to have chemotherapy. Second-order denial involves the inferences the client draws from his illness. An example of this is the acceptance of the diagnosis but a lack of acknowledgment that this diagnosis implies death. Third-order denial or "middle knowledge" is used to describe a state of fluctuation somewhere between acknowledgment of terminal illness and the rejection of that same status. Although the client may make arrangements for his own death and recognize a shortened life expectancy, there is a vacillation toward life-saving measures, such as the introduction of a new medication or procedure. Nurses have long been educated as to the negative function of denial; however, denial cannot be defined in a concrete fashion. Denial is not always dysfunctional. Lazarus and Folkman (1984) describe situations in which denial is functional. For example, denial or denial-like processes can be adaptive in situations in which the client has no ability to overcome the threat. Parts of a threatening situation can be effectively denied such as in the case of the diabetic who may take his insulin or follow his diet yet at the same time adaptively deny the possibility of neuropathy, blindness, or peripheral vascular disease that might occur in the future. In this case, adaptation is facilitated by the client's ability to cope within a present time frame. Concurrently, the timing of the denial is critical. Denial during the onset of insulin shock could prove to be fatal if the client chose to delay necessary treatment. Thus, it becomes clear that nurses need to ascertain what is being denied and whether there are favorable or unfavorable outcomes resulting from the use of denial or denial-like processes. Recognition of denial as health promoting in certain situations will prevent needless confrontations with clients who "won't accept the fact that they are dying."

To understand the world of the dying client, it is also necessary to consider the social context in which the client exists. Glaser and Strauss (1972) in their early work with dying clients describe four contexts of awareness: closed awareness, suspicion, mutual pretense, and open awareness. Although the current emphasis is on open dialogue between client and health care professional, personality traits, coping style, situation, and other social factors influence participants in the dying process and their ability to communicate. The contexts of awareness provide a framework from which to assess levels of communication; however, it would be a mistake to rigidly pidgeonhole clients and/or families into a specific category. Open communication can be useful to clients and families. Yet it would be simplistic to think that everyone is willing to and capable of addressing their impending death with unreserved forthrightness. The box on this page presents the contexts of awareness as described by Glaser and Strauss.

Although the literature has provided nurses, physicians, families, and dying clients with the much-needed impetus to bring the issue of dying out of the closet, we cannot assume that each client, each health care provider, or family member will communicate openly. The interrelationship of factors such as personality, previous coping methods, the illness itself, past communication style—all influence the client/nurse/family interaction. To expect clients to alter established patterns of interaction at this critical juncture in life is unrealistic. To acknowledge these behaviors and to offer possible alternatives is a more feasible goal.

A 45-year-old housewife was readmitted to the oncology unit following a six-month remission of her ovarian cancer. Her husband and two young daughters visited daily, yet neither client nor her husband openly discussed her terminal status. Her weight loss increased, fatigue became more pronounced, and she finally became unable to move about without assistance from others. Throughout this time period, the oncologist informed the husband that the client was not responding to the treatment regimen. The client would periodically joke with her husband, stating, "I've always

---

Contexts of awareness

CLOSED AWARENESS

Avoidance of direct conversation about nature of terminal illness. Outright lies avoided; "safe" information exchange directed by health professionals. Occurs on unconscious level for most part.

SUSPICION

Client suspects terminal outcome from other sources, i.e., overheard comments from aides, technologists, social workers, or from physician to family, other physicians, or overheard from one staff member to another; from changes in medications, treatments, physical location (intensive care unit; hospice care); altered response about future plans from significant others; signals from one's own body such as increasing fatigue, weight loss. Unstable context—will become either mutual pretense or open awareness.

MUTUAL PRETENSE

Both client and staff are aware that client is dying, but each pretends that this is not so. Utilized commonly and is adaptive in certain situations to maintain emotional stability. May help staff to keep some distance while at the same time permitting the client to exercise some control over his life.

OPEN AWARENESS

Open acknowledgment of the client's situation by both client and staff. Essential facts are discussed. Allows client to prepare for death through such activities as planning the funeral, making out the will, saying goodbye to significant others.

---

been a little overweight—now I'm thin enough to wear one of those skinny bikinis this summer at the beach." Several days later, a staff member found a notepad with instructions for funeral arrangements written in the client's own hand.

In summary, the accurate appraisal of the client's level of awareness as well as the social context in which he and she must exist are critical to the development of effective intervention strategies. It is not the goal of nursing to "tie up" all the emotional loose ends. This is an unrealistic expectation and diverts energy that could be utilized to facilitate the client's achievement of a dignified death. The recognition of how each client copes with his own death—whether through the use of denial, avoidance, rationalization, intellectualization, or some other form of defense mechanism—as well as the effectiveness of these strategies must be considered.

Sociocultural aspects of dying and death

Culture influences the kind of comfort measures and care that are given to a dying individual and the context in which the individual dies. For example, Mexican-Americans view the illness of one member of the family as a primary concern to the others. When possible, terminally ill people die at home among their family members and in familiar surroundings rather than in hospital settings (Gonzales, 1975).

Rural or elderly black Americans, Chinese-Americans, and Native Americans may equate admission to a hospital for treatment with going there to die. Early diagnosis and treatment are resisted; an individual eventually enters the hospital on an emergency basis or in a terminally ill state, which reinforces the belief that hospitals are a place to die. Cultural orientation is reflected in the belief that individuals should not be alone at a time of trouble and one should be surrounded by family members at the time of death.

Hispanics often view illness and pain as a *castigo*, or punishment from God, for their sins. Suffering can then be equated with penance, in which case comfort measures and pain medications are refused during the dying process to atone for sins (Baca, 1969).

Culture also influences individuals' attitudes about death as well as funeral practices and care of the body. Native Americans may view death to be the result of the violation of cultural taboos, while Haitians believe that voodoo can cause sudden death. Violent death such as suicide is often viewed

as less acceptable than other forms of dying. For example, traditionally Roman Catholics who committed suicide were not permitted to be buried in consecrated ground. (For further discussion of suicide, see Chapter 22.)

Care of the body after death is determined by cultural beliefs. Muslim beliefs dictate that bodies must not be cremated or be used as teaching cadavers. Organs cannot be donated, and an autopsy cannot be done. The Orthodox Jewish faith holds that the body should be buried intact; thus cremation, embalming, and any cosmetic processes are not permitted. Some cultures view death as a part of life that needs to be prepared for. For example, Amish women sew the white burial garments for themselves and their family members. Instructions are left with friends and other relatives regarding the care of the body and the burial itself.

Spiritual aspects of dying and death

Spiritual and cultural aspects of dying cannot be easily separated. Often culture influences the spiritual beliefs that an individual considers most important. During the bargaining stage, clients may bargain with God or some other omnipotent being for more time to see or do "one last thing." Nurses need to consider spiritual beliefs or the lack thereof as they are working with dying clients and their families. For example, a client's spiritual background can help in preparing for death, through prayer, quiet meditation, or chanting or song. Family members may wish to have a quiet time each day with their loved one so they may pray together—saying the rosary or other appropriate prayers. Spiritual beliefs of clients and families can easily be overlooked when physical needs are present. Nurses need to be cognizant of clients' and families' desire for spiritual comfort through the visits of ministers, priests, or rabbis. Family members may wish to have their own clergyperson, or they may feel comfortable with the hospital chaplain. It is necessary to assess spiritual beliefs on death as well as to recognize the importance of religious rituals for family and clients. It might be determined that the client or the family has no need or desire for consideration of spiritual beliefs. Nurses need to respect the right of clients to refuse spiritual counseling. Spirituality can take the form of a belief in a supreme being rather than a belief in God. Spiritual beliefs in whatever form deserve the respect of health care professionals as a component of a holistic nursing approach.

Paranormal experiences

Death is a physically degenerative process, yet there is evidence that suggests a radical alteration of consciousness and perception of reality that cannot be perceived by the five physical senses, or "paranormal experiences." Hine (1982) hypothesizes that "it is possible that a gradual spiritualization of consciousness is what life is all about and that the altered states of consciousness observed at many deathbeds are simply the final and rapidly accelerating stages of the process." Grof and Halifax-Grof (1976) describe the knowledge gained from working with persons who have had near-death or paranormal experiences. These authors do not view deathbed hallucinations and visions as the delusions of an overmedicated client. They believe that the altered, higher state of consciousness is so overwhelming that it occurs outside the logical sequence of language as well as outside linear time and space. For example, often a client describes the experience of viewing all the events of his or her life as if they were occurring simultaneously— "my life flashing before my eyes." A client can also experience segments of his or her life juxtaposed but not in a chronological or rational manner. An example of this is a client's description of having been traveling with people who have long been dead. The experience is often confused by the perception that the events are real.

Clients report hearing health care professionals pronounce that they are dead yet having no sense of the loss of reality or the alteration of consciousness. A frequently described experience of clients who have undergone cardiac arrest is the feeling that they are watching the activities being performed as if they were outside of their bodies—a phenomenon known as autoscopic observation. Clients after near-death experiences describe following the body to the operating room, noting the details of the operation, and later being able to identify the staff members involved. During a client-support

group for individuals with life-threatening arrhythmias, one woman stated that while undergoing cardioversion in the electrical studies laboratory, she perceived that she was watching everyone try to resuscitate her. She did not remember feelings of terror or panic but simply a warm, comforting sense that everything would be all right even if she died. Another client in the support group shared a similar experience during a cardioversion but remembers trying to shout down to himself, "Wake up!"

Another near-death experience, similar to autoscopic observation, is transcendental observation, whereby the mind leaves the body and the environment and is transported to another place and time. For example, a client describes returning to the scene of an accident, after having been taken to the hospital, and observing the activities at the accident scene (Oakes, 1981).

Those who have had near-death experiences describe the mind being moved either through a tunnel or through darkness to a place of warmth, love, and brightness. The mind may be invited to enter the warm place or may be told not to enter because earthly activities have not been completed. The mind is then rapidly propelled backward and is reunited with the body, which is often accompanied by pain or discomfort. Negative apparitions in the form of hell-fire or monsters can occasionally occur.

The caregiver and the dying client

Kastenbaum in 1976 described a quest for "healthy dying." The characteristics of this process included criticism of extensive life-support measures without consideration for the beneficence factor and, second, the need for health professionals and families to create and execute a "good" death—whatever that may be. Martocchio (1987) indicates that the current quest is to achieve a healthy and meaningful *living* of life. The reframing of the context of dying permits the client to remain in the realm of the living. When a client is labeled as "dying," his or her role changes as do the roles of significant others around him or her. What is this new role? Clients describe feelings of ambiguity, conflict, dissonance, anxiety, and an incompatibility with others' wishes. A feeling of being in limbo between life and death results. Health professionals may "expect" on an unconscious level the client to die within a "scheduled" time frame. Frustration may be expressed, particularly on a covert level by staff members and families when dying does not occur "when it should." Choices may be taken away, leaving the client with little or no social identity other than as a dying person. The client has moved from a well-established role as wife or husband, businessperson, housewife, son, or daughter to the "person who is dying." All focus is directed toward the dying rather than the living process. Martocchio notes that the reconceptualization of the process of dying into a process of living maximizes potential capabilities of client, family, and

health professional. She describes four concepts that are the keys to the development of genuine relationships: authenticity, self-representation, emotional closeness, and belonging (see Table 6-10). She believes that these factors can enable clients and families to emerge from the grieving process in a more healthy frame of mind. Loss is reconceptualized as a gain when clients and families are able to make decisions regarding the quality of their lives. The tragedy of life is not the process of dying but rather what dies in a person while he is still alive. Clients then are encouraged through genuine committed relationships to experience their lives through the full range of emotions that each of us has as a human being.

Authentic relationships permit the expression of

TABLE 6-10 Martocchio's relationship concepts

Concept	Nursing implications
Authenticity—foundation from which one makes career choices; sense of autonomy; ability to appraise reality of illness situation; evaluation of new choices; recognition of new self within context of current situation	Assist client in overcoming immobilization; determine what client wants to know, what information is necessary; respond with feelings; clarify meaning of events, i.e., biopsies, treatments; ask clients how they envision nurse and others helping them at this time
Emotional closeness—based on open bonding and trust, not exclusion; basic elements include sharing of joy and suffering; knowledge of own weaknesses and struggles is critical for both nurse and client	Create an atmosphere of closeness not friendship; accept painful emotions as a growing experience; permit honest expression of feelings; share own feelings and weaknesses within an objective context
Belonging—emerges from open sharing of feelings between client and nurse; feeling at home with certain people at certain times—never completely achieved; dependent upon client's previous experiences with concept—may evoke either positive or negative feelings	Affirm ownership of one's feelings as authentic; enable client to express true feelings and hopes; allow self-representation to occur within context of current situation
Self-representation—honest presentation of how one wishes to live and to die; how one plans to achieve goals; each person is different in ability to confront reality and make choices	Enable clients to express what they want in their living and dying; what their agendas are; assist client in identifying own agenda—what it is that they want at any given point in time; assist client in sharing agenda with significant others
Uniqueness of situation is critical—agendas will change based on family circumstances, course of disease, emotional state	Recognize that each individual (client and nurse) experience different feelings at different times yet there is *always* meaning; understand that dying clients may require values that are more relevant to memories of an active life rather than a participation in occupations or other more active pursuits

feelings and enable a sense of belonging; there is a sense of future, no matter how small—seconds, minutes, hours, days, or years. Those who are dying are perceived as having unique personalities with specific goals. Nurses and families can facilitate the development and expression of meaningful agendas. To do this, clients must have accurate information about their well-being so as to make decisions before care is given. Information must be honest and understandable. Dying individuals must be permitted to choose what decisions they wish to take part in as well as those which they do not. The choice of style of dying is critical and must be supported by those around the dying client, including family members and caregivers. Agendas may vary dependent upon situation and the client's own value system. For example, a primary agenda may be the inclusion in a social network such as family or community. The client may actualize this agenda by requesting family to be present as much as possible, by sharing memories through family albums. The client may wish to revisit homes or places that hold special significance. Unfortunately in many instances these wishes are denied because the client is deemed "too ill" or the experience would be "too taxing." Other agendas may include the desire to remain autonomous—to not be a burden on family members or others. It is often more acceptable for the client to enter a hospital or nursing home because he or she would feel less of a burden there than to be cared for at home. Another agenda might be the need to maintain an attractive appearance or a desire to seek a higher spiritual meaning to one's life. Whatever the agenda, it belongs to the client and has significant meaning. The nurse and family must maintain a neutral position to permit the client to actualize that agenda. This may be difficult, since the perspective of family and nurse may be quite different from the client—the vision of one more sunset from a favorite beach holds a very different meaning for a client whose future is more finite than that of his family or caregivers.

Martocchio notes that the importance of the four concepts she has described lies in the fact that caregivers and families can facilitate and share in authentic relationships with those who are dying. Dying is no longer simply an end but a beginning of

another process of the life-cycle. Authentic relationships allow clients to experience meaning and personal achievement. Caregivers and families gain awareness of their own agendas; share their weaknesses and struggles; and develop an inner sense of strength through their relationship with the dying individual.

Dugan (1987) also notes the importance of support—emotional, spiritual, and ethical for clients, families, and caregivers. He raises the issue that caregivers found it difficult to listen to painful emotions expressed by dying clients. Often they would respond by identifying client statements as being suicidal. The need on the part of the caregiver was to "improve" the client's emotional state. The message to the client was to "not feel those emotions." The dying process often aroused unresolved personal loss on the part of the caregiver; thus, the caregiver may attempt to resolve these losses through the relationship with the dying client. Dugan suggests that caregivers can enable clients to release emotional pain through verbal as well as nonverbal communication. Should a client say, "I would truly rather be dead," a supportive response on the part of the nurse would be, "Tell me more about your feelings." This statement conveys permission to share emotional pain rather than deny its existence. Statements such as, "You should be braver for your family" or "Other people in your position at least make an effort," only serve to block further communication. Emotional support on the part of the nurse permits the client to rant and rave, shout, cry, or laugh as a means of tension relief. The nurse's emotional availability is a great therapeutic resource. The emotional well of nurses who work with dying clients can be replenished through the ongoing mechanism of collegial support where acceptance and honesty characterize relationships.

Dugan describes the provision of spiritual support as a challenge similar to the provision of emotional support. He defines it as a "loss of one's personal integrity, a fragmenting of one's sense of internal togetherness." Often the client is left feeling confused and immobilized, unable to respond. Dugan makes the point that clients need to be accepted, their spiritual pain acknowledged. It is not helpful to counter painful expressions by attempts to instill faith or hope. Spiritual support is not inappropriate; however, it may be offered too quickly. Nurses need to hear and understand what the client is saying. Experiencing this current time of loss with the client facilitates spiritual growth; it implies moving beyond the stage of denial and distinguishing symbolic from literal communications.

Last, Dugan notes the need for ethical support of dying clients and their families. Nurses may facilitate ethical support by permitting clients to participate in the decision-making process regarding medical and nursing treatments. Dialogue between client and nurse is essential to determine quality of life as defined by the client—not by the nurse or the medical establishment. Options involving life-preserving measures must be carefully considered by the client as well as by significant others. The concept of beneficence, the right to health care that maximizes benefits while minimizing suffering, is viewed in a broader perspective that includes social, cultural, emotional, spiritual, and financial factors. Ethical dilemmas occur most frequently when the client is unable to determine what he feels is best for him or her. Nursing support is directed toward facilitating decision making about treatment procedures, life-support measures, tube feedings, risks and benefits of various options before the client is unable to do so. Open, listening-oriented communication is required to actualize the decision-making process. Nurses should be aware that the establishment of an atmosphere that is conducive to the expression of emotional pain is critical. The management of the client's emotional pain often becomes intertwined with the nurse's own unresolved losses. Rather than attempt to resolve past loss situations within the context of the client's dying, nurses should permit the client to live—and to die as he or she chooses with the support of family, friends, and health care professionals.

Working with dying clients and their families also involves the assessment of physical needs, toward which, as mentioned previously, nurses generally direct most of their energies. Comfort measures, such as providing adequate pain management, positioning clients appropriately, and maintaining sufficient hydration, can be instituted by the nursing staff on the basis of assessment of the client and in collaboration with the physician.

Hospice care for the dying client

Hospital care has traditionally been organized around the central goal of saving lives—and recently through the use of high technology. However, Knaus et al. (1983) concluded that high technology incurs as many burdens and is extremely expensive. Results from their study of ICU admissions over a 30-month period demonstrated that there was little evidence to suggest that intensive care units improved quality of life or survival rates. The question arises as to the influence of high-technology medicine and its impact on dying. Is there a dearth of health resources for that population that needs it most—the elderly? If this is the case, are these resources being disproportionately distributed to intensive care medicine? In part due to the conflict in values regarding care of the dying and allocation of scarce resources, the movement toward hospice care began. Davidson (1988) defines the hospice movement as a variety of programs that facilitates the dying process of terminally ill individuals for whom intensive medical treatment regimens are no longer appropriate. Although origins of the hospice movement can be traced back as far as 238 BC, the most well-known inspiration came in the person of Dr. Cicely Saunders. Dr. Saunders initiated the first hospice, St. Christopher's, in 1967 outside the city of London. Over 30 hospice programs exist in Great Britain at present. Each hospice shares a common philosophy—that of providing compassionate care for the terminally ill.

Hospice programs in the United States have modeled themselves after St. Christopher's, but none duplicate it in totality. Davidson (1988) identifies several models that have been adopted in this country: wholly volunteer programs; home care programs; freestanding, full-service, autonomous institutions; hospital-based palliative care units; and continuum-of-care subacute units. The volunteer program functions as a self-help model where individuals from the community provide services wherever needed, i.e., getting medical equipment, acting as client advocate, initiating bereavement support services. Home care programs provide similar services to the terminally ill as the volunteer program; however, they also provide comprehensive nursing care. Freestanding institutions can be most closely aligned with the

TABLE 6-11 Piagetian theory and the understanding of death

Piaget's periods	Concepts	Developmental period/era
Preoperational cognitions (2-7 years)	Reversibility External causation (poison, falls, violent acts) Revival is possible	Preschool years
Concrete operations (7-11-12 years)	Physical function ceases Irreversibility Universality Internal causation Simple beliefs, i.e., heaven or hell; afterlife regarding death	Early school years Middle childhood Preadolescence
Formal operations (11/12 years and older)	Religious and philosophical theories about the nature and existence of death	Adolescence

St. Christopher model. This type of hospice allows clients to remain at home for as long as possible but also makes provisions for those who may need inpatient hospitalization as well as inpatient day care where clients receive care during the day and go home at night. The difficulty inherent in this type of program is the lack of coordination between the hospice and other facilities necessary to the survival of the program. Hospital-based palliative care units are able to utilize hospital resources such as laboratory facilities and the sound financial foundation that the hospital has established. However, in the United States, little success has been achieved with this model due to utilization review restrictions and reimbursement procedures. Last, Davidson describes the subacute continuum-of-care unit. The model provides a range of coordinated services such as the movement from one health care facility to another that can be accomplished expeditiously. Treatment goals are achieved through the separation of acute and hospice units, although they may exist in one institution. Centralized administration and budgeting permit specialized care to be offered in a cost-effective manner.

Although there are several models of hospice, the central goal remains constant—provision of care to the terminally ill. Gonda and Rouark (1984) describes six functional elements of hospice care: client and family are considered the "client"; home care services are coordinated with inpatient services; an interdisciplinary team inclusive of nursing, medicine, social work, clergy, volunteers, and ancillary staff provides care; the skills of these health care providers are available 24 hours a day; bereavement care is provided for significant loved ones; and emotional support to all hospice staff is provided on an ongoing basis. Gonda and Rouark also states that the relief of physical symptoms is at the center of hospice care. The effective management of pain, decreased appetite, nausea, and other physical complaints is accomplished through an understanding of pain and its interactional effects. Each individual is respected as unique, with his or her own dying trajectory, priorities, and methods of coping with the singularly most difficult task of life—death.

Children, adolescents, and death

The understanding of death moves in an orderly progression concurrent with the development of language and thought processes. Wass, Berardo, and Niemeyer (1988) note that the understanding of death can be paralleled with Piaget's model of cognitive development. Table 6-11 presents children's and adolescents' concepts of death. (Wass et al., 1988).

Wass et al. (1988) indicate that there is little substantive data to support the notion that infants conceptualize about death. Gonda and Rouark (1984) suggest that separation anxiety relative to significant caretakers most closely parallels an infant's awareness of death as an event. The loss of a parent during this period can have a profound effect on the child in later developmental stages.

Wass et al. (1988) also note that variations in understanding and assimilating concepts of death may depend upon demographic variables. For example, children in lower socioeconomic groups tended to comprehend the irreversibility of death at an earlier age. Wass and Scott (1978) found that early adolescents with college-educated parents were more likely to formulate their own theories of life and death than adolescents from parents with a high school education. Reilly, Hasazi, and Bond (1983) conducted a study which found that children who had lost a family member had a more mature understanding of death at younger ages than those who had not experienced that type of loss. From these studies and others, it would seem that children and adolescents understand death through the maturation of the cognitive processes. However, certain loss experiences have a significant impact on this understanding of death that reaches far beyond the maturational level of the child.

From a sociocultural perspective, it is important to understand how the ideas, values, and norms of culture relative to death are transmitted in our society. The parental system has a strong influence on beliefs, behaviors, and values regarding death. Yet each individual exists within the context of society where a variety of messages regarding death are conveyed on a daily basis—some of which are conflictual in nature. For example, television brings violence into the home through news broadcasts, cartoons, feature-length movies, and weekly series. The young child who sits for 3 hours on Saturday morning watching cartoons is subjected to six times as much violence as a one-hour adult show (Gerbner, Morgan, and Signorelli, 1982). Wass and Stillion (1988) concluded from the analysis of 1,500 commercial television programming that over 80% of the deaths were caused by violent means. The report from the National Institute of Mental Health (1982) condemns the use of violence on television, stating that observed violence is then condoned by society, which in turn gives children

the message that violence and aggression are acceptable.

Preadolescents and adolescents are greatly influenced by rock music and the music videos widely seen on MTV. Death and violence are implicitly or explicitly conveyed through the music media. Themes of suicide, nuclear war, murder, and drug and alcohol use appear in the hard-rock expression of negativism. It has been suggested that regulatory measures be instituted to reduce the expression of violent themes. However, there is no empirical evidence to suggest that there is a correlation between hard rock and future violent or aggressive behaviors. The significant influence of music on adolescents is apparent. The need is to determine to what extent attitudes and behaviors are influenced.

Consider the games children and adolescents play. The favorites include cops and robbers, cowboys and Indians, or the traditional war games. In each situation, someone is "killed." A 1980s game "Photon" or "Tracer" is a variation of laser tag. An arena is set up where teams search out and destroy members of the opposition. Computer games also involve the use of the "killer" and the "victim" where children are socialized into aggressive roles. It would be foolish to attempt to curtail some of these traditional games; however, it becomes society's as well as parents' roles to monitor the use of such games and to recognize the impact they have on children's perceptions of death and violence.

THE DYING CHILD AND ADOLESCENT

How does the child deal with the notion of his or her own death? Bluebond-Langner (1978) found that children move through five stages of understanding and knowledge relative to their own demise. Information is gained through communication with parents and health care professionals and through everyday experience. Changes in self-concept occur in parallel fashion as the illness progresses and the child becomes aware that death is inevitable. The adolescent views death more as the adult does with an understanding of its finality. Yet the unfairness of the situation prompts feelings of anger, denial, resentment, anxiety, fear, and guilt. Adolescents who wish to share these feelings are often confronted with parents and others who are uncomfortable with this level of communication. Often the dying adolescent will put up a front to protect his parents from having to deal with his anger, depression, or whatever he is experiencing. For example, a 17-year-old young woman with leukemia was describing her relationship with her parents to her primary nurse. "My parents are wonderful, but every time I want to talk about my funeral or other feelings I have, they change the subject to something else. I've finally just about given up trying, and I really feel badly. There's so much I want to say to them before I die, but I think they feel if they talk about my dying, then it will surely happen. It's going to happen, I know that, but how can I convince them that they need to hear me—because soon I won't be here to talk to them. I feel as though I have to protect them from this dreaded occurrence." The sense of frustration as well as the role reversal is apparent. Health care professionals can facilitate the grieving process by encouraging open communication between parents and children. This may be accomplished through a gradual process accompanied by ongoing support of the parents as well as the dying child or adolescent. Families can be assisted to express their rage and resentment in an atmosphere of support and understanding.

The process of caring for the dying child and adolescent is a critical one for health care professionals. It is an emotionally charged process fraught with questions of justice and fairness. How can nurses provide effective nursing intervention? The following serves as a guideline for intervening with the dying child.

1. Consider the cognitive level of the child/adolescent when presenting information.
2. Determine what information is important to the client.
3. Establish a positive climate for communication through eye contact and touching, allowing sufficient time for discussion.
4. Allow the client to tell as much as he or she wants at any given time.
5. Present information in an honest, supportive manner.
6. Encourage the client to ask questions and share negative feelings about the current situation.
7. Ascertain to what extent the client can participate in making decisions regarding the direction and type of treatment.
8. Utilize other methods to facilitate communication, such as play therapy with dolls or other toys; through art or writing a short story, letter, or play. These methods are less likely to be hindered by defense mechanisms and allow children to reveal perceptions of relationships with family members, friends, and others. Comic strip simulations can also be utilized by allowing the child or adolescent to express thoughts and feelings through the comic strip format.
9. Encourage the family to participate in a dialogue of feelings to maintain an open-awareness social context.
10. Always support the notion of "hope" for clients and families.
11. Offer option of peer sharing for adolescents who are experiencing similar concerns.
12. Define support systems and functions they can provide for both client and family.

A 13-year-old boy was admitted to the pediatric unit following a recurrence of his Hodgkin's disease. This was the third admission in 6 months. Two days after admission, his primary nurse found him sitting alone in the playroom staring out the window.

Nurse Jack, you've been sitting there so quietly—may I join you?

Jack Yeah sure—I don't have a lot to say; I'm pretty boring.

Nurse I'm not sure what you mean (as she sits down with him).

Jack Nobody seems to want to talk to me—my parents come in and talk about what everybody is doing at home and in school; life is just rolling along.

Nurse What would be important for you to talk about right now?

Jack I don't know—everything, nothing—I'm just so confused.

Nurse I feel a sense of frustration and perhaps some anger there—it's alright to feel those kinds of things.

Jack Everybody else is going to have a life—I'm not; I know I'm not getting any better, but no one will talk to me about it.

Nurse I'd like to hear what you have to say.

Jack *I'd like to be able to make some choices about what's going to happen to me.*

Nurse *Do you mean in terms of your treatment?*

Jack *Yes—but also what I can do with my friends and my brothers. My parents always want me to be careful and not get hurt.*

Nurse *Would it help to be able to tell your parents these things?*

Jack *Yeah—but I'd also like to tell them to stop being afraid to talk to me about what I've got and what might happen to me.*

Nurse *Well, I think I can share some of your feelings with them and then we can set up a time for all of us to get together.*

In this situation the nurse provided an opportunity for the adolescent to express his feelings and his concerns about dying. She validated the normalcy of this expression without minimizing its significance. She also respected his need to feel a part of the decision-making process. Since the parents seemed to be having some difficulty in communicating openly, the nurse recognized the need to clarify their needs and feelings prior to discussing the situation with the child. To facilitate open dialogue, the nurse must be aware of the parents' patterns of communication as well as how they perceive the illness as it currently exists.

CHILDREN AND ADOLESCENTS WHO EXPERIENCE THE LOSS OF A PARENT

The loss of a parent may have profound ramifications for the future development of the child. As noted previously, even at the early stage of infancy, the child experiences a separation anxiety when there is the loss of a parent. The understanding of the meaning of death is again dependent upon the cognitive maturation of the child. Wass et al. (1988) state that most early parental deaths are sudden, leaving the remaining parent in a state of shock, often unable to respond to the emotional needs of the child. Zambelli et al. (1988) suggest that an interdisciplinary bereavement program is necessary to provide services for the child as well as the parent. Zambelli found that creative arts groups for children accompanied by companion groups for the surviving parent were useful in facilitating juvenile grief reactions. The key factor as noted by the authors was that children who had a parent participating in the companion group had more successful outcomes than those who did not.

The range of emotions felt by children and adolescents following the death of a parent is wide. Regressive behavior may occur as a protective mechanism and to elicit care-taking responses from others in the environment. Open, honest communication is essential. Gonda and Rouark (1984) indicate that children feel more comforted when included in the mourning rituals rather than excluded. They fear being abandoned by others and may seek constant attention. Mutual sharing of feelings is important; if intense displays of emotion are a natural part of the cultural response to death, the child should not be shielded from them. Difficulties may arise when the surviving parent becomes emotionally dependent upon the child. In this case, psychiatric referral may be necessary. Last, nurses may provide the necessary support to children and adolescents to strengthen their emotional reserves and to permit them to continue their own lives.

Nursing Intervention
PRIMARY PREVENTION

Although there has been an emphasis on understanding the process of dying and death, the provision of care to the dying client and his family remains a challenge. There is a greater level of sophistication of the American public toward the phenomena associated with death that has come about through the printed media as well as through television and film. Legal, ethical, moral, and social issues relative to the right to die have emerged as a result of this "thanatological" revolution. We have, however, been unable to abolish death; instead, there has been an increased impetus to define death. The role of the nurse as a primary provider of physical as well as psychological support is a critical element in the care of dying clients and their families.

What are the elements of primary prevention in the care of dying clients? The role of the nurse can be defined as encompassing the following:

1. Facilitation of an environment that fosters dying as an integral part of the life-cycle.
2. Provision of anticipatory guidance.
3. Education of clients, families, and significant others relative to the dying process.

4. Validation of the normalcy of feelings associated with the dying process.
5. Consultation and education with schools, communities, and other health professionals.

To actualize the role of health care provider, the nurse must consider his or her own knowledge base as well as values and belief system regarding life and death. Support groups for health professionals and values-clarification exercises can facilitate the nurse's ability to provide educational and supportive services.

SECONDARY PREVENTION

Crisis intervention skills are useful in meeting the needs of the dying client and his family and significant others. Interventive strategies are directed toward assisting the client in achieving an appropriate death as defined by the client and his family as well as facilitating the family's adaptation to role changes incurred by the client's death.

Nursing process

The nursing process provides the framework for the development, implementation, and evaluation of nursing strategies. It is critical that nurses assess their own values and beliefs relative to the legal, ethical, moral, social, and psychological issues that have arisen around the dying process. The following issues may confront nurses working with dying clients:

A. Inability of nurse to accept client's current stage of dying
   1. Nurse encourages client to give up denial before he or she is ready, which increases denial and anxiety.
   2. Nurse responds to client's anger with anger, avoidance, or punitive action.
   3. Nurse doesn't accept decathexis and tries to reinvolve client in world.
   4. Nurse doesn't respect client's philosophy regarding life and death, tries to force own values on client.
   5. Nurse has not recognized own feelings about death, avoids dying clients.
   6. Nurse has not resolved moral and ethical

questions regarding euthanasia and allowing terminally ill client to discuss issues of ending life.
   7. Nurse doesn't understand client's cultural and religious orientations toward death. This leads to misunderstanding and violation of client's and family's wishes regarding kind of care given, setting in which client dies, care of body after death, and funeral practices.
   8. Nurse has not resolved own feelings about death, tries to avoid emotional pain of witnessing client in process of dying, tries to shield client from knowledge of own impending death or reinforces client's denial.
   9. Nurse attempts to work through his or her own past experiences with the dying process—e.g., encouraging client and family to discuss dying before they are ready, because of own past experience with family members who allowed person to die without discussing feelings.

B. Inability of nurse to respond appropriately to near-death experiences
   1. Nurse pushes or probes for account of near-death experiences—if client can't recollect, may fabricate an account; if client can recollect, pushing and probing may make client back off from giving account until he or she can find person whom he or she can trust and who will allow him or her to proceed at own pace.
   2. Nurse views client's account as delusional, fanatical, or a scam, which blocks communication of near-death experiences and increases client's anxiety and fear of abandonment.
   3. Nurse is very task-oriented and focuses on life-support systems to the neglect of personalized care, which increases client's anxiety and sense of depersonalization.
   4. Nurse does not support client in recounting near-death experiences to family, which increases family's disbelief of client or leads to family reacting with emotional

outburst; blocks communication of near-death experiences and increases client's anxiety and fear of abandonment.

ASSESSMENT

The nurse facilitates an environment of trust and respect for one's needs at whatever level through the therapeutic use of self and through the knowledge of the dying process; familiarity with social, legal, moral, and ethical issues; and the desire to assist the client to an appropriate death. Accurate data collection from client as well as family and significant others is critical to the development of a comprehensive care plan.

ANALYSIS OF DATA

The analysis of data leads to the formulation of nursing diagnoses. Through the interpretation and appraisal of the data, the nurse is able to identify client strengths such as positive sense of self, posi-

tive experiences with loss in the past, strong support systems, desire to participate in the treatment process, and knowledge of the disease process, treatment, and outcomes. Data analysis also identifies areas of difficulty that may or may not be identified by the client. Prior to the identification of nursing diagnoses, it is important that client and nurse review the data and mutually determine goals and the priority of each. Strategies to achieve goals will be identified and mutually discussed.

PLANNING AND IMPLEMENTATION

Planning is based on a realistic appraisal of each individual client. The nursing care plan that follows presents nursing diagnoses that are frequently made for dying clients and their families. Each diagnosis is followed by a plan of care that reflects a realistic approach to secondary preventive intervention. Dependent upon the situation, goals may be adjusted.

NURSING CARE PLAN

Terminally Ill Clients

Long-term Outcomes	Short-term Outcomes	Nursing Strategies
Nursing diagnosis:	Anticipatory grieving related to impending death (NANDA 9.2.1.2; DSM-III-R V62.89)	
Achieve an "appropriate death"	Identify and describe feelings of loss Recognize stages of the dying process Identify potential and actual situations that precipitate feelings of loss Develop adaptive coping measures to facilitate grieving process Communicate sense of loss (present and future) to significant others Identify past experiences with loss and impact on current situation Identify maladaptive coping measures	Establish a relationship where client feels free to express feelings of anger, rage, guilt Assess stage(s) of dying process Evaluate success of client's coping strategies Support client's use of denial Assist client in effective problem-solving techniques Explore meaning of death with client Encourage client participation in treatment regimen and other decision making Support client's need to limit social interactions as desired Support expression of NDE (near death experiences) by acknowledging their place in client's perception of death Provide access to other resources, i.e., spiritual, social, financial Identify own values re dying and impact on nursing care

Long-term Outcomes	Short-term Outcomes	Nursing Strategies

Nursing diagnosis: Social isolation related to withdrawal secondary to diagnosis of terminal illness (NANDA 3.1.2.; DSM-III-R V62.89)

Long-term Outcomes	Short-term Outcomes	Nursing Strategies
Maintain social interaction with family and significant others Increase ability for optimal levels of communication within the context of the client	Identify and describe feelings of rejection, abandonment, and being unable to meet people's expectations Identify and describe situations that precipitate these feelings Identify factors that contribute to the absence of a satisfying relationship Identify times when it is adaptive to distance from others	Provide an atmosphere that facilitates the expression of feelings Explore feelings of abandonment, rejection, loss of all ties Discuss the impact of this illness on social interactions Describe feelings that arise in relationship to changes in body image, mental deterioration, chronic pain, fatigue, and their influence on interactions Encourage client to evaluate own behaviors that might be socially isolating Assist client to prioritize social interactions when energy is limited Support client in his need to limit social interaction as dying progresses Educate family and friends as to changes in social interaction as dying progresses Encourage family and friends to maintain social interaction that is based on open awareness Suggest support groups where clients can share feelings with others in similar situations

Nursing diagnosis: Spiritual distress related to questioning of basic value and beliefs systems (NANDA 4.1.1.; DSM-III-R V62.89)

Long-term Outcomes	Short-term Outcomes	Nursing Strategies
Achieve a satisfactory level of spiritual strength	Identify basic spiritual beliefs Describe changes in spiritual value system incurred by dying process Develop measures of faith that can be utilized during dying process Identify spiritual support resources Participate in defined religious rituals as appropriate	Provide an atmosphere where client can share feelings Encourage evaluation of current belief systems in relation to current situation Assist client in identifying blocks to communication resulting from own belief system Encourage client to explore alternative beliefs compatible with one's own developmental stage Avoid imposing one's own belief system on the client Provide access to spiritual care, i.e., communion, taking client to chapel Encourage discussion of the meaning of life and death for client Discuss religious rituals that client wishes for his death Identify dysfunctional religious convictions that prevent client from grieving in an adaptive manner

Continued.

NURSING CARE PLAN—cont'd

Terminally Ill Clients

Long-term Outcomes	Short-term Outcomes	Nursing Strategies
Nursing diagnosis: Knowledge deficit in relationship to the treatment regimen, alternatives to care, and/or of the disease process itself (NANDA 8.1.1.; DSM-III-R V62.89)		
Increase level of knowledge re disease process, treatment plan, and alternatives	Identify areas where honest information is needed Communicate need for further clarification Seek out other resources for information, i.e., Make Today Count, Reach for Recovery, etc.	Provide climate where client can feel comfortable asking questions Assess areas where knowledge deficit exists Assess level of readiness to learn Assess factors that may affect reception of information, i.e., increased anxiety, fear, dysfunctional denial Clarify with client areas where distortions or myths are present Recognize that client will assimilate knowledge at own pace Present information honestly without destroying sense of hope Encourage client to utilize increased knowledge in relationship to problem-solving strategies Encourage family and significant others to share information honestly Reevaluate periodically the client's need for further knowledge

---

EVALUATION

Evaluation of intervention strategies occurs within the context of the nurse-client relationship. The client may be the individual who is dying, or it may be the family and/or significant others as a "collective" client. Evaluation should reflect a positive direction, i.e., family's increased ability to accept role changes incurred by terminal diagnosis; increased knowledge base relative to the disease process. During the evaluation process, the nurse and client address goals that have been accomplished and modification of those still to be achieved.

Referral to other health professionals who have more advanced knowledge in the field of thanatology may be necessary. Community resources such as support groups for clients as well as support groups for families of the terminally ill can provide an environment where clients and family members can share their concerns. Strategies of coping that have been effective for group members can be tested out by others in a nonthreatening, supportive environment.

Last, nurses must reflect on their own philosophy of life and death; their value systems regarding the definition of death; and the moral, ethical, and legal dilemmas that have emerged as a result of high-technology medicine. To define death is no longer a simple matter. To effectively use self as a therapeutic tool, nurses need to be keenly aware of their biases and beliefs to provide quality nursing care. Nonverbal communication of beliefs that are in conflict with client choices may act to block any further intervention strategies. Values clarification is useful in facilitating the confrontation of one's own negative perceptions regarding specific grieving behaviors, philosophy of life, feelings relative to organ donation, and other feelings that may be encountered when working with dying clients and their families.

Long-term Outcomes	Short-term Outcomes	Nursing Strategies

Nursing diagnosis: Ineffective family coping styles related to changes in roles (NANDA 5.1.2.1.2; DSM-III-R V61.80)

Long-term Outcomes	Short-term Outcomes	Nursing Strategies
Increase level of family coping skills Develop roles appropriate to changes occurring in family system	Identify and describe role changes precipitated by terminal illness Identify and describe feelings associated with role changes Develop more effective adaptive measures to cope with role changes Identify support resources to facilitate adaptation to role changes	Establish a climate where client and family can share feelings Assess family strengths and limitations related to role changes Encourage members to share painful feelings such as frustration, resentment, anger, anxiety Facilitate discussion as to how changes in role can be accommodated in the family system Set limits on inappropriate behaviors, i.e., scapegoating Assist family in allowing client to maintain an active role in family system Evaluate expectations family has of dying client's role Educate family members as to changes in role that accompany dying process Assure that role distribution occurs in a fair and equitable manner Give family permission to be away from the client to replenish themselves and to take care of other children and other household activities Assist family to cope with each day as a singular event Encourage family and client to discuss such issues as where the client would like to die, i.e., hospice, home, hospital; funeral arrangements, etc. Educate family about the physical process of dying, i.e., cooling of the body, breathing difficulties, coma Prepare family for role changes following client's death Assist family to maintain a realistic sense of hope Refer family members who experience prolonged difficulty with loss to appropriate resources

TERTIARY PREVENTION

The principal focus of tertiary prevention is the identification of those individuals who utilize dysfunctional denial and other defense mechanisms that inhibit an adaptive grieving process. Crisis intervention with clients and families has resulted in limited improvement in coping with the loss; thus, further provision of ongoing services is necessary. Clients who are unable to cope with the diagnosis of terminal illness may be referred to a psychiatric mental health clinical specialist, a clinical thanatologist, or other health care professionals, including clergy who have advanced levels of knowledge and clinical expertise. Families may also be incorporated into the therapy if members are unable to adjust to the potential loss of the family member. Tertiary prevention may include support groups that can assist clients and families in coping with loss and role change. Support groups can provide an arena where issues can be shared and new strategies learned.

Nurses may also identify chronic dysfunctional patterns of coping with loss within the family system, such as suicidal ideation and depression. In this case, direct care may be provided by the nurse, or the client may be referred to appropriate resources that can facilitate the achievement of an optimal level of function for each client and/or family.

CHAPTER SUMMARY

The process of personality development can be viewed from many perspectives. We have presented for discussion the many factors that influence this process.

There are numerous theories regarding the sequence of development. Our intention has been to present four major developmental theories, as well as to discuss Maslow's theory of the hierarchy of needs. It is essential that nurses assume an eclectic approach. The ultimate goal is to recognize each client as a unique human being. When a nurse keeps this fact in mind, a nursing assessment will reflect an accurate appraisal of all the elements that combine to form an integrated human being.

Dying and death have been presented as an integral component of human development, and strategies for providing holistic nursing care to dying clients—both children and adults—and to their families have been discussed.

SELF-DIRECTED LEARNING

Sensitivity-Awareness Exercises

1. Obituary exercise*
   a. Procedure
      (1) Write an obituary for your pet, for a significant other, for yourself.
      (2) For each obituary include the following:
         (a) Day, month, year of death
         (b) Age at which individual or animal died
         (c) Cause of death—lengthy illness, illness of short duration, accident
         (d) Scene of death—home, hospital, elsewhere
         (e) Type of service or arrangements for funeral—e.g., flowers, visiting hours, mass or other type of religious service
         (f) Accomplishments and/or merits of deceased
         (g) Who survives the deceased
   b. Purposes of exercise
      (1) Assists you in clarifying feelings about death and meaning of life and death; addresses the questions of how and when one would choose to die, which will ultimately affect perceptions of how others choose to die

      (2) Progression from a pet to a significant other to yourself enables you to gain some insight into the ability to confront the reality of death
      (3) Facilitates discussion of the meaning of death
2. "Where do I stand" exercise† (for use with a group)
   a. Procedure
      (1) On a blackboard draw the following continuum:

My body will be disposed of in an efficient manner and people will not mention me when I am dead.

I want everyone to grieve for me every day of the rest of their lives.

      (2) Go to the board and write in where you fit on the continuum.
   b. Purposes of exercise
      (1) Explores expectations an individual has of

---

*Rationale adapted from Koestenbaum (1976).
†Adapted from Epstein (1975).

SELF-DIRECTED LEARNING—cont'd

others in regard to his or her own death yet gives indirect clues as to how that individual would like to be treated should he learn he is dying

(2) Decreases the possibility of confusing your own needs and desires regarding death with those of the client—believing you are doing what the client wants when in fact you are doing what you would like to have done yourself

3. "Confronting the conflict" exercise† (for use with small groups)
   a. Procedure
      (1) On a blackboard draw the following continuum:

It is ridiculous to suppose that
anyone might obtain satisfaction
from caring for a client who
dies shortly.

         Great satisfaction can be
         derived from treating a client
         who dies shortly.

(2) Mark the point at which you seem to fit.
(3) Write a brief statement describing the level of satisfaction you believe would be derived from caring for a dying client. List specifics when possible.
   b. Purposes of exercise
      (1) Assists you in identifying conflicting feelings regarding your role in promoting health as well as in facilitating a good death
      (2) Enables you to recognize some of the possible satisfactions involved in relating to a dying client

Questions to Consider

1. The directing of unacceptable libidinal energies into more socially acceptable channels is termed:
   a. denial
   b. projection
   c. sublimation
   d. rationalization

2. A husband who is angry at his employer criticized his wife for not having dinner ready when he arrived home from work. This is an example of which defense mechanism?
   a. rationalization
   b. displacement
   c. projection
   d. compensation

3. Libidinal energy is shifted from the anal to the genital area in which developmental stage?
   a. oral
   b. latency
   c. genital
   d. phallic

4. According to Kubler-Ross, which of the following behaviors is most characteristic of the first stage of the dying process?
   a. bargaining for more time
   b. anger and rage
   c. depression
   d. denial

5. A six-year-old child's understanding of death is characterized by which of the following concepts?
   a. reversibility
   b. cessation of physical function
   c. universality
   d. internal causation

Match the following theorists with the appropriate concepts:

6. Freud	a. Pre-operational thought
7. Sullivan	b. Ego, id, superego
8. Erikson	c. Tools and tasks
9. Piaget	d. Generativity vs stagnation
10. Maslow	e. Self-actualization

Answer key

1. c	6. b
2. b	7. c
3. d	8. d
4. d	9. a
5. a	10. e

REFERENCES

Baca JE: Some health beliefs of the Spanish-speaking, Am J Nurs 69:2172-2176, 1969.

Baldwin AL: Theories of child development, New York, 1967, John Wiley & Sons, Inc.

Barton D: Dying and death, Baltimore, 1977, The Williams & Wilkins Co.

Bluebond-Langner M: The private worlds of dying children, Princeton, 1978, Princeton University Press.

Bowlby J: Attachment and loss: separation, anxiety, anger, vol 1, New York, 1973, Basic Books.

Corr C and McNeil J: Adolescence and death, New York, 1986, Springer Publishing Co.

Davidson G: Hospice care for the dying, In Wass H, Berardo F, and Neimeyer R, editors: Dying: facing the facts, ed 2, Washington DC, 1988, Hemisphere Publishing Co.

Dugan D: Death and dying, J Psychosoc Nurs 7:21-29, 1987.

Duvall E: Family Development, ed 4, Philadelphia, 1971, JB Lippincott Co.

Epstein C: Nursing the dying patient, Reston, Va, 1975, Reston Publishing Co.

Erikson E: Childhood and society, ed 2, New York, 1950, WW Norton & Co.

Erikson E: Identity: youth and crisis, New York, 1968, WW Norton & Co.

Escalona S and Leitch M: Early phases of personality development: a non-normative study of infant behavior. Monographs of the Society for Research in Child Development 17(1):33-49, 1953.

Flavell J: Developmental psychology of Jean Piaget, Princeton, NJ, 1963, D. Van Nostrand Co.

Freud S: A general introduction to psychoanalysis, New York, 1916, Liveright Publishing Co.

Gerbner G, Morgan M, and Signorelli N: Programming health portrayals: what viewers see, say, and do, In Pearl D, Bouthilet L, and Lazar J, editors: Television and behavior: ten years of scientific progress and implications for the eighties, Washington, DC, 1982, US Government Printing Office.

Glaser B and Strauss A: Awareness of dying, Chicago, 1965, Aldine.

Gilmore M and Gilmore D: Machismo: a psychodynamic approach (Spain), Psychol Anthropol 2:281-299, 1979.

Gonda T and Rouark J: Dying dignified: the health professional's guide to care, Menlo Park, Cal, 1984, Addison-Wesley Publishing Co.

Gonzales H: Health care needs of the Mexican-American, In Ethnicity and health care, NLN Publication # 14-1625, New York, 1925, National League for Nursing.

Grof S and Halifax-Grof J: Psychedelics and the experience of death, In Toynbee A and Koestler A, editors: Life after death, New York, 1976, McGraw-Hill Book Co.

Hauck B: Differences between sexes at puberty, In Evans ED, editor: Adolescence: readings in behavior and development, Hinsdale, Ill, 1970, Dryden Press.

Hine VH: Holistic dying: the role of the nurse clinician, Topics Clin Nurs 3:45-54, 1982.

Hoy WK and Applebury T: Teacher-principal relationships in 'humanistic' and 'custodial' elementary schools, J Experiment Ed 2:161-170, 1970.

Jahoda M: Current concepts of positive mental health, New York, 1953, Basic Books.

Knaus WA: The use of intensive care: new research initiatives and their implications for national health policy, Milbank Memorial Fund Q 61:561-583, 1983.

Kastenbaum P: Is there an answer to death? Englewood Cliffs, NJ, 1976, Prentice-Hall, Inc.

Kubler-Ross E: On death and dying, New York, 1969, Macmillan, Inc.

Kubler-Ross E: Death: the final stage of growth, Englewood Cliffs, NJ, 1975, Prentice-Hall, Inc.

Lazarus R and Folkman S: Stress appraisal and coping, New York, 1984, Springer.

Lidz T: The person, New York, 1968, Basic Books, Inc.

McCandless B and Evans E: Children and youth: psychosocial development, New York, 1973, Dryden Press.

Malinowski B: Sex and repression in a savage society, New York, 1957, Harcourt Brace.

Martocchio B: Authenticity, belonging, emotional closeness, and self-representation, Oncol Nurs Forum 14(4):32-27, 1987.

Maslow A: Motivation and personality, New York, 1954, Harper & Row.

Metcalf CW: Humor, life and death, Oncol Nurs Forum 14(4):19-21, 1987.

Nagy M: The child's theories concerning death, J Genetics Psychol 73:3-27, 1948.

National Institute of Mental Health: Television and behavior: ten years of progress and implications for the eighties, vol 2: technical reviews, Washington, DC, 1982, US Government Printing Office.

Neugarten BL: Adult personality: toward a psychology of the life cycle, In Neugarten BL, editor: Middle age and aging: a reader in social psychology, Chicago, 1968, University of Chicago Press.

Oakes AR: Near-death events and critical care nursing, Topics Clin Nurs 3:61-78, 1981.

Rando, T: Grief, dying, and death: clinical intervention for caregivers, Champaign, Ill, 1984, Research Press Co.

Reilly T, Hasazi JE, and Bond L: Children's conceptions of death and personal mortality, J Pediatr Psychol 8:21-31, 1983.

Sapir, E: Cultural anthropology and psychiatry, In Selected writings of Edward Sapir in language, culture, and personality, Berkeley, 1963, University of California Press.

Satir V: Conjoint family therapy, Palo Alto, Cal, 1967, Science and Behavior Books.

Satir V: Peoplemaking, Palo Alto, Cal, 1975, Science and Behavior Books.

Shalom, Melissa, Nursing 88, 18(6):52-57, 1988.

Stone LJ and Church J: Childhood and adolescence: a psychology of the growing person, ed 2, New York, 1968, Random House.

Sullivan HS: The collected works of Harry Stack Sullivan, New York, 1953, WW Norton & Co.

Thompson R: Culture and personality, In Psychology and culture, Dubuque, Ia, 1975, Wm. C. Brown Co.

Veatch R: The definition of death: problems for public policy, In Wass H, Berardo F, and Neimeyer R, editors: Dying: facing the facts, ed 2, Washington, DC, 1988, Hemisphere Publishing Co.

Waechter EH: Children's awareness of fatal illness, Am J Nurs 71:1168-1172, 1971.

Wass H, Berardo F, and Niemeyer R: Dying: facing the facts, ed 2, Washington, DC, 1988, Hemisphere Publishing Co.

Wass H and Scott M: Middle school students' death concepts and concerns, Middle School J 9:10-12, 1978.

Wass H and Stillion J: Death in the lives of children and adolescents, In Wass H, Berardo F, and Niemeyer R, editors: Dying: facing the facts, ed 2, Washington, DC, 1988, Hemisphere Publishing Co.

Weisman A: On dying and denying, New York, 1972, Basic Books.

Weisman A and Worden J: Psychosocial analysis of cancer deaths, Omega 6:61-75, 1975.

Whiting C: Child training and personality: a cross-cultural study, New Haven, Conn, 1953, Yale University Press.

Zambelli G et al: An interdisciplinary approach to clinical intervention for childhood bereavement, Death Stud 12:41-50, 1988.

Zigler E: Social class and the socialization process, Rev Ed Res 4:120-135, 1970.

ANNOTATED SUGGESTED READINGS

McClowry S et al: The empty space phenomenon: the process of grief in the bereaved family, Death Stud 11:361-374, 1987.

Interviews of 49 families who had experienced a death following childhood cancer were conducted 7 to 9 years postdeath for the purpose of determining long-term responses. Contrary to traditionally held bereavement theories, it was found that many parents and siblings experienced a sense of loss 7 to 9 years after the death. The authors suggested that the loss of a child leaves an "empty space" for surviving members. Three patterns of grieving were described: "getting over it," "filling the emptiness," and "keeping the connection." The authors explored similarities and differences of the patterns as well as the significance of the relationship to the grieving process. Implications for further research in this area were also proposed.

Fulton R: The many faces of grief, Death Stud 11:243-256, 1987.

The author explored three areas: the sociologic conditions under which people die, the contemporary understanding of the grief process, and the concept of anticipatory grief and its relation to the "Stockholm Syndrome." He addresses in particular those individuals who provide care to those most likely to die—the elderly. He notes the challenge for caregivers in today's society to make the connection—to respond to the client as a whole person. Fulton also identifies the profound emotional response that is felt by the caregiver when the client dies. The article raises several pertinent issues relative to the dying client and to those who care for the dying.

Parkes C: Models of bereavement care, Death Stud 11:257-261, 1987.

This article reviews the pros and cons of the three traditional models of bereavement care: professional care, mutual help, and hospice care. The author then suggests a fourth model, which has been developed by the British organization Cruse. The author presents a discussion of the Cruse model, which utilizes individual and group counseling through a national network of trained volunteers who are supported and backed by professional caregivers.

Phipps, W: The origin of hospice care, Death Stud 12:91-99, 1988.

This article describes the origins of hospice, from its beginning as an outgrowth of the teachings of Jesus to its current-day status. The author notes the distinction between hospice and hospitals in terms of the philosophy of care for the dying client. St. Christopher's, initiated by Cicely Saunders in 1967, is considered by Phipps to be the model for hospice care today. He also suggests that the hospice concept—that of caring for the dying—has added much to the positive position of Christianity.

Zambelli G et al: An interdisciplinary approach to clinical intervention for childhood bereavement, Death Stud 12:41-50, 1988.

The authors describe the use of creative arts therapy groups for children who have lost a parent. Companion parents groups are run concurrently. The goal of these groups is to provide a social sanction for childhood grief, which may be accomplished through the use of activities. Children in the group are encouraged and supported in their attempt to express their feelings. The parent group provides an arena where the surviving parent can dialogue with other parents in relation to their own loss and the subsequent change in role to widowed parent. The article presents data from a bereavement intervention program that has been in existence since 1984. The authors note that the success of the child is related to whether a parent is involved in the companion group. It was concluded by the authors that to provide effective intervention, the child who is grieving must be considered within the context of the family system.

FURTHER READINGS

Junge M: The book about daddy dying: a preventive art therapy technique to help families deal with the death of a family member, Art Ther 2(1):a4-9, 1988.

Ley D: Spirituality and hospice care, Death Stud 12:101-110, 1988.

Roy D: Is dying a matter of ethics? Death Stud 12:137-145, 1988.

Strom-Paiken J: Studying the NDE phenomenon, Am J Nurs 4:420-421, 1986.

CHAPTER 7

Human sexuality

CHAPTER FOCUS

To provide a holistic approach to nursing care, nurses must respond to the sexual health needs of their clients. Knowledge of normal human sexual response patterns and the development of sexuality throughout the life cycle are necessary to the understanding of individuals as sexual beings. Equally critical to the success of nursing intervention is self-awareness. Nurses must be aware of their own values and beliefs regarding sexuality and the impact these may have on nursing care.

The chapter presents a discussion of the various explanatory theories of sexual dysfunctions as well as appropriate treatment modalities. Alternative sexual life-styles and the effects of illness on sexuality are also discussed. Last, sexual health care as a function of the nursing process is described within the context of primary, secondary, and tertiary levels of prevention.

HISTORICAL PERSPECTIVES

Human sexuality may be considered a multifaceted dimension of each individual. As noted in Chapter 6, sexuality in its broadest sense incorporates the biologic, psychologic, intellectual, spiritual, and sociocultural subsystems of the individual. The concept of one's sexuality influences roles in society, how one views self as well as how others perceive them. Sexuality cannot be separated from self. Cantor (1980) notes that self-esteem is related to how one feels about one's body and the pleasure that is derived from one's body. Feeling comfortable about one's body is then connected to the abil-

196

ity to experience sexual pleasure. Thus it may be said that sexuality is a component of one's self-esteem and sense of identity. Hartmen (1968) noted that early in development the child gains significant amounts of pleasure and displeasure from others' responses to self and body. Continued negative reinforcement tends to result in lowered self-esteem. Derogatis (1980) pointed out that body image is the first point of contact with others; it creates the image of a private world as well as acting as an expressive instrument of one's own individuality. It becomes crucial for nursing to recognize the significance of sexuality as it relates to the health and illness of clients. Sexual health needs will not disappear because we ignore them. Throughout the life cycle, sexual health issues emerge as factors influencing the growth and development of individuals. Biologic factors may in fact dictate sexuality, particularly one's roles as mother and father. However, psychologic, sociocultural, spiritual, and intellectual factors impact on sexuality. Sex roles are influenced by societal mores, for example, expected sexual behaviors. In today's society sex-role options are increasing. Females are entering professions that have been dominated historically by males, such as medicine, law, and business. Men are assuming more of the traditionally held female roles such as homemaking and child rearing. There is also an increase in joint ownership of such roles as housekeeping, food shopping, cooking, and child rearing. The percentage of women in the work force is on the rise—perhaps forcing the joint ownership of these roles. The role of primary provider is being shared by both male and female in the household. The provision of child care, formerly the domain of the female, is now occurring in areas other than the home (see Chapter 5 for further discussion). Childbearing is often being put off until later in relationships. The concept of "DINK"—Dual Income No Kids—is appearing on the horizon with further implications for the traditional male and female roles.

Sexual health is a right of clients in all settings. For nurses to provide comprehensive mental health care, human sexuality must be considered in all its dimensions. The first section presents factual information on the male and female sexual response cycles. This is followed by a discussion of sexuality throughout the life cycle, including normal growth and development as well as sexual health issues pertinent to each life cycle. Cultural and religious implications as well as alternative life-styles must be understood. Theories of sexual dysfunction and classification of dysfunction will be explored. Last, sexuality and illness, the effects of drugs on sexuality, and the nursing role in the promotion and maintenance of sexual health will be explored.

HUMAN SEXUAL RESPONSE PATTERNS

To meet the sexual health needs of clients, nurses must first possess a knowledge of sexual response patterns. Woods (1984) notes that a critical prerequisite to intervention with sexual health issues is a sound understanding of the physiologic phenomena associated with male and female sexual responses. It was not until Masters and Johnson introduced specific data regarding the sexual response that a knowledge base for education and counseling of clients emerged. Concomitant psychologic responses were also described by Masters and Johnson to further broaden the scope of knowledge relative to the sexual response pattern. Kaplan (1974) described the human sexual response as a "highly rational and orderly sequence of physiological events, the object of which is to prepare the bodies of two mates for reproductive union." She notes that sexual intercourse can be considered analogous to other bodily functions such as sleeping and eating in that certain changes must occur physiologically for these functions to be carried out successfully.

In their initial work, Masters and Johnson (1966) divided the human sexual response for both male and female into four stages. The first stage is that of excitement. This stage is characterized by erotic feelings as well as erection in the male and vaginal lubrication in the female. Vasocongestion and myotonia are present. Heart rate and blood pressure increase; breathing becomes heavier. Penile erection occurs in this stage concurrent with a thickening of the scrotal sack. In the female, genital and general vasocongestion are present. Breasts begin to enlarge, and nipples become erect. A thick transudate forms on the walls of the vagina within 10 to

30 seconds of sexual stimulation. The clitoris may at this time become erect, although this does not occur in all women. The uterus rises from the pelvic floor while the vagina enlarges to accommodate the penis. During the plateau or second stage, Masters and Johnson describe a more advanced state of arousal that precedes orgasm. The local vasocongestive response is at an optimal level. This vasocongestive response is responsible for the physiological changes that occur in both the male and the female. The testicles are engorged and are 50% greater than their resting size. The penis is distended to its maximum capacity. Skin mottling is apparent in both sexes at this time. In the female there is a swelling of the labia minora as well as a deep burgundy coloration. The uterus completes its rise, and the vagina enlarges fully. The clitoris retracts into a flat position behind the symphysis pubis. The third stage, orgasm, is noted to be the most pleasurable. Ejaculation occurs with the emission of semen at .8 second intervals. Masters and Johnson (1966) described the phenomenon of "ejaculatory inevitability," which is characterized by the rhythmic contractions of the penile urethra and the perineal muscles. Following orgasm, the male experiences a "refractory" period, or a time of rest before ejaculation can occur again. During this stage the female also experiences .8 second rhythmic contractions of the circumvaginal and perineal muscles. Kaplan (1974) noted that there is much controversy over whether women experience vaginal or clitoral orgasm. She asks the question from a different frame: Does vaginal or clitoral stimulation produce orgasm? Initially, Freudian theory hypothesized that clitoral orgasm was a precursor to the more mature psychosexual phase of vaginal orgasm. Many theorists now believe that the clitoris is critical in the ultimate stimulation of female orgasm. It must also be noted that there is no refractory period for females. Women retain the ability to experience multiple orgasms throughout their lifetime. During the last stage, resolution, the physiologic responses in both the male and the female begin to decrease. The penis returns to its flaccid state, while the clitoris returns to its normal position. The cervical os begins to close, and the uterus returns to its resting state. The burgundy coloration of the labia minora changes as the blood drains from the area.

These stages provide a knowledge base for assessment and education of clients. Thus, it is important to understand that these are only guidelines. Not every person will experience these changes in each stage. Situationally, responses may differ. Through the education process nurses can allay anxiety and dispel myths regarding what one "should" experience and permit each individual to develop as a sexual being at one's own comfort level.

Kaplan (1974) put forth the notion that the sexual response is biphasic in nature. The four-stage process as described by Masters and Johnson is actually composed of two independent and distinct phases. This premise has implications for the assessment and treatment of sexual disfunctions. Briefly, Kaplan's premise suggests that vasocongestion resulting in penile erection and vaginal lubrication occurs as a result of parasympathetic stimulation. Ejaculation is found to be a sympathetic function, as is orgasm. Treatment procedures would be different based on the area of innervation. Kaplan would also conclude that dysfunction in one area would not necessarily involve dysfunction in the other.

Masters and Johnson described subjective experiences of both males and females. These are subjective experiences, however, and must be considered as such. They noted that women characteristically experienced a three-phase orgasmic response. Initially orgasm was described as a sensation of "stoppage" or "suspension" with a concurrent sense of bearing down. The second phase involves a warm feeling that begins in the genital area and moves throughout the body. Last, the woman experiences a feeling of vaginal contraction and pelvic throbbing. Males described an initial feeling of ejaculatory inevitability followed by the sensation of urethral contractions and expulsion of seminal fluid.

SEXUALITY THROUGHOUT THE LIFE CYCLE

Although human development was covered in great depth in Chapter 6, certain characteristics relative to the development of self as a sexual being will be addressed. Sexual health issues considered by the authors to be pertinent in today's society will also be explored.

Birth through adolescence

Money and Erhardt (1972) proposed a model of psychosexual differentiation that reflects an integration of biological, psychological, and sociocultural dimensions. Initially, the XX or XY chromosomal dyad determines the development of ovaries or testes at approximately the fifth to sixth week of life. The role of fetal gonadal hormones further influences the differentiation of the testes and ovaries, particularly that of fetal androgen. Without androgen, male genitalia will not develop. Thus, in the absence of fetal androgen, female reproductive organs will begin to develop. There is little evidence to indicate that estrogen plays a significant role in genital development. By the seventh to twelfth week, biologic sex has been determined. Money and Erhardt term this development *genital dimorphism*—the development of external and internal sex organs correspondent with chromosomal sex. Estrogen is not necessarily essential for further development of the female reproductive tract, although it is secreted in the embryo. The production of testosterone in the male embryo acts to offset the production of female hormones. Money and Erhardt indicate that at this critical juncture, testosterone acts on the brain, a process referred to as *sex typing of the brain.* The brain that is acted on by testosterone will in turn activate the acyclic or male pattern, releasing gonadotropins. A cyclic pattern is stimulated in the female-typed brain.

In conclusion, based on the premise put forth by Money and Erhardt, there are two critical periods in the development of gender identity. The first is the point in the prenatal period at which the development of the genitalia is initiated in the male embryo. The second occurs either in prenatal life or early childhood whereby sex-typing of the brain is completed. The term *core gender identity*—that feeling of maleness or femaleness—has been utilized by Money and Erhardt to correlate with biological sex. It is their belief that the sense of one's biological sex is firmly established by the age of 3. At this point sex reassignment for any reason has little chance for success.

At birth, the impact of learning and environment influences the development of sex roles. Bardwick (1971) suggests that the sex-typing of the brain is correlated with qualities that are rewarded by significant others in the environment based on sex-role appropriate behaviors. These behaviors, even in early infancy, are learned in response to parental cues. The process of identifying oneself as male or female becomes part of social learning. Infants are dressed in pink or blue; toys are sex appropriate, such as stuffed footballs or baby dolls; the manner in which the nursery is decorated; and the choice of a name are examples of sex-role identification. Reflected appraisals from the significant others in the environment facilitate the development of self-concept and its component, body image.

Controversy exists as to the extent of influence of innate factors, social learning, and cognition. Kohlberg (1966) proposed in his cognitive view that once the child has categorized himself or herself as male or female, the child then values objects and behaves consistently with that gender identity. Cognitive judgment then serves as the foundation for gender identity early in development. Gender identity is maintained with little influence from social reinforcements. Cognitive consistency leads the child to select experiences that will be consonent with his or her gender identity. Mischel (1966) postulated that sex-typed behavior is reinforced by significant others in the environment, beginning in infancy as noted above. Based on this theory, the infant seeks rewards, is rewarded by significant others for either male or female behaviors, then assumes the gender identity that is consistently reinforced.

Based on research data it must be concluded that innate biological factors, social learning, and cognition have a profound and interactive effect on the development of gender identity. How much each of these factors influences development continues to be in question and awaits further research.

Issues of sexual health in infancy relate to the development of core gender identity. The lack of a stable sense of being male or female in infancy and early childhood has been related to the development of transsexualism in later life. Money and Erhardt note that there may be a biologic error in the differentiation of gender in early life. This error may be consistent with inadequate neural differentiation either before or immediately following birth. Lack of comfort with societal expectations of sex-role behavior may also be a relative factor in the development of transsexual behavior.

The development of healthy sexuality rests on the foundation that is set in childhood by both parents and society as a whole. Sexuality as part of one's self-esteem must be addressed directly and age-appropriately for children to evolve as mentally healthy adults. Children in this age group are curious about sex and are interested in beginning to understand their own bodies. Masturbation may begin in both sexes and may be accompanied by fear as well as excitement. It is important to recognize that this is natural exploration. Heterosexual play begins with the childhood games of "doctor" and "playing house." Facilitation of an understanding of normal sexual development within the family setting assists the child in developing a sound sense of self. Human-sexuality curricula in elementary school settings can provide information regarding normal growth and development, development of healthy self-esteem, and the establishment of family and peer relationships.

The advent of adolescence is a critical period for both parents and adolescent. Biologic changes occur—menstruation, the emergence of secondary sex characteristics. Social and emotional tasks involve the establishment of a sense of identity and a place in society. Peer group is particularly important and has a profound effect on the development of relationships. Adolescents may feel pressure to engage in sexual activities before they are ready due to peer response. Sexual activities such as petting may occur within the context of adolescent relationships and act as a precursor to adult relationships. Masturbation in both males and females may also be used as a method of sexual release. Tumultuous emotions are often experienced in the adolescent phase. Fear of not being sexually attractive or not having a significant relationship can seriously affect how the individual perceives him or herself. Promotion of sexual health in adolescence should provide information regarding sex-role expectations, the development of positive social relationships, the need for self-respect and the ability to make responsible decisions based on one's own values and beliefs. Responsible decision making as it relates to sexual behavior must be the thrust of parent and societal education. The threat of AIDS

today will have a significant influence on current and future sexual behaviors of young adults. Federally mandated sex education programs will present information to adolescents relative to "safe sex" as well as risk behaviors. There is a belief on the part of some that the sexual permissiveness experienced in society today will see a retrenching with a trend toward monogamous relationships. Theresa Crenshaw, President of AASECT, in her comments on ABC's 20/20 indicated that young adults in particular must realize that AIDS is a life-threatening illness that is relative to one's sexual life-style. Changes in sexual life-style must be considered to decrease one's risk of contracting the AIDS virus.

Young adulthood through the older years
YOUNG ADULTHOOD

As noted in Chapter 6, this stage is characterized by the development of intimate relationships, the establishment of one's self in the work force, and the need to make choices regarding marriage and having children. Current trends indicate that more women are in the work force and are choosing to have children later in life or are not having children at all. Sexual behaviors are influenced by societal forces, again, notably the threat of AIDS. Sexual health in this developmental phase is reliant upon open communication between partners. Open discussion of feelings and needs is the foundation upon which a healthy sexual relationship is based. Kaplan (1979) noted that inhibited sexual desire, a persistent and pervasive inhibition of sexual desire, may occur as a result of several factors: a lack of communication between individuals, educational deficits, inhibitions regarding appropriate sexual behaviors, or physiologic problems. It would be interesting to determine the effect of dual careers on sexual desire and the expression of one's sexual needs within the context of the dual-career couple.

MIDDLE AGE

Physiologic changes occur in both men and women during the middle years. Menopause heralds the cessation of menstruation and the onset of various physical symptoms as a result of changes in hormonal level. Thinning of the vaginal mucosa occurs with resulting tearing upon intercourse. Lubrication decreases, and a shortening of the vaginal canal may also be evident. Men experience physical changes, including impotence, which may be related to certain disease states and to medication usage. Normal physiological changes such as delay in attaining an erection, loss of ejaculatory volume, and decrease in seminal fluid are to be expected. Both sexes experience feelings of concern for sexual attractiveness. Women often associate sexual attractiveness with the ability to bear children. Once this ability has been removed either by surgery or menopause, there is a belief that one may not be sexual. Although there is no hormonal change in the male, there may be an increased need to promote one's self as an attractive sexual being. This need may also be confounded by changes in self-esteem resulting from retirement, change in financial status, and change in physical status. Men may attempt to compensate for what they perceive as decreased sexual attractiveness by having an affair or even divorcing their spouse of many years for a younger woman. At this stage of development, there is an increased need for communication between partners as both are feeling the onset of the aging process and concern for their own sexual attractiveness. An understanding of the normal physiological changes that occur in both partners is essential to promote a healthy ongoing relationship. Pfeiffer, Verwerdt, and Davis (1974) noted in a study of 261 males and 241 females between the ages of 46 and 69 that as high as 70% of the women described sexual interest as moderate to strong, while as high as 91% of the men described their sexual interest as moderate to strong. Factors influencing sexual interest and activity related to previous sexual experiences, availability of a socially appropriate partner, physical status, and desire for sexual intimacy. Positive sexual relationships can be encouraged by nurses through an understanding of the individual's comfort level with sexual health issues, a provision of information regarding normal physiological changes, and a recognition that sexuality is a component of positive self-esteem.

THE OLDER YEARS

Sexuality in the older years moves from a genital focus to one that is more diffuse. There is a need for physical touching and closeness—a sense of companionship and intimacy that is enjoyed by older couples. This does not mean that older individuals are not capable of intercourse. Pfeiffer, Verwerdt, and Davis (1974) noted that men and women can enjoy sexual intercourse well into their seventies dependent upon physical status, availability of partners, and previous positive experiences. Often adult children negatively view their parents' need for companionship and discourage positive sexual relationships based on their own discomfort. Health professionals working with older adults can implicitly convey their own beliefs about sexuality in the older adult by simply neglecting to address the issue in the comprehensive health history. LaTorre and Kear (1977) indicate that a facilitation of sexuality as a component of self-esteem is imperative in the older population. It is important to note that in the desire to provide an atmosphere where sexuality is valued, nurses lose sight of the cultural mores and values of this generation. Education and counseling of the older population must consider what options for healthy sexuality would be considered appropriate by their clients. The suggestion of masturbation as a sexual alternative may frighten or repulse a client who has grown up with the belief that this is wrong. Thus, it is important to assess the values and beliefs of the target population. A summary of sexuality across the life span is presented in Table 7-1.

SOCIOCULTURAL CONTEXT
Sexuality, culture, and religion
SEXUALITY AND CULTURE

Each society has a culture of sex. Sex is a part of embryonic life; its biological existence impacts upon consciousness as a force reflecting its instinctive nature. Yet enculturation provides the form and meaning necessary to define sexuality. Sexual standards and behavior vary from one society to the next as well as from generation to generation within one society.

Davenport (1977) suggests that the culture of sex is anchored in two directions. At one end, it is linked to the potentialities and limitations of biological inheritance. On the other end, it is tied to the logic and internal consistency of the total culture. As one aspect of the total culture undergoes

TABLE 7-1   Sexual function, sexual self-concept, and sexual relationships across the life span

	Sexual function	Sexual self-concept	Sexual role/relationship
Infancy	Orgasmic potential present Erectile function present	Gender identity reinforced Association of sexuality and good/bad Distinction between self and others	
Childhood	Genital pleasuring and exploration Sensual activity (e.g., hugging)	Core gender identity solidified (by age 3)	Sex role differences learned Discrimination between male and female role models Sexual vocabulary learned
Preschool	Sex play—exploration of own body and those of playmates Self-pleasuring (masturbation)		Sex roles learned Parental attachment and identification
School age		Curiosity about sex Sexual fears and fantasies Interest in aspects of sexual development Self awareness as sexual being	Same-sex friends
Adolescent, prepubertal	Menarche Seminal emissions	Concerns about body image	Same-sex friends Sexual experiences as part of friendship
Early adolescence	Awkwardness in first sexual encounter (50% not sexually active) Masturbation, petting	Sexual thoughts, fantasies Anxiety over inadequacy, lack of partner, virginity	Appropriate sex friendships Dating
Late adolescence	May or may not be sexually active	Responsibility for sexual activity	Intimacy in relationships learned Sex-role behaviors, lifestyles explored
Young adult	Experimentation with sexual positions, expression Exploration of techniques	Responsibility for sexual health, e.g., contraception, sexually transmitted disease prevention Development of adult sexual value system, tolerance for others	Giving and receiving pleasure learned Long-term commitment to relationship developed
Middle adult	Adaptation to altered sexual function, e.g., vaginal dryness of menopause, slower erections	Accept body image changes related to aging	Adjustment of relationship as roles change
Late adults	More gradual sexual function	Accept slowed sexual response cycle without ending sexual aspects of relationship	New ways of sharing sexual pleasure and intimacy developed Adaptation to loss or illness of partner

From Woods NF: Toward a holistic perspective of human sexuality: alterations in sexual health and nursing diagnosis, Holistic Nurs Prac 1(4): p. 4, 1987. Reprinted with permission of Aspen Publishers, Inc. Based on data from Mims F and Swenson L: Sexuality: a nursing perspective, New York, 1980, Appleton-Century-Crofts, pp. 62-77.

change, so must all the others. However, there are some inherent limitations because biological parameters cannot be exceeded. He further notes that *to understand one culture of sex, it is necessary to know how sexual performance is conceptually joined to the total culture.*

Traditions regarding intercourse, menstruation, contraception, and gender identity vary from culture to culture. For example, the pre–World War II Manus in Papua New Guinea considered intercourse between husband and wife as sinful and degrading. Women believed intercourse was something to be endured until a child was born. Intercourse outside the marriage was a crime that brought on supernatural punishments. Menstruation was such a well-kept secret that Manu men denied that women experienced monthly cycles.

The Polynesian cultures consider sexuality in a much different light. Infants and young children are encouraged in their expressions of sexuality, as are adolescents and young adults. In the latter group, members of both sexes are encouraged to masturbate and have premarital sex. The expression of sexuality is highly prized within the culture.

A culture that applies a negative connotation to sexuality is that of the Gusii of southwestern Kenya. The act of coitus itself implies hostility and antagonism. The man is expected to overcome the woman's resistance and, in fact, inflict pain and humiliation. Intercourse becomes a sort of ritualized rape, with some of the affective components as well. Women are expected to frustrate men by sexually taunting them. Overt expression of sexuality is punished from childhood throughout adolescence. Extramarital relationships bring on heavy punishment from the gods. An adulterous Gusii wife who continues to have intercourse with her husband may put him in mortal danger if he becomes ill or is injured in any way.

The Dobu, who constitute another Papua New Guinea society, believe that women are sorceresses. Husbands are particularly vulnerable to sorcery during intercourse; therefore males must constantly decide between sexual gratification and the risk of sorcery.

Erotic codes vary from culture to culture as well. Acts such as the sharing or offering of food can be

tinged with sexual meaning. In East Bay, a Melanesian society of the southwest Pacific, an act of sexual intimacy is the sharing of betel nuts and pepper between members of the opposite sex.

The use of language can be erotically stimulating as well. Davenport (1977) notes that Hawaiians clearly make sexual allusions through metaphor, pun, and multiple meanings. In addition, he identifies similarities between the Hawaiians and the Iban of Sarawak, whose issuances of compliments, scoldings, and expressions of respect and insult are couched in erotic terms.

The development of gender identity is also influenced by culture. Gilmore and Gilmore (1979) discuss male social impotence (lack of social power on the part of males) and gender identity conflict among men in the lower class in Spain. In the early life experience of males in this socioeconomic group, there is little or no contact with their fathers on a daily basis. Most time is spent in the "female" sphere, which is studiously avoided by the fathers, who spend much of their time in bars or taverns. Little socialization occurs between fathers and sons, even in adolescence. The dominant figure is female, in the form of mother, grandmother, or both. Power resides with the female, who is dispenser of all material goods as well as love and affection. Allowances are given by maternal figures, permission is granted to participate in activities by maternal figures, and maternal figures confer with teachers and other external authority figures. Further strengthening the female influence was the fact that, during the Franco period, working class women often were more able than men to maintain gainful employment, particularly in the service of wealthy and powerful employers. Therefore, the wife was often not only in control of the "private" sphere, or home life, but was also superior economically in her position as wage earner. Thus, as Gilmore and Gilmore suggest, there has been an increasing degree of sex-role reversal and confusion as perceived by lower class males. Further evidence of the gender identity conflict has been noted by the authors during the festival *carnavale*. The upper class does not participate, considering it to be brutish and uncivilized. The lower class as a whole acts in ways that are normally unacceptable. Women drink and smoke, while men dress in female garb, often that of an old grandmother. It is the latter feature that is striking in relation to gender-role identity. It seems that this ritualized transvestism may be symbolic of the underlying gender identity conflict—the male's inability to control or satisfy the powerful maternal figure. Lower-class males then must compensate for a fragile male identification. The "macho" reputation is achieved in young adulthood by severing emotional and physical ties with the "female" sphere, thus producing the distant or absent father figure. The cycle is perpetuated as male children are brought into a world influenced predominantly by females.

Sex-role stereotyping has been perpetuated throughout the years by both males and females. Neither group has been willing to risk being identified as "different." Sex roles are defined by characteristics representing masculinity and femininity. These categories emerge from the sociocultural framework inherent in each society. Traditionally, characteristics such as competitiveness, aggressiveness, and intelligence have been considered masculine in Western cultures. Female traits have included gentleness, warmth, and passivity, as well as tendencies toward being understanding and showing emotion.

Recently theorists in the field of human sexuality have suggested the concept of androgyny—the possession of human traits rather than those identified as either masculine or feminine. This concept, which involves a blurring of sex roles, can be viewed as a step toward positive mental health, because it does not require that a person be given a label based on whether a characteristic is appropriate. There is, however, concern that the concept of androgyny may increase the difficulty a child experiences in developing a sound sense of identity. It is important that children be clearly given the message that they are male or female to prevent ambiguity in core gender identity. They can then be encouraged to select from traits that are identified as "human" rather than "male" or "female." It is indeed important for nurses, counselors, sex educators, and other professionals to recognize that androgyny can be a threatening concept—an unknown. For example, a boy growing up in a tough neighborhood may feel extremely uncomfortable about assuming characteristics not acceptable to his

group. He cannot be expected to assume traditionally feminine traits if he is going to be harassed by his peers. Thus the assimilation of human, rather than sex-linked, traits must occur over a period of time, because positive reinforcement from one's cultural group is a necessary ingredient in the process. It can be said, then, that the goal of mental health care is the introjection and expression of human traits.

Sex roles play a part in determining what is considered appropriate or inappropriate behavior. It is not possible to separate sex roles, sexual attitudes, and sexual behavior from one another. Each is interrelated with the others to produce a unique, complex, sexual human being. Likewise, one cannot separate biological, psychological, and sociocultural factors in the determination of gender identity. Each variable reinforces the others; one variable does not operate to the exclusion of the others. It is difficult to separate a biological imperative from one that is imposed by a culture.

As culture impacts on expression of sex role, so does it influence the definition of sexual dysfunctions. One may note the emergence of inhibited sexual desire as sexual dysfunction. In the society of today, lack of sexual desire constitutes consideration as a dysfunction, since desire is a valued component of a relationship. Incidence of a dysfunction is then based on its definition as noted by society. Another example of the cultural influence on definition of dysfunction is described by Messinger (1971) in his discussion of Irish culture. Restricted views of female sexuality in Irish culture place little if any emphasis on female orgasm; thus, the prevalence of anorgasmia in that culture tends to be higher. In Mangaaian culture the prevalence of anorgasmia is close to zero, however, because the culture holds a more liberal view of sexuality.

RELIGION AND SEXUALITY

It has been noted in the literature that religion does play a role in one's beliefs about sexuality and one's sexual practices. Different religions share different views as to what is considered sexually moral. Kinsey (1948) in his early studies indicated that religiosity, defined as the acceptance of the teachings of a particular religion, has a more profound effect on sexual behavior.

Hogan (1982) indicated that Orthodox Judaism, traditional Catholicism, and traditional Protestantism continue to condemn masturbation, abortion, and homosexuality. They view sexual intercourse in any setting other than the marital relationship as being unacceptable behavior. However, it is important to note that there are various groups within each larger religious denomination that share views that may be in direct contradiction to the teachings of that religion. The Catholic Church, for example, is experiencing a widening gap between what is put forth as doctrine and what is actually practiced—in relation to abortion, birth control, and homosexuality, to name a few. Many theologians as well as practicing Catholics feel that the gap must be bridged to meet the needs of Catholics in today's society. Authors of the much-criticized book written by the Catholic Theological Society recognized sexuality as a viable part of life that needs to be reaffirmed rather than hidden away. They also noted that a blanket condemnation of homosexuality, contraception, and masturbation was inappropriate. A perspective based on a broader view of society as it exists today requires an update of traditional sexual ethics that would address the development of oneself throughout the life cycle.

Modern Judaism has also noted changes in its perspectives on sexuality. Most congregations support the notion of contraception and planned parenthood. Abortion is considered an alternative in selected circumstances; however, it is not to be used as a contraceptive method. The role of women in Judaism is emerging in the form of female rabbis and a more active role in the leadership of the congregation. The family is considered the focal point of life where children are viewed as blessings.

Many differences exist in the various sects of the Protestant religion. Early Protestant teachings, Puritanism in America, stated that sex was evil and was not to be discussed. Hogan notes that this Puritanical perspective remains to some extent; however, there is a trend in the Protestant church as a whole to be more sensitive to the needs of their congregation in today's society. Thus, teachings are no longer taking a negative perspective but rather are presenting sexuality as a healthy component of life as a whole. Sex-education programs for teenagers that facilitate the development of a positive attitude regarding one's self as a sexual being are being incorporated into religious education.

Within the context of the various religious perspectives, it is important to note that nurses be aware of the value clients place on their religion or religious beliefs as they relate to their sexual self. There are no standard guidelines or rules as to who believes what. Surveys of sexual mores often reveal contradictory data. Those individuals who respond to surveys may not be considered representative of the larger population. In any case, nurses must acknowledge that religious views may play a role in the client's presentation of self as a sexual being. Nurses may also subtly condemn clients' behavior due to the conflict created by the nurse's own religious views. It is imperative that nurses reassess their value system to be able to accept others as they present themselves. More important, nurses can enhance the client's potential as a human being by recognizing the impact of religion on the actualization of one's sexual self.

ALTERNATIVE SEXUAL LIFE-STYLES

The concept of sexual orientation refers to an individual's sexual object choice. The orientation may be directed toward an inanimate object, as in fetishism, or may be heterosexual, homosexual, bisexual, or ambisexual. Choice of life-style in our society may be freely made when consenting adults commit to a relationship that is satisfying to each partner. Sexual behavior may not be used, on the other hand, to abuse or take advantage of another individual. Thus, homosexual, bisexual, and lesbian relationships may be considered appropriate alternatives.

Homosexuality

Historically, homosexual behavior has been traced back to ancient Greece where homosexuality was viewed as natural in many segments of society. Plato's *Symposium* extolled the virtues of homosexual behavior and indicated that homosexual lovers would make the best soldiers (Masters and Johnson, 1986). Boswell (1980) in his book *Christianity, Social Tolerance, and Homosexuality* states that homosexuality was not considered socially deviant behavior as previously noted in earlier works. He further suggests that it was not until Thomas Aquinas and St. Augustine that homosexuality was actually denoted as being unnatural as it did not lead to conception. Homosexual behavior continued to be condemned until the medical community began to evaluate homosexuals as being "ill"; this occurred during the latter part of the nineteenth century. It was not until 1980 with the DSM-III-R that homosexuality was considered to be an alternative sexual life-style rather than a deviant behavior. Unfortunately in many cases even in the medical community, views on homosexuality remain skewed toward the belief that homosexuality is an unnatural sexual behavior.

The theories underlying the development of homosexual behavior are many. The traditional psychoanalytic perspective suggests that a dysfunctional parent-child relationship, particularly the inadequate resolution of the Oedipal phase, may result in adult homosexuality. Research findings showed mixed results: Bieber (1969) noted that homosexual males tended to have dominant, aggressive mothers, while fathers were weak and passive and had poor relationships with their sons. Others found that not relevant. Bell, Weinberg, and Hammersmith, in their 1981 study, concluded that there were no significant data to support Bieber's earlier beliefs. Data to date show no evidence that homosexuality emerges solely as a result of ineffective parenting.

There is a belief on the part of some theorists that homosexual behavior may be a learned response. Thus, positive experiences with early homosexual behavior can influence the direction of sexual orientation as can negative experiences with heterosexual relationships. This premise would be supported by behaviorists, who believe that early sexual experiences play a role in the development of adult sexual dysfunctions as well. There is also some support for a biological basis of homosexuality. Proponents of this theory suggest that the individual has no choice in sexual orientation. In 1952, Kallman found a 100% concordance rate for homo-

sexuality in identical twins; however, studies to date do not support this finding. There is little scientific data to conclude that there is a direct relationship between prenatal hormonal influence and homosexual behavior. Rather there are many conflicting reports as to the biological etiology of homosexuality. In conclusion, homosexuality as a sexual orientation is not a direct result of one factor but rather must be viewed from a holistic perspective. The intent is not to treat homosexual behavior as deviant but rather to understand its dimensions from various perspectives.

Ms. White, the head nurse on the psychiatric unit, was approached by one of the staff nurses regarding the behavior of a newly admitted client. Data indicated that the client was a homosexual and that his lover frequently visited. During visits, the curtains in the two-bed room were closed. The staff nurse was irate that this "kind of behavior" was occurring on her unit. Ms. White set up a client care conference for the next morning for staff of all three shifts. At the conference, Ms. White initiated the discussion of concerns staff might have in relation to this particular client. Few staff responded. Ms. White shared her feelings: "I was first frightened when I realized that the client was a homosexual—I don't know what I thought would happen to me if I took care of him—perhaps I would become a homosexual. I knew these fears were irrational but they still affected how I felt." Another staff nurse stated: "I'm not frightened—I think homosexual behavior is disgusting and there must be something wrong with this person." Another member of the group stated: "He's really a nice person—no different from any of us, although I must admit I'm not completely comfortable with his behavior." Another pointed out that "he shouldn't have closed the curtains when his lover came because that wasn't right." Ms. White facilitated the group discussion and encouraged staff to share as they felt comfortable and reinforced the need to acknowledge these feelings as valid. She suggested that meetings with the psychiatric liaison nurse would be helpful in facilitating sexual attitude reassessment to examine their perceptions of sexual differences and the potential impact on nursing care.

Homosexual behavior cannot be pigeonholed into one particular life-style. Homosexuals may commit to one partner for an extended period of time as do heterosexuals; they may also "play the field" as do heterosexual males. In past history, many misconceptions have entered the public perspective regarding homosexual behavior. Evelyn Hooker's (1965) longitudinal study of a matched sample of heterosexual and homosexual males concluded that raters could not distinguish characteristics of either group, indicating that the homosexual sample was not dysfunctional to any greater degree than the heterosexual sample. Bell and Weinberg (1978) note that a typology of sexual experiences exists which includes: close—coupled relationships with one other partner; open-coupled—one partner with some outside relationships; functional—no specific partner; dysfunctional—no coupling and sexual problems; and, asexual—no coupling with little sexual desire. Although studies of homosexual behavior may not provide data related to the etiology of homosexuality, they do indicate that homosexual behavior, as heterosexual behavior, has many and varied patterns of relationships.

Bisexuality

Masters and Johnson (1986) note that little research exists related to bisexuality. They found that individuals move into bisexual relationships as a means of experimentation or as a means of availability. In most cases, however, bisexuals do have a preference for one gender. In the early seventies as a response to the permissiveness of society, individuals turned to bisexuality as a means of expressing their freedom of choice. In the eighties, with the threat of AIDS, this alternative has been severely curtailed. Masters and Johnson (1986) also include a category—ambisexual—those individuals who have no preference for gender and have no commitment to relationships whatsoever. These individuals select sex partners on availability and physical need. The authors further indicated that bisexual behavior may emerge out of several situations. First, the individual may be involved in a close relationship with a same-sex friend that develops into more intimate behaviors. Homosexuals may experiment with a close friend of the opposite sex. Bisexual behavior can also be an offshoot of group sex. Last, bisexual behavior may be a result of one's own personal belief system as in the case of

those involved in the women's movement. This is certainly not to state that all those involved in the women's movement are bisexual; however, in some cases, women may be drawn to one another by virtue of their compelling belief in their cause. Suffice it to say, there are very few data to suggest any conclusive information relative to the development of bisexual behavior.

Lesbianism as a form of homosexual behavior has not received the attention that male homosexuality has. Moses and Hawkins (1982) indicate that lesbians tend to have more stable, one-partner relationships. They exist within the community, carrying out their daily activities with little harassment. Little research has been conducted on the etiology of lesbian behavior. Literature suggests that an indifferent mother and distant or absent father may also be significant characteristics.

Transsexualism

Transsexual behavior is often linked with and confused with homosexuality. A transsexual is an individual who feels trapped in the body of the wrong sex. It is believed to relate to the ineffective development of one's core gender identity in early childhood. Money and Wiedeking (1980) state that the transsexual believes that he or she has the mind of the opposite sex and is intent upon changing sex legally and surgically. The phenomenon was first noted in 1953 with Christine Jorgensen, who converted his sexual appearance to that of a female amidst worldwide controversy. Since then the number of transsexuals who have completed sex reassignment are in the thousands. Masters and Johnson (1986) note that the number of males who request sex reassignment are much larger than females. Initially, many transsexuals may cross-dress in their attempt to actualize their role as a member of the opposite sex. Social stigma attendant upon cross-dressing is often overwhelming and causes the individual much distress. Those individuals who choose sex reassignment are evaluated stringently and often require intensive psychotherapy to determine whether this option is the most viable for each candidate. Surgery is done in stages, and hormones are a component of the treatment. Success of the treatment is also dependent upon the support of significant others in the environment. Masters and Johnson (1986) note that there is serious question as to the effectiveness of surgery by the researchers at Johns Hopkins University. They indicate that there is little evidence of significant psychological benefit to those who have undergone surgery versus those who have not.

Few theories exist to explain the phenomenon of transsexual behavior. Some support the relevance of organic factors, while others believe that psychological factors have a greater impact. The consensus of opinion, however, suggests that multiple factors must be considered.

Ms. N., a 22-year-old male-to-female transsexual, was admitted to the psychiatric unit for depression. Initial orders included one-to-one observation daily. During morning report, one of the nurses stated, "I'm not going to take care of him or her, whatever it is—she deserves what she gets." Another staff member joined in, stating, "No wonder she wants to kill herself—she probably doesn't like being a girl either." Mrs. F., the head nurse, noticed that the client overheard the comments while sitting in the dayroom and had begun to cry. Ms. D., a graduate student on clinical rotation, also noted the client crying and offered to be the primary nurse. She approached the client, offering her a tissue and put her hand on Ms. N.'s arm.

Ms.D.   *Let me sit with you a while.*

Ms.N.   *No one understands why I did this—I'm happy as a woman—that has nothing to do with why I'm here.*

Ms.D.   *I'd like to hear what brought you here.*

Ms.N.   *I've been happier as a woman than I ever was as a man (starts crying again).*

Ms.D.   *It must be hard to talk about.*

Ms.N.   *I had what I thought was a wonderful relationship with a man, but I had not told him about my sex change. When I told him, he looked at me as though I was a degenerate of some kind. . . . I really loved him.*

Ms.D.   *How long had he known you?*

Ms.N.   *About three weeks—he was the first relationship I've had since the sex change.*

Ms.D.   *What kind of response did you expect when you told him?*

Ms.N.   *I don't know—I guess I thought if he loved me—he'd love me no matter what.*

Ms.D.   *Have you been in contact with him since you have been hospitalized?*

Ms.N.   *No, this happened last week—he's put messages on my machine, but I don't want to talk to him. He'll only hurt me.*

Ms.D.   *It might be that he was caught by surprise and didn't know how to respond. . . .*

Ms.N.   *We had just started to become intimate, and I thought it best to tell him even though I've had vaginal surgery.*

Ms.D.   *It might be that intimacy is also a threatening issue— perhaps he has not had a successful intimate relationship.*

Ms.N.   *I didn't think of that aspect—I assumed it was me as a transsexual.*

Ms.D.   *I think that that is also an issue that needs to be explored. My primary concern at the moment is your feelings about yourself as a person—including your concept of yourself as a sexual being.*

EXPLANATORY THEORIES OF SEXUAL DYSFUNCTION

Historically, individuals experiencing difficulty with sexual expression were directed toward psychoanalysis, incorporating a lengthy review of past relationships. Emphasis was on resolution of the unconscious conflicts that were at the root of sexual dysfunction. However, Kaplan and others believe that other causative factors must be considered to provide comprehensive treatment. Earlier in this chapter, Kaplan's premise of the biphasic nature of the sexual response suggested that understanding and treatment of sexual dysfunction must reflect the differentiation of stimulation from the parasympathetic and sympathetic nervous systems. In this discussion, the biologic, psychologic, and cognitive dimensions of sexual dysfunctions will be explored.

Biologic theory

Kaplan (1974) noted that the first area of assessment of sexual dysfunction must be physiology— biologic soundness of the sex organs as well as potential organic influences. She indicated that estimates of organically based sexual dysfunction ranged between 3% and 20%. Organic factors included undiagnosed diabetes, alcohol and drug abuse, neurological disease, and undetected pathology of the genital organs. Before further discussion, it must also be noted that organic factors may cause variable symptoms from individual to individual; thus, careful assessment of organic factors is necessary.

Endocrine disorders may be related to sexual dysfunction resulting from alterations in pituitary or gonadal functioning. The androgen levels are decreased, which in turn may cause a decrease in sexual desire in both sexes and affect erectile capacity in males. Kaplan indicated that support for this hypothesis can be found in recent research findings. Testosterone levels tend to fluctuate based on stress experienced by the individual. Depression of testosterone levels appeared to be correlated with chronic stress; once stress had been reduced, testosterone levels returned to within normal limits for that individual.

Neurological impairment may have various effects dependent upon the area affected. Surgical intervention that affects the parasympathetic or sympathetic nervous system will alter sexual response. Tumors of the spinal cord that impinge on sensory and motor transmission to the reproductive organs as well as infections and malnutrition have profound effects on male and female sexual response. Diabetes in particular has been found to alter erectile function in the male by decreasing the neural transmission to the genital area. Concurrently, the effects of vascular damage on sexual response must be addressed. Since vasocongestion is necessary for erection, any impairment of vascularity to the penis will affect erectile ability. Local thromboses, for example, may decrease vascular flow and impact on erection.

General physical health is an important consideration in the assessment of sexual response. Conditions that affect the system as a whole such as malignancy, systemic infection, chronic lung disease, renal disease, or any other disease that causes chronic pain affects sexual desire, motivation, and function. Generalized pain resulting from arthritis, for example, can prevent the actualization of sexual intercourse. Specific genital disorders such as imperforate hymen, pelvic inflammatory disease, poor episiotomy repair, and vaginal infections may affect desire as well as sexual expression. A thorough nursing assessment will provide information that can be utilized to effect resolution of specific sexual dysfunctions.

The effects of medication on sexual response relate to their impact on the autonomic nervous system. A broad discussion of these effects will be presented here. Generally, those drugs which affect the brain itself will impact on sexual desire, while drugs which affect the peripheral nervous system will impact on erection or orgasm or both. The assessment of the influence of drugs on sexual response is complicated by the multiple factors that can have an effect on that response. It is also difficult to assess and document the effects of drugs, particularly in the case of the female sexual response.

Central nervous system depressants such as alcohol, sedatives, barbiturates, and other drugs that may depress psychomotor responses have an effect on sexual libido and response. Those drugs which generally have a depressive response on the brain center itself will tend to have a depressing effect on sexual response as well. Kaplan notes that narcotics in particular have a profound effect on the sex drive. Addicts have been found to experience a diminished desire and loss of erectile capability.

Anticholinergic medications, which block parasympathetic response, have an effect on vasocongestion, thus impairing erectile function. Antiadrenergic drugs block sympathetic response, which in turn affects ejaculatory response. Antihypertensive medications are best known for their impact on sexual response. Newer antihypertensive medications are more successful in reducing the negative effects on sexual function.

Last, many psychotropic medications may not have a direct influence on sexual functioning, yet indirect benefits may result from reduction in anxiety and depression. Individuals recovering from a depressive response may also experience a reawakening of sexual desire. Manic individuals in a hypomanic phase describe a decrease in sexual urgency as they respond to the effects of lithium control. Haldol seems to have a direct affect on the brain center with a diminished sexual desire and decreased potency (Kaplan and Sadock, 1981).

Psychological theory

To understand the interrelationship of the many factors that influence sexual responsiveness, the psychological components of sexual function must be considered. Historically, it was thought that sexual dysfunction was a result of unresolved conflicts in childhood. Intrapsychic conflict remains as one of the theories to be understood in relation to the development of dysfunction. Freud's concept of the unconscious conflict between enjoying the sexual experience and fear of punishment for doing so has been presented as the basis for sexual dysfunction in later adult life. The psychoanalytic model postulates that the adult is victimized by unconscious childhood fears that impact on erectile or orgastic ability. The mechanism of repression acts to control anxiety relating to sexual behavior—all of which acts on an unconscious level. The presence of unresolved Oedipal conflict also plays a dominant role in the understanding of the role of psychoanalytic theory in the development of sexual dysfunction. Kaplan (1974) notes that the importance of childhood experiences cannot be understated in its relevance to sexual dysfunction. Sexual responses in the form of pleasing erotic fantasies and impulses occur in early childhood. The response from parents and significant others in the environment at that time is significant in personality development and the emergence of a sound feeling of self-worth. The resolution of the critical Oedipal period remains a cornerstone in psychoanalytic theory. Unresolved Oedipal conflicts in the male may result in an individual who develops shallow emotional relationships that are a forum for the expression of his own narcissistic behavior. Females may also develop shallow emotional ties but are also noted for their castrating personalities. In either case, the individual is unable to experience a lasting emotional experience. Kaplan (1974) notes that the concept of unresolved conflict is an important one but must not be considered unilaterally. Many factors act in concert in the development of dysfunction. She also notes that it is not clear as to the mechanism of translation of unconscious conflict into sexual dysfunction.

Cognitive theory

As intellectual beings, individuals are unable to function adequately without appropriate information. Such is the case in the development of healthy sexual relationships. Two partners in a sexual relationship need information regarding the needs of one another as well as knowledge of the sexual response cycle. Many times individuals feel uncomfortable asking for information and operate on false information or myths. Our culture has not permitted individuals to question their own sexuality, nor has it encouraged individuals to communicate their sexual needs to their partners until recently. Kaplan found that most couples were sexually ignorant and were too frightened or plagued by guilt to ask. Couples had little understanding of the sexual response cycle, physiology, or the effects of age, medication, or emotional state on their sexual response. There may be a lack of knowledge regarding how to give sexual pleasure as well as unrealistic expectations of performance.

Sexual anxiety as described by Kaplan and others may be considered an immediate cause of sexual dysfunction. Fear of failure, particularly in males, can initiate a cycle that results in a chronic state of impotence. One temporary experience can stimulate an ongoing concern for future success in achieving erection. Spectatoring, described by Masters and Johnson as "observing one's sexual reactions as though outside one's self," can be concomitant with fear of failure. Individuals who most often experience fear of failure are those who are insecure or who feel the need to compete and achieve even in the sexual arena. Anxiety may be created by an excessive need to please one's partner, which ultimately results in disappointment and self-deprecation. Demand for performance in the male also acts as a negative reinforcer and often leads to erectile and orgastic dysfunction. Immediate causes may be seen in isolation; however, insecurity and poor feelings of self-worth may also be related to unresolved unconscious conflicts. A thorough sexual health history will assist the nurse in assessing the causative factors and enable him or her to develop an appropriate plan of intervention.

Kaplan suggests that marital discord may be at the root of sexual dysfunctions. Relational factors, which may have their base in childhood or in previous sexual relationships, can impact on sexual response outside the awareness of the couple. Kaplan indicates that two dynamics are most apparent: rage toward the partner and fear of rejection. A fear of rejection can prohibit the development of a satisfying sexual relationship. If the partner feels that the other individual is not trusting, then sexual expression is inhibited. The need to protect one's self from embarrassment or ridicule is paramount. Fear of failure may accompany a lack of trust. Kaplan notes that performance anxiety is directly related to a lack of trust. An understanding partner who permits less than optimal performance creates an atmosphere of acceptance that facilitates a healthy sexual relationship. Power struggles between partners and lack of fulfillment of unconscious contracts act as a stimulus for sexual dysfunction. Struggles that relate to earlier childhood experiences with parental figures may give way to distorted adult sexual relationships. An individual's need to dominate may be reflected in the inability to submit to the pleasure of sexual arousal. The concept of the unconscious marital contract is also an important determinant of a healthy sexual relationship. Either partner may have unconscious expectations such as sexual reward for certain behaviors within the context of the relationship. If expectations are not communicated yet are expected to be fulfilled, one or both partners may experience feelings of rage, rejection, or disappointment. A healthy sexual relationship is dependent upon the explication of these expectations and their impact on the couple.

Learning theory does not present causative factors, yet it has specific implications for understanding sexual dysfunction. The basis for learning theory in general supports the belief that symptoms are learned through conditioning and reinforcement from the environment. The experience of orgasm or erection may continually be followed by rejection or humiliation of some kind. Over time this negative reinforcer leads the individual to inhibit sexual responsiveness so as not to experience the negative reinforcer. Eventually the individual avoids all sexual experiences. Certain dysfunctional behaviors may also be rewarded because these behaviors cause distress for the other partner. For example, premature ejaculation may cause anger on the part of the female partner but may enable the male to punish her on an unconscious level. For whatever reason, learned negative sexual responses can be very damaging to the relationship. Kaplan further states that learning theory and psychoanalytic models are synergistic rather than contradictory. Resolution of negative sexual symptoms can be accomplished in many cases through behav-

ioral techniques or tasks that enable the couple to experience positive rewards for healthy sexual behavior.

Systems theory

One must note that to understand sexual dysfunction, a multidimensional view of the person must be considered. Masters and Johnson's studies (1986) show a conservative estimate that approximately half the marriages in this country either currently are experiencing sexual dysfunction of some kind or will in the near future. Further studies demonstrate that fewer than 20% of sexual dysfunctions are purely physiologic. Thus, the importance of assessment of sexual health in the overall nursing history and physical is critical in the identification and treatment of potential and actual sexual dysfunction (see Sexual Health Assessment on p. 222).

COMMON SEXUAL DYSFUNCTIONS

The following discussion will present the most common male and female sexual dysfunctions as described by DSM-III-R. The first category— orgasm-phase disorders—includes premature ejaculation, retarded ejaculation, and impaired female orgasm.

Premature ejaculation is the ejaculation of semen before the partners reach a state in which mutual enjoyment is experienced. DSM-III-R describes premature ejaculation as "occurrence of ejaculation before the individual wishes it, because of recurrent and persistent absence of reasonable voluntary control of ejaculation and orgasm during sexual activity. The judgement of 'reasonable control' is made by the clinician's taking into account factors that affect duration of the excitement phase, such as age, novelty of the sexual partner, and frequency and duration of coitus" (p. 280). It is one of the most common of the male sexual dysfunctions and is most easily treatable. Kaplan noted that the most crucial factor is not how quickly the man ejaculates but rather his inability to control the response. There is no definitive time limit for ejaculation, yet the lack of ability to control the ejaculatory response may cause frustration and unhappiness for both partners. During early sexual experiences, particularly in the teenage years, a quick ejaculation became a conditioned response. Masters and Johnson concluded that men who had little regard for the satisfaction of their partners were most consistently found to prematurely ejaculate. Control of the ejaculatory response was determined to be closely related to the man's inability to attend to sensory feedback. Inattention may be due to guilt, fear, or performance anxiety.

Retarded ejaculation is the inability to ejaculate although erection does occur. DSM-III-R describes retarded ejaculation as "the recurrent and persistent inhibition of the male orgasm as manifested by a delay in or absence of ejaculation following an adequate phase of sexual excitement" (p. 280). This supports Kaplan's notion of a biphasic sexual response. The erectile function is unimpaired; vasocongestion occurs, yet the individual is unable to ejaculate. Varying degrees of inhibition range from situational inability to ejaculate to the inability to experience ejaculation under any circumstances. The latter category is infrequently seen. Often retarded ejaculation is found in the older male and should be considered a normal part of aging. Effects of retarded ejaculation may be noted in the couple's level of sexual satisfaction. Women tend to feel rejected or responsible for their partner's inability to ejaculate. In turn, successive experiences of retarded ejaculation may lead to secondary erectile dysfunction.

Impaired female orgasm, last of the orgasm-phase disorders, is described by DSM-III-R as the "recurrent and persistent inhibition of the female orgasm as manifested by a delay in or absence of orgasm following a normal sexual excitement phase during sexual activity that is judged by the clinician to be adequate in focus, intensity, and duration" (p. 279). Kaplan (1983) notes that these women are not "frigid," as previous literature has indicated, but rather are unable to achieve orgasm although they do experience desire and excitement. In earlier works, Kaplan (1974) described orgasm as occurring along a continuum. At one end, women may have an orgasm in the presence of erotic fantasy without any physical contact of the clitoral area. Approximately 30% of the female population is able to achieve orgasm through coitus without any direct stimulation of the clitoral area. Next there are those women who can achieve orgasm only if coitus

is accompanied by clitoral stimulation. Moving along the continuum, we find women who cannot achieve orgasm with a partner through coitus with clitoral stimulation. However, this group can achieve orgasm with self-stimulation. Last, at the extreme end of the continuum are those women who have never experienced orgasm of any kind. There is controversy over whether women who cannot experience orgasm with vaginal penetration alone should be treated as having a sexual dysfunction. DSM-III-R indicates that most professionals at this time do not consider such a response abnormal. Thus one can understand that the responses to this dysfunction are widely varied. Often it is the male partner who feels more uncomfortable with the situation than the woman. Kaplan (1983) notes that coitally anorgastic women can acquire a coital orgasm, but that remains the woman's choice and should not be forced upon her. Treatment is the option of the woman rather than a response to societal and partner pressures. A complete physical examination is necessary to determine if in fact the genitalia are intact. Several theories have been proposed related to physiological causes for anorgasmia such as clitoral adhesions, weakened pubococcygeal muscles, or lack of stimulation of the "Grafenberg" or "G" spot. Ladas, Whipple, and Perry (1982) suggested that the stimulation of the "G" spot will incur swelling with resultant orgasm and "female ejaculation." The latter supposition lacks scientific supporting data and only serves to increase the anxiety of women who cannot or do not "ejaculate."

The second area of psychosexual disorders as described in DSM-III-R includes disorders of the excitement phase: impotence or erectile dysfunction and impaired female excitement.

Erectile dysfunction or impotence is a result of lack of sufficient vasocongestion. DSM-III-R describes impotence as the "recurrent and persistent inhibition of sexual excitement during sexual activity, manifested by partial or complete failure to attain or maintain erection until completion of the sexual act" (p. 279). Kaplan (1974) noted that erectile dysfunction may be considered primary or secondary. Primary impotence includes those individuals who have never experienced erections with women yet are able to achieve an erection with masturbation. Individuals with secondary impotence have had success in achieving erections up until the time of the initial onset of erectile difficulties. Males of all ages can experience erectile dysfunctions; perhaps at least half of the male population will experience secondary impotence at some point in their lives. Erectile dysfunction does vary in degree and frequency. The duration of the symptoms has a direct effect on the successful outcome of treatment. Kaplan found that the prognosis for secondary impotence is significantly better than for those individuals who had never experienced an erection with a partner. Situations in which impotence occurs vary widely. Some males, for example, may achieve erection only during foreplay. Others cannot achieve erection when the partner is physically aggressive or when performance is expected by the partner. In many cases individuals are able to experience an erection with an individual other than their wives or significant others. Last, some may achieve an erection only when engaging in variant sexual behavior such as fondling women's underwear, watching women undress, or dressing in feminine clothing. It must be noted that erectile dysfunction in general has a profound psychological effect on the individual. Depression is often noted with lowered self-esteem and feelings of worthlessness in relation to self and others. Feelings of masculinity have historically been tied to one's ability to achieve an erection, i.e., locker room discussions of how many times an individual is able to achieve that symbol of masculine prowess. Unlike the female, the male is unable to "pretend" or "fake it." The inability to achieve an erection cannot be hidden from one's partner and is very devastating on an emotional level.

Impaired female excitement is described by DSM-III-R as "a recurrent and persistent inhibition of sexual excitement during sexual activity, manifested by partial or complete failure to attain or maintain the lubrication-swelling phase of sexual excitement until completion of the sexual act" (p. 279). Kaplan (1983) notes that women who experience this syndrome feel the desire for lovemaking and enjoy sex. Orgasm can be reached by intense stimulation, yet lubrication is absent. Intercourse can then be painful and unpleasant and result in other disorders such as dyspareunia and vaginismus as well as inhibited sexual desire. This disorder can

be seen most frequently in women who are experiencing menopause where estrogen deficiency is apparent. A relatively small number of women do experience inhibited excitement as a result of psychogenic causes; however, as Kaplan (1983) indicates, most women lose their interest in sex or have orgastic difficulties rather than experience inhibited excitement.

The third category of psychosexual disorders—desire-phase disorders—includes impaired sexual desire, the paraphilias, and ego-dystonic homosexuality. DSM-III-R describes psychogenic deficient sexual desire as the "persistent and pervasive inhibition of sexual desire. The judgement of inhibition of sexual desire is made by the clinician's taking into account factors that affect sexual desire such as age, sex, health, intensity and frequency of sexual desire, and the context of the individual's life" (p. 278). Masters and Johnson (1986) state that individuals with inhibited sexual desire (ISD) generally present complaints of low interest in sexual activity and are not receptive to initiatives made by their partners. Occasionally these individuals will acquiesce to having sex just to meet the other partner's needs. Individuals with ISD are generally physically able to engage in sexual activities. It has been found that there may also be associated sexual dysfunctions, although it is questionable whether the sexual dysfunction occurred as a result of ISD. ISD may vary according to situation and may be either primary or secondary. The incidence of ISD seems to be on the rise, although scientific data have not been made available to support this premise. Kaplan (1987) suggests that individuals experiencing ISD have a fear of intimacy rather than a fear of sex itself. She further proposes that these individuals fear enjoyment of sexual pleasure—that this is not psychologically "safe." Frieda Stuart (1987) indicates that to consider women who have low sexual desire abnormal would be remiss. Research by Stuart comparing women with ISD with those having normal sexual desire found that those with ISD are not greatly different in psychological makeup from those with normal sexual desire. Further conclusions from this study indicated that a woman's sexual desire is greatly influenced by the quality of her marital relationship and impact of parental attitudes and values regarding sex and affection. Masters and Johnson (1986) found that ISD is not a conflictual situation in all relationships. Often partners can work out an acceptable accommodation that meets the needs of both partners. An important consideration in the evaluation of ISD is the effect of dual-career coupling—sharing household responsibilities and the general pace of life in society today. Perhaps we must consider that low sexual desire or inhibited desire may initially result from a lack of time spent with one's partner due to conflicting business schedules, pressure of professional or corporate success, the arrival of an infant, or other factors that may impact on a couple's intimacy. Inhibited sexual desire may in fact be the result of our current societal values and mores. The young, upwardly mobile professional or "Yuppie" may be confronted with the issue of ISD as a concomitant of status in society.

The paraphilias are described by DSM-III-R as "disorders in which unusual or bizarre imagery or acts are necessary for sexual excitement" (p. 266). The eight paraphilias are presented as they appear in DSM-III-R:

fetishism   "The use of nonliving objects (fetishes) is a repeatedly preferred or exclusive method of achieving sexual excitement" (p. 269).

transvestism   "Recurrent and persistent cross-dressing by a heterosexual male" (p. 270).

zoophilia   "The act or fantasy of engaging in sexual activity with animals is a repeatedly preferred or exclusive method of achieving sexual excitement" (p. 270).

pedophilia   "The act or fantasy of engaging in sexual activity with prepubertal children is a repeatedly preferred or exclusive method of achieving sexual excitement" (pp. 271-272). As adults these individuals tend to prefer sexual activities with children of the same sex.

exhibitionism   "The essential feature is repetitive acts of exposing the genitals to an unsuspecting stranger for the purpose of achieving sexual excitement, with no further attempt at sexual activity with the stranger" (p. 272).

voyeurism   "The individual repeatedly observes unsuspecting people who are naked, in the act of disrobing, or engaging in sexual activity and no sexual activity with the observed people is sought. The observing is the repeatedly preferred or exclusive method of achieving sexual excitement" (p. 273).

sexual masochism   "A preferred or exclusive mode of producing sexual excitement is to be humiliated, bound, beaten, or otherwise made to suffer" (p. 273).

sexual sadism   "The essential feature is the infliction of physical or psychological suffering on another person in order to achieve sexual excitement" (p. 274).

The last category includes atypical paraphilias such as coprophilia (feces); urophilia (urine); frotteurism (rubbing); and necrophilia (corpses), to name a few.

Ego-dystonic homosexuality is considered by DSM-III-R as a category within the disorders of sexual desire. Kaplan (1983) supports this inclusion by stating that this population has a low or absent desire for and gratification from heterosexual partners in a committed relationship as well as a normal desire and gratification in variant sexual arousal situations. Within the context of the DSM-III-R, ego-dystonic homosexuality is described as the "desire to acquire or increase heterosexual arousal, so that heterosexual relationships can be initiated or maintained, and a sustained pattern of overt homosexual arousal that the individual states has been unwanted and is a persistent source of distress" (p. 281). In this category, the critical factor is the desire of the individual to experience heterosexual relationships and to enjoy a normal family life. Those homosexuals who are comfortable with their life-style should not be forced into treatment, yet treatment for those who are not should be made available and encouraged.

The final category of psychosexual disorders is that of sexual pain and disorders associated with genital muscle spasm. This category includes dyspareunia, uterine muscle cramps, vaginismus, and ejaculatory pain. Kaplan (1983) notes that dyspareunia includes sexual pain with the exception of pain caused by involuntary spasm of the genital muscles such as orgasmic uterine cramps, vaginismus, and ejaculatory pain. DSM-III-R describes dyspareunia as "recurrent and persistent genital pain, in either the male or the female" (p. 280). Pain can be present during orgasm, excitement, or intercourse and should not be considered a normal consequence of sexual activity. Physical factors must be evaluated due to the fact that numerous physical conditions can cause a painful experience.

This is not to say that psychogenic factors must not be considered; however, individuals may feel the need to bear their pain rather than reveal its effects. Dyspareunia may result from inadequate lubrication in the female, pathological penile anatomy, and various lesions and infections of the reproductive tract.

Kaplan (1983) notes that orgasmic uterine cramps occur primarily in postmenopausal women. It has been related to estrogen deficiency, which in turn causes the individual to experience spasms following orgasm. This can be most readily treated by counseling and information giving.

DSM-III-R characterizes vaginismus by a "history of recurrent and persistent involuntary spasm of the musculature of the outer third of the vagina that interferes with coitus" (p. 280). In the case of normal sexual arousal, vaginal muscles relax; however, in this case, vaginal muscles tighten, which virtually prevents penetration unless it occurs forcibly, which in turn causes pain. Kaplan (1983) indicates that women may experience sexual desire, lubrication, and orgasm, yet penetration of any type is difficult. Physical factors must be evaluated; in some cases the tightness of the vaginal muscles may prevent entry for examination. Reassurance can reduce anxiety and promote relaxation to permit entry. Psychogenic factors may range from a single precipitating situation to a more severe neurotic conflict.

TREATMENT MODALITIES

Sexual dysfunction in some form will affect over half of the couples in the United States (Fogel, 1979). Yet sexuality itself remains a taboo subject in many instances, which restricts the discussion and treatment of sexual difficulties. Masters and Johnson in their early works gave credence to the emerging concern for sexuality and the right to sexually satisfying experiences. Professionals in the field of psychiatry such as Helen Singer Kaplan, Domeena Renshaw, and Harold Lief, to name a few, have instituted programs whereby couples are treated in a holistic environment and encouraged to develop healthy sexual relationships. Students in medicine, nursing, and social work as well as the clergy are educated to provide comprehensive sexual health care as it is appropriate for their clients.

The issue of sexual health spans a lifetime. Clients need permission to be sexual and to have their questions and concerns addressed at whatever level is comfortable for each individual. Health professionals have the obligation to demystify sex by providing accurate and appropriate education regarding the sexual response cycle, a range of acceptable behaviors within the context of societal norms, and the freedom to ask for information to make responsible choices. It must be pointed out that not all health professionals feel comfortable with discussions regarding sexuality. Often lack of basic knowledge of the sexual response cycle—its physiological and psychological dimensions—causes anxiety on the part of the health professional. Watts (1979) states that the sexual health history can be considered a functional part of the reproductive health history. Questions regarding sexual function may be asked concurrently with those related to urinary and reproductive function. Detection of possible dysfunctions can be accomplished through a thorough sexual history.

Therapy, whether it be individual or group, requires specific knowledge and skills. Annon (1976) suggests a model that denotes the level of intervention and the skills required for each. PLISSIT can be described as a four-level model—P stands for permission to be a sexual being with questions and issues whether implicit or explicit; LI is limited information—factual information is presented to clients based on their specific concerns; SS is specific suggestions—techniques to assist the client to overcome sexual difficulties; IT is intensive therapy. The last two areas of intervention require a more advanced level of professional preparation. Nurses must have a more in-depth knowledge of sexual dysfunctions and treatment modalities. They must also be keenly aware of their own values, fears, concerns, and vulnerabilities when confronting the sexual health issues of others. When areas of discomfort arise or more intensive therapy is required, the nurse may refer to other appropriate resources.

Individual therapy

Sexual dysfunction can arise from multiple causative factors—physiologic, intrapsychic, relational, behavioral, sociocultural; thus, therapy must be consistent with this premise. Kaplan notes that insight can now be coupled with techniques that can effect a resolution of the unconscious conflict as well as modify destructive sexual behaviors. The blend of therapeutic approaches may be utilized to meet the varying needs of clients.

Psychoanalytic therapy focuses on the unconscious conflicts generated in childhood that now impact on adult sexual behaviors. Powerful systems of irrational beliefs create guilt, fear, and overwhelming anxiety. The desire to experience fulfillment in a sexual relationship is countermanded by fear of punishment for doing so. The goal of psychoanalytic therapy is to resolve specific underlying conflicts, particularly those early incestuous feelings generated in the Oedipal period. Psychoanalysis is a long-term, one-to-one relational process that does not focus on specific techniques to change sexual behaviors but rather on the exploration of unresolved childhood conflicts.

Masters and Johnson are best known for their couples approach to sexual dysfunction. For the most part, treatment takes place at their clinic, which requires a commitment of two weeks during which a comprehensive physical and psychological history is completed. The presence of pathophysiology is ruled out, and factors that impact on healthy sexuality are considered. Several basic tenets are incorporated in Masters and Johnson's treatment program. They believe that sexual behavior is a learned response that can either be positively or negatively reinforced. If negatively reinforced, anxiety, fear, and guilt can result from experiencing pleasurable sexual relationships. Couples can learn to overcome negative attitudes and develop more healthy responses to the sexual experience. Masters and Johnson also believe that the couple is the client rather than each individual as a separate entity; thus, clients are treated by dual-sex therapy teams. Lack of knowledge is considered a major factor in sexual dysfunction as is a lack of appropriate communication skills. The goals of therapy then are to educate clients, to improve verbal and nonverbal communication skills, and to experience satisfying sexual relations within an interpersonal context. Sensate focus exercises are utilized to encourage couples to experience nongenital sexual pleasuring through the use of nonverbal communication skills. Although the requirement of

two weeks for both partners is prohibitive in many situations, the success of the Masters and Johnson therapy approach has been well documented and continues to play a major role in the treatment of sexual dysfunction.

Helen Singer Kaplan has developed a mode of therapy that is a blend of psychoanalysis, marital dynamics, sex therapy, and behavioral and systems theory. She believes that the determination of causality is the most critical factor in the evaluation of sexual dysfunction. If organicity is ruled out, the assessment of psychological factors must be completed in a thorough manner. Kaplan's premise of the biphasic nature of the sexual response cycle serves as a foundation for the treatment of sexual dysfunctions. Kaplan (1983) notes that the immediate psychological causes or the current disruptive sexual behaviors and destructive interactions and emotions are the initial focus of the therapy. The following is a presentation of the specific disorder and the identified treatment modality as described by Kaplan (1983).

IMPAIRED FEMALE ORGASM

Orgasm by manual self-stimulation of the clitoris coupled with erotica and fantasy is the initial step. Movement toward orgasm with a partner either through self-stimulation or stimulation of the clitoris by a partner follows. Orgasm through intercourse is the next step; if this is unsuccessful, a "bridge maneuver" is utilized whereby one partner stimulates the clitoris while the penis is in the vagina up to the point of orgasm. Penile thrusting then takes over stimulation of orgasm. If a couple experiences clitoral orgasm solely yet their sexual relationship is a positive one, reassurance must be given that clitoral orgasm is not second best.

EJACULATORY INCOMPETENCE OR RETARDED EJACULATION

Behavioral methods are utilized to desensitize systematically "in vivo" or in the client's bedroom. Initially the client is instructed to ejaculate under any circumstances with the ultimate goal being intravaginal ejaculation. Erotic fantasies and activities may be incorporated as they apply in each individual situation to enhance ejaculatory competence. Sexual tasks are assigned that are performed and then reported in therapeutic sessions. Through these sessions, the therapist is able to assist the couple in identifying and resolving conflicts and resulting marital issues.

PREMATURE EJACULATION

Kaplan (1974) notes that the primary objective of the therapeutic sexual tasks is to get the male to focus his attention consistently on the sensations of impending orgasm while making love to his partner. This approach teaches the individual to clearly perceive his erotic preorgastic sensations and to avoid distraction by the process of sexual intercourse. The "stop-start" technique, initially used by Semans, has been modified by Kaplan. The couple is instructed to engage in limited foreplay; the woman stimulates the male, while the male focuses solely on the erotic sensations coming from the stimulation of the penis. He is stimulated until he feels the urge to ejaculate, at which point he tells his wife to stop. This process is repeated four times, and at this time he does ejaculate. After three to six extravaginal sessions, intercourse is suggested. The female superior position is encouraged in conjunction with the male guiding the partner's pelvic thrusting. The stop-start technique is again utilized intravaginally until the fourth time, at which point the male is permitted coital ejaculation. In most cases, Kaplan reports success with the utilization of this method.

ERECTILE DYSFUNCTION (IMPOTENCE)

The primary objective of therapy is to reduce the anxiety related to the achievement of erection. Restoration of confidence in the ability to achieve an erection is a critical factor. A series of sexual tasks is assigned as follows: nondemand pleasuring with no coitus and ejaculation; dispelling of fear of failure through techniques that permit the male to achieve an erection by means of fondling; distraction from obsessive thoughts of failure through erotic fantasy during lovemaking; permission to be selfish and enjoy the sexual response; coital experience after erectile confidence has been established. The emphasis of the therapy is to enhance the erotic factors

within the context of the relationship and to reduce those factors which inhibit the sexual response.

INHIBITED SEXUAL DESIRE

Kaplan (1979) suggests that the basic premise in the treatment of desire disorders is the modification of the individual's tendency to inhibit erotic tendencies and to allow feelings to emerge freely and naturally. The treatment utilizes insight therapy as well as active confrontational techniques. Sexual tasks are again assigned and reviewed with the therapist. Critical to success with ISD patients is the awareness of "why" they do not want to have sex—what earlier conflicts are contributing to their current perceptions. Sensate focus exercises are initially prescribed with the goal of a positive coital experience. Reassurance and acceptance by the therapist is an important factor throughout the therapeutic process. The couple may also be confronted with the destructive effects of the current behavior on the relationship. Desire disorders cannot be treated as other simpler genital-phase disorders. Kaplan further notes that individuals with desire disorders may benefit more from long-term individual and marital therapy rather than brief therapy, although few data support this premise.

VAGINISMUS

The objective in the treatment of vaginismus is gradual dilatation of the vagina. A sequence that involves reducing the conditioned spasm of the muscles surrounding the vagina may be utilized beginning with the actual visualization of the vaginal opening and moving slowly through digital dilatation to penile insertion to penile insertion with thrusting.

The treatment of sexual dysfunctions is dependent upon multiple factors. Recognition of a potential or actual sexual dysfunction is a primary function of nursing. Dependent upon knowledge, experience, and comfort level, the nurse will either intervene at an appropriate level or refer to a health professional with the necessary skills and knowledge. The crucial factor is the awareness of the individual as a sexual being who may in fact be experiencing a sexual dysfunction.

EFFECTS OF ILLNESS ON SEXUALITY

Sexuality is an integral component of each unique individual. As illness affects one's physical sense of being, so does it impact on one's sense of self-worth—one's body image. Yet sexual health issues may be ignored. The very awareness of and subsequent information that a client receives regarding the illness has an impact on the client's existing perception of self. The emotional investment attached to a particular body part and/or its function is a critical factor. For example, a woman who considers her breasts important in actualizing her role as a sexual being may experience a great sense of loss of self-esteem and value as a sexual partner following a mastectomy. It has also been noted in the literature that women who have had hysterectomies often indicate that they feel less feminine and less attractive sexually. Clients who have experienced heart attacks may initially fear engaging in sexual activity, believing that sex may stimulate another attack.

Mr. Smith, a 45-year-old male airline pilot, has been hospitalized for cardiac evaluation of his ventricular tachycardia, a lethal arrhythmia. Following completion of the evaluation, his physicians indicated that he will no longer be able to fly. During the night, Ms. K. was checking Mr. Smith's temperature when he reached out and touched the nurse on her breast. Startled, Ms. K. moved back from the bedside. Mr. Smith, chagrined by his actions, began to cry.

Ms. K. *Can you tell me what you're feeling right now (putting her hand on his arm)?*

Mr. Smith *I'm so sorry—I don't know what's wrong with me.*

Ms. K. *I can see you're sorry—I appreciate your apology. Perhaps we can talk about what might have precipitated this.*

Mr. Smith *I don't feel like the same person I was yesterday—I know that sounds strange, but I can't explain it any differently.*

Ms. K. *Are you saying that something or someone has changed who you are?*

Mr. Smith *A major part of my life was flying—enjoying the world—being in the company of women—now that's all over.*

Ms. K. *I think I hear you saying that perhaps you as a man—as a sexual being—have changed or that others may perceive you as having changed.*

Mr. Smith *Well, I probably won't be able to have the same level of sexual activity as I did before.*

Ms. K. *Can you describe what your previous level of sexual activity was—that will be helpful information for me in order to answer some of the questions you have.*

Mr. Smith *Although I didn't have one single relationship, I have had a continuing relationship with three different women—I would say I have sexual intercourse three to four times weekly.*

Ms. K. *During sexual activity did you experience any chest pain or other cardiac symptoms?*

Mr. Smith *No, but I'm afraid I might.*

Ms. K. *Would you consider your relationship with three different women as being stressful to you?*

Mr. Smith *No, why do you ask that?*

Ms. K. *A critical factor in sexual activity with cardiac clients is that of stress—if there is a fear of being "found out," there is an increased risk of cardiac symptoms occurring. What I would like to do is set up a meeting with your cardiologist, you, and myself to discuss your cardiac status and its relationship to your sexual activity. If necessary, we can also discuss possible alternatives to your current sexual activity that can be as satisfying to you and your partners. Your sexual health is equally as important as your cardiac status. Would this be acceptable to you at this point in time?*

Mr. Smith *Yes, although it seems strange to be discussing my sexual activity—I don't think I realized that I might have been having concerns about it, but I guess that I was.*

Individuals with cancer report that loved ones may distance themselves at a time when intimacy and caring are most needed. Renal disease causes fatigue and lack of sexual desire. In many instances male clients experience impotence. Diabetes may also cause impotence as a result of decreased vasocongestion. Surgical procedures such as ileostomy, colostomy, vulvectomy, or amputation alter body image and may impact on client and partner. Whatever the situation, the impact of altered body image must be considered and addressed. Treatment procedures such as radiation, chemotherapy, and dialysis may also impact on one's perception of self as a whole and sexual being.

Mr. Rudy, a 35-year-old married black male, has been on dialysis three times weekly for three months. During daily treatment he generally is talkative and friendly. However, Ms. D., his primary nurse, noticed that for the last two treatments Mr. Rudy has been withdrawn and tearful. Ms. D. approached Mr. Rudy before the completion of his current treatment.

Ms. D. *Rudy, you seem to be upset.*

Mr. Rudy *You're damn right! They told me that once I was on dialysis I'd start feeling better about things.*

Ms. D. *Can you tell me what 'things' in particular you're concerned about?*

Mr. Rudy *Well—I'd be less tired and I'd—well, I'd be able to be more like the man I used to be.*

Ms. D. *I'm still not completely clear. . .*

Mr. Rudy *My wife and I had a great sexual relationship until I started having these kidney problems six months ago. My family doctor told me "no problem—you'll be fine." That's not happening.*

Ms. D. *I do understand your concern. First the dialysis should improve your kidney function which should then begin to decrease your feelings of fatigue. Second, we need to talk about what it is that you specifically expect in regard to your sexual activity. Your sexual health is an important factor as well. Do you have any questions right now about your sexual health?*

Mr. Rudy *No—but it felt better to just say that to someone and have it matter. I think if I could talk about my feelings and my dialysis—my anger, frustration, feeling like half a man.*

Ms. D. *You have a right to have those feelings—the way you feel about yourself has an impact on your physical, emotional, social, and sexual self. We can also clarify any concerns you have regarding your physical state and its impact on your sexual activity.*

Adaptation to changes in body image is dependent upon the significance of the alteration, the effectiveness of coping measures, previous experiences in coping with loss, the support of significant others, and the desire to participate in one's own care as it is possible. Responses may vary—often ranging from denial to a complete inability to function. Nurses can provide an atmosphere where permission is given to clients to acknowledge their loss and to recognize the clients' needs to express concerns regarding their body image, inclusive of sexual health concerns. By facilitating clients' expression of feelings of abandonment, loss of affectional

ties, loss of adequacy in the sexual role, need for touching and emotional closeness, fear of changes in interpersonal relationships, nurses reaffirm the significance of sexual health needs. A simple statement such as, "Often women express a fear that their partners won't love them following their hysterectomy" validates the feelings they are experiencing as normal and provides a forum for further discussion. A client may say, "I'm not going to be the person I used to be after my mastectomy (prostatectomy, colostomy, amputation)." This statement indicates a change in perception of self and a need for further assessment. Concern for self as a sexually healthy and active individual may be covert. By the nurse's recognizing potential sexual health concerns, encouraging open discussion, and providing appropriate factual information, positive adaptation to the changes created by the illness can be facilitated.

Nursing Intervention
PRIMARY PREVENTION

With the advent of increased awareness of sexuality, including sex roles, attitudes and behaviors, it becomes imperative that nurses take an active role in the promotion of sexual health. The World Health Organization in 1975 defined sexual health as "the integration of the somatic, intellectual, emotional and social aspects of a sexual being in ways that are positively enriching and that enhance one's personality, communication and love. Every person has the right to receive sexual information and to consider accepting sexuality for pleasure as well as procreation" (p. 10). Recommendations from the World Health Organization Committee indicate that sexual health services should be incorporated into other health services and reimbursed in a similar fashion. Furthermore, health care providers should be able to provide counseling for individuals and couples.

Support for the nursing role has been documented in the literature. Mims (1975) indicated that nurses must begin to integrate sexual health care in comprehensive treatment plans as it relates to the mental, social, and physical well-being of the

client. Woods (1984) clearly defined seven major components of this role:
1. Facilitation of an environment that fosters the client's sexuality as valid.
2. Provision of anticipatory guidance.
3. Validation of the normalcy of behaviors, thoughts, and feelings.
4. Education of clients.
5. Provision of intensive therapy when appropriate.
6. Counseling of clients.
7. Consultation with schools, community groups, and other health professionals.

To actualize the role as sexual health care provider, the nurse must consider his or her basic knowledge level, attitudes, and comfort level relative to sexuality. The nurse must be keenly aware of self—individual value systems, fears, concerns, and vulnerabilities—when confronting the sexual health needs of others. Values clarification and desensitization through sexual attitude reassessment programs are often effective in helping health professionals to become more aware of their own belief systems and biases.

How do I assess my sexual beliefs and values? What issues are important for me to consider? Questions nurses might ask themselves include the following:
1. What do I consider "male" and "female" traits? Is there a dichotomy between the two?
2. What is "normal" sexual behavior to me? How do I feel about masturbation and oral-genital sex? What are variants of sexual behavior? How do I achieve sexual gratification?
3. How do I feel about alternative sexual lifestyles such as homosexuality, lesbianism, and transvestism?
4. How comfortable do I feel discussing sexual issues with a client? How comfortable do I feel discussing sexual issues with my partner?

SECONDARY PREVENTION

Short-term therapy and crisis intervention are utilized to treat identified sexual dysfunctions such as premature ejaculation, retarded ejaculation, and anorgasmia. Interventive strategies are also directed toward the facilitation of increased sexual satisfaction with one's partner as well as toward the development of a positive sense of worth as a sexual being.

Objectives for secondary prevention include:
1. Early identification of sexual dysfunctions
2. Seeking prompt and effective treatment
3. Assessment of community resources available for sexual dysfunctions; sex education for sexually transmitted diseases.
4. Participation with schools, community agencies, and churches to provide appropriate resources.

Casefinding

School nurses, community health nurses, as well as staff nurses are in a critical position to identify situations where sexual health may be compromised. Hospitalized clients may be experiencing changes in physical function and/or appearance that may affect sexual function or perceptions of self as a sexual being. Lack of knowledge regarding contraception may lead to teen pregnancy. Community health nurses are able to provide factual information about birth control as well as supportive counseling. Couples, both heterosexual and homosexual, who are experiencing interpersonal conflict within the context of a relationship can benefit from counseling designed to increase effective communication skills.

The following are principles of secondary prevention:
1. The focus should be client-centered, whether an individual or a couple.
2. Individual symptoms and behaviors may be defense mechanisms utilized to reduce anxiety.
3. A trusting, noncritical environment is necessary to facilitate effective problem resolution.
4. Behavior of one individual within the context of a relationship has a direct effect on the other.
5. Nursing intervention should be directed toward alleviating symptomatic behavior and developing more effective communication skills.

6. Nurses must develop an awareness of their own values and attitudes regarding sexuality and sexual behavior. This awareness is critical to effective intervention with clients experiencing sexual health problems.

Nursing process

The nursing process provides the framework for the development, implementation, and evaluation of nursing strategies. To effectively utilize the nursing process in the area of sexual health, it is critical that the nurse assess his or her values and beliefs regarding sexuality and sexual behavior.

ASSESSMENT

The use of self to create an environment where sexual health is perceived as an integral component of the comprehensive history and physical is most critical. Mims (1975) stated that it is imperative that nurses create an atmosphere where the sexual health history can be incorporated into the overall health history. A sense of trust and a feeling that one's concerns regarding body image, sexual choice, lack of sexual desire or satisfaction, or request for information relative to alternative methods to enhance sexuality must be facilitated by the nurse to ensure that the client's perceptions, feelings, and needs are validated as real. Accurate data collection relies on the ability of the nurse to create an environment where it is *expected* that there will be sexual health issues and concerns. Krueger et al. (1977) noted that women with reproductive cancer wanted the nurse to provide information regarding sexual adjustment following surgery. This same group of women also urged that nurses initiate the discussion of sexual health issues rather than wait for the client to raise concerns. Since the screening of sexual health issues in data collection is a significant component, the following are guidelines for the facilitation of a comfortable climate for the nurse-client interview.

1. Utilize an honest, matter-of-fact approach that acknowledges the client as having sexual concerns and questions.
2. Maintain eye contact and sit comfortably close to the client.

3. Provide a sufficient amount of time for discussion—don't "run in and run out."
4. Utilize broad, general, open-ended questions to elicit information regarding sexual knowledge, perceptions of the impact of illness on sexuality, methods of sexual gratification, and attitudes relating to sexual issues.
5. Do not push the client into a discussion of sexuality. Leave the issue open for further discussion at a later time. (Also, do not assume that because there are no questions, there are no concerns.)
6. Concerns about body image, activities of daily living, and return to preillness functioning can act as precipitants for discussion of sexual health issues. For example, statements that reflect general concern among all clients can be utilized: "Many people in your situation express concern about resumption of sexual activity."
7. Observation of the client during successive interactions provides information regarding comfort level (which issues are discussed and which are avoided), anxiety levels, unrealistic expectations of self or partner, guilt and shame, and level of psychosexual development.
8. Ask for clarification of unclear verbal and nonverbal communication: "When listening to you talk about your sexual preferences, I'm not sure what you are saying. Can you be more clear? I want to understand what this means for you."
9. Initiation of the discussion of sexual health issues acknowledges an individual as a sexual being and makes it possible for questions and concerns to emerge (see Sexual Health Assessment on p. 222).

ANALYSIS OF DATA

The analysis of data leads to the formulation of the nursing diagnosis. Through the interpretation and appraisal of the data, the nurse is able to identify client strengths such as good physical health, willingness to increase his/her knowledge level, positive sense of self, and having a positive relationship with a significant other. Data analysis also reveals areas of difficulty that may or may not be identified by the client. Prior to the identification

Sexual health assessment

BIOLOGICAL SUBSYSTEM

1. Neurological system
   a. CVA
   b. Spinal cord injuries/tumors
   c. Multiple sclerosis
   d. Surgery related to sympathetic/parasympathetic function
2. Cardiovascular system
   a. Coronary artery disease
      1. Bypass grafts, transplantation
   b. Peripheral vascular disease
   c. Hypertension
   d. Circulatory disorders—leukemia, lymphoma, sickle cell anemia
3. Endocrine system
   a. Diabetes
   b. Thyroid dysfunction
   c. Obesity
   d. Pituitary/gonadal dysfunction
4. Reproductive system
   a. Onset of menstruation; menarche; PMS syndrome; contraceptive history; number of pregnancies (live and stillbirth).
   b. Ability to achieve an erection or orgasm; ability to ejaculate; pain, bleeding secondary to sexual activity; current sexual activity level/any recent changes in sexual activity level secondary to present illness and/or hospitalization or treatment.
   c. Surgical history: mastectomy, hysterectomy, sterilization, prostatectomy, orchiectomy.
   d. Cancer: ovaries, uterus, cervix, vulva, breasts. Type of treatment, frequency, duration.
5. Genitourinary system
   a. Urinary tract infections; pelvic inflammatory disease; sexually transmitted disease; penile/vaginal discharge; itching; scarring; cystic disease.
   b. Benign prostatic hypertrophy; prostatic cancer.
6. Gastrointestinal system
   a. Ulcers; gall bladder; excessive flatus/bloating; diarrhea; constipation.
   b. Cancer of GI tract; colostomy.
7. Medications currently taking? Prescribed/recreational?
8. Average alcohol consumption?
9. Perceived changes in sexual activity level?
10. Family history of sexual health problems?

PSYCHOLOGICAL SUBSYSTEM

1. Perceived life stressors at present (change in job status, recent relocation, death of significant other, separation/divorce, birth of a child).
2. Perception of self as a sexual being (body image, satisfaction with sexual activity level, ability to satisfy partner, positive/negative experiences with sexual satisfaction.
3. Specific feelings generated by sexual experiences: anxiety, frustration, anger, repulsion, pleasure, other.
4. Changes you would like to make in your sexual relationships?
5. Attitudes regarding alternative sexual lifestyles.

SOCIOCULTURAL SUBSYSTEM

1. Perceptions of traditional sex roles—male involvement in childrearing/household activities; female in the work force.
2. Family values re expression of affection, handholding, kissing, hugging. Are partner's values similar?
3. How does ethnic background influence yours and your partner's expression of sexuality?
4. How would you describe your experience with sexual relationships?
5. How would you describe your comfort level in discussing sex with your partner, your siblings, your parents, your children?

SPIRITUAL SUBSYSTEM

1. What are your basic beliefs regarding the place of sexuality in your life? (i.e., sexual intercourse is only for procreation, etc.)
2. Are your beliefs related to a specific spiritual upbringing? Are these beliefs consonant with your partner's?
3. What do you generally do when your beliefs are in conflict with others?
4. Do you feel a sense of fulfillment through your sexual experiences?

INTELLECTUAL SUBSYSTEM

1. What is your knowledge of the male/female sexual response cycle?
2. What is your knowledge of male/female anatomy and physiology? Do you generally use anatomically correct terms for body parts? If not, what words do you use?
3. Are you aware of the various factors that can affect sexual response/satisfaction, i.e., drugs, alcohol, fatigue, previous experiences?
4. How do you feel about learning other measures to enhance your sexual experiences?

of nursing diagnoses, it is important that both client and nurse review the data so that mutually determined problems are identified.

PLANNING AND IMPLEMENTATION

Goals can be established that the client perceives as important and is willing to work on. Strategies to achieve these goals will be identified and mutually discussed. The nurse's expertise will influence the type of intervention, such as referral to more appropriate resources, i.e., a certified nurse sexual counselor. Planning must reflect a realistic appraisal of each individual client's situation and presenting problem. Lastly, goals must be prioritized by both client and nurse to ensure commitment to their accomplishments.

Following are nursing care plans that reflect a realistic approach to secondary preventive intervention. The nurse may initially establish goals, but as therapy progresses, the client should enter into goal setting to ensure commitment to accomplishing these goals.

NURSING CARE PLAN
Clients with Sexual Dysfunction

Long-term Outcomes	Short-term Outcomes	Nursing Strategies

Nursing diagnosis: Sexual dysfunction secondary to inability to achieve a satisfactory ejaculatory response related to values conflict with partner (NANDA 3.2.1.2.1; DSM-III-R 302.75)

To experience a satisfying ejaculatory response within the context of the relationship with partner. To explore personal value systems as it relates to sexual behavior	To establish working relationship with nurse. To develop more effective communication skills with partner. To participate in sensate focus exercises with partner. To utilize "stop-start" or "squeeze" technique	Provide an atmosphere that permits clients to be sexual. Complete a detailed sexual history. Discuss the need for accountability to perform exercises. Follow process for "stop-start" or "squeeze" technique. Discuss potential and actual problems encountered with therapy. Identify current stressors that may be related to personal value system. Describe measures for mediating stressors

Nursing diagnosis: Pain related to normal physiological changes accompanying the aging process (NANDA 9.1; DSM-III-R 302.90)

To develop a positive sense of self as a sexual being	To clarify distorted perceptions of sexuality in older persons. To verbalize feelings regarding changes incurred by aging process	Provide quiet atmosphere without interruption. Use touch and warmth as appropriate. Assess client's previous sexual experiences within the context of own value system. Assure client that sexual health is an integral part of his or her life

Continued.

NURSING CARE PLAN—cont'd

Clients with Sexual Dysfunction

Long-term Outcomes	Short-term Outcomes	Nursing Strategies

Nursing diagnosis: Pain related to normal physiological changes accompanying the aging process (NANDA 9.1; DSM-III-R 302.90)—cont'd

Long-term Outcomes	Short-term Outcomes	Nursing Strategies
To achieve a satisfactory level of sexual expression	To identify sexual experiences that precipitate discomfort To experience decreased discomfort during sexual intercourse.	Explain the normal physiological changes associated with aging Discuss sources of discomfort associated with sexual activity Encourage sharing of feelings regarding sexuality Discuss measures to decrease discomfort (i.e., K-Y jelly as lubricant, different positions, time of day of sexual activity) Discuss importance of direct genital stimulation Encourage verbalization of concerns regarding change in role, being without partner Encourage sharing of feelings with partner to enhance mutual sexuality

Nursing diagnosis: Increased anxiety related to fear of public awareness of homosexual orientation (NANDA 9.3.1; DSM-III-R 302.0)

Long-term Outcomes	Short-term Outcomes	Nursing Strategies
Develop a positive sense of self as a sexual being Demonstrate a decreased anxiety level	Identify precipitators of anxiety Explore personal value system regarding homosexuality Discuss myths regarding homosexuals and their lifestyle	Demonstrate acceptance of choice of homosexual orientation Suggest specific literature on homosexuality to increase knowledge base Encourage exploration of personal beliefs regarding homosexual behavior Discuss client's perceptions of cause of anxiety Explore methods to reduce anxiety Test out strategies through role play Encourage use of support groups for homosexuals and lesbians

Nursing diagnosis: Knowledge deficit related to impact of chronic illness on sexual function resulting in inability to achieve satisfactory level of sexual arousal (NANDA 8.1.1; DSM-III-R 302.11)

Long-term Outcomes	Short-term Outcomes	Nursing Strategies
To develop a positive sense of self To achieve a level of sexual desire that is satisfying within the framework of the chronic illness	To establish a working relationship with nurse To clarify distorted information related to impact of chronic illness on sexual health To explore alternative measures to enhance desire To participate with partner in support group designed for specific chronic illness	Provide an atmosphere where sexuality is viewed as important Discuss normal range of sexual responses Discuss impact of illness on self-esteem Discuss misconceptions regarding impact of chronic illness Encourage client to share fears with partner regarding sexual activity Discuss alternative methods of sexual expression Act as a referral for community resources (i.e., support group)

EVALUATION

Evaluation of sexual counseling and intervention occurs within the context of the nurse-client relationship. The client in this case may be the individual or may be a couple, depending upon the nature of the dysfunction. Evaluation should reflect a positive direction, for example, a reduction in anxiety; an increase in sexual satisfaction; a decrease in ejaculatory incompetence. During the evaluation process, nurse and client identify goals that need to be modified and goals that are to be met in the future. Due to the sensitive nature of sexual health, the nurse must be attuned to the comfort level of the client in regard to specific interventions. If clients are not comfortable with proposed interventions, they may refuse to participate in the plan of care at any time.

Referral to other health professionals who have more advanced preparation in the field of sexual counseling may be necessary. In the case of specific sexual dysfunctions, advanced clinical knowledge and experience is a must and should not be undertaken by individuals without the necessary level of expertise. Community resources such as support groups for gays and lesbians as well as support groups for those with chronic illnesses (i.e., diabetes, cardiovascular disease, renal disease) can provide an arena where sexual health issues can be discussed among those with similar concerns. Strategies to cope with common stressors can be tested out in a supportive nonthreatening environment.

Last, evaluation must reflect an appraisal of the nurse. In the area of sexual health, the nurse's comfort level with his or her own sexuality is a critical factor. Depending on the nurse's own value system regarding sexuality, intervention with clients may precipitate feelings of disgust, vulnerability, anger, fear, or pity. Nonverbal communication of these feelings may inadvertently block effective intervention. Ongoing evaluation of one's own feelings, values, beliefs, and the ability to confront one's own negative perceptions is necessary to provide supportive intervention. Values clarification with other health professionals is a worthwhile tool to increase one's own effectiveness in providing these interventions (see Self-directed Learning on pp. 227-228).

TERTIARY PREVENTION

The principal focus of tertiary prevention is the provision of ongoing services to those individuals and/or couples who have demonstrated limited improvement as a result of brief psychotherapy or crisis intervention. Dysfunctional sexual behavior may be rooted in early childhood experiences that prevent full reconstitution without further goal setting and ongoing therapy. Such dysfunctions as premature ejaculation respond readily to brief psychotherapy where both individuals in the couple system actively engage in directed exercises. However, the complex nature of one's self-esteem and belief system regarding sexuality may preclude the success of short-term psychotherapy. Psychoanalysis may be necessary to facilitate the resolution of unconscious childhood conflicts that are impacting on adult sexual behaviors.

The provision of services at the tertiary level may vary. Nurses prepared with advanced knowledge and practice in sex therapy may conduct individual and couples therapy. Nurses may also act as resource persons who can provide referrals to other sources that can enhance the reconstitution process. From the broad perspective of sexuality that incorportates more than just a genital focus, tertiary prevention can include such groups as Parents without Partners, widows/widowers groups, as well as singles groups. These groups provide a forum where issues relevant to one's perception of self can be discussed. The idea of being without a partner whether it be a result of death, divorce, or lack of availability is often a topic of concern. The individual in this case is often left without the necessary reflected appraisals from significant others that are so critical to one's positive sense of self. Through support groups individuals may begin to reaffirm their sense of self as human beings with sexual needs. The perspective from which we as nurses must come is the consideration of sexuality as an integral component of one's healthy sense of self-esteem.

Nurses may also identify chronic dysfunctional patterns of sexual behavior in children, adolescents, and adults who have not received treatment. In this case, direct care may be provided by the nurse, or referrals may be made to appropriate resources that can assist these clients to an optimal level of function.

CHAPTER SUMMARY

Sexual health has historically received little attention from health professionals. Although human sexuality was incorporated into medical school and nursing curricula as early as the 1970s, it remains questionable whether practitioners are integrating sexual health issues into plans of care. The concept of human sexuality remains to a great extent shrouded in antiquated myths. Many authors such as Woods, Mims, Fogel, and Watts have documented the role of the nurse in providing sexual health care across the developmental cycle at all levels of prevention. This chapter further emphasizes the need for nurses to recognize the significance of sexuality as it relates to the health and illness of their clients.

Knowledge of normal male and female sexual response patterns as well as the conceptual development of sexuality throughout the life cycle is provided as a baseline of information. The role of various cultures in the definition of sexuality is described as are religious influences. Sexual dysfunctions are presented as a result of multiple inter-

related factors. Assessment reflects a consideration of the biologic, psychologic, intellectual, spiritual, and cultural dimensions. These factors act as a foundation for subsequent nursing diagnoses, client outcomes, and nursing strategies. The nurse may act as the actual provider of sexual health care or may act as a referral source for those individuals who would benefit from sex therapy.

A primary focus of the chapter is the importance of the awareness of one's own values and beliefs as they relate to human sexual behavior. The success of interventive strategies relies to a great extent on the nurse's ability to provide an atmosphere where clients feel they have permission to be sexual and to have sexual health needs. The area of sexual health remains an emotionally charged one that requires ongoing evaluation of one's beliefs—whether toward particular life-styles or toward activities of particular age groups. A subtle but negative appraisal of a client's sexual value system may impair effective communication.

Nurses play a critical role in the promotion of sexual health through the provision of accurate knowledge and the facilitation of the development of a positive sense of self-worth. Through interventions at all levels, nurses enable clients to attain and maintain an optimal level of sexual functioning.

SELF-DIRECTED LEARNING

Sensitivity-Awareness Exercises

The purposes of these exercises are to:

- Develop a sensitivity to one's own values and attitudes regarding sexuality.
- Develop an awareness of one's responses to sexual practices and alternatives different from one's own.
- Describe how sexual roles are portrayed through the media and influence societal role expectations.

Exercises

1. While watching TV identify one TV show that portrays the healthy expression of sexuality in the older couple. What is your response to this portrayal?
2. Describe how female and/or male sexuality is portrayed through TV commercials. Identify both positive and negative points.
3. Discuss how the media (newspapers, TV, radio) reinforce traditional male and female sex roles.
4. Describe how male and female sex roles are actualized in your own life: in your family; in your dorm or other living arrangement; with your significant other; with your friends.

Values Clarification*

1. This exercise sets two beliefs at the opposite end of a continuum. Place an X at the point that most closely corresponds with your beliefs.
   a. What do you feel about premarital/extramarital sex?
   It's ok under any con-   It's wrong in any sit-
   ditions. _____   uation. _____
   b. How do you feel about individuals who choose a sexual preference different from your own?
   I am totally against   I think it can
   it. _____   be meaningful and posi-
                          tive. _____

   c. How would you feel if your partner suggested that you both use erotic material during lovemaking to enhance arousal?
   I am totally against   It would turn me
   it. _____   on. _____
   d. Older individuals should be permitted to engage in sexual activities in residential nursing facilities.
   I am totally against   I think it could
   it. _____   be meaningful and pos-
                          itive. _____

2. Describe briefly what you would say and how you would feel in the following situations. These exercises can be used in small group settings after some level of trust has developed among group members.*
   a. A stranger of the opposite sex walks up to you and says "I would like to know you better—you're sexually attractive to me."
   I would feel . . .
   I would say . . .
   b. Your date for the evening has been making sexually oriented statements and finally reaches over and touches your genitals.
   I would feel . . .
   I would say . . .
   c. Your husband/wife of ten years tells you that he/she has never had an orgasm during lovemaking with you.
   I would feel . . .
   I would say . . .
   d. Your significant other suggests that the two of you be part of a group sex encounter with houseguests who have come for the weekend.
   I would feel . . .
   I would say . . .
   e. Your spouse tells you that he/she has had an affair, but it is now finished.
   I would feel . . .
   I would say . . .

*It is important to note that these exercises cannot be used effectively unless group members feel a reasonable level of trust.

*Adapted from Read D: Healthy sexuality, New York, 1979, Macmillan Publishing Co., Inc.

Continued.

Values Clarification—cont'd

3. This group of unfinished sentences can be used to stimulate discussion in a small group. It is important that each person share his or her initial reaction to each statement.

"Sexually I am. . ."

"Self-stimulation in any form is. . ."

"Feelings about sexual intercourse include. . ."

"At this point in time my sex life is. . ."

"Alternative sexual preferences are. . ."

"The idea of group sex is. . ."

"In my wildest dreams I would. . ."

"Sexually I could never. . ."

Questions to Consider

1. All of the following statements about human sexual response are true except:
   a. Men and women respond somewhat differently to similar stimuli.
   b. Men and women are sexually aroused by erotic material.
   c. Men generally have a greater sex drive than women.
   d. There is greater individual variation among the same sex in relation to sexual response.

2. Explanatory theories relative to the development of homosexual behavior include:
   a. Environmental
   b. Alteration in sex-hormone balance
   c. Genetic factors
   d. All of the above

3. Premature ejaculation is *most* successfully treated by:
   a. Psychoanalysis
   b. "Squeeze" technique
   c. Marital therapy
   d. Couples therapy

4. For older couples to enjoy a more satisfying sexual experience, anticipatory guidance by the nurse should include the following factual information:
   a. Foreplay is not a necessary apsect of sexual activity for this age group.
   b. Water-soluble (K-Y) jelly is useful for vaginal lubrication to reduce the risk of vaginal tearing.
   c. Ejaculatory force is the same in the older male as it is for the young adult male.
   d. The primary thrust of sexual expression in the older adult continues to be genital sex.

5. The primary causative factor in the development of sexual dysfunctions as noted by Masters and Johnson is:
   a. Psychological
   b. Genetic
   c. Physical
   d. Spiritual

6. The vasocongestive phase of the human sexual response cycle is characterized by:
   a. Vaginal lubrication and erection.
   b. Refractory response following ejaculation.
   c. Skin mottling and swelling of labia minora.
   d. Flaccidity of the penis and decreased blood pressure.

7. Kaplan's notion of a biphasic sexual response suggests that:
   a. Treatment for all sexual dysfunctions is primarily long-term.
   b. Women experience vaginal lubrication as a result of sympathetic innervation.
   c. Treatment of sexual dysfunctions would be determined by area of innervation.
   d. Orgasm and ejaculation are primarily parasympathetically stimulated.

8. Transvestism is defined as:
   a. Using nonliving objects to achieve sexual excitement.
   b. Exposing one's genitals to strangers to achieve arousal.
   c. Changing one's sex through surgical procedures.
   d. Cross-dressing by a heterosexual male.

9. One's biologic sex or the sense of maleness or femaleness one possesses is termed:
   a. Core gender identity
   b. Sex role
   c. Androgyny
   d. Sexual orientation

10. Effective nursing intervention in sexual health issues should include all of the following except:
    a. Referral of all clients to a qualified sex therapist.
    b. Development of an awareness of one's own values and beliefs.
    c. Gaining a knowledge base in the area of human sexuality.
    d. Completing a comprehensive sexual health history for all clients.

Answer key

1. c	6. d
2. d	7. c
3. b	8. d
4. b	9. a
5. a	10. a

REFERENCES

American Psychiatric Association: Diagnostic and statistical manual III-R. Washington, DC, 1987.

Annon JS: The behavioral treatment of sexual problems: brief therapy, New York, 1976, Harper & Row.

Bardwick J: Psychology of women: a study of biocultural conflicts, New York, 1971, Harper & Row.

Bell A and Weinberg M: Homosexualities, New York, 1978, Simon-Schuster.

Bieber I: Homosexuality, Am J Nurs 69(2):37-41, 1969.

Boswell J: Christianity, social tolerance, and homosexuality, Chicago, 1980, University of Chicago Press.

Bradley B: Lack of interest: a common complaint in sexual treatment, Kansas City Star, November 8, 1987.

Cantor P: Self-esteem, sexuality and cancer-related stress, Frontiers Therapy Radiation Oncol, Karger-Basel, 14:51-54, 1980.

Crenshaw T: The impact of AIDS on sexual behavior, Interview on ABC's "20/20", February 1987.

Davenport W: Sex in cross-cultural perspective, In Beach F, editor: Human sexuality in four perspectives. Baltimore, 1977, Johns Hopkins University Press.

Derogatis L: Breast and gynecologic cancers, Frontiers Radiation Therapy Oncol, Karger-Basel, 14:1-11, 1980.

Feldstein I: Transsexualism and sex reassignment, Oxford, 1986, Oxford University Press.

Fogel CI: Sexual dysfunction: etiology and therapy, In Woods N, editor: Human sexuality in health and illness, St Louis, 1979, The CV Mosby Company.

Freud S: Three essays on the theory of sexuality, In The complete psychological works of Sigmund Freud, vol 7, London, 1953, Hogarth Press.

Gilmore M and Gilmore D: Machismo: a psychodynamic approach (Spain), J Psychol Anthropol 2:281-289, 1979.

Hauck B: Differences between the sexes at puberty, In Evans ED, editor: Adolescence: readings in behavior and development, Hinsdale, Ill, 1970, Dryden Press.

Haroran S, McIlvenna E, and Pomeroy W: Sexologists suggest manifesto of basic sexual rights, Sexuality Today, 7(12):1, 1984.

Harrison R: The institutionalized mentally ill, In Gochros H, Gochros J, and Fisher J, editors: Helping the sexually oppressed, Englewood Cliffs, NJ, 1986, Prentice-Hall, Inc.

Hogan R: Human sexuality: a nursing perspective, New York, 1982, Appleton-Century-Crofts.

Hooker E: An empirical study of some relations between sexual patterns and gender identity in male homosexuals, In Money J, editor: Sex research: new developments, New York, 1965, Holt, Rinehart, Winston.

Kaplan HS: The new sex therapy, New York, 1974, Bruner-Mazel.

Kaplan HS: Disorders of sexual desire and other new concepts and techniques in sex therapy, New York, 1979, Simon-Schuster.

Kaplan HS: The evaluation of sexual disorders, New York, 1983, Bruner-Mazel.

Kaplan H and Sadock B: Comprehensive textbook of psychiatry, IV, Baltimore, 1984, Williams & Wilkins.

Kinsey A, Pomeroy W, and Martin C: Sexual behavior in the human male, Philadelphia, 1948, Saunders.

Kohlberg L: A cognitive developmental analysis, In Maccoby E, editor: The development of sex differences, Standford, 1966, The Stanford University Press.

Krueger J et al: Relationship between nursing counseling and sexual adjustment after hysterectomy, Nurs Res 28:145-150, May-June 1977.

Ladas AK, Whipple B, and Perry J: The G spot and other recent discoveries about human sexuality, New York, 1982, Holt, Rinehart, & Winston.

LaTorre R and Kear K: Attitudes towards sex in the aged, Arch Sexual Behavior 6:203-204, 1977.

Lion E, editor: Human sexuality in the nursing process, New York, 1982, John Wiley & Sons.

Malinowski B: Sex and repression in a savage society, New York, 1927, Harcourt Brace.

Marshall DS: Sexual behavior on Mangaia, In Marshall DS and Suggs RC, editors: Human sexual behavior, New York, 1971, Basic Books.

Masters W and Johnson V: Human sexual response, Boston, 1966, Little Brown & Co.

Masters W, Johnson V, and Kolodny R: Masters and Johnson on sex and human loving, Boston, 1986, Little Brown & Co.

Messinger JC: Sex and repression in an Irish folk community, In Marshall DS and Suggs RC, editors: Human sexual behavior, New York, 1971, Basic Books.

Mims F: Sexual health education and counseling, Nurs Clinic N Am, 10:187-191, September 1975.

Mischel W: A social learning view of sex differences, In Maccoby E, editor: The development of sex differences, Stanford, 1966, The Stanford University Press.

Money J and Erhardt A: Man and woman, boy and girl, Baltimore, 1972, The Johns Hopkins University Press.

Money J and Wiedeking C: Gender identity role: normal differentiation and its transpositions, In Wolmann B and Money J, editors: Handbook of human sexuality, Englewood Cliffs, NJ, 1980, Prentice-Hall, Inc.

Moses A and Hawkins R: Counseling lesbian women and gay men: a life issues approach, St. Louis, 1982, The CV Mosby Co.

Pfieffer E, Verwerdt A, and Davis G: Sexual behavior in middle life, Am J Psychiatr 128: 1262-1267, 1974.

Qualls CP, Wincze J, and Barlow D, editors: The prevention of sexual disorders: issues and approaches, New York, 1978, Plenum Press.

Roesel R: The nurse's role in primary prevention in sexual health, Imprint 27:27, December 1980.

Stuart F: Inhibited sexual desire in today's society, Kansas City Star, September 23, 1987.

Watts RJ: Dimensions of sexual health, Am J Nurs 79:1568, September 1979.

Woods NF: Human sexuality in health and illness, ed 3, St. Louis, 1984, The CV Mosby Co.

World Health Organization: Educational treatment in human sexuality: the training of health professionals, Report of WHO meeting No 572, Geneva, 1975, The Organization.

ANNOTATED SUGGESTED READINGS

Baggs JG: Sexual counseling of women with coronary heart disease, Dimensions Critical Care Nurs 16(2):154-159, 1987.
This research, conducted on a sample of 58 women with coronary heart disease, found that generally no one approached these women to offer counseling regarding return to sexual activity. Subjects agreed that it was the health care professional's responsibility to initiate counseling and were very positive about counseling when it was offered. Recommendations for further research included: exploring the effect of counseling on the rate of return to sexual activity; identifying what form of counseling would be most effective; and exploring the information levels and attitudes of nurses and physicians. The author noted the need for the inclusion of sexual health in the education of physicians and nurses to maximize cardiac rehabilitation.

Bozett F, editor: Holistic sexuality, Holistic Nurs Prac 1(4):V1-89, 1987.
This journal addresses many issues relevant to the concept of human sexuality: cultural influences; sexuality through the life span; attitudes toward sexuality in nursing texts; sexual identity and human diversity; male sexuality in the childbearing years; body image disturbance and adolescent sexuality; and alterations in sexual health with related nursing diagnoses. Each article incorporates implications for nursing in areas of assessment, intervention, and evaluation.

LaChat M: Religious support for the domination of women—breaking the cycle, Nurse Practitioner 13(1):31-34, 1988.
This article explores the relationship of religious imagery to female subordination to males. The author notes that nurse practitioners, whether conscious or not, are products of religious traditions that have shaped values and attitudes. The religious legacy has also shaped expectations of what nurses should be in the public eye—"servanthood; selfless giving and caring." The author also questions whether this has disenfranchised women from political, social, and economic power. Last, the author explores the role religious attitudes play in legitimizing cultural attitudes toward family violence. Nurses can more effectively deal with the results of this violence by becoming active in educating the public as to its prevention. The need for nurses to become aware of negative imagery and its impact on practice as well as on the definition of victims of abuse is also emphasized.

Muscari M: Obtaining the adolescent sexual history, Pediatr Nurs 13(5):307-311, 1987.
The article identifies the importance of one's own sexual attitudes and preferences and the recognition of personal biases when assessing adolescent sexuality. The author presents the need to provide a private atmosphere that facilitates the discussion of sexuality as a valid health issue. The author discusses specific guidelines for adolescent sexual health assessment, including areas that should be addressed, i.e., masturbation, fantasies, coital history, homosexuality, substance abuse, and sexual abuse.

Shipes E: Sexual function following ostomy surgery, Nurs Clin North America 22(2):303-310, 1987.
This article provides a brief examination of normal sexual function as well as the potential sexual problems of the ostomy client. Of particular importance is the discussion of nursing strategies that can alleviate sexual problems.

FURTHER READINGS

Campbell M: Sexual dysfunction in the COPD patient, Dimensions Crit Care Nurs 6(2):70-74, 1987.

Cardin S: Nursing's role in the sexual counseling of critical care patients, Dimensions Crit Care Nurs 6(2):67-68, 1987.

Chapman J et al: A model for sexual assessment and intervention, Health Care Women Internat 8(1):87-99, 1987.

Cohen JA: Sexual counseling of the patient following myocardial infarction, Crit Care Nurse 6(6):18-19; 22-24; 26-29, 1986.

DeSantis L et al: Parental attitudes toward adolescent sexuality: transcultural perspectives. . . Cuban and Haitian beliefs and practices, Nurse Practitioner 12(8):43-48, 1987.

Durie B: Drugs and sexual function, Nurs Times 83(32):34-35, 1987.

Glass JC et al: Knowledge and attitudes of health-care providers toward sexuality in the institutionalized elderly, Educat Gerontol 12(5):465-475, 1986.

Klink K: Dyspareunia, an uncomfortable topic, Pat Care 21(17):57-59, 1987.

Manley G: Diabetes and sexual health, Diabetes Educat 12(4):366-369, 1986.

Owen P: Recovery from myocardial infarction: a review of psychosocial determinants, J Cardiovasc Nurs 2(1):75-85, 1987.

Shuman N et al: Nurses' attitudes towards sexual counseling, Dimensions Crit Care Nursing 6(2):75-81, 1987.

Travis S: Older adults' sexuality and remarriage, J Gerontol Nurs 13(6):8-14, 1987.

Webb C et al: Nurses' knowledge and attitudes about sexuality in health care—a review of the literature, Nurse Educator Today 7(2):75-87, 1987.

Young E: Sexual needs of psychiatric clients, J Psychosoc Mental Health Serv 25(7):3032, 1987.

CHAPTER 8

Stress and anxiety

CHAPTER FOCUS

Adaptation, stress, anxiety—these are terms of significance for the health care team as well as for clients. The concepts these words represent will very often be the basis for clinical assessment and intervention.

A person's mental health fluctuates according to his or her ability to adapt to stress. Through the process of adaptation an individual meets needs dictated by internal and external factors. Adaptation may be equated with survival. The degree of ability to adapt inevitably influences the ability to survive. Adaptation may also be viewed as the changes an individual experiences as a reaction to stress. These changes act as a defense system by which a person attempts to deal with stress—whether by limiting its impact or by neutralizing its effects. Thus, adaptation permits the whole person to continue to function in an effective manner. It promotes forward movement by reducing or alleviating the negative aspects of change. Adaptation can be viewed as a lifelong process that is neither permanent nor static; it involves constant change.

The nurse's role is unique. The nurse can be instrumental in helping a client to develop successful adaptive mechanisms in both the psychosocial realm and the physiological realm. Nurses are in a position to facilitate the efforts of the client to deal with obstacles that may interfere with the ability to respond appropriately and realistically to the demands of environment, situation, or condition.

UNDERLYING DYNAMICS OF STRESS

Adaptation theories

Selye (1976) describes stress as nonspecific and requiring a person to make some type of change. It is often perceived as negative and the source of all of life's miseries. Yet stress is a normal and useful response of the human system. In some cases stress is excessive and damaging, resulting in the need to avoid such situations.

The term *nonspecific* as used by Selye enables one to differentiate stimulus from response. The body's response is termed *stress*, while those demands on the body that cause stress are termed *stressors*. Every demand made on the body is specific, yet the body's response to stressors is nonspecific. For example, drugs exert specific actions on the body. Insulin reduces the blood glucose level, and diuretics increase the production of urine—each is a specific response. At the same time there is a common *nonspecific* response. Differing specific results occur, yet the nonspecific effects are similar. Both require adaptation even though the initiating stressors are different. It is unimportant whether stressors are positive or negative, pleasant or unpleasant; the nonspecific effect depends upon the adaptive demands made upon the body.

PHYSIOLOGICAL ADAPTATION

What occurs on the physiological level during a stress reaction? Stress stimulates the release of adrenocorticotropic hormone (ACTH) from the anterior lobe of the hypothalamus. Continued stimulation causes the production of cortical hormones. These hormones have various effects on the body, one of which is to act on the pituitary, when necessary, to reduce the production of ACTH. Stress acts first on the brain and then on the sympathetic nervous system to stimulate the production of norepinephrine and epinephrine. How is this hormone activity perceived by the individual? The body prepares itself for the stressor by increasing the heart rate and respiratory activity; the pupils dilate to provide a wider range of vision; the skin may become cold and clammy and the person may become pale; "butterflies," muscle stiffness, weakness, increased perspiration, and chest pain often occur as well. Norepinephrine stimulates arteriolar

vasoconstriction to increase blood pressure; the adrenal glands produce epinephrine, which stimulates the release of glucose by the liver; and peristaltic activity is slowed. Blood is diverted from the gastrointestinal tract to the cardiovascular system for the purpose of "fight or flight." The parasympathetic system may act simultaneously to produce diarrhea and excessive urination. (See Table 8-1).

Let us briefly look at Selye's (1976) general adaptation syndrome (GAS) as a correlate of the sympatho-adreno-medullary response to stress. Selye divides adaptation into three states or stages (see Table 8-2): Stage I is the initial "call to arms," which serves to alert the sympathetic nervous system. Stage II is the stage of resistance and prolonged abnormal physiological functioning in an attempt to deal with the stressors. Stage III is the final stage—exhaustion. Selye's emphasis on the pituitary-adrenal mechanism as a response to stress serves as a foundation for his concept of "diseases of adaptation." He sees stress—rather than inherent physiological defects—as responsible for the various disease states.

PSYCHOLOGICAL ADAPTATION

To effectively enable clients to cope with stressful situations, the nurse must understand the process of psychological adaptation. The three stages of adaptation that make up Selye's general adaptation syndrome can be correlated with a psychological model of adaptation. The alarm stage, which corresponds to a mild or +1 level of anxiety, alerts the system to stress. The client is able to perceive data. He or she can visualize connections, and he or she can engage in problem solving. However, the client may not be able to relieve the anxiety by his or her normal adaptive mechanisms. In such a case, anxiety increases and less adaptive types of behavior occur (for example, irritability, anger, withdrawal, denial, and silence). During the second phase, the resistance stage, characteristics of the moderate level of anxiety are apparent. Ego adaptive mechanisms may be called into action if anxiety continues to heighten. The mechanisms utilized are sublimation, rationalization, displacement, and compensation. Should these mechanisms fail, the client moves into the exhaustion stage, in which mechanisms of a more disintegrative nature are utilized for adaptive purposes. Unless the client

TABLE 8-1   Stress-related signs and symptoms

↑ Gluconeogenesis ⟶	Diabetes mellitus
↓ Gluconeogenesis ⟶	Hypoglycemia
↓ Excretion of intracellular potassium ⟶	Cardiac arrhythmias
↑ Vasoconstriction ⟶	Hypertension
↑ Anti-inflammatory response ⟶	Infectious diseases
↓ Immunity ⟶	Cancer
↑ Blood clotting ⟶	Coronary thrombosis
↑ Myocardial contractions ⟶	Altered cardiac demands
↑ CNS stimulation ⟶	Confusion, disorientation, thought disturbances

TABLE 8-2   General adaptation syndrome

Alarm stage
  Stimulation of hypothalmus→stimulation of anterior pituitary→ ↑ adrenocorticotropic hormone (ACTH)
  Catecholamine release→sympathetic nervous system activity→ ↑ epinephrine and ↑ norepinephrine
  Posterior pituitary releases antidiuretic hormone (ADH)
  Sympathetic response:
    ↑ anti-inflammatory response
    ↑ respiration
    ↑ muscle tonus
    ↑ free fatty acids
    ↑ blood pressure
    ↑ cardiac rate
    Pupils dilate
    ↑ metabolism
  Parasympathetic response:
    Pupil dilation fixes
    ↓ cardiovascular output
    ↓ Muscle tonus
    Depletion of metabolic reserves
    Respiratory difficulty
Resistance stage
  Tissue anabolism
  ↑ antibody production
  ↑ hormonal secretion
  Hemodilution occurs
Exhaustion stage
  Repeated GAS responses deplete body reserves, leading to increased risk of physical or emotional illness. Psychological exhaustion in the form of panic can result from prolonged anxieties and may incur psychotic episodes.

changes his or her behavior, the client may become chronically ill and may even die. The exhaustion stage is correlated with a severe state of anxiety (+3 to +4); the client's attention is either focused on one particular detail or directed toward many scattered details. Adaptive mechanisms in this phase may include hallucinations, compulsive behavior, or severe psychophysiological illness.

Valiga and Frain (1979) have defined four levels of stress to assist nurses in their assessment of clients experiencing stress.

Level I—everyday living; use of energy to respond to habitual tasks

Level II—mild; new or less routine events (e.g., job interview); usual modes of coping alleviate stress

Level III—moderate; persistently stressful event; previous repertoire of coping strategies does not effect resolution; person expresses feelings of powerlessness, exhibits denial, depressive-elative mood swings, decreased social interaction, and decreased verbal communication; assistance from others to facilitate problem solving is helpful

Level IV—severe; exhaustion phase of GAS; events are perceived as life-threatening; person exhibits extreme discomfort, purposelessness; if not controlled can lead to ulcers, asthma, psychosis; intervention focuses on development of intact resources of the individual (e.g., when physical reserves are currently unavailable, draw upon psychological strengths)

CULTURAL ADAPTATION

To live productively, individuals develop patterns of living and relationships with others that allow them to interact with the physical environment rather than be controlled by it. Cultural systems provide parameters for behavior and physiological functioning yet permit individual diversity. They allow individuals to adapt to various situations and problems and to be informed about the environment.

Adaptive changes often have been achieved through genetic, physiological, and constitutional means and have then been transmitted for generations through natural selection or conditioning by a culture.

Cultural adaptation in regard to mental health and mental illness may take place in a variety of ways. For example, modification of the environment may enable a client to adapt to a condition that interferes with optimum health.

Culture plays an important role in determining a client's definition of stress and how he or she responds to that stress. Alland (1970) views evolution of human behavior, or rather how one adapts, in light of Darwin's theory of biological evolution. Alland argues that there is an interrelationship between organic and social life that is significant to the understanding of adaptation.

Two types of cultural adaptation are significant. Inward-directed adaptation, including internal homeostasis or integration, results in continuous change and/or motion. Outward-directed adaptation is the result of encounters between a person and his or her environment. The total of these interactions results in the development of an effective self-regulatory system, one that is capable of functioning within a variety of environments.

The interaction between evolutionary concepts (the development of effective feedback or self-regulatory systems) and cultural concepts results in a change in the human system in the direction of a better environmental "fit." For example, organisms with higher developmental levels of homeostatic mechanisms will produce more offspring, leading to increased populations of these more highly adapted organisms. Eventually, less adaptable organisms will be overshadowed by organisms that more readily "fit" the environment.

It is important to note that both inward-directed adaptation and outward-directed adaptation have physiological, environmental, and cultural modes. Thus, cultural adaptation is as much a biological process as the inherent genetic process is.

How does this fact relate to the development of a "disease process"? Individuals are in a constant state of interaction with the environment. In the study of human stress, then, it is impossible to negate cultural and environmental factors, because they are interrelated with specific biological stressors. When the human organism adapts to reduce stress of biological origin, the organism also moves toward consonance with environment and culture.

Cognitive appraisal theory

Cognitive appraisal can be described as the activity that takes place between stimulation of the stress response and the individual's response to that stressor. Selye demonstrates that a physiologic response occurs as a result of stress. Later theories indicate that there are other factors that must be considered in the stress response. Lazarus and Folkman (1984) delineate three categories of stress response: harm-loss, where evaluation of loss occurs; threat, which includes anticipation of loss; and challenge, which includes the appraisal of situations for loss as well as for growth. The response to stress at whatever level is considered to be mediated by cognitive processes. Subjectivity is inherent in cognitive appraisal. The meaning an event has for one individual may be very different from the meaning another individual has for the same event. There may also be differences in perception of the stressful nature of an event for the same individual at a different point in time. For example, a student is caring for a dying infant in the intensive care nursery. She gains great satisfaction from interacting with the parents, providing them with ongoing support and information. Several weeks later she is assigned to a 45-year-old man who is dying of pancreatic cancer. The student finds that she is making excuses for not spending time with the man's wife and two daughters. She also notices that on the days she is caring for the client, she has no appetite and often experiences diarrhea. During the postconference discussion group, her instructor asked if the student might have had any similar experiences that could be impacting on her care and creating a stressful situation. The student was able to connect her stress response to the fact that her own father had died one year earlier after a long bout with cancer. Thus, the situation of working with the dying infant was not perceived as stressful, yet working with a dying client similar in age to her own father generated a high level of stress for this student.

Lazarus and Folkman note that several factors must be considered within the context of cognitive process that affect the perception of a stress response. These factors include stimulus-response chains, motivation, perception of potential success or failure, response availability, and variety of responses available at the given time of a stress reaction.

Lowery (1987) notes that there are questions regarding the efficacy of the cognitive appraisal model, specifically, is the appraisal consistent with reality. It is possible to consider denial as an inaccurate appraisal, yet denial might be effective in mediating stressful situations. Hackett and Cassem (1970) described a high incidence of denial in myocardial infarction patients that was correlated with longer survival rates. Other studies, however, indicate that expression of feelings of anxiety post myocardial infarction did not lead to increased stress levels. Thomas et al. (1983) concludes that denial is not necessarily more healthy in post myocardial infarction patients.

Other theorists such as Dohrenwend et al. (1982) and Billings and Moos (1984) have developed models of stress that account for other variables that influence the stress response. Such variables include ego strength, age, developmental level, general health status—sleep patterns, exercise, and leisure habits, physical aspects of the environment. Dohrenwend et al. indicate that social resources provide individuals with emotional support as well as with tangible support such as financial resources, etc. The authors raise the issue as to how much support is actually provided to those experiencing stress and to what degree support is utilized. Scheier and Carver (1985) suggest that optimism

plays a significant role in the interpretation of stress. They found that those individuals who were optimistic tended to utilize active goal-directed coping strategies that were more successful than mere emotional discharge. Breznitz (1986) concludes that hope plays a role in the mediation of stressful responses; however, further research is necessary to provide supportive data. Last, Lowery (1987) notes that stress may also be defined as behavioral, affective, physiological responses to an environmental stressor. Two factors—the stimulus characteristics (situational context and perception of control) and the internal resources of the individual (intellect, repertoire of coping strategies, and genetic predisposition)—interact to result in the perception of the stress itself.

Life change theory

Holmes and Rahe (1967) propose that life events, whether positive or negative, result in stress and require adjustment by the individual. A list of 43 events was compiled, scaled, and used to correlate the occurrence of events with incidence of physical illness. Points were assigned to each life event in order of severity (see Chapter 9, Table 9-2, for Life Change Unit scale). Determination of life changes was made retrospectively for 1 year. High scores were considered indicative of an 80% probability of physical illness within the next 2 years. Criticism of this tool and other life-event scales is noted by several researchers. Lowery notes that little consideration is given to the context within which the stressor occurs or to the individual's perception of that stressor. Paykel (1987) indicates that quantification of life events is difficult. The lack of clear definition relates to the personal meaning attributed by individuals to a stressful event at the time of the occurrence. The definition may at best be limiting; therefore, it may not be applicable to the general population. Paykel suggests the use of a life-review interview based on a list of life events so as to include significant points. Definitions of events are presented, and the interview is organized into ten discrete areas. In an attempt to quantify stress as a construct, Derogatis (1987) developed a self-report inventory to measure stress (Derogatis Stress Profile—DSP). Rather than utilize a single construct such as life events, Derogatis derived the DSP from Lazarus's interactional theory of stress. The DSP reflects three major components: environmental events, personality mediators, and emotional responses. Thus, the concept of stress can be measured more accurately through a three-dimensional perspective.

Lowery (1987) notes the need for further nursing research, particularly in the area of outcomes or consequences of actual or potential stress-producing situations. Assumptions are made that increased stress results in negative outcomes. Lowery suggests that further studies be conducted to determine whether stress inoculation techniques—the exposure to stressful situations—does in fact facilitate the proactive mastery of stressful situations.

The key factor in understanding stress is understanding the perception of the event by the individual (which determines coping strategies and the impact on self-worth). Research and practice have indicated that health care professionals must direct their efforts toward prevention—helping clients to manage stress rather than become seeming victims of circumstance. To be effective, the nurse must be able to

1. understand the concept of stress
2. recognize its signs and symptoms
3. identify factors influencing perceptions of stressors and those altering effective coping with stress
4. identify and implement strategies to reduce stress
5. educate individuals about the management of stressors (e.g., nutritional and health counseling, use of relaxation techniques, biofeedback, methods of effecting change in lifestyle)

STRESS IN THE NURSING PROFESSION

Stress has been identified as an integral component of societal structure. Each living organism experiences stress through the process of living; excessive stress can be harmful, yet at moderate levels stress acts as an initiator of action, a promoter of growth. Stress incorporates the physical charac-

teristics of the environment as well as the sociocultural and psychological facets, all of which are part of the context of the nurse-client relationship. Thus, stress can arise from *within* the context of this multidimensional relationship. In addition, stress can be a product of the broader environment as well as a product of specific relationships within that environment—with clients' families, other health care professionals, and so on. In short, the stress that a person experiences as a result of being part of a helping profession must be addressed.

Environmental stressors

Donovan (1987) notes that a cross-national study of job conditions and mental strain found that nurses were more prone to occupational stress due to the excessive emotional and physical work load imposed on them by the day-to-day patient care activity level. Donovan also indicates that nurses felt powerless in their environment; responsibility for patient care was predominantly in their domain, however, physicians and hospital administrators were the most active decision makers. Job dissatisfaction was identified by nurses as the primary reason for leaving the profession, and recent studies by Reed (1983) reflected an escalating percentage of nurses who were addicted to narcotics and other medications.

Occupational stress is manifested not only in job dissatisfaction but also in several other characteristic behaviors such as absenteeism, depression, anxiety, rapid turnover, decreased job performance, frustration, and other maladaptive coping behaviors such as overeating, smoking, and increased alcohol and drug consumption. Stress in the work environment then becomes a critical factor. Menaghan and Merves (1984) report that stress caused by one's occupation is less likely to be mediated by the individual's coping strategies. The support or lack of support within the work environment is a significant variable in the effectiveness of coping strategies. Individual coping strategies do not seem to be effective in a stressful work environment. Pearlin and Schooler (1978) note that job stress is intertwined with the social structure and organization of the work environment. Thus, collective measures that address the sources of stress are more likely to be effective than those measures which are directed toward the management of individual stress.

Very often the units in which nurses function are too small or their physical layouts are inappropriate. Long corridors, too little storage space, overcrowding resulting from the presence of equipment, and absence of windows are examples of possible stressors in the environment. Having a private space for nurses has been identified by one staff member of a very busy cardiac unit as being instrumental in reducing stress. In this particular situation there had been little space at the nurses' station, and the only other available area had been in the crowded locker room. It had been necessary to spend only several minutes in this windowless "closet" to understand why staff members did not utilize this area. Support from the head nurse as well as other administrators led to the construction of a space for nurses alone, indicating their importance in the hospital hierarchy.

Large intensive care units do not usually provide individual cubicles; clients and their nurses are separated by thin curtains. Although curtains can be drawn, there is very little sense of privacy. Every staff member is aware of what the others are doing. As one staff member of such a unit has noted, she doesn't have to ask for help; someone is always right there to offer. However, other staff members have expressed feelings of being in a "fish bowl"—a sentiment expressed by clients as well. Some nurses from this same intensive care unit have expressed a preference for individual rooms because then only those people who were involved in a client's care would be at the bedside.

Other physical factors in the environment can act as stressors. Noise levels in busy intensive care units were the first factor to be recognized as possibly contributing to stress. Turner, King, and Craddock (1975) found that the average minimum noise level exceeded 60 decibels. This level was noted during the early morning hours. Maximum levels, occurring between 1 PM and 7 PM, reached nearly 90 decibels. This is roughly the intensity of an automobile horn. According to these authors, daytime noise exceeding 50 decibels is perceived as annoying. Thus, it is not difficult to understand why clients complain about noise and feel as though

they are getting no rest. Nurses may complain of headaches upon leaving a busy unit at the end of the day, possibly because of the increased noise level.

Light can also be a factor in contributing to a stressful environment. It is not a question of enough light but often the type of lighting, as well as glare, that becomes an issue. Often there are no windows to provide natural lighting, or windows face directly onto other buildings. A semidark, artificially lighted environment can lead to sensory deprivation and generalized feelings of lethargy and depression. For example, the gynecology-oncology unit of one large urban hospital is located on the ground floor of a building between several other buildings. Each window faces onto another building. It is impossible for staff or clients to determine what is happening in the outside world. This further isolates an already-isolated staff and client population. Nurses in this unit have expressed feelings of being "second-class citizens," being in the "dungeon," and being the "death ward." They have identified their physical location as contributing to their lack of identity as a viable part of the hospital and ultimately to the development of stress in the unit.

Scheduling can also be a stressor. Much of the work force in the business world operates on a "9 to 5," Monday through Friday work week. Nurses, however, must provide 24-hour care to clients; someone must work during the evening and night-time hours, seven days per week. New graduates must spend their allotted time on evenings and nights, while "veterans" may, in some institutions, work days permanently. Nurses may work 1 month of days, then 1 to 2 months of evenings or nights. It is difficult to adapt to any one shift when shift rotation occurs frequently. The Stanford study (Steffen, 1980) concluded that staff members who do shift rotations (including nurses) exhibit greater incidences of digestive difficulties, disturbed sleep patterns, accidents, high anxiety levels, depression, and generalized dissatisfaction with life than do staff members who work regular hours.

Shift rotation not only affects the individual nurse but also has a profound impact on families and friends.

Several young nurses were discussing the demands of the nursing role with a psychiatric liaison clinical specialist. Many in the group spoke to the issue of being "out of synch" with the rest of the world. One young woman who was newly married voiced her concern for her marriage: "If I work days, I usually don't get off work exactly at 4:30—it's not due to disorganization but is usually due to a client being admitted right at change of shift, or a client's family having one last question. My husband is supportive but doesn't really understand why I can't leave when it's 4:30. In his world, what doesn't get done today will still be there tomorrow! When I work off-shifts, there may be two or three days when I don't even see him. I can understand how difficult it must be to have a family, be a wife, and pursue a career in nursing."

This is just one example of the impact shift rotation has on nurses and their significant others. Stress arises when men or women attempt to meet the demands of a schedule that may be changing monthly while concurrently attempting to maintain stable relationships with others.

A male nurse in a medical intensive care unit described the stress he experienced having to work evenings and leave his pregnant wife alone. She taught school; he worked evenings and every other weekend. He had chosen to work evenings to continue his professional education during the day. After consultation with a psychiatric nurse liaison, he decided to change to a unit that required him to work only Monday through Friday, 9 AM to 5 PM. Although he was relinquishing a job he prized highly, he found it necessary to select a different type of position to decrease his own personal stress. As was noted in the Stanford study (Steffen, 1980), shift rotation can exact a physical as well as psychological toll from the staff.

Internal stressors

Larson (1987), in her article "Helper Secrets: Internal Stressors in Nursing," presents a cogent discussion of internal stressors or "helper secrets" as identified in a study of 495 nurses. She found that nurses, engaged in an ongoing struggle to be competent, caring individuals, were often confronted by uncomfortable and stress-generating feelings. Eight categories delineated by Larson include the following themes: inadequacy characterized by feelings of being an imposter or lacking the expertise to function in a competent manner; feelings of one-way giving, which includes feelings of wanting to be appreciated and to be taken care of instead of always being the caretaker; too many demands including those at work as well as in other aspects of life such as being a mother, a wife; anger, which is characterized by frustration and impatience with clients, family members, other staff, and hospital administration; overinvolvement, including feelings of helplessness and of being overwhelmed; emotional and physical distancing characterized by attempts to distance self from clients and families to reduce stress, which often acts to increase stress levels; wishing for a client's death, which then precipitates feelings of anger, guilt, and distress; and, last, the desire to leave the profession, including feelings of negativism and lack of the ability to make an impact on clients, families, and society in general. These internal "secrets" may have a negative impact on the individual's ability to perceive self as a valued contributor to society. Pennebacker (1985) notes that the inability of nurses to express thoughts and feelings relative to the stress created by their work environment increases the risk of long-term illness and is related to chronic obsessing about the event. He found that the inability to communicate may be more damaging than actually having experienced the event. Lack of communication may result in stress-related illness as well as eventual burnout and the desire to leave the profession.

NURSING AS A FEMALE PROFESSION

Various authors have noted that the nursing profession has emerged concurrently with the growth of the women's movement. Changes in roles and expectations have had a profound impact on the nurse as a professional being. The concept of the nurse as a career person is coming to the fore. Nursing is involved in the process of professionalization. More and more, individuals are entering nursing with a commitment to a career. The number of "washing machine" nurses is decreasing somewhat. These individuals have moved in and out of nursing, often on the basis of personal economic need. Excellent nursing care has still been provided, yet a conflict has been created between nurses who have felt that their profession is a career and requires a commitment and those who view nursing as a job with little future orientation.

Although the number of male nurses is increasing, nursing is still predominantly a female profession. Change is occurring slowly; the problems noted by Lavinia Dock (1920) are very similar to those seen today. She pointed out that the status of nursing has depended in large part upon the status of women. In the past, women were not expected to make career commitments, nor were they rewarded for such commitments. Women were the nurturers and caretakers, assuming a passive, submissive role. Men were the breadwinners, the dominant force in the family. These same roles were often actualized in the hospital environment, with the doctor assuming the dominant role. Male physicians made decisions, wrote orders, and asked for charts and seats in the nursing station. Nurses followed orders, provided care, and were compassionate to their clients. Power and decision making were ascribed to the male; independence was viewed as being unfeminine. Thus, today nurses still tend to experience difficulty in asserting themselves, in actively participating in decision making, and in effecting conflict resolution.

MEN IN NURSING

In a profession dominated by women, the male nurse is often viewed as unique or uncommon. Bush (1976) suggests that male nurses are suspected of being homosexual. Men who consider a career in nursing are frequently discouraged by parents and friends. During discussions of their career plans, they are often less able than other students to tell others about their occupational preference.

Male nurses experience stress in relation to role expectation. Traditional male attributes include assertiveness, self-control, and aggressiveness, yet the nursing role implies nurturance and warmth. How does the male nurse reduce the dissonance and act out his role? As the number of male nurses increases, perhaps the nursing profession will be able to deal more effectively with the issue of role expectation for both men and women.

It has been noted by Gulak (1981) that male nurses receive higher salaries than female nurses and that a larger proportion of them occupy administrative positions. However, male nurses sometimes feel that they are being "used" for their size or their strength rather than being considered nurses.

It seems that there are sources of stress for the male nurse in a female-dominated profession that arise out of being male with certain ascribed masculine characteristics. Female nurses, while accepting and valuing their male counterparts, can also resent their ability to generate higher incomes. In addition, women may fall back into the traditionally prescribed role of submissive responder and encourage male nurses to assume the initiative in decision making and conflict resolution. In any case, stress for both male and female nurses may be the result of a lack of role integration in the profession as a whole.

SUPPORT GROUPS AS A STRESS-REDUCING TECHNIQUE FOR NURSES

Support groups are a useful mechanism in reducing stress. A support group provides a place where members of a particular unit or floor can meet to share information about clients, to discuss ways of meeting the needs of particular clients, and to share feelings and frustrations concerning their work. In this type of group, a sense of acceptance exists and members receive comfort from sharing both positive and negative feedback without fear of repercussion. A feeling of "I'm not in this alone" allows individuals to explore various options without decreasing their senses of self-worth. Larson (1987) suggests that meetings be used for catharsis, to help nurses to recognize and deal with their own feelings and limitations, and to identify strategies of intervention for clients (as well as for the solving of organizational conflicts).

Active support groups can be successful in mediating the effects of stress by encouraging a problem-solving approach to situations. Various issues can arise, depending upon the nature of the group; new graduates have different concerns from a group of management-level nurses. A support group does not provide therapy, nor should it be a "bitch" session. Gripes are a part of life; members need to express their feelings and then seek to resolve the issues.

Support systems are an essential component of the context of the nurse and his or her environment. Nurses must define their support resources—their peers, their administrators, and other health care professionals. Support must be drawn upon and returned in a mutual relationship. Through this process personal and professional growth is facilitated.

STRESS MANAGEMENT

Stress management involves an active approach to determining the course of one's life. Stressors may be personal or individual; interpersonal, as within the context of a family, a nursing unit, or a classroom; or a complex interrelationship of both personal and group or professional. Assume, for example, that a nurse has not had much sleep prior to coming to work because she was up with her young baby during the night. She enters her unit to find that there have been several emergency admissions, two staff members have called in sick, and one client is near death. She experiences an overwhelming sense of lack of control and snaps out at a ward clerk who asks her where the operating room schedule is. In this situation, the nurse's lack of sleep and her possible concern over her young child's sleep habits increased her vulnerability when she was confronted with the scene in the unit. Initial problem-solving measures were not instituted. Stepping back and reviewing the events, possible stressors, and perceptions of the situation would enable the nurse to mobilize actions that would more effectively reduce stress.

The following techniques of stress management can be used by individuals who are encountering stressful situations:

1. Identify stressors you are experiencing ("self-monitoring"). Check your own feelings, and recognize symptoms of stress. Ask yourself, "Is this stress work-related, home-related, or both? Am I anxious most of the time?"
2. Examine your behavior to determine what you are doing that might increase your stress level ("What triggers my stress? Unrealistic

expectations of self? 'I must/should do . . .' rather than 'I would like to . . .'? Do I resist change?")
3. Examine coping strategies (avoidance, confrontation, etc.) and determine their effectiveness.
4. Identify what can be lived with and what cannot—set *priorities*. Is this a stressor that merits attention or one that takes care of itself?
5. Decide which stressors are within your control and which are not at this current stage. Identify what can realistically be changed and what cannot—don't waste energy on unrealistic goals.
6. Avoid use of overgeneralizations such as "I *always* make mistakes" or "Nothing will *ever* change."
7. Assume a positive frame of reference—i.e., "I can" rather than "I can't." Negative frames of reference use more energy and are less productive; reframe your thoughts from "This is terrible" to "What can I do, what are my choices?" Assume control rather than being the "victim"—manipulate the environment (e.g., change jobs, change activities or routine way of doing things, rearrange priorities, *make* choices and recognize consequences of actions). Controlling involves risk-taking—be a risk-taker! Utilize a problem-solving, action-oriented approach.
8. Use lists. When you can't cross something off in a reasonable period, reevaluate.
9. Use thought stopping. Monitor negative thoughts and actually instruct yourself to stop negativism.
10. Concentrate on "quick recovery." You can wallow in bad feelings for however long you choose to, or you can return to rational thinking and decision making.
11. Use mental diversion. Prepare information as you need it (for a test, a presentation, etc.), and then focus on a favorite activity.
12. Take care of yourself. Focus on positive things that have been accomplished rather than on all negatives. Make appropriate use of leisure time and vacation days. Ensure appropriate nutrition: How do you eat?

What do you eat? Ensure sufficient sleep: Are your sleep habits regular? Do you often feel fatigued? Get sufficient exercise. Make use of biofeedback, relaxation measures, guided imagery, transcendental meditation, or momentary relaxation ("quickie") to reduce stress.

Other measures to reduce stress
BIOFEEDBACK

Brallier (1988) describes biofeedback as a mechanism that encourages an indepth awareness of self and a high degree of responsibility for one's own health. Biofeedback enables clients to gain voluntary control over some facets of the mind-body interaction through the use of electrical, audiovisual, tactile, or other sensory modalities. She notes that while biofeedback is considered as instrumental conditioning of visceral responses, it is enriched by the cognitive experiences and processes that the individual brings to the feedback process. Reduction of blood pressure and pulse rate, as clinical examples, have been effected through the use of biofeedback measures.

GUIDED IMAGERY

Guided imagery is an exercise involving the teaching of positive outcomes relative to their stressful situation. One example of guided imagery is assisting the client to imagine a peaceful scene of his own choosing, i.e., a mountain lake, the beach. The client is then asked to utilize all his senses—to smell the ocean, to feel the sun and the wind, to hear the birds, the ocean waves, and to touch the warm sand. Through this mechanism, the individual can create in his own mind a quiet mental repose. Through repeated use of the imagery, the individual can rapidly generate the scene and reduce stress in as little as 15 seconds. Vines (1988) notes that guided imagery may be used by nurses to assist clients in losing weight, in stopping smoking, in preparation for surgery, and in the process of delivery. She also suggests the use of imagery with children in relation to wound-healing processes, use of chemotherapy, and burn debridement. The use of imagery capitalizes on the world of imagination that children often exist in. Vines does caution

about the use of imagery by those who are not comfortable with or capable of responding to the emotions generated by the tapping of unconscious unresolved conflict.

PROGRESSIVE RELAXATION

Titlebaum (1988) notes that the literature does support the usefulness of relaxation therapy. Relaxation therapy as described by Jacobsen (1978) involves a progressive muscle relaxation program that helps individuals to sequentially tense and relax muscle groups, beginning with the neck and head and moving through the extremities. This exercise program takes about 20 to 30 minutes and should be done two to three times weekly. It must be reinforced regularly for it to be effective in stress reduction. Titlebaum has found that relaxation can be utilized by nurses to reduce anticipatory anxiety, to increase concentration, to increase sense of control, to energize clients, to increase suggestibility, to slow heart rate, to reduce pain, and to warm or cool parts of the body.

HUMOR

Humor has been described by Ruxton (1988) as a viable option for patient teaching, for clients who are facing life-threatening situations, for children and adults who are experiencing anxiety about hospitalization, and for those who are in isolation. Humor may be utilized in a variety of situations; however, Ruxton notes that timing, receptiveness, and content must be considered. Humor is inappropriate if it is utilized in a crisis situation by a caregiver who is unfamiliar with the client. The effectiveness of humor has been demonstrated by data which suggests that humor has been instrumental in reducing stress in high-stress units. It has also been noted that humor between staff and clients and between clients is effective in alleviating anxiety and stress.

PET THERAPY

The use of pet therapy or animal-facilitated stress management is emerging as a new measure of stress reduction. Davis (1988) notes that although the benefits of animal-facilitated therapy are not clear at this point, clinical nursing research can contribute empirical data to support the use of pet therapy as an effective means of stress reduction. Conflicting studies report the benefits as well as the lack of benefits in such groups as the bereaved. Pet therapy may in fact reduce loneliness, isolation, and the incidence of physical illness through the animal's presence as a social support mechanism. However, Davis indicates that the following issues must be addressed to validate pet therapy as a stress-management technique: are there neuro-chemical and social correlates of the pet-person affective interaction; do physiology and mood vary with different types of pets; does reminiscing affect physiological and affective response. As the questions are answered, the value of animal-facilitated therapy as a strategy of stress reduction will be determined.

GROUP THERAPY

Group resolution of stressors may also be a method of stress management. It rests on the group's commitment to direct, open communication. Individuals must be assertive—both in the expression of anger and in the expression of affection—yet be respectful of others as human beings. There must also be a mutual willingness to resolve interpersonal issues, to reach shared goals, and to explore conflicts. When a group is unable to resolve a stressful situation, a consultant may be helpful in suggesting solutions.

Nurses are in a position in health care settings to assist clients to identify stressors, to implement strategies to reduce stress, and to evaluate their effectiveness. The nursing assessment of a client reveals psychological, physiological, and social history, as well as information relevant to the client's stress response: When does it occur? Is it rational? Is it a conditioned response to a specific stimulus? What demands are made on the client? What resources are available to the client? Planning and implementation of specific stress-reduction techniques will depend upon the data gathered as well as the client's preferences and usual coping strategies. Evaluation of the strategies can initially be done by the nurse, with the eventual goal being to have it done by the client.

In summary, the goals of stress management can be succinctly stated: to help individuals learn to be responsive to themselves, to alter their responses to stress, and to alter their environments to reduce stress.

THEORIES OF ANXIETY

Anxiety is a result of stress. Engel (1962) describes anxiety as the psychological response to great amounts of energy running unchanneled as a result of a stressful situation. As was previously stated, stress is the inducer, not the effect, of an action. Anxiety is often described as a feeling of apprehension, of impending doom. The behavior of a person who is experiencing anxiety can run the gamut from maintenance of a state of alertness to panic of such severity that the individual either becomes immobilized or attends to every minute cue in his or her environment. Anxiety is a subjective experience that results from a fear of an undetermined nature. Anxiety may have its roots in past experiences, or it may be produced by a threatened or perceived loss of inner control or by a threat to self-esteem. Feelings of isolation, helplessness, and insecurity are associated with anxiety.

Anxiety can be described as a motivating force; it activates an individual to make changes and to grow. Without mild to moderate levels of anxiety, an individual might remain in a static state with little energy to confront the daily issues of life. An individual who copes successfully with an anxiety-producing situation emerges feeling a greater sense of worth and competence. Successes only serve to reinforce a personal pride in one's problem-solving abilities. Anxiety at this level acts to promote a sense of well-being. This is not to say that in the process one does not feel uncomfortable, nervous, or threatened; however, the long-term result is a renewed confidence in oneself.

Psychoanalytic theory

Freud used the term *anxiety* to refer to that anxiety which results from the trauma of the birth process itself. Then, throughout the developmental span, anxiety is generated by conflict between the id and the superego. The ego acts as referee between the two conflicting forces. Freud (1936) proposed that anxiety acts as a signal system, warn-

TABLE 8-3   Levels of anxiety

Mild (+1)	Moderate (+2)	Severe (+3)	Panic (+4)
Person is alert; sees, hears, grasps more than he would ordinarily; goal-oriented learning is enhanced; recognizes anxiety May protect self by limiting close interpersonal relationships Uses coping mechanisms to relieve tension, such as nail biting, walking, crying, sleeping, eating, laughing, smoking, drinking Anxiety is controlled with little conscious effort	Perceptual field is narrowed, but person can attend to more if directed to do so (person makes use of selective inattention—i.e., directing attention to a primary focus with little attention to the periphery) Increased powers of concentration Problem-solving capacity still available	Perceptual field greatly reduced Person may become preoccupied with one detail or focus on many details simultaneously ("scattering") Selective inattention continues to be operative Physical and emotional discomfort increases: nausea, vomiting, dizziness	Attention is narrowed severely, or speed of scatter is sharply increased Feelings of awe, dread, terror are common; delusions and hallucination can appear Exhaustion and death occur if panic continues for prolonged period

Data adapted from Peplau, H: A working definition of anxiety, in Burd S and Marshall M, editors: Some clinical approaches to psychiatric nursing, New York, 1963, Macmillan Inc; and Menninger K: The vital balance, New York, 1963, Viking Press.

ing that a conflict may become overwhelming. He also believed that the object of anxiety is unconscious and related to earlier object loss. Freud differentiated fear from anxiety by arguing that fear has its origins in a threatening external event. It is an acute response whose precipitating factors are real and immediate, while anxiety has its origins in intrapsychic conflict. According to Freudian theory, ego-defense mechanisms defend the ego against anxiety. These mechanisms operate outside the level of conscious awareness, acting to repress all material that is anxiety producing (see Chapter 6 for a discussion of defense mechanisms).

Psychodynamic theory

Sullivanian, or interpersonal, theory proposes that anxiety is a tension state that is transmitted through an empathic process from mother to infant, with the infant responding as though mother and self were one. For this process to occur, the ego must have some awareness of the environment.

Sullivan (1953) believes that the infant fears disapproval from the mothering figure and that later experiences with significant others thus can generate feelings of anxiety if the individual perceives that his or her behavior will not receive approval. The lack of parental approval during childhood therefore affects adult interpersonal situations.

Peplau (1963) bases much of her theoretical framework on Sullivan's theory. She defines four levels of anxiety, which are summarized in Table 8-3.

Learning theory

Learning and behavioral theorists propose that anxiety is a learned response based on the primary drive aroused by pain. Dollard and Miller's (1950) classical work on the arousal of anxiety can be summarized as follows: Anxiety is a motivating factor; anxiety is a reinforcer of behaviors for future pain reduction, and anxiety is related to neutral cues that evoke a stimulus-response cycle. As a motivator of behavior, learning theorists suggest that anxiety may have either a positive or negative influence. Prior to an important examination, a mild to moderate level of anxiety acts to increase concentration and attention to task. Anxiety may also be generated by an unpleasant experience such as being stung by a bee. Once stung, an individual may experience anxiety when he is exposed to bees in anticipation of being stung again. Avoidance behaviors are then utilized to protect the individual from being stung. These behaviors may become maladaptive; the individual may choose to remain indoors; anxiety levels may reach panic proportions if the individual is forced to go out. The following diagram demonstrates the stimulus-response cycle as outlined by Dollard and Miller:

Stimulus (pain) → **Learned drive** (fear) → **Behavior** (avoidance, crying, hitting) → **Anxiety reduction** (reinforcer of behavior)

The response cycle becomes a habitual response to painful stimuli, and anxiety-reducing behaviors are automatically called into action. As long as the anxiety-reducing behaviors are effective, these mechanisms will be reinforced.

Dollard and Miller note that stimuli may generate conflicting behavioral responses. In this case, conflict resolution may involve four discrete behavioral responses. The individual may choose to pursue two incompatible goals that are equally desirable. The individual may be forced to choose between two undesirable goals. Third, the individual may exhibit ambivalence regarding conflicting stimuli. Last, the individual may simultaneously wish to avoid and to achieve a goal. The authors conclude that the strength of the drive influences the tendency to avoid or to achieve a goal and the tendency to avoid a goal increases as one approaches the goal. When considering anxiety level, nurses must be cognizant of learned responses to reduce anxiety when planning appropriate nursing strategies to facilitate client coping.

Existential theory

Rollo May is best known for his treatise on the experiential meaning of anxiety. May (1977) describes anxiety as apprehension generated by a threat to one's values, beliefs, or mores. Anxiety is considered by the existentialists to be a valid part of life, particularly in relation to one's sense of authenticity. Threats to authenticity are perceived as threats to one's very existence, which in turn arouse anxiety. There is a need then to confront one's self and determine the value of one's life and to accept the strengths and limitations that one brings to one's existence.

Within the framework of existential theory, anxiety may arise as a result of conflict over the freedom of personal choice and the allegiance to one's societal group. The individual may be encouraged to reach a resolution that reflects a sense of personal choice that remains within the context of societal values and norms.

In summary, each theory presents cogent support for the development of anxiety. However, it is important to note that anxiety does not emerge in a linear manner; rather, anxiety may result from the simultaneous interaction of several dynamics. Table 8-4 presents a summary of theories and selected nursing implications for practice.

General characteristics of anxiety, then can be identified as: (1) energy that cannot be directly observed, while its effects on behavior can be; (2) a subjective experience; (3) a physical, emotional, intellectual, sociocultural, and spiritual experience; (4) an emotion without a specific object; and (5) something interpersonally communicated.

Certain physiological and psychological changes occur as a result of anxiety. Physiological changes involve primarily the autonomic nervous system. Mild or moderate anxiety tends to increase physiological functioning, while severe levels slow down functioning and can ultimately result in death.

Physiological changes	Psychological changes
Tachycardia	Tension
Palpitations	Apprehension
Tremors	Indecisiveness
Muscle tension	Oversensitivity
Diarrhea	Tearfulness
Frequent urination	Agitation
Diaphoresis	Irritability
Dry mouth	Dread
Cold, clammy skin	Panic
Pallor	Powerlessness
Dilated pupils	Low self-worth
	Poor reality testing (delusions, hallucinations)

TABLE 8-4 Anxiety theories and nursing implications

Theory	Nursing implications
Psychoanalytic Freud	Nurses assist clients to identify and resolve underlying conflicts that generate anxiety through the use of the transference process. Nurses educate clients about the use of effective coping strategies to meet needs.
Psychodynamic Sullivan Peplau	Nurses facilitate the identification of areas that threaten security. Nurses educate parents about the need to validate and affirm children through interpersonal relationships. Nurses assist parents to understand that anxiety is transmitted through the relational process.
Learning Dollard and Miller	Nurses educate clients about the nature of learned response to anxiety. Nurses assist clients to learn more effective responses to anxiety. Clients are assisted to learn conflict resolution strategies.
Existential May	Nurses assist clients in the process of values clarification to determine those values which are most significant to an authentic existence. Nurses encourage clients to confront ambiguous situations through active decision making.

Clients express anxiety in a variety of ways, many times quite subtly. For example, a client may describe admission to the hospital in terms of feeling "shaky" and "nervous." Other client responses to anxiety-producing situations include: "My heart is pounding," "I have a lump in my throat," and "My body felt cold and I was perspiring a lot."

Mild levels of anxiety can help a person to cope with a stressor. For example, a student is preparing for an examination and notices details and logical connections she had not noticed previously. She describes herself as being "on edge." This mild anxiety facilitates her use of problem-solving strategies, which enhance her learning.

However, a moderate level of anxiety may prevent a person from noticing connections between details:

Mr. A has been receiving an anticoagulant for approximately 1 year. He has been hospitalized for a pulmonary embolism and has been receiving appropriate treatment.

Nurse *Mr. A., I'd like to spend some time discussing your anticoagulant medication before your discharge.*

Mr. A. *Just tell me what I need to know—I've never been on any medication before (fumbling with his sheets, swinging his legs over the side of the bed).*

Nurse *I want to go over the signs of bleeding that you should be aware of as well as aspirin usage and regular blood work.*

Mr. A. *I don't know if I can handle all of this—I've never done this before.*

Nurse *You look uneasy—can you tell me what you're experiencing right now?*

Mr. A. *I'm not sure—I don't know what to expect.*

Nurse *I am going to go over the signs of bleeding you should be aware of so you can let your doctor know.*

Mr. A. *O.K. let's get started.*

The nurse reviews signs of bleeding and then discusses the need for regular bloodwork and the use of aspirin while on anticoagulant medication. She then begins to review this information with the client.

Nurse *Mr. A., I'd like you to tell me how often you should have blood work done.*

Mr. A. *Ah, I don't know; I don't remember what you said—can you repeat that again.*

Nurse *All right (reviews blood work protocol).*

Mr. A. *I don't think I can remember all this; I know when I have to take the medication but all the rest of this is making me confused.*

Mr. A is able to recognize and respond to a limited amount of information. Some pieces of information assume great importance, to the exclusion of other significant information. This client's anxiety needs to be reduced to a mild level and then utilized in the problem-solving process.

Severe and panic levels of anxiety drastically impair functioning in all realms. Connections between details may no longer be apparent. Physical and emotional discomfort increase; feelings of dread, apprehension, and terror ensue. Thought processes are affected; loose associations, delusions, and hallucinations are called into operation to create a reality that is less threatening than the existing one. An individual may also exhibit dissociative responses, obsessive-compulsive behavior, conversion, or psychosomatic responses to severe levels of anxiety. At this point anxiety has gone beyond its service to the individual; the inability to cope appropriately with mounting levels of anxiety leads to the development of pathological behavior. Anxiety, then, can be viewed as the underlying dynamic of emotional illness. Symptoms of anxiety, as mentioned above, are attempts to control anxiety. The symptoms of anxiety also represent, at a symbolic level, an unresolved inner conflict.

Mild levels of anxiety are handled with little conscious thought or effort. Menninger (1963) has listed a number of coping mechanisms that are utilized to relieve the tension of day-to-day living:

Overeating
Drinking
Smoking
Self-discipline
Laughing, giggling
Crying
Cursing
Boasting
Sleep
Hobbies
Talking it out
Thinking things through
Physical exercise
Acting to alter
Fantasy formation and daydreaming
Dreaming
Use of religious faith
Symbolic substitutions (i.e., going on shopping spree)

It is important to note that one must distinguish between the "normal" use of coping mechanisms in everyday living and the misuse of them. Coping mechanisms are only effective insofar as they permit individuals to live in a reality-based environment. (For further coping strategies, see the section on stress management, earlier in this chapter.)

Moderate, severe, and panic levels of anxiety require greater effort and energy to control the effects on self. These coping strategies can be divided into task-oriented and ego-oriented behaviors.

Task-oriented behaviors involve the use of one's cognitive abilities. Problem-solving activities are used to confront a situation and meet the needs presented. Assertive behavior is an essential component of problem-solving. Individuals are respected for their beliefs, and an outcome that is satisfactory for all those involved is the long-term goal. Compromise is not a win-lose situation but rather a strategy that implies gains on both sides. Task-oriented behaviors vary; in fact, they can be destructive when rights of others are violated in the process of meeting a need or solving a problem. In such a case, one individual's anxiety might be reduced at the expense of another's.

Ego-oriented behaviors are those mechanisms utilized by the ego to protect the self. Task-oriented behaviors may not be sufficient to resolve a situation. Ego-defense mechanisms then protect the individual from experiencing feelings of overwhelming inadequacy and the resulting loss of self-worth. These mechanisms are used with mild and moderate levels of anxiety. However, as the degree to which they are used and the frequency of use increase, distortion of reality may become apparent and interpersonal relationships may be disturbed. For the most part, these mechanisms are out of the realm of conscious control; therefore, monitoring of reactions becomes difficult. (For further discussion of ego-defense mechanisms, see Chapter 6.)

FEAR AND ANXIETY

The terms *anxiety* and *fear* are frequently used synonymously. Fear, however, is aroused by the presence of an actual threat, of a danger that is currently present. Fear and anxiety differ in that fear is relatively self-limiting. For example, a person might fear skiing down a mountain for the first time. He or she would perceive the situation as fearful, yet it is doubtful that the event would cause a prolonged feeling of loss of self-worth. The physiological symptoms aroused by a frightening situation are similar to those generated by mild to moderate levels of anxiety. The cognitive and emotional changes attributed to anxiety are not usually experienced by a person who is frightened.

CATEGORIES OF ANXIETY

Free-floating anxiety can be associated with panic-arousing feelings of terror and dread that cannot be connected with a particular causative factor. Individuals experiencing this type of anxiety have the sensation that it invades every inch of life, exerting its influence on every aspect of life. Relief behaviors include withdrawal, phobic responses, ritualism, and dissociative responses.

State anxiety is precipitated by an event or situation that is perceived by the individual as being outside of his or her realm of control. An example of a precipitant of state anxiety would be learning that a close female friend has been assaulted by a rapist. The situation can be identified as anxiety provoking; this is different from free-floating anxiety.

Some individuals experience, or are predisposed toward experiencing, high levels of anxiety simply as a result of their personalities. Often the underlying conflict that generates the anxiety has occurred early in development yet continues to recur. Such individuals—who are said to have habitual anxiety, or *trait anxiety*—are likely to respond to many situations by exhibiting behaviors indicative of moderate to severe anxiety.

An understanding of state and trait anxiety can be helpful in predicting and assessing a client's responses to stressful situations. Measuring tools such as the State-Trait Anxiety Inventory can be used to assist the nurse in establishing a relationship that will enable the client to successfully alleviate anxiety.

The Freudian conception of anxiety—that it is generated by instinctual drives approaching the ego, creating a sense of danger—is known as *signal anxiety*. If the id-based instinctual drives cannot be satisfied by the ego in an appropriate manner, the intrapsychic defense mechanisms are called into action by the ego.

A young woman in her thirties complained of nervousness, insomnia, palpitations, and gastrointestinal disturbances. She described her life as being quite miserable, her husband being the major source of that misery. Her description of her past experiences revealed that she had had a cool, rejecting mother and an alcoholic father whom she adored. Her husband, on the other hand, was a much more giving, loving person. At the time when her 8-year-old daughter began to develop a close relationship with her father, a reemergence of the woman's need for a relationship with her own father occurred. She experienced overwhelming feelings of anxiety as the original conflict reappeared, and she lashed out at her husband.

Separation anxiety is the anxiety that occurs when an individual is confronted with the impending or feared loss of a person who is considered significant. Children at various stages of development, such as the infant of 8 to 9 months, the toddler, and the school-age child, can experience this type of anxiety when facing separation from a parent or significant adult. "School phobia," a related condition, may be described as an anxiety response to being away from home for even short periods of time, rather than as an aversion to school per se.

Anxiety has been defined in several different ways. It is important to note that anxiety may be categorized to delineate the various constructs relative to anxiety in a more clear manner. Table 8-5 presents the five major categories of anxiety.

In addition to being described in terms of levels (mild, moderate, and so on) and types (separation, signal, and so on), anxiety can be described in terms of duration. *Acute anxiety* has a sudden onset and may last from a few hours to a few weeks. Symptoms can be severe, such as rapid heart rate and pounding in the chest, increased respiratory rate, tachycardia, tremors of the extremities, nausea, diarrhea, and headache. Feelings of loss of control, apprehension, inadequacy, irritability, and decreased problem-solving ability occur as well. *Chronic anxiety* has no sudden onset but rather generates a constant, generalized feeling of apprehension or nervousness. Symptoms are much less pronounced than in acute anxiety yet may exert more impact on body systems because of their chronic nature. Chronically anxious individuals are *always* waiting for something to happen to them, always worrying about everything. Life is never fully enjoyed but is actually ruminated over. Chronic anxiety can be a combination of state, trait, and signal anxiety.

TABLE 8-5 Categories of anxiety

Category	Characteristics
Free-floating	Panic-arousing feelings of terror and dread lacking connection to specific causative factor; perceived to impact on every aspect of life
State	Precipitated by event or situation outside of realm of control of individual
Trait	Unresolved conflicts continue to generate anxiety in later development; habitual anxiety is present; individuals often respond by exhibiting behaviors indicative of moderate to severe anxiety
Signal	Freudian concept of anxiety generated by instinctual drives impacting on the ego creating a sense of danger
Separation	Anxiety that occurs when an individual is confronted with impending or actual loss of significant person; often described in relation to the anxiety experienced by a child when facing separation from a significant adult

PRIMARY AND SECONDARY GAIN

The concepts of primary and secondary gain need to be discussed in relation to anxiety and relief behaviors. The primary gain resulting from phobic behavior, obsessive-compulsive responses, withdrawal reactions, and so forth is the reduction of anxiety, which is generated by internal sources as well as environmental forces. A secondary gain is an advantage an individual experiences as a result of the primary symptom or symptoms. For example, a mother of five children is hospitalized for hysterical paralysis. The symptoms prevent her from carrying on her responsibilities as wife and mother. Therefore, underlying dependency needs are met that otherwise might have been expressed in other, more destructive ways. Secondary gains include not only relief from responsibilities but also a mechanism by which to seek attention and a means by which to control others in the environment.

Although relief of anxiety is of great importance, secondary gains are often equally important. Secondary gains can interfere with the client's wish to recover and in some cases prevent recovery.

Although anxiety has a negative connotation, mild to moderate levels act in the service of the ego to promote learning. Without some level of anxiety, there would be no need for change. Anxiety acts as a motivating agent; it disrupts equilibrium sufficiently to promote the initiation of coping strategies or relief behaviors. Life would certainly be boring without some type of energizing force. Therefore, anxiety and the adaptation that it brings forth serve as the foundation from which each person develops and preserves his or her sense of identity. The most healthy person is the one who has confronted anxiety-provoking situations and has actively taken steps to resolve them. Thus, repeated experiences with anxiety in limited amounts have growth-promoting potential. Anxiety serves to provide the energy necessary for adaptation.

Anxiety that is perceived as a threat can give rise to relief behaviors that protect or distance an individual from his or her anxiety. Intrapsychic defense mechanisms such as denial, projection, rationalization, and displacement can operate as part of a cluster of relief behaviors. These mechanisms can control anxiety for a limited period of time; however, at some point anxiety must be experienced as an energizing force that can be utilized as a growth-promoting force. When anxiety is continually avoided or denied, more severely dysfunctional behaviors occur, such as hallucinations, delusions, or other forms of psychotic behavior.

Stress, as an inducer of anxiety, may be seen as a precipitator of very individualistic responses on the part of clients, families, and nurses themselves. There continue to be unanswered questions: Why do some people respond in a psychophysiological manner while others respond in a phobic or compulsive manner? Why are some people able repeatedly to meet life's challenges with seemingly little difficulty while other people have great difficulty? In the next section, nursing intervention will be presented.

Nursing Intervention
PRIMARY PREVENTION

Primary prevention is a critical concern for nursing. A person's ability to respond to anxiety depends on the person's ability to identify potential stressors in his or her life situation. Anxiety can stimulate a positive growth response. Continued anxiety, however, causes exhaustion and the eventual development of psychopathology or pathophysiology. The goal of primary prevention is to help people develop healthy patterns of coping with anxiety during the early years of life to prevent later maladaptive responses. The family becomes the unit of focus. Intervention with the family directs the family's attention toward (1) the development of a positive self-concept, including healthy feelings toward one's own body; (2) the facilitation of interaction with others in the environment; (3) the sharing of feelings in an open, honest, caring manner; (4) the utilization of the problem-solving process to resolve disagreements; and (5) the acceptance of each individual as a separate being with unique behavior. A healthy family environment provides an atmosphere in which members can communicate their needs and identify potential stressors without feeling ashamed or afraid of repercussions. Each member feels unique and important. To minimize the effects of stressors and resulting anxiety, family members support one another in their attempts to plan their lives. Children grow up feeling confident in their ability to cope and are able to reach out for support from others when it is necessary.

Adult clients can be educated to recognize potential life stressors. Nurses and other members of the health care team can assist clients in managing their own environments through anticipatory planning—that is, by helping them to determine the number and types of stressors they can cope with comfortably. Education, role modeling, and supportive counseling with families and individuals are primary nursing measures for promoting effective coping patterns and healthy adaptation.

SECONDARY PREVENTION

The nursing process provides the framework for secondary prevention.

Nursing process
ASSESSMENT

Nursing assessment of a client experiencing anxiety is based upon presenting behaviors, including the client's subjective description of feelings, previous experiences with similar anxiety-producing situations, effectiveness of coping strategies, and current support systems.

These questions will be helpful in the assessment process: Is the client's reaction to the stressor appropriate to the situation? If it is inappropriate, are cognitive functions impaired? What is the client's level of anxiety? Has the client repeatedly attempted the same coping strategy and failed? How does his or her behavior reinforce the anxiety? Are coping strategies effective or destructive? Is the anxiety acting in the service of learning and promoting growth? What is the effect of the client's family on his or her anxiety level? Are expectations of the family consistent with those of the client or in conflict? What function does symptomatic behavior (for example, psychosis) play in the family? What happens when symptomatic behavior decreases? What coping strategies are used by the family to resolve anxiety? What secondary gains can be attributed to symptomatic behavior? What sources of support, other than the family, are available to the client? Formulation of nursing diagnoses will be specific to the level of anxiety. Severe and panic levels of anxiety may result in distortion of thoughts, feelings, and behavior.

A complete nursing history is critical to the formulation of nursing diagnoses reflective of the issues facing the client. Anxiety affects cognitive ability, interpersonal relationships, physiological and psychological function, and sense of self-worth.

ANALYSIS OF DATA

Assessment of presenting symptoms, stimulus situations, maladaptive coping responses, and holistic health factors leads to an increased understanding of the client within the context of his or her current situation. After a thorough analysis of data, nursing diagnoses are formulated.

Those clients experiencing severe to panic levels of anxiety frequently need to be hospitalized. They are unable to care for themselves physically or participate in realistic decision making and activities of daily living. Nursing diagnoses reflect the need to reduce severe anxiety levels as rapidly as possible and to protect the client from self and others.

PLANNING AND IMPLEMENTATION

Following are nursing care plans that reflect a realistic approach to secondary preventive intervention. The nurse may initially establish goals, but as therapy progresses, the client should enter into goal setting to ensure commitment to accomplishing these goals.

NURSING CARE PLAN

Client with Anxiety

Long-term Outcomes	Short-term Outcomes	Nursing Strategies
Nursing diagnosis: Severe level of anxiety related to loss of a child (NANDA 9.3.1; DSM-III-R 313.00)		
To work through the conflicts that are arousing anxiety To learn to effectively cope with stressful life situations so that a panic level of anxiety is not generated	To learn to identify and describe feelings of anxiety To identify and describe the precipitating stressful life situation and the associated feelings To relate the precipitating stressful life situation to situations in the past that aroused similar feelings To reevaluate the potency (in terms of stress) of the precipitating stressful life situation To develop more effective coping behaviors To avoid excessive use of secondary gain	Be directive with the client—for example, "I am going to move you into a quieter space; I will stay with you until you're feeling more calm." Listen with the intent to *hear*—use the "third ear." Stay with the client while respecting his or her need for space. Acknowledge overwhelming feelings of awe, apprehension, terror, or fear of "going crazy" as being *real* to the client. Present a calm, honest approach that affirms your ability to provide control when the client is unable to do so. Provide a protective environment, meeting physical needs until the client is able to do so: Proper diet, high protein • Encourage fluids • Small, frequent feedings • Establish a routine of eating, sleeping, elimination • Symptomatic relief of diarrhea and gastric hyperactivity Reduce environmental stimuli by removing the client from situations that increase anxiety, such as a crowded day room. Assist the client in identifying what stressor he or she feels comfortable dealing with. Support present coping strategies rather than removing defenses prematurely. Current defenses *do* relieve anxiety even though they may be inappropriate. Criticism of defenses may lead to increased anxiety. For example, ritualistic behavior should not be interrupted initially. Set limits on inappropriate coping strategies once anxiety has been reduced and a trusting relationship has been established.

Long-term Outcomes	Short-term Outcomes	Nursing Strategies

Nursing diagnosis: Severe level of anxiety related to loss of a child (NANDA 9.3.1; DSM-III-R 313.00)—cont'd

		Encourage participation in activities:
		• Support the use of gross motor activities that require little concentration or problem-solving.
		• Work individually with clients rather than involve them in group activities.
		• Involve family members in activities.
		Determine what types of comfort measures are preferred by the client—for example, warm milk, hot bath, soft music, favorite quilt or afghan.
		Reduce the number of demands made on the client, since decision making is difficult. Allow choices in treatment, diet, and daily activities when appropriate.
		Cautiously use tranquilizing medications; monitor for untoward effects.
		Distinguish between anxiety and physical symptoms such as those of cardiac arrhythmias and myocardial infarctions.
		NOTE: It is critical that severe to panic levels of anxiety be addressed rapidly by the nurse. Once anxiety has been decreased to more manageable levels, nursing intervention is directed toward enabling clients to develop more effective ways of resolving stressful situations. This effort cannot be accomplished when clients are experiencing severe levels of anxiety.

Nursing diagnosis: Moderate level of anxiety related to impending cataract surgery (NANDA 9.3.1)

Long-term Outcomes	Short-term Outcomes	Nursing Strategies
Develop more effective ways of coping with anxiety. Develop positive sense of self.	To learn to identify behavioral responses that are indicative of anxiety in a given situation. To participate in the scheduled set of activities each day for 2 weeks. To learn to identify potentially anxiety-producing situations. To learn to remove self from situations that potentially will increase anxiety levels	Help the client recognize that he or she is anxious by acknowledging signs and symptoms you observe in him or her—for example, "You look uneasy, upset, or concerned." Connect the observable behaviors with the feeling of being anxious—for example, "After you spoke to your mother this morning, you paced for about twenty minutes and seemed to lose your concentration. How would you describe your feelings then?" Refrain from giving false reassurances such as, "Don't worry—you'll feel better later" or a similar empty cliché. Explore possible causative factors of anxiety: "Can you tell me what was happening before you started to feel anxious?" Direct intervention toward connecting the perceived stressor with possible underlying conflict. Assist the client in identifying previous coping strategies and their effectiveness.

Continued.

NURSING CARE PLAN—cont'd

Client with Anxiety

Long-term Outcomes	Short-term Outcomes	Nursing Strategies
Nursing diagnosis: Moderate level of anxiety related to impending cataract surgery (NANDA 9.3.1)—cont'd		

Support the client's use of effective coping strategies.

Identify maladaptive use of coping strategies; point out the client's responsibility for his or her behavior and support the client's ability to mobilize effective coping stategies. Provide comfort.

Assist the client in the appraisal of threatening situations—that is, within the context of past and current relationships.

Use the educative-supportive nature of the nurse-client relationship as the forum for the testing out of new behaviors and the provision of appropriate feedback.

Encourage the use of physical exercise, such as walking, jogging, and bicycling, to relieve anxiety.

Offer other methods of tension reduction as options—for example, progressive relaxation, yoga, meditation, biofeedback, or guided imagery.

NOTE: The use of the problem-solving process is an integral component of nursing intervention to reduce moderate levels of anxiety. The use of an insight-oriented, educative approach helps the client to define anxiety and its causes and to utilize adaptive methods to resolve anxiety-producing situations. The nurse can then explore the motivational aspects of mild anxiety, that level of anxiety which acts to promote growth and prevent stagnation. As noted previously, a client who succeeds in reducing anxiety enhances his or her repertoire of coping strategies and increases his or her sense of worth as a human being.

EVALUATION

The client and, whenever feasible, the client's family and significant others (for example, housemate, very close friend) should be included in estimating the client's progress toward attainment of goals. Any evaluation should encompass the following areas:

1. Estimation of the degree to which conflicts have been worked through
2. Estimation of the degree to which goals have been achieved and client functioning has improved (demonstrated by a decrease in maladaptive coping behavior and the learning of more effective coping behavior)
3. Identification of goals that need to be modified or revised
4. Referral of the client to support systems other than the nurse-client relationship
   a. People in the client's social network who are willing to serve as a support system
   b. Community organizations, church groups, civic organizations, self-help groups, and

neighborhood support groups that can assist in the maintenance of coping strategies
5. Analysis of cost-effectiveness of stress-management programs
6. Estimation of risk-benefit ratio of interventions

TERTIARY PREVENTION

The focus of tertiary prevention is on the assessment of maladaptive responses to anxiety, alterations in body image, lengthy immobility, painful stimuli, or situations that generate a sense of loss. Intervention at this level is directed toward helping the client to resolve maladaptive coping measures and to minimize further effects of these maladaptive measures.

CHAPTER SUMMARY

Each individual is in a continual state of flux, always responding to internal and external cues. Adaptation is the series of changes that occurs in response to stressors. The way an individual adapts to stress is influenced by cultural, physiological, and psychological factors. If a stressor is not perceived as very threatening, anxiety levels are mild. Mild anxiety can be utilized in the service of learning. As anxiety levels increase, however, problem-solving capacities become impaired and previously successful coping behavior becomes inadequate. If severe anxiety continues for a prolonged period, physical exhaustion and maladaptive patterns of behavior result. Recognition of anxiety levels and their implications for nursing intervention are critical to the process of healthy adaptation.

Several commonly encountered stressors that pose varying degrees of threat to self-concept have been presented. Key concepts in the understanding of these stressors include the perception of the event and the degree and type of coping mechanisms utilized. In some instances a change, such as an increase in body size, is both a stressor and the *result* of a stress response. Nurses need to keep in mind the difference between *stressor* and *stress response*.

Primary, secondary, and tertiary preventive measures in relation to stress, anxiety, and adaptation have been presented. Primary prevention directs its efforts toward identification and management of potential stressors. Secondary prevention involves the early detection of actual stressors and the implementation of nursing strategies to cope with them. Tertiary prevention deals with the assessment of maladaptive responses arising from prolonged periods of uncontrolled anxiety and intervention to keep these maladaptive responses from becoming permanent.

Evaluation of these three levels of intervention is an integral component of nursing practice. Nurses need to be aware of the implications of the stress response and the attendant anxiety levels—both for themselves and for their clients. One goal of the nurse-client relationship is the identification of motivators of behavior. An understanding of anxiety and its effects on behavior enables nurse and client to explore present and future coping mechanisms. The nursing diagnosis and the subsequent nursing intervention should reflect this understanding. Nursing care of the person experiencing stress includes all areas of prevention—primary, secondary, and tertiary.

SELF-DIRECTED LEARNING

Sensitivity-Awareness Exercises
Stress-reduction measures
1. Progressive relaxation*
   a. Procedure
      (1) Lie very quietly in a comfortable position.
      (2) Loosen clothing.
      (3) Allow yourself to be relaxed; assume a mental posture that permits relaxation.
      (4) Follow a sequence beginning with the upper extremities and moving down through the trunk and lower extremities, tensing each group of muscles twice for 30 seconds and relaxing each group twice for 60 seconds. Produce tension in one group at a time. Do not tense muscles after they have become relaxed. (These instructions are often given on tape so that they may be followed more easily.)
      (5) Progressive relaxation should be practiced regularly, once a day each day. When it has been mastered, it can be used at any time as a self-regulatory measure. It does *not* work for everyone.
   b. Purpose: to help you note the difference between muscle tension and muscle relaxation. You will also be able to remember what it feels like to release the tension. Recall may then be used to effect muscle relaxation.
2. Breathing exercise†
   a. Procedure
      (1) Sit in a chair in a comfortable position, with loose clothing.
      (2) Control your breathing so that it is slow, deep, and regular.
      (3) Close your eyes and exhale slowly while pulling your abdomen in.
      (4) Inhale quickly through your nose, bringing in as much air as you can so as to fill the rib cage.
      (5) Draw in your abdomen and push the air out through your mouth.
      (6) Repeat steps 3 to 5 ten times.
      (7) Inhale slowly through your nose. Hold your breath for 10 seconds.
      (8) Exhale slowly through your mouth until your lungs are empty.
      (9) Repeat steps 7 and 8 five times.
   b. Purpose: to reduce stress by controlling your breathing. Tension and relaxation are mutually exclusive; therefore by focusing on relaxation you cannot be tense. This measure, as do the others, enables you to feel more in control of your situation, which also serves to reduce stress.
3. Guided imagery*
   a. Procedure
      (1) Find a quiet, comfortable place to sit.
      (2) Close your eyes and imagine a peaceful scene that has special meaning for you—a place where you have been or would like to go.
      (3) Visualize this scene in as much detail as you can. Imagine the smells, sounds, and "feels" of this place, such as the sun, the breeze, the scent of flowers, the trickling of a brook.
      (4) Experience the pleasure of this scene for a few minutes, and then slowly open your eyes.
   b. Purpose: to respond to symbolic stimuli, enabling you to feel as if you are *actually* experiencing the restful scene. You feel the effects of the imagery and stress is lessened.

Guide for developing your own stress profile†
Take a little time to reflect on the following questions as a guide to self-exploration.
1. How often do you feel tense, anxious, irritable?
2. How often do you eat, drink, or smoke to relieve tension?
3. Do you feel that you have more to do than you can accomplish each day? Do you always feel rushed?
4. Do you enjoy what you are doing? Are your daily tasks a source of pleasure and satisfaction?
5. Do you find time to relax regularly every day?

*Adapted from Jacobsen (1978).
†Adapted from Ulene (1978).

*Adapted from Ulene (1978).
†From Sutterley, DC: Stress and health: a survey of self-regulation modalities, Topics in Clinical Nursing, 1:1, 1979.

SELF-DIRECTED LEARNING—cont'd

6. Do you have difficulty sleeping?
7. How would you rate your general state of health at present?
8. Do you consider your present weight to be a problem?
9. Do you eat a nutritious balanced diet (free from the excesses that can become "stressors")?
10. Do you exercise regularly?
11. Do you believe you are getting adequate exercise and do you enjoy it?
12. Do you believe you are physically fit? (Is your resting pulse rate above 80/min?)
13. Calculate your life change index; is it more than 300 for the year?
14. Do you try to recognize tension in yourself? (And how do others see you expressing your stress and tension?)
  Ask yourself:
• What kind of tension you feel and under what circumstances.
• What were you thinking or feeling and how did you respond when under heavy stress?
  Keep a log or diary to assist you in a self-examination to identify your own sources of stress (what bothers you).
  Try to recognize your own manifestations of stress and tension (others may need to help you).

Questions to Consider

1. Accurate assessment of +3 (severe) level of anxiety reveals which of the following characteristics?
   a. Sharp reduction in scattering of thought
   b. Increased power of concentration
   c. Enhanced learning potential
   d. Sharp reduction of perceptual field
2. When anxiety is manifested by a conscious fear over a pending medical procedure, which of the following would be *least* reassuring?
   a. A simple explanation of what is to be done
   b. Assurance that the procedure will be painless
   c. Minimal discussion and doing the procedure quickly
   d. Suggesting to the client that anxiety is a normal response at this time

Match each of the following terms with the statement associated with it:

3. Separation anxiety
4. Free-floating anxiety
5. State anxiety
6. Trait anxiety
7. Secondary gain

a. A painful feeling that cannot be connected with a particular causative factor
b. Anxiety that is precipitated by an event or situation perceived as outside of one's control
c. Habitual anxiety that is related to baseline personality
d. Anxiety generated by impending loss
e. Relief from routine responsibilities
f. Long-term anxiety

Answer key
1. d
2. b
3. d
4. a
5. b
6. c
7. e

REFERENCES

Alland A: Adaptation in cultural evolution: an approach to medical anthropology, New York, 1970, Columbia University Press.

American Psychiatric Association: Diagnostic and statistical manual of mental disorders (DSM-III-R), Washington, DC, 1987, The Association.

Billings A and Moos R: Coping, stress, and social resources among adults with unipolar depression, J Personality Soc Psychol 46:877-891, 1984.

Brallier L: Biofeedback and holism in clinical practice, Holistic Nurs Prac 2(3):26-33, 1988.

Breznitz S: The effect of hope and denial in coping with stress, paper presented at the University of Pennsylvania School of Nursing Research Symposium, Philadelphia, 1986.

Burd S and Marshall M, editors: Some clinical approaches to psychiatric nursing, New York, 1963, MacMillan, Inc.

Bush P: The male nurse: a challenge to traditional role identities, Nurs Forum 4:390, 1976.

Davis J: Animal-facilitated therapy in stress mediation, Holistic Nurs Prac 2(3):75-83, 1988.

Derogatis L: The Derogatis stress profile: quantification of psychological stress, In Fava G and Wise T, editors: Research paradigms in psychosomatic medicine, New York, 1987, Karger.

Dock L: A short history of nursing, New York, 1920, Putnam.

Dohrenwend B et al.: Report on stress and life events, In Elliott G and Eisdorfer C, editors: Stress and human health: analysis and implications of research, New York, 1982, Springer.

Dollard J and Miller N: Personality and psychotherapy: an analysis in terms of learning, thinking, and culture, New York, 1950, McGraw-Hill.

Donovan R: Stress in the workplace: a framework for research and practice, Soc Casework: J Contemporary Soc Work, May 1987, pp 259-266.

Engel G: Psychological development in health and disease, Philadelphia, 1962, WB Saunders Co.

Freud S: A general introduction to psychoanalysis, New York, 1936, Pocket Books.

Gulak R: Nurses' salaries: just begining to catch up, RN 44:40-42, 1981.

Hackett T and Cassem N: How do patients react to heart disease? Med Insight 2:79-81, 1970.

Holmes T and Rahe R: The social readjustment scale, J Psychosom Res 11:213-218, 1967.

Jacobsen E: You must relax, ed 5, New York, 1978, McGraw-Hill.

Larson D: Helper secrets: internal stressors in nursing, J Psychosoc Nurs 25(4):20-27, 1987.

Lazarus R and Folkman S: Stress appraisal and coping, New York, 1984, Springer.

Lowery B: Stress research: some theoretical and methodological issues, Image: J Nurs Scholarship 19(1):42-44, 1987.

McLane A, editor: Classification of nursing diagnoses, St. Louis, 1987, The CV Mosby Co.

May R: The meaning of anxiety, ed 2, New York, 1977, WW Norton Co.

Menaghan E and Merves E: Coping with occupational problems: the limits of individual efforts, J Health Soc Behav 25:406-423, 1984.

Menninger K: The vital balance, New York, 1963, The Viking Press.

Paykel E: Methodology of life events research, In Fava G and Wise T, editors: Research paradigms in psychosomatic medicine, New York, 1987, Karger.

Pearlin L and Schooler C: The structure of coping, J Health Soc Behav 19:12-20, 1978.

Pennebacker J: Traumatic experiences and psychosomatic disease: exploring roles of behavioral inhibition, obsession, and confiding, Canadian Psychol 26:82-95, 1985.

Peplau H: Interpersonal techniques: the crux of psychiatric nursing, Am J Nurs 62:53-54, 1962.

Peplau H: A working definition of anxiety, In Burd S and Marshall M, editors: Some clinical approaches to psychiatric nursing, New York, 1963, MacMillan, Inc.

Reed M: The dependent nurse, Nurs Times (79):12-13, 1983.

Ruxton J: Humor intervention deserves our attention, Holistic Nurs Prac 2(3):54-62, 1988.

Scheier M and Carver C: Optimism, coping, and health: assessment and implications of generalized outcome expectancies, Health Psychol 4:219-247, 1985.

Selye H: The stress of life, New York, 1977, McGraw-Hill Co.

Steffen S: Perceptions of stress: 1800 nurses tell their stories, In Claus K and Bailey J, editors: Living with stress and promoting well-being, St. Louis, 1980, The CV Mosby Co.

Sullivan H: Interpersonal theory of psychiatry, New York, 1953, WW Norton Co.

Sutterly DC: Stress and health: a survey of self-regulation modalities, Topics Clin Nurs, 1979.

Thomas S et al: Denial in coronary care patients, Heart Lung 12:513-526, 1983.

Titlebaum H: Relaxation, Holistic Nurs Prac 2(3):17-25, 1988.

Turner A, King C, and Craddock J: Measuring and reducing noise, Hospitals 49:85-89, 1975.

Ulene A: Feeling fine, New York, 1978, Ballantine Books.

Valiga T and Frain M: The multiple dimensions of stress, Topics Clin Nurs, 1979.

ANNOTATED SUGGESTED READINGS

Fagin C: Stress: implications for nursing research, Image: J Nurs Scholar 19(1):38-41, 1987.
This article explores stress research as it relates to the field of nursing. Fagin reviews the history of stress research and identifies the emerging role of nursing as it parallels the evolution of stress research. She explores such issues as biologic responses and behavioral responses to illness-induced stress and highlights areas for future clinical nursing research.

Larson D: Helper secrets: internal stressors in nursing, J Psychosoc Mental Health Serv 25(4):20-27, 1987.
Larson presents a unique view of those feelings that nurses are generally unable to share with their peers or others. She reports data from a study of 495 nurses that were then categorized into eight major themes. Larson discusses the negative

effects that result from the lack of sharing of these internal stressors and suggests the peer group support method of coping with those stressors which seem to be particular to the nursing population.

Lowery B: Stress research: some theoretical and methodological issues, Image: J Nurs Scholar 19(1):42-44, 1987.

Lowery presents some of the current theoretic and methodologic concerns in regard to stress research. She identifies potential stressors and mediators of stress and their role in a stress continuum. She points out the need for further study of emotional and physiologic reactions when coping strategies fail as well as understanding the immediate and sustained reactions that might have a significant impact on nursing interventions.

Stokes S and Gordon S: Development of an instrument to measure stress in the older adult, Nurs Res 37(1):16-18, 1988.

This article discusses the results of a study conducted to evaluate a tool to measure stress in adults 65 years of age and older. Fifty-one stressors were identified and categorized into 13 major areas. Additional stressors were included as a result of input from experts in the area of gerontology. The authors piloted the tool with 43 subjects. They conclude that the tool is valid and reliable as a predictor of stress. The authors note the usefulness of this tool, which can serve as a diagnostic aid for the development of appropriate intervention strategies.

FURTHER READINGS

Allanach E: Perceived supportive behaviors and nursing occupational stress: an evolution of consciousness, Adv Nurs Sci 10(2):73-82, 1988.

Clark S: Nursing diagnosis: ineffective coping, Heart Lung 16(6):649-652, 1987.

Dewe P: Investigating the frequency of nursing stressors: a comparison across wards, Soc Sci Med 26(3):375-380, 1988.

Earl W: Relaxation groups and the aging: suggestions for longevity, Nurs Homes 36(5):16-19, 1987.

Munn V: Nurses' perceptions of stressors in pediatric intensive care, school-aged children, and adolescents, J Pediatr Nurs 2(6):405-411, 1987.

O'Malley P et al: Relationship of hope and stress after myocardial infarction, Heart Lung 17(2):184-190, 1988.

Pasternak I: The effects of primary care nursing and feelings of isolation/depersonalization of the critical care nurse: background for the study, Nurs Manage 19(3):112-114, 1988.

Scalzi C: Role stress and coping strategies of nurse executives, J Nurs Admin 18(3):34-37, 1988.

Snyder M: Relaxation, In Fitzpatrick J, Taunton R, and Benoliel J, editors: Annual review of nursing research, vol 6, New York, 1988, Springer.

White J: Toughing with intent: therapeutic massage, Holistic Nurs Prac 2(3):63-67, 1988.

CHAPTER 9

Commonly encountered stressors

CHAPTER FOCUS

Illness creates a crisis for individuals and their families. The ability to adapt to these situations fluctuates according to the individual's ability to cope with stress in a healthy manner. Chapter 8 presented the concepts of anxiety and stress and their relationship to an individual's ability to develop and to maintain adaptive mechanisms.

Chapter 9 explores four commonly encountered stressors: pain, body image, immobilization, and loss. Each stressor is discussed in terms of theoretical foundation and impact on life-style and coping strategies. Stressors are conceptualized within the framework of the three levels of prevention. Utilizing the nursing process, relevant nursing diagnoses, long- and short-term outcomes, and nursing strategies are presented to illustrate each stressor.

The nurse's role in addressing these stressors is unique. The provision of psychosocial care to clients in all settings—general hospital, ambulatory care, home, hospice, and nursing homes—is essential. The mutual interaction of physical and psychological factors impacts on clients of all ages and in every phase of development. Nurses can assist clients through anticipatory guidance to resolve losses in a healthy manner. Nurses can facilitate the integration of body image changes to promote a positive sense of self. Nurses can reduce the negative effects of sensory overload and deprivation. Through an understanding of the impact of stressors, nurses can maximize the potential for healthy adaptation.

STRESSORS
Body image

As was discussed in Chapter 6, body image is an integral part of self-concept. Body image is reflective of the attitudes one holds about one's body. Related to body image is sense of identity—one's perception of one's strengths and weaknesses and one's relationships to others.

Body image can be altered by the addition of artifacts or by a threat to body integrity. The disruption of body image can be caused by many situations, including weight loss or gain, surgical intervention, and pathophysiological and psychopathological conditions. Because certain areas of the body hold more meaning for an individual than others, threats to these areas may be considered more significant and require more action by the individual. Throughout the life cycle, varying dimensions of body image are developed and redeveloped. Feelings of self-worth may correlate with positive body image. An individual who has difficulty developing an integrated self-concept has a corresponding difficulty relating to others. It is only after the development of positive feelings about self that an individual seeks to invest in others.

Many factors contribute to the development of body image. The most pertinent factors include responses from others in the environment (such as parents and peers), one's own attitudes and emotions regarding the body, one's degree of independence and motivation, physical appearance, how well the body functions, and perception of body territoriality. Body image thus is multidimensional rather than unidimensional. Nursing assessment and intervention must include a survey of the various factors in an effort to develop a realistic appraisal and plan of action. Clients' feelings about particular aspects of body image depend on whether they perceive them as functional tools or as central personal attributes. For example, dentures may be accepted as a tool rather than as a central attribute, while hair may be viewed as essential to one's identity.

A sense of body space and self-concept emerge during the first year of life. As the child moves through the developmental stages, changes occur in the physical aspects of the body. During adolescence, the body is viewed as a social tool; however, as middle age and old age approach, the body becomes wrinkled, skin sags, and sensory functions decrease. As the actual physical appearance of the body changes, the feelings one has about oneself may also change. Therefore, it is important that nurses assess the impact that disturbances in body image have on an individual and his or her relationships with others.

Kolb (1959) groups body image disturbances into five categories: (1) neurological dysfunctions that affect sensorimotor status, such as paraplegia or hemiplegia; (2) metabolic dysfunction, such as thyroid disease or obesity; (3) dismemberment, such as loss of a limb; (4) personality dysfunctions, such as neuroses, psychoses, and psychophysiological diseases; and (5) dysfunctions related to progressive deformities, such as arthritis. Body image is a vulnerable entity. It may be distorted, as in a person experiencing pain, or diminished, as in a person with decreased sensory function. Although a client in pain often focuses attention on the area of pain, the whole self is consumed by the pain.

Threats to body image are sources of stress because body image is related to various areas of function. The choice of a life's work, sexual behavior, the ability to respond appropriately to stress, and relationships with others are related to the concept of self and body image.

Surgical removal of a body part (for example, amputation of a limb or removal of the gall bladder) or alteration of a body function (for example, colostomy or ileostomy) often constitutes a threat to body image. Gross changes in body size and shape may also serve as threats to one's self-concept. Changes result, for example, from the increases in weight caused by pregnancy or overeating and from excessive weight loss. Finally, pathological processes, such as coronary artery disease, cause changes in the functioning of critical body parts, such as the heart. Even though there may be no outward manifestation that the body is not functioning properly, one's self-concept is definitely altered.

Surgical removal of a body part such as a breast or a limb often causes the client to perceive himself or herself as no longer being whole. Breast cancer is on the rise in the United States, and its impact is being felt in all social classes. The changes in self-concept that result from a mastectomy depend upon the significance a woman places on the breast and her perception of the seriousness of the threat posed by the loss of a breast. Various values are placed on the breast—it is a symbol of femininity for many, and it is often closely linked with sexual functioning. Loss of a breast may mean loss of a job, if performance in the job relies on use of the whole body, as in modeling. With the loss of a breast, a woman comes face to face with her feelings of self. She will depend on the reactions of significant others to help her assimilate the change in body image into the self-concept. The loss of a limb causes a similar disturbance in body image. The degree of the threat to self-concept that results from such a loss depends upon the value placed on the limb and the ability of the individual to successfully adapt to the loss.

A colostomy or an ileostomy often poses a threat to body image and self-concept. Defecation and urination traditionally have been considered private functions. Feces have often been considered dirty, both literally and figuratively, and odors and sounds related to bowel function have been considered taboo. Thus, to release feces into a small plastic bag that may leak or smell is often regarded as repulsive, and clients may display a tendency toward social isolation to protect their self-concepts. Very often they resist accepting the reality of body image change. However, the changes—the stoma, the odor, the plastic bag—need to be incorporated into a restructured body image.

Coronary artery disease is frequently described as a psychophysiological response to stress. Coronary artery disease therefore may be viewed both as a threat to body image and self-concept—a stressor—and as a *result* of maladaptation to stress. The heart is the "organ of choice" (refer to Chapter 19). It is important to recognize this dual position that coronary artery disease holds. The disease process is commonly interpreted in nursing assessments as being stress-induced; however, it is equally important to assess the impact that coronary artery disease has on body image and self-concept. (Coronary artery disease as a psychophysiological response to stress is discussed further in Chapter 19.)

An increase in body weight is one of the prominent changes that occurs during pregnancy. Women often speak of feeling "like a balloon." A woman's body space enlarges, possibly restricting her movement through territory that had originally been familiar and accessible. Everyday functions such as bending down to tie shoes, driving a car, and turning around in a small space are no longer as easy to accomplish. The increased size may result in a disturbance in body image and a threat to self-concept, depending upon a woman's feelings toward the pregnancy.

Thus it is critical that a nurse determine the impact of a client's body size on body image and self-concept. The physical changes that an individual experiences may result in increased anxiety levels and the utilization of pathological defense mechanisms.

Several commonly encountered stressors that may cause disturbance in body image and alteration of self-concept have been presented. In a nursing assessment, it is important to determine the client's perception of the meaning of a threat and its implications for his or her life-style. It is also important to note that age affects perception and adaptation to change in body image. For example, a young child might have fewer adjustment problems to a crippling illness than an adult. The client calls varying levels of defense mechanisms into action, depending on the seriousness of the threat. The goal of nurse and client is to recognize the implications of the alterations and to maximize the client's adaptive capacities.

The following is an example of a nurse-client interaction related to an alteration of body image.

Jeffrey, a 17-year-old high school senior, has had an above-the-knee amputation of the right leg following a car accident. This interaction takes place three days following the surgery.

Nurse   Hi, Jeff, I'd like to change the dressing on your stump today.

Jeff   Well, go right ahead—pretend I'm not even here; I don't even want to know what it looks like.

Nurse   You sound as though you have some really strong feelings about what's happened.

Jeff   How would you like it if your leg was just cut off—now what am I going to do?

Nurse	*I'm sure I wouldn't like it either. Can you tell me what bothers you most?*
Jeff	*I'm going to be a freak—every one in school is going to stare at me.*
Nurse	*Do you think people might feel you're a different person?*
Jeff	*I guess so—but I am different and now I can't do anything.*
Nurse	*Yes, your body might look different and there may be some things that you can't do right now. It takes a while for a person to cope with those differences but I think with a little time it's possible for you to adjust in a positive way to what has occurred. I'd like you to think about taking a look with me at your leg.*
Jeff	*I don't know—I guess I could try but I don't want to take care of that thing.*
Nurse	*We won't do that today, but soon I'm going to help you with "taking care of that thing" too.*

The interaction demonstrates the client's initial lack of acceptance of the body image alteration. The nurse's ultimate goal is to assist the client in physically caring for the wound as well as to facilitate the development of healthy coping strategies that will enhance acceptance of the change in body image.

Pain

Pain is in many ways an essential part of everyday life. Burkholz (1987) notes that the ancients saw pain as a scourge from the gods; pain in Greek and Latin means punishment, yet it was accepted as part of the order of existence. Pain in today's society has been described by Dr. John Bonica as affecting over one-third of all Americans and costs upwards of 70 billion dollars each year in medical costs and lost employment time (Burkholz, 1987).

Orshan (1988) notes that many of the theories of pain reflect the controversy between the holistic perspective of health care and mind-body approach. One of the most well-known and earliest theories of pain is that of the gate-control hypothesis proposed by Melzack and Wall in the early 1960s. Information regarding pain stimuli is transmitted through the autonomic nervous system and spinal cord, leading ultimately to the brain. Pain stimuli travel on small nonmyelinated fibers to the substantia gelatinosa, which acts as a gateway be-

tween stimuli and the brain. Nonpain stimuli travel more rapidly on large-diameter myelinated fibers. Faster impulses then are capable of closing the gate and preventing pain impulses. Strong painful impulses, however, can override and reopen the gate, thus allowing painful stimuli to reach the brain and be perceived as pain. This theory did not account for the individual's perception of pain as a subjective experience. Melzack and Wall (1982) expanded the gate-control hypothesis to incorporate individual perception of pain. They proposed that pain impulses travel to the limbic system, center of emotions. Response to pain thus reflects individual perception, previous experience with pain, and previous coping strategies. Feldman (1984) further supports this theory, stating that the theory provides an integrative model of cognitions, sensory discrimination, motivation, and evaluation of stimuli.

Immunomodulators, endogenous opiate-like substances, have been discovered in the limbic system as well as the thalamus and the substantia gelatinosa—centers for pain transmission. Orshan (1988) notes that there are two types of immunomodulators: endorphins and enkephalins. Although research in this area is limited, these substances seem to exert an inhibitory influence on pain, possibly by closing the gate to pain stimuli.

Last, McKean (1986) presents the concept of bradykinin—a substance developed by John Stewart that is produced whenever the body is injured. Bradykinin has been identified as the most potent pain-producing chemical known. Stewart believes that bradykinin can be utilized as a pain killer based on its action as an initiator of pain response. Bradykinin acts by causing neurons to fire, sending information to the brain that damage has occurred. It then activates the inflammatory response and encourages further development of bradykinin, which facilitates the feedback loop of pain and inflammation until the injury has been resolved.

Taylor (1987) indicates that further research is needed in the area of pain transmission, perception, assessment, and management. The complex nature of the pain response requires more effective measurement tools as well as an understanding of the impact of health care providers' values regarding pain and its expression.

FACTORS INFLUENCING THE PAIN RESPONSE

What influences the behavior of a person experiencing pain? Does each person respond according to a predetermined "set"? Because cultural, physical, and psychological factors influence the pain response, it is important to recognize that a client may not fit into any specific category of responses.

Pain coping strategies may then be described as a set of behaviors particular to each individual. These behaviors are activated as a response to pain or injury. Individuals exhibit coping strategies that reflect their perception of self, their previous experience with pain, and their expectations of staff management of their pain. Table 9-1 is a summary of five models of coping behavior. To develop a comprehensive nursing care plan, nurses must be cognizant of factors influencing the pain response and client coping strategies. The following factors are presented as guidelines for nursing assessment and intervention.

The duration and intensity of pain will be reflected in client behavior. For example, the chronic pain involved in terminal cancer is best described as all-consuming. The focal point of behavior is relief of pain. Superficial pain, on the other hand, prepares the body for "fight or flight." Additional factors that affect the perception of pain are sensory restriction and prolonged loss of sleep. Clients often experience more pain during the night than they do during the day because the number of incoming stimuli decreases during the night, and their type and pattern change. The body responds to stimuli of lesser intensity during periods of quiet, such as nighttime; during the day the number and variety of stimuli bombarding the client are greater. The other factor, sleep deprivation, lowers the adaptive capacity of the client, thus intensifying the perception of pain. The client who has been undergoing a rigorous series of diagnostic tests, the preparations for which preclude normal sleep, may cry pitifully following the pinprick for a blood sample. This is not irrational behavior. It should be expected in light of our understanding of pain perception.

Traumatic life experiences can initiate or sustain pain or increase its intensity. Past experiences with pain will also influence pain perception. Increased experience with pain will often lead to an increased perception that pain is threatening, which in turn leads to increased sensitivity to pain. Powerlessness regarding the cause of illness and the resulting pain reinforces an increased sensitivity to painful stimuli. Often the presence and attitudes of others influence pain perception. For example, a client who experiences annoyance from health care professionals regarding his or her expression of pain can have a more intense subjective experience with pain and a resulting fear of pain.

The client's perception of pain as a threat to life must be considered. As the perception of a threat to life, life-style, or body image increases, concurrent increases in anxiety, depression, pain intensity, and complaints about pain will occur. Subsequently, there will be an observable increase in the intensity of behavioral responses to pain.

Religious beliefs may have an impact on the meaning pain has for clients. Pain may be perceived as a punishment for not having followed God's teachings, or it may be accepted as part of God's plan—a component of life that is nonnegotiable but one that must be taken along with the good aspects of life. Clients who perceive pain as a punishment may pray for forgiveness, while those who perceive pain as a part of God's plan may pray for the ability to tolerate that pain.

The social acceptability of the body part involved influences clients' verbalization of pain. Pain experienced in the genitals or the rectum is frequently not expressed, because clients are embarrassed and do not know proper terminology to describe the location of the pain. In such a situation, a client will often select a health care professional on the basis of age, sex, occupational title, and ethnic background to discuss pain perceptions with—someone who is as similar as possible to himself or herself. For example, an older man may experience difficulty discussing his hemorrhoids with a young female nurse who is close to the age of one of his granddaughters. He may feel much more comfortable sharing his pain perceptions with a male attendant.

Culture may dictate very detailed and specific responses to pain. Reactions to pain vary according to a person's age, sex, and occupation. Culture may

TABLE 9-1 Coping model

Pain/self-image	Language	Self situation	Coping with pain	Client expectation
TYPE ONE				
Pain Powerful Coper: Passive victim	Merciless Cosmic Overwhelming Continuous Irrevocable Irreparable Irrational	Fragile Helpless Dread-filled Abandoned Alone Suffering	Skepticism Fate Ritual Magic	"Nothing will be effective."
TYPE TWO				
Pain: Invading Coper: Combat- ant	Episodic Strong Sharp Dominating Testing	Fighter Coper Survivor Soldier Confronter	Counterpain* Muscle lan- guage Delegates Assigns tasks Armamentarium	"Staff will help me to control pain."
TYPE THREE				
Pain: Reality Coper: Respon- sive	Testing Demanding Mysterious Hidden Cosmic	Confronter Endurer Suffering Analyzing Strategizing	Meditating Focusing Searching for meaning	"Meaning of pain is impor-tant to me. Staff treatment may intrude on my internal resources."
TYPE FOUR				
Pain: Cunning Coper: Reactive	Hidden Faceless Sneaky Sly Invading Degrading	Watcher Waiter Monitor Vigilant Ready	Anticipating Rehearsal Review Early warning Not risking Avoidance	"Staff will help me to avoid pain."
TYPE FIVE				
Pain: Demanding Coper: Interactive	Intense Persistent Sharp Probing Treacherous Ill-tempered Strong	Cooperator Collaborator Communicator Contractor Dependent Reporter Consumer	Contractual Arrangement Permission Compliant Bonding Rule keeper Sets limits	"I will enter into pain-control treatment plan. If pain management is effective, a bond is formed between me and the staff."

*Counter irritant, e.g., pinch, rub, etc., the pain area.
First four columns from Copp LA: Pain coping, In Copp L, editor: Perspectives of pain (Recent advances in nursing series), Edinburgh, 1985, Churchill-Livingstone Co.

also determine whether curative or palliative treatment is sought and whether the intensity and duration of pain are sufficient to merit reporting. Recognition of cultural influences allows a nurse to understand the significance of pain for each individual client as well as the overt response to that pain. Nurses thus can develop a wide range of approaches when intervening in the process of pain perception.

Since there are many ethnic groups within American society, nurses need to identify the influences that the culture has upon pain expectancy and pain acceptance. Zborowski (1969) has done extensive work in the field of pain perception and its cultural components. McCaffery (1979) supports Zborowski's belief that cultural background exerts more influence on behavioral response than the pain situation itself.

Each culture defines its own parameters of pain response, determines the necessity for pain relief, and dictates the type and duration of use of defense mechanisms employed to control increased levels of anxiety. For example, the "old Americans," typically third-generation Americans of white, Anglo-Saxon background, do not often verbalize pain. Their reflex response to pain is to withdraw rather than to cry out. These clients are frequently future-oriented and optimistic about treatment plans. They are often labeled "good" patients because they rarely ask for assistance. This type of behavior can be misleading to the nurse and can discourage the sharing of feelings regarding the pain experience.

Members of another group, Jewish-Americans, may describe pain as being "terrific" or "unbearable." Tolerance or acceptance of pain is usually low. Outward expressions of the stress of a pain experience are considered acceptable. Crying and moaning elicit sympathetic responses from others and serve to draw others close to the client. Jewish-Americans are future-oriented yet pessimistic about their treatment plans. They may seek several medical opinions.

Latin Americans and Americans of a Mediterranean background respond in a manner similar to that of Jewish-Americans. A low tolerance for pain exists, along with the need to verbalize one's inner response to a painful experience. There is, however, an orientation to the present; palliative relief is sought immediately.

Irish-Americans present another distinct response to the pain experience. The client is stoic, almost to the point of being unable to admit to experiencing pain. Withdrawal behavior is the means most frequently utilized to control overt responses. Pain is viewed as something one must face with the attitude of "grin and bear it." This group is future oriented, and its members accept the validity of information provided by the health care team.

Black Americans also have parameters of pain response. There is a denial of the existence of pain until it reaches an emergency state. Clients describe pain in general terms, and there is a reluctance to seek pain relief.

Each cultural group has its own parameters of pain tolerance and response behavior. The goal of a nursing assessment is not to rigidly categorize each client's subjective pain experience on the basis of ethnic group. However, as Larkin (1977) points out, "The experience of pain defies explanation in purely physiologic or biological terms; the sociocultural aspect of pain must be taken into account. The patient's cultural background influences not only attitudes towards pain but his response to it as well."

An important consideration in the assessment of the expression of pain is the reward or gain that a client derives from that expression. For example, clients who verbally express pain may elicit a sympathetic response from family, staff, and friends. They are placed in a dependent, "sick" role that releases them from the responsibilities of the adult-parent-spouse role. Clients who need to receive such a reward for the expression of pain may be attempting to adapt to a situation that has become excessively stressful, such as the increased responsibility associated with a new job, marriage, or parenting.

Pain is a subjective personal experience. Pain responses are altered by physical and physiological factors as well as by cultural and psychological determinants. To decide upon and implement a plan of action, a nurse should consider the overt as well as covert expressions of pain and their implications. "Bad" clients are not necessarily the ones who are most vocal about their pain, nor are the "good" clients necessarily the ones who stoically keep their complaints to themselves. Observation of responses to the pain experience will promote the accurate assessment of the implications of that experience for each client.

Nursing intervention may be based on an understanding of the theories of pain transmission. For example, Orshan (1988) notes that reflexology, Shiatsu, massage, and effleurage are strategies that function on the principle of ascending action that can close the pain gate. Other strategies that close the gate via descending action include meditation, relaxation techniques, hypnosis, imagery, humor therapy, and music. The following is a sample interaction of a client experiencing chronic pain.

Ms. Kay, a 28-year-old secretary, presented at the ambulatory care clinic with complaints of lower back pain for a two-week period. She has been unable to work, and her husband has been caring for the house and their 8-month-old daughter. Her husband has accompanied her to the clinic.

Nurse *I'd like to spend the next few minutes having you describe the pain for me—when it occurs, what it feels like, how it affects you.*

Client *It just seemed to begin about a month ago—so much was going on at that time. My parents had come to visit for two weeks and I was very busy getting ready for that.*

Nurse *Was there anything that you did that might have injured your back?*

Client *I was doing a lot of shopping and getting the house ready but nothing specific is apparent to me.*

Nurse *Had you had any previous back pain?*

Client *No, well once I did but that was several years ago.*

Nurse *Would you say there were any similarities between the pain that brought you here now and the pain then?*

Client *I was just starting my new job—I remember being very anxious about doing well.*

Nurse *Would you say that having your parents visit may generate some anxiety for you?*

Client *No, but I do like for everything to go well—they don't visit very often; my father doesn't like to travel very much.*

Nurse *Were you able to visit with them when they did come or was the back pain interfering with the visit?*

Client *I did visit but it wasn't much fun for them—they had to take care of the baby and prepare some of the meals. That wasn't what I had planned.*

The interaction continued with assessment of physical characteristics of the pain and implementation of strategies to meet the physical needs of the client. Further intervention with the client and husband would be directed toward identification of potential difficulty in expressing angry feelings as well as development of more effective strategies of coping with dependency needs.

Immobilization

Immobilization commonly causes stress that may affect all areas of function—physical, emotional, sociocultural, and cognitive. Prolonged immobilization has a profound impact on the psyche. Feelings of powerlessness occur. A reorganization of territory results. There may also be a redefining of self from young, strong, active, vigorous, and productive to weak, vulnerable, inactive, and nonproductive. There is a decreased physical ability and decreased energy level; full-time work is prohibited, yet there is little recreational ability available either. Clients perceive a sense of downward mobility, which in turn leads to a sense of loss of control and a decreased sense of self-worth.

To discuss the concept of immobilization as a stressor, we must consider the effect of immobilization on sensory status. When an individual is immobilized, multiple changes occur in the patterning and variation of incoming stimuli. One of the primary nursing actions is to identify each client's sensory status to maintain perceptual and responsive function. There is no clear-cut mechanism to determine at what point sensory overload or deprivation begins. But it is certain that there are gross changes in behavior when overload or deprivation occurs.

What occurs as a result of sensory overload or deprivation? The client experiences a decrease in the ability to solve problems. The ability to perform tasks requiring eye-hand coordination is decreased, as is perceptual alertness. Often there is disorientation to time, and the client feels as though his or her body parts were floating. Hallucinations and illusions are described vividly by clients who have spent extended periods of time in intensive- or coronary-care units, where restrictions regarding visitors, flowers, clocks, and reading materials are imposed. In these units, sensory overload may be experienced because of the constant humming of monitors or other types of machinery and the constant lighting, whether it be day or night. Clients rapidly lose orientation to time and place, since the familiar objects that act as cues are absent. Clients who are isolated in such units, as well as those who are restricted to their own homes or rooms, often experience a sense of overwhelming anxiety and depression.

Who fares well in these situations? Does everyone respond similarly, or are there persons who do not develop behavioral changes? The person who needs to be amused continuously—to be on the go or always engaged in some kind of activity—is the type of client who adapts poorly to sensory deprivation or overload. It has been found that, as in many other situations, clients who have developed successful adaptation mechanisms before their illnesses and whose egos are sound are better able to cope with the multiple effects of sensory deprivation or overload. This is not to say, however, that such clients rely solely upon their own resources for the development of adaptation mechanisms. Nursing intervention to prevent or reduce the effects of sensory deprivation or overload will be presented later in this chapter.

Immobilization and sensory deprivation or overload are stressors that are interwoven with one another. Each system of the body responds differently to prolonged periods of immobility. Often, immobilized clients must deal with many crises at once. For example, associated with immobilization are often changes in body image as well as in such normal bodily functions as breathing, urinating, and defecating. Concurrently, clients experience profound changes in emotional, social, and cognitive status. Nursing measures therefore must be directed toward identifying these changes as stressors and mobilizing clients' resources to help them adapt to their new situations.

Loss and change

In recent research, loss and concurrent changes have been identified as predominant stressors; they have been shown to precipitate varying degrees of anxiety. Life changes correlate with major health disruptions. Individuals who experience many changes over a short period seem to be more susceptible to illness. Toffler (1970) believes that too much change in too short a period can cause adverse physical as well as emotional reactions. Although this statement is not necessarily true for all individuals, it is imperative that nurses recognize the correlation between change and illness.

Holmes and Rahe (1967) developed a "social readjustment rating scale" on which are ranked stressful life events of both a positive nature (such as marriage, pregnancy, and promotion) and a negative nature (such as death of a spouse, divorce, or illness). Each event is rated in "life change units" (LCU's); the number of LCUs ranges from 100 to 19. Holmes and Rahe's hypothesis was that the greater the number of LCUs, the greater the probability of a client experiencing a health crisis. Table 9-2 lists the various stressful events and their corresponding numbers of LCUs.

The scale ranks life events according to their "stress value"—that is, the amount of coping that is required to adapt to them. The stressors listed include those which are threats to physiological integrity as well as those which are threats to self-esteem. Clients perceive stressful events differently, depending on their past experiences and their current emotional and physical health. By observing clients' responses to stressors, nurses can formulate comprehensive nursing care plans. (For further discussion of stress, see Chapter 8.)

Why do some people become ill as a result of stress while others are much more capable of adapting to stress with a minimal amount of health change? Are some people more vulnerable as a result of certain variables? Do some individuals have better outside support systems, more optimistic outlooks on life, or better health habits? McNeil and Pesznecker (1977) sought to discover whether good health habits, strong support systems, and a positive outlook could act as forces in assisting people to adapt to increased change. They noted that although the above variables made slight differences in the likelihood that major illness would occur, change was still the most significant factor. There are many ways in which a nurse, particularly in a community setting, can intervene on the primary level to help persons experiencing stress. The

TABLE 9-2 Social readjustment rating scale

Rank	Life event	Mean value
1	Death of spouse	100
2	Divorce	73
3	Marital separation	65
4	Jail term	63
5	Death of close family member	63
6	Personal injury or illness	53
7	Marriage	50
8	Fired at work	47
9	Marital reconciliation	45
10	Retirement	45
11	Change in health of family member	44
12	Pregnancy	40
13	Sex difficulties	39
14	Gain of new family member	39
15	Business readjustment	39
16	Change in financial state	38
17	Death of close friend	37
18	Change to different line of work	36
19	Change in number of arguments with spouse	35
20	Mortgage over $10,000	31
21	Foreclosure of mortgage or loan	30
22	Change in responsibilities at work	29
23	Son or daughter leaving home	29
24	Trouble with in-laws	29
25	Outstanding personal achievement	28
26	Wife begin or stop work	26
27	Begin or end school	26
28	Change in living conditions	25
29	Revision of personal habits	24
30	Trouble with boss	23
31	Change in work hours or conditions	20
32	Change in residence	20
33	Change in schools	20
34	Change in recreation	19
35	Change in church activities	19

Reprinted with permission from Holmes T and Rahe R: The social readjustment rating scale, J Psychosomatic Res 11:213-218. Copyright 1967, Pergamon Press, Ltd.

goal is to help individuals become managers of their own life changes rather than simply to help them cope with the crises that occur as a result of those changes.

Loss, like change, cannot be avoided during a lifetime. As individuals move through the life cycle, they are continuously experiencing some degree of loss—the loss of instant gratification of all demands, the loss of total dependence through learning to crawl and to walk, the loss of control over the environment through illness, the loss of hearing and sight, the loss of close friends through separation or death, the loss of independence through the aging process, and, finally, the loss of their own lives. How well individuals adapt to new losses depends, to a great extent, on past experiences with loss. If they have been positive, an individual can successfully assimilate new losses and changes. However, the more negative past experiences with loss have been, the greater the potential that a person will have difficulty in adapting to current losses.

This concept can be stated in another way: Early modes of adaptation to loss are the foundation of future patterns. To cite an example, the infant who is being weaned from the breast may receive nonverbal messages that this is a traumatic experience, and the experience may therefore be a negative one. For a more positive picture, consider the situation of a school-age child who moves away from his best friend. He and his parents discuss his feelings as well as theirs. There are open lines of communication and a sense of honesty. There is an understanding of the meaning of the loss to all involved. The child develops healthy patterns of adaptation, which are supported by his parents. The course has been set for the continuation of these healthy mechanisms in the future.

Nursing Intervention
PRIMARY PREVENTION—PAIN

The focus of primary prevention is the development of healthy patterns of coping with stress to increase the client's ability to cope with pain and decrease anxiety associated with the anticipation and aftermath of pain. The client will then be better able to recognize and to seek help for pain.

SECONDARY PREVENTION—PAIN

The focus of secondary prevention is the accurate assessment of pain for clients across all levels of development. Nurses must recognize factors influencing pain perception and expression, including social, psychological, and cultural imperatives that affect clients' identification and expression of pain. Nurses must also be cognizant of their own values and beliefs regarding the nature and expression of pain. Assessment and intervention are subsequently affected by one's own perceptions of pain and its management.

Nursing process

The nursing process is the mechanism that provides the framework for therapeutic intervention.

ASSESSMENT

Assessment is directed toward eliciting the following information: nature, duration, and type of pain; what relief measures are useful; meaning and perception of this pain experience; previous experience with pain; cultural and spiritual influences on pain expression; congruence of verbal and nonverbal expression of pain.

ANALYSIS OF DATA

Following a thorough assessment of client perception and response to pain, nursing diagnoses can be formulated as they relate to specific situations.

PLANNING AND IMPLEMENTATION

The following nursing care plan reflects a realistic approach to secondary preventive intervention. The nurse may initially establish goals; but as therapy progresses, the client should enter into goal setting to ensure commitment to accomplishing these goals.

PRIMARY PREVENTION—BODY IMAGE

The development of a positive self-image, including a positive attitude toward one's own body, is a critical focus of primary prevention. Positive feelings about one's body image permit open, direct, honest communication and the expression of feelings with others in the environment. Perceptions about body image emerge in the first year of life. Education of parents regarding the importance of reinforcing a positive body image through interaction with their children is an important function of nursing as a primary preventive measure. A positive sense of self develops as a result of affirming appraisals from the environment, particularly from parents and significant others.

NURSING CARE PLAN

Client With Chronic Lower Back Pain

Long-term Outcomes	Short-term Outcomes	Nursing Strategies
Nursing diagnosis: Chronic pain related to torn lower back ligaments (NANDA 9.1.1.1)*		
Establish effective methods of pain reduction Develop sense of positive self-worth with control over environment	To learn to identify the nature and duration of painful stimuli To learn to verbalize painful experiences within the context of his or her society and culture To develop more effective coping skills, which will reduce the effects of painful stimuli	Recognize that the pain experience is real to the person who is describing it. Explore the meaning of the pain experience with the client. Perhaps a desire for gain or reward is an important aspect of his or her behavior. Remain with the client during the painful experience. Perceptions of pain increase during the night or at other times when the client is left alone to focus on the pain. Reduce environmental stimuli of a noxious nature, such as excessive lighting and noise. Often a quiet, slightly darkened room serves to alleviate pain. Provide periods of rest and relaxation. It has been noted that fatigue potentiates the pain experience. Educate the client as to the various pain relief measures that are available; this enables the client to maintain a sense of control over his or her pain. Pain relief measures include breathing exercises, relaxation techniques, and guided imagery. Touch the client. Touching and other means of sensory input often reduce pain perception. Observe verbal and nonverbal expressions of pain. Are they congruent with one another? For example, does the client describe excruciating pain while lying casually on the bed watching television? Does the client deny pain even though he maintains a rigid posture while in the supine position? After careful observation of pain behavior, administer analgesics in a prudent manner. Document pain relief and attendant behavior. Behavior modification and hypnosis are used successfully in the management of pain. Surgery such as chordotomy may be indicated in the case of intractable pain. Assist the client to determine positions that reduce the pain.

*DSM-III-R diagnosis of idiopathic pain disorder applies if no physical findings of pain are evident—307.80. Other NANDA diagnoses for pain may include ineffective individual coping 5.1.1.1; anxiety 9.3.1; powerlessness 7.3.2.

SECONDARY PREVENTION— BODY IMAGE

The focus of secondary prevention is the accurate assessment of the effect of changes in body image on the client in relation to self-esteem, role function, and impact on life-style and implementation of strategies to facilitate the client's achievement of a higher level of well-being.

Nursing process

The nursing process is the mechanism that provides the framework for therapeutic intervention.

ASSESSMENT

Assessment reveals the meaning body image holds for the client and how his or her perception may change regarding self, depending upon the extent, duration, location, nature, and visibility of a body alteration. It is also important to note previous experience with successful coping strategies, availability of rehabilitation programs, availability of support networks, age of the client, degree of impact on life-style, and rapidity of onset of the change. The client's perception of body-image changes is a key factor in assessment. Since each individual is unique, this perception can vary from client to client.

ANALYSIS OF DATA

Assessment of presenting symptoms as well as coping strategies, changes in life-style, and perception of body-image changes leads the nurse to formulate a nursing diagnosis. The following diagnosis is intended to serve as a prototype for other changes in body image.

PLANNING AND IMPLEMENTATION

The following nursing care plan reflects a realistic approach to secondary preventive intervention. The nurse may initially establish goals; but as therapy progresses, the client should enter into goal setting to ensure commitment to accomplishing these goals.

PRIMARY PREVENTION— IMMOBILIZATION

The foci of primary prevention are to facilitate the client's adaptation to immobilization and to enable the client to maintain a positive sense of self.

SECONDARY PREVENTION— IMMOBILIZATION

The focus of secondary prevention is the assessment of the impact of immobilization on client behaviors and coping strategies within the framework of the nursing process.

Nursing process

The nursing process is the mechanism that provides the framework for therapeutic intervention.

ASSESSMENT

Assessment focuses on identification of physical, perceptual, and social deficits caused by immobility; the meaning of immobilization to the client; assessment of coping strategies; onset and duration of immobilization; previous experiences with immobilization; age at onset; and the availability of support systems.

ANALYSIS OF DATA

The assessment should provide an understanding of the presenting symptoms and their interrelationship with family dynamics, precipitating factors, and client coping strategies. Nursing diagnoses will reflect situation-appropriate changes in mobility.

PLANNING AND IMPLEMENTATION

The following nursing care plan reflects a realistic approach to secondary preventive intervention. The nurse may initially establish goals; but as therapy progresses, the client should enter into goal setting to ensure commitment to accomplishing these goals.

NURSING CARE PLAN

Client With Disturbed Body Image

Long-term Outcomes	Short-term Outcomes	Nursing Strategies
Nursing diagnosis:	Body image disturbance related to the surgical amputation of a limb (NANDA 7.1.1)*	
Integrate body change into current perception of body image. Develop positive sense of self incorporating change in body image	Observe stump 3 to 5 days postoperatively Identify and describe feelings associated with body-image changes Implement more effective coping strategies as necessary Participate in dressing changes 5 to 7 days postoperatively Identify changes in life-style resulting from alteration in body image	Identify areas of concern to the client by listening and observing for nonverbal messages. Explore feelings and validate the client's statements in relation to his or her changed body image. Rather than probe directly into this emotionally charged area ask open-ended questions. Emphasize the client's areas of strength—accentuate the positive! By mobilizing his or her own strengths, the client begins to regain a sense of worth and a more positive self-concept. Encourage physical movement, since it enhances the client's ability to integrate body changes into a new body image. The client develops competence through mastering his or her own body again. Facilitate the interaction of the client with others in his or her environment. Provide an atmosphere in which the client can gradually resume previous social roles as well as develop new ones. It is imperative that nurses allow the client to progress at his or her own pace. It is often helpful for the client to discuss feelings with others who have experienced similar alterations. Nurses can act as resource persons by contacting support groups as is necessary. Include the client in self-care activities that will increase the client's opportunities to become reacquainted with his or her body. Such activities as looking at a wound, participating in dressing changes, feeling the bandages or cast, and handling equipment (for example, colostomy bags, prostheses) are crucial in the restructuring of body image and self-concept. Recognize that the client will take cues from the nurse's reactions to his or her changed body image. The client is acutely aware of responses from the environment, and the client assimilates those responses into newly developing body image. Facilitate the expression of unresolved feelings such as anger, fear, hopelessness, and dependence by providing open lines of communication at all times. Include family and significant others in all aspects of the client's course of recovery. Encourage the sharing of feelings and concerns that they may have regarding the care of the client and his or her eventual resumption of previous roles (or assumptions of new ones). As was previously noted, responses from significant others are crucial.

*DSM-III-R diagnoses such as conversion disorder (300.11) and other somatoform disorders as appropriate. Other appropriate NANDA diagnoses may include impaired social interaction 3.1.1; altered role performance 3.2.1; altered sexuality patterns 3.3; ineffective individual coping 5.1.1.1; impaired physical mobility 6.1.1.1; anxiety 9.3.1; self-esteem disturbance 7.1.2; personal identity disturbance 7.1.3.

NURSING CARE PLAN

Client With Impaired Physical Mobility

Long-term Outcomes	Short-term Outcomes	Nursing Strategies

Nursing diagnosis: Impaired physical mobility related to full body cast secondary to spinal surgery (NANDA 6.1.1.1)*

Long-term Outcomes	Short-term Outcomes	Nursing Strategies
Develop effective methods of coping with immobilization Maintain a positive sense of self	Identify and describe feelings associated with immobilization Identify successful coping strategies to resolve sensory overload and/or deprivation Select options that will facilitate participation in activities of daily living	Provide such physical activities as turning and moving of unaffected parts of the body within the confines dictated by the client's situation. Movement helps the client to determine his or her own body space, which may have been altered by the immobilization. Activity also serves to reduce the severity of the negative physiological effects of prolonged immobilization. Identify individual effects of sensory overload or deprivation. For example, while one client may quietly accept all the medical procedures being done for him or her, another client may evidence hypersensitivity to the environment by being acutely aware of and involved in all of these activities. This type of client needs to feel a sense of control over the environment. The nurse can facilitate this control by providing information and including the client in the care process. Maintain sensory-perceptual stimulation by means of newspapers, television, radio, and visitors. Reduce environmental stimuli of a monotonous nature, including noise, lighting, and personnel impinging on the client's space. Identify adaptation mechanisms, along with their efficiency levels, in the current situation and in past situations of a similar nature. What are similarities and differences? Accentuate ego strengths. How can they be developed in the client's best interest? Describe the client's immediate environment, and explain the various sights, sounds, and smells. This enables the client to understand the patterns of what is going on around him or her. Allow the client to resume activities at his or her own pace. Introduce changes in routine slowly and with brief explanations of rationale. Structure the environment and activities so that the client is not expected to accomplish tasks that require in-depth problem-solving processes. Sensory overload or deprivation decreases his or her capacity to learn and to solve problems.

*DSM-III-R diagnoses such as conversion disorder (300.11) may be applicable if there is psychogenic basis for immobilization. Other appropriate NANDA diagnoses may include ineffective individual coping 5.1.1.1; impaired social interaction 3.1.1; altered patterns of sexuality 3.3; altered role performance 3.2.1; sensory/perceptual alterations (specify) 7.2; body image disturbance 7.1.1.

Long-term Outcomes	Short-term Outcomes	Nursing Strategies

Nursing diagnosis: Impaired physical mobility related to full body cast secondary to spinal surgery (NANDA 6.1.1.1)*—cont'd

When you consider a roommate for an immobilized client, it is often wise to place the immobilized client with a person who is oriented toward and involved with the environment.

Provide an atmosphere of open communication whereby the client may verbalize concerns or fears relating to immobilization.

Point out inappropriate responses, such as prolonged hallucination, hostility, withdrawal, or belligerence, to the nursing team. Consultation with a psychiatric nurse-clinician or a physician may be necessary.

Include family members and significant others in the nursing care plan of the immobilized client. Assist them to recognize and understand the effects of prolonged immobilization (for example, sensory overload or deprivation). They may also be instrumental in enabling the client to resume former social roles or to develop new ones.

The primary goal of nursing care is to recognize situations that may cause sensory overload or deprivation and the clients who are potentially at risk. Nurses should consider not only those clients who are physically immobilized but also those who have social, emotional, or cognitive impairments. Individuals in mental institutions or orphanages, the elderly, the blind, the deaf, and the mute—these are just a few of the target populations that are at high risk in regard to the effects of sensory overload or deprivation.

PRIMARY PREVENTION—LOSS

Primary prevention focuses on the early development of adaptive strategies to effect a healthy resolution of the crises of change and loss. Within the family setting, children can be encouraged to grieve openly and to share the positive and negative aspects of change and loss. It is imperative that individuals learn methods of coping in the early phases of life, since change and loss characterize every stage of the life cycle. Those who have learned effective strategies and have experienced successful resolution of the crises of loss and change will be less likely to experience major difficulties in coping with these crises in later life.

SECONDARY PREVENTION—LOSS

The focus of secondary prevention is the accurate assessment of the effect of loss and change and to implement strategies that facilitate the client's achievement of a higher level of well-being.

Nursing process

The nursing process is the mechanism that provides the framework for therapeutic intervention.

ASSESSMENT

Assessment focuses on the client's strengths and the client's ability to make active choices regarding the course of his or her life. The client needs to prepare for change and constructively resolve issues of loss. The following are areas to consider in the assessment: previous life changes (within past year), effectiveness of coping strategies, presence of maturational crises, level of helplessness or hopelessness, level of ego strength, presence of support systems, previous experiences with loss, phase of grief, and perception of life following loss.

ANALYSIS OF DATA

The assessment should reflect the client's responses to loss, presenting symptoms, level of integration, and use of coping strategies as well as the impact of family and environmental dynamics. Nursing diagnoses will be formulated on the basis of individual situations. The following nursing diagnosis serves as a protocol for individuals experiencing loss.

PLANNING AND IMPLEMENTATION

The following nursing care plan reflects a realistic approach to secondary preventive intervention. The nurse may initially establish goals; but as therapy progresses, the client should enter into goal setting to ensure commitment to accomplishing these goals.

NURSING CARE PLAN

Client with Job Loss

Long-term Outcomes	Short-term Outcomes	Nursing Strategies
Nursing diagnosis: Altered role performance related to loss of current employment status (NANDA 3.2.1)*		
Resolve loss through appropriate grieving process Integrate changes resulting from loss	Verbalize anger, helplessness, and other feelings related to loss Identify and develop successful methods of coping with loss Mobilize available resources to assist in coping with loss	Encourage the verbal expression of feelings of anger, helplessness, fear, or hopelessness by maintaining open lines of communication. Support the client yet allow the client time to grieve. Be there when the client feels the need to relate to another human being. (See Chapter 22 for further discussion of grief.) Facilitate participation in activities of daily living. Support attempts to engage in such new behavior as managing the checkbook or putting on the storm doors. Gradually encourage the client's reinvestment in new object relationships. Since this process often reemphasizes the sense of loss, it should be paced cautiously. Identify ego strengths. Help the client to perceive himself or herself as a worthwhile human being who is capable of experiencing life to its fullest in spite of loss. Direct the client in anticipatory planning by preparing him or her for what changes and/or losses lie ahead. Persons who are most in need of such planning include expectant parents, couples contemplating mar-

---

*Other appropriate NANDA diagnoses may include anxiety 9.3.1; impaired social interaction 3.1.1; ineffective individual coping 5.1.1.1; impaired adjustment 5.1.1.1.1; powerlessness 7.3.2.

EVALUATION

The client and family and significant others should be included in evaluating the client's progress toward achievement of long- and short-term outcomes. A comprehensive evaluation should incorporate the following criteria:

1. Evaluation of the degree to which conflicts have been resolved
2. Evaluation of the degree to which goals have been accomplished and client functioning has improved as demonstrated by a decrease in maladaptive coping behaviors and utilizing effective strategies of coping
3. Identification of goals that need to be modified

4. Referral of the client to other support systems:
   a. Network of support in client's environment who are willing and capable of acting as support persons
   b. Community agencies that provide resources to assist clients in living with changes incurred by the stressor, i.e., ostomy clinics and enterostomal therapists
   c. Centers that specialize in assisting clients to cope with specific stressors, i.e., pain clinics
   d. Support groups, self-help groups that can provide ongoing support such as ostomy groups, amputee groups

Long-term Outcomes	Short-term Outcomes	Nursing Strategies

Nursing diagnosis: Altered role performance related to loss of current employment status (NANDA 3.2.1)*—cont'd

		riage, adolescents who are experiencing maturational crises, clients in low-income housing projects, individuals whose spouses have chronic or terminal illnesses, couples that are separating or divorcing, clients who move frequently, clients who are about to experience menopause, and individuals who are about to retire. To focus on these groups before the onset of illness is a major nursing priority.
		Assess the client's previous life changes in light of adaptive mechanisms used—their effectiveness or ineffectiveness in coping with the stress incurred as a result of the change or loss. What symptoms does the client have?
		Educate the client—on either an individual or a group basis. The client learns through relationships with group members and nursing staff how to become a manager of his or her own life. The client need not wait for a major health crisis to occur. Instead, the client's preparation for and understanding of change and loss enable him or her to develop successful adaptation mechanisms. Pressures of life will no longer seem insurmountable. Some changes may be delayed while the client is adapting to those of higher priority. The goal of intervention is the recognition of changes and their impact on life-style.
		Refer to community resources that may help the client adjust to changes in life-style.

TERTIARY PREVENTION

The focus of tertiary prevention is on the assessment of ongoing maladaptive responses to alterations in body image, immobilization, chronic pain, and situations that generate loss and change. Intervention at the level is directed toward facilitating client resolution of maladaptive coping strategies and minimizing further effects of these maladaptive strategies.

CHAPTER SUMMARY

Four commonly encountered stressors—alterations in body image, pain, immobilization, and loss and change—have been presented. These stressors pose varying degrees of threat to self-esteem and the ability to cope in an adaptive manner. Key concepts to the understanding of these stressors in-clude the perception of the event and the degree and type of coping mechanisms utilized.

Primary, secondary, and tertiary preventive measures in relation to these stressors have been presented. Primary prevention directs its efforts toward the identification and management of the potential effects of the stressors. Secondary prevention involves the implementation of nursing strategies. Tertiary prevention is the assessment of those chronic maladaptive responses and the implementation of efforts to minimize permanent detrimental effects.

Evaluation of all levels of intervention is an integral component of the nursing process. Through a mutual evaluation by client and nurse, ongoing effective intervention is maintained until the client reaches his or her highest level of functioning.

SELF-DIRECTED LEARNING

Self-Awareness Exercises

1. Types of exercises
   a. Think about your body, its appearance and functioning. Identify one body part that you view as central to your body image. Next, imagine yourself with that body part mutilated or dysfunctioning.
      (1) What feelings are evoked?
      (2) How do you think this change would affect your relationship with significant others? Your interaction with strangers?
      (3) What effect do you think it would have on your ability to establish a meaningful sexual relationship? At what point in the relationship would you disclose or discuss the alteration in your body?
      (4) What influences have your family, your society, and your religious and ethnic heritage had in the formation of your attitudes and feelings about this body part and your anticipated reaction to the alteration?
   b. Recall an incident in which you experienced pain that lasted a minimum of several hours. This pain may have been from something as common as a toothache or a severe headache or from something more complex (such as surgery, an accident, or an illness).
      (1) Describe the pain both verbally and pictorially (the picture may be abstract or concrete).
      (2) How old were you when you experienced this pain?
      (3) What were your feelings during your pain experience?
      (4) What occurrences or factors seemed to increase your perception of pain? Decrease your perception of pain?
      (5) What were your responses to your pain?
      (6) How long did your pain last?
      (7) What were your feelings and responses when your pain was over?
      (8) Ask family and friends to tell you their perceptions of your reactions during and after your pain experience.
      (9) How do your responses to pain compare with the responses of your family members to pain? With the responses of other mem-

bers of your religious or ethnic group to pain?

c. Spend an entire day in a wheelchair or immobilized in bed (this means you cannot ambulate and can only change position with assistance). Keep a diary of the day. (The entries in your diary may be written or may be made on a tape recorder. If you discontinue the exercise before the day ends, discuss why you made that decision.) Your diary entries should discuss the following:
   (1) How immobilization affects your physical, perceptual, and social functioning
   (2) How immobilization changes your lifestyle
   (3) Your feelings
   (4) The mechanisms you use to cope with immobilization
   (5) Assistance you receive from others
   (6) The reactions of others to your immobilization
   (7) Factors in the physical and social environment that facilitate or make more difficult your attempts to cope with immobilization

2. Purposes of the exercises:
   a. To facilitate the development of insight into factors that influence one's own perception of, interpretation of, and response to altered body image, pain, and immobilization
   b. To facilitate the development of sensitivity to clients who are experiencing altered body image, pain, or immobilization
   c. To increase understanding of the effect that one's family, ethnic heritage, religious affiliation, and society have on the perception of, interpretation of, and response to altered body image, pain, and immobilization

Questions to Consider

1. During the second night following admission, an elderly client complains about intense abdominal pain. The day staff indicate that this is different from her pain behavior during the day. The increase in response to pain during the night is based on the principle that:
   a. People do not have pain as frequently during the day
   b. The body responds to stimuli of lesser intensity at that time
   c. There are more staff available to respond to client needs
   d. Endorphins are stimulated more readily when the body is at rest

2. An individual who copes with pain by assuming the role of passive victim may describe the role of the staff in pain management by which of the following statements?
   a. "No one can help the pain."
   b. "The staff can help me control the pain."
   c. "The staff will take away my ability to control my pain."
   d. "Staff will help me to avoid my pain."

3. Which of the following nursing strategies best illustrates the concept of primary prevention when working with clients who are experiencing stress associated with loss and change?
   a. Recommend the use of minor tranquilizers to lower stress levels
   b. Encourage clients to minimize the effect change has on daily life
   c. Assist clients to understand the meaning that loss has on future response to loss
   d. Engage clients in psychoanalysis to reduce unresolved conflicts, which produce stress

4. Successful intervention with a client who has experienced body image changes as a result of physical illness or trauma includes
   a. Limited physical movement of the affected part
   b. Recognizing that denial is an unhealthy factor in the healing process immediately following the trauma
   c. Facilitating the client's interaction with others in the environment
   d. Referral to a psychotherapist

Select the answer from the second column that best matches the group in the first column.

5. Anglo-Saxon	a. Future-oriented; pessimistic
6. Jewish-American	b. Future-oriented; withdrawn; stoic
7. Latin-American	c. Present-oriented; low tolerance; increased verbalization
8. Irish-American	d. Future-oriented; optimistic; "good" patient
	e. Reluctant to seek treatment until emergency exists

Answer key

1. b	3. c	5. d	7. c
2. a	4. c	6. a	8. b

REFERENCES

American Psychiatric Association: Diagnostic and statistical manual of mental disorders (DSM-III-R), Washington, DC, 1987, The Association.

Burkholz H: Pain: solving the mystery, New York Times Magazine Part II, September 27, 1987, pp. 16-19, 32, 34-35.

Copp LA: Pain coping model and typology, Image: J Nurs Scholarship 25(3), 1985.

Feldman H: Psychological differentiation and the phenomenon of pain, Adv Nurs Sci 6(2):50-57, 1984.

Holmes T and Rahe R: The social readjustment scale, J Psychosom Res 11:213-218, 1967.

Kolb L: Disturbances of the body image, In Arieti S, editor: American handbook of psychiatry, vol 1, New York, 1959, Basic Books, Inc.

Larkin F: The influence of one patient's culture on pain response, Nurs Clin North Am 12(4):156-162, 1977.

McCaffery M: Nursing management of the patient with pain, ed 2, Philadelphia, 1979, JB Lippincott Co.

McKean K: Pain, Discover 7, (10):82-92, 1986.

McLane A, editor: Classification of nursing diagnoses, St. Louis, 1987, The CV Mosby Co.

McNeil J and Pesznecker B: Keeping people well despite life change crises, Pub Health Rep 92(4):343-348, 1977.

Melzack R and Wall P: The challenge of pain, New York, 1982, Basic Books.

Orshan S: Pain and stress management in nursing: controversy and theory, Holistic Nurs Prac 2(3):9-16, 1988.

Taylor A: Pain, Ann Rev Nurs Res, vol 5, 1987.

Toffler A: Future shock, New York, 1970, Random House.

Zborowski M: People in pain, San Francisco, 1969, Jossey-Bass, Inc.

ANNOTATED SUGGESTED READINGS

American Pain Society: Relieving pain: an analgesic guide, Am J Nurs, pp 815-826, 88, 1988.

This continuing education presentation was developed by the American Pain Society to bridge the gap between knowledge of pharmacology and its application in clinical practice. Relevant information includes the differences between acute and chronic pain, the principles of analgesic therapy, the differences between physical and psychological dependence and tolerance, and the stepwise management of pain.

Donovan M, editor: Pain control, Nurs Clinics N Am 22(3), September 1987.

This volume present a selection of articles that represented a variety of topics relevant to pain—its definition, management measures, ethical dilemmas, and assessment factors. The authors provide various perspectives and explore current research including both qualitative and quantitative data. It is important to note that these authors seem committed to improving patient care across all levels of development. It is the goal of this symposium to alert nurses to the issue relevant to pain, to provide alternative solutions, and to direct research for the future.

Larkin D and Zahourek R, editors: Stress, coping, and pain. Holistic Nurs Prac, 2(3), May 1988.

This volume explores the issues of pain and its relationship to the concept of stress. Present theories of pain are presented, and relevant nursing strategies are identified. The concept of holism acts as a central theme for the discussion of pain and stress management, biofeedback, touch, humor intervention, relaxation, guided imagery, and therapeutic storytelling. This volume may also be applicable to Chapter 8, Anxiety and Stress.

FURTHER READINGS

Camp L et al: Comparison of medical, surgical and oncology patients' descriptions of pain and nurses' documentation of pain assessments, J Adv Nurs 12(5):593-596, 1987.

Favaloro R: Adolescent development and implications for pain management, Ped Nurs 14(1):27-29, 1988.

Gauvin-Piquard A et al: Pain in children aged 2-6 years: a new observational rating scale elaborated in a pediatric oncology unit—a preliminary report, Pain 31(2):177-188, 1987.

Geach B: Pain and coping, Image: J Nurs Scholarship 19(1):12-15, 1987.

Hurley A: Cognitive development and children's perception of pain, Ped Nurs 14(1):21-24, 1988.

Martin B et al: Influence of cultural background on nurses' attitudes and care of the oncology patient in Africa and in Midwest America, Cancer Nurs 9(5):713-716, 1986.

Platzer H: Body image—a problem for intensive care nurses, part I, Intensive Care Nurs 3(2):61-66, 1987.

Platzer H: Body image: helping patients to cope with changes—a problem for nurses, part II, Intensive Care Nurs 3(3):125-132, 1987.

Whipple B: Methods of pain control: review of research and literature, Image: J Nurs Scholarship 19(3):142-146, 1987.

Basic concepts of communication

CHAPTER FOCUS

Communication is a process involving three levels of interaction: verbal, kinesic, and proxemic. Just as language varies from culture to culture, kinesic behavior and proxemic behavior are also culturally variable. When members of different cultures interact, dissimilar verbal, kinesic, and proxemic cues can contribute to misunderstandings and disruption of role relationships. Therapeutic communication involves more than learning a body of interviewing skills. It involves understanding the process of communication and the influence of culture on communication.

Communication is the social matrix of psychiatry. Until recently, health workers have focused primarily on verbal communication. Now they are beginning to recognize the importance of nonlinguistic communication—kinesics, the use of body parts in communication, and proxemics, the use of space in communication.

Meaning is communicated each time one member of a society interacts with another member. This is known as a *cultural event*. For instance, think of all the verbal and nonverbal ways that people communicate the message of dominance-submission.

The United States is a nation of immigrants. Its population is an ethnic mix. Even though most of its people speak English, they use ethnically patterned kinesic and proxemic behavior. Even when people speak the same language, it cannot be assumed that there is shared meaning. Communication may be misunderstood; communication problems may arise. Knowledge of the process of communication and the influence of culture on communication may prevent the development of communication barriers and may help to establish therapeutic communication.

Communication is the act of imparting and exchanging ideas, information, and feelings with others. People communicate through both verbal and nonverbal expression. Verbal communication is spoken language: the words we use and the way we use them. Nonverbal communication embraces kinesics and proxemics: the way we move body parts and the way we use the space around us. The two modes of communication—verbal and nonverbal—are neither separate nor unrelated. Instead, they are different *levels* of communication that systematically interrelate to reinforce, supplement, or contradict one another. This chapter will discuss some classic studies in linguistic and nonverbal communication as well as more recent communication studies.

VERBAL COMMUNICATION

"In the beginning was the word...." Verbal communication refers to spoken language, to the sounds (paralanguage) and words we use when we communicate. Language influences the way people perceive, interpret, and respond to the world around them. For instance, the grammatical forms of American Indian languages influence Indians' perception of relatedness. Many of these languages do not contain coersive or possessive words. The Wintu Indians of California cannot say "I have a child" or "I took my child to the doctor." Wintu language does not permit such expression. Instead, the Wintu say, "I live with the child" or "I went with the child to the doctor." Similarly, the Navaho Indians of Arizona and New Mexico guide rather than command their children to observe numerous Navaho taboos. Navaho parents do not speak of teaching children to obey or of punishing children. Instead, they explain that when a taboo is broken, a specific unpleasant consequence follows. When a child violates a taboo, parents view it as a mistake that the child must rectify and not as a consequence of something that parents either did or did not do. Thus language plays an important role in reinforcing the concepts of permissiveness and personal

integrity that are central to the interpersonal relationships of many American Indians.

Any group of people can create arbitrary meanings for words and phrases. An ethnic group, an age group, a social class, or an occupational group may have its own vocabulary (Ervin-Tripp, 1977). For example, the abbreviation "S.O.B." has a different meaning to nurses than to the general public. The shared meaning and understanding of language help to create and maintain a sense of identity, belonging, and exclusivity. To understand the way people communicate verbally, we must have some knowledge of the properties of spoken language.

Properties of spoken language

In this section, we will utilize some classic linguistic studies in discussing the properties of spoken language. The basic components in the structure of language are phonemes, morphemes, and syntax. Phonemes and morphemes form the basic units of the expressive system (sound system) of language. A phoneme is a minimal unit of sound that distinguishes one utterance from another. For example, the /p/ sound in the word "pet" is a phoneme. In addition, there may be variants of a phoneme. For example, the aspirated /k^h/ is a variant of the unaspirated /k/, as in /ski/ (s<u>k</u>y) versus /k$^{\overline{h}}$e/ (key) (Gleason, 1961). Immigrants may have difficulty learning the phoneme variants of the language of the host country. This sometimes causes communication difficulties and stress.

A school nurse–teacher noticed that a 10-year-old Cuban girl who had immigrated three years before frequently came to the infirmary with complaints of headache and upset stomach. During a conference with the girl's teacher, the school nurse learned that although the girl was conversant in English, she had difficulty with phoneme variants. When she spoke in class, her classmates would laugh. The girl would then become embarrassed, quiet, and withdrawn. The school nurse recognized that the language problem was causing the girl stress and that it might undermine her self-concept. The school nurse therefore referred the girl to the school's speech therapist.

TABLE 10-1 Properties of verbal language

Unit	Behavior	Example
Phoneme	Utterance	/p/ sound
Morpheme	Meaningful utterance	/p/ sound combines with other sounds to give meaning to the utterance, as in "pin" vs. "nip"
Syntax	Utterance of phrases and sentences	"The sky is blue"

A morpheme is a *meaningful* sound that cannot be broken down into smaller meaningful sounds. Root words such as "walk" and "trot" and affixes such as "ed," "ing," and "s" are examples of morphemes. In addition, morphemes, like phonemes, can have variants. For instance, /z/ is a variant of the affix /s/, as in /sk ez/ (skis) versus /räks/ (rocks). Phonemes and morphemes are related because every morpheme is composed of phonemes (Gleason, 1961.)

Syntax, the third component in the structure of language, refers to structural cues and the arrangement of words into phrases and sentences. Syntax tells how a sentence should fit together (Bloomfield, 1933). In English, the usual order is subject-verb-object.

Types of structural cues include intonation, transition, and pitch. Taken together, pitch, intonation, and transition usually mark off phrases and sentences and tell us about their construction. For example, sentences that terminate with a rise in pitch are usually questions, whereas those which drop in pitch are usually declarative statements (Gleason, 1961). Table 10-1 outlines the properties of spoken language just discussed.

Although spoken language changes, the rate of change is usually slow enough so that speakers of the same language are able to communicate. When linguistic variations cause communication difficulties between speakers of the same language, we say that the people speak different dialects (Bloomfield, 1933; Jesperson, 1967).

Culture and spoken language

Spoken language is culturally specific. The relationship between language and culture can be divided into the following two areas of exploration:

1. World view, which looks at whether culture is influenced by language or whether language influences culture
2. Sociolinguistics, which studies the relationship between language and the social context in which it occurs (Eastman, 1975)

WORLD VIEW

Some linguists believe that language structures thought and defines experience, thereby determining world view. Because members of a language community share a similar perception of the world, any given reality, whether physical or social, can be structured in various ways. Different languages utilize different structures. Therefore, there is no universal reality but many different realities. By understanding the meaning of a people's language, we learn about their thought process, culture, and perception of reality (Whorf, 1956; Sapir, 1964; Lucy and Shweder, 1979).

Antilanguage is an example of language emerging from, creating, and reinforcing the social structure of society, in this case an "antisociety" (a society that runs counter to society-at-large). The role and function of antilanguage is to create an alternative reality that emphasizes certain "anti" aspects of society. Antilanguage words refer to the central activities of the counterculture and they express meanings and values that are not shared by the rest of established society. Antilanguage thus creates and maintains an alternative reality and an alternative social structure with its own system of values, sanctions, rewards and punishments (Halliday, 1976).

A nurse began working in an adolescent treatment program. Most of the youths in the program had been referred there because of drug abuse and juvenile delinquency. The nurse discovered that the youths had their own language, a language that he did not understand. For instance, there were many new words for police, drugs, and acts of vandalism. The nurse soon realized that this language served a dual purpose for the youths. It created and described the reality of their counterculture and, because it was not understood by members of "straight" society, it acted as a boundary-maintenance mechanism.

However, some anthropologists do not agree with the view that separate realities are generated by different language systems. These anthropologists argue that there is a universal reality and that different societies segment this reality differently. Language and the number of words in a language that refer to specific concepts permit the members of a language community to be more aware of and more articulate about certain aspects of their environment but do not create separate realities (Fishman, 1960; Berlin and Kay, 1969).

SOCIOLINGUISTICS

Some linguists seek to identify and describe the characteristics of and the interrelationships between language varieties, the functions of language, and the speakers. The basic unit of analysis is a speech community. A speech community is a social group that shares a similar understanding of the speech and rules of at least one dialect of the several dialects or languages that may be found within a particular locale (Fishman, 1971; Hymes, 1972).

Sociolinguists have found that people who speak a common language often use different rule systems. This sometimes leads to misinterpretation of communication. Two rules, the violation of which may cause misunderstandings, are the rules of alternation and co-occurrence (Ervin-Tripp, 1972). *Alternation rules* establish the alternatives available to a speaker, such as whether to address a person by title, first name, surname, or any combination of these options (Ervin-Tripp, 1972).

In one unit of a hospital, clients called student nurses by their first names and graduate nurses by their surnames. However, clients usually addressed the clinical nurse specialists by their titles and surnames (for example, Dr. Traube).

Ervin-Tripp points out that social categories such as kinship, sex, status, age, and type of interpersonal relationship influence the range of alternatives available to a speaker.

Rules of co-occurrence mandate the use of the same level of structure, be it lexical or syntactic (Ervin-Tripp, 1972). For example, the rule of co-occurrence is followed when a bilingual client uses Spanish syntax and pronunciation when speaking Spanish and English syntax and pronunciation when speaking English. Conversely, the rule is violated when a bilingual client uses the syntactic order of one language and the vocabulary of another language.

Bilingual ethnic groups may reveal diverse forms of consciousness through language choice. The choice of language may reflect perceptions about one's own ethnic group as well as perceptions of the dominant society. Factors influential in patterns of linguistic choice include interclass relations and the politicoeconomic position of one's ethnic group within society. *Codeswitching*, the juxtaposing of elements from different language systems, may occur. Some ethnic groups may engage in codeswitching within a single turn of talk; others may compartmentalize language and speak their native language in the private sphere and the dominant language in the public sphere. Patterns of language choice reflect attitudes not only about language but also about the people, activities, social solidarity, and power relations associated with a particular language (Gumperz, 1982; Woolard, 1985; Myers and Myers, 1985; Gal, 1987).

A community health nurse served a catchment area that had a sizeable Hispanic population. The English-speaking population resented the influx of Hispanics and openly voiced the belief that if Hispanics wanted to live in the United States, "they should at least learn to speak English.'' The community health nurse noticed that in the shops owned by English-speaking shop-keepers and in the neighborhood health station, where many of the nurses were bilingual, Hispanic clients spoke English. They explained to the community health nurse that they would never ''make good'' in the United States unless they learned English. However, at home and at solely Hispanic social gatherings, Spanish was spoken.

Politicoeconomic factors made it advantageous for Hispanics to speak English in the public sphere. English was associated with social and economic status. Codeswitching (language compartmentalization) was perceived as essential for assimilation and upward mobility.

Spoken language is part of any communication system. It communicates needs, feelings, and intentions. The properties of verbal communication can be identified, described, and analyzed. In looking at the communication value of speech, we have seen the importance of understanding the interrelationship between language and the context in which it occurs. We will now explore another level of human communication: nonverbal communication.

NONVERBAL COMMUNICATION

Nonverbal communication is any type of communication other than verbal. We will focus on two areas of nonverbal communication: kinesics and proxemics. *Kinesics* refers to the way we use body parts when we communicate, and *proxemics* refers to the way we use space when we communicate. Observation will show that body movements and spatial arrangements *do* communicate significant information. We can think of kinesics as body language and of proxemics as space language.

Kinesics

Birdwhistle (1963, 1970), a pioneer in the field of kinesics, recognized certain similarities between spoken and written language and body language. His research was guided by two basic assumptions: that individuals are constantly maneuvering to ac-

commodate the presence and activities of other individuals and that the system of kinesic movement is learned and ultimately analyzable. To understand the way people communicate kinesically, we must have some knowledge of the properties of kinesic behavior.

PROPERTIES OF KINESIC BEHAVIOR

Kinesic behavior is most often unconsciously performed. It is found both among primates and among other mammals. Socialization plays an important role in transmitting kinesic systems from generation to generation. Body movements are responsive to an individual's biopsychocultural state and usually vary in form and meaning according to ethnic background, sex, age, and social class (Birdwhistle, 1970; Scheflen and Scheflen, 1972; Argyle, 1975; Vargas, 1986).

The point of origin, speed, and destination of a gesture, empathic assessment, a person's psychophysiological state and cultural backgound, and the context in which a gesture is made are all involved in the way a person reads and responds to the body movements of another. For example, when a man with whom we are conversing raises his arm, we rapidly and unconsciously ask ourselves, "What is he doing? Is he friend or foe? What do I mean when I do that? What has happened in similar situations when someone has raised his arm like that? Who is he aiming at?" The interpretation we arrive at and the way we respond will vary greatly—they depend on our answers to these questions. Certainly the raising of an arm by a stranger on the street has a different meaning from the same gesture performed by a friend at a cocktail party, an opponent in a sports arena, or a person receiving physiotherapy.

Body movements, then, are very important to our understanding of others and to being understood by others. Just as individuals have the physical capacity for producing thousands of sounds, but are limited by language to the use of only a very few, each individual, on the basis of culture, uses only a relatively small number of the many motions available for communication. Kinesic behavior can be classified according to function. Three types of body movement aid in communication: markers, reciprocals, and territorials. (Scheflen and Scheflen, 1972; Krivonos and Knapp, 1975; Knapp et al., 1975).

Markers act as punctuation points and indicators:

During a group therapy session, it was observed that participants lowered their heads, eyebrows, and hands at the end of statements, but raised one or all of these body parts when they asked questions. Moreover, when one participant accused another of monopolizing the session, he pointed his head and right hand in the direction of the accused and said, "Harry doesn't give any of us a chance to get a word in edgewise."

Can there be any question that these group members were using their bodies to clarify or dramatize situations?

When people make one gesture as they say one word and another gesture as they speak the next word and so on, we say that they are using markers of speech. Gestures are also used to mark the beginnings and endings of sentences. For example, at the end of a sentence, people not only lower voice pitch but also lower their hands and heads. On the other hand, when people ask a question, they raise their voices, heads, and eyebrows. When people have completed an idea, they usually signal this fact by shifting their eyes and heads and changing their posture. When they begin to express another idea, they again shift kinesically.

Whereas markers of speech involve only the speaker, markers of discourse involve both speaker and listener. People try to obtain speaking rights in one of several ways, depending on the situation. They may stand, as when making a formal presentation. They may remain seated, but lean forward and extend one or both hands into the space in front of them. They may lean back in their seats and either steeple their fingers or place the palms of their hands behind their heads. These latter types of posturing often indicate that the people about to speak have some status, and the posturings are usually differentiated by sex. Women tend to steeple, while men tend to place the palms of their hands

behind their heads. Meanwhile, listeners are looking in the direction of the speaker, occasionally making eye contact with the speaker, and intermittently making such listening movements as nodding. In addition, if speaker and listeners are in rapport, they indicate this by posturing and moving in synchrony. Finally, when discourse is completed, a terminal marker signals the end of the encounter. Participants lower their eyes and engage in some parting ritual such as shaking hands, kissing, or palm brushing.

Reciprocals indicate affiliation between people. Reciprocals include bond-servicing behavior (behavior that reinforces interpersonal bonds, such as exchanging food and drink or giving affection and attention) and empathic behavior (such as looking sympathetic or exchanging winks and smiles).

Courtship behavior and quasicourtship behavior are also reciprocals. Courtship behavior is characterized by increased muscle tonus and preening. A message of intimacy is conveyed. Women protrude their breasts and display their wrists or palms. Men display their chests by straightening up, contracting abdominal muscles, and squaring their shoulders. Voices are kept low so that conversations will not be overheard. Quasicourtship behavior, on the other hand, contains qualifiers or metacommunication signaling that courting should not be taken seriously. Voices may be loud enough for conversations to be overheard. References may be made as to the inappropriateness of the situation for courting, or an incomplete postural-kinesic configuration may be given. For instance, participants may be facing each other, but their torsos may be turned toward other people or their eyes may dart around the room.

Quasicourtship behavior has a systems-maintenance function. In situations in which one participant either withdraws or is excluded, quasicourtship behavior calls back the errant participant and thereby maintains the interaction. Quasicourtship behavior thus facilitates rapport and sociability, necessary elements in group cohesion.

To avoid misunderstanding communication, nurses must be able to distinguish between courtship and quasicourtship behavior.

A student nurse observed a psychiatrist interacting with a 23-year-old female client in the sitting room of a large hospital. They were facing each other, with their bodies turned toward the staff in the nurses' station. The client frequently brushed hair away from her face, presenting the palm of her hand to the psychiatrist. The psychiatrist adjusted his tie several times. They were speaking loudly enough so that the student nurse could hear that they were discussing plans for the young woman's imminent discharge.

The student misinterpreted this quasicourtship behavior for courtship behavior and felt that the psychiatrist was encouraging his client's "seductive behavior." After talking the situation over with her instructor, the student was able to identify the behavioral qualifiers that signaled the message that courting should not be taken seriously (participants' torsos were turned away from each other and toward the rest of the staff, they were talking in a large sitting room and in the midst of other people, and they were speaking loudly enough so that their conversation could be easily overheard.)

Occasionally, individuals inadequately learn either the courtship behavior or the behavioral qualifiers. Since both sets of behavior are essential for quasicourtship, deviance or pathological behavior ensues when *either* set is performed in the absence of the other. Persons with schizophrenia often use courtship behavior without including behavioral qualifiers. Instead of quasicourting, they court. We usually say that they are exhibiting inappropriately seductive behavior. Or an individual may be unable to deal with quasicourtship behavior and respond by "decourting"—withdrawing or criticizing. This type of behavior is often associated with sexual dysfunctions (Scheflen and Scheflen, 1972).

Scheflen states that misinterpretation of quasicourtship behavior results, at the individual level, in a loss of courtship readiness and rapport and, at the social level, in a loss of group cohesion.

Other types of reciprocals, those of dominance and submission, indicate status. A dominant male may place his hands on his hips, scowl, or place the palms of his hands behind his neck. A dominant female may steeple her fingers. The person in the

submissive position will usually "reciprocate" by lowering his or her head. It is important for a nurse who is working with a submissive client to avoid assuming a dominant role either verbally or kinesically. By being aware of reciprocals of dominance and submission, the nurse can be more attuned to patterns of dominance and submission in the nurse-client relationship.

Unlike reciprocals, *territorials* frame an interaction and define a territory. When people want to pass through or intrude on other people's territories, certain behavior patterns are displayed. The intruders will bow their heads, curl their shoulders inward so that their chests do not protrude, keep their arms at their sides, and look downward. In addition, they may mumble a "pardon me."

A nurse noticed that whenever Mrs. Bowens walked past the library section of the sitting room, she looked downward and curled her shoulders inward. The nurse mistakenly assumed that Mrs. Bowen was intimidated by Mr. Jackson, who usually spent his free time in the library. After discussing the situation with another nurse, who was more knowledgeable about kinesics, the first nurse recognized that, since Mr. Jackson had staked out the library section as his territory, Mrs. Bowen was displaying normal behavior for passing through or intruding on another's territory.

Table 10-2 outlines the kinesic signals that help interacting participants recognize what is happening. We will now explore the regulatory nature of kinesics.

REGULATORY NATURE OF KINESICS

Nonverbal behavior, especially kinesic behavior, serves to regulate the pace of a relationship and to monitor deviant behavior (Scheflen and Scheflen, 1972; Vargas, 1986). Regulatory behavior occurs many times during an interaction. When deviance appears, a new pattern of behavior may emerge to monitor the deviant behavior; it will continue until the deviant behavior ceases.

TABLE 10-2 Properties of kinesic communication

Unit	Behavior	Example
Marker	Gesture	Pointing to a person or object under discussion
Reciprocal	Bond servicing; empathic behavior	Exchanging food or smiles among friends
	Courtship behavior; quasicourtship behavior	Preening and whispered conversation among lovers (courtship); preening that is accompanied by conversation loud enough to be overheard by others (quasicourtship)
	Dominance behavior; submission behavior	Scowling teacher with hands on hips (dominance) and student with lowered head (submission)
Territorial	Interactional framing; territorial defining	Sitting couple have outstretched legs and bodies oriented toward one another; people who pass between them look down and say "excuse me"

A nurse-therapist had received a family's permission to videotape its family therapy session. After the session, the nurse studied the videotape and tried to identify group dynamics. She noticed that every time the husband-father leaned in to speak to her, he would lower his voice. This excluded the rest of the family from the interaction. The wife-mother and two daughters would then cross their legs and rub their noses. At the appearance of this behavior, the husband-father would lean back in his chair and raise his voice, so that the rest of the family could hear what he was saying. By interrupting any alliance with the nurse that excluded other family members, the wife-mother and the two daughters were monitoring the husband-father's behavior.

Thus we see how monitoring gestures and signals can occur synchronously among members of a group and can serve to check deviant behavior.

Whenever we try to interpret the meaning of kinesic behavior, we have to look beyond the individual or the group to the interrelationship between behavior and context. This is what is meant by a systems approach to understanding behavior.

Kinesic behavior is learned and passed on from generation to generation. Scheflen and Scheflen (1972) point out that the nuclear family or household is the first group to which a person belongs. It is here that most kinesic behavior is learned. Family or household members function interdependently to obtain food, affection, status, and self-esteem. Should a member deviate from culturally defined behavior, some of these ministrations can be withheld as a sanction. Therefore, at one and the same time, family interactions physically sustain a young child while servicing social bonds and teaching culturally approved values and behavior.

As individuals grow to maturity, they belong to other groups and expand their social networks. In each of these groups, they play specific roles. Should they deviate from expected role behavior, metacommunications occur that serve to discipline and reindoctrinate them or to keep them out of the mainstream of society. Bateson (1955) defines *metacommunication* as communication that tells how verbal communication should be interpreted.

A community health nurse was visiting with a woman who was the mother of a toddler and an infant. The nurse was discussing sibling rivalry with the mother. The toddler was sitting at the kitchen table eating cookies and drinking milk. As the toddler reached for a cookie, he knocked over the glass of milk. The mother jumped up and said sweetly, "Don't worry, Johnny—accidents will happen." However, from the frown on her face and her brusque behavior in cleaning off Johnny's wet clothes, both the community health nurse and Johnny were very aware that the mother was annoyed with Johnny's behavior.

The behavior that communicated the message of annoyance contradicted the verbal message; it indicated how the verbal message should be taken. This is the function of metacommunication. It can support or contradict verbal communication and thereby reinforce the values, behavior, and standards of society. Interactions continue in their customary manner, and unusual experience and information are kept to a minimum.

Taken together, metacommunication, marking, and territorial and reciprocal behavior serve to clarify ambiguous communication, signal deviance in an interaction, and bring about a return to conventional behavior. It is primarily through this regulatory function of kinesics that social order is maintained.

CULTURAL INFLUENCES ON KINESIC BEHAVIOR

Communication specialists like Birdwhistle (1970), Scheflen and Scheflen (1972), and Vargas (1986) believe that kinesic behavior is culturally variable.

For example, considerable time has been spent exploring the culturally specific form and meaning of eye movements. Ashcraft and Scheflen (1976) have found that while most British-Americans seek eye contact as a means of establishing affiliation and rapport, West Indians and Afro-Americans usually avoid direct eye contact, for such behavior invites the escalation of hostility. British-Americans often misinterpret the black American's avoidance of eye contact as being indicative of submissiveness or of having something to hide. Black Americans often misinterpret British-American eye contact as either a put-down or a confrontation. Hispanic women tend to hold eye contact slightly longer than women from other ethnic groups, and this behavior is often interpreted by non-Hispanic people as seductive.

Hall (1966) has found that even in the "British-American world" eye contact differs. The British tend to blink their eyes to show they are listening and understanding conversation, while Americans, who have conventions against staring, do not look directly into people's eyes. Instead, Americans indicate attentiveness by nodding and making listening noises. While an American's gaze wanders over the face and sometimes off the face, an Englishman's gaze is fixed on the eyes.

Needless to say, the cultural variability of the form and meaning of eye movements can result in many misunderstandings.

A young Hispanic nurse was assigned as primary nurse to an Irish-American male client. The client had been hospitalized for treatment of a myocardial infarct. The nurse spent much time listening to the man's fears, explaining his diet to him, and helping him to establish a prescribed exercise program. Because the young man was unaccustomed to women maintaining prolonged eye contact except when inviting or involved in intimate encounters, he interpreted the nurse's slightly prolonged eye holding as seductive behavior. He responded by inviting her out for a date. To the nurse, whose behavior was customary for someone from her Hispanic culture, the client's behavior was unwarranted. She could not see why this young man had acted as he had. In talking the situation over with a nurse-anthropologist, she was able to identify the kinesic behavior that had resulted in the misunderstanding. Once she understood the cultural dynamics of the situation, she was able to explain to the client that she was not trying to establish a social relationship and to point out why he might have thought that she was. The confusion was resolved, tension between them was lessened, and a more therapeutic relationship was established.

Misinterpretation of the culturally specific form and meaning of another's kinesic behavior can cause misunderstandings and produce barriers to communication. Without effective communication a therapeutic relationship cannot be established.

The cultural specificity of kinesic behavior is also revealed in the form and meaning of gestures. Scheflen and Scheflen (1972) have noted that British-Americans tend to gesticulate less frequently than persons from Mediterranean countries and Eastern European Jews. When British-Americans do gesticulate, they usually keep their forearms in fixed positions and move either or both hands from the wrist in a circle approximately 6 inches in diameter.

Effron's (1942) classic study found that, in day-to-day communications, Italians tend to use their hands, faces, arms, and shoulders to emphasize and illustrate their words. Gestures can become so flamboyant that Italians need approximately an arm's length of lateral space to avoid striking things with their sweeping arms. Eastern European Jews tend to use motions to "support" words. Instead of the sweeping arm movement of Italians, which starts at the shoulder and involves the entire arm, they tend to hold the upper arm close to the body and use only the lower arm to gesture. Eastern European Jews usually stand within touching range as they converse. They are able to poke, pull, and push as they embellish, punctuate, and accent their conversations.

Scheflen and Scheflen (1972) observed that black Americans tend to gesticulate much like British-Americans but that working-class blacks often use more gestures than middle-class blacks. Black Americans generally gesticulate with the index finger and also display their palms more frequently than do British-Americans.

One might wonder of what import this knowledge of the cultural specificity of gestures is to nursing. We will look at two examples.

Ms. Galiano, a nursing instructor, was a second-generation Italian-American. After several years of teaching, she found herself becoming increasingly tense during clinical seminars. One day, she sat down and tried to identify the dynamics of the situation. Everything was similar to previous semesters with one exception: This semester her clinical group was sitting in a tight circle with barely 6 inches of space between the chairs. Ms. Galiano suddenly realized what was happening. Her clinical group was composed of British-American students and Eastern European Jewish students, none of whom needed lateral space for body movements. Ms. Galiano, however, used the gesticulatory behavior common to her ethnic group. To kinesically communicate, she needed lateral space. Without such space, her body language was being stifled. As a result, she was becoming tense. She explained the dynamics of the situation to the group. They spread open their circle and allowed Ms. Galiano the space she needed to gesticulate. The problem was solved. Both students and teacher had received a first-hand lesson in the role of kinesic behavior in the process of communication.

Ms. Thompson, a 60-year-old British-American, had been admitted to a psychiatric hospital. A student nurse established a one-to-one relationship with her. The student became concerned about Ms. Thompson's lack of body movement during their interactions. He told his instructor: "Either Ms. Thompson is scared to death of me or she's catatonic. She never moves." His instructor helped the student to look at the dynamics of the interaction. The student was of Eastern European Jewish extraction and used much gesturing and touching during conversation. Ms. Thompson was British-American and accustomed to little gesturing. Her behavior was neither rooted in fear nor pathological. It was completely normal for someone of her ethnic background.

Postures and gestures thus can have various causes and various meanings. Form and meaning are influenced by cultural context. Probably because culturally specific behavior is unconscious and not formally learned, it is one of the last types of behavior to be acculturated. As a result, when people of different ethnic backgrounds interact, misinterpretation of behavior may cause misunderstandings.

Body language, then, like speech, is very much a part of any communication system. Kinesic behavior communicates needs, feelings, and intentions that are universal, but the form and meaning of body movements are culturally specific. In looking at the communicational value of kinesic behavior, we have seen the importance of understanding the interrelationship between kinesic behavior and its context. We will now explore another level of human communication: proxemics.

Proxemics

The proxemic level of communication—the use of space—has only recently become an area for study. Hall (1966) was a pioneer in proxemic research. Scheflen and Ashcraft (1976) see space as neither thing-defined nor people-defined. They refer to bounded space as territory that is framed and used by people but that does not consist of people. Instead, it surrounds people or exists between them. It is defined by a relationship or pattern of behavior and movement. Therefore, a "territory" is more than just a space. It is a space that has been claimed by a person through body language, and the claim has been acknowledged by others. People claim space either through the direction in which they orient their bodies or by the way they project their gazes or voices. Even though claims may be of a temporary nature, once a space has been claimed and the claim has been acknowledged, a territory has been established.

Mr. Jefferson was recovering from abdominal surgery. He spent a great deal of time in bed watching television. The television set was located on a shelf on the wall opposite his bed. Any time that a nurse came in to care for the person in the next bed, he or she had to walk through the space between Mr. Jefferson's bed and the television set. Each time that the nurse did this, if Mr. Jefferson was watching television, the nurse said, "Excuse me." By orienting his body and his gaze toward the television set, Mr. Jefferson had claimed this territory, and the behavior of the nurse acknowledged the claim.

PROPERTIES OF HUMAN SPACING

Scheflen and Ashcraft (1976) have been pioneers in the examination of the properties of space. By studying territories of orientation, these researchers have shown how we can better understand the ways in which human beings organize space.

Scheflen and Ashcraft use the term *point behaviors* to refer to the way in which body parts move within a space and orient themselves in some direction. For example, the gaze of an instructor's eyes may be directed toward a student to warn, reprimand, or focus attention upon the student. A nurse's head may be cocked so that it can be oriented toward a client. The small space that becomes the object and extension of point behavior is called a "spot."

Positional behaviors involve four body regions: head-neck, upper torso, pelvis-thighs, and lower legs-feet. These regions may be oriented in the same direction or in different directions. When saying a fast "hello" to classmates, a student may orient head, chest, and arms toward the classmates while orienting the lower part of the body in the direction in which he or she is walking. When a single body region or a cluster of body regions is pointed in a specific direction, it claims a space beyond that occupied by the body region. People usually avoid looking into or walking through this space. It is through such acknowledgment that a space is claimed and a territory established.

Besides being organized by identifying spatial orientations, space can also be organized by degree of affiliation. In Scheflen and Ashcraft's terminology, people who are affiliated ("with" one another) share *"with" space*. In "with" spaces, participants use body parts and regions to show that they are affiliated and that they share a similar spatial orientation. For example, a nurse and a client may, during the course of their interaction, assume congruent body positions or mirror-image stances ("bookending") and thereby define a common focus of attention. In addition, people show they are affiliated by leaning toward each other, forming links through touching, and using arms and legs to demarcate spatial boundaries.

In *"non-with" spaces*, participants use body parts and regions to show that they have different spatial orientations and that they are unaffiliated with one another. For example, during a nurse-client interaction, the nurse and the client may assume stances that show that they are affiliated but may position their extremities to form a barrier between themselves and others. They are indicating that they are temporarily unaffiliated with the others.

So far we have looked at how body parts and regions define spatial orientation and organization. However, body parts and regions belong to and are part of the total body. When looking at the orientation of the total body in space, we are describing relationships. People may commit all or only part of their bodies to an interaction. We will now look at patterns of low commitment and patterns of high commitment.

While *low-commitment configurations* may result in the dissolution of a relationship, *high-commitment configurations* reinforce a relationship. Low-commitment configurations are characterized by the involvement of only one body part, the positioning of a body region so that a person is only partially oriented toward the focus, the maintenance of maximal interpersonal distance, the crossing of extremities, or the covering or immobilization of body regions so that body movements are minimal. High-commitment configurations are characterized by the involvement of several body regions, the positioning of body regions toward the focus of orientation, the maintenance of minimal interpersonal distance, the uncrossing of extremities, and the display of mutual point and positional behavior. In the following hypothetical situation, patterns of both high and low commitment affect an interaction.

Ms. Zender, a student nurse, was sitting outdoors with her client, Mr. Morrow. They were seated on chairs and facing each other. Each was leaning forward as they talked. After about 20 minutes, Ms. Zender gazed over at a softball game that was being played nearby. Within minutes, not only was she looking at the game but her head and upper torso were turned away from Mr. Morrow and toward the softball field. A silence fell between nurse and client. Five minutes later, Mr. Morrow said he had nothing more to say. He got up and left. Ms. Zender was frustrated and confused. She told her nursing instructor that the interaction had been going "so well and then suddenly Mr. Morrow got up and left." The instructor had been sitting outside and had observed the changing behavioral configurations. In the beginning of the interaction, both Ms. Zender and Mr. Morrow were engaged in high-commitment configurations. When Ms. Zender turned her gaze and her body toward the softball game, she changed her spatial orientation and assumed a low-commitment configuration. From that point on, the interaction deteriorated. Once the student became aware of her behavior, she stopped blaming Mr. Morrow for interrupting the interaction and recognized how her own spatial orientation had affected the interaction.

Spatial orientations and relations do not exist in isolation. They are formed by people who cluster together at a given time. Scheflen and Ashcraft (1976) use the term *formations* to refer to these clusters of people and the term *sites* to refer to the spaces these formations define and occupy.

One type of site, a solo site, is the space occupied when a person is alone or with very few other people. The size of a solo site is determined by such factors as ethnicity, age, affiliation, role, activity,

social class, and sex. Scheflen and Ashcraft (1976) have found that a British-American or Afro-American man, when standing and conversing with acquaintances, usually occupies a site of approximately 1 square yard. Since persons from the Mediterranean area and from Eastern Europe are inclined to stand closer together, each person's site tends to be smaller than the site occupied by a British-American or a black American. Latin Americans stand even closer together than Mediterraneans. Since Cubans stand only about 18 inches apart when conversing, their sites tend to be even smaller than those of Mediterraneans or Eastern Europeans.

Another type of spacing, unaffiliated rows, is found when strangers sit side by side in a public area (for example, when strangers sit on a park bench). They may try to separate themselves from others by maintaining space around themselves, orienting themselves in different directions, or erecting temporary barriers.

On the other hand, persons who know each other may show affiliation by huddling together and maintaining a distance from others, erecting barriers to separate themselves from others, and orienting themselves toward each other and away from the strangers present.

Obviously, it is important for nurses who work with clients of various ages, social classes, and ethnic backgrounds to recognize how these variables influence the way people occupy and use space and show affiliation.

A nurse was explaining hospital visiting regulations to a Cuban client. Both nurse and client were standing in a face-to-face formation. The nurse, who was British-American, suddenly began feeling very uncomfortable. She started moving around, side-stepping, and taking occasional steps backward. Every time she moved, the client would take a step toward her. Each person was doing a "distance dance." The British-American nurse was trying to maintain slightly more than an arm's length of space between herself and her client. The Cuban client was trying to maintain a much smaller (approximately half an arm's length) interpersonal space. Each was trying to establish and maintain the interpersonal distance that was common to his or her ethnic background, and each was confused by the distancing maneuvers of the other. Had the nurse been aware of what was occurring, she might have felt less uncomfortable and she might have been able to use her energy to interact more effectively with her client. Unfortunately, she did not have this awareness. Because she felt uneasy, she terminated the interaction prematurely.

Up to now, we have been focusing on relationships. Scheflen and Ashcraft (1976) have shown that another way to examine the properties of space is to look at the characteristics of fixed spaces and built spaces. Because it sets a focus of orientation, provides a place in which to interact, and defines what is going to happen, furniture establishes *fixed spaces*. For instance, wheeling a medicine cart into a hospital room, building a nurses' station in the center of a hospital unit, or placing a television set in the sitting room of a day hospital sets a focus and defines the type of activity that is going to occur.

Built spaces are bounded by such physical structures as curbs, walls, and fences. Areas may be marked off by lines or low barriers across which people can see and interact, or they may be marked off by walls through which participants cannot see one another. The latter type of built space obviously provides a greater degree of privacy.

The use of fixed and built spaces has many implications for nurses. For example, in the 1960s Sommer (1969) observed that in a certain state psychiatric hospital all chairs were arranged in straight lines against walls. Although people sat side by side, rarely in the course of a day did they engage in more than two brief conversations. Sommer hypothesized that conversation was inhibited by the fact that clients had to turn their heads at a 90-degree angle to talk to persons sitting alongside. As a result, clients usually sat quietly, staring at the floor or ceiling. Sommer wondered why the chairs were arranged side by side and arrived at the following answers:

1. The arrangement made it easier to clean the room.
2. It was easier for nurses to supervise the unit.
3. The arrangement was a function of "institutional sanctity." Since the furniture had always been arranged that way, it had become a fixed routine.

Rather than the environment being arranged to meet the needs of the people inhabiting it, the people had been arranged to fit the environment. Sommer received permission to rearrange the furniture. He began by placing chairs around square tables. He chose square tables because the boundaries of a square table can be determined and demarcated more easily than those of a round table. Shortly after the furniture was rearranged, client interactions increased in both number and duration.

We have seen how built and fixed spaces, point behavior, and positional behavior occur within some larger pattern of behavior. Table 10-3 outlines the properties of these patterns of human spacing. Types of behavior are hierarchically arranged and occur within a broad context that is both temporally and spatially defined. Now we will look at the way culture influences the meaning, ordering, and use of space.

CULTURE AND PROXEMICS

The organizational, social, and symbolic meaning and use of space have been explored by archeologists, social anthropologists, psychologists, geographers, and ethnographers.

Hall (1966) has looked at people's perception of space. He sees people as surrounded by expanding and contracting perceptual fields that at all times provide them with information. He believes that people interact in four spatial zones: intimate, personal, social, and public (Refer to Table 10-4.)

The *intimate zone* is the zone of physical contact. This is the zone of lovemaking and comforting. Americans feel uncomfortable if forced into the intimate zones of strangers. For instance, when crowded onto an elevator, Americans respond by becoming immobile, holding their arms at their sides, fixing their eyes on some spot, and tensing their bodies. Many nurses have experienced this same response when comforting clients with whom they have not established rapport, trust, and confidence.

The *personal zone* is sometimes visualized as a "bubble" that a person keeps between self and others. The bubble expands and contracts according to circumstances. At a small personal distance, one

TABLE 10-3   Properties of human spacing

Unit	Behavior	Example
Point behavior	Moving and orienting body parts within space	Turning your head and looking at a person to get that person's attention
Positional behavior	Orienting body regions within space	Turning your body toward an approaching person with whom you want to talk or away from a person with whom you do not want to talk
"With" or "non-with" space	Using body parts and regions to show degree of affiliation	"Book-ending" and leaning toward a friend with whom you are engrossed in conversation ("with" space); standing with your back to someone whom you do not know ("non-with" space)
Commitment configuration	Using body parts, orienting body regions, and maintaining interpersonal distance to show high or low involvement in a relationship	Sitting close to and turning all body regions toward a person who is discussing a topic that interests you (high commitment); shifting away from the person and looking around the room when the topic of conversation no longer interests you (low commitment)
Formation	Clustering to show degree of affiliation	Sitting with book between you and the stranger sitting next to you on a park bench (unaffiliated); huddling on a bench with friends at a football game (affiliated)
Fixed space	Using furniture to focus interaction	Turning on a video cassette recorder sets one focus for interaction; turning on a stereo sets another focus for interaction
Built space	Using physical structures to define degree of interaction	Leaving a door ajar invites more interaction and affords less privacy than closing the door

can hold and touch another person. At a great personal distance, one is just within reach when both parties extend their arms. During a nurse-client interaction, participants usually maintain personal distance.

Social distance is the distance at which most business is conducted; it is also the distance maintained by student and teacher during a classroom lecture.

Public distance separates public figures from the public. It is used in formal situations. This is the distance maintained between student and lecturer in a large lecture hall.

These zones of interaction are neither static nor absolute. They are related to the way people organize their senses, a process that is culturally determined. What is considered intimate distance in one society may be considered personal or public distance in another society.

Although there are areas of cultural similarity among societies of the Western world, there are also many areas of cultural difference. People who are unaware of these differences risk misunderstanding others and being misunderstood. Behavior that differs from that of the dominant culture is usually interpreted as rudeness, ineptness, or apathy. We will now explore some proxemic differences among cultures.

TABLE 10-4   Spatial zones

Zone	Distance	Characteristics
Intimate	0–18 inches from the body	Sight is blurred or distorted; perception of odors, heat, and breath from another's body is heightened; voice either is not used or kept to a whisper
Personal	18 inches to 4 feet from the body	Vision is undistorted; texture of hair, pores in the skin, and the three-dimensional quality of an object are visible; breath and body heat of another person are imperceptible; voice level is moderate
Social	4–12 feet from the body	People are unable to touch one another; condition of hair, skin, and clothes is visible; voice level is raised so that it can be easily heard by people standing nearby (close phase) or people in an adjacent room (far phase)
Public	12–25 feet from the body	Fine details of another's body are lost; the three-dimensional quality of an object is lost; voice level is loud but not full volume (close phase) or needs amplification (far phase)

Scheflen and Scheflen (1972) have observed that when people place themselves in a vis-à-vis position for the purpose of communication, the amount of space between them depends on their ethnic background, their degree of intimacy, their previous relationship, the reason they assembled, and the amount of available physical space. Should the people interacting come from different ethnic backgrounds or have different ideas about the purpose and circumstances surrounding the interaction, they will have difficulty agreeing on the distance between them. They might do a "spatial dance" until they arrive at a spatial compromise. For example, Englishmen and British-Americans usually arrange themselves just beyond touching distance, and they touch very little while interacting. Latins and Eastern European Jews tend to position themselves within easy tactile range and to use varying degrees of touching during conversation. A nurse who has been culturally conditioned to use little touching while conversing may be made very uncomfortable by the small interpersonal distance and the use of touching by a client or a colleague, and vice versa.

Use of space is also influenced by social class. For example, Scherer (1974) found that while middle-class children maintain greater personal space than lower-class children, there tend to be no differences in the personal spacing of middle-class black and white children nor in the personal spacing of lower-class black and white children.

As we have seen, we all have a sense of territoriality that is operative in our daily lives. As we interact with others, we both acknowledge other people's claims to space and expect them to acknowledge our claims. Problems arise when the use of different spacing signals results in ambiguous or disputed claims. When this occurs, we do not realize that a claim has been made and therefore do not respect it.

DEVIANT PROXEMIC BEHAVIOR

We have discussed how the use of space can be misinterpreted by persons of differing backgrounds. However, some people exhibit behavior that is deviant even by the standards of their own ethnic, economic, or regional groups. Such people might touch persons with whom they do not have tactile rights, or they might fail to touch persons with whom they have such rights. They may orient their bodies away from persons with whom they are interacting, or they may stand at distances that are too close even for their own ethnic backgrounds. Such deviant territorial behavior is called "distance maneuvering."

Ashcraft and Scheflen (1976) have advanced several possible explanations for deviant territorial behavior. One is decreased living space. As population density has increased, we have developed behavior to try to ensure some modicum of privacy. Such territorial behavior includes not only actions that stake out private areas but also actions that show respect for privacy. Rooms in a house or an apartment are arranged so that a person goes from communal areas to increasingly private areas. The central hallway and the living room are open to guests, but access to the kitchen is usually only by permission. In fact, sometimes the kitchen is even off limits to certain family members. How often is a family member shooed away by a mother so that she may work in "her" kitchen? Bedrooms are very private areas. In fact, adolescents often mark this privacy with "no trespassing" and "keep out" signs. Rooms thereby become a means of ensuring some degree of privacy.

However, crowding can be defined only by looking at the context in which it occurs. For instance, Ashcraft and Scheflen (1976) have observed that children are better able to tolerate sleeping in a crowded bedroom if they can study and play in another room. Ashcraft and Scheflen have also found that crowding is culturally defined. While black Americans and British-Americans tend to disperse throughout the available space in a house, Puerto Ricans tend to cluster in one room. While Italian-Americans, British-Americans, black Americans, and Jewish Americans usually define being "alone" as being physically removed from *family members* (they go outside or into another room), Puerto Ricans usually define being alone as being physically separated from *strangers* but being among their families.

In light of such information, nurses need to recognize that the crowded and cramped living conditions of ghetto apartments have conceptually different meanings to people of different ethnic groups.

If a British-American nurse suggested to a harried Puerto Rican mother that she try to get some rest and privacy by relaxing in her bedroom away from the noise and activity of family members, the nurse would be imposing his or her concept of privacy on someone whose definition of privacy might be very different. The Puerto Rican mother might view the idea as strange and unworkable. The nurse, unless aware of the ethnic variation in the definition of privacy, would not even realize that he or she was being ethnocentric. A misunderstanding might result as both nurse and client become frustrated in working toward their goal of decreasing the mother's sense of fatigue and harassment.

Patterns of proxemic communication vary. By looking at these patterns, nurses can discover cultural frames that influence the structure of a person's perception of the world. Since a person's perceptual structuring of the world influences his or her definitions and interpretations of the use and meaning of space, people of differing ethnic backgrounds often misinterpret the meaning of each other's proxemic behavior. Territorial intrusion occurs, and conflicts of varying intensity develop. When we study proxemic communication, we are studying how people of different cultures use their senses to screen perceptual data, admitting some information and filtering out other information. Culture therefore serves as a medium for proxemic communication.

RELATIONSHIPS AMONG LEVELS OF COMMUNICATION

We have heuristically examined all three levels of communication: verbal, kinesic, and proxemic. We will now consider how these levels are interrelated. For years, communication specialists have realized that the process of communication involves more than speech. Until recently, however, they have lacked the tools to study the nonverbal aspects of communication. They therefore have focused their attention on the aspect of communication that they have had the tools to study—the verbal aspect.

Scheflen and Scheflen (1972) explain that as language evolves and attempts are made to clarify and punctuate speech, specific body motions such as gestures, posturing, and spacing behavior begin to be used. Interactions thus come to involve the interpretation of kinesic and proxemic behavior, both as autonomous means of communication and as mechanisms integrated with speech.

The investigation of the relationships between various levels of communication probably owes its inception to the collaborative efforts of Traeger, Smith, Hall, and Birdwhistle. Fromm-Reichman later joined them. Research commenced on kinesics, proxemics, and metalinguistics. The process of communication was defined as including three co-existing levels: verbal, kinesic, and proxemic.

Out of this early research, interest was stimulated in communication as a system of interrelated levels. Birdwhistle (1972) recalls that "circum-

speech" behavior was identified. Circum-speech includes such behavior characteristics of conversation as instrumentals, interactional behavior, markers, demonstratives, and stress kinesics. Instrumentals are such task-oriented movements as walking, smoking, eating, and knitting. People often carry on these activities while they are speaking. Interactional behavior is found in both verbal and nonverbal interactions. It includes shifts or movements of all or part of the body that increase, decrease, or maintain space between interacting individuals. Remember the "spatial dance" that people do when trying to adjust the distance between them? Markers are body movements that illustrate ambiguous words. For example, hand sweeps that indicate direction and accompany such

TABLE 10-5 Communicative functions

Function	Definition	Example
Instructional	Use of language to convey information	Nurse explains actions and side effects of a psychotropic medication to a client and the client's family; the nurse's communication imparts information to the client and the family
Relational	Use of metacommunication to establish, maintain, or change the interpersonal contract	Nurse states that client may express angry feelings to the nurse; when the client begins to express anger, the nurse's tone of voice and kinesic and proxemic behavior convey the message "I am afraid of anger"; the nurse's metacommunication changes the contract to one where anger can not be expressed in the nurse-client relationship
Identity	Use of communication in the presentation of self and in the facilitation of identity of interacting others	Nurse verbally points out strengths and accomplishments of a client and respects client's claims to territory and privacy; the nurse's communication behaviors promote development of positive self-esteem in the client
Regulative	Use of communication as a mechanism of social control	Nurse uses a firm but nonpunitive approach when explaining to a client the rules of the therapeutic community and the consequences of rule infractions; the nurse's communication is directed at controlling the social environment and regulating the client's behavior

Sources consulted include Scheflen and Scheflen (1972), Scheflen and Ashcraft (1976), Blake and Haroldsen (1975), Goffman (1981), and Kasch (1984).

phrases as "here" or "there" and head nods that clarify pronominal references are all markers. Demonstratives, like gestural mapping, are actions that accompany and illustrate speech. When people indicate with their hands that a toddler has grown "this tall" or that a melon is "this big," they are using demonstratives. The term stress kinesics refers to movements of the hand, head, or eyebrow that serve to mark the flow of speech; these movements generally coincide with linguistic stress patterns. When students raise their eyebrows as well as the pitch of their voices to state in amazement, "I received an 'A' on my nursing process paper," they are using a stress kineme.

Until recent years, we paid little attention to the interrelationship of linguistics, kinesics, and proxemics. Anthropologists, psychologists, and nurses focused almost all of their attention on verbal communication. What people said and how they said it were analyzed extensively. It was not until the 1950s that kinesic behavior became the object of study. Proxemic behavior was not studied until the late 1960s.

COMMUNICATION AND NURSING PRACTICE

Verbal, kinesic, and proxemic communication are the means for establishing nurse-client relationships. It is therefore important for nurses to be knowledgeable about communication. Kasch (1984) suggests that for nurses to be effective practitioners, they need to develop communication competency in four areas of communicative function: regulative, relational, identity, and instructional. Table 10-5 describes these communicative functions.

Because effective nursing practice is dependent, in part, on knowledge of communication, nursing research needs to explore communication and communication competence. Areas of research should include (a) specific communication strategies used in nurse-client interaction, (b) sociocultural influences on the communication behaviors of nurses and clients, (c) influence of institutional roles on nurse-client communication behaviors, (d) communication behaviors that characterize the various stages of the nurse-client relationship, and (d) impact of situational factors such as rules, norms, and routines of specific clinical settings on communication behaviors of clients and nurses (Bernstein, 1974; Delia, 1980; Kasch, 1984).

CHAPTER SUMMARY

People from different cultures not only speak different languages but also inhabit different sensory worlds. Selective screening of sensory data admits some information and filters out other information. An experience that is perceived through one set of culturally patterned sensory screens is quite different from the same experience perceived through another set. An encounter or interaction is one type of experience. When members of different cultural groups use dissimilar verbal, kinesic, or proxemic cues, assumptions, and orientations, misunderstandings can occur and role relationships can be disrupted. A sense of nonrelatedness to the members of the other cultural group can develop. Culturally influenced and acceptable behavior that is different from that of the dominant culture can be mistaken for deviant or pathological behavior. Because communication is an integral part of nursing practice, nursing research needs to explore communication and communication competence.

SELF-DIRECTED LEARNING

Sensitivity-Awareness Exercises

The purposes of these exercises are to:
- Develop awareness of communication behaviors
- Develop sensitivity to verbal and nonverbal cues
- Develop awareness of inferences that you make on the basis of nonverbal cues
- Develop awareness of the interrelationship between verbal and nonverbal communication

1. Sit in a public gathering place, such as your school cafeteria or a hospital waiting room, and observe the people there. What can you infer about their interpersonal relationships (e.g., commitment, status, affiliation) from their body movements, postures, facial expressions, and use of space?
2. Watch segments of a soap opera, a situation comedy, and a talk show on television with the sound turned off.
   a. What can you infer about what is happening from the kinesic and proxemic cues?
   b. How do the three television shows differ in the frequency and type of nonverbal behavior used?
   c. Turn the sound on. What circum-speech behaviors are used and when?
3. Watch a foreign language program and an English language program on television with the sound turned off.
   a. What can you infer about what is happening from the kinesic and proxemic cues?
   b. How do the two segments differ in the frequency and type of nonverbal behavior used?
   c. With the sound turned on, observe the foreign language program for instances of code-switching.
4. Take your favorite comic strip and identify a morpheme, a phoneme, a phrase, and a sentence.
   a. What kinesic and proxemic cues accompany these speech properties?
   b. How do the nonverbal cues reinforce, modify, or contradict the verbal message?

5. Observe a hospital room, a classroom, a restaurant, and your bedroom.
   a. How do furniture and physical structures establish fixed and built spaces?
   b. How do these fixed and built spaces set a focus and define a type of activity?
   c. How do the four settings differ in the use of fixed and built spaces?

Questions to Consider

1. A nurse noticed that when a Hispanic client spoke with her family members, she spoke Spanish. However, when she spoke with the hospital staff, she spoke English. This is an example of
   a. Quasi-courtship behavior
   b. Codeswitching
   c. Antilanguage
   d. Metacommunication
2. During a nurse-client interaction, the nurse and the client were seated with their bodies oriented toward one another and they appeared engrossed in conversation. Their nonverbal behavior indicates
   a. Non-with spacing
   b. A low commitment configuration
   c. A high degree of affiliation
   d. Metacommunication
3. After class, a student went up to the teacher and asked if the teacher would explain several parts of the lecture. The teacher frowned, tossed a piece of chalk she had in her hand on the desk, and said, "Of course. What is confusing you?" The student felt uncomfortable and said, "Well, maybe I can get the notes from one of my friends. If not, I'll come to your office hours." The teacher's nonverbal behavior contradicted the teacher's verbal behavior. This is an example of
   a. Circum-speech
   b. Codeswitching
   c. Instrumental language
   d. Metacommunication

Continued.

SELF-DIRECTED LEARNING—cont'd

Questions to Consider—cont'd

4. A _____ is a meaningful utterance.
   a. Marker
   b. Phoneme
   c. Morpheme
   d. Reciprocal
5. Antilanguage is a term used to refer to _____.
   a. Language that creates and maintains an alternative reality and alternative social structure.
   b. Language cues that tell how verbal communication should be interpreted.
   c. Language alternatives available to a speaker.
   d. Language compartmentalizing.
6. Nurses need to develop communicative competency in four areas of communicative function: relational, identity, regulative, and _____.
   a. Circum-speech
   b. Instructional
   c. Codeswitching
   d. Instrumental

Match each of the following terms with the statement that is associated with it:

7. Built space
8. Personal zone
9. Fixed space
10. Social zone

   a. Distance at which most business is conducted
   b. Furniture focuses interaction
   c. Physical structures define interaction
   d. Distance for most nurse-client interactions

Answer key

1. b	6. b
2. c	7. c
3. d	8. d
4. c	9. b
5. a	10. a

REFERENCES

Argyle M: Bodily communication, New York, 1975, International Universities Press.

Ashcraft N and Scheflen A: People space: the making and breaking of human boundaries, New York, 1976, Anchor Press.

Bateson G: The message, "this is play," In Schaffner B, editor: Group processes, Madison, NJ, 1955, Madison Printing Co.

Berlin B and Kay P: Basic color terms: their universality and evaluation, San Francisco, 1969, University of California Press.

Bernstein B: Class, codes and control: theoretical studies towards a sociology of language, New York, 1974, Schocken Books.

Birdwhistle R: Some relationships between American kinesics and spoken American English, paper presented at the annual meeting of the American Association for the Advancement of Science, 1963.

Birdwhistle R: Kinesics and context, Philadelphia, 1970, University of Pennsylvania Press.

Birdwhistle R: A kinesic-linguistic exercise: the cigarette scene. In Gumperz JJ and Hymes D, editors: Directions in sociolinguistics: the ethnography of communication, New York, 1972, Holt, Rinehart & Winston.

Blake RH and Haroldsen EO: A taxonomy of concepts in communication, New York, 1975, Hastings House, Publishers.

Bloomfield L: Language, New York, 1933, Holt, Rinehart & Winston.

Delia JG: Some tentative thoughts concerning the study of interpersonal relationships and their development, West J Speech Commun 44:97-1-3, 1980.

Eastman CM: Aspects of language and culture, San Francisco, 1975, Chandler and Sharp, Publishers, Inc.

Effron D: Gesture and environment, New York, 1942, King's Crown Press.

Ervin-Tripp SM: Language and thought, In Tax S and Freeman LG, editors: Horizons of anthropology, 1977, Chicago, Aldine Publishing Co.

Fishman JA: A systemization of the Whorfian hypothesis, Behav Sci 5:323-339, 1960.

Fishman JA: Readings in the sociology of language, The Hague, 1968, Mouton.

Fishman JA: Sociolinguistics: a brief introduction, Boston, 1971, Newbury House Publishers.

Gal S: Codeswitching and consciousness in the European periphery, Am Ethnol 14(4):637-653, 1987.

Gesell A and Amatura G: The embryology of behavior, New York, 1946, Harper & Row.

Gleason Jr HA: An introduction to descriptive linguistics, New York, 1961, Holt, Rinehart & Winston.

Goffman E: Forms of talk, Philadelphia, 1981, University of Pennsylvania Press.

Gumperz JJ: Conversational codeswitching. In Discourse strategies, Cambridge, 1982, Cambridge University Press.

Gumperz JJ and Hymes D: Directions in sociolinguistics: the ethnography of communication, New York, 1972, Holt, Rinehart & Winston.

Hall ET: The hidden dimension, Garden City, NY, 1966, Doubleday & Co., Inc.

Halliday MAK: Anti-languages, Am Anthropol 78:570-584, 1976.

Hediger H: Wild animals in captivity, London, 1950, Butterworth & Co.

Hediger H: Studies of the psychology and behavior of captive animals in zoos and circuses, London, 1955, Butterworth & Co.

Hediger H: The evolution of territorial behavior, In Washington SL, editor: Social life of early man, New York, 1961, Viking Fund Publications in Anthropology, No. 31.

Hymes D: Models of the interaction of language and social life, In Gumperz JJ and Hymes D, editors: The ethnography of communication, New York, 1972, Holt, Rinehart & Winston.

Jesperson O: Causes of change, In Hayden DE, Alorth EP, and Tate G, editors: Classics in linguistics, New York, 1967, Philosophical Library, Inc.

Kasch CR: Interpersonal competence and communication in the delivery of nursing care, Adv Nurs Sci 6(2):71-88, 1984.

Knapp ML et al: The rhetoric of goodbye: verbal and nonverbal correlates of human leave-taking, Speech Monographs 40:182-198, 1975.

Krivonos PD and Knapp ML: Initiating communication: what do you say when you say hello? Central States Speech J 26:115-125, 1975.

Lucy JA and Shweder RA: Whorf and his critics: linguistic and nonlinguistic influences on color memory, Am Anthropol 81:581-615, 1979.

Myers GE and Myers MT: The dynamics of human communication, New York, 1985, McGraw-Hill Book Co.

Sapir E: Conceptual categories in primitive languages, In Hymes D, editor: Language in culture and society: a reader in linguistics and anthropology, New York, 1964, Harper & Row, Publishers, Inc.

Scheflen AE and Ashcraft N: Human territories: how we behave in space-time, Englewood Cliffs, NJ, 1976, Prentice-Hall, Inc.

Scheflen AE and Scheflen A: Body language and social order: communications as behavior control, Englewood Cliffs, NJ, 1972, Prentice-Hall, Inc.

Scherer SE: Proxemic behavior of primary school children as a function of their socioeconomic class and subculture, J Personal Soc Psychol 29:800-805, 1974.

Sommer R: Personal space, Englewood Cliffs, NJ, 1969, Prentice-Hall, Inc.

Traeger GL: Paralanguage: a first approximation, In Hymes D, editor: Language in culture and society: a reader in linguistic anthropology, New York, 1964, Harper & Row, Publishers, Inc.

Vargas MF: Louder than words: an introduction to nonverbal communication, Ames, 1986, The Iowa State University Press.

Whorf BL: Language, thought and reality, In Carroll JB, editor: Selected readings of Benjamin Lee Whorf, New York, 1956, John Wiley & Sons, Inc.

Woolard K: Language variation and cultural hegemony: toward an integration of sociolinguistic and social theory, Am Ethnol 12(4):738-748, 1985.

ANNOTATED SUGGESTED READINGS

Kasch CR: Interpersonal competence and communication in the delivery of nursing care, Adv Nurs Sci 6(2):71-88, 1984.
The author notes that there has been little research on the articulation between communication and the delivery of nursing care. After exploring factors that have impeded such a systematic study, the author proposes that the area of interpersonal competence offers an adequate example for guiding nursing communication research.

Myers GE and Myers MT: The dynamics of human communication, New York, 1985, McGraw Hill Book Co.
The book takes both a theoretical and experiential approach to all levels of human communication. The authors also look at interrelationships among the different levels of communication.

Vargas MF: Louder than words: an introduction to nonverbal communication, Ames, 1986, The Iowa State University Press.
The author examines such aspects of nonverbal communication as kinesics, proxemics, and paralanguage within a social and cultural context. This book is designed to sensitize readers to the complexity of nonverbal communication. Experiential learning activities at the end of each chapter aim at helping readers analyze, organize, and utilize new learning.

FURTHER READINGS

Bavelas JB: Situations that lead to disqualification, Hum Commun Res 9(2):130-145, 1983.

Bowers JW: Does a duck have antlers? some pragmatics of transparent questions, Commun Mon 49(1):63-69, 1982.

Dance FEX, editor: Human communication theory: comparative essays, New York, 1982, Harper & Row.

Knapp ML: Essentials of nonverbal communication, New York, 1980, Holt, Rinehart Winston.

Shanon B: Semantic representation of meaning: a critique, Psychological Bul 104(1):70-83, 1988.

Smith B J and Cantrell PJ: Distance in nurse-patient encounters, J Psychosoc Nurs 26(2):22-27, 1988.

CHAPTER 11

Therapeutic communication and the nursing process

CHAPTER FOCUS

The nursing process is the framework for nursing practice. Nurses and clients explore client experiences, nurses sustain clients in those experiences, and nurses communicate their assessments, plans, and evaluations to other health team members. The focus of therapeutic communication is the client's here-and-now experience. The task of the nurse is to sustain the client in that experience. The cultural backgrounds of nurses and clients influence their perceptions and interpretations of experiences, their responses to experiences, and their responses to communication cues. In addition, behavioral concepts relating to sexuality, privacy, humor, empathy, and touching figure prominently in the nurse-client relationship and in the ability of nurses to sustain clients.

THE NURSE-CLIENT RELATIONSHIP
Nurse and client as components of the relationship

Client and nurse bring the five dimensions of the self (biological, intellectual, psychological, sociocultural, and spiritual) to the therapeutic relationship. Together, client and nurse explore what the client is presently experiencing that is of import or concern to the client.

The elements of any experience are perception, interpretation, and response. The way people view an event or a situation and the meaning it has for them affect the way in which they react. Many factors may influence one's perception, interpretation, and, ultimately, one's response to an event. These factors may be categorized as follows:

Biophysical factors
1. Organs or systems involved or affected by the event or situation
2. Degree of involvement: partial or total
3. Nature of onset: sudden or gradual; age at onset
4. Duration of involvement: short-term or long-term

Psychosocial factors
1. Past experience with similar events or situations
2. Values, attitudes,* and beliefs (influenced by religion, social class, ethnicity, and acculturation)
3. Present emotional state
4. Habitual ways of coping and problem-solving
5. Personality traits, such as rigidity, flexibility, introversion, extroversion
6. Situational factors, such as sick leave, insurance benefits, and supportive social networks.

The influence that any given factor or combination of factors has on one's perception, interpretation, and response varies not only from situation to situation, but also from person to person. Thus, a symptom such as occasional chest pain may be experienced differently by different people.

Client A, a 50-year-old Hispanic man, immigrated to the United States 10 years ago. He is married, and he has a 15-year-old son and a 10-year-old daughter. Although he understands English, client A speaks only Spanish at home. For the past 5 years, he has worked as a factory piece-worker. When he does not work, client A does not get paid. He has no health insurance.

Although client A knows that his father died in middle age, he does not know the cause of his father's death. When client A began experiencing chest pain, he initially ignored it. When the pain persisted, he consulted an espiritista (a Puerto Rican native healer) and he also prayed and did "good works." When client A finally decided to consult a physician, he sought a middle-aged, Hispanic doctor who spoke Spanish.

• • •

Client B is a 59-year-old second-generation Hispanic-American. He is married, and he has two married chil-

dren. Although client B knows Spanish, he speaks English at home. For the past 10 years, he has been employed as a dairy manager in a supermarket. Client B belongs to a union whose benefits include 10 days of sick leave and health insurance.

At the age of 60, client B's father died from "heart trouble." When client B began experiencing occasional chest pain, he was certain that he was developing the same type of heart trouble that had killed his father. Client B went to his family doctor, an American "who doesn't rush you in and out. Who spends time with you. Who asks about the family, and who isn't prejudiced against Spanish people."

• • •

Client C is a 37-year-old third-generation Hispanic-American. He is married, and he has a 10-year-old daughter and a 7-year-old son. Client C understands very little Spanish. English is the only language that he speaks. Client C is a junior executive with a bank. He has 30 days of sick leave, health insurance, and disability insurance that pays his salary if he is unable to work because of serious illness.

There is no history of heart disease in client C's family. Three weeks before his pre-promotion physical examination, he began experiencing occasional chest pain. Client C initially rationalized that the chest pain was "indigestion" and that it was caused by the anxiety he was experiencing about his upcoming promotion. He tried to relax by "unwinding with a few drinks at lunch and at home in the evening." When client C did seek medical attention, he went to "a young American doctor with up-to-date knowledge and the newest in office equipment."

These hypothetical situations illustrate the effects of biophysical and psychosocial factors on the perception and interpretation of an event and the response to it. In these vignettes, such factors as age at onset of chest pain, past experience with people who have experienced chest pain, coping patterns, type of employment, presence or absence of sick benefits, cultural background, and degree of acculturation influenced the frames of reference from which the three clients approached a similar event—occasional chest pain.

Likewise, when nurses and clients approach situations from different frames of reference, their perceptions, interpretations, and responses may differ. Nurses may identify certain client needs as priorities, but clients may not share this view. Also,

---
*Refer to Chapter 4 for a discussion of values, beliefs, attitudes, and attitude clarification.

nurses may have definite expectations about how clients experiencing a particular crisis should respond. If nurses are unaware of the factors that affect the experience, they may react with frustration and anger toward clients whose responses differ from their own.

A client, accompanied by his wife and two daughters, was brought into the emergency room. The client, a 47-year-old man, was having intermittent chest pain and he was experiencing severe anxiety. His family was crying and begging the physician and nurse to "do everything that can be done. Just don't let him die." The nurse felt that the client and his family were "overreacting." A diagnosis had not been made, and the nurse did not believe the client to be in immediate danger of dying. The nurse became annoyed and responded with impatience to both the client and his family.

The nurse was unaware that at the age of 47, both the client's brother and his father had died from heart attacks. To the client and his family, the client's intermittent chest pain was viewed as yet another family member suffering a heart attack that would probably result in death.

Had the nurse been aware of their frame of reference, the response of the client and his family may not have been viewed as an overreaction but as an appropriate response given the circumstances. Instead, because the nurse and the client and family had different frames of reference, the nurse responded with frustration and impatience and was unable to sustain the client and his family in their experience.

To cope with and profit from an experience, one must be able to learn from that experience. Learning is an active process that uses intellectual and perceptual capacities and acquired knowledge to explain events, to engage in problem solving, and to plan and implement change.

Both client and nurse bring intellect, perception, knowledge, and experience to the therapeutic process. Together, they explore the client's perception of events that the client regards as important or as matters of concern. Although occasionally comparisons may be made with past experience or remi-

niscing may occur, the *focus* is on the here and now—what the individual is presently experiencing. Clients can thus talk about events of concern or importance to them with assurance that only subject matter that they are psychologically able to tackle will be explored. Should the nurse introduce a topic, he or she might inadvertently select one that is traumatic to the client (Sayre, 1978). Nurses encourage clients to take the initiative in setting the focus by offering such broad opening questions as, "What have you been thinking about?" or "What's been going on with you?"

Behavioral concepts and the nurse-client relationship

The *task* of nurses is to sustain clients in their experiences. Sustaining refers to all nursing interventions that are designed to help clients cope with and learn from their experiences. Attitudes and feelings about sexuality, privacy, humor, empathy, and touching figure prominently in the nurse-client relationship and in the ability of nurses to sustain clients.

SEXUALITY

Since people are sexual beings, the sexuality of nurses and clients may influence the nurse-client relationship in many ways. Feelings and beliefs about sexuality contribute to attitudes about sex. These sexual attitudes in turn may either promote or inhibit therapeutic communication and the ability of nurses to sustain clients in their experiences.

A holistic view of sexuality* stresses the following concepts:

1. Human sexuality includes more than the act of intercourse. Sexuality integrates the physical, emotional, intellectual, sociocultural, and spiritual dimensions of human beings. The expression of sexuality enriches personality, communication, and love.
2. Authenticity and effective communication enrich human sexual functioning.

---

*Refer to Chapter 7 for an indepth discussion of human sexuality

3. Human sexual behavior involves three aspects:
   a. Fantasy—mental images of engaging in sexual behavior alone or with others
   b. Emotion—subjective feelings and sensations that may be manifested by such observable signs as flushing, rapid pulse, and increased respiratory rate
   c. Behavior—sexual activity engaged in alone or with others
4. Sexuality is an integral part of the human condition. It continues throughout life and does not disappear as one ages.
5. Human sexuality is influenced by a person's sociocultural background, especially by ethnicity, religion, and social class. For example, sociocultural factors may influence a person's conception of what is masculine behavior and what is feminine behavior. This conception often results in sex-role stereotypes. Sociocultural factors may also influence what a person views as appropriate sexual expression and appropriate sex objects.
6. At some point in most people's lives, they experience stress that is related to sexuality (Whipple and Gick, 1980).

The conceptions, feelings, and values that people have about human sexuality are often reflected in their attitudes about sex. Sexual attitudes include what people regard as "normal" and "abnormal" sexual behavior and how they feel about their own sexuality (Blondis and Jackson, 1982).

An understanding of human sexuality and the development of self-awareness about and comfort with their own sexuality is necessary before nurses can help clients deal with sexual concerns. Nurses are primarily involved with activities of education, counseling, case finding, and referral. For example, when educating and counseling parents about human sexuality, nurses may assist them to foster in their children guilt-free attitudes about sex, thereby helping the children to incorporate their sexuality into their self-systems.

When counseling clients who have suffered disturbances of body image,* nurses may
1. explore client attitudes about their sexuality

---

*Refer to Chapter 9 for further discussion of body image.

2. explore family relationships, support systems, and religious and ethnic heritages that have influenced client attitudes about sex
3. explore how altered body image is affecting clients' senses of self as sexual beings as well as their sexual relationships and sexual functioning

If sexual conflicts and sexual problems (for example, inorgasmia, impotence) are identified that are beyond the nurse's therapeutic expertise, referral should be made to sex therapists or to sex clinics.

When working with clients who are institutionalized for prolonged periods of time (for example, nursing home residents), nurses should try to ensure clients' privacy so that they can fulfill their sexual needs through either self-gratification or other means (this approach has also been suggested by Blondis and Jackson, 1982).

If nurses are uncomfortable with their own body images and sexuality and are unaware of their own attitudes about sex, barriers to therapeutic communication may develop. For example, some nurses may feel embarrassed when discussing sex and they may avoid opportunities for client education and counseling (Whipple and Gick, 1980).

A nurse in an oncology clinic was conducting an intake interview with a woman who 5 months before had had a mastectomy. The nurse was trying to determine how the woman was tolerating chemotherapy and how she was coping with her altered body image. Suddenly the woman began to cry as she told the nurse, "I dread having sex with my husband. The pressure of him leaning on my chest makes me feel like the left side of my chest is caving in, and when he penetrates me, I feel like I'm being torn apart. I even have some vaginal bleeding afterwards." The nurse became flustered and said, "You should discuss this with your gynecologist."

The nurse's comment blocked communication; the client no longer talked about her sexual concerns. The nurse's embarrassment prevented exploration of the client's feelings about herself as a sexual being after her mastectomy. The nurse's embarrassment also prevented client counseling concerning alternative coital positions that might avoid pressure on her chest and the importance of foreplay and nonhormonal vaginal lubricants in counteracting the drying effect of chemotherapy on the vaginal mucosa.

Sometimes the embarrassment that nurses may feel about sex may lead them to misinterpret or fail to understand client behavior.

Geoffrey White was scheduled to have an orchidectomy later in the week. He seemed unconcerned about the surgery and very jovial. He continuously joked about "hoping the doctor would sleep well the night before surgery and would have a steady hand." He also told many jokes about sex, and many of his comments to the nurses contained sexual innuendos. The nurses felt very uncomfortable with Mr. White. They tried to avoid going into his room. When they did have to interact with him, the nurses often were sarcastic or brusque with him.

The nurses' embarrassment about the client's sexual behavior interfered with their understanding of the meaning of his behavior. The nurses did not recognize that through sexual acting-out the client was expressing concerns about his scheduled orchidectomy and about his sense of masculinity. Instead of trying to help the client explore his feelings and fears, the nurses' behavior conveyed rejection and disapproval of the client's sexuality.

This does not mean that nurses should not set limits on the sexual acting-out of clients. It is possible to recognize and intervene in the situation underlying sexual acting-out behavior while explaining to the client that it is inappropriate for him to try to place the nurse in the role of sexual partner (Blondis and Jackson, 1982). The nurse may also assess whether the client knows how to relate to a person of the opposite sex in a way other than on an overtly sexual level. If the nurse discovers that the client has difficulty in relating nonsexually with members of the opposite sex, this might be an area to work on during nurse-client interactions. By taking these approaches, the nurse is dealing with the client's sexual acting-out behavior in a therapeutic, nonjudgmental, and nonpunitive manner.

Nurses may be judgmental and punitive about sexual behavior that is different from their own.

For example, they may view masturbation or homosexuality as "sinful" or sex-change operations as "unnatural," and they may convey these attitudes verbally and nonverbally to clients.

Judgmental attitudes and punitive behavior present barriers to therapeutic communication. To promote therapeutic communication and to sustain clients in their experiences, nurses need to feel comfortable with their own sexuality. Nurses also need to evaluate the sexual behavior of a client on the basis of its meaning for the client and its appropriateness to the nurse-client relationship. These principles should guide nurses in their interactions with clients, both males and females, heterosexuals and homosexuals.

PRIVACY

The way in which nurse and client define privacy and the types of privacy mechanisms they use may very much affect the nurse-client relationship. Privacy is a culturally specific concept. What is regarded as intrusive behavior by one ethnic group may not be regarded as intrusive behavior by another ethnic group.

A traditional American definition of privacy stresses individualism and the restriction of personal responsibility to the nuclear family (Altman, 1975). However, many first- and second-generation ethnic Americans (for example, Hispanic-Americans, Chinese-Americans, Italian-Americans) tend to be extended-family oriented; their sense of responsibility includes the extended family of real and/or fictive kin.* This difference in orientation toward privacy may lead some ethnic clients to stereotype American health care practitioners as "cold" and "aloof."

A first-generation Cuban-American woman was very unhappy with the quality of antepartum and postpartum care that she had received when she had her first child. Physicians and nurses had taken health histories and had given health counseling to her and her husband, but they had viewed her parents and mother-in-law as "outsiders" and had not included them in the family unit. This woman confided to a nurse-anthropologist that "the American doctors and nurses were

---

*Refer to Chapter 5 for a discussion of real and fictive kin.

ference, the nurses determined that self-disclosure to Colin was not therapeutically indicated. Then the nurses discussed how they would handle Colin's questions in the future. One nurse felt comfortable saying, "I wonder why you are always asking me about my personal life?" Another nurse decided to honestly tell Colin that "I feel uncomfortable when you ask me personal questions." A third nurse said she had found it helpful to refocus the conversation whenever Colin started asking about her personal life. She would say, "You were telling me about . . ." or "What is the reason that you changed the subject?"

The above vignette demonstrates different strategies that nurses may use to handle situations where self-disclosure to clients is inappropriate. The different techniques all serve to reinforce the boundaries of nurse-client interaction.

Most nurses also need time away from clients and the families of clients so that they can be alone or with colleagues. This time is necessary for them to integrate their experiences with clients and for them to express their emotions (for example, feelings about working with an angry client or about caring for a terminally ill client).

A recognition that, while all people have privacy needs, different people have different concepts of privacy and different ways of regulating privacy is essential to therapeutic communication and to the effective functioning of the nurse-client relationship.

HUMOR

Humor can decrease social distance by encouraging rapport, by decreasing anxiety, and by making the social structure of the health care setting seem more relaxed and flexible. However, humor can also be a means of expressing such feelings as aggression, hostility, and depression. It is, therefore, important that nurses understand the functions and purposes of humor so that they can use it to facilitate therapeutic communication and to sustain clients in their experiences.

Situations that produce humor vary from culture to culture, and there is no universal agreement on a definition of humor. However, humor is usually generated by the incongruous, the ludicrous, or the unexpected. In our culture, humor is characteristically described as follows:

1. It can be verbally or nonverbally communicated.
2. It is an indirect form of communication.
3. A continuum of laughter exists, ranging from laughing at to laughing with.
4. A sense of humor is a sign of mental health and maturity; it demonstrates an ability to laugh at one's *minor* misfortunes and to see oneself as one is seen by others (Robinson, 1970; Moody, 1978; DuBois, 1979).

The United States is a multiethnic society. It is therefore important for nurses to understand that although humor is found cross culturally, both the style and the form of humor are culturally variable. For example, the style of British humor is usually viewed by Americans as understatement, while the style of American humor is usually viewed by the British as overstatement, exaggeration, or slapstick. Both the British and the Americans tend to view the style of Oriental humor as subtle and characterized by degrees of amusement.

The form that humor takes tends to reflect ties with other aspects of the culture. For example, one theme in traditional Hispanic culture is male dominance and female submissiveness. A man's good name is maintained through the reputations of the women to whom he is related (wife, sisters, daughters). Women are supposed to be virginal and faithful, and men are supposed to demonstrate their *machismo* through the consumption of alcohol, by engaging in premarital and extramarital sexual liasons, and by protecting the family (Murillo-Rhode, 1976; Gilmore and Gilmore, 1979; Pasquali, 1982). Hispanic humor often reflects this cultural theme. For example, "loose women" are frequently the object of jokes.

The purposes and functions of humor operate on both the individual and the societal levels. On the level of the individual, humor may

1. decrease anxiety, stress, and tension
2. release angry, aggressive, or hostile feelings in a socially acceptable way
3. deflect emotionally painful conflicts and situations. Repeated joking about a topic may indicate conflict concerning the topic; joking

may be the way the person is trying to cope with feelings generated by conflict.

4. facilitate learning
5. reflect self-acceptance, an adequate self-image, and sound mental health
6. indicate underlying pathology. Inappropriate, aberrant, or uncontrollable laughter may be symptomatic of pseudobulbar palsy, amyotrophic lateral sclerosis, or gelastic epilepsy. Inappropriate silliness is often found in people with Alzheimer's disease, Pick's disease, and hebephrenic schizophrenia.
7. alleviate physical pain and stress, strengthen the immune system, and produce a sense of euphoria or physical well-being. It has been suggested that by stimulating the production of T-lymphocytes laughter strengthens the immune system and that by stimulating the endocrine system (especially the pituitary gland) to release endorphins,* laughter decreases pain and produces a sense of well-being (Abeles, 1982; Goldstein, 1982; Pasquali, 1980; Watson, 1988).

The following vignette illustrates how humor may operate on the level of the individual.

A nurse was trying to teach an adolescent boy with diabetes to give his own insulin injections. The boy was very angry about having diabetes, and he was resistant to the idea of daily insulin injections. The nurse began sharing with the client cartoons that dealt with people's feelings and attitudes about chronic illness and injections. The cartoons provided an avenue of release for the boy's angry feelings, and he was able to laugh at some of his fears about injections. He soon was finding cartoons that dealt with chronic illness and injections to share with the nurse. The humor that the nurse and client shared facilitated trust and decreased the client's anxiety. This relaxed atmosphere facilitated the young man's sharing of his concerns and learning about his diabetes.

---

*Laughter stimulates the manufacture of catecholamines (for example, epinephrine, norepinephrine, and dopamine). The catecholamines in turn stimulate the release of endorphins, which act as natural opiates.

On the societal level, humor serves to lessen intergroup conflict and to promote social solidarity:

1. Humor provides a means of expressing feelings and attitudes that might otherwise be difficult to express and permits these feelings and attitudes to be expressed in a socially acceptable manner.
2. Humor decreases social distance by functioning as a leveling mechanism. If people flaunt success, others may tease them or play down their successes.
3. Humor provides a means for individual feelings and concerns to be shared, thereby facilitating consensual validation and camaraderie.

The societal functions of humor may sometimes be institutionalized. For example, the anthropologist Radcliffe-Brown (1952) was one of the first to describe one type of institutionalized humor, the joking relationship. A joking relationship refers to a relationship between two people where custom allows or, sometimes, prescribes the teasing or ridiculing of one or both participants in the relationship. When one person teases the other and the other person accepts the teasing good-naturedly and without retaliating, the joking relationship is said to be asymmetrical. This contrasts with a symmetrical joking relationship, in which each of the participants teases and ridicules the other.

When a man marries a woman, he forms relationships with her family. However, prior to the marriage, he had been considered and had considered himself an outsider to her family group. Although this situation may be modified, it is not totally changed by marriage. Similarly, although after marriage a woman usually maintains ties with her family, these ties are altered by her new and close relationship with her husband. Thus, marriage results in both attachment and separation, in both social conjunction and social disjunction. While social conjunction requires the avoidance of hostility, social disjunction involves divergence of interests and thus contains the seeds of conflict. The joking relationship permits the release of antagonisms that may be engendered by social disjunction, while the custom requiring that teasing be accepted good-naturedly avoids the eruption of serious conflict.

Thus, the joking relationship serves both as a social release and as a social control.

Joking relationships are common in Africa, Asia, Oceania, and North America. In the United States, mother-in-law jokes and nurse-doctor jokes are forms of asymmetrical joking relationships. For example, nurses may tease some doctors about the "aseptic aura" that doctors seem to think they have. The joking relationship permits the nurses to release their irritation about the physicians' poor aseptic techniques, while the custom that such bantering be accepted good-naturedly avoids serious conflict between the nurses and doctors involved in the joking relationship and allows them to continue working together.

Another type of institutionalized humor is the intercultural jest. Intercultural jesting serves to express aggression toward an outgroup or to express cultural conflict among acculturating groups. Intercultural jesting may have as its theme the pitting of folk medicine against medical science. These jests often reflect the rejection that acculturating people may feel for their folk culture as well as the antagonism that they may feel toward American culture and what they perceive as uncaring American health care providers. Intercultural jesting thus helps to express the conflicts engendered by acculturation (Apte, 1985).

In Anglo-American society, jokes are also often made about modern medicine, especially about technology and medicine or about inept or callous health care givers. For example, comic strips abound with illustrations of nurses taking a client history while the client is bleeding to death, of interns administering intravenous fluids through the wrong orifice, and of people whose pacemakers need battery transplants or whose "tiny timepieces" all explode at the same time. These comic strips not only try to familiarize Americans with the new technology in health care but also reflect the feelings and fears that many Americans may be experiencing about health care (Pasquali, 1980).

Only when nurses understand the many purposes and functions that humor serves can they begin to understand the implications that humor has for the nurse-client relationship. Certainly a shared joke can strengthen the relationship if the humor occurs within an atmosphere of caring and respect. Also, because humor can serve as a release for emotion, can facilitate learning, and can alleviate physical pain and strengthen the immune system, nurses might creatively incorporate humor into their care plans.

A mental health nurse was giving grief counseling to a woman whose spouse had died 3 months earlier. In addition to helping the client work through her feelings of grief, the nurse was concerned about the woman's vulnerability to illness. Aware that the level of T-lymphocytes is lowered during grief reactions and of research suggesting that humor may stimulate T-lymphocyte production, the nurse helped the client to select two television programs that made her laugh real "belly laughs" and encouraged the client to watch these programs daily.

However, if nurses want to use humor therapeutically, they need to consider the cultural backgrounds of their clients. What is suitable for joking in one culture may not be suitable in another culture. In addition, a joke may not be understood.

A cartoon that showed a dog dressed as a preppie and acting very "cool" was hung on a nursing school bulletin board. All the students thought it was "cute and funny." However, a first-generation Lebanese-American faculty member did not see the humor in the cartoon. Instead, he became upset because he interpreted the cartoon to mean that in the United States students are treated like dogs.

Clients may joke about situations that are emotionally painful to them or that are causing them conflict. Humor may be one way in which clients try to cope with feelings that are generated by conflicts.

A client who had hypertension and a family history of strokes was advised by her doctor to stop smoking and to lose 50 pounds. The client ignored the physician's advice. She joked, "I live to eat, not eat to live," and she teased friends and relatives who were dieting, saying that they were "trying to live forever." The client also told many jokes about people outliving their doctors.

The client's humor, explored in the context of her other behavior, suggested the presence of a problem. The client's compulsive smoking and eating, juxtaposed with her family history of cerebral vascular accidents, was engendering conflict. Her joking was one way that she attempted to cope with the anxiety generated by this conflict.

Institutionalized clients (for example, clients in hospitals or nursing homes), often engage in jocular griping among themselves about their low status in the health care hierarchy, about institutional routines, or about embarrassing and tension-producing procedures.

Three clients who shared a hospital room joked about "vampires [laboratory technicians] who come in several times a day to suck our blood [take blood samples]" and about the nurses who wake them at 5 AM to take vital signs and again at 11 PM to give them sleeping pills. The clients enjoyed cutting out and sharing comic strips that ridiculed hospital routines, and they frequently exclaimed, "We'll have to go home to get some rest."

By joking about their displeasure with hospital routine, individual complaints became shared and collective complaints. Not only does this facilitate consensual validation and camaraderie, but, in the process, people are able to step outside themselves and to laugh at the discomforts that they share with others (Pasquali, 1980).

Family and friends of clients may also use humor to handle their feelings about a loved one's serious illness, emotional instability, or imminent death. Humorous get-well cards are one vehicle for the expression of this humor, although many times these cards may seem unfeeling to seriously ill clients or to clients who are trying to cope with altered body image or impending death.

It is not enough for nurses to recognize that humor is serving a purpose for clients and for the families and friends of clients. Nurses need to listen for the messages (or themes) that underlie the humor. Once themes have been identified, nurses can use the nursing process to intervene.

Often nurses and other health team members can use humor to handle their own reactions to serious illness and to death. Sometimes the humor may be macabre. Macabre humor may be found among staff members in such high-stress situations as emergency rooms, operating rooms, and special care areas (for example, psychiatric units, oncology units, and cardiac care units). Although humor is one way of expressing their feelings, staff members need to learn to cope with feelings surrounding client care in more authentic ways. Nurses and other health team members also need to be very careful that clients and their relatives and friends do not overhear macabre humor and interpret it as callousness or lack of concern for clients.

An understanding of the functions and purposes of humor is important if nurses are to use humor to facilitate therapeutic communication and to sustain clients in their experiences. Table 11-3 summarizes criteria for appropriate use of humor in client care.

EMPATHY

Empathy increases the ability of nurses to sustain clients in their experiences. Effective counselors are more empathetic with clients than are ineffective counselors.

Nurses may ask, "What is empathy? What is the relationship between empathy and understanding?" Understanding refers to a cluster of *intellectual* assessments of client behavior.

During an intake interview, a nurse noted that the client cried easily, was withdrawn, appeared disheveled, and complained of insomnia and appetite loss. The client's history revealed that his wife had died recently.

This level of understanding helps nurses to describe and analyze client behavior.

In contrast, empathy involves viewing a client's experience as the client perceives it and "borrowing" or tuning into the client's feelings (Bradley and Edinberg, 1982). Thus, empathy is the ability to

TABLE 11-3   Criteria for determining appropriateness of humor in client care

Criterion	Determinants
Timing	Humor is appropriate when anxiety is mild to moderate, when it helps a client cope more effectively, or when it facilitates learning; humor is inappropriate when anxiety is severe or panic level, when it reinforces ineffective coping, or when the client needs to focus energy on dealing with and resolving an anxiety-producing situation
Humor style	Humor is appropriate when it conforms to a client's humor style; humor is inappropriate when it disagrees with a client's humor style; nurses need to assess a client's humor quotient (e.g., role humor plays in client's every day life; types of humor enjoyed such as comic strips, situation comedy shows, jokes, funny stories)
Themes	Humor is appropriate when it laughs *with* people, decreases social distance, reduces tension, or puts situations in perspective; humor is inappropriate when it laughs *at* people (put-down humor), increases social distance, increases tension, or is used to avoid dealing with emotions or a problem

Sources consulted include Lathrop (1981) and Apte (1985).

use imagination and will to project oneself into the emotions and thoughts of another person without losing one's objectivity. The avoidance of subjective involvement and value judgments is an important component of empathy (Forsyth, 1980). Empathy facilitates an "I-thou" rather than an "I-it" relationship.

One way of projecting oneself into a client's phenomenological world is to develop an internal frame of reference (Brammer and Shostrom, 1982). This means that the nurse tries to view a client's phenomenological world as the client perceives it. When the nurse uses an internal frame of reference rather than an external frame of reference, he or she begins feeling *with* the client rather than feeling or thinking *about* the client.

A nurse was counseling a recently widowed woman. The client was very upset about her husband's death. The nurse assumed an internal frame of reference and thought, "How does this woman view her husband's death? What does she see as the difficulties? How would she like to resolve those difficulties? How can I help her to clarify her thinking so that she can resolve the difficulties?"

Compare the above situation with the following example:

A nurse was counseling a recently widowed woman. The client was very upset about her husband's death. The nurse assumed an external frame of reference and thought, "What are the problems that I can identify? What solutions can I find for these problems? How can I help the client to recognize these problems and accept my solutions?

Obviously, an internal frame of reference rather than an external frame of reference facilitates tuning into a client's phenomenological world and increases a nurse's understanding of a client's experience.

Empathetic therapists seem better able to establish and maintain warm and accepting relationships with clients than are nonempathetic therapists. Empathy helps nurses to establish therapeutic communication with clients and to sustain clients in their experiences by

1. cutting through the deep sense of aloneness often experienced by clients.
2. increasing nurses' knowledge of client difficulties.
3. enabling nurses to give clients clues about how they (clients) may be feeling and how they (clients) are coming across to others (Blondis and Jackson, 1982; Bradley and Edinberg, 1982).

An empathetic response to a client not only gives the client a sense of being understood but also facilitates the client's self-exploration, thereby promoting client growth.

A nurse walked into a client's room and found her forlornly looking at a negligee that had been a gift from her husband. The client had recently had a mastectomy. The nurse placed a hand on the client's shoulder and said to her, "You look so sad." The client began to cry and told the nurse, "I wonder if I'll ever be able to wear this again?" The nurse sat down next to the client and answered, "Perhaps you would like to talk about your sadness." The client began to tell the nurse that she felt she had lost her femininity.

The nurse's ability to tune into the client's phenomenological world not only made the client feel that the nurse understood her concern but also gave the client feedback about how she was coming across to others. The nurse's sensitivity and accurate therapeutic understanding helped the client to express her thoughts and feelings, validate her experience, and minimize her sense of aloneness.

However, there may be obstacles to empathetic response. Language may be a barrier. Even when people speak the same language, different people may attach different meanings to the same words.* Therefore, nurses need to clarify with clients the meanings they attach to words and concepts. For example, a client may be referring to anger when talking about being "upset," while a nurse may associate anxiety with feeling upset.

Differences in life experience may also interfere with empathetic response. The discussion of experiential differences earlier in this chapter has implications for the development of empathy. When nurse and client are of different sexes, ages, or races or when they have different cultural or socioeconomic backgrounds, obstacles to empathy may be present. For example, a 22-year-old nurse who has never been seriously ill may have difficulty understanding the reaction to hospitalization of an 80-year-old, chronically ill client. Such experiential

differences make it very important for nurses to focus consciously on the client's perception of the situation. This approach will help nurses to avoid making value judgments about a client's life-style or coping behaviors. Judgmental attitudes may lead nurses to reject or avoid a client and may contribute to closing nurses off from therapeutically understanding a client's experience.

Sometimes, similarities in life experience between client and nurse may lead to a nurse overidentifying with and sympathizing with a client. For example, a nurse may begin to feel sorry for or pity a client, or a nurse may become angry at the people with whom the client is angry. When this occurs, the nurse becomes very subjective and may be unable to help the client cope with the experience.

In direct contrast to the nurse who overidentifies and sympathizes with a client is the nurse who is reluctant to tune into a client's phenomenological world for fear of being exposed to the client's emotional pain. Should a nurse be afraid to "borrow" a client's emotional pain, then the nurse may wall himself or herself off from the client's experience.

Any of these obstacles may lead nurses to assume an external frame of reference, may block therapeutic understanding, and may produce an "I-it" relationship. Likewise, the ability of nurses to assume an internal frame of reference and tune into the phenomenological worlds of clients facilitates therapeutic communication.

TOUCHING

Touching is one way of communicating. By touching, people express such emotions as love, sympathy, hostility, and fear. Nurses often use touching to communicate care and empathy to clients. Holding a fearful client's hand or placing one's hand on the shoulder of a crying client may communicate more empathy or concern than any words might offer. Therefore, it is not surprising that many nursing activities incorporate touching. These activities range from such comfort measures as bathing clients and giving backrubs to such caregiving measures as changing dressings and irrigating ostomies.

Touching is also a means of exploring one's environment (Blondis and Jackson, 1982). Toddlers are

---

*Refer to Chapter 10 for a discussion of language and meaning.

always touching objects—furniture, toys, flowers, and so on. They are learning about the world they live in. As people mature, they continue to use touching to familiarize themselves with new environments. For example, clients who have only recently been admitted to a hospital unit may stroke, finger, or grasp bedcovers, arms of chairs, and magazines in an attempt to familiarize themselves with the objects in their environment and to become spatially oriented. Nurses need to become aware of the significance of touching and not to view it as random or meaningless movement.

Bradley and Edinberg (1982) point out that, for many nurses and clients, the high degree of touching that is customary in the nurse-client relationship can be at variance with the degree of touching that they have been conditioned to consider "normal" in social interaction. These nurses and clients may feel uncomfortable with the degree of touching involved in comfort- and care-giving nursing activities and with tactile communication of feelings. For example, some nurses and clients may interpret touching as aggressive or intrusive rather than as evidence of empathy and caring.* Generally, people who speak Latin-derived languages use more touching and are more comfortable with touching than are people who speak Anglo-Saxon–derived languages. On the cultural continuum of touching, Scandinavians tend to fall midway between Latins and Anglo-Saxons. However, even within the same cultural groups, there may be a great deal of variation (Montagu, 1971).

Therefore, to avoid misinterpreting the use of touching, nurses need to be aware of both their own attitudes about touching and the attitudes of their clients. The self-assessment guide (opposite) might help nurses gain insight into their own attitudes abut touching.

Communication themes

A communication theme is a recurrent idea or concept that underlies communication and ties it

---

*Clients who are suffering from some psychiatric disorders, such as schizophrenia, may have difficulty with ego boundaries. In such instances, touching should be used judiciously. Refer to Chapter 25 for further discussion.

Touch self-assessment guide

1. How much touching is customary among members of my family? My ethnic group?
2. In what context(s) do I and my family most use touching? Least use touching?
3. Among people of which age groups and/or which sex do I consider touching most acceptable? Least acceptable?
4. How do I feel when, during conversation, people touch me?
5. Does my reaction to being touched vary according to the part of my body being touched (for example, limb vs. trunk vs. genitals)?
6. Does my reaction to being touched vary according to the person doing the touching (for example, family member, lover, friend, professional care giver) and the sex of the person doing the touching?
7. How do I feel (or imagine I would feel) when I am the recipient of personal care (for example, a backrub, a bath, a dressing change, an ostomy irrigation)?

together. Communication themes provide part of the data base for identifying client behavioral responses that require nursing intervention. Peplau (1953, 1954) and Ujhely (1968) have pioneered in helping nurses listen for the meaning or messages being conveyed—the themes of communication. There are three types of communication themes: content theme, mood theme, and interaction theme.

The *content theme* is the idea that underlies or links together seemingly disparate topics of discussion. It is the "what" of communication.

Elvira Johnson, 31 years old, was hospitalized after an attempted suicide. She had been married for 3 years to Stuart Johnson, a successful insurance agent. Barbara, a student nurse, began meeting biweekly with Mrs. Johnson to talk about her concerns. After 3 weeks, the student nurse became very disheartened and frustrated. She believed that Mrs. Johnson was using the time to socialize and that she was only talk-

ing about superficial topics. Barbara's verbatim notes showed that Mrs. Johnson frequently spoke as follows: "When I was younger, I had several girl friends. None of us were any beauties. We would go bowling or out for pizza. We had a lot of laughs. We didn't need boyfriends to have a good time."

"My husband is an insurance agent, and many of his clients are pretty young student nurses like you. They take out professional liability insurance." Then she would laugh and ask, "Do you think I can trust him with those students?"

"I had a beautiful wedding. Many friends were invited. My sister was my maid of honor, and my husband's best friend, Jeff, was his best man. They really are good friends—best buddies they call each other. I think if my husband had to choose between the two of us he would choose Jeff."

In discussing this interaction with her instructor, Barbara began to see that low self-esteem was a recurrent theme. Mrs. Johnson saw herself as an unattractive woman. She felt threatened by her husband's young clients and believed that her husband preferred his male friend to her. Mrs. Johnson had not been engaging in superficial conversation. The underlying message or theme in her interactions was that of low self-esteem. Once this theme was identified, nursing intervention could be planned.

The *mood theme* is the affect or emotion a person communicates. To identify the mood theme, one needs to listen for speech patterns and tone of voice. In addition, gestures, facial expressions, posture, and personal appearance should be observed. The mood theme reflects an individual's affect. Is the person angry? Hopeless? Apathetic? Any adjective describing a mood may be a possible mood theme. The mood theme is the "how" of communication.

Mrs. Barnes had recently been diagnosed as diabetic. A community health nurse was counseling her in diabetic care and helping her work through her feelings about being diabetic. The nurse noticed on each of her visits that Mrs. Barnes' 14-year-old son, Matthew, appeared listless. His face was expressionless. Regard-

less of what was happening or what he was speaking about, Matthew's face remained expressionless and his voice was monotone.

The community health nurse identified Matthew's mood as apathetic. She recognized that this flatness of affect or apathy might be an indicator of deep emotional conflict. The nurse referred Matthew to a neighborhood counseling center.

By identifying the mood theme of apathy and recognizing its import, the community health nurse was able to make an appropriate referral.

The *interaction theme* is the idea or concept that best describes the dynamics between communicating participants. Are the partners in communication relating to one another in a pattern of dominance-submission? Collaboration? Power struggle? Parallel play? If the interaction theme is reinforcing well-established patterns of pathology or if it is destructive of therapeutic communication, it may need to be identified so that the problem can be resolved.

After a 1-year stay in a psychiatric hospital, John Toomey was discharged to his home. Carlos Rodriquez, a psychiatric nurse, visited John on a weekly basis. Carlos' purpose was to help John readjust to living in the community. The focus of these visits was to assist John in finding employment, to teach him to shop for and prepare meals, and to help him to budget his money. Whenever John had to make a decision or initiate a plan of action he would ask Carlos, "What do you think I should do?" Carlos would usually respond with his assessment of the best course of action. After several visits, Carlos realized that the interaction theme had become one of dominance-submission. He had taken the dominant role, and John had assumed the submissive role. Once Carlos had identified these dynamics, he pointed out to John the pattern their interactions had taken. Carlos explained that in the future he would help John explore alternatives and arrive at a decision but would not make the decision.

Had Carlos failed to identify the interaction theme, he might have continued to reinforce unhealthy patterns of communication and behavior.

These vignettes illustrate what is meant by content, mood, and interaction themes. Although these hypothetical examples have been drawn from nursing situations, any one or a combination of themes can be identified in any sequence of communication, be it social or therapeutic.

THE NURSING PROCESS

Identifying predominant communication themes and helping clients learn appropriate and effective coping behaviors require that nurse and client actively explore a client's experience within the framework of the nursing process.

Steps in the nursing process

The steps in the nursing process have been delineated in various ways by various authors. Basically, each way has been a form of the scientific method. Briefly outlined, the steps are as follows*:

1. Making an assessment—collecting data about a client;† aim: to gather information from the verbal and nonverbal communication of the client, the client's family and/or significant others
   a. Gather the following information systematically and continuously from one-to-one interactions, group therapy sessions, and recreational and unit activities:
      (1) The client's, the client's family's, and significant others' perceptions of the situation or problem
      (2) The client's intrapersonal, interpersonal, and sociocultural strengths and limitations
      (3) The client's verbal, kinesic, and proxemic behavior
      (4) The client's status: biological, intellec-
      tual, psychological, sociocultural, and spiritual
      (5) Factors that predisposed the client to the situation or problem
      (6) Factors that precipitated the situation or problem
      (7) The client's present environment (both social and physical)
      (8) The interaction of yourself and the staff with the client, the client's family, and significant others
   b. Verify the data.
      (1) Confirm observations and perceptions by obtaining consensual validation or additional information from the client, the client's family, significant others, and/or other sources (for example, records, psychological tests).
      (2) Communicate assessment information to other staff members, verbally and through charting. A particular form of charting may be done at the time of admission—the admission assessment. The following information is usually charted on admission:
         (a) The event that precipitated hospitalization
         (b) Prior psychiatric problems
         (c) Past school and childhood relationships; relationships with parents and siblings
         (d) Sexual and marital history
         (e) Relationships with children
         (f) Job; vocational and avocational history
         (g) Any special physical conditions
         (h) History of allergies
         (i) Medications taken recently or within the past 2 or 3 weeks (does the client have any medications with him or her *now?*)
         (j) Blood pressure, temperature, pulse and respiratory rates, weight and height
         (k) List of clothing and valuables
         (l) Phone number of family member or friend

---

*Adapted from National Council of State Boards of Nursing, Inc., 1980; Atkinson and Murphy, 1980; American Nurses' Association, 1982.
†Although the singular "client" is used throughout the discussion of the nursing process, it should not be interpreted as referring only to individuals. The term "client" also encompasses social units such as families and couples.

2. Analyzing the data—making inferences based on the collected data;* aim: to understand the meaning of the client's behavior patterns
    a. Identify predominant themes and the interrelationship among these themes.
    b. Identify predisposing and precipitating factors, the client's overall health status, and the client's perception of the situation or crisis.
    c. Formulate a nursing diagnosis that states the behavioral response (or potential response) and its related factor (for example, dysfunctional grieving related to loss of spouse [NANDA 9.2.1.1]: anxiety related to culture shock [NANDA 9.3.1]).
3. Planning client care—establishing outcomes and developing intervention
    a. Aim: to develop a plan of action for initiating change or for enabling the client to better cope with the existing situation
        (1) Determine whether the locus of decision making is predominantly with the nurse, predominantly with the client, or shared between nurse and client.†
        (2) On the basis of the locus of decision making, facilitate or encourage the participation of the client, the client's family, and/or significant others in setting outcomes and in establishing priorities among outcomes (several outcomes may be pursued simultaneously; highest priority outcomes relate to preventing a client from harming self or others).
        (3) State projected outcomes as observable behavioral changes to be achieved
        (4) Differentiate between long-term and short-term outcomes.
    b. Aim: to design and modify a client care plan that is based on psychiatric nursing

principles, the psychiatric literature, and the nurse's own experience with effective approaches to specific behavior problems
        (1) Anticipate client needs on the basis of the priority of outcomes.
        (2) Include the client, the client's family, and/or significant others in the development of intervention strategies.
        (3) Plan care that is congruent with the client's age, sex, locus of decision making, religion, and culture.
        (4) Identify nursing approaches that should be followed for specific behavioral problems.
    c. Aim: to cooperate with other health team members in the delivery of health care
        (1) Design a care plan that is consistent with the total therapeutic regimen.
        (2) Coordinate the client's treatment program (for example, unit, recreational, and occupational activities; group and one-to-one therapies).
        (3) Report and/or chart information that is pertinent to client care.
4. Implementing the care plan—instituting and completing nursing actions that are necessary for the achievement of established goals and the facilitation of growth-promoting behavior
    a. Aim: to counsel the client
        (1) Help the client to identify stressors and to develop effective means of stress management.
        (2) Facilitate the client's relationships with family, health team members, and/or significant others.
        (3) Inform the client about or ensure that the client is informed about mental health status, confidentiality, and, when applicable, retention status.*
        (4) Refer the client to appropriate community resources (for example, Alcoholics Anonymous, Alatot, Alateen, Alanon).

*This step of the nursing process may be facilitated through clinical supervision—either with the help of a teacher or supervisor or through "peer supervision," which implies a mutual exchange of ideas and suggestions among co-workers.

†Refer to Chapter 1 for a discussion of the locus of decision making.

*Refer to Chapter 3 for a discussion of retention status and confidentiality.

b. Aim: to provide care that will facilitate the accomplishment of therapeutic outcomes
   (1) Establish a physical and social milieu that ensures the client's safety.
   (2) Provide a physical and social milieu that promotes rapport, verbalization, the development of insight, and the trying out of more adaptive coping behaviors.
   (3) Provide care that compensates for gaps in the client's perception, interpretation, or response.
   (4) Encourage the client to participate in and follow the therapeutic regimen.
   (5) Modify care according to the client's needs or priorities.
   (6) Provide care that encourages self-actualization and emotional interdependence.
   (7) Supervise and coordinate the work of health team members for whom you are responsible.
   (8) Report and chart nursing actions and client responses to nursing actions.

5. Evaluating the care plan—determining the degree of outcome achievement; aim: to include the client in estimating the client's progress toward the attainment of outcomes
   a. Estimate the degree to which outcomes have been achieved, crises have been resolved, and coping behaviors have become more effective.
   b. Identify outcomes that need to be modified or revised.
   c. Evaluate the effectiveness of nursing actions or approaches.
   d. Identify aspects of the milieu and/or nursing approaches that need to be modified or revised.
   e. Bridge the client to support systems other than the nurse-client relationship.
      (1) People in the social environment (for example, friends, relatives, clergy) who are willing to serve as support givers
      (2) Community agencies that offer help with problems that may arise in the future

The following vignette illustrates how the nursing process is used in mental health nursing.

Toby Jackson, a 69-year-old woman, was hospitalized for congestive heart failure. Because of her physical condition, for the past year her physical activity had been severely restricted. John, a student nurse, met biweekly with Mrs. Jackson. John had noticed that Mrs. Jackson took little interest in her physical appearance and rarely spoke with her roommate. Mrs. Jackson had told John, "When I was younger, I took care of my children and my home. I was widowed when I was 31, and I had to earn a living and support and raise those children all by myself. I was always busy. I took care of everyone. Now I can't even take care of myself. I'm no good to anyone." John replied, "It sounds like you define your value as a person by what you can do for yourself and others." Mrs. Jackson answered, "That's right. You have to keep busy and be useful. Otherwise, you're no good to anyone, even yourself."

John had gathered the following data about Mrs. Jackson:
1. restricted physical activity
2. little interest in her physical appearance
3. little social interaction with her roommate
4. productive and independent most of her life
5. accustomed to caring for others
6. feels worthless

In supervision with his instructor, John looked at the meaning of the data he had collected. He identified low self-esteem as one of Mrs. Jackson's predominant content themes. At this point, John was able to develop a nursing diagnosis. Then John determined that the locus of decision making could be shared between him and the client. Thus John, in collaboration with Mrs. Jackson, established the nursing care plan shown on p. 318.

John decided that his evaluation would encompass the following areas:
1. The degree of interest Mrs. Jackson took in her personal appearance (e.g., attending to personal grooming, coordinating her clothes)
2. The degree that Mrs. Jackson conversed with her roommate

NURSING CARE PLAN

Client with Low Self-Esteem

Long-term Outcomes	Short-term Outcomes	Nursing Strategies
Nursing diagnosis: Self-esteem disturbance related to a decreased sense of productivity (NANDA 7.1.2)		
Accept both strengths and deficits Develop insight into sources of low self-esteem Develop feelings of adequacy and security	Recognize that low self-esteem is causing discomfort Identify current situations that arouse feelings of low self-esteem Identify some positive qualities in the self Develop skills/talents that will build self-confidence Set realistic goals Engage in activities that provide a sense of accomplishment	Convey to client that she is a worthwhile person Accept but do not condone feelings of worthlessness Assess social and self-care skills, support systems, and interests Encourage client to do all she can for herself Do things with, not for, client whenever possible Provide activities that client can accomplish and that will interest her Do not make situations so easy that success is achieved with little effort Encourage and support social interaction with roommate, family, and friends

3. The degree to which Mrs. Jackson was able to identify personal strengths
4. The degree to which Mrs. Jackson was able to communicate positive feelings about herself
5. The degree of participation by Mrs. Jackson in activities that provided her with a sense of accomplishment

By the time the relationship between John and Mrs. Jackson was terminated, the client had begun to brush her hair each morning and to hold it in place with some brightly colored combs that her daughter had brought her. She also had begun to knit a sweater for her grandson. Mrs. Jackson and her roommate occasionally talked about her knitting. Mrs. Jackson told John, "If I can't help take care of my grandchildren, at least I can knit them some winter clothes. That will help my children with the clothing bills. That makes me feel good." Just prior to her discharge from the hospital, John referred Mrs. Jackson to a clinical nurse specialist in private practice who would work with Mrs. Jackson to accomplish more fully the established goals. In addition, John helped Mrs. Jackson to identify two people in her social environment, her clergyman and her oldest daughter, to whom she could express her concerns and on whom she could count for support.

The nursing principles on which the above client care plan was based are as follows:

1. Negative appraisals have contributed to Mrs. Jackson's feeling of low self-esteem. It is important to provide an environment that is nonjudgmental. The nurse should accept Mrs. Jackson's negative as well as positive attributes.
2. When an individual sets unrealistically high goals, the result will be failure. When failure consistently occurs, feelings of inadequacy are reinforced. The setting of challenging but realistic goals will help Mrs. Jackson to overcome some of her feelings of inadequacy.
3. Feelings of neglect tend to reinforce feelings of low self-esteem. It is important to approach Mrs. Jackson in a consistent, accepting manner and to make her realize that the nurse considers her a worthwhile person.

The nursing process also involves the *charting of observations* of client behavior. In most mental health facilities, the nurse is not the only team member who charts observations. All team members are expected to record observations of clients with whom they work. The purposes of charting are as follows:

1. To facilitate the sharing of information among the entire staff
2. To provide information for planning and revising a treatment plan
3. To keep a record of changes in a client's behavior that may lead to a better understanding of client problems
4. To provide a legal record of client problems, nursing assessments, the treatment plan, and client response to the treatment plan

Nurses should observe the following basic principles of charting:

1. Record accurately, using concise, simple language.
2. Be objective and nonjudgmental.
3. Give concrete examples. For instance, what was the *behavior* that suggested hostility? What *intervention* was taken? What *effects* did the intervention have?
4. Quote *exactly* what a client says. This is especially important in reporting delusions and hallucinations. Use quotation marks.
5. Sign, date, and record the time of each entry.
6. If a mistake is made, cross through it and initial.

Guide for assessment of mental health

The following guide has been designed to assist students to assess a client's mental health status, to establish goals and develop nursing strategies consistent with a client's perceptions and orientations about health and illness, and to communicate (verbally and through charting) information about a client's condition to other health team members. Examples of primary NANDA nursing diagnoses related to a range of maladaptive responses are included after each behavioral category.

1. Demographic data
   a. Name
   b. Address
   c. Age
   d. Sex
   e. Education
   f. Ethnicity (optional)*
   g. Religion (optional)*
   h. Living arrangements
   i. Marital status
2. Admission data
   a. Date and time of admission
   b. Manner of admission
      (1) Self
      (2) Relatives
      (3) Police
      (4) Other (describe)
   c. Form of retention (if hospitalized)
      (1) Informal retention
      (2) Voluntary retention
      (3) Involuntary retention
      (4) Emergency
      (5) Comments
   d. Reason for admission
   e. Client's primary complaint
   f. Client's premorbid personality
3. History of psychiatric problems
   a. Previous condition: date; problem
   b. Assistance sought: native healer; therapist; agency; clergyman; other (describe)
   c. Current levels of functioning and coping
4. Thought patterns
   a. Delusion: grandeur; persecution; somatic; self-accusatory
   b. Obsession
   c. Ideas of reference
   d. Phobia
   e. Looseness of association
   f. Flight of ideas
   g. Fugue
   h. Impaired judgment
   i. Impaired insight
   j. Impaired orientation to time, place, or person
   k. Impaired memory
   l. No observable thought disturbance
   m. Comments

---

*Legislation protects people from being required to reveal ethnicity and religion.

Example of primary NANDA nursing diagnosis: altered thought processes

5. Sensory processes
   a. Hallucination:
      olfactory; auditory; tactile; gustatory; visual
   b. No observable sensory disturbance
   c. Comments

Example of primary NANDA nursing diagnosis: sensory/perceptual alterations: visual, auditory, kinesthetic, gustatory, tactile, olfactory

6. Speech patterns
   a. Blocking
   b. Word salad
   c. Echolalia
   d. Circumstantiality
   e. Irrelevancy
   f. Confabulation
   g. Mutism
   h. Neologism
   i. Perseveration
   j. Stuttering
   k. No observable speech disturbance
   l. Comments

Example of primary NANDA nursing diagnosis: impaired verbal communication

7. Affect
   a. Elation
   b. Depression
   c. Ambivalence
   d. Apathy
   e. Anger and hostility
   f. Anxiety
   g. No observable disturbance of affect
   h. Comments

Examples of primary NANDA nursing diagnoses: dysfunctional grieving; hopelessness; anxiety; powerlessness; spiritual distress; potential for violence: self-directed or directed at others

8. Motor activity
   a. Hyperactive
   b. Hypoactive
   c. Stereotypical: persistent; aimless; repetitive
   d. Perseveration
   e. Catalepsy: stupor; waxy flexibility
   f. Compulsion
   g. No observable disturbance in motor activity
   h. Comments

Example of primary NANDA nursing diagnosis: impaired physical mobility

9. Level of consciousness
   a. Confusion
   b. Stupor
   c. Delirium
   d. Alert
   e. Comments

Examples of primary NANDA nursing diagnoses: altered thought processes; altered role performance

10. Physical appearance
    a. Posture
       (1) Sagging
       (2) Rigid
       (3) Curled into fetal position
       (4) Bent
       (5) No observable disturbance in posture
       (6) Comments
    b. Facies
       (1) Drooping or sagging: deflected eyes; lusterless eyes; drooping eyelids; deep nasolabial folds

(2) Uplifted or retracted: smiling; retracted brow; wide open eyes; darting eyes
(3) Blank: staring into space; distant expression in eyes
(4) Mask-like or ironed-out
(5) Facial tic
(6) No observable disturbance in facies
(7) Comments
c. Mode of dress
(1) Overly neat
(2) Disheveled
(3) Bizarre
(4) Appropriate
(5) Comments

Examples of primary NANDA nursing diagnoses: impaired physical mobility; ineffective individual coping

11. Physical status
   a. Vital signs: pulse; temperature; respiration; blood pressure
   b. Physical condition
      (1) Medical problems: acute; chronic
      (2) Physical aids (describe)
      (3) Medications: date and time of last dose
      (4) Allergies (describe)
      (5) Physical signs and symptoms: skin rash; edema; sore throat (phenothiazine side effect?); unusual gait, fine hand tremor, or any extrapyramidal symptom
      (6) Comments

Examples of primary NANDA nursing diagnoses: fluid volume excess; impaired skin integrity; impaired physical mobility

12. Patterns of daily living
   a. Sleep patterns: restlessness; insomnia; narcoplexy; average number of hours of sleep
   b. Personal hygiene: kempt; unkempt

c. Eating patterns: number of meals a day; compulsive eating; anorexia
d. Drinking patterns: beverage; quantity consumed; frequency of consumption
e. Sexual patterns: sexual orientation or preference; attitudes about sexuality; sexual activity
f. Elimination patterns: constipation; diarrhea; urinary frequency; urinary retention
g. Social patterns: recreation; work; intimacy; community involvement
h. Comments

Examples of primary NANDA nursing diagnoses: sleep pattern disturbance; sexual dysfunction; urinary retention; impaired social interaction; social isolation

13. Level of self-care
   a. Personal hygiene
   b. Activities of daily living
   c. Comments

Examples of primary NANDA nursing diagnoses: bathing/hygiene self-care deficit; dressing/grooming self-care deficit; altered growth and development

14. Cultural orientation
   a. Place of residence: interethnic neighborhood; ethnic enclave
   b. Family organization: nuclear; extended; members composing family unit; members vested with authority; members involved in child rearing; sense of obligation of family members to one another
   c. Sex-defined roles: stereotyped male and female roles; amount of independence permitted men and women; degree of intimacy permitted between married men and women, unmarried men and women
   d. Communication patterns: language spoken at home; language spoken outside

home; use of touching and gesturing; interpersonal spacing

e. Type of dress: traditional ethnic dress; Western-style dress

f. Type of food: ethnic food; American food

g. Relationship to people: individualistic; group-oriented; egalitarian; authoritative

h. Relationship to time: past-oriented; present-oriented; future-oriented

i. Relationship to the world: personal control; goal directed; fatalistic

j. Health care patterns: ideas concerning causes of mental illness; ideas concerning treatment of mental illness; people consulted for treatment of mental illness (e.g., family member, native healer, mental health therapist, other [describe])

k. Comments

Examples of primary NANDA nursing diagnoses: impaired verbal communication; altered role performance; impaired social interaction

---

15. Effective social network
    a. Family
    b. Household members (if different from family)
    c. Friends
    d. Associates: employer; coworkers; neighbors; others
    e. Religious affiliates: clergyman; church elders; congregants
    f. Comments

Examples of primary NANDA nursing diagnoses: impaired social interaction; ineffective family coping: disabling; ineffective family coping: compromised; family coping: potential for growth

---

16. Stressors
    a. Culture shock
       (1) Communication (foreign verbal, kinesic, and proxemic systems)

(2) Mechanical environment (e.g., different types of food, housing, clothing, utilities)

(3) Social isolation from family and friends

(4) Foreign customs, standards, and/or values

(5) Different or new role relationships

b. Life changes
   (1) Affectional: marriage; birth; death; divorce; abandonment
   (2) Socioeconomic: promotion; demotion; unemployment; change of employment; change of residence; increased responsibilities
   (3) Biophysical: serious illness (acute or chronic); surgery; accident; loss of body part; sexual trauma (e.g., rape, incest)

c. Other (describe)

d. No significant stress

e. Comments

Examples of primary NANDA nursing diagnoses: impaired verbal communication; impaired social interaction; social isolation; altered role performance; rape-trauma syndrome

---

17. Coping mechanisms
    a. Coping mechanisms used (describe)
    b. Effectiveness of coping mechanisms
    c. Client's perception of mechanisms that are effective in reducing stress
    d. Comments

Examples of primary NANDA nursing diagnoses: ineffective individual coping; ineffective family coping: disabling; ineffective family coping: compromised; family coping: potential for growth

---

18. Resources
    a. Personal: interests; leisure time activities; physical and mental abilities; educational achievement; other
    b. Social: interpersonal networks; economic support systems (e.g., health insur-

ance, sick leave, union benefits); food, shelter, clothing; other

c. Comments

Examples of primary NANDA nursing diagnoses: altered health maintenance; impaired social interaction; social isolation

---

19. Candidacy for active involvement in treatment program
    a. Developmental level
    b. Interactional ability
    c. Willingness to participate in treatment program
    d. Locus of decision making
    e. Client problems, plans, ideas, hopes, or complaints that may impact on the treatment plan or progress
    f. Areas of anticipated need for assistance from nursing staff
    g. Comments

Examples of primary NANDA nursing diagnoses: altered growth and development; noncompliance (specify)

Operation of the nursing process throughout the nurse-client relationship

The various steps of the nursing process tend to be associated with definite phases of the nurse-client relationship.

The nurse-client relationship is characterized by three phases: orientation, working, and termination. Initially a client may speak about many different areas but will not delve deeply into any one area. This is to be expected. During this stage, which is called the *orientation phase*, the nurse and the client are getting to know one another and the client is mapping out areas of concern. At this time, the nurse begins to collect data about the client. At some point, the client will begin to repeat areas and will assume a high commitment configuration and/

or postures of affiliation. This should indicate to the nurse a readiness to discuss these areas in greater detail. This repetition also signals the beginning of the next step in the process of exploration: description and clarification. This step is also referred to as the *working phase* in a therapeutic relationship.

As a client observes and describes what he or she perceives of his or her experiences, the nurse assists the client in this description. The nurse encourages the client by saying, "Start at the beginning and tell me what happened" or "Tell me more about that." Occasionally the nurse might assist the person to clarify thoughts by seeking to clarify speech. We have all had the experience of being unable to put something into words until we have thought it out clearly in our heads. Therefore, when a client uses vague pronouns, speaking of "them," "they," "he," "she," or "it," the nurse needs to seek clarification. The nurse may ask, "Who is 'she'?" or "Who are you referring to when you speak about 'all of them'?"

Mr. Graff, a 62-year-old man, had been admitted to the hospital after slipping in the bathtub and fracturing his leg. Following surgery to reduce the fracture, Mr. Graff was resting in his hospital bed. When his meal was served, he became very upset. He could not eat because he did not have his dentures. Repeatedly he ranted, "How do you expect me to eat when they took my teeth?" Nurses and aides hastily looked through his bedside stand and in his closet but found no dentures. Yet the hospital record indicated that he had been wearing dentures when he was admitted. The staff activity seemed only to further aggravate Mr. Graff. He continued to rant, "They took my teeth." Finally a nurse asked, "Mr. Graff, who took your teeth?" Mr. Graff answered, "My daughter and son-in-law took my teeth home with them. They were afraid they'd get lost or broken if left here. Now how am I going to eat?" Once the situation was clarified, a phone call was made to the daughter, and she brought Mr. Graff's dentures to him. The problem had been resolved.

Occasionally during the process of exploration, a nurse may have to provide information to compensate for some lack in a client's ability to perceive or to correct a client's tendency to subjectively and selectively perceive and interpret an experience. For example, a nurse might give concise instructions to a person experiencing moderate to severe anxiety or might try to help a client perceive an experience more objectively by expressing doubt as to the reality of a perception and asking, "Isn't that a bit unusual?" However, a nurse must be careful to word such an expression so that it does not threaten the client, increase the client's anxiety, and further distort the client's perception of reality.

Once a client has described and clarified an experience, he or she is ready to progress to the next step of exploration. It is at this point that the nurse and client *together* look at the data. They try to place events in sequence, to determine in what way the experience is similar to or different from other events, and to evaluate the impact of the experience on the individual. In helping a client explore an experience, a nurse might inquire, "What happened first?" or "In what way was this the same as (or different from) . . .?"

A 70-year-old woman, Mrs. Rich, had just completed the first week in a home for the aged. She appeared lonely and explained, "I feel so alone and afraid. I don't know anyone here. I have no one to talk to. I've never been in a place like this before. I've never even been in a hospital. I had all my children at home." A nurse inquired, "Was there ever a time in your life that you had some of these same feelings?"

Mrs. Rich thought a while and said, "Yes, when I was first married. My husband brought me to this small town where he had found work. I didn't know a soul, and all my family lived miles away. I felt so alone—I thought I'd never feel like I belonged. I'd go for long walks, and before long I'd begin to see some of the same faces. I'd sort of smile, and they'd smile, and before you'd know it we would be talking."

The nurse had assisted Mrs. Rich to find similarities between the present experience of loneliness and a past experience.

Once nurse and client have sifted through the data, putting events in sequence and establishing similarities to and differences from other experiences, the client is ready to draw conclusions and to

formulate the meaning of the experience. The nurse assists the client in this process by facilitating summarization or by suggesting a tentative conclusion. The nurse might say, "Then what you are saying is . . ." or "What do you conclude from all this?" or "It sounds like what you're saying is . . .. Does that sound right to you?" In the case of Mrs. Rich, once she had made the comparison between her experience as a bride and her present experience in the nursing home, the nurse would be able to ask, "Might you be able to handle this new experience in a similar way?" Ideally, Mrs. Rich would state that it might be possible and would agree to give it some thought.

Now the client is ready to decide whether events should be allowed to progress as they have been or whether new behavior is needed to better cope with the experience. The nurse might inquire, "The next time this happens, what might you do?" By asking a client to consider what behavior might be more appropriate in the future, the nurse encourages the client to formulate a plan of action. In the example of Mrs. Rich, once she had recognized similarities between her past and present experiences, the nurse would be able to help Mrs. Rich deal with the situation. Mrs. Rich might decide that since, in the past, taking long walks had helped to familiarize her with her new neighbors, she might start strolling around the nursing home and into scheduled activities.

"Perhaps," Mrs. Rich stated, "taking walks will help me get to know people." The nurse agreed that this plan was worth a try and suggested that they evaluate the results after a week. At the end of the week, Mrs. Rich proudly reported that she had made one "pretty nice friend" and that several other people were stopping and chatting with her.

Thus during the working phase, the nurse assesses and analyzes client data, helps the client plan a course of action, supports the client in trying out the plan, and assists the client in evaluating how effectively the plan has helped him or her cope with the situation. Should the evaluation show the new behavior to be ineffective, nurse and client need to

TABLE 11-4 Therapeutic communication strategies

Strategies	Example
Anxiety reduction	Allow client to proceed at his or her own pace; do not introduce a highly anxiety-producing subject; teach progressive relaxation techniques
Open-ended questioning	Ask questions that begin with "where, what, or when" (e.g., "What did you do this weekend"); avoid questions that can be answered by "yes" or "no"
Clarification seeking	Attempt to make clear client's ambiguous or global statements (e. g., "Who do you mean when you say that nobody likes you?")
Confrontation	Attempt to point out client's ambivalent or discrepant statements (e.g., "You told me that you want to go to college, but now you are saying that you want to get a job." or "You are telling me how happy you feel, but you look sad.")
Consensual validation	Determine if what you understand is what the client means (e.g., "It sounds like you are feeling lonely. Is that correct?")
Empathic understanding	Tune into the client's feelings and perceptions by asking oneself such questions as, "How does the client see the problem? How does the client feel about the situation? How would the client like to resolve the problem?"
Environmental manipulation	Modify the physical and/or social environment (e.g., respect client privacy; allow client quiet time; teach client assertiveness skills so he or she has an increased sense of self control; modulate the noise level)
Here-and-now focusing	Set the focus of interactions on immediate events or current feelings (e.g., "Tell me what you are feeling now.")
Information giving	Make available to client facts that will aid him or her in perceiving, interpreting, or responding to a situation
Leading	Help client describe events and feelings in greater detail and depth (e.g., "Tell me more about how you feel about your divorce.")
Mirroring	Observe client's behavior and give client this feedback (e.g., "You look anxious" or "You sound angry.")
Reality orientation	Correct client's distorted perceptions of reality (e.g., "That is a shadow. It is not a dog," or "I don't hear any sirens.")
Cognitive restructuring	Help client focus on the positive aspects or accomplishments of his or her life; help client reframe events so that they contribute to self-esteem
Expressing doubt	Let client know that you do not perceive events in the same way as the client (e.g., "Isn't that a bit unusual?")
Verbalizing the implied	State directly what the client has inferred (e.g., "You said that you are angry with everyone. Are you angry with me?")
Summarizing	Express in one statement several ideas or feelings and/or their relationship to one another (e.g., "Today you talked about your role as a parent and how it makes you feel needed.")

Adapted from Anderson (1983).

identify the reasons why it does not work and to develop a new course of action. Refer to Table 11-4 for a summary of therapeutic communication techniques.

The *termination phase* is the conclusion of the nurse-client relationship. It is often characterized by such relationship stalls as client avoidance of interactions (either missing sessions or leaving early) or client attempts to extend the relationship.

Because it was the end of the semester, Judith Johanson was terminating her relationship with both of her clients. Judith had told her clients at their very first meeting that their last interaction would be on May 7, and she had, in recent interviews, reminded them that their last interaction was imminent. Each client responded to termination differently. While for the past two sessions one client had made such excuses as being too tired or too busy to meet with the student nurse, the other client had told Judith, "You have helped me so much. I really appreciate it. Can I have your address so I can keep in touch with you?"

Judith discussed her clients' reactions to termination with her instructor. Judith decided to confront her first client with his behavior, and the client told Judith that he always had difficulty saying goodbyes. Judith also explained to her second client that extending the relationship was not part of their original agreement and would change the relationship from a therapeutic to a social relationship.

In addition to the actual saying of good-bye between client and nurse, during the termination phase the nurse and the client summarize the problems that have been worked upon and discuss the degree of goal accomplishment. The nurse helps the client to assess the motivation and effort used in problem solving. This is also a time when the nurse might give feedback to a client about the client's strengths, therapeutic accomplishments, and areas to continue to work upon. The nurse might also share with the client something that the nurse has gained from their interactions. For example, a nurse might tell a client, "You have shown me that life experience is an important source of learning" or "You have helped me to better understand what it is like to experience such a life crisis." Time should also be set aside for the client to express feelings about the relationship—for example, what was helpful and not helpful, what areas were easier to talk about than other areas, feelings about termination. The nurse should discuss his or her feelings about termination with a colleague or supervisor. Finally, the nurse should help the client establish networks of support other than the nurse-client relationship (for example, significant others, rap groups, self-help groups) that may be of assistance

TABLE 11-5 Nursing process throughout nurse-client relationship

Phase of the nurse-client relationship	Steps of the nursing process
Orientation	Assessment (begin to collect data)
Working	Assessment (continue to collect data, verify data)
	Analysis of data; planning of client care, implementation of the care plan, evaluation (begin to evaluate and revise care plan as needed)
Termination	Evaluation (continue to evaluate—goals attained, outcomes achieved, and effectiveness of nursing actions; bridge client to other support systems)

in coping with problems that might arise in the future.

Thus, the termination phase focuses on the nursing process step of evaluation, and this phase ideally occurs over several weeks. When termination occurs prematurely because of the sudden discharge of a client from the health care setting, both the client and the nurse may have a sense of frustration and of unfinished business.

The operation of the nursing process throughout the nurse-client relationship is summarized in Table 11-5.

GUIDELINES FOR PROMOTING THERAPEUTIC COMMUNICATION

Using the nursing process and establishing and maintaining a therapeutic relationship require therapeutic communication. To therapeutically communicate with clients, it is necessary for nurses to understand psychiatric nursing principles, to use the supervisory process, to be knowledgeable about the "do's" of therapeutic communication, and to recognize barriers to therapeutic communication.

Principles of psychiatric nursing

Some of the important principles* underlying psychiatric nursing intervention include:

1. Freud's dictum that *all behavior is meaningful* and that most behavior, in the complex human organism, is designed to satisfy several needs. For example, an individual who strives to do a job well may be attempting to satisfy the following needs:
   a. The need for approval
   b. The need for security
   c. The need for affection and companionship
   d. The need for self-respect
   e. The need for increased knowledge
   f. The need to create and to express creativity

   Several other needs could be added to the list. Pathological behavior also may represent attempts to satisfy needs. For example, a person who maintains a delusion of being persecuted by the FBI or the CIA may be satisfying the following needs:
   a. The need to disown one's negative and aggressive thoughts and to project them onto the outside world
   b. The need to feel important (as a result of being singled out)
   c. The need to provide some reasons for the existence of a chaotic inner world and thus restore some measure of order to that world

2. Maslow's hierarchy of needs (Maslow, 1967). A person tries to meet the most pressing needs first and, in doing so, may not recognize other important (perhaps even life-supporting) needs. For example, a person who is in a manic state seeks immediate release of tension through physical exertion. Sometimes the need for rest and adequate food are completely ignored in deference to the need for physical release of energy. Individuals whose needs have been satisfactorily met in the past are generally able to tolerate delays in the satisfaction of present needs.

3. The humanistic-existential stance that *all human beings have potential for growth.* Many psychiatric clients have led chaotic lives in the past and are experiencing a multitude of severe problems in the present. A feeling of hopelessness about a situation can become contagious, affecting even the nurse, or it can take the form of a self-fulfilling prophecy. To be truly helpful, the nurse must appeal to, cultivate, and reinforce the client's "healthy part." This belief in an individual's potential for change and for growth is also an antidote for any other dissatisfaction that can arise out of the nurse's own hopelessness.

4. The use of "themes" as a way of collecting and organizing data about the needs, problems, and goals of a client.

In interaction with psychiatric clients, *consistency* is important. When there is intrapsychic turmoil, a consistent, fairly well-ordered outer world can be a calming influence that provides the client some security. A person who has the painfully low self-esteem that is so common with psychiatric clients may automatically blame himself or herself for inconsistency on the part of others.

Acceptance as a worthwhile human being is what we are all looking for. Because of traumatic past experiences, the need of the psychiatric client for acceptance is extreme. However, acceptance of a client does not include automatic acceptance of all of the client's behavior. Self-destructive acts or aggressive acts that constitute a danger to other people are some obvious examples of behavior that cannot be accepted. *Limit setting* may be necessary to control some types of behavior, but the setting of limits can be done in a respectful, accepting manner that is therapeutic and not destructive of the client's self-esteem.

For example, when a nurse is involved in a one-to-one interaction with a client, and another resident of the unit keeps interrupting their conversation by trying to be included, some action is necessary.

---

*In the 1960s, Matheney and Topalis (1965) compiled a very useful and concise list of psychiatric nursing principles that are still pertinent. Several of them have been incorporated into this discussion.

A student and a client, Derrek, were engaged in their biweekly interaction. They were sitting in Derrek's room talking when Derrek's friend, John, walked into the room. John sat on Derrek's bed and started to tell Derrek and the student about his weekend at home. At this point, the student said, "John, this is the time that Derrek and I spend together. The conversation is private. We will be finished at 10:30. I will have some time then, if you would like to talk about your weekend at home." Derrek said, "Yes, I would like to hear about your weekend too, after I'm finished here."

The student was firm in setting limits on John's behavior, explaining to John that the conversation was private. The student also made an appointment for a one-to-one conversation with John in the very near future. Such a response by the student recognized the needs of both John and Derrek. It fostered self-respect and respect for others, and it helped promote Derrek's trust in the student.

When they first begin to work with psychiatric clients, nurses are often reluctant to employ any form of limit setting. This reluctance probably arises out of the fear that setting limits may hurt the client, whom they view as having suffered sufficiently already, and also out of the nurse's need to be accepted. *Therapeutic limit setting*, however, is not harmful, and it can be very beneficial for clients who are unable to exercise control over their own behavior. The validity of this statement has been demonstrated by the case of a young woman who, after having recovered from a period of confusion and florid psychosis, thanked her nurse for having set limits on some of her bizarre behavior.

In dealing with *unacceptable behavior*, nurses need to remember some important points. First, is the behavior truly unacceptable? The ability to express negative feelings verbally is a necessary part of living. Verbal expression of anger is more mature and socially acceptable than physical expression of anger. Therefore, the expression of negative feelings, although it can be threatening to the nurse, should be encouraged and supported. Nurses do, however, sometimes need to protect other clients—especially *vulnerable* clients—from verbal abuse.

When behavior is truly *unacceptable* or when

safety requires that some amount of physical force be used, the least amount possible should be employed. An example of a situation that might prove very distressing to a nurse working with psychiatric clients would be the need for several staff members to restrain a client who simply must be given medication.

A small, frail-looking elderly woman who had a severe heart condition and who was also psychotic was expressing her psychosis with hyperactivity that was threatening her life. Sedation was absolutely necessary; the woman had only recently been admitted, and the behavior was a continuation and escalation of what had been happening at home. Since she refused all medication and exhibited a degree of strength that was extraordinary for her age and size, it was necessary for several staff members to restrain her while an injection was administered.

While it was not possible in this case, many such situations could be avoided through judicious use of medication *before* anxiety has escalated. A cooperative nurse-client relationship that facilitates good communication and close observation can alert staff and client to a build-up of anxiety or aggression that might be alleviated by appropriate use of sedative medication.

The legitimate goals of psychiatric nursing intervention allow for acceptance of individuals as they are and for the fostering of personal growth. Control of behavior, while sometimes necessary, is never completely benign, and it is certainly not one of the main goals.

In interacting and communicating with clients, *nurses use themselves as therapeutic tools.* But they should keep some important points in mind. Responding to clients' emotional or mental problems with an appeal to logic is usually not much help. If clients were able to be logical about their inner turmoil, they probably would not be in the hospital or clinic and under psychiatric care. Murray Bowen (1976), a noted family therapy theorist, points out that persons who are most vulnerable to emotional illness live in a feeling-dominated world in which it is often impossible to distinguish feeling from fact.

Sometimes clients deny or feel guilty about their real feelings. "They aren't logical" is a common remark. Allowing for the expression of feelings is probably the best course at such a time. For some clients, the ability to take a more logical stance toward their problems may be a longer-term goal. This is particularly true of acutely ill psychiatric clients.

Giving advice, like appealing to logic, usually is not helpful. If we could simply visit every psychiatric unit and hospital and advise clients of the best courses of action for their future, we could probably empty most of these facilities. Not only is giving advice a naive approach but also it does not allow for differing value systems. It would be better to remember that when people are troubled and looking for answers to their problems, they often have most of those answers inside their own heads. The way to help is to facilitate the process of getting to those answers. This is why *listening* can be such a valuable tool.

The nurse generally should avoid raising client *anxiety levels* unnecessarily. An increase in anxiety level will only exacerbate symptoms because the symptoms of psychopathology are exaggerations of the normal defense mechanisms used to control anxiety. There are times, however, when some provocation of anxiety may be justified to facilitate growth. Encouraging a client to begin to participate in group therapy may be an example of such justified provocation. For clients who have had difficulty learning to relate to others at all and for clients who have never had a "group experience," the thought of participating in a group can be frightening. The nurse can help by *supporting* clients through the necessary stages. Clients can develop increased self-respect and optimism as a result of having accomplished a difficult task.

Support and reassurance, in the situation just described and indeed in any situation, must be given in a realistic manner and with authenticity if they are to be effective. Telling the truth is the best approach; sometimes the amount of information or detail may need to be modified, but for a nurse to lie to clients to protect their self-esteem is not a good idea. For example, a nurse who praises a client falsely or intentionally loses games to bolster a client's self-esteem is participating in self-defeating

behavior. The client is likely to spot this dishonesty, and it may destroy any trust the client had in the nurse and result in a *decrease* in the client's self-esteem.

In using the nursing process in the psychiatric setting, the nurse often needs to analyze client behavior. The goal of this analysis is to try to understand what clients are attempting to communicate or what some of their needs may be. The analysis is done in the nurse's head, and the behavior should *not* be interpreted to clients. There are several reasons for this:

1. The nurse may indeed be right on target with interpretations that are made to clients, but clients may not be emotionally ready to accept the information or knowledge about their underlying motivations. Information of this kind can exacerbate psychotic or neurotic symptoms.
2. The nurse may be wrong in the interpretation.
3. Communications that even hint at mind reading are not helpful. Many psychiatric clients have habitually used unclear communication patterns, and verbalized interpretations of their behavior serve to reinforce these faulty communication patterns. In addition, some clients have delusions that other people can read their minds, and it is thus not therapeutic to reinforce these delusions through communications that might suggest mind reading.

Countertransference is a universal phenomenon in helping relationships. It can be a helpful tool in understanding clients, or it can be a significant nursing problem. Countertransference is experienced by the therapist; *transference* is experienced by the client. Both are intrapsychic concepts. Transference, as it occurs in the helping relationship, has been defined as "those feelings and attitudes that were originally experienced with regard to significant others in the past but are now displaced or projected upon the therapist" (Saretsky, 1978). Countertransference has been defined as

. . . the emotional process present in the therapist [that] . . . (1) is in relationship to the patient, (2) has a bearing on the therapeutic process, (3) involves unconscious feelings of the therapist, (4) has a component of conscious or unconscious anxiety, and (5) represents a blending of appropriate, defensive and fixated responses (Eisenbud, 1978).

A nurse must ensure that countertransference becomes an effective agent for, rather than an obstacle to, understanding and relating to a client. A nurse's acceptance and awareness of countertransference are the first steps in avoiding some of its pitfalls. To use the self as a therapeutic tool, one should know as much as possible about the tool. *Reasonable objectivity* is the ideal, but this does not mean cold underinvolvement (what was referred to years ago in nursing as "being professional"). Therapeutic use of self is not effective unless a nurse is open to involvement and committed to going beyond the imparting of learned skills. Underinvolvement may be as damaging and as useless as overinvolvement. There are three factors from which underinvolvement may arise: the need of the nurse for a facade, lack of knowledge of how to be effectively therapeutic, and apathy toward and dissatisfaction with one's work.

There is, therefore, an optimum level of involvement between nurses and clients in psychiatric settings. Maintaining that level is rather like walking a tightrope, with overinvolvement on one side and underinvolvement on the other. Perhaps a better way to describe the situation would be to refer to the "art" of psychiatric nursing—this branch of nursing is characterized by a dynamic state of relative equilibrium, as far as involvement with clients is concerned. How does the nurse reach this state of relative equilibrium? One thing that can help is the availability of an objective person with whom the nurse can discuss clinical work and problems—in other words, a person with whom the nurse can establish a supervisory relationship.

The supervisory process

Ideally, anyone involved in therapeutic relationships with psychiatric clients should also be involved in a supervisory relationship. Problems of countertransference, overinvolvement, manipulation, or mutual withdrawal between staff members and clients may all be dealt with through a supervisory process. In addition, increased self-awareness—a necessary and important goal for the nurse working in a psychiatric setting—can be promoted through the supervisory process. It is also helpful to have another source of ideas for modifying a care plan.

The supervisory process can be part of scheduled staff meetings or team conferences, or it can be the focus of separate meetings. Regardless of which format is used, meetings held on a regular basis, with sharing of clinical material and with peer supervision, can help to meet the goals of supervision. Where a fairly open and trusting atmosphere exists, interpersonal conflicts among staff members are appropriate topics for discussion. Otherwise, the effects of staff conflicts may be projected onto clients, and certain clients may even act out some of the conflicts.

Constructive supervision that involves the sharing of information can facilitate a dynamic, creative approach to carrying out the nursing process in a psychiatric setting.

"Do's" of therapeutic communication

It is not uncommon for students or for beginning practitioners to be fearful of "prying" or of "saying the wrong thing." All too often, principles and techniques of interacting abound with "don'ts." *Don't* pry! *Don't* ask questions merely to satisfy your own curiosity! *Don't* give personal information to clients! *Don't* push for too much too soon! Certainly, such don'ts are important to keep in mind, but a therapeutic relationship should not be based solely on them. There are also a great many "do's." During an interaction, it is just as important, if not more important, to be mindful of these positive guidelines. In fact, if nurses can focus on such positive parameters, they may find that they are better able to establish therapeutic relationships and more confident in establishing them. The following are some important "do's" of therapeutic communication:

1. *Do* select a quiet, private area in which to hold interactions. Imagine how it may feel to discuss personal feelings and problems within hearing range of others or in a place subject to frequent intrusion.

2. *Do* provide for comfortable seating arrangements. Standing is not conducive to in-depth interaction. People cannot stand for long in one place without becoming tired and restless. Also, sitting on a bed in a client's room is neither comfortable nor conducive to therapeutic interaction. The nurse should be seated in a chair. This enables the nurse to see the client without staring and without blocking the client's avenue of egress. It is often a good idea to sit down first and let the client arrange his or her chair so that he or she feels comfortable with the seating arrangement. Remember that staring may heighten anxiety. The client is already carrying around enough anxiety. The interview situation should not add to it.

3. *Do* provide an avenue of egress. An already anxious person frequently leaves an interview situation to get a cigarette or a drink of water. Whatever the reason given for a client's physical departure from the interview situation, leaving provides the client with an opportunity to gain both physical and emotional distance from what might be perceived as a stressful situation. Keep in mind that by providing an area of "escape" the nurse is also providing an area of reentry. If a client does not have to climb over people and furniture, he or she is much more likely to return to an interview.

4. *Do* be aware that behavior usually satisfies several needs at the same time. For example, bragging serves to build the braggart's self-esteem, but, by making others feel insecure, it may also serve to manipulate and control people. Eating is another example of multipurposeful behavior. When people eat during a time of stress (for example, exam week), they may be meeting not only a physiological need but also a psychosocial need. Food symbolizes love and security. From infancy on, many people associate being fed with being cared for. Everyone has a special "security" food. For some, it may be chocolate; for others, warm milk. While eating such foods, people gain a sense of security and well-being.

5. *Do* keep in mind that when people are trying to satisfy a need that is of primary importance to them, they may either ignore or fail to recognize that other needs exist. Many community health nurses have encountered parents who must devote almost all of their time and energy to earning enough money to keep food on the table and a roof over their heads. As a result, these parents may give a lower priority than does the nurse to such preventive health measures as immunizations and annual physical examinations. This is an example of focusing on a felt primary need and ignoring other needs.

6. *Do* recognize that people should be accepted as they are. To accept people as they are means to recognize that they have strengths and weaknesses and positive and negative emotions. For instance, when clients are angry, allow them to express anger. Saying, "Calm down," "Be more rational," or "Put it all in the past and forget it" is not only fruitless but also ignores the reality and importance of their feelings.

7. *Do* allow people to proceed at their own pace. The less threatened people feel, the more quickly rapport can be established. People will also be better able to look at their experiences and to learn from them.

A student nurse had established a pattern of asking a client questions about her family. The student was "pushing" the client to talk about an area that was not of her own choosing. The client would tersely answer these questions and then fall silent. The student soon became frustrated because the client would not "open up." One day the student developed laryngitis. Student and client agreed they would spend the allotted time sitting together. The student would listen to whatever the client wanted to talk about. Much to the student's amazement, the client began to talk about the difficulties she had experienced on her last weekend pass home!

Once the pressure to talk about traumatic material was lifted, the client was able to discuss areas that were meaningful to her.

8. *Do* observe client behavior. Are clients depressed? Elated? Apathetic? Do they appear alert? Confused? Hyperactive? Pay attention to physical appearance. Are clients appropriately dressed? Bizarrely dressed? Slovenly dressed? Do they hold themselves in a sagging posture? Do they move rigidly? What are their facial expressions? Physical appearance reflects how people feel about them-

selves. Nurses may learn much about their clients' emotional states by observing behavior and physical appearance.

9. *Do* remember that nonverbal behavior can only be understood in its context and that it may either reinforce or contradict the verbal statements or behaviors of either nurses or clients. Scheflen (1973) found that the following metabehaviors or metacommunications are frequently encountered in psychotherapeutic relationships:

   a. Nose wiping. The back of one's index finger is run laterally between one's nostrils and upper lip. This behavior is often used when a person is lying or exaggerating or when a person is monitoring the deviant behavior of another person.

   b. Mouth covering. One's hand is placed over one's mouth. This behavior characteristically occurs when a speaker is told to keep quiet or when a person says something that is prohibited or embarrassing or that should not have been divulged.

   c. Eye covering. The palm of the hand is used to cover the eyes. This behavior may be a monitoring behavior, or it may indicate that a person is trying to understand an idea or gain insight.

   d. Eye pointing. The index finger is used to point to one's own eye. This behavior usually tells others to "pay attention."

   e. Lint picking. The index finger and thumb are used to pick lint (real or imaginary) off one's clothes. This behavior often signifies that a person is saying something that would normally elicit censure from the lint picker but that, at the time, the lint picker feels it would be inappropriate to censure the speaker.

   f. Looking up. One looks up at the ceiling and then down at an individual. This behavior usually signifies that a person is going to say something that he or she considers significant.

   g. Eyebrow raising, shoulder shrugging, deadpan facial expression. These behaviors characteristically are used to discredit unrealistic conceptions.

10. *Do* be consistent when interacting. Consis-

tency facilitates the establishment of security, rapport, and trust in a relationship.

A nurse and a client decided that between 4 PM and 5 PM each day they would talk over the events of the day and assess how the client had dealt with them. One day, the client was particularly talkative and continued talking beyond the agreed-upon limit. The nurse reminded the client of their agreement and helped the client summarize and terminate their conversation.

Thus the nurse was consistent in maintaining the boundaries of their relationship. To talk an hour one day, half an hour the next day, and perhaps 2 hours another day would create an ambience of uncertainty. The client might begin wondering: "What is expected of me? How long will the nurse stay with me today? How much time do I have to discuss my problems?" As such feelings of uncertainty grow, it is very likely that the client will question the nurse's reliability. Certainly, if a particular need arose, a nurse and a client might agree to extend their time together. By doing so, they would be acknowledging that the situation warranted an exception to their usual arrangement. By maintaining the boundaries of the relationship, consistency and trust are reinforced rather than undermined.

11. *Do* try to keep client anxiety to a minimum. High anxiety decreases one's ability to perceive, and learning is less likely to occur. The nurse needs to help clients decrease their anxiety. Altering the environment may have a therapeutic effect. By controlling the noise level and avoiding overcrowding, the nurse can make the environment less stressful. For instance, in a crowded unit, it is important to provide a quiet area. It is not uncommon for very anxious individuals in a psychiatric unit to request some time in a seclusion room. The individuals recognize that by limiting external stimuli they may decrease their stress levels. A nurse's availability to anxious clients so they can verbalize their concerns may also help reduce anxiety. Finally, a nurse should remember that physical activity, such as gardening and partici-

pating in sports, serves to dissipate anxious energy and to help anxious individuals feel more comfortable.

12. *Do* explain routines and procedures in terms that people can understand. A nurse needs to assess the levels of anxiety and levels of understanding of clients, evaluate the influence of past experiences, and explain technical terminology. For example, when a nurse is establishing a therapeutic relationship, a client's past experiences with psychotherapy may have a great influence on the client's present experience. If a client has participated in a relationship in which a nurse pushed the discussion into an area that the client was not yet ready to explore, the client may be reluctant to enter into a new therapeutic relationship. In addition, if a nurse orients a client to the purpose of a therapeutic relationship by saying, "We are entering into a one-to-one relationship, and you can discuss your problems during these interviews," the client may hesitate to talk with the nurse for several reasons. The client may not understand what is meant by a "one-to-one relationship." The client may associate the word "interview" with probing questions. The client may be frightened by the focus on "problems." The client may feel that he or she does not have enough "problems" to fill up the "interview" time. When a nurse explains that during an interaction clients may discuss anything that is of interest or concern in their daily lives, the nurse is using vocabulary that is more understandable and less threatening.

13. *Do* offer clients realistic reassurance. To give false reassurance or to reassure clients before their situation has been explored blocks communication. For example, to reassure a crying person that everything will be "all right" before you know why the person is crying cuts off communication. To tell someone who has had mutilating surgery, "Things will look brighter once you get out of the hospital" is to deny that there will be difficult times ahead. By acknowledging that there will be some difficult times but that rehabilitation and psychotherapy will help with readjustment, a nurse offers realistic reassurance. The nurse thereby provides clients with opportunities to explore their concerns and also points out treatment modalities that will assist

them in dealing with the stress caused by their situations.

14. *Do* remember that there is always potential for growth. There are no "hopeless," "hardcore" individuals. People who do not show progress or seem resistant to therapy may not yet be ready to change. Readiness to profit from therapy is not much different from readiness to learn how to walk or talk. People must see a need for change before change can take place. Also, it is possible that the staff may need additional knowledge of therapeutic tools to help clients work through difficulties. If client and nurse are ready and able to grasp an opportunity for therapy, there is potential for growth.

The process of therapeutic communication focuses on client experience. By helping clients to learn more appropriate and effective coping behavior, nurses encourage them to move beyond mere tolerance of a stressful situation to understanding and profiting from it.

Barriers to therapeutic communication

Up to now we have primarily concentrated on the unimpeded process of therapeutic communication. Therapeutic principles have functioned as guides to effective interaction. However, the process does not necessarily progress from stage to stage without some difficulties being encountered. Difficulties may arise out of characteristics of the client, the nurse, or both. We will describe some of the most frequently encountered barriers to the therapeutic process. It is important to note that these barriers are not restricted to the therapeutic process; they may be found in any situation in which two or more people interact.

EGOCENTRISM

Egocentrism is the attitude that one's own mode of living, values, and patterns of adaptation are superior to all others. This attitude is often accompanied by contempt for life-styles that differ from one's own. Egocentrism tends to manifest itself in superior, proselytizing, moralizing, rejecting, hostile, or aggressive behavior.

When a nurse and a client have different values,

especially if one or both are unaware of how strongly they are influenced by these values, conflict may result.

A community health nurse had been visiting the Smith household to assist Mrs. Smith in the care of her 72-year-old mother-in-law. The mother-in-law had suffered a stroke that had left her aphasic and that had paralyzed her right side. After several weeks, Mrs. Smith confided to the nurse that she found it very time-consuming and fatiguing to take care of her mother-in-law. Mrs. Smith said, "My primary responsibility is to my husband and children, and now I feel like I have no time or energy left for them." She feared that the strain was also being reflected in her children. She pointed out that her 5-year-old son had begun bed-wetting and that her 8-year-old daughter, complaining of stomach aches, had seen the school nurse three times in the past 2 weeks. Mrs. Smith said that she and her husband were considering placing her mother-in-law in a nursing home.

The nurse had strong feelings about the duty of children to care for their aged parents. In fact, he came from a family background that regarded it as disgraceful to place parents in a nursing home. He responded to Mrs. Smith, "Oh, that would be such a shame. I'm sure you'll be able to manage once you get a routine. After all, you have to remember that you're setting an example for your children. The way you treat your mother-in-law is probably the way your children will treat you when you're older."

The community health nurse inadvertently was imposing his values on the client.

Sometimes it is the client's values and attitudes that function as a barrier to therapeutic interaction.

Marcia Henderson, 22 years old, went to a neighborhood mental health center for counseling. Ms. Henderson complained of feeling "tired and sad." She added that she cried easily and had no appetite. During a subsequent session, Ms. Henderson asked the nurse, "What is your religion?" The nurse responded, "Catholic. Why do you ask?" Ms. Henderson replied, "Oh, no reason, I'm just nosy I guess." At the following session, Ms. Henderson requested another nurse, ex-

plaining, "I'm living with a man whom I have no intentions of marrying. I can't talk about this to someone who's Catholic. I don't want any moralizing at my expense."

The client's values and attitudes led her to assume that the nurse would pass judgment on her. The client erected a barrier to the therapeutic process and terminated the relationship.

Thus problems may arise when a nurse and a client have different value systems. Conflict is especially apt to result when participants are unaware of the influence their values exert on them. Even the most self-aware people have values that operate outside their full awareness. Only as nurse and client become more aware of the values that influence their thoughts and feelings can they begin to free themselves from subjectivity and to accept that another person's value system can be adaptive. (See Chapters 4 and 6 for discussion of attitudes.) Egocentrism then ceases to exist as a barrier to effective communication, and nurse and client can begin to set mutually agreed-upon goals.

DENIAL

Denial is the unconscious evasion or negation of objective reality. Denial functions to reduce anxiety, to stabilize and define relationships, and to retain or regain a sense of autonomy.

When either nurse or client uses denial, a barrier to the therapeutic process is erected. Eventually, the nondenying participant becomes bored, frustrated, or angry with the other's systematic avoidance of certain topics and may respond either by ignoring the pattern of denial or by confronting the use of denial. Ignoring the pattern of denial serves to reinforce its use. Confronting denial too early or too severely almost certainly will threaten the denying individual, provoke anger in the individual, and cause the individual to try to cope with reality by further reliance on denial. The therapeutic process then becomes characterized by anxiety.

A student nurse, Marty Hendricks, was working with Julie, a verbally and physically abusive adolescent girl. Without any observable warning, Julie would sud-

denly lash out at people. Recently she had severely scratched her psychiatrist's face.

During supervisory conferences, Marty consistently assured his instructor that he felt comfortable in Julie's presence, that he trusted Julie, and that he did not think Julie would strike out at him. The more his instructor questioned him about his feelings, the more adamantly he asserted that he was unafraid. The instructor believed that Marty was denying reality and decided to stop challenging his description of his feeling and instead to be increasingly supportive of him during this experience. As Marty began to feel more comfortable with his instructor and less threatened by possible recriminations from her, he began to talk about how he felt "uneasy" with Julie.

Thus, challenging people's use of denial can cause them to feel threatened and to rely increasingly on denial as a way to cope with reality. When attempts are made to alleviate the anxiety underlying denial, the need to use denial usually decreases.

RESISTANCE

Resistance is conscious or unconscious reluctance to bring repressed ideas, thoughts, desires, or memories into awareness. By preventing the entry of such threatening material into consciousness, resistance functions to maintain an individual's security or self-esteem.

Therapeutic intervention involves helping clients explore experiences that are of concern to them. If clients try to avoid material that threatens their self systems, attempts to help them verbalize feelings, evaluate patterns of behavior, or examine interpersonal relationships may be met by resistance. Should a nurse fail to recognize clients' use of resistance and try to force them to talk about painful areas from which they feel a need to retreat, the nurse may only succeed in increasing their anxiety.

Peter Mulally had been experiencing auditory hallucinations. The nurse assigned to work with Peter noticed that whenever she questioned him about the content of these hallucinations, he would change the subject. The nurse became very impatient with his behavior and began pressuring him to talk about the hallucina-

tions, explaining, "I can't help you unless I know what's troubling you." Peter began rocking back and forth in his chair. Instead of changing the subject, he got up and walked away.

Resistive behavior, then, can escalate when a nurse does not recognize that resistance is being used to avoid extremely anxiety-producing material. Had the nurse allowed the client to retreat from the areas that were painful to him, the client's anxiety might have decreased rather than increased. At the same time, the nurse would have contributed to an atmosphere of trust. The client might eventually have felt free to explore threatening material without fearing loss of security or self-esteem.

The use of resistence is not restricted to clients. Sometimes nurses use resistance.

Joan Bellows, a student nurse, was consistently absent the last day of each clinical experience. During her community mental health experience, her instructor pointed this pattern out to her. Joan responded, "I'm coming down with a cold and don't want to talk about it right now." The instructor said, "Maybe you'll feel like discussing it some other time."

As the day for terminating with her client approached, Joan's instructor again pointed out her habit of being absent on the last day of each clinical experience. Joan explained, "One time I was sick. Another time I had car trouble—and the last time the alarm clock didn't ring and I overslept." The instructor replied, "Sometimes good-byes are difficult to say."

The next time Joan and her instructor discussed Joan's plans for termination with her client, Joan began to cry. She explained that she never could say good-bye to anyone and would do anything to avoid good-byes. She was ready to talk about an area that until then had been too painful to explore.

Given an accepting relationship, individuals can be helped to deal with previously resisted material. By gradually calling attention to their resistive behavior and slowly and nonjudgmentally exploring or pointing out possible reasons for the behavior, a nurse can facilitate the resolution of resistance. Individuals can then begin to deal with the threatening material. It is important to remember that since resistance is a mechanism used to maintain security and self-esteem, attempts should not be made to pointedly confront people using resistance or to argue them out of resistance.

• • •

Characteristics of the client, of the nurse, or of both may set up barriers to the therapeutic process. Egocentrism, denial, and resistance are three frequently encountered barriers. However, they need not be insurmountable. If they are recognized and understood, steps can be taken toward resolution of the difficulties and reestablishment of the therapeutic process.

Listening is essential for effective communication. Listening requires moving beyond the words used in order to hear the meaning or messages (themes) being conveyed. In the process of therapeutic communication the focus is on the client's experience as the client perceives it. Client and nurse become actively involved in moving beyond mere tolerance of the experience and toward an increased understanding of the situation and a plan for developing appropriate and effective coping behavior. During this exploration, some barriers to therapeutic communication may arise. Once these barriers have been understood, they can be sur-

mounted and therapeutic communication can be reestablished.

CHAPTER SUMMARY

Therapeutic communication involves more than learning a group of interviewing skills. It involves understanding the process of communication and the role that nurse and client play in establishing and maintaining therapeutic communication. The focus of therapeutic communication is the client's here-and-now experience. The task of the nurse is to sustain the client in that experience. The nurse and the client actively explore the client's experiences within the framework of the nursing process. The cultural backgrounds of nurse and client affect their perceptions and interpretations of experiences, their responses to experiences, and their responses to communication cues.

Many factors may influence therapeutic communication and the ability of nurses to sustain clients in their experiences. Chief among these factors are behavioral concepts relating to sexuality, privacy, humor, empathy, and touching. With this knowledge, barriers to effective communication may be avoided and therapeutic communication may be promoted.

SELF-DIRECTED LEARNING

Sensitivity-Awareness Exercises

The purposes of these exercises are to:
- Develop insight into some of your own customs and communication behaviors
- Develop awareness of the customs and communication behaviors of others
- Develop sensitivity to differences in customs and communication behaviors that may contribute to culture shock in immigrants and culture conflict in ethnic Americans
- Develop awareness of the impact of culture on the nurse-client relationship

1. Look at the kinesic and proxemic patterns used by you and your family in the following situations:
   a. At the dinner table
   b. Standing and conversing
   c. Sitting and conversing
   Especially note interpersonal distances maintained, how territorial boundaries are established and acknowledged, and the degree to which gestures and touching are used.
2. When conversing with your family or friends, alter your usual kinesic and proxemic patterns in the following ways: use more gesturing and touching; use less gesturing and touching; increase your interpersonal space by 6 inches; decrease your interpersonal space by 6 inches.
   a. How did you feel with each of the above alterations in your usual nonverbal communication pattern?
   b. How did the people with whom you were conversing react? (For example, they tried to reestablish spatial distance; they withdrew when

SELF-DIRECTED LEARNING—cont'd

you tried to touch them; they moved further away to give you more room to gesture.)
  c. Ask the people with whom you were interacting how they felt.
  d. What cultural factors might have influenced the reactions and feelings of the people with whom you were interacting?
3. Role play that you are visiting a foreign country. You become ill and you go to a hospital. You are not familiar with the language or customs of the country. Try to make your symptoms or discomfiture known to the "health practitioners" without using verbal language. Remember that your life may depend on your ability to make yourself understood. At the end of 5 minutes, look at:
  a. Your feelings during the experience
  b. The behavior you demonstrated
  c. The behavior and reactions of the "health practitioner." Ask the "health practitioner" what his or her feelings were.
    Now reverse roles and reenact the exercise. How do reactions compare with the first enactment?
4. Examine a relationship that you have established with a client. Look at the effects that attitudes about sexuality, privacy, humor, empathy, and touching have on the relationship.
5. Analyze and describe how your cultural background (for example, ethnicity, religion) influences or may influence your perception, interpretation, and response in such health-related experiences as physical illness, emotional illness, and hospitalization. How might your perception, interpretation, and response affect your ability to sustain clients having similar experiences?

Questions to Consider

During their interactions together, a student noticed that a client had drooping facies, lusterless eyes, and was sitting bent over, with her hands in her lap. The student also observed that the client was softly crying. The student said, "You look sad." The next two questions refer to this situation.

1. The student's observations provided partial data for identification of the
  a. Content theme
  b. Communication theme
  c. Mood theme
  d. Interaction theme

2. The student's statement is an example of which of the following communication techniques?
  a. Mirroring
  b. Leading
  c. Confrontation
  d. Summarizing
3. During a supervisory conference, a student discussed ways of instituting and carrying out nursing actions designed to achieve specific behavioral outcomes. The student was engaging in which step of the nursing process?
  a. Assessing
  b. Analyzing data
  c. Planning client care
  d. Implementing the care plan
  e. Evaluating the care plan
4. A client was visiting with his family. The client and the family spoke softly. The man in the next bed and his visitors could not overhear the client's conversation. The client was most probably
  a. Depressed and withdrawn
  b. Aloof and alienated
  c. Erecting an interpersonal privacy barrier
  d. Erecting a physical privacy barrier
5. Humor is an *inappropriate* nursing intervention when it
  a. Laughs with people
  b. Laughs at people
  c. Helps a client cope more effectively
  d. Decreases social distance

Match each of the following terms with the statement that is associated with it:

6. Physical privacy barrier
7. Leading
8. Clarification seeking
9. Empathy
10. Interpersonal privacy barrier

  a. Modulating one's voice
  b. "Who do you mean by they?"
  c. A closed door
  d. "Tell me more about that."
  e. "Tuning into" a client's feelings

Answer key

1. c	6. c
2. a	7. d
3. d	8. b
4. c	9. e
5. b	10. a

REFERENCES

Abeles JH: Letters, The Sciences 22:3, 1982.

Altman I: The environment and social behavior: privacy, personal space, territory, crowding, Monterey, 1975, Brooks/Cole Publishing Co.

Altman I, Nelson PA, and Lett EE: The ecology of home environments, Catalog of Selected Documents in Psychology 2:65, 1972.

American Nurses Association Division on Psychiatric and Mental Health Nursing Practice: Standards of Psychiatric and Mental Health Nursing Practice, Kansas City, 1982, ANA Publications.

Anderson ML: Nursing interventions: what did you do that helped? Persp Psychiatr Care 21(1):4-8, 1983.

Apte ML: Humor and laughter: an anthropological approach, Ithaca, NY, 1985, Cornell University Press.

Ashcraft N and Scheflen AE: People space: the making and breaking of human boundaries, Garden City, NY, 1976, Anchor Press/Doubleday.

Atkinson L and Murphy ME: Understanding the nursing process, New York, 1980, MacMillan, Inc.

Auvil CA and Silver BW: Therapist self-disclosure: when is it appropriate? Persp Psychiatr Care 22(2):57-61, 1984.

Blondis MN and Jackson BE: Nonverbal communication with patients: back to the human touch, New York, 1982, John Wiley & Sons, Inc.

Bowen M: Theory in the practice of psychotherapy. In Guerin PJ, editor: Family therapy, New York, 1976, Gardner Press, Inc.

Bradley JC and Edinberg MA: Communication in nursing, New York, 1982, Appleton-Century-Crofts.

Brammer LM and Shostrom EL: Therapeutic psychology: fundamentals of counseling and psychotherapy, Englewood Cliffs, NJ, 1982, Prentice-Hall, Inc.

DuBois R: Introduction. In Cousins N: Anatomy of an illness as perceived by the patient: reflections on healing and regeneration, New York, 1979, W.W. Norton & Co., Inc.

Eisenbud R: Countertransference. In Goldman G. and Milman D, editors: Psychoanalytic psychotherapy, Reading, Mass, 1978, Addison-Wesley Publishing Co., Inc.

Fiedler FE and Senior K: An exploratory study of unconscious feeling reactions in fifteen patient-therapist pairs, J Abnormal Soc Psychol 47:446-453, 1952.

Forsyth G: Analysis of the concept of empathy: illustration of one approach, Adv Nurs Sci 2:33-42, 1980.

Freud S: Jokes and their relation to the unconscious, In Strachey J, editor: The complete psychological works of Sigmund Freud (orig. 1928), London, 1961, Hogarth Press.

Gilmore MM and Gilmore DD: Machismo: a psychodynamic approach (Spain), J Psycholog Anthropol 2:281-299, 1979.

Goldstein JH: A laugh a day—can mirth keep disease at bay? The Sciences 22:21-25, 1982.

Hall ET: The hidden dimension, Garden City, NY, 1969, Doubleday & Co., Inc.

Hsu FLK: Americans and Chinese: reflections on two cultures and their people, Garden City, NY, 1970, Doubleday Natural History Press.

Johnson MN: Self-disclosure, J Psychiatr Nurs 18:17-20, 1980.

Lathrop DD: Laughing away the CIA (and other paranoid delusions), Voices: Art Sci Psychother 16(4):7-9, 1981.

Maslow AH: A theory of metamotivation: the biological roots of the value of life, J Human Psychol 7:93-127, 1967.

Matheney R and Topalis M: Psychiatric nursing, ed 4, St. Louis, 1965, The CV Mosby Co.

Montagu A: Touching: the human significance of the skin, New York, 1971, Harper & Row, Publishers, Inc.

Moody Jr RA: Laugh after laugh: the healing power of humor, Jacksonville, Fla, 1978, Headwaters Press.

Murillo-Rhode I: Family life among mainland Puerto Ricans in New York City slums, Persp Psychiatr Care 14:174-179, 1976.

National Council of State Boards of Nursing, Inc: National Council Licensure Examination for Registered Nurses, Chicago, 1980, The Council.

Pasquali EA: Comic strips in the classroom, In Mirin SK, editor: Teaching tomorrow's nurse: a nurse educator reader, Wakefield, Mass, 1980, Nursing Resources, Inc.

Pasquali EA: Assimilation and acculturation of Cubans on Long Island, Ph.D. dissertation, State University of New York at Stony Brook, 1982.

Peplau H: Themes in nursing situations, Am J Nurs 53:1221, 1953.

Peplau H: Utilizing themes in nursing situations, Am J Nurs 54:325, 1954.

Radcliffe-Brown AR: Structure and function in primitive society, New York, 1952, The Free Press.

Robinson VM: Humor in nursing, In Carlson CE, editor: Behavioral concepts and nursing intervention, Philadelphia, 1970, J.B. Lippincott Co.

Saretsky L: Transference, In Goldman G and Milman D, editors: Psychoanalytic psychotherapy, Reading, Mass, 1978, Addison-Wesley Publishing Co., Inc.

Sayre J: Common errors in communication made by students in psychiatric nursing, Persp Psychiatr Care 4:175-183, 1978.

Scheflen AE: Communicational structure: analysis of a psychotherapy transaction, Bloomington, 1973, Indiana University Press.

Ujhely G: Determinants of the nurse-patient relationship, New York, 1968, Springer Publishing Co., Inc.

Watson MJ: Facilitate learning with humor, J Nurs Educ 27(2):89-90, 1988.

Weiner M: Therapist disclosure: the use of self in psychotherapy, Boston, 1978, Butterworth.

Westin A: Privacy and freedom, New York, 1970, Atheneum.

Whipple B and Gick R: A holistic view of sexuality-education for the health professional, Topics Clin Nurs 1:91-98, 1980.

ANNOTATED SUGGESTED READINGS

Anderson ML: Nursing interventions: what did you do that helped? Persp Psychiatr Care 21(1)4-8, 1983.
This author discusses some advantages and disadvantages of general labeling to describe nursing interventions. The author then presents a list of therapeutic communication techniques with their descriptions, which the author believes is a way of more specifically labeling nursing interventions.

Auvil CA and Silver BW: Therapist self-disclosure: when is it appropriate? Persp Psychiatr Care 22(2):57-61, 1984.

This article looks at self-disclosure from psychoanalytic, humanistic, and behavioral orientations; discusses the nursing implications of self-disclosure; provides guidelines for the appropriate use of self-disclosure in nurse-client interaction; and offers communication techniques for deflecting client questions when self-disclosure by the nurse is inappropriate.

Blondis MN and Jackson BE: Nonverbal communication with patients: back to the human touch, New York, 1982, John Wiley & Sons, Inc.

The authors discuss the role that nonverbal communication plays in nurse-client interaction. Special attention is given to the interpretation of nonverbal cues and to the use of nonverbal techniques for more effective nurse-client interaction. Included in the book are such topics as pediatrics and parenting, sexual behaviors, geriatrics, death and dying, crisis intervention, and the nursing process.

Bradley JC and Edinberg MA: Communication in nursing, New York, 1982, Appleton-Century-Crofts.

This book takes both an experiential and a theoretical approach to nurse-client interaction. Vignettes and verbatim excerpts of conversations illustrate topics dealt with, such as interviewing techniques, communication stalls, and empathy. Situations and suggestions that facilitate experiential learning are included.

Watson MJ: Facilitate learning with humor, J Nurs Ed 27(2):89-90, 1988.

The author looks at the role of humor as a teaching strategy. She discusses ways of helping students to "think" humor and suggests such humor activities as "caption the picture," "dress-up," and "you turn my button."

FURTHER READINGS

Flaslerud JH: A proposed protocol for culturally relevant nursing psychotherapy, Clin Nurse Specialist 1(4):150-157, 1987.

Jess LW: Investigating impaired mental status: an assessment guide you can use, Nurs 88 18(6):42-50, 1988.

Jones MP: The nursing process in psychiatry, Nurs Times 76:1273-1275, 1980.

Karshmer JF: Rules of thumb: hints for the psychiatric nursing student, J Psychosoc Nurs Mental Health Stud 20(3):25-28, 1982.

Norris J and Kunes-Connell M: A multimodal approach to validation and refinement of an existing nursing diagnosis, Arch Psychiatr Nurs 2(2):103-109, 1988.

Podrasky DL and Sexton DL: Nurses' reactions to difficult patients, Image 20(1):16-21, 1988.

Rosie J: The therapist's self-disclosure in individual psychotherapy, Can J Psychiatr 25:469-472, 1980.

Simon JM: Therapeutic humor: who's fooling who? J Psychosoc Nurs Mental Health Stud 26(4):9-12, 1988.

Wheeler K: A nursing science approach to understanding empathy, Arch Psychiatr Nurs 2(2):95-102, 1988.

UNIT 3

Therapeutic settings and modalities

This unit focuses on types of therapeutic settings and modalities. Chapter 12 introduces the concept of the therapeutic milieu and discusses the interrelated and sometimes overlapping roles and functions of the members of the mental health team. The role of the nurse is explored, and, in keeping with the holistic health systems approach of this book, the client-system is viewed as an integral part of the mental health team.

Chapters 13, 14, and 15 focus upon nursing functions in relation to group therapy, family therapy, and crisis intervention. In Chapter 16, community mental health services are presented as a system of interacting health and welfare subsystems. These subsystems are oriented toward a defined community, or catchment area. It is emphasized that community mental health services should not only address the psychosocial needs of the community served but also should consider the sociocultural background of its residents. The history and the current status of the community mental health movement are explored. In addition, the organization of community mental health services is discussed in terms of primary, secondary, and tertiary prevention, and the roles and functions of community mental health nurses are described.

CHAPTER 12

The therapeutic milieu

CHAPTER FOCUS

In addition to relationship therapy, the nurse who works in a psychiatric setting is usually involved in important elements of milieu therapy. According to Fann and Goshen (1977), milieu therapy is "a therapeutic approach to hospital psychiatry in which the entire hospital environment is designed to facilitate rehabilitation. This includes occupational therapy, recreational therapy, team approach, work assignments and education of all who work in the hospital and participate in the care of patients." Although Fann and Goshen specify a hospital setting, milieu therapy can also be provided in various outpatient settings.

While professional nurses carry the greatest responsibility for maintaining a therapeutic milieu, they work cooperatively with other members of the interdisciplinary health team. In working as collaborative members of interdisciplinary teams, nurses find that their functions and responsibilities often overlap or even duplicate those of other team members. Because of the nature of nursing education and clinical nursing experience, nurses bring some unique attributes and abilities to team participation. Health teaching from a holistic point of view is a prime example. In psychiatric settings the natural tendency is to focus on psychosocial problems. But a human being is also a biological organism. The nurse, with knowledge of physiology, psychology, sociology, nutrition, pharmacology, and health in general, can be the catalyst that helps the team members to approach the client as a whole person. In addition, nurses are the only professional members of the team who are always present in the milieu—24 hours a day, 7 days a week. Indeed, maintenance of the therapeutic milieu is a prime

343

responsibility of the nurse. The nurse can be instrumental in managing the milieu in a way that facilitates a consistent progression in the psychosocial growth of the client.

The mental health team within a therapeutic milieu operates differently from the traditional hierarchical or authoritarian structure found in many health facilities, in which decisions are made at the top and passed down. In the mental health team concept, authority and accountability are shared by team members, although the responsibilities that define professional practice are retained by the specific professionals. The client is considered to be an important, participating member of the team; the "community meeting" or "staff-client meeting" is one vehicle for accomplishing this in a therapeutic milieu.

Treatment modalities used in milieu therapy include art, music, poetry, movement therapy, and psychodrama. Each of these adjunctive therapies will be discussed in this chapter. Individual, family, and group therapy—also crucial elements of a milieu—are discussed in subsequent chapters.

HISTORY AND DESCRIPTION

"Milieu" is the French word for "middle" or "middle place"; in English we use it to mean "environment."

Milieu therapy implies use of the *whole environment* as a therapeutic agent—hence Maxwell Jones' term "the therapeutic community."

A useful definition of milieu therapy is "scientific manipulation of the environment aimed at providing changes in the personality of the patient" (Cumming and Cumming, 1962).

The concept of therapeutic community, or milieu therapy is a spin-off of Maxwell Jones' work (1953) in Britain. Jones, a Scottish psychiatrist who has also done a great deal of work in America, developed a treatment modality that uses the environment—its physical facilities, various therapies, and interpersonal relationships—to foster a healthy personality. A therapeutic community is a protective setting. It provides relationships that will help its residents learn more effective and more socially

acceptable means of coping. The therapeutic community becomes a microcosm of society. The individual is helped to look at how he or she interacts and functions in this small and specially structured segment of society. Individuals who are acting out their inner conflicts with their hostility, alienation, manipulation, insensitivity, lack of responsibility, and poor judgment are confronted by the entire community.

UNDERLYING ASSUMPTIONS

Maxwell Jones outlined what he saw as five basic principles of a therapeutic community:

1. Responsibility for treatment belongs not only to physician and staff but also to the residents.
2. Social distance between staff and residents is reduced; this may permit free discussion of the behavior of staff members as well as the behavior of residents.
3. A democratic atmosphere is cultivated.
4. Open communication in the form of shared feelings and information is strongly encouraged.
5. Deviant behavior is controlled and social learning takes place through the mechanism of resident-staff meetings (adapted from Erickson, 1982).

Skinner (1979) has further delineated the underlying assumptions of a therapeutic community:

1. Staff members focus on residents' assets in order to encourage growth.
2. Each interpersonal interaction is seen as an opportunity to improve communication skills.
3. Participation in unit government provides (a) a vehicle for helping clients to meet their needs for autonomy and (b) a structure for meeting the needs of the group as a whole.
4. Individuals are responsible for their own actions.
5. Peer pressure is the medium through which the community itself develops and which enforces community behavioral norms.
6. Inappropriate behaviors are examined and dealt with as they occur.
7. Group discussion and the use of temporary

seclusion (to protect the rights of others) are techniques that are favored over punishment and prolonged restriction.

A therapeutic community is characterized by a team approach. Residents are part of the team and share in the responsibility and the process of decision making. They are included in the planning and implementation of treatment approaches and in the evaluation and reevaluation of their effectiveness. All aspects of the therapeutic community are seen as presenting opportunities for residents to examine their behavior and, when indicated, to grow in the direction of more socially acceptable behavior. There are three phases to treatment in a therapeutic community:

1. Adjustment to the setting
2. Observation, examination, and discussion (often confrontation) of adaptive and maladaptive responses (socially acceptable and unacceptable behavior)
3. Development of new, socially acceptable patterns of coping and communicating

Residents are included in all phases of treatment (both planning and implementation). Many different types of therapy may be used to facilitate change in behavior: encounter therapy, sociodrama, recreational and work activities, educational therapy, and community government.

Community government is an outstanding characteristic of a therapeutic community. Jones (1953) and Cumming and Cumming (1962) view community government as a primary means of implementing the goals of milieu therapy. Meetings are used to inculcate the social standards, values, and behavior that may never have been internalized by acting-out individuals. Community government provides opportunities to explore behavior, try out new roles, make decisions, and engage in problem solving. In the process, group identification is fostered. The following description illustrates some of the principles and techniques of a therapeutic community.

Late one afternoon, Jean was admitted to a therapeutic community that worked with drug abusers. After a brief orientation to the house in which the community members lived, Jean was introduced to the residents and staff. Then she was shown to the room that she would share with two other girls. Jean settled in, had dinner, and then attended a group "sing." Residents played guitars, sang, and generally had fun. After the sing, Jean was told to help others clean up. She was directed, rather than asked, to take some responsibility for the evening's recreation. After helping with the clean-up she went to bed.

At 6 o'clock the following morning, a bell rang. The residents got up and busied themselves with washing, dressing, and straightening their rooms. During orientation Jean had been told that unless her section of the room passed morning inspection, she would not be able to join others at breakfast. Jean was hungry, so she quickly tidied up her dresser and made her bed. Then she went down to breakfast.

After breakfast, everyone attended a community government meeting. The "president" presided. She led a discussion of jobs that needed to be done in the house, activities that had to be planned, and problems that had arisen. Then she read a list of names of people who have been repeatedly ignoring rules. Each person was permitted to speak in his or her own defense. However, anyone attempting to rationalize or manipulate was "blown away." This means that in front of the entire group one of the several staff members who had formerly been addicts would verbally attack the offender's behavior. Then the community would decide how to handle the situation. It is important to emphasize that the person's behavior, not the person, was attacked. Next, the president read the names of those residents whose behavior had improved and who were eligible for privileges. The entire group, including the person under consideration, decided whether privileges had been earned. Then work assignments were made. The community's house was run entirely by the staff and the residents. Community members were assigned to groups for cooking, doing laundry, shopping, and housekeeping. Jean was assigned to the housekeeping group.

Thus the residents are fully involved in every aspect of life in a therapeutic community. From the very first, Jean was included in the routine and incorporated into the process of community socialization. This example illustrates a therapeutic community or milieu for drug abusers. Interaction themes of these clients often include *manipulation*, *rationalization*, and *denial*. Confrontive techniques and rules that may seem too rigid for other clients are deemed appropriate here—the goal is to foster increased responsibility for self. This goal is appropriate for all clients, but in a therapeutic milieu for schizophrenic clients, for example, the means for reaching the goal would differ. Depending on the degree of regression and fragility in the residents, the approach would be less confrontive and more nurturing and supportive. Similarly, an appropriate milieu for chronically ill, regressed schizophrenics would not reach the same degree of self-government that a therapeutic community for substance abuse clients might.

According to one writer (Abroms, 1969) the goals of milieu therapy are the same as those of any other form of psychiatric care: to *set limits* on symptomatic behavior and to foster the learning of some basic *psychosocial skills.*

Psychosocial skills

Abroms has organized the teaching of psychosocial skills into four broad categories: orientation, self-assertion, occupational activities, and recreational activities.

Orientation can be as basic as the adjustment to time, place, and person that is necessary for a confused person. It can be as general or as extensive as the fostering of an understanding of the workings of an institution's social system, which would be appropriate to a tertiary-care, transitional-service setting.

Self-assertion implies the learning or relearning of direct, self-regulated ways of expressing feelings or attitudes—for example, learning to "talk it out" in the encounter groups of a therapeutic milieu for drug abusers. The adoption of such socially accepted behavior is evidence of growth from a stage in which chemical substances were used to avoid the pain of interpersonal relationships.

Occupational activities can include the learning of basic skills for managing one's life, such as the ability to adhere to a schedule. These activities may also include formal occupational or vocational counseling, training, and placement.

Recreational activities are important to help clients develop the ability to engage in various leisure pursuits, to enjoy them, and to cooperate with others in enjoying them. The development of such

ability helps to increase a client's self-confidence and self-esteem.

Setting limits

In discussing the types of behavior that necessitate limit setting, Abroms described "five Ds" of pathology and listed them in order of decreasing severity:

1. *Destructiveness*—suicide, homicide, and other forms of behavior that harm persons or property
2. *Disorganization*—for example, the autistic and bizarre behavior and thinking of an acutely psychotic person
3. *Deviancy*—for example, acting-out behavior, illegal activities, and rule breaking
4. *Dysphoria*—for example, depression, hypochondriasis, schizoid detachment, elation, obsessions, and phobias
5. *Dependency*—avoiding responsibility for one's own feelings, thoughts, and actions

PHYSICAL STRUCTURE OF A THERAPEUTIC MILIEU

Structure and physical surroundings are important in enhancing therapy—ideal hospitals and units are set up in such a way as to provide a homelike, attractively decorated setting for the clients. Nursing stations are open and accessible and are not "cages" where staff members can retreat and withdraw from clients. The use of street clothes instead of uniforms by staff members has been part of the effort to minimize interpersonal barriers between staff and clients. The present-day architecture of psychiatric settings has the same purpose. Furniture is arranged to promote increased socialization among clients and between clients and staff. Fortunately, the large, barren day room with chairs rigidly placed against the wall has, for the most part, disappeared. Safety is considered without the obvious accoutrements of an old-style "asylum." For example, instead of barred windows, the newer facilities use a special break-proof glass in a tamper-proof window. Rooms are designed with the goal of maximum utility. Pleasant day rooms convert from sitting rooms to dining rooms to recreation rooms to group therapy rooms. Often the clients' bedrooms are designed to look more like comfortable and attractive motel rooms than hospital "sick rooms." Paint colors that help to promote emotional tranquility are chosen. Children's psychiatric facilities are designed in family-type arrangements—units are set up to resemble a home living situation as closely as possible, with a central living room, a kitchen, several bedrooms, and an outside yard.

PROGRAM OF A THERAPEUTIC MILIEU

Several important elements that are usually integral parts of the program of a therapeutic milieu include:

1. Some form of *self-government*. Self-government can be accomplished in the form of structured meetings such as client-staff meetings, large community meetings, and clients' business meetings. An expectation in many facilities is that clients or residents will have some input into all of the unit activities. Some units expect clients to participate in team decisions about their fellow residents, around such issues as weekend passes, discharges, and changes in status while in the hospital. Meetings may provide a healthy, open forum for the discussion of everyday living problems in the unit. For example, at a meeting in one facility, the staff members' habit of not knocking before entering clients' rooms during the daytime hours was brought up by some of the annoyed clients. Feelings were expressed, ideas were exchanged, and clients and staff were able to work through a potentially milieu-destructive situation in a growth-enhancing manner. Usually community meetings are held on a once-a-week basis, and, because all members of the community should have an opportunity to participate, they tend to run longer than other group meetings (1½ to 2 hours). Six techniques for running a constructive therapeutic community meeting, as outlined by Russakoff and Oldham (1982), follow.

   a. *Roll call* or *attendance* is taken. The unexplained absence of a staff member or a client may provoke fantasies of danger unless it is explained. New members of the community may be introduced at this time. Embarrassing questions about "why they are here" are avoided so that new residents can adjust comfortably to the milieu.

   b. *An agenda* is created openly, within the meeting; this prevents the development of a potentially disorganizing "secret agenda." Too many or too few items on the agenda can lead to a discussion as to possible meanings (for example, excessive silence may indicate the clients' reluctance to talk about an earlier, upsetting event). "Emergency" issues can be given high priority in the agenda.

   c. *Information gathering* is an important process. There should be no reliance on secrecy; relevant information should be presented openly. Interpretation of issues is avoided before the information-gathering process has been adequately addressed. Reality issues are clarified *before* proceeding to fantasy; this is particularly important when there are psychotic clients in the community, in which case it is best to maintain a concrete focus in the discussion. Information is best solicited from the entire community rather than singling out specific clients (for example, "What do members of the community understand about this?"). This helps maintain the focus as a *community* meeting.

   d. An issue is brought to a conclusion before another topic is introduced. This helps the more disorganized clients to follow the proceedings.

   e. *Separation experiences* are addressed. For example, clients who are being admitted or discharged are noted. This is especially important for psychotic clients, for whom issues of separation are of primary concern.

   f. *A supportive beginning and a supportive ending* to each meeting are necessary. Disruptive endings defeat the efforts of some disorganized clients to involve themselves in this important socializing event. Disruptive endings also may affect the behavior of clients after the meeting, while ending with a fairly benign issue helps clients to maintain social attitudes.

2. *Graded responsibility.* Treatment plans often

reflect the principle of allowing the client to proceed at his or her own pace. Graded responsibility is a system that can demonstrate to the client his or her own progress in a very real way when passing through "levels," "groups," or other structures for conveying status. This system also allows a reduction in responsibility for the client who needs a situation in which to temporarily regress. For example, a client may sometimes need a "quiet room" for isolation to meet a need for fewer stimuli. A quiet room, if it is to be a therapeutic experience, must be used by staff and clients in a way that is protective of self-esteem and that does not imply any sort of punishment by the staff. (However, it should not provide clients with a means of avoiding responsibility.) Some units have "open charting" systems wherein clients may read their own charts at any time—the belief is that this practice fosters trust in the staff and the expectation of responsibility for oneself.*

3. *Sufficient stimulation and activity.* To prevent regression, most units or hospitals use recreational and occupational therapy situations and activities to maintain the clients' link between hospital and community.

4. *Individualization of treatment.* Overall rules and regulations are necessary to run any sort of community. However, since the needs of clients vary, their treatment must be individualized.

5. An *optimistic philosophy.* The philosophy underlying one therapeutic milieu may differ from that of another milieu, depending on the client population served. The needs of acutely psychotic or confused clients differ from the needs of acting-out, sociopathic individuals. The needs of adolescents differ from those of a geriatric population. Maxwell Jones did his original work with sociopathic individuals, but the basic principles can apply to several settings. One part of any milieu's philosophy, however, remains crucial: there needs to be

an air of optimism about the prognosis for mental disorders.

6. An *adequate communication system for staff.* It is to be hoped that optimum communication will help resolve conflicts among personnel and prevent any harmful projection of staff problems onto the clients. Staff members need to feel secure in their positions, and they need to obtain job satisfaction. A staff member who feels good about self and job is a much more effective therapeutic agent than one who does not have these feelings. Adequate communication among staff members regarding the problems, progress, and daily activities of clients is likewise important. The *confidentiality* principle that operates within a therapeutic milieu is *not* one of confidentiality between client and single therapist. While the client must be assured that no personal information will leave the unit, client–single therapist confidentiality is not compatible with the fact that each staff member must be an actively involved member of the therapeutic team. Complete and full communication among staff members is crucial to a program's success. Since observation of clients' behavior is an important and valuable part of milieu therapy, the results of observation need to be shared with all staff members for maximum benefit to the client. Such information can be used effectively to modify treatment plans, and it can also help dilute possible distortions resulting from negative countertransference situations (see Chapter 11 for discussion of transference and countertransference). Some important ways of communicating among staff members include report meetings, weekly case conferences, and charting of observations.

SPECIAL THERAPIES WITHIN THE MILIEU

In addition to the more conventional forms of individual and group therapy, other types of therapy are used in a therapeutic milieu. Among these special types of therapy are poetry therapy; psychodrama; art therapy; graffiti therapy; dance, exercise, and yoga groups; music therapy; and video-

---

*However, clients in psychiatric facilities may not be automatically entitled to access to their records. For example, in New York state, it is the law that, in addition to consent by the client, consent by the Commissioner of Mental Health is required before a facility can allow access.

tape therapy. A brief description of each of these modalities follows.

Poetry therapy

Poetry is a useful tool for reaching many psychiatric clients. Poetry therapy can be handled in more than one way. A single poem may be chosen ahead of time by the leader for the group members to react to in a personal way. The leader may choose a poem that he or she thinks is particularly meaningful to many of the clients in the group, that addresses the problems, feelings, and life-style of the group members. It is hoped that the feelings the poetry evokes will be communicated and discussed by the group members. Many of Robert Frost's and Walt Whitman's poems seem ideally suited to such a purpose, but the choice is as wide as the therapist's experience with poetry. Kobak and Neinken (1984) recommend that abstract works be avoided since poems should be readily understandable.

Another way of proceeding is for the leader to present several poems, representing different themes, to the group and have each member choose the one that is most meaningful to him or her and discuss it in a personal way. Still another method is to have the members write their own poetry—an activity that can have the added benefit of increasing an individual's self-esteem through creativity.

Whichever method is used, the poetry serves to stimulate self-understanding (perhaps even catharsis), self-expression, and interpersonal interaction and to increase self-esteem. According to Arthur Lerner (1973), the important qualities of an effective poetry therapist are an acquaintance with a wide variety of poems, a genuine concern for people, an authentic love of poetry, and sensitivity and openness to the possible meanings of the poems. Hirsch Silverman (1986) adds another essential for therapists who would use poetry therapy: "It is best used by therapists who know their own values and how they may influence their perception of the patient."

Silverman also points out that an individual in despair may read a poem of despair and hopelessness and experience even greater depression. He believes that poems with sad themes can be useful for catharsis or identification but that they must also contain stanzas that reflect optimism as a balancing factor.

Some therapists (Kobak and Neinken, 1984) have effectively combined poetry with drama by using an "acting out" technique that involves clients directly in the poetry. For example, a poem about power and the self is made personal by having the clients hold that "power" in a cupped hand. Role playing about power and dominance can also be used. A more complicated form of drama as therapy is *psychodrama*.

Psychodrama

Psychodrama, a form of group therapy that was originally developed by the late Dr. Jacob Moreno (Van Servellen, 1984) is becoming widely used in short-term psychiatric units and in such places as alcoholism rehabilitation centers. Various institutes and continuing education courses train professionals in psychodramatic techniques, which focus on dramatizing an individual's conflicts, problems, and past and present relationships. A therapist directs the scene, and other clients or staff members play key roles or act as "alter egos" (roughly, persons who provide uninhibited versions of what the client is saying). There are opportunities for insight development through such methods as role reversals and for catharsis through such activities as conversations with a dead parent. The therapist keeps the action rolling as a stage director does, steps in to protect when necessary, interprets at times, and intentionally reduces group anxiety at the end through the use of a low-key "sharing session." Warm-up techniques and gimmicks are used at the beginning of the session to promote group and individual interaction.

Some schizophrenic clients have reacted adversely to psychodrama with an increase in psychotic symptoms. Clients should be assessed carefully before participation in this modality. When schizophrenic clients do participate, the process should be modified to prevent any literal interpretation of the content of acting sessions as reality and for a possible threat to the ego that the awareness of previously unconscious and unacceptable material might present.

Psychodrama is a powerful tool and should not be used in psychiatric settings except under the supervision of a trained person.

Art therapy

Art therapy is useful in three ways:
1. It can be used as a tool for stimulating self-expression in a client (particularly clients who have difficulty expressing their feelings—for example, regressed schizophrenics or children before they can express feelings or conflicts verbally).
2. It can be used as a diagnostic tool from which modifications in a treatment plan can be made.
3. It can provide opportunities for increasing self-esteem and for promoting sublimation and personal growth.

Deep, analytical interpretation of a person's conflicts can be made on the basis of the art he or she produces. Interpretation, of course, should only be done by persons who have extensive knowledge of psychoanalysis and art therapy and diagnosis. However, using art therapy to stimulate expression, provide recreation and sublimation, increase interpersonal interaction, and enhance self-esteem is an appropriate method for nurses who work with psychiatric clients. Various materials may be used—water colors, oil paints, crayons, modeling clay, felt-tipped pens. Felt-tipped pens are particularly useful—they are easy to store and use, inexpensive, and colorful. Sometimes a group leader will offer a theme to the group and ask the members to draw their responses to it (for example, "What do you look forward to?" "What was your happiest time?" "When do you feel sad?"). Group members usually need a good deal of encouragement and support—an invariable complaint is "I simply cannot draw at all!" They need to be reassured that artistic ability is not a requirement; it often helps if the leader is willing to participate in the project as a member of the group. Each drawing is viewed by the group, and discussion follows. Any interpretation of a drawing is best given by the person who

produced it. Another way of using art therapy is to have the group participate in the production of a large mural or collage. Such an activity promotes cooperation and interaction among members.

A specialized form of cooperative art therapy is *graffiti therapy*, which is a way of stimulating clients' expressions of self and communication with others. Participants are provided with a large piece of brown paper or a blackboard, and they are given pencils, crayons, chalk, or other writing instruments with which to scribble messages and comments. Clients are free to write whatever they choose (as long as it is socially acceptable to the community) and to remain anonymous. Themes or topics may be suggested, and staff *and* clients are encouraged to participate.

Movement therapy

Several forms of movement therapy are used in psychiatric settings; dance, exercise, and yoga are examples. Movement therapy provides several benefits. It can increase physical well-being and self-esteem and reduce anxiety. Exercise and dance can be particularly helpful to those depressed clients who tend to immobilize themselves in despair. Such group activities can also encourage interpersonal interaction—and, to put it simply, they can be fun. Rhythmic dance movements to music have been found to be especially beneficial for psychotic children—such movements help them to improve body coordination (Gunning and Holmes, 1973). Many nurses working in psychiatric settings who have had training in dance, yoga, or calisthenics—or who simply have an interest in these arts—are participating in movement therapy groups.

Music therapy

Music therapy has a long history in psychiatric care. The ancient Greeks believed that music could be a healing agent for persons in disturbed emotional states (Manfreda and Krampitz, 1977). In the seventeenth century, music was a specific part of the treatment of madness.

The goals of music therapy include increased self-esteem through pride in achievement, increased interpersonal relating, improved abilities

also be a built-in mechanism for avoiding the "woodwork client" phenomenon—the not-so-interesting client becoming lost in the shuffle. The phenomenon of the "problem client," whose taxing behavior elicits avoidance from staff, is another situation that might be prevented through primary nursing. Certainly, it has been reported that primary nursing can lead to increased job satisfaction. Psychiatric nursing, with its long tradition of therapy involving one-to-one relationships, seems especially compatible with a primary nursing philosophy. Because the benefits may be as numerous as the problems in adapting the primary nursing model to milieu therapy, what is needed is a creative blending of the goals of primary nursing with the requirements for an effective and therapeutic milieu. *Primary care* that is flexible in its administration and not arbitrary in its assignment could be one aspect of the total milieu that enhances the effectiveness of treatment.

Liaison nursing: reaching out from the therapeutic milieu

Liaison nursing has become an important part of the health care system. Clinical specialists in psychiatric nursing act as liaisons by providing consultation services for their nursing colleagues in medical-surgical, parent-child, and geriatric settings. They also provide these services to other professionals, such as physicians and social workers. Another aspect of liaison nursing is the giving of care directly to clients in settings outside of the psychiatric unit. For example, the anxious client awaiting life-threatening surgery, the severely depressed victim of a stroke, or the family of a dying person may all be included in the case load of a psychiatric nurse involved in liaison nursing.

The liaison nurse may be called in to conduct group sessions for staff members who are working in high-stress environments such as terminal care units, intensive care units, or pediatric units. The goal of these sessions is to help staff members to discuss and express their feelings about the difficult and painful aspects of their work and to provide group support for individuals who are experiencing stress.

Thus, the functions of the psychiatric nursing clinical specialist who performs liaison work may include consultation; client assessment; teaching of staff, clients, and their families; and direct intervention with clients. In a hospital, a good deal of this intervention with clients may be in the form of crisis intervention.

THE MENTAL HEALTH TEAM

People are treated for mental illness in a variety of settings—for example, community mental health clinics, day-care centers, psychiatric hospitals, and psychiatric units of general hospitals. These facilities become part of the social network or support system of an individual, and they are social systems in and of themselves. Some people (for example, workers and "outpatients") spend part of the day within such a system, while others ("inpatients") spend all their time there. Each of these systems is rather like a self-contained society; subcultures may evolve with their own customs, rules, and mores (Goffman, 1961). Goffman and the Cummings (1962) are among many social scientists who have studied the psychiatric facility as a social system.

In most psychiatric facilities the formulation of treatment plans for clients is the responsibility of several different health care workers. The way this group of individuals works together as a team can be crucial to the success of a treatment plan. A relationship based on mutual respect and equality not only facilitates the team's functioning but also promotes the well-being of the client.

In a therapeutic milieu or community a certain amount of blurring of the distinctions between the roles of the various team members is considered appropriate. This role blurring may include the designation of an interdisciplinary team leader. While some agencies follow the medical model, in which a psychiatrist serves as team leader, other agencies allow any member of the helping professions to fill the role. Role blurring is based on the belief that the best person to help an individual is one who has developed a meaningful relationship with him or her. This belief does not negate the fact that each of the disciplines brings something unique to the team and to the overall care plan for a client. The nurse, as a cooperating member of the team, needs to have an understanding of the roles and functions of the other persons who make up the team.*

The most crucial member of the team is the client. It is important for nurses or any health professional to remember that no amount of treatment can be successful if the client is not engaged as a responsible partner in a therapeutic alliance. In the last analysis, it is the client who will, in one way or another, decide the outcome of therapy. Today, in many enlightened treatment centers, this fact is acknowledged through efforts to include the client in the process of making decisions about treatment or about goals for the future. Unfortunately, however, this philosophy is not always carried through; too often the client's views are considered *after* the ideas of other team members.

Most units and facilities allow clients some form of self-government within the overall treatment plan. The amount of self-government varies considerably. In some units clients participate only in once-a-week "client-staff" or "community" meetings that deal with here-and-now situations affecting staff and clients. In other units clients are expected to be responsible for many day-to-day decisions. Such decisions may involve the planning of recreational events and outings, the granting of weekend passes, and changes in the status of individual clients. In such units, clients also may be involved in decisions about discharge. In some alcoholic rehabilitation units, before clients are readmitted to the community, they must meet with the entire treatment staff to discuss what the clients see as their problems and their goals, as well as their potential degree of commitment to their treatment plans. Some facilities have "open charting"— clients are allowed to read their own charts at any time. All these policies are based on the belief that encouraging an individual to be responsible for himself or herself and to assume responsibility for his or her peers will facilitate recovery and growth.

Inspired in part by the "radical therapists" (see Chapter 25), consumer advocacy* is beginning within the ranks of the mentally ill—or, more accurately, among recovered, or formerly mentally ill, persons. Advocacy takes energy, and someone in the midst of trying to cope with severe mental illness has little strength to spare. A significant portion of this advocacy is also carried out by relatives of clients, and they have been successful in making some major changes in large state-run facilities. Their efforts have caused federal and state funds for certain mental health institutions to be withheld until services and facilities were improved.

Clients have won some important court cases concerning their rights to freedom and to adequate and appropriate treatment while under psychiatric care. In addition to the right to treatment, other rights are being promoted by advocacy groups, including the following:

1. The right to the least restrictive form of housing
2. The right to education (particularly in the cases of mentally handicapped and emotionally ill children)
3. Employment rights, including restrictions on the use of institutionalized persons to perform labor without receiving *at least* the minimum wage as well as protection against discrimination in employment in the community
4. The right to live in the community without being subject to discriminatory zoning ordinances
5. The right to refuse treatment (Trotter, 1975)

The roles and functions of each member of the health team will vary according to the needs of the population being served and the organization of the particular agency.

Certain professional responsibilities, however, may not be divided among the members of the mental health team. The physician, for example, always retains professional responsibility for such functions as prescribing medications. The nurse

---

*For a detailed description of the roles of the various team members, see Chapter 1.

*Advocacy and the community as a client are discussed in Chapter 16, the nurse's role as a client advocate is discussed in Chapter 3.

shares with the physician the responsibility for the administration of drugs and the evaluation of their effectiveness and side effects.

But many aspects of psychiatric treatment can be provided by all professionals and by some paraprofessionals. Individual and group therapy and maintaining a therapeutic milieu are some examples. It is in these areas, in which there is an overlapping of professional roles and responsibilities, that the professional expertise and experience of particular team members determine who is responsible for intervention. For example, a nurse with training and experience in crisis intervention or psychodrama would be the team leader when these therapeutic modalities are employed. Or a member of the team who is of the same ethnic group as a client may be more effective than other team members when ethnicity is an important consideration in therapy. Evaluation of client behavior and of the effectiveness of treatment plans are additional areas in which team leadership may shift from one team member to another.

In addition to the crucial ingredients of personal identity and integrity, the effective interdisciplinary team member has the ability to

1. accept the perspectives of others
2. trust the knowledge and expertise of members of other disciplines
3. function in an interdependent manner
4. form new attitudes, values, and perceptions when necessary
5. negotiate roles with other members of the team
6. tolerate a constant review and challenge of ideas
7. take risks
8. accept a "team" philosophy of health care
9. be problem and client oriented rather than status or profession oriented (Given and Simmons, 1977).

CHAPTER SUMMARY

Because of the nature of nursing education and nurses' clinical experience, milieu therapy is probably the area in which the responsibility of the nurse is most evident. The nurse brings a background in science and the humanities, as well as an understanding of psychiatric nursing principles, to the mental health team.

Milieu therapy usually includes some form of self-government for clients, such as community or client-staff meetings. Therapeutic limit-setting and graded responsibility are also important elements of the milieu.

Milieu therapy for clients who are experiencing emotional or mental problems often includes art, poetry, music, movement therapy, and psychodrama. Nurses who work in psychiatric settings are involved in varying degrees in these treatment modalities.

Ideally, members of the mental health team work together to engage the client in cooperative, goal-oriented involvement in his or her own treatment. Team members share in the evaluation of clients and in planning, implementing, and evaluating treatment programs. Team leadership may shift or rotate among team members, depending upon which member has the greatest expertise in a given situation or the most information about a given client.

Within the milieu, efforts are directed toward fostering responsibility for self and others and toward facilitating growth.

SELF-DIRECTED LEARNING

Sensitivity-Awareness Exercises

The purposes of these exercises are to:

- Develop an awareness about your own attitudes and feelings toward participating in some of the treatment modalities used in milieu therapy
- Develop a sensitivity toward some of the possible uses and abuses of milieu therapy
- Develop an awareness about the subjective experience of clients residing in therapeutic communities

1. Choose a poem that you find particularly meaningful. Write down all the thoughts and feelings that the poem arouses in you.
2. Choose, at random, a poem from an anthology of poetry. Write down the thoughts and feelings that this poem arouses in you. If you have difficulty relating to the poem for some reason, write down your thoughts and feelings about that.
3. Obtain a videotape of the movie "One Flew Over the Cuckoo's Nest." Write a description of the milieu depicted in this movie.
4. For a group:
   Bring in sheets of paper and several magic markers of various colors to your clinical group conference, seminar, or class. Pick a theme (e.g., "How do you feel when you come to a new clinical agency for the first time?"). Have the members of the group translate their thoughts and feelings into a picture.
5. Some therapeutic communities for substance abuse clients hold monthly "open house" sessions to which the public is invited. If there is such an opportunity in your community, arrange to attend it. Discuss what you learned there and some of your own thoughts and feelings with your clinical group/class.

Questions to Consider

1. Ideally, the mental health team:
   a. shares authority and accountability with one another
   b. follows traditional hierarchical structure in decision making
   c. allows responsibilities that define professional practice to be a part of role blurring
   d. take sole and total responsibility for their client's growth
2. You have just found John (a resident in a substance abuse therapeutic community for the past two months) smoking in a restricted area. John apologized profusely, looked very upset, and asked you not to report him because if he loses his leave privileges, he won't be able to go for a planned job interview on Saturday. You, as a member of the mental health team, know how difficult it was to arrange this interview in the first place. You also know that John has been very upset because of the recent divorce of his parents.
   The first action to take in this case is:
   a. accept his apology in a straightforward manner and negotiate a contract between the two of you that would include no further infractions on the rules
   b. inform John that he has broken a rule and that you will report it to the residents' committee for their decision on the matter
   c. tell John that you are *very* disappointed in his behavior and ask him if he is aware of why he did it. Explore his feelings about the divorce
   d. sit down with John and discuss the matter. Make any decision about how you will handle the situation after you have learned what the basis for the rule breaking was
3. Roll call, or attendance-taking, at a community meeting in a therapeutic community is important because: (choose the best answer)
   a. it keeps the meeting from becoming too disorderly
   b. it reinforces the rules and the importance of attending meetings
   c. it provides a structure for staff members who may rotate as leaders
   d. it helps to introduce new members to the group

Match the term with the name:

4. "Stress" groups   a. Jacob Moreno
5. Psychodrama   b. Maxwell Jones
6. Milieu therapy   c. Art therapy
7. Graffiti therapy   d. Liaison nurse
8. The program of a therapeutic milieu usually includes:
   a. graded responsibility and sufficient stimulation and activity to prevent regression
   b. strict therapist-client confidentiality
   c. standardized treatment plans for all clients
   d. some form of hierarchical government for clients

Answer key

1. a	5. a
2. b	6. b
3. d	7. c
4. d	8. a

REFERENCES

Abroms G: Defining milieu therapy, Arch Gen Psychiatr 21:553-560, 1969.

American Nurses' Association Division on Psychiatric-Mental Health Nursing Practice: Standards of Psychiatric-Mental Health Nursing Practice, Kansas City, Mo, 1982, ANA Publications.

Cumming J and Cumming E: Ego and milieu, New York, 1962, Atherton Press.

Erickson R: Viewing the therapeutic community through Adlerian spectacles, J Group Psychother 32:201-216, 1982.

Fann W and Goshen C: The language of mental health, ed 2, St. Louis, 1977, The CV Mosby Co.

Given B and Simmons S: The interdisciplinary health-care team: fact or fiction? Nurs Forum 16(2):165-184, 1977.

Goffman E: Asylums: essays on the social situation of mental patients and other inmates, Garden City, NY, 1961, Anchor Books.

Gunning S and Holmes T: Dance therapy with psychotic children, Arch Gen Psychiatr 28:707-714, 1973.

Jones M: The therapeutic community: a treatment method in psychiatry, New York, 1953, Basic Books, Inc., Publishers.

Kobak D and Neinken E: Poetry therapy with hospitalized mentally ill patients, J Group Psychother, Psychodrama Sociometr 37(3):134-136, 1984.

Lerner A: Poetry therapy. Am J Nurs 73(8):1336-1338, 1973.

Manfreda M and Krampitz S: Psychiatric nursing, ed 10, Philadelphia, 1977, FA Davis.

Parriot S: Music as therapy, Am J Nurs 69(8):1723-1726, 1969.

Russakoff L and Oldham J: The structure and technique of community meetings: the short-term unit, Psychiatry 45:38-44, 1982.

Silverman H: Poetry therapy, Arts Psychotherapy 13(4):343-345, 1986.

Skinner K: The therapeutic milieu: making it work, J Psychiatr Nurs–Mental Health Serv 17(8):38-44, 1979.

Smith C: Primary nursing care—a substantive nursing care delivery system, Nurs Admin Q 1(2):1, 1977.

Trotter RJ: Open sesame: the Constitution and mental institutions, Sc News, vol. 108, July 12, 1975, p. 31, 1975.

VanServellen G: Group and family therapy: a model for psychotherapeutic nursing practice, St. Louis, 1984, The CV Mosby Co.

ANNOTATED SUGGESTED READINGS

Baker B: The use of music with autistic children, J Psychosoc Nurs Mental Health Serv 20(4):31-34, 1982.
The author describes four phases of intervention into isolation patterns of autistic children through the use of music therapy: Phase I (breaking the shell), Phase II (shifting awareness), Phase III (building competence), Phase IV (building relationship with others). The interventions to break patterns of isolation include repetition; continuity in the environment; use of musical and rhythm instruments; imitative games; and bridging trust between the child and significant others.

Benfer B: Defining the role and function of the psychiatric nurse as a member of the team, Persp Psychiatr Care 18(4):166-177, 1981.
Benfer presents a clearly organized delineation of the variables that affect the functioning of the interdisciplinary mental health team, with particular attention to the functioning of the psychiatric nurse. Phases of group development in relation to interdisciplinary teams are reviewed, and the topic of "organizational politics" is briefly discussed.

Carser D: Primary nursing in the milieu, J Psychiatr Nurs Mental Health Serv 19(2):35-41, 1981.
Definitions of primary nursing and of milieu therapy are included as well as a brief historical overview of the concepts. The relationship between the two concepts is examined, with some discussion of potential problems and solutions.

Devine B: Therapeutic milieu/milieu therapy: an overview, J Psychiatr Nurs Mental Health Serv 19(3):20-24, 1981.
This is a historical and current overview of milieu therapy and its application to particular patient populations. A review of some research findings on therapeutic communities is provided, and some issues in milieu therapy are touched upon.

Islam A and Turner D: The therapeutic community: a critical reappraisal, Hosp Com Psychiatr 33(8):651-653, 1982.
This provides a critical assessment of the concept of the "therapeutic community." As a "protest movement" the authors believe that the therapeutic community has achieved some degree of success. However, they suggest that its therapeutic value should be reassessed in light of recent research and presently changing social conditions.

Lockwood R: Pet-facilitated therapy grows up, The Humane Society News, Spring, 1986:4-8, 1986.
The history and development of this approach is outlined and some of the important therapeutic advantages to various groups of people are discussed. The author also explores some of the past and present threats to the animals' welfare, and he suggests methods and guidelines for preventing these.

Phillips D: Photography's use as a metaphor of self with stabilized schizophrenic patients, The Arts in Psychotherapy 13:9-16, 1986.
Working with schizophrenic clients is described. Photography is seen as: 1. Enhancing self-esteem through mastery of the skill; 2. Providing stable outer boundaries through its "consistent" properties that may help to counteract chaotic inner boundaries; 3. Facilitating feelings of shared interaction between client and therapist; 4. Providing insight into the client's inner world through the understanding of choice of photographic subject as a metaphor for that inner world; and 5. Providing a bridge between the client and the outer world.

Puskar K: Structure for the hospitalized adolescent, J Psychiatr Nurs Mental Health Serv 19(7):13-16, 1981.
This article notes the various types of structure available to the hospitalized adolescent. The "six c's" of structure for the adolescent are reviewed: consistency, communication, clear rules, clear consequences, clear roles, and consultation-education for the staff. Strengths and weaknesses of an approach based on the six c's are briefly discussed.

Robinson L: Psychiatric consultation liaison nursing and psychiatric consultation liaison doctoring: similarities and differences, Arch Psychiatr Nurs 1(2):73-80, 1987.

While discussing the differences in approach to consultation/ liaison work between the medical and nursing professions, this article also provides a history of its development and of the subsequent development of psychiatric consultation/liaison nursing.

FURTHER READINGS

Byrne A et al: Graffiti therapy, Persp Psychiatri Care 9(1):34-36, 1972.

Challela M: The interdisciplinary team: a role definition in nursing, Image (Sigma Theta Tau) 11(1):9-15, 1979.

Ciske K: Accountability—the essence of primary nursing. Am J Nurs 79(5):890-894, 1979.

Fink P et al: Art therapy: a diagnostic and therapeutic tool, Int J Psychiatr 11(1):104-125, 1973.

Fitzgerald R and Long I: Seclusion in the management of severely disturbed manic and depressed patients, Persp Psychiatr Care 11(2):59-64, 1973.

Hyde N: Play therapy: the troubled child's self-encounter, Am J Nurs 71(7):1366-1370, 1970.

Leone D and Zahourek R: 'Aloneness' in a therapeutic community, Persp Psychiatr Care 12(2):60-63, 1974.

Lewis A and Levy J: Psychiatric liaison nursing: the theory and clinical practice, New York, 1983, Prentice-Hall, Inc.

Lyon G: Limit setting as a therapeutic tool, J Psychiatr Nurs Mental Health Serv 8(6):17-21, 1970.

North M: Personality assessment through movement, Boston, 1972, Plays, Inc.

Pesso A: Movement in psychotherapy, New York, 1969, New York University Press.

Romoff V and Kane I: Primary nursing in psychiatry: an effective and functional model, Persp Psychiatr Care 20(2):73-78, 1982.

CHAPTER 13

Group therapy

CHAPTER FOCUS

Group therapy is a well-established treatment modality in psychiatric inpatient units, in outpatient clinics, and in community mental health centers. It originally received the impetus for its growth from economic factors during World War II (more people could be treated at one time), but it soon became apparent that group therapy provided important therapeutic benefits that were different from and in addition to those of individual psychotherapy.

In accordance with their various levels of educational preparation, professional nurses working in psychiatric settings have assumed the roles of group leader, group therapist, and co-therapist. The role of group therapist is the responsibility of the master's-degree clinical specialist in psychiatric nursing.

This chapter focuses on the curative factors inherent in group therapy, the types of groups, definitions relevant to group dynamics, some guidelines for intervening as an effective group leader, and some important phenomena that occur in therapy groups. Guidelines for group therapy with minority group clients and a discussion of the short-term psychiatric unit group are also included.

A knowledge of group dynamics can aid the nurse in working with colleagues and as a team member in any setting. A guide for the assessment of group process is included, and the use of the nursing process within a group situation is outlined.

Cartwright and Zander (1967) have defined groups in general. They describe a group as being made up of members who

1. engage in frequent interactions
2. define themselves as members of the group
3. are defined by others as belonging to the group
4. share norms with other group members
5. participate in a system of interlocking roles
6. identify with one another through role models or ideals held in common
7. find rewards within the group
8. pursue interdependent goals
9. have a sense of group unity
10. tend to act in a unitary way toward the environment

Therapy groups are a specific type of group. They differ from social groups (such as clubs, fraternal organizations, and lodges) in that they are specifically aimed at changing the maladaptive coping behavior of their members. A definition of group therapy has been provided by Kaplan and Sadock (1972). They describe it as a type of treatment involving two or more clients participating together in the presence of one or more therapists, who facilitate both emotional and rational or cognitive interaction to effect changes in the maladaptive behavior of the group members.

Group therapy came into existence at the turn of the century when a Boston physician, Dr. Joseph H. Pratt, used it to enhance the medical treatment of tuberculosis patients by attempting to deal with their emotional problems. During and immediately after World War II, when there was a shortage of psychiatric personnel, group therapy was seen as an economical form of psychotherapy. Eventually, a body of theory developed surrounding group treatment, and it became quite evident that in addition to its economic advantages group therapy had other important advantages over individual therapy. These advantages include provision of a protective environment for trying out new patterns of behavior, opportunities for learning new patterns of behavior, and the availability of a role model for interpersonal relating (the leader or leaders and other group members). There is also the opportunity for multiple transference situations (see

Chapter 11) within the group, which can lead to the development of greater insight.

CURATIVE FACTORS IN GROUP THERAPY

One authority (Yalom, 1975) has delineated the curative factors that group treatment can offer:

1. *The instillation of hope.* Seeing the progress of others in the group, a group member feels hopeful about receiving similar help.
2. *Universality.* When a group member sees that others in the world share similar feelings or have similar problems, anxiety is decreased.
3. *Imparting of information.* Interpersonal relating, developmental tasks and stages, medications and other somatic treatments, and the structure of the setting are only a few areas in which information may be shared.
4. *Altruism.* The opportunity to support and to help increase self-awareness in another group member gives the helping individual increased self-esteem. It also encourages a preoccupied individual to become less self-focused.
5. *Corrective recapitulation of the primary family group.* Multiple transference opportunities are available in group treatment to help develop insight into one's background and its effects on present relationships. (The individual displaces and projects feelings and attitudes onto the therapist *and* onto other group members.)
6. *Imitative behavior.* The group leader, a recovering group member, or a group member who has already mastered a particular psychosocial skill or developmental task can be a valuable role model.
7. *Interpersonal learning.* The group offers many and varied opportunities for relating to other people on a here-and-now basis.

TYPES OF GROUPS

There are several ways of using group therapy and many ways of describing groups.

Play therapy groups are specifically used for

therapy with children because children have limited verbal abilities. Conflicts and problems are acted out in play, and interpersonal learning takes place.

Psychoanalytically oriented group therapy is an "uncovering" type of therapy aimed at helping group members delineate and understand their intrapsychic and interpersonal conflicts and problems. The group and the leader may follow any one of the various theoretical schools of psychoanalysis, such as Freudian, Sullivanian, or Jungian. This type of group therapy is most often done in an outpatient setting, with clients who are neurotic rather than psychotic and who are functioning on an adequate level of adjustment.

Repressive-inspirational group therapy provides the framework for such self-help groups as Alcoholics Anonymous and Overeaters Anonymous. Repressive-inspirational groups try to alter socially unacceptable behavior while developing and emphasizing socially acceptable qualities. These groups, which consist exclusively of acting-out (socially deviant)* or formerly acting-out individuals, usually meet in a community setting.

Michele had been overweight for as long as she could remember. Even in kindergarten she had been taunted by other children, who gave her the nickname "fatty." She had been on and off diets all of her life. She would lose 50 or 60 pounds and then regain them. Now that Michelle was the mother of two children, she was afraid that her children would follow her poor eating habits and develop weight problems. She joined Overeaters Anonymous. With the support of the group members, all of whom either had been or were presently overweight, she was able to acknowledge her problem—that she ate when she was unhappy and that eating was a means not only of satisfying hunger but also of feeling secure. Michelle and another member of Overeaters Anonymous were teamed as "buddies." When one of them experienced an uncontrollable craving for food, she called her buddy and "talked it out." If necessary, the other person came to the house and stayed with her buddy until the craving for food passed. In this way, food binges were avoided.

---

*Refer to Chapter 20 for further discussion of acting-out or socially deviant behavior.

It is obvious that a fundamental idea behind repressive-inspirational therapy is that with the help of persons who have experienced the same problem, acting-out individuals can face up to their socially unacceptable behavior, vow not to repeat it, and help others who are struggling with the problem.

Although nurses may not be directly involved in repressive-inspirational groups, they do play important roles as facilitators and resource persons. In hospitals, self-help groups such as Alcoholics Anonymous and Narcotics Anonymous frequently hold meetings for people who are potential members. Nurses who have established some degree of rapport with acting-out individuals can be influential in encouraging them to attend a meeting of the appropriate group. When nurses provide members with adequate time, privacy, and space for meetings, they give people the message, "This is important therapy." In the community, community health nurses, occupational health nurses, and school nurse–teachers serve as important sources of information. In their role as case finders, these nurses come in contact with many people who may be in need of but unaware of existing self-help groups. It is often through the encouragement and support of such nurses that acting-out individuals make their initial contacts with these groups.

Encounter groups, or T-groups (the "T" stands for "training in human relations"), originated with Kurt Lewin in 1946. Lewin had been asked by the Connecticut Interracial Commission to help resolve some of the state's interracial problems. He and his colleagues assembled some of Connecticut's black and white leaders in an attempt to help them resolve their differences. Lewin appointed four observers to record the group process. After each session, these recorders discussed the group's dynamics with the group's leaders. Group members insisted on being present at these "postmortems." Lewin found that the conferees learned more from these feedback sessions than from the group meetings themselves. This was the inception of encounter group therapy.

Encounter groups focus on the here and now—on what group members experience as they meet. Members are urged to be completely candid and to shed their facades of adequacy, competence, and self-sufficiency. These groups are peer-oriented rather than leader (authority)-oriented. Members are encouraged to tell one another how they come across to others (that is, to provide feedback). Brutal verbal attacks often develop. Encounter group therapy seems to crack the shell of maladaptive communication patterns used by acting-out individuals. They then can begin to develop insight and to change their behavior. An encounter group thus functions as a microcosm of society.

Yablonsky (1965) describes an encounter group session at Synanon, the original therapeutic community for drug addicts in the United States. The meeting becomes an emotional battlefield. Complete candor is the order of the day. Maladaptive defenses and socially unacceptable behavior of members are repeatedly attacked. The encounters are designed to help acting-out persons see themselves as society sees them. They are forced to see both their strengths and their weaknesses.

Although nurses do not usually participate in encounter sessions, it is important for them to understand the therapeutic function of what might appear to be destructive group techniques.

A student nurse was trying to establish a therapeutic relationship with Jamie, who had been using alcohol since elementary school and drugs since he began high school. Jamie, aged 16, was now part of a therapeutic drug community. One of the treatment modalities used by this community was encounter group therapy. After a session in which the group had "attacked" Jamie's behavior and attitudes, Jamie complained to the student nurse. The student, who was not acquainted with encounter therapy, sympathized with Jamie and told him that it sounded as though he was being scapegoated. She explained, "They are probably ganging up on you so that no one will focus on them."

When the student recounted this episode to her instructor, the instructor explained the therapeutic rationale underlying the group's approach. After that, the student was able to support Jamie through the experience by helping him listen to what the group was saying. She also helped him realize that although his socially unacceptable behavior was under attack, he as a person was not being rejected.

As members of health teams, nurses need to be involved in developing and implementing therapeutic goals. It is also the function of nurses to sustain acting-out individuals during their experiences with encounter therapy. Moreover, because nurses work closely with families, it is important for nurses to understand the therapeutic rationale underlying encounter group therapy so that they can explain it to family members. Otherwise, the families of acting-out individuals could become alarmed at what might appear to be a brutally destructive or punitive group process.

The approaches of all health team members must be coordinated to ensure that the therapeutic goals of encounter group therapy are implemented and that socially acceptable behavior is promoted.

Activity group therapy* is task oriented. A variety of recreational and occupational forms of therapy is used for the purpose of assessing and developing social and leisure skills. Activity groups are found in both hospital and community settings. The goals of activity group therapy are as follows:

1. To encourage communication
2. To facilitate the expression of feelings
3. To provide opportunity for decision making
4. To increase a person's concentration span
5. To teach a person how to cooperate, share, and compete

Activity group therapy is especially well suited for acting-out individuals. Such persons are action oriented—they try to cope with inner conflicts by doing and not by talking. Activities necessitating gross physical movements therefore provide socially acceptable outlets for the hostility and aggressiveness that underlie most acting-out behavior. Woodworking, sports, and arts and crafts are only a few of the activities that are suitable for acting-out individuals.

A group of student nurses brought construction paper and paints to a unit for newly admitted acting-out individuals. One young man had been admitted after he

---

*See Chapter 12 for a discussion of various types of activity group therapy.

had taken LSD and experienced a "bad trip." He would not talk about the experience. Midway through a session in which the clients were using the art supplies, the young man sat down at the table. He picked up a piece of green construction paper and, using the colors yellow, purple, orange, red, and black, drew a demonic face. One student asked, "Who is that?" the young man answered, "That's how I felt—just like a devil." He was beginning to admit his experience and to assimilate it into his self system.

Activity therapy thus can facilitate communication and the expression of emotion. In addition, when people set up the equipment for an activity, share materials and tools, and put everything away afterward, they are engaged in interaction, interplay, and interdependency.

Few formal demands are made on activity group members. In this relatively nonthreatening atmosphere, they can "do" to things rather than to people. This is an important phase in the treatment of acting-out behavior. It serves the dual purpose of redirecting and sublimating aggression and hostility. New, socially acceptable behavior can supplant the older, socially unacceptable behavior.

Multifamily therapy groups and *couples groups* are composed of more than one family unit. These groups help members to work with the problems of intrafamily communication and relationships. Individuals and families help one another in a supportive, learning atmosphere. For example, the multifamily therapy group is commonly used to help the families of clients who are hospitalized with schizophrenia to be supportive factors in the clients' recovery.

In *groups for persons with special problems*—for example, colostomy groups, laryngectomy groups, and mastectomy groups—feelings are expressed and support and suggestions are offered in a way that helps members adjust to and accept their changed body images and decreased ability to function. Members are encouraged to function at their maximum potential levels. These groups can be "self-help" groups, or they can have varying degrees of professional leadership or involvement.

Other groups found in community and hospital settings include *sensory awareness groups, trans-*

actional analysis groups (based on the theory of Eric Berne [1967]), and *problem-solving* or *brainstorming groups*, which are found in business and used by the staff members of health care facilities.

Therapy groups may be short-term, open-ended groups—the type most often formed in the psychiatric units of general hospitals—or they may be of the closed, long-term type found in community outpatient settings. "Open-ended" simply means that as one group member is discharged and leaves the group, another member may be added. The composition of the group is flexible and always changing. A closed group begins with a certain composition, and if someone leaves the group, no additional member is added. And while a closed group may be long term, there is often a specific time at which it is to disband.

DEFINITIONS

The following section will define and discuss some concepts important to the understanding of group dynamics and group therapy.

Group norms

Group norms help to identify and define the group; they define the limits within which member behavior is considered acceptable. They act as guides for individuals and thus they reduce ambiguity in the group. Group norms can help the group to attain its goals (but some norms may also inhibit work toward goals). Norms may evolve from the goals of a group. The following are some examples of group norms:

1. Cooperation among group members is expected here.
2. Openness is essential to the group process.
3. Competition between group members is not acceptable.
4. Competition between group members is necessary.
5. Everyone should participate in the group discussion.
6. We should be on an informal basis with one another.

7. We won't talk about certain things.
8. Don't trust anyone from the staff.

Group norms can be *explicit* (stated norms). For example: "We always start and end the group session on time." They may be *implicit* (unspoken). Implicit norms often develop because members may have preconceived ideas about what is appropriate for discussion in a group. They may also develop through the leader's role modeling (Corey and Corey, 1982). A norm that a leader would likely want to foster through example is "mutual respect for one another." Group norms can serve a *group task function* or they can serve a *group maintenance function.* In serving a task function, they allow a group to function in a smooth, coordinated manner to accomplish tasks. In the area of group maintenance, they help the group to survive (Sampson and Marthas, 1981). Some examples of group maintenance norms are

1. the rules for dealing with absences
2. standards concerning group members' personal relations with one another
3. mechanisms for resolving members' conflicts

Norms are necessary therefore to help the group reach its goal or goals and to survive as a group. Each group exerts pressures on members toward *conformity* to the norms. This pressure includes subtle and direct means of positive and negative reinforcement (Northern, 1969). The size of the group; the style of leadership; the personal characteristics of group members, and the intragroup relationships (e.g., family members?; mental health team members?, fellow inpatients?) are some of the variables affecting conformity to norms. A good definition of a norm is: ". . . . a rule or standard to which the members of a group are expected to adhere. A set of norms defines the range of behavior that will be tolerated within the group" (Northern, 1969, 33-34).

Group boundaries

A definition of a boundary is: "physical or psychological factor that separates relevant regions in the group structure. An external boundary separates the group from the external environment . . . an internal boundary distinguishes the group lead-er from the members" (Kaplan and Sadock, 1972, VII). In any group, individual members are constantly struggling with the polarity of their individual autonomy and the pull to merge with the group. Boundaries in a group limit merging, and they limit freedom to the extent that they define the lines across which one cannot go. Boundaries are necessary for the group to have structure and to function. Boundaries of a group include "what will and will not happen, who will and will not be included and how the process will be executed in space and time" (Van Servellen, 1984, 114). Group growth is fostered through the creation, maintenance, and transformation of boundaries. Boundaries can be physical (e.g., the four walls of the room where the group meets); temporal—the time when group sessions occur, psychosocial—implicit rules between members concerning the amount of intrusion that is tolerated. They may even be intrapsychic (Foulkes and Anthony, 1968). An example of the latter would be the result of a clinical decision not to foster awareness of unconscious conflict in schizophrenic clients.

An important aspect of group leadership is *boundary control.* The leader of a therapy group for psychiatric inpatients might, for example,

1. prevent nongroup members from entering the room while group is in session
2. start and end the group on time
3. interrupt one group member who is interrogating another in a much too intrusive manner
4. foster norms and use techniques that do not increase awareness of unconscious conflicts.

Group conflict

Conflict between one group's values and those of other groups to which a person belongs is common. Conflict in a group of people is inevitable (Corey and Corey, 1982, 98), and it is a necessary catalyst for change and growth. It is also necessary for stimulation of interaction among group members. The basis of conflict may be differences in the goals, values, norms, and interests of the group members.

Conflict may be realistic or unrealistic. Realistic conflict is part of a rational goal, and the conflict is

TABLE 13-1 Group member roles according to function

Group maintenance	Group task	Individual goals
Encourager—praises others; agrees with and accepts the ideas of others; open to differences within the group *Harmonizer*—mediates and reconciles intragroup differences *Compromiser*—operates to resolve conflicts; seeks a compromise that all can accept	*Initiator*—offers new ideas, suggests solutions *Elaborator*—gives examples, develops meanings and explanations *Evaluator*—relates the group standards to any problem *Coordinator*—clarifies relationships among ideas and activities of the group	*Aggressor*—acts negatively with hostility towards others; jokes aggressively; attacks the group and its members *Recognition Seeker*—calls attention to own activities; boasts about achievements; redirects conversation toward self *Help Seeker or Confessor*—uses group to express non-group oriented feelings and thoughts; uses group to gain sympathy; expresses insecurity and self-deprecation *Dominator*—asserts authority and manipulates individuals and the group as a whole

around the means used for reaching the goal. Unrealistic conflict comes from the irrational, emotional processes of the group members, and it tends to become an end in itself. Most group conflicts have both rational and irrational elements, and they may be both functional and dysfunctional at the same time.

Groups control conflict, subtly or directly, through the following processes:

1. *elimination*—forcing the opposing individual or subgroup to withdraw
2. *subjugation*—the dominant member or subgroup's view is accepted by others
3. *compromise*—relatively equal factions each give up something to safeguard a common area of interest
4. *alliance*—individuals or subgroups form alliances, each maintaining independence but combining to achieve a goal
5. *integration*—a group may reach a solution that is satisfying to each individual and more creative and productive than any other solution

This latter process is the highest achievement in a group (Northern, 1969).

Group roles

Benne and Sheats (1948) have described the types of roles that emerge in groups. These roles are categorized by Van Servellen (1984) under three types of functions as follows:

1. contributing to group maintenance
2. contributing to group task or tasks
3. contributing to individual goals, irrespective of the needs of the group as a whole

Table 13-1 summarizes some of the group member roles according to function, using Benne and Sheats's descriptions (adapted from Marthas and Sampson, 1977).

Group cohesiveness

The accomplishment of group cohesiveness is essential to the success of any group (Corey and Corey, 1982). The members of a cohesive group tend to be more open to change and growth, and they are more supportive of one another. They are also more likely to internalize the norms of the group (Olmstead and Hare, 1978). A group doesn't focus its full energy on the common task until cohesiveness has been achieved (Kaplan and Sadock,

1972). A definition of group cohesiveness is: "The total field of forces which act on members to remain in the group." (Festinger et al., 1950).

This definition by Festinger is a widely quoted and concise description of the concept. Kaplan and Sadock's definition of cohesiveness is: "Effect of the mutual bonds between members of a group as a result of their concerted effort for a common interest and purpose."

Cohesiveness, then, is a very important element in the group process. Some of the indications that cohesiveness is beginning to operate in a group (adapted from Corey and Corey, 1982) include the following:

1. cooperation among members is evident and increasing
2. attendance patterns reflect commitment to the group
3. members are punctual
4. the members demonstrated trust—this is reflected in their willingness to take risks and share inner experiences
5. members demonstrated a degree of initiative that indicates responsibility for the group process
6. members are supportive to one another

Following are some ways of fostering group cohesiveness by the group leader (adapted from Corey and Corey, 1982; Olmstead and Hare, 1978):

1. Cooperation rather than competition is emphasized.
2. An atmosphere of mutual respect for one another is modeled.
3. A democratic rather than an authoritarian or laissez-faire atmosphere is maintained.
4. The leader's self-disclosure is demonstrated in the here-and-now of the group.
5. Goals are developed by members and the leader and are clearly stated.
6. The group is attractive to the members (e.g., it deals with matters that interest the members; the atmosphere is supportive; the members feel respected).
7. An open, honest exchange between members, including positive and negative reactions, is encouraged.

8. All group members are invited but not forced to participate actively in the group process.
9. The leadership role is shared by all members. (In an inpatient group this would be modified somewhat, but it can still be accomplished by encouraging "member-to-member" interactions, not always "leader-to-member" or "member-to-leader" ones.)

Group process and group content

Group process refers to *everything* that happens within a group—who talks to whom, who "pairs" with whom, who sits where, the tone and atmosphere of the group, who acts as "assistant therapist," the "norms" of the group, the degree of group cohesiveness, and any conflict in the group. *Group content* simply refers to *what* is discussed.

PHASES OF A GROUP

As in individual treatment, there are phases to the life and natural history of a group. Most ongoing groups will proceed from the *orientation phase* through the *working phase* toward *termination*. Testing of the therapist and the group norms tends to occur in the early, orientation stage, which is generally characterized by only superficial discussion of the group's area of concern. The emerging group responsibility, cooperative therapist-client efforts, and identification with the leader occur in the working phase. Group cohesiveness then becomes evident.

According to Van Servellen (1984), the working phase is generally heralded by the members accepting responsibility for their own interpersonal problems—they become more open to other ways of viewing relationships, and they are ready to explore different ways of finding support and resolving dilemmas. *Resistance* also appears in the working phase as members begin to experience the fear of facing oneself honestly.

As in individual treatment, the termination phase requires that the leader prepare the group well ahead of the group's ending. A summary of the group's history and progress and the formulation of any future plans for individuals are appropriate during this phase.

The leader assists the group (and the leader) to deal with the loss of the group experience in termination.

Levine (1979) has delineated four phases in a group's development according to the directionality of relationships among the group members and the therapist: the parallel phase, the inclusion phase, the mutuality phase, and the termination phase (see Figs. 13-1 to 13-3). A change in the direction of relationships represents the evolution from one phase to another. Levine has also outlined the three recurring crisis themes in the life of a therapy group: authority, intimacy, and separation.

The parallel phase is the phase in which all relationships tend to be directed toward the group leader or therapist. The name is derived from the concept of "parallel play" in childhood social development. The amount of time spent in this phase depends on the level of psychosocial development of the individual members. For instance, an outpatient group of clients with neurotic problems may move rapidly to the next stage, whereas a group of

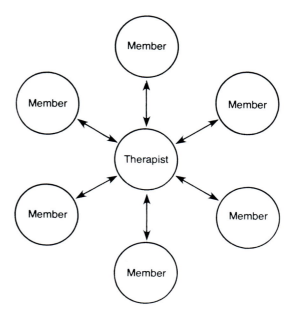

Fig. 13-1 Lines of relationship in parallel phase (extreme situation). (From Levine B: Group psychotherapy: practice and development. © 1979. Reprinted by permission of Prentice-Hall, Inc., Englewood Cliffs, N.J.)

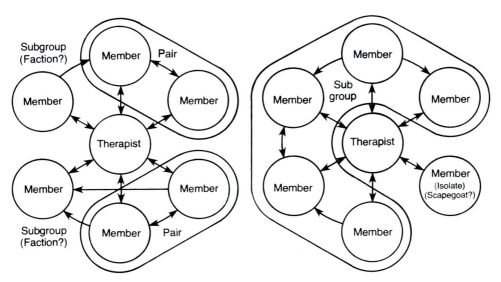

Fig. 13-2 Two of many possible patterns of relationship during inclusion phase. (From Levine B: Group psychotherapy: practice and development. © 1979. Reprinted by permission of Prentice-Hall, Inc., Englewood Cliffs, N.J.)

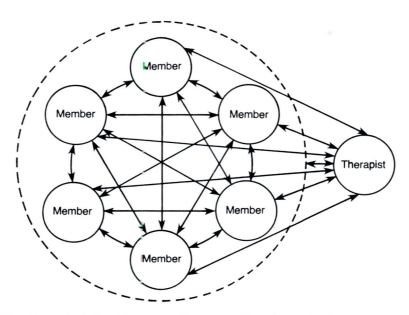

Fig. 13-3 Lines of relationship in mutuality phase. (From Levine B: Group psychotherapy: practice and development. © 1979. Reprinted by permission of Prentice-Hall, Inc., Englewood Cliffs, N.J.)

clients who are chronically suffering from schizophrenia may spend the entire existence of the group in the parallel phase. This phase corresponds to the *orientation phase* described above.

During the inclusion phase there is a decrease in the centrality of the therapist in group relationships, and member-to-member relationships tend to increase. Members are beginning to share a more equal distribution of power within the group. For example, a group of adolescents becomes capable of and involved in some degree of self-government within the group. This inclusion phase occurs in the first half (roughly) of the *working phase* described earlier.

In the mutuality phase, relationships extend from most or all members to most or all members and the therapist. Everyone feels accepted and included, and there is a sharing of power. Initial empathy is developing and being facilitated. While members feel emotionally linked to one another, they also feel free to express themselves. Less work is expended on the group as a system and more on accomplishing the therapeutic task. The mutuality phase occurs in the latter half of the *working phase*.

The termination phase is mostly a phenomenon of closed groups but can also be associated with members leaving an open-ended group. The direction of relationships changes as members disengage from other members and the therapist and move toward outside relationships. Ideally, therapeutic goals have been reached. The nature of this phase may reflect the degree to which the crises of authority, intimacy, and separation have been resolved.

These crises are interrelated with all other forces operating in the group. Crises can occur at any phase, but some are usually associated with specific phases. *Authority crises* usually arise at the onset of a group's existence, and they are challenges to the power of the therapist. The resolving of the first authority crisis usually marks the transition from the parallel phase to the inclusion phase. Authority crises can recur at any time during the life of the group.

Intimacy crises occur as intimacy develops

Group therapy **369**

among group members. Although these crises tend to recur throughout the group's existence, often the first resolution of an intimacy crisis occurs at the beginning of the mutuality phase. Pseudointimacy may be appropriate in adolescent groups, where peer conformity pressures are phase appropriate, but pseudointimacy in adult groups may signify a premature forcing of intimacy on the group by the therapist. This could be detrimental to individual members, who might believe that the other group members actually experienced a degree of intimacy that they only simulated and are actually incapable of at this time.

Separation crises occur during various phases; they are often brought on by absences of members or therapist or by fears of members or therapist. These crises are not resolved if members continue to deny and repress their feelings about separation. Members of an effective therapy group tend to develop effective ways of resolving separation crises throughout the evolution of the group.

COMPOSITION OF A GROUP AND FREQUENCY AND DURATION OF MEETINGS

The size of a group and the frequency and duration of meetings can, of course, vary greatly. As a general rule, however, an ongoing therapy group meets once a week, its optimal size is eight to ten members, and a session lasts an hour to an hour and a half.

A group may be *homogeneous*—that is, composed of people who share characteristics such as age, sex, diagnosis, or particular problem—or it may be *heterogeneous*. There are advantages to each situation, and which is chosen generally depends upon the goals of the group.

Clients whose special needs tend to be best met within a homogeneous structure include adolescents, acute psychotics, alcoholics, isolated elderly persons, and seriously handicapped persons (Fried, 1972). In contrast, middle-aged parents and young adults who are having difficulty bridging the generation gap in their own families may be able to improve communication and increase empathy through experiences in groups that are heteroge-

neous in terms of age. Heterogeneity and homogeneity of groups are concepts that can be related to the holistic health status of the client, and any of the five subsystems of the person (biological, intellectual, psychological, sociocultural, and spiritual). For example, homogeneity in regard to physical status can be an important consideration in the composition of a group of postmastectomy clients, while heterogeneity in regard to sociocultural background can provide a cross-fertilization that stimulates personal growth in group members.

Scheidlinger (1982) points out that in addition to heterogeneity and homogeneity, the concept of *balancing* is an important one. He cites as examples of unbalanced groups those comprising one man and several women, those comprising one withdrawn, socially constricted individual in a group of impulsive personalities, and those comprising members who are all withdrawn and constricted.

PHENOMENA OCCURRING IN GROUPS

Various communication problems are encountered in groups. One such problem is *monopolizing*. Group meetings have definite time limitations, and a person who monopolizes the conversation uses it up and deprives the other group members. This can lead to a sense of injustice in the group members and anger toward a group leader who fails to intervene (Sampson and Marthas, 1981). The evident signs of the monopolizer are:

1. incessant, compulsive talking
2. inability to listen
3. interrupting others
4. finishing others' thoughts and sentences
5. a tangential, confusing style of talking
6. a "dream quality" to what is being said
7. restlessness and inattentiveness among the other group members
8. symptoms of frustration and anger in other group members, especially against the leader

Ways of intervening with the monopolizer include:

1. verbally reflecting the behavior

2. interpreting the underlying meaning of the behavior (for example, relating it to anxiety)
3. reflecting the group feelings about it
4. confrontation of the group in regard to their reasons for allowing the monopolizing (Sampson and Marthas, 1981)

Intellectualizing tends to occur in a client who has difficulty dealing with feelings. Intellectualizing all group topics is a way of defending against internal conflicts and the emotional reactions that may be attached to them. Talking in the abstract and generalizing about everything are signs of intellectualizing. An atmosphere that encourages expression and exploration of feelings and direct confrontation of the group member's tendency to intellectualize are ways of intervening.

Using a *semantic argument* is one way for a member to attempt to control the situation (including control of others). Laborious discussions about exactly what is meant and philosophizing in general are ways of avoiding real issues, internal conflicts, and painful feelings. It is best to confront the individual and bring the topic back to the individual's feelings (for example, "But how does all of that apply to you and your feelings?" "In what way do you find these things affecting your life personally?").

Circumstantiality is a tendency to digress into numerous and unnecessary details and inappropriate thoughts before getting to the main idea. The effects of circumstantiality are similar to those of monopolizing—and, indeed, circumstantiality can result in monopolizing. Often the individual who communicates this way in group does so in other areas of life and is unaware of the devastating effects on interpersonal relations. Gentle but direct and consistent confrontation is usually helpful.

Tangentiality is a disturbed communication pattern in which the group member is unable to express ideas directly. Instead, the individual goes off on "side trips" with other, loosely related ideas. The main idea is not expressed. This way of communicating can be very confusing to the other group members. For this reason and because the individual is often unaware of the detrimental effects on interpersonal relating, there needs to be direct, consistent confrontation when tangentiality occurs in a group session.

Another type of problem in groups is *scapegoating*, which is the "tendency of human groups to project onto others such emotions as fear, aggression, and guilt—emotions they must negate in themselves . . ." (Scheidlinger, 1982). Scapegoating may be carried out against a group member who is present at a meeting, or it may be directed toward an individual who is not present. The leader must protect the scapegoated individual, point out what the group is doing, and use the phenomenon as a means of increasing the self-awareness of individual group members.

Transference can be directed toward the leader or toward other members of the group. Within any one group there may be transference reactions based on past or present relationships with mother, father, siblings, husband, wife, children, or boss. If one person's transference reaction is based on two or more relationships, the phenomenon is called *multiple transference*.

Relationships among group members can take several forms. For example, there may be pairing, subgrouping, or polarization. Such developments can be destructive if they interfere with honest and constructive confrontation or if they result in scapegoating or infighting. *Pseudomutuality* within a group can also interfere with honest relating and communicating. Sometimes *sadomasochistic* relationships will erupt between group members. Such relationships are often reflections of the way members relate outside of the group, and they can be used as learning opportunities. Some group members may display their tendencies to *withdraw* and *isolate* themselves or to *conform* as a pattern of relating.

Catharsis, an outpouring of emotional tension through verbalization or display of feelings, can occur in any group session. It can be a tension-reducing and growth-enhancing phenomenon. A cathartic release of pent-up emotions has been known to be a crucial turning point in a group member's life. In addition, an individual's strong expression of emotions has effects on the other group members; it is a vital part of the group process. It may be instrumental in producing group cohesiveness (Yalom, 1975).

Group members, as discussed earlier in this chapter, often assume various *roles* within the group. These roles serve various functions for the group, and they also may serve an unconscious, intrapsychic function for the individual assuming the role. Examples of some other roles seen frequently in therapy groups include *the peacemaker, the group catalyst, the leader, the protector, the attacker, the interpreter*, and *the assistant therapist*. The group member who assumes the role of assistant therapist or that of group catalyst can be very helpful to a leader. Often this individual is insightful and able to confront constructively and appropriately. However, this behavior may also be an attempt to avoid looking at one's own personal problems and to avoid being exposed to the group process.

A group leader should be aware of *seating arrangements*. Where an individual sits in relation to the leader may be an important clue to his or her personality. Members who always sit next to the leader may be indicating a need to associate with the leader for some reason—perhaps for protection. Habitually sitting directly opposite the leader may indicate a desire to engage in direct communication or confrontation with the leader. That "pairing" has occurred between two group members may be demonstrated by their choice of seats. The need to withdraw or isolate oneself or the feeling of being threatened by the group may result in placing one's seat at a point *outside* the group circle. While all group members are expected to sit within the circle, an exception to the rule may need to be made for a threatened and timid schizophrenic client (Berne, 1966, 56).

It is sometimes helpful for co-therapists to sit opposite one another to maximize nonverbal communication between them and to enlarge their view of the nonverbal communication of other group members.

GROUP LEADERSHIP

Group treatment may be based on any of the many schools of psychotherapy (Freudian, Sullivanian, transactional analysis, gestalt, Jungian, and so on), or it may be based on an eclectic viewpoint. Leadership style varies: it may be directive or nondirective, authoritarian or democratic, or laissez-faire.

As a general rule and for most group therapy situations, it is best for a leader to start out in a somewhat authoritarian role (authoritarian only in the sense that the leader gives the group its basic ground rules and perhaps states some goals for the group sessions). As the members begin to express trust and confidence in the leader, the leader gradually relinquishes this moderately authoritarian role by fostering interaction among the group members. The goal of the leader is to become a "facilitator," a "referee," a "consultant," or a "clarifier," or to assume any combination of these roles.

Characteristics of a group leader

Carl Rogers was the originator of "client-centered" psychotherapy. He viewed the therapeutic process as allowing the client to grow through increased understanding of self. The therapist uses a nondirective technique of consistently reflecting the client's feelings. Rogers also applied this philosophy to group therapy; he saw the leader as a facilitator of the group's own potential for self-discovery and growth. Rogers (1971) described several characteristics of an effective group leader.

1. The leader is a *facilitator* rather than a *director* of the therapeutic process; he or she works toward becoming a participant and toward being able to move comfortably back and forth between the stances of leader and participant.

2. The leader is responsive to *meaning* and *feelings*, which are more important than the details of *what* happened to the group member. However, it may be necessary to explore these details before getting to the meaning.

3. The effective leader accepts the group where it is *now*. This implies an acceptance of the individual group member and the member's degree of participation. The group may not accept a particular member's degree of participation, but the leader must. The silence of a member is acceptable if it is not unexpressed pain.

4. Sympathetic understanding of the individual member's intellectualizations and generalizations and the ability to select the self-referent

meanings of these and respond to them are crucial.

5. The facilitating leader operates in terms of his or her own feelings but with a degree of caution. A leader who is *too* expressive *too* early in the group's evolution may be unaware of these feelings and may be doing a kind of "acting-out" by expressing feelings without adequate thought.

6. The leader should confront appropriately and provide constructive feedback without attacking a group member's defenses. The group leader should use his or her *own* feelings responsibly and therapeutically in confronting group members and providing them with feedback.

7. An effective leader is able to use self-disclosure in a manner that is tempered by professional conscience and that serves a therapeutic purpose.

8. An effective leader avoids excessive planning and group "gimmicks." Gimmicks are used only as a last resort, because they rarely work.

9. A leader who is successful at being therapeutic tends to avoid interpretive comments, which only serve to make group members self-conscious. Commenting on group process *can* be helpful sometimes but should not be overdone.

Functions of a group leader

Scheidlinger (1982) believes that in functioning effectively, the group leader

1. structures the composition of the group (time, meeting place, remuneration procedures)
2. structures the rules of the session concerning such matters as confidentiality, physical contact, social contacts outside the group
3. accepts each member empathetically and believes in each person's capacity for growth
4. encourages open expression of feelings and concerns
5. fosters a group atmosphere that accepts dif-

ferences in feelings and behaviors among the members
6. fosters group norms of interpersonal scrutiny and self-awareness
7. encourages all members to participate
8. controls tension, anxiety, and drive expression within acceptable limits
9. balances the needs of the individual member with the needs of the group as a whole
10. uses verbal interventions from simple observations to confrontations that are aimed at the development of reality testing, insight, and self-awareness in the group members

Co-leadership

There are advantages to the co-leadership method in group therapy. According to Van Servellen (1984) there are advantages for members *and* for leaders.

For group members:

1. Co-leadership enables the leaders to cover more area with more clients. This is not to be interpreted as "bigger groups" or "more clients" because this has been found to be ineffective. What is meant here is that the two leaders each offer more to each client and also there are two authority figures with whom to identify.

2. The primary family group is reproduced for transference purposes in the therapist dyad—family conflicts re-emerge and past difficulties that may be causing present problems can be worked through.

3. The two therapists provide the model for a good relationship and communication through their interactions with each other.

For the leaders:

1. Co-leadership promotes growth in the leaders because it provides continual peer interaction for professional growth and better insight into each other's behavior.

2. It permits co-workers to validate individual perceptions of client's interactions and group process.

3. It permits co-workers to gain support from one another for any therapeutic interventions within the group.

Van Servellen has developed a helpful questionnaire (see the box below) for co-leaders to use after each group session:

APPROACHES TO GROUP THERAPY

The following are some techniques that are effective in group therapy.

1. Provide a safe, comfortable atmosphere.

Generally, when people feel secure, they are able to participate more easily in self-disclosure. Putting group members "on the spot" and attempting to force self-disclosure are the actions of an inexperienced and misinformed group leader. An exception to this is the highly confrontational format used by groups of clients who abuse drugs or alcohol.

Names of group leaders/therapists _____
_____
_____

COTHERAPY QUESTIONNAIRE

Session number _____
Date _____
Please complete a cotherapy questionnaire following each session of your group or family work.

1. How many members did you expect to appear at this session?
   _____

2. How many actually appeared? _____ Who did not appear?
   _____

3. For group therapy sessions, group cohesiveness may be defined as the extent to which the group experiences a sense of solidarity or "we-ness." How cohesive would you judge your therapy subsystem to be at this session? (Please check response that describes your judgment.)

Highly	Moderately	Slightly	Not at all	Unable to
_____ cohesive	_____ cohesive	_____ cohesive	_____ cohesive	_____ determine

   Comments: _____
   _____
   _____

4. Did members demonstrate high levels of self-disclosure of personal feelings, thoughts, fears, and concerns?

Yes, very high	Yes, moderately high	No, only slightly	Not at all self-disclosing	Unable to determine
_____	_____	_____	_____	_____

   Comments: _____
   _____
   _____

5. Briefly state what you think were the main overt structural or process themes of the therapeutic system (that is, what did they talk about; what did you talk about with them).
   _____
   _____
   _____

From Van Servellen G: Group and family therapy: a model for pschotherapeutic nursing practice, St. Louis, 1984, The CV Mosby Company, pp. 266-267.

Continued.

COTHERAPY QUESTIONNAIRE—cont'd

6. Briefly state what you think were the main covert (structural or process) themes (that is, what do you think was going on in the interactions between members or between members and therapists).

_____

_____

_____

7. Which adjectives describe the chief ways(s) members responded to you? (Please circle those which describe your members.)

Compliant (who: _____) Noncompliant (who: _____)
Friendly (who: _____) Hostile (who: _____)
Cooperative (who: _____) Resistant (who: _____)
Trusting (who:_____) Suspicious (who: _____)

If other descriptions, please specify behavior and who demonstrated the behavior.

_____ _____ _____

_____ _____ _____

_____ _____ _____

8. What would you judge was the affect or mood(s) the family/group communicated in this session?

_____

_____

_____

9. What is your feeling(s) in response to what happened in the therapeutic subsystem?

_____

_____

_____

10. In your judgment, what progress (or lack of progress) was made in meeting the overall objectives of your group/family therapy?

_____

_____

_____

11. Given your responses to the above questions, which level of congruence is expressed in your coleadership/cotherapy dyad?

Very	Moderately	Slightly	Not at all	Unable to
_____ high	_____ high	_____ congruent	_____ congruent	_____ determine

12. Based on this appraisal, which steps would you take?

_____

_____

_____

2. As a general rule, focus on the "here and now." While some discussion of past events can be helpful, a client's obsession with them may be his or her way of avoiding current problems in living. Berne (1967) has described this game played in group therapy situations as "archeology."

3. Use any transference situations, as they become evident, as learning and insight-development opportunities. Point out the *differences* between the transference object and the group member's significant other. The increasing ability to be aware of one's own distortions is a sign of improving mental health.

4. Whenever necessary, protect individual members from verbal abuse or from scapegoating. This is an *important* role of the leader, and it also enables the leader to act as a model for constructive communication and interpersonal relating.

5. Whenever appropriate, point out any change a group member has made. For example, one group member in an inpatient unit was not able to tolerate sitting with her group for an entire session. But with encouragement she gradually became able to stay for the entire session and then even began to participate. Another group member, who was prone to using a good deal of circumstantiality, was able, after participation in the group, to control this behavior effectively. In both of these situations, positive reinforcement provided ego support and encouraged future growth.

6. Handle *monopolizing, circumstantiality, hallucination,* or *disclosure of delusional material* in a manner that protects the self-esteem of the individual but that also sets limits on the behavior to protect the other group members. Other group members may feel threatened by psychotic behavior because they do not know how to respond to it, because they are afraid that they, too, may come to such a point, or both. Disclosure of delusional material is particularly threatening to other group members. Quite often, the delusional beliefs have *not* been totally accepted by the individual and thus are somewhat open to therapeutic intervention. Since there is usually this doubt on the part of the delusional client, it often helps to connect the beliefs to real feelings—of fear, anxiety, anger, and so on. For example, a leader might say, "Sometimes when we get frightened or feel insecure, we become suspicious of other people." The next step is to avoid dwelling on or exploring the delusional material in the group session. These steps on the part of the leader can help decrease the anxiety within the group, which is partially the result of members not knowing how to respond to their fellow group member.

7. Develop the ability to intuitively recognize when a group member (particularly a new member) is "fragile." Chances are that the member is indeed in a precarious mental and emotional state and should be approached in a gentle, supportive, and nonthreatening manner.

8. Use silence effectively, to encourage self-responsibility within the group. Silence should not be allowed to continue when it is nonproductive or when it becomes too threatening to the group members. A good rule of thumb is that usually the most anxious person in the group will break the silence—sometimes it is the leader.

9. Laughter and a moderate amount of joking can act as a safety valve and at times can contribute to group cohesiveness.

10. The "assistant therapist" in the group can be a useful phenomenon. A group member may assume this role, and is often extremely insightful in providing valuable feedback and suggestions. The group leader should be able to use this help without allowing the assistant to completely avoid group attention or to avoid dealing with personal problems.

11. Role playing and role reversals can sometimes be useful in short, modified versions. They may help a member develop insight into the ways he or she relates to others.

12. The promotion of interaction among group

members is one of the main goals. Some techniques include:

   a. Reflecting or rewording comments of individual group members

   b. Asking for group reaction to one member's statement

   c. Asking for individual reactions to a member's statement

   d. Pointing out any shared feelings within the group

   e. Amplifying an individual situation to include either some or all of the group members

   f. Summarizing at various points within the session and at the end (Smith, 1970)

13. Encourage the cohesiveness of the group. Group cohesiveness includes all of the factors, both evident and subtle, that interplay to encourage individuals to remain in the group. The following factors may enhance group cohesiveness:

   a. The ability of the members to be *interdependent*

   b. A uniformity of standards among group members concerning behavior, communication, goals, and so on

   c. A mutually supportive attitude

   d. An attitude of responsibility toward one another

   e. An atmosphere that is protective and that enhances security and self-esteem

The following factors may contribute to group dissolution:

   a. Frequent absenteeism of members or leader

   b. Loss of a leader

   c. Addition of new members without adequate preparation

   d. Canceled meetings

   e. Structural changes—time, day, size of group

   f. Subgrouping, pairing, or polarization

Ethnic factors in group process

Tsui and Schultz (1988) have developed some guidelines that are helpful to remember when conducting group therapy with members of different ethnic and racial backgrounds:

1. Group workers must be in touch with their own prejudices or biases toward any particular ethnic group before beginning work with a new therapy group.

2. Group leaders should foster group norms that are generally in accord with the different cultural backgrounds and personal expectations of the group members.

3. Leaders should educate group members about functioning in the group—behavior expected and the nature of member's relationship to the leader and to fellow members is included.

4. Leaders should acknowledge and validate the member's unique life experience arising from the interplay between cultural heritage and the realities of living in a multi-racial, culturally diverse society.

5. Group workers should avoid treating ethnic group members as representatives or spokesmen for their ethnic groups; other group members should be helped to avoid this situation also.

6. Leaders should be neither overprotective nor overly confrontive with the client; projection on the part of leaders around their own vulnerability or of ethnic stereotypes can foster this problem.

The short-term psychiatric unit group

Group therapy in short-term psychiatric units differs from that of traditional outpatient groups (Nudleman, 1986; Yalom, 1983). The issues, phenomena, methods, and particularly the validity and value of this type of group therapy is receiving much attention from group workers (Brabender, 1985; Klein, 1985; Nudleman, 1986; Yalom, 1983).

The life of a short-term unit group is very short indeed—as short as one session. Yalom, an authority on this type of group, believes that the group has a single-session time frame. The short-term psychiatric unit group is the one that nurses are most apt to be involved with. Following are some of the attributes of these groups (adapted from Yalom, 1983, 50-51 and 82-83):

1. Rapid client turnover—the length of stay on the units is usually 1 to 3 weeks. Some cli-

ents attend a group meeting for only one or two sessions. There isn't any time to work on phase-related tasks—this is especially true of any termination. In an open-ended, short-term group, someone is terminating in each session so that to focus on termination would consume all of the group's time.

2. The groups are composed of people with varied diagnoses (for example, psychosis, neurosis, substance abuse, major affective disorder, adolescent adjustment problem, geriatric adjustment problem, characterological disturbance), all in one group.

3. Clients are acutely uncomfortable—resolution of psychosis and relief from deep depression are more often the individual's goal rather than the personal growth and self-awareness goals of long-term groups. The severity of distress affects the group experience. Hospitalized clients are more deeply troubled, and they usually lack environmental supports more often than the clients of outpatient groups.

4. Some group members may be quite unmotivated—they may not even want to be in the group—they may be psychologically unsophisticated, and they may not have the energy to be curious about themselves.

5. There is little or no time to prepare or screen clients for group therapy.

6. Group composition is not usually in the control of the therapist.

7. Clients often see the group leader in other roles on the unit throughout the day.

8. There is little therapist stability—the leader role changes with changing schedules of staff members.

9. Group therapy is only one of many other therapies within the unit's milieu, and a client will participate in these other therapies with some of the same clients and the same therapist.

10. Group cohesiveness is difficult to develop because of the time limitation that makes it more difficult for clients to learn to care for or trust one another.

11. The gradual recognition of the more subtle interpersonal problems, their "working through," and the transfer of group experi-

ence and learning to the "outside" are difficult because of time limitations.

12. This type of group is not an independent entity as is most often the case with outpatient groups. It is part of a larger treatment system, and events of the larger system can significantly influence group process.

13. As is the case for milieu therapy (see p. 348), traditional rules about confidentiality must be modified. The clients are being treated by a team of professionals and nonprofessional workers. The issue of confidentiality becomes one of confidentiality to the unit, not "therapist-client" or "client-group."

14. Group members in an outpatient group have little contact between sessions—group members in inpatient groups live together and are continually interacting with one another.

15. An inpatient group therapist has access (through charts, team meetings, histories) to much more information than that supplied by the client in group sessions.

These groups have evolved out of problematic situations, but they have proven to be of real value to inpatients (Brabender, 1985; Klein, 1985; Yalom, 1983), and there are some important goals related to this type of therapy (adapted from Klein, 1985; Yalom, 1983):

1. the engagement of the client in a two-fold process: (a) the short-term group and the therapeutic milieu, (b) the outpatient course of treatment—another group, ongoing individual therapy, etc.

2. the amelioration of distress—a reduction of the discomfort of symptoms

3. prompt re-establishment of a client's previous emotional equilibrium

4. helping the clients to realize that talking about oneself and one's problems can help and that they are not the only ones facing problems (Yalom's principle of *universality*)

5. problem spotting—to help individuals learn about their maladaptive interpersonal behavior

6. the alleviation of iatrogenic anxiety—the discomfort that arises from the fact that there is a need for hospitalization and from other aspects of the hospitalization itself (e.g., fears of

stigmatization; fear of other psychotic clients; unrealistic expectations of the staff)

7. promotion of efficient use of client resources (e.g., sense of control or mastery, aiding behavioral changes, and encouraging social effectiveness)
8. assisting the client's understanding of the current crisis and increasing coping skills for the future
9. preparation for longer-term outpatient therapy

Some helpful strategies in short-term inpatient group therapy*

1. The time frame is single-session, the group composition is continually changing—some clients will attend only one or two sessions. Efficiency of process and a high level of activity in the leader is necessary.
2. This type of group requires structure. A nondirective leader may be helpful for some outpatient groups but not for confused or frightened inpatient clients in crisis. It takes time for group norms to develop on their own—in this case, the leader must provide the norm structure. The leader is directive but also flexible to meet the needs of a rapidly changing group. For example, some may become tangential, confused, belligerent, delusional, or otherwise disruptive in group, and the group members need to know that the leader can deal with this occurrence decisively, therapeutically, and safely.
3. The spatial-temporal boundaries should be protected—there should be as few interruptions as possible to provide an atmosphere of stability. In groups of severely withdrawn or highly anxious clients, some may need to know that they can leave the session if they begin to panic. This "out" will usually help to avoid the panic.
4. It will be helpful to the leader if there is a pregroup session with a member or members

*Adapted from Yalom, 1983.

of the unit staff to provide additional information about the group members—particularly new admissions to the unit.

5. The group atmosphere should be more supportive than confrontive, and any confrontations should be very gentle, noncritical and not angry. The therapist who is positive, nonjudgmental, and accepting will be the most effective in this group. Clients are in crisis and in too much distress to work through negative transference feelings in relation to the leader's behavior.
6. Acknowledgment of the group members' contributions is important. This can range from complimenting one member's thoughtful support of another to acknowledging that a frightened group member was able to stay in the group for an entire session.
7. Encourage positive behavior—any development of self-awareness, support of others, the healing occurrence of catharsis—whenever it manifests in the group.

THE NURSING PROCESS IN GROUP THERAPY

An understanding of the phases of group development, the crises that occur in the life of a group, the various phenomena that can occur in groups, and some ways of intervening in groups can help the nurse to apply the nursing process to group therapy. This section will deal with assessing, analyzing, planning care, implementing the plan, and evaluating the effectiveness of the plan.

1. Making an assessment; aim: to gather information from verbal and nonverbal communication of the group and of the individuals within the group
   a. Gather the following information about group dynamics systematically and continuously from group therapy sessions:
   (1) Individual clients' perceptions of their situations or problems (content themes)
   (2) Predominant themes of the group as a whole (content *and* process themes)

(3) Kinesic and proxemic behavior of individuals within the group (process themes)

(4) The predominant theme of the present group environment (for example, hostility, parallel play, resistance, cooperation)

(5) Biological, intellectual, psychological, sociocultural, and spiritual similarities and differences among group members (holistic health status)

(6) Factors predisposing individuals within the group to their particular situations or problems

(7) Factors precipitating particular situations or problems within the group

(8) Strengths of individuals within the group

(9) The directionality of relationships: leader to members, members to leader, among members

(10) The particular phase of group development (for example, orientation, working, termination *or* parallel, inclusion, mutuality, termination)

(11) Various types of phenomena occuring within the group process (for example, pairing, scapegoating, monopolization)

(12) Current crises of group development (for example, authority, intimacy, separation)

(13) The degree of power held by the leader as opposed to the members. This changes in accordance with the phase of the group's development and/or the influence of group crises

(14) The interrelationships among group phenomena, roles, behavior, interpersonal relationships, content themes, phases, and crises

b. Verify the data

(1) Confirm observations and perceptions by obtaining consensual validation from individuals within the group, through group consensus, and/or through other sources (records, psy-

chological tests, pregroup and post-group meetings with others, such as co-leaders and staff members)

(2) Communicate assessment information to the other staff members verbally, in post-group sessions, in written group reports, and through charting on individual clients' records. Group session reports are written assessments of the therapy session that usually include:

(a) Identification of predominant group themes

(b) Identification and description of individual "content" themes

(c) Identification and description of individual verbal and nonverbal "process" themes

2. Analyzing the data; aims: to understand the nature of individuals' situations or problems and to understand the structure and developmental phase of the group and current themes and crises

a. Formulate nursing diagnoses that state the predominant themes of individuals and their relationships to contributing factors (for example, low self-esteem and unexpressed anger related to an impending divorce and the earlier loss of mother—precipitated in current group session through absences of regular group leader)

b. Formulate a nursing diagnosis that states the predominant social environment of the group and its relationship to contributing factors (for example, group resistance and hostility related to absence of regular leader during vacation time)

3. Planning client care

a. Aim: to develop goals (individual and group) and a plan of action for initiating changes in individuals that will enable them to better cope with their existing situations and/or problems

(1) Depending on your assessment of the distribution of power within the group (centrality of leader vs. greater degree of "shared" power within the group) and/or group crises, help and encour-

age the group and individuals to set goals and establish priorities among goals (for example, need to discuss feelings and impending discharge of one member vs. need to plan for social event next week).

(2) Differentiate between long-term goals and short-term goals.

(3) State projected outcomes to the group.

b. Aim: to identify and modify group goals, taking into consideration individual capabilities, strengths, and weaknesses and the group status. Modifications should be based on group theory, group therapy principles, psychiatric literature, and the group leader's own experience with effective approaches to group interaction and development.

(1) Anticipate group and/or individual needs based on the priority of goals.

(2) Include all members of the group in the development of group interaction.

(3) Plan and work toward goals that are appropriate for the group members in terms of age, sex, locus of decision making, and intellectual, sociocultural, biological, psychological, and spiritual subsystems.

(4) Identify group therapy interaction techniques that are helpful for specific group phenomena.

c. Aim: to cooperate with other health team members in the delivery of health care

(1) Provide a group atmosphere that is consistent with the total therapeutic environment.

(2) Allow for flexibility to meet the varied needs of individuals within the group.

(3) Report and/or chart information that is pertinent to client care and to smooth functioning of the therapeutic milieu.

4. Implementing the care plan; aim: to facilitate group interaction and movement toward established group and individual goals.

a. Promote the individual's and the group's experience and use of the curative factors in group therapy (for example, universality, instillation of hope).

b. Facilitate interaction among group members through knowledge and use of some of the techniques of group psychotherapy.

c. Follow guidelines for effective leadership in group therapy.

5. Evaluating the care plan

a. Aim: to include the client in estimating the client's progress toward attainment of goals

(1) Toward the end of session, summarize and ask for summarizing input from the group regarding themes and phenomena of that particular group session.

(2) For ongoing groups, schedule periodic individual sessions for group members to evaluate individual progress.

b. Aim: to evaluate the effectiveness of the current care plan in group therapy

(1) Periodically evaluate the development and changes in the group in regard to crises.

(2) Participate in pre-group and post-group sessions with other staff members and with co-therapists.

PREGROUP AND POSTGROUP STAFF MEETINGS

To facilitate an effective use of the nursing process in a group therapy session, it is helpful for staff members to meet, share information, and plan possible strategies for intervention. The pregroup meeting is generally in the form of a report that is given by staff members to the group leader or leaders. Each group member's history and present status are reviewed, and any potential problems of interaction between group members and/or between group members and the staff are discussed. Any known group trends or crises can also be addressed at this time.

Postgroup sessions are useful in helping the staff to evaluate the whole group process. Staff members can share and discuss their observations and interpretations about the group and the individual members, and some problem solving may be done at this time. The postgroup session also provides an opportunity for "peer supervision" and learning. Feedback about staff members' participation is available while it is still fresh in the minds of the participants.

The following guide has been developed to aid nurses both in making an assessment and in establishing goals for group therapy.

GUIDE FOR ASSESSMENT OF GROUP PROCESS

1. Description of group
   a. Type of group (e.g., activity, encounter, remotivation, psychodrama)
   b. Theoretical framework
   c. Goals of group
   d. Size of group
   e. Composition of group
      (1) Age of members
      (2) Sex of members
      (3) Ethnic backgrounds of members (optional)*
      (4) Physical health status of members
      (5) Behavior exhibited by members
      (6) Educational levels of members
      (7) Communicational levels of members (e.g., verbal; mute; speak a foreign language)
      (8) Reality testing levels of members
      (9) Other (describe)
2. Physical setup of group (describe)
   a. Furniture (e.g., table and chairs or chairs only)
   b. Ventilation (Smoking vs. nonsmoking may be a group issue.)
   c. Distractions (noise from other areas; privacy)
3. Characteristics of group
   a. Group phase or stage (orientation, work-

ing, termination *or* parallel, inclusive, mutuality, termination)
   b. Level of cohesiveness
   c. Level of anxiety
   d. Level of conflict
   e. Level of resistance
   f. Crisis theme (authority, intimacy, separation)
   g. Other (describe)
4. Patterns of group interaction
   a. Communication patterns
      (1) Silence
      (2) Semantic argument
      (3) Intellectualization
      (4) Monopolization
      (5) Scapegoating
      (6) Other (describe)
   b. Behavior patterns
      (1) Physical activity
      (2) Withdrawal
      (3) Detachment
      (4) Cooperation
      (5) Competition
      (6) Other (describe)
   c. Social patterns
      (1) Group norms
      (2) Group rules
      (3) Roles (e.g., peacemaker, assistant therapist, leader, protector, attacker, interpreter)
      (4) Alliances among members (subgroups)
      (5) Conflict between alliances
      (6) Other (describe)
5. Patterns of leadership
   a. Approach of leader(s)
      (1) Laissez-faire
      (2) Democratic
      (3) Power struggle
      (4) Authoritarian
      (5) Other (describe)
   b. Competence of leader(s)
      (1) Provides relaxed, nonjudgmental atmosphere
      (2) Protects group members from disruptive communication patterns (scapegoating)

---

*Legislation protects people from being required to reveal ethnic background.

(3) Accepts all feelings, attitudes, and ideas as valid themes for group discussion
(4) Responds to verbal and nonverbal communication
(5) Facilitates communication and problem solving by:
    (a) Encouraging group members to clarify and describe feelings, attitudes, and ideas
    (b) Summarizing as needed
(6) Facilitates group cohesiveness by:
    (a) Asking for feedback and validation
    (b) Giving responsibility to the group
    (c) Encouraging the group to make decisions
    (d) Permitting the group to review and revise goals as indicated
    (e) Developing leadership among group members
(7) Other (describe)

CHAPTER SUMMARY

Group therapy is a valuable treatment modality. Nurses who work in psychiatric settings are involved, according to their educational preparation, as group leaders, group therapists, and co-therapists.

Some of the therapeutic benefits of group therapy may be similar to those of individual treatment, while other benefits are unique to group therapy. The curative factors of group therapy have been delineated, and the important characteristics that facilitate effective group leadership have been outlined.

It is possible to recognize a group's phase of development, current "crises" facing the group, and the emergence of various phenomena within the group. Effective use of the nursing process within a group situation is based on knowledge and sensitive understanding of these dimensions of the group process.

SELF-DIRECTED LEARNING

Sensitivity-Awareness Exercises

The purposes of these exercises are to:
- Develop awareness of some of the ways a group operates and evolves
- Develop sensitivity to the subjective experience of others as they function in a group setting
- Develop awareness about your own functioning in a group

1. Choose a group to which you already belong (e.g., clinical group, seminar group, fraternity/sorority group, club, church group, etc.) Observe it and analyze it according to the following dimensions:
  a. Task of the group:
  b. Norms:
    (1) explicit
    (2) implicit
  c. Boundaries:
    (1) physical
    (2) temporal
    (3) psychosocial
  d. Conflicts:
    (1) realistic (related to the task)
    (2) unrealistic (emotional and irrational)
    (3) group's method of resolving conflicts
  e. Identify any roles manifested in the group (see Table 13-1)
  f. Is the group a cohesive one? Identify any signs of cohesiveness that you observe in the group.
2. (To be done as a *group exercise*—with a clinical group, seminar, or class). Time required: approximately 2 hours.
  a. choose a task (theoretical or real)
  b. select a group leader or two co-leaders (random selection, assignment, or volunteer)
  c. assign roles to group members using roles described by Benne and Sheats (see Table 13-1)

(random selection, volunteer choice, or assigned by the leader)

   d. carry on a group discussion about the group's task and ways of achieving it for exactly 45 minutes

   e. (for the final 45 minutes after the discussion) discuss as a group, the thoughts and feelings of each member in relation to their own "roles" and their reactions to the "roles" of others. Include the reactions that members had to "participating" in a group.

3. Visit an *open meeting* of Alcoholics Anonymous, Overeaters Anonymous, or Gamblers Anonymous for a view of a repressive-inspirational group in action.

Questions to Consider

1. *Imitative behavior* in groups is:
   a. counterproductive to the group task
   b. a curative factor in group therapy, according to Yalom
   c. according to Benne and Sheats, it is necessary for the avoidance of role playing
   d. usually leads to a consistent lack of self-disclosure in group members

2. Group cohesiveness is evidently developing when:
   a. individual group members do not take the initiative in accepting responsibility for group process
   b. competition becomes an accepted norm
   c. group members are punctual and seldom miss meetings
   d. trust is reflected in a conscientious avoidance of risk-taking in the group

Match the following terms:

3. Group process   a. time, place, and psychosocial restraints

4. Group boundaries   b. everything that happens within a group

5. Group norms   c. rules and standards of the group

6. Group maintenance   d. group compromiser

7. Joe is a man of 56, married with two sons—ages 17 and 19. He has been hospitalized on the psychiatric unit of a general hospital for 2 weeks. He has been diagnosed as suffering from a Major Depression: single episode (DSM-III-R 296.2x). Joe is beginning to feel better since participating in the activities of the unit's milieu and since beginning a regimen of antidepressant medication. He has been a member of the unit's therapy group that meets three times a week. In the particular session he is *monopolizing* and *intellectualizing* about how "the younger generation doesn't accept any responsibility." You are assisting the clinical nurse specialist who is leading the therapy group. You would like to respond therapeutically to Joe—your best response in this situation would be to:
   a. do some client teaching with the goal of resolving intergeneration conflict
   b. ask Joe how his comment that "younger people don't accept responsibility" relates to him specifically
   c. ignore Joe's persistent referrals to the younger generation, since he has already taken up too much of the group's time. In this way you are helping to control group boundaries
   d. confront Joe with his monopolizing behavior and let him know of the group's anger about this

Answer key
1. b   5. c
2. c   6. d
3. b   7. b
4. a

REFERENCES

Benne K and Sheats P: Functional roles of group members, J Soc Issues 4(2):42-49, 1948.

Berne E: Principles of group treatment, New York, 1966, Oxford University Press, Inc.

Berne E: Games people play: the psychology of human relationships, New York, 1967, Grove Press, Inc.

Brabender V: Time limited inpatient group therapy: a developmental model, Int J Group Psychother 35(3):373-390, 1985.

Cartwright D and Zander A: Group dynamics: research and theory, ed 3, New York, 1967, Harper & Row, Publishers, Inc.

Corey G and Corey M: Groups: process and practice, ed 2, Monterey, Calif, 1982, Brooks/Cole Publishing Company.

Festinger L et al: Social pressures in informal groups, New York, 1950, Harper.

Foulkes S and Anthony E: Group psychotherapy: the psychoanalytic approach, Middlesex, England, 1968, Penguin Books, Ltd.

Fried E: Basic concepts in group psychotherapy, In Kaplan H and Sadock B, editors: The evolution of group therapy, New York, 1972, E. P. Dutton & Company, Inc.

Kaplan H and Sadock B, editors: The origins of group psychoanalysis, New York, 1972, E. P. Dutton & Co., Inc.

Klein R: Some principles of short-term group therapy, Int J Group Psychother 35(3):309-326, 1985.

Levine B: Group psychotherapy: practice and development, Englewood Cliffs, NJ, 1979, Prentice-Hall, Inc.

Northern H: Social work with groups, New York, 1969, Columbia University Press.

Nudleman E: Group psychotherapy, Nurs Clin North Am (Psychiatric/Mental Health Nursing), 21(3):505-514, 1986.

Olmstead M and Hare A: The small group, ed 2, New York, 1978, Random House.

Rogers C: Carl Rogers describes his way of facilitating encounter groups, Am J Nurs 7(2):275-279, 1971.

Sampson E and Marthas M: Group process for the health professions, ed 2, New York, 1981, John Wiley & Sons, Inc.

Scheidlinger S: Focus on group psychotherapy: clinical essays, New York, 1982, International Universities Press, Inc.

Smith AJ: A manual for the training of psychiatric nursing personnel in group psychotherapy, Pers Psychiatr Care 8(3):106, 1970.

Tsui P and Schultz G: Ethnic factors in group process: cultural dynamics in multi-ethnic therapy groups, Am J Orthopsychiatr 58(1):136-142, 1988.

Van Servellen G: Group and family therapy: a model for psychotherapeutic nursing practice, St. Louis, 1984, The CV Mosby Company.

Yablonsky L: Tunnel back synanon, New York, 1965, MacMillan, Inc.

Yalom I: Inpatient group therapy, New York, 1983, Basic Books, Inc. Publishers.

Yalom I: The theroy and practice of group psychotherapy, ed 2, New York, 1975, Basic Books, Inc., Publishers.

ANNOTATED SUGGESTED READINGS

Dublin R: Concurrent Group and Family Treatment for Young Adults, Social Casework 62(10):614-621, 1981.
This article discusses some of the benefits of concurrent group and family treatment for young adults with serious emotional problems. Case material on individual clients is presented, as well as the interrelationships with family dynamics and family treatment. Family treatment is seen as a natural outcome of the increased self-awareness and self-esteem that is inherent in involvement in group process.

Ernst C, Vanderzyl S, and Salinger R: Preparation of psychiatric inpatients for group therapy, J Psychiatr Nurs Mental Health Serv 19(7):29-33, 1981.
This article reports and discusses a study of the effectiveness of formally structuring the preparation of group participants in an inpatient setting. In this method clients and therapist discuss purpose, goals, plans, and the roles of members and leader. Any preexisting attitudes toward therapy and therapy groups are also explored. Instructional aids in the form of a film and written material are used. A review of the literature supporting a planned program of preparation for potential group members is included in this article.

Mackey R: Developmental process in growth-oriented groups, Social Work 25(1):26-29, 1980.
The author examines how the changes that take place in individuals within a group occur. Several definitions of the term group process are discussed, and studies of group process by well-known group theorists are reviewed. A five-stage model of group development (Garland, Jones, and Kolodny) is presented. This includes (1) preaffiliation, (2) power and control, 3) intimacy, (4) differentiation, and (5) separation.

Marcovitz R and Smith J: Patients perceptions of curative factors in short-term group psychotherapy, Int J Group Psychother 33(1):21-39, 1983.
A study of the mechanisms of change as perceived by clients in inpatient group psychotherapy is presented. The Yalom (1975) Curative Factor Q-Sort was used to determine the most helpful mechanisms of change (as perceived by clients). The author concluded that (1) a here-and-now orientation is best, (2) the teaching of concepts and the clear delineation of goals are important, (3) clients benefit from being encouraged toward self-responsibility and responsibility toward others, (4) sufficient time for expression of feelings is crucial, (5) it is important to foster an attitude of acceptance and respect in regard to differences within the group, and (6) praising risk-takers may encourage others to do the same.

Nudelman E: Group psychotherapy, Nurs Clinics N Am (Psychiatr/Mental Health Nurs), 21(3):505-514, 1986.
This presents an overview of the modality of group therapy. Historical backgrounds, benefits of group therapy, types of groups, group phases, beginning a group, and evaluation are all summarized. A helpful table on group phase/group characteristics/therapist role is included.

Rogers C: Carl Rogers describes his way of facilitating encounter groups, Am J Nurs 71(2):275-279, 1971.

This excellent article describes Carl Rogers's philosophy of working therapeutically with groups. It is particularly helpful for nurses leading or participating in group therapy sessions in the psychiatric units of general hospitals. Appropriate use of self and self-disclosure is discussed.

Tsui P and Schultz G: Ethnic factors in group process: cultural dynamics in multi-ethnic therapy groups, Am J Orthopsychiatr 58(1):136-142, 1988

This article presents clinical material and a framework for practice that is based on work with Asian clients in predominantly Caucasian therapy groups. Cultural differences in perceptions of power, interpersonal boundaries, and the role of the family have an impact on group dynamics. The authors believe that the issues encountered and the guidelines developed are applicable to group work with clients from other ethnic minorities.

Yalom I D: Inpatient group therapy, New York, 1983, Basic Books, Inc., Publishers.

Short-term psychiatric inpatient group therapy is an art unto itself. This excellent primer for clinicians who work with inpatient groups includes appropriate goals, common problems (e.g., rapid turnover of group members), and specific goals and techniques for different levels of functioning.

CHAPTER 14

Family dysfunction and family therapy

CHAPTER FOCUS

The family is a system and has the properties of any social system. As the family system operates within its context, it may become vulnerable to stressors that affect family structure and family function. Alterations in family membership, sociocultural strains, maturational events, and disordered family relationships may stress the family system into dysfunction.

Nurses need to be aware of the models of family theory and family therapy that can be used in treating dysfunctional families. Among these models are the structural model, the interactional model, the multigenerational model, and the ecosystem model. Nurses should also recognize that cultural presuppositions may be inherent in some aspects of these family models. Therefore, as nurses engage in primary, secondary, or tertiary prevention of family dysfunction, they should strive to keep their assessments, interpretations, and goals from being value laden.

Throughout the United States, there is a growing tendency to view the family, rather than the individual, as the client of choice for the delivery of health care. Nurses, whether they are general-duty nurses, mental health nurses, occupational health nurses, or community health nurses, are becoming increasingly involved with the mental health needs of families. To effectively work with families, nurses need to become knowledgeable about family dysfunction and family therapy.

DYSFUNCTION WITHIN THE FAMILY SYSTEM
Stressors on the family system

As the family system interacts with other social systems, it may become vulnerable to any number of stressors that may impair its structure and function. Chief among these stressors are:

1. Changes in family membership—loss of a family member through divorce, separation, death, chronic illness, or hospitalization or addition of a family member through birth, adoption, or incorporation (for example, grandparents move into the household)
2. Sociocultural strains—environmental pressures such as inadequate support systems, community disorganization, discrimination, inadequate housing, culture shock, overcrowding, and economic difficulties
3. Maturational events—transitions between developmental stages, such as marriage, entrance of a child into school, and retirement
4. Disordered family relationships—imbalance in the internal structure of the family, caused by such factors as double-bind communication, parental overburdening, overbonding to the family, and psychosomatogenesis.

The degree of stress that may be engendered depends on the nature of the stressor and the family's perception, interpretation, and response to the stressor. The following discussion focuses on the ways in which some of these stressors contribute to family dysfunction.

CHANGE IN FAMILY MEMBERSHIP

Vulnerability factors associated with a change in family membership include the ages of family members at the time of the change,* the emotional make-up of family members, and the nature of relationships among family members.

The addition or loss of a family member may force a reorganization of the family system and may engender stress in the family system. This stress may threaten the emotional, social, and interpersonal security of individual family members, and it

_____
*Refer to Chapter 6 for a discussion of human development.

may influence their ability to accomplish developmental tasks.

During the infancy period, the infant's primary relationship is with the care giver (who is usually the mother). Loss of this relationship not only can result in decrease in the quality and quantity of the infant's nurturing, but also can contribute to later difficulties with attachment or object permanence (Critchley, 1981).

However, it is during the preschool period that children are very vulnerable to the emotional, social, and interpersonal insecurities associated with change in family membership. For example, the birth of a sibling may engender jealousy in a preschool child. The hospitalization of a parent or parental divorce may cause a preschool child to experience separation anxiety and fear of abandonment. In addition to these reactions, a preschool child may respond to the loss of a parental relationship with repression and denial. The inability of the still present parent to authentically express feelings in front of the child may reinforce the child's denial and repression. Preschool children may also become regressed, withdrawn, hyperactive, and anorexic, and they may have temper tantrums, gastrointestinal upsets, and sleep disturbances. These responses are usually transient; there is no cause for alarm unless they become permanent. Since this is the stage in which children normally lay the foundation for satisfactory object relations, parental depression, overprotectiveness, or anxiety (parental responses to change in family membership) may interfere with the ability of preschool children to form object relationships (Critchley, 1981).

It is during the school-age stage that children face the developmental tasks of industry and autonomy. At this time children become very involved with friends and with school activities. The involvement of children with the family is usually minimal. Change in family membership reinvolves children with the family, and this reinvolvement may interfere with childhood achievement of industry and autonomy.

If a change in family membership is due to the death of a family member, children may experience guilt feelings about having been unkind to or having wished for the demise of the family member. If a child dies, parents may idealize the dead child, and they may create an unrealistic model for surviving children to follow. School-age children may respond to the stress of change in family membership with guilt, withdrawal, sadness, hostility, anxiety, and/or poor school grades. The persistence or intensification of any of these reactions, or the development of somatization, socially deviant behavior (lying, stealing), or depression, may signal the onset of a psychopathological condition* (Wallerstein and Kelly, 1980; Critchley, 1981; Wallerstein, 1983).

Young school-age children usually have difficulty using such coping behaviors as fantasy, denial, and structured activities to deal with the emotions engendered by a change in family membership. If the change was produced by divorce, a child may develop problems associated with strong and conflicting loyalties to both parents. For example, the loss† through divorce of a relationship with father may be experienced by a child as rejection, loss of security, and paternal deprivation. The child may respond to this situation by blaming and becoming angry with his or her mother. At this age, resignation to parental divorce usually occurs within 1 year. Young school-age children achieve this resignation by increasing their psychological distance from both parents, thus coping with the turmoil engendered by conflicting parental loyalties (Wallerstein and Kelly, 1980; Wallerstein, 1983).

Because older school-age children are better able to use coping behaviors of fantasy, denial, and structured activities and are better able to understand the situations surrounding changes in family membership, they are usually better able to cope with family membership changes than are younger school-age children. However, the increased ability of older school-age children to cope with family membership changes does not mean that difficulties do not arise. For example, an older school-age child may feel shame about parental divorce. He or she may evidence such symptoms as headaches and stomachaches, as well as depression, poor self-esteem, school problems, and anger toward the

parent he or she perceives as causing the divorce. Age-appropriate tasks of identity formation and the development of mutuality and reciprocal support in interpersonal relationships may be undermined. If the parents use the parent-child relationship to decrease their own loneliness and insecurity, the child may become overburdened with adult responsibilities. This overburdening may interfere with the child's ability to form peer relationships. Such difficulty in relating to peers may lead some older school-age children to precociously engage in sexual experimentation in an attempt to form close interpersonal relationships (Wallerstein and Kelly, 1980; Critchley, 1981; Wallerstein, 1983).

When adolescents experience a change in family membership, they may try to cope by distancing themselves from the family. They may also perceive parents, irrespective of their actual involvement, as unavailable. This seems especially true of children's perceptions of their fathers after divorce. Adolescence is the developmental stage when children try to achieve independence from their families through a high degree of participation in school, work, and social events, and if a change in family membership occurs at this time, involvement in these activities may intensify more than is usual. Danger may be signaled when adolescents use excessive sexual activity or socially deviant behavior as a means of accomplishing family distancing (Critchley, 1981; Johnson, Klee, and Schmidt, 1988).

Sometimes late adolescents and young adults (aged 18 to 25 years) become overly concerned about family financial problems that result from change in family membership, concerned about the effect of family membership changes on younger siblings, or concerned about their parents' future. Other times, they assume a disproportionate responsibility for household tasks or they become confidants to their parents. Any of these situations may produce overburdening. By interfering with the ability of late adolescents and young adults to establish their own identities, to enter into intimate relationships with other people, and to become interdependent, this overburdening may hinder their ability to accomplish the developmental task of this life stage—intimacy vs. isolation. Family stability therefore continues to be an important factor

---

*See Chapter 17 for a discussion of psychopathology in children.

†Refer to Chapter 22 for further discussion of loss and grief.

in adjustment even into young adulthood (Critchley, 1981; Cooney et al., 1986).

Family membership changes also affect adults and their ability to accomplish developmental tasks. The tasks of the adult stage of life is generativity as opposed to stagnation. This is the period of life when the capacity to enter into a sharing relationship develops. A dyadic relationship may be formed, and the relationship may be extended by the addition of children. The birth of a child, especially of a first child, may arouse feelings in the parents of anxiety, inadequacy, and disenchantment with the parenting role. The death of a child may transform a family triad back into a dyad. If a spouse is lost, the sexual dyad itself is disrupted. Loss of family members may lead adults to question their life goals and to feel that they have not been successful in life. For example, after a divorce, the adults involved may feel anxious, depressed, angry, helpless, or insecure, and they may try to cope with their loneliness and insecurity by using one of their children as a confidant. When parents lose a child, they may respond to the child's death by engaging in self-blame. They may feel that they should have been able to prevent the child's death, and they may view the child's death as evidence of their failure to successfully perform their parenting roles (Critchley, 1981; Arnold and Gemma, 1983).

The final phase of development* is ego integrity as opposed to despair. Older adults who are faced with family dismemberment may experience many of the same reactions as do young and middle-aged adults. However, for some older adults, in reviewing their lives, the loss of a family relationship may become a cause for despair. For example,

---

Mr. and Mrs. Rockford were in their sixties. When their son, who had been married for 10 years, announced that he was getting a divorce, the Rockfords were shocked. After the divorce, their daughter-in-law obtained custody of the children, and she moved out of the state. Mr. and Mrs. Rockford had been very close to their grandchildren, and they were accustomed to seeing them on a weekly basis. They knew that they would now only see their grandchildren infrequently

---

*Refer to Chapter 18 for a discussion of conflict and stress among the elderly.

and that they would not be part of their grandchildren's growing up. They despaired over what might have been.

• • •

Mrs. Fulicetti, who was 70 years old, lived with her daughter, her son-in-law, and their children. When Mrs. Fulicetti's son-in-law died, she felt sad and she despaired. At the funeral and in the days afterward, Mrs. Fulicetti frequently said, "I'm an old lady. God should have taken me. I've lived my life. My son-in-law had his life ahead of him and a family that needed him."

Yet some older adults respond to family dismemberment with sadness and anxiety but without despair. They have had much experience with the establishment, maintenance, and termination of relationships. They are able to look at the loss of a family member within the perspective of a life that has contained both positive and negative happenings, and they do not despair over what might have been. Table 14-1 summarizes the effects of change in family membership on a family.

SOCIOCULTURAL STRAINS

In families that are characterized by overcrowding, scarcity of resources (food, fuel, money, clothing), or instability (for example, inadequate support systems, interrupted interpersonal relationships, or lack of routine in daily living), parental overburdening may develop. Minuchin (1974) refers to these families as disorganized or disadvantaged families. In such families, parents may only have sufficient time and energy to fulfill their children's needs for physical nurturing. Children's psychosocial needs may not be recognized. Parents may view discipline only as a means of controlling children and not as a way of teaching and guiding children in socially acceptable behavior. Thus, although undesirable behavior may be punished, desirable behavior may go unacknowledged and unrewarded. As a result, the children from these family systems may experience the following problems:

1. An inability to recollect events so that they can be drawn upon for guidance in similar life situations.

TABLE 14-1 Change in family membership

Age group of family member	Developmental task	Response to change in family membership
Infancy	Trust vs. mistrust	Change in quantity and quality of nurturing and/or later difficulties with attachment or object permanence
Preschool	Autonomy vs. shame and doubt	Separation anxiety, fear of abandonment, repression and denial of feelings, regression, hyperactivity, anorexia, sleep disturbances, temper tantrums, and/or gastrointestinal upsets
School-age	Industry vs. inferiority	Interference with achievement of industry and autonomy, guilt feelings, withdrawal, sadness, hostility, anxiety, poor school grades, somatization, anger, and/or precocious sexual experimentation (in older school-age children)
Adolescence	Identity vs. role diffusion	Overinvolvement with nonfamily activities, socially deviant behavior, and/or sexual acting out
Young adult	Intimacy vs. isolation	Role overburdening, interference with achievement of intimacy
Middle age	Generativity vs. stagnation	Anxiety, inadequacy, role disenchantment, questioning of life goals, anger, self-blame, inadequacy, insecurity, and/or loneliness
Old age	Ego integrity vs. despair	Reactions of young and middle-aged adults, acceptance, and/or despair

2. An inability to recognize subtle variations in interpersonal behavior. The behavior of others is either interpreted as aggressive or not understood at all.
3. An inability to respond to situations with moderation. The children are either passive or aggressive, intensely involved or totally uninvolved.

Sociocultural stress is also experienced by many ethnic families.* Ethnic families often try to become acculturated to American society while at the same time attempting to preserve ethnic traditions, customs, and behaviors. Ethnic parents may give their offspring a self-contradictory message: Become successful in American society, but maintain strong ties with your ethnic group. If ethnic parents

have experienced discrimination, they may become overly protective in their attempts to protect their children from discrimination. In addition, ethnic children, who in school are exposed to American life-styles, often become acculturated more rapidly than their parents. The children may then assume the tasks of acculturating their parents. This role reversal may produce overburdening in the children, a situation that may not only produce tension in intrafamilial relationships but may also deprive the children of opportunities to successfully compete in American society and to develop the social skills necessary to relate to people outside the ethnic group (McGoldrick et al., 1982).

Sociocultural stress may be further experienced when ethnic persons marry outside their ethnic groups. The ethnic identities of the interethnic

*Refer to Chapter 4 for further discussion of ethnicity.

couple may weaken. For example, an ethnic language may not be spoken at home and ethnic foods may not be prepared. For the offspring of interethnic marriages, ethnic identity may become more optional than ascriptive. Children may opt to identify more with the ethnic heritage of one parent than with the heritage of the other parent, or they may ignore the ethnic heritage of one parent. The parent whose ethnic heritage is not chosen may feel slighted or resentful.

In addition, differing concepts of male-female relationships may cause tension in interethnic marriages. For example, while Mediterranean and Latin American male-female relationships are often strongly influenced by a tradition that includes a double standard and male domination of women, American male-female relationships are usually more egalitarian. Therefore, during the early years of marriage, interethnic couples may have to make many adjustments concerning sex-defined role expectations and behaviors (Pasquali, 1982; McGoldrick et al., 1982).

Different definitions and concepts of "family" may also create tension in interethnic marriages.* For instance, the extended family is a central force in the lives of many people of Asian, Hispanic, African, and Mediterranean descent. Should such a person marry someone with a nuclear family orientation, the spouse may become resentful, impatient, or jealous of the degree of involvement with extended family members.

A Hispanic man who had married a British-American woman complained: "My grandparents, aunts, uncles, and cousins have always been a very important part of my life. When we first came to the United States from Cuba, we all lived together. Even when we all had enough money to get our own places to live, we lived near each other. We still have a close-knit family. I feel secure knowing that no matter how bad things get, I have any number of people who will help me and who care about me. With my wife, it's a very different situation. Her idea of a family is her mother and father and her sister and brother. She has aunts and uncles and cousins, but she's not as close to them as I am to my

relatives. My wife always thinks my family is taking advantage of me. She doesn't understand how it is with us—how we all feel responsible for each other."

Thus, because of different conceptualizations of male-female relationships and of the family, tension and conflict may be engendered when people with different ethnic backgrounds marry. This tension and conflict may be compounded if offspring opt to identify more with the ethnicity of one parent than with the ethnicity of the other parent.

MATURATIONAL EVENTS

Events that mark the transitions between developmental stages can produce stress and tension in the family system. Marriage, parenthood, the entry of a child into kindergarten, and retirement are only a few of the maturational events that may force a reorganization of the family system. There may need to be a reassignment of family roles, a reordering of status positions, a reassessment of values, a re-channeling of communication, and a restructuring of ways to fulfill the needs and expectations of family members (Van Servellen, 1984). The tension and disorganization that accompany these changes lead to maturational crises. Maturational crises* are predictable developmental events that occur at transition points in the life cycle.

A classic study by Klein and Ross (1965) of children's entry into kindergarten illustrates how a maturational event can generate stress within the family system. Klein and Ross found that the entry of a child into kindergarten was marked by tension within the family and by altered patterns of behavior. The way in which tension was expressed varied from family to family and even differed among members of the same family. The following reactions were observed in children: (1) physical complaints such as anorexia, fatigue, and nausea; (2) increased use of or regression to such behaviors as bedwetting and thumb sucking; (3) hyperirritability, expressed in fighting with siblings or other children, talking back to parents, and uncooperativeness; (4) increased reliance on their mothers; and

---

*Refer to Chapter 5 for a discussion of family forms.

*Refer to Chapter 15 for a discussion of maturational crises.

(5) such miscellaneous signs of stress as appearing "worried" or "keyed up," not wanting to attend school, and being either very talkative or very quiet.

Klein and Ross noted that parents usually experienced a sense of loss when their children entered kindergarten. Kindergarten entry also led to parental concern about value conflicts between the school and the family in the following three areas: (1) individuality vs. group comformity; (2) control of aggression vs. assertiveness and self-defense; and (3) learning to relate to the opposite sex vs. premature heterosexual interest.

Discomfit with shifts in parental roles was also evidenced. Many parents became annoyed when their children looked to the teacher as an authority figure and role model. Parents frequently experienced feelings of inadequacy about their ability to motivate and discipline their children as compared to the teacher's ability.

Klein and Ross also observed that at the same time that family members were reacting to the entry of a child into kindergarten, they began to display such growth behaviors as increased independence from the family, assumption of responsibility for oneself, and development of interests and activities outside of the family milieu.

Thus, the entry of a child into school, just like other maturational events, may engage families in role shifts, value reassessments, and other changes that alter family equilibrium, generate tension, and force a reorganization of the family system.

DISORDERED FAMILY RELATIONSHIPS

The way in which children are socialized within the family helps to mold their subsequent behavior as adults. Children learn from adult family members patterns of communication, means of coping with conflict, and ways to tolerate stress and alleviate anxiety.

Lucy grew up in a family that focused on health and illness to an extreme degree. When Lucy's father came home from work each evening, he would feel her forehead to see if she had a fever. This ritual of "feeling" Lucy's forehead replaced the kiss that is a common form of parent-child greeting in other families. In

addition, whenever there was conflict between Lucy's parents, the conflict would be put aside when one parent complained of a severe headache. Lucy cannot ever remember her parents sitting down and trying to resolve a conflict. As Lucy grew into early adolescence, she began experiencing severe "migraines." These headaches were usually triggered by parental dissension. Extensive neurological examinations could uncover no physiological basis for Lucy's headaches.

The intrafamilial coping patterns of Lucy's family have been described by Minuchin, Rosman, and Baker (1978) as being characteristic of a psychosomatogenic family.* In the psychosomatogenic family, children learn from adults that not only is psychophysiological dysfunction a concern common to all family members but also that it is a way to deal with conflict in the family. Instead of engaging in problem solving that would lead to conflict resolution, the family avoids the conflict by focusing on psychophysiological symptoms.

When intrafamilial behavior patterns deviate consistently and markedly from society's standards, family dysfunction may be engendered and family members may encounter difficulties interacting with their social environment. The primary reasons for intrafamilial behavior patterns that deviate significantly from social norms are parental overburdening and family overbonding.

Parental overburdening may be found most often in nuclear and single-parent families. Because these families are often both emotionally and geographically distant from extended family members, there may be too few adult family members to effectively care for children and to provide adults with whom children can identify. The total burden of child rearing then falls on the parents.

Searles (1965) and Scheflen and Scheflen (1972) were among the first to see in parental overburdening the seeds of family dysfunction. Family members who remain in these families without avenues of mobility may develop overbonding to and overdependency on the family. There are three pat-

*See Chapter 19 for further discussion of the psychosomatogenic family and coping through psychophysiological responses.

terns that overbonding and overdependence may take: (1) Clinging, overdependent children, who are afraid to be separated from the family, often develop phobias, hypochondriasis, or psychophysiological dysfunctions. (2) Children who are so strongly bonded to the parent of the opposite sex that they develop sexual attachment to that parent may become frozen in their emotional growth. They are often referred to as having unresolved Oedipus complexes. (3) Family members of any age who are overbonded to the family may become alcoholics or drug abusers. They may use alcohol or drugs to become assertive and confident enough to break away from the family, function independently, and relate to outsiders. However, they inevitably experience failure, lose confidence, and return to the family. Alcohol or drug abuse may at this point make them so helpless that the family takes them back and protects them.

Overbonded persons are often the identified clients in family systems. However, in all instances of overbonded, overdependent clients, we find that this is not solely the problem of the identified clients. Other family members are also locked into this overbonded relationship. In addition, these heavily bonded people tend to be vulnerable to double-bind situations,* in which they are confronted with paradoxical alternatives that can be neither resolved nor avoided (Hoffman, 1981).

Disordered family relationships that generate identified clients are disappointing and destructive to all members of the family because:

1. The behavior of the identified client shatters the hopes of family members, especially of parents, to impress the community with the family's ideals.
2. The angry and rebellious behavior of the identified client can destroy parental expectations that their child will like them.
3. The socially deviant behavior of the identified client can be devastating to parents who look to their child to fulfill their own ambitions.
4. The behavior of the identified client may emphasize marital conflicts and divide the fami-

ly, putting children in the position of having conflicting attachments and loyalties.
5. The identified client not only internalizes parental marital conflicts but continues to act out the family drama with other men and women long after the parents have died.
6. The identified client's labeling by the family as sick, bad, or different contributes to the development of low self-esteem in the client.
7. The identified client (and often other family members) is inadequately prepared to cope with life outside the family system. Family, especially parental, perceptions, interpretations, and responses to the environment tend to be incongruent with what members of other families experience. Since facts have to be consistently modified to meet emotionally determined needs, the family provides training in irrationality (Hoffman, 1981; Madanes, 1984; Van Servellen, 1984).

Vulnerability of families to dysfunction

To summarize the discussion of family dysfunction, it may be helpful to borrow the concept of "balancing factors" from Aguilera and Messick (1989). The interrelationship between such balancing factors as the way a family perceives a stressor (which is influenced by the stage of the domestic cycle occupied by the family, the cultural heritage of the family, and the ages of family members), the adaptability of the family social system, and the nature of family patterns of relating and communicating can either throw a family system into disequilibrium and dysfunction or contribute to a family system's maintenance of equilibrium and sound functioning. These opposing processes are diagramed in Fig. 14-1.

Although an entire family may experience a stressor or a series of multiple stressors, many factors may determine why one family member develops severe impairment of functioning while others do not. Chief among these factors are the ages and developmental levels of family members; parental preference for one sex; parental reactions to fretful,

*See Chapters 10 and 25 for further discussion of double-bind situations.

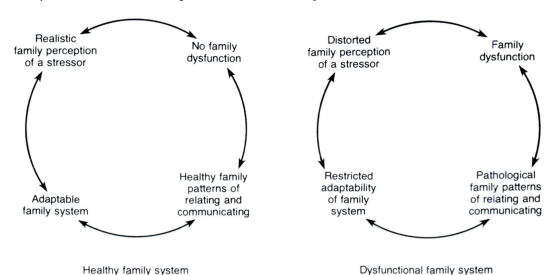

Fig. 14-1 Interrelationship of family balancing factors.

colicky behavior in infants; nonresponsiveness of an infant; a high level of anxiety between spouses; a low degree of emotional involvement between spouses; and the holistic health status of family members. In addition, *pathological patterns of relating* may increase a family member's vulnerability to dysfunction. Table 14-2 summarizes some pathological patterns of relating.

Sample interaction 14-1: coalition across generational boundaries

Child: (Eight-year-old boy who has been playing outside runs into the house). Daddy, can I have money for ice cream? The ice cream man is outside.

Father: No, it's 15 minutes before your supper!

Child: (Goes into the next room where his mother is preparing supper). Mommy, can I have money for ice cream?

Mother: (Might answer in one of the following ways:)
a. No, your father is right; it's too close to supper.
b. Ok, here's the money, but let's not tell Daddy.
c. I don't agree with Daddy, and I will tell him so—here's the money.

Response "a" is probably the healthiest; it indicates agreement among the spouses about child rearing.

Response "c" indicates a certain amount of marital discord, disagreement over child rearing. However, "c" is a healthier response than response "b," because the conflict is out in the open and the child is not engaged by one parent in a conspiracy against the other parent.

Sample interaction 14-2: double-bind communication

Child: (Drops a glass of milk on the floor).

Mother: (Has just finished washing the floor, frowns, and says angrily) That's ok. Don't worry about it, honey. Mommy will clean it up.

• • •

Son: I've been thinking about college and where I want to go to college.

Father: Son, your mother and I want you to be an independent person who makes his own decisions, so we have decided that you should go to a school out of town.

• • •

Daughter: I love you and Dad.

Mother: If your father and I were drowning and you could only save one of us, which one would it be?

TABLE 14-2 Pathological patterns of relating

Behavior pattern	Description
Scapegoating	Process of consciously or unconsciously singling out one family member (often a child) to be the carrier of family problems. Possible explanations for a family member's acceptance of this role include the fear of annihilation of the family system if he or she does not accept the role and the desire to defend against unconscious incestuous feelings.
Emotional divorce	Process that occurs when emotional investment between spouses has been withdrawn. Spouses may be "staying together for the children" or for any number of other reasons, but there is little real involvement with one another.
Pseudomutuality	Pattern of relating among family membrers in which there is surface harmony and a high degree of agreement with one another. This pattern of relating is a facade that masks overt and covert conflict and confusing communication.
Coalition across generational boundaries	Conspiracy or alliance exists between a parent and a child. Such a conspiracy, which is usually against the other parent, undermines the marital relationship and instills guilt and fear in the child, who has a self-perception of betraying one parent and being too close to the other parent (see Sample Interaction 14-1).
Vagueness	Unclear ways of communicating, with a tendency to use global pronouns (e.g., "they") and loose associations, lead to ambiguity and confusion on the part of a listener.
Tangentiality	Association disturbance characterized by the tendency to digress from one's original topic of conversation. This "going off on tangents" confuses a listener, who is not sure whether a question has been answered or, if it has been answered, what the response was.
Double-bind communication	Communication pattern involving the giving of two conflicting messages at the same time. One message may be verbal and the other nonverbal or both messages may be verbal (see Sample Interaction 14-2). A person who receives such a message is usually not consciously aware that it contains two conflicting messages, but the conflicting nature of the messages serves to immobilize and confuse the listener (refer to Chapter 25 for a discussion of double-bind communication and schizophrenia).
Family myth	Communication pattern involving the construction of myths that serve to deny the reality of the family situation. For example, a father who is an alcoholic tyrant may have a wife who denies this fact to the world and to herself and insists that her children participate in the myth that the father is a sober and loving person. Any attempts by a family member to state the real facts or to discuss feelings about them are met with strong denial and guilt-producing accusations.
Mystification	Communication process that may include vagueness, tangentiality, double-bind communication, and family myths. Mystification serves to maintain the equilibrium of a family system even while it confuses family members. The following are some key characteristics of this communication process: (1) children being mystified do not realize that the family uses faulty communication patterns and thus blame themselves for their confusion, (2) children unconsciously sense that to question these patterns would threaten the equilibrium of the family system and their security, (3) the family continually uses these patterns of communicating.

Communication "a" contains conflicting verbal and nonverbal messages; communication "b" contains two conflicting verbal messages; communication "c" is a "damned-if-you-do and damned-if-you-don't" message. All three communications are examples of double-bind communication.

FAMILY THERAPY

Family systems theory and family therapy began in the mid-1950s. In the United States, individuals and groups initially worked independently in the area of family treatment. They eventually began to communicate with each other, and a body of theoretical knowledge evolved. Today, family therapy is an effective tool for alleviating emotional problems. Graduate psychiatric nursing programs include family systems theory and clinical courses in family therapy as parts of their curricula. Psychiatric nursing clinical specialists are often actively involved as family therapists; many have increased their understanding and knowledge through participation in workshops and enrollment in family therapy institutions throughout the country.

Family therapists

In conducting family therapy, the goals of the therapist are to clarify and improve *family communication patterns* and *family relationship patterns*. The family itself is viewed as the client. It is thought that through reinforcement of healthy, clear boundaries between individuals, family members will be able to relate to one another in a meaningful way—in a way that protects healthy individual autonomy. There will not be the threat of loss of self through engulfment *or* the need to defend against this threatened loss through destructive distancing maneuvers. When necessary, the family therapist protects family members who are potentially scapegoats and acts as a role model for more mature functioning in the family environment. The therapist *clarifies* and *educates* and thus *facilitates* healthier functioning within the family system. In working with a family, a therapist usually wants to know something of the family history of both the husband and the wife. This information is helpful in assisting the family members to connect their past experiences to the present situation and to gain insight into their tendencies to use certain patterns of communicating and relating.

On the basis of how therapists work with families, two types of family therapy approaches have been identified: (1) verbal exchange ("talking through" a problem by facilitating insight, personal disclosure, confrontation, etc.) and (2) tasks and activities (using behavior modification, visualization exercises, genogram development, family drawing, etc.). Regardless of the approach that a therapist uses, the therapist's *use of self* is an important aspect of family therapy. Not only do therapists need to work through the relationships in their own families of origin and procreation, but they also need to work through their own ethnic identities. This helps therapists to resist being "triggered" by problematic relationships and ethnic characteristics found in their own backgrounds. In addition, when therapists learn about the orientation of the cultural groups from which they draw clients, they are less likely to be ethnocentric about values, attitudes, and behaviors that are different from their own (McGoldrick, 1982; Sturkie, 1986).

Models of family therapy

Conceptual approaches devised by Jones and Dimond (1982) and Hoffman (1981) will be used to discuss models of family therapy.

STRUCTURAL MODEL

The family is viewed as an open system whose impetus for change arises from two sources: (1) biopsychosocial alterations in family members, and (2) interactions with other social systems. To fulfill family functions, the family group may differentiate into subsystems on the basis of age, sex, interest, or abilities (subsystems can consist of one or more family members). For example, in a given family the following subsystems may exist to carry out specific family functions: (1) the spousal subsystem, to fulfill conjugal functions; (2) the parental subsystem, to fulfill parenting functions; and (3) the sibling subsystem, to facilitate peer socialization. In addition, family members follow scripts or "transactional patterns" that regulate their lives and their relationships. These scripts are reinforced by systems of constraints. General rules that order family organization are known as *generic constraints*. For instance, in most families, parents have more authority in family matters than do children. The ways in which generic constraints are modified by a family are referred to as *idiosyncratic constraints*. For example, how parents specifically carry out their authority in the family and how parental authority differs from the authority of children may vary from family to family.

Minuchin (1974) and his followers are structural therapists. They view the demands for change that constantly face the family as potentials for family dysfunction. When faced with demands for change, individual family members, family subsystems, and the family as a whole may respond either with growth behaviors or with maladaptive behaviors. Maladaptive behaviors are dysfunctional transactional patterns for organizing family life and family relationships. The *goal* of therapy is to help the family learn new, alternative scripts or transactional patterns.

Parents came to a nurse–family therapist with complaints about their 8-year-old daughter destroying books. The mother was a university professor, and she spent much time reading and preparing lesson plans. The father was a law student, and he spent many hours studying. The nurse–family therapist found that the parents were not spending enough time with their daughter. The child tore up books when she was left to her own devices because her parents were busy reading or studying.

The nurse–family therapist assigned the parents the task of setting time aside each day for the purpose of teaching their daughter about the proper use of books. They might read aloud to one another, go to the library together, or, by following instructions in a book, create something (such as baking cookies or constructing a kite).

The activity of teaching their daughter about the appropriate use of books became an avenue for the parents to learn to spend time with their daughter. Thus, a new script was developed for family relationships.

INTERACTIONAL MODEL

The family is viewed as a communication system composed of interlocking subsystems (the individual family members). The process of family interaction, including rules that regulate relationships, is the focus of analysis. Family dysfunction occurs when the rules that govern family interaction become vague and ambiguous. This leads to confusion about what family members can expect from one another. Satir (1972), Haley (1976) and their followers are interactional therapists. The *goal* of therapy is to help the family clarify the rules that govern family relationships.

The Browns sought help for their 7-year-old son Peter. Peter's behavior at school had become disruptive. He teased his classmates, talked in class, and "resisted settling down to work."

After talking with Peter and his parents, a nurse-therapist determined that Peter's disruptive behavior was an attempt to unite his parents. Peter had learned that when his parents focused their attention on his disruptive behavior, they would stop arguing. The nurse-therapist therefore helped the Browns to focus on their marital relationship—not on Peter's behavior or on their parenting behavior. Central to the discord in their marital relationship was ambiguity in their communication of expectations. For example, Mrs. Brown "expected" that, since she had recently taken a job outside the home, her husband would help with the housework. Mr. Brown "assumed" that, if his wife wanted his help, she would ask for it. Neither person had ever clearly communicated what was wanted or expected from the other.

The nurse-therapist helped the Browns to see that each of them operated as if the other were a mindreader. Messages were not clearly stated, and, because they did not communicate the expectations and wishes of the sender, the messages were incomplete. The nurse-therapist then helped the Browns to learn to communicate more clearly and completely with one another. Once the Browns learned to deal with their communication problems, their son Peter no longer needed to use disruptive school behavior to try to unite his parents.

The activity of clarifying rules for family interaction and of communicating expectations clearly to one another became an avenue for dealing with family dysfunction.

MULTIGENERATIONAL MODEL

Because Bowen's (1978) multigenerational model focuses on reciprocal role relationships *over time* and thus takes a longitudinal approach to family therapy, Jones and Dimond consider it a quasidevelopmental model. Bowen views the family as an emotional system. Change in one family member leads to change in other family members in a predictable, chain-reaction pattern. By using the following set of interrelated concepts, family dysfunction may be explained. If there is a high degree of *differentiation of self* among family members, family members are able to cope with changes and stress without being emotionally ill. Well-differentiated family members are characterized by authenticity in interpersonal relationships and by an ability to distinguish between thoughts and feelings. They are able to have "I" positions (ideas, plans, beliefs, and goals) that are their own and not their family's. They therefore can participate in the family system without being an "emotional domino" in the system. People who have low levels of differentiation of self become fused with those with whom they have intimate relationships. Much of their energy is devoted to finding affection and approval. Decisions tend to be based on feelings and cues from the family rather than on independent, objective thinking. People who have low degrees of differentiation of self tend to have high degrees of unresolved emotional attachment to their parents or to experience *emotional cutoff* (emotionally withdrawing from or denying the importance of one's parents, thereby creating an emotional disconnectedness between parents and child). In addition, the *sibling position profiles* (personality characteristics for each sibling position) of people with poor self-differentiation often are more typical of sibling positions other than their own. For example, an oldest child may exhibit the profile usually associated with a youngest child.

Generally, a person takes as a spouse someone with a similar degree of differentiation. The *nuclear family emotional system* refers to patterns of interaction and emotional functioning among parents and children in the nuclear family. These patterns are often "replicas" of what has happened in one's family of origin. Within the nuclear family, relationships are composed of interlocking *triangles*, the fundamental building blocks of the family. A triangle can be composed of a dyad that holds inside, comfortable positions and a third person, issue, or organization that holds an outside position. When relationships in the triangle become tense, the "outsider" may be brought into a closer position, or a family member holding an inside position in the triangle may try to avoid stress and obtain comfort by moving into the outside position. The classic family triangle is the mother-father-child triangle, and the tensions in this triangle, as in any triangle, are usually in flux (see Fig. 14-2).

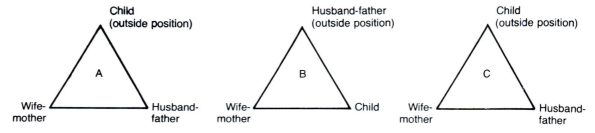

Fig. 14-2 Dynamic tensions of triangulation. Triangle A illustrates family triangle with spouse-parents holding inside positions and child in outside position. As tension increases between spouse-parents, child moves into inside, "confidant" relationship with mother, and father escapes from marital tension to outside position in triangle (triangle B). Later, when child engages in behavior unacceptable to both parents, wife-mother and husband-father realign themselves, and child again holds outside position in triangle (triangle C).

Within the nuclear family, spouses may try to control ego fusion in any of the following ways: through overt conflict between spouses; through functional impairment of one of the spouses (for example, through alcoholism, physical illness, obesity, schizophrenia); or through functional impairment of one or more "triangulated" children (for example, through socially deviant behavior, physical illness, schizophrenia). This last method of controlling ego fusion among family members is referred to as the *family projection process.* When it is carried out over generations, it becomes the *multigenerational transmission process;* patterns of interacting and coping (for example, priorities, goals, attitudes) and unresolved issues can be passed down from generation to generation and can cause stress in the family members on whom they are projected. Illness thus is viewed as the transmission of insufficient differentiation across generational lines. The *goal* of therapy is to help family members attain a higher level of differentiation.

Larry was the identified client in the family. During several interviews with the family, the nurse-therapist learned that Larry's parents and grandparents had always valued education. In addition, it was customary in the family for parents to decide what careers their children would pursue.

Larry's father, his two uncles, and his grandfathers were lawyers. When they went to law school, they had attended local universities and had lived at home. Larry's father said this was because they were a close-knit family.

Larry's parents had brought Larry up with the expectation that he would attend college. Larry wanted to be a veterinarian, but his parents did not want him to go out of town to veterinary school. Instead, they decided he would attend a local university that had a law school. Larry would become a lawyer like his father.

Although Larry was unhappy with his parents' decision, he fulfilled his parents' expectations. Years later, Larry told a therapist, "I still wonder how my life would have been if I could have become a veterinarian like I wanted. But I also wanted to please my parents. If I had said 'No,' all hell would have broken loose. My parents would have thrown me out of the house and probably disowned me. Then what would have become of me?"

Larry had taken on the expectations and wishes of his parents. This was a behavior pattern that had been occurring in the family for generations, and it was a consequence of a low degree of differentiation. The therapist's goal would be to help Larry and his family attain higher levels of self-differentiation so that the lack of differentiation that had been transmitted over generations to Larry would not be projected onto Larry's children.

ECOSYSTEM MODEL

The family is viewed as an open system within a broad social field of other social systems. Interacting subsystems that need to be considered are extended family members, professionals, community figures, and social institutions (e.g., health delivery system, welfare system). The focus of the ecosystem model is on the here and now. Auerswald (1968), one of the pioneers of the ecological model of family therapy, stressed that if contextual integrity was to be maintained, then the limitations of time and space imposed by professionals had to be eliminated. Toward this end, Auerswald insisted that community psychiatry agencies should be open 24 hours a day and that mobile mental health teams should respond to problems wherever the problems arise (e.g., at home, at school).

The ecosystem model takes a holistic approach to treatment. Biological, psychosocial, and environmental factors are considered and the family therapist becomes part of the ecosystem (Keeney, 1979). Therapists are sensitive to the layering of contexts and to systems other than the family. Maladaptive behaviors are thought to be metaphorical communication about the ecology of the family's social network. Change in one set of network relationships will generate change in other sets. The *goal* of therapy is to help mobilize family and/or network resources or to minimize stressors that have intensified the crisis.

Mr. Peterson sought help for his depressed wife, Helga. Helga had become depressed after the birth of their second child. The nurse-therapist convened the family but also directed them to bring all the significant people in Helga's life to the meeting. This included Helga's friends as well as her parents, aunts, uncles, and cousins. The nurse-therapist helped Helga and

TABLE 14-3 Comparison of family therapy models

Family therapy model	Focus of analysis	Goal of therapy
Structural	Dysfunctional transactional patterns	Help family learn new, alternative transactional patterns (scripts)
Interactional	Vague and ambiguous rules governing interactions	Help family clarify rules governing family relationships and interactions
Mutligenerational	Transmission of insufficient differentiation across generational lines	Help family members attain a higher level of differentiation
Ecosystem	Ecology of relationship systems	Help family members attain more effective interaction with their social networks

her network identify pressures in Helga's life and ways that network members could help decrease those pressures or help Helga cope with them more effectively. It was revealed that shortly before the birth of their second child, Mr. Peterson had lost his job. Recently, he had been looking for work and was out of the house most of the day job hunting. The social service department was contacted and food stamps were obtained for the family. A friend who owned a gas station offered Mr. Peterson a part-time job until he could find permanent work. Several network members agreed to take turns supervising Helga's child care until Helga was able to function without supervision. Other network members offered to babysit a few hours each week so that Helga could have some time free of child care. Helga stated that for the first time since the baby was born "I don't feel like I'm drowning all alone. Now I feel people know I'm drowning and they are throwing me a rope."

The activity of mobilizing network resources became an avenue for dealing with family dysfunction. Table 14-3 compares the different models of family therapy.

Cultural influences and family therapy

FAMILY DYNAMICS

The point was made in Chapter 5 that family organization and family dynamics vary according to cultural context. Although many family therapists are becoming increasingly aware of cultural variability, family theory and family therapy models are often culture bound and predicated on the family model of a "normal" middle-class, white, urban, nuclear family (Miller, 1981; McGoldrick et al., 1982).

The assessments and goals of many family therapists tend to reflect this ethnocentrism. For example, self-direction, self-disclosure among family members, trusting in others, and independence are viewed by many family therapists as goals for a "healthy," well-functioning family system regardless of its cultural orientation. Yet self-direction and self-disclosure are characteristics that tend to be found in and valued by mainstream middle-class and upper-class families. These families usually have a sense, born out by experience, that their opinions, decisions, and actions can influence their fate. However, family therapists need to recognize that not all family systems encourage self-direction and self-expression and that this does not necessarily make them dysfunctional family systems. Some ethnic groups, such as the Chinese, do not encourage open expression of feeling among family members (Lee, 1982). Also, many families in the lower stratum of American society often have a "nonintrospective orientation" (Miller, 1981; McGoldrick et al., 1982).

Similarly, family styles of relating to others may also be culturally influenced. For example, in Italian-American families, loyalty to the family, suspicion toward those outside the family, and family honor are stressed. On the other hand, Irish-American families tend to have great respect for personal boundaries and for family members' rights to privacy (Rotunno and McGoldrick, 1982; McGoldrick, 1982).

It is therefore important for family therapists to be aware of the cultural variability of family organization and family dynamics so that their assessments, interpretations, and goals will not be value laden.

FAMILY HEALING SPECIALISTS

All societies have healing specialists. In contemporary American society, psychiatric clinical nurse specialists, psychiatric social workers, psychologists, and psychiatrists can be trained as family therapists. In other cultures, such a role might be assumed by native healers, including *curanderos* (Central Americans), root doctors or *hoodoo* men (Afro-Americans), shamans (native Americans and Eskimos), and *babalawos* (Cubans and Yorubas).

The difference between family therapists and native healers is not as great as it may appear at first glance. We will now look at some of the similarities between family therapists and native healers.

▶ Identifying and labeling the problem

A family therapist may speak of family fusion or of a closed family system as a source of family distress. A native healer may identify violation of a taboo or spirit possession as the source of family distress. In either case, identifying the problem conveys to the client-family that someone understands and cares. The very act of labeling the problem implies that it can be treated. Moreover, underlying the process of labeling is the assumption that, since the family therapist or native healer can identify and place the problem within a framework that the family can understand, he or she must share the client-family's world view. When world view is not shared between the therapist or native healer and the client-family, treatment is usually ineffective.

The parents of a Mexican-American girl were told by an Anglo-American family therapist that their daughter's depression and listlessness were related to their dysfunctional marital relationship. Therefore, the parents should become involved in marital therapy. The parents knew that their daughter was suffering from susto *(magical fright). They consulted a* curandero, *who performed the necessary* limpia *(spirit-cleansing ritual).*

An Anglo-American family would have found referral to a *curandero* as irrelevant as this Mexican-American family found the family therapist's approach.

▶ Personal qualities of the specialist

Among family therapists, empathy, authenticity, and nonpossessive warmth are important to the therapeutic process. Few studies have been done on the personal qualities of native healers; however, because people from different cultural groups conceptualize health and illness differently, the personal qualities of healers probably also vary. As was mentioned before, though, the ability of family therapists and native healers to share (or at least to understand) the world view of their client-families is a quality that is important to both.

▶ Expectations of client-families

Client-families usually have expectations in regard to the treatment they seek. In the vignette about the Mexican-American family, the family's expectation was that a *limpia* ritual would be performed to treat the daughter. Family therapists and native healers contribute to the expectations of client-families. For example, both family therapists and native healers are specialists in their societies, and some portion of client-family expectation is based on this expertise. In Western society, family therapists are accorded the status of professionals. Native healers are revered and sometimes feared because of their unique knowledge and power, a power that followers often believe is mystical or occult.

In addition, both family therapists and native healers have completed training programs. Family therapists either have finished graduate programs that focus on family therapy or have taken courses in family theory and have had supervised clinical practice. Native healers, such as *babalawos* and *espiritistas** have had a long preparatory period. This period is devoted to obtaining knowledge about herbs, learning rituals and divining procedures, and acquiring self-knowledge and self-control.

► **Techniques of family therapists**

Family therapists try to ease family tension and resolve family conflicts. Family therapists use techniques to define the strucure of the family, facilitate family process, enhance personal and interpersonal awareness, and/or improve family communication. Table 14-4 gives examples of techniques that facilitate these aims. Below we outline the nursing process as it applies to the family in the following case study:

Babalawos are high priests of Santería. *Espiritistas* are spiritists of Espiritismo. These belief systems embody healing aspects.

The Hogan family is referred to a nurse-family therapist because Elizabeth, who is 15 years old, has been experiencing severe stomachaches. A physical workup has shown no physiological disorder. Because of her stomachaches, Elizabeth has not been able to attend school for the past 2 weeks. There are three younger daughters in the family, aged 12, 9, and 7. During the initial family interview, the mother and father begin to argue and derogate each other. Mr. Hogan states that the family's problems began when "my mother-in-law came to live with us four weeks ago. The rest of us were never consulted. My wife made the decision that her mother would move in with us and that was that. She always makes the decisions and then thinks we should just go along with them." Mrs. Hogan retorts: "You never want to get involved. Maybe if you weren't so afraid to make a decision, I wouldn't have to decide everything." Elizabeth immediately begins to cry and begs her parents not to fight with each other. Elizabeth's three sisters sit quietly and look at the floor.

TABLE 14-4 Family therapy techniques

Technique	Explanation	Purpose
Sculpting	Construction of a live family portrait that depicts family alliances and conflicts.	Define family structure and facilitate interpersonal awareness
Projective drawing	Spatial depiction of relational patterns among family members.	Define family structure and facilitate interpersonal awareness
Blindman's walk	Family members take turns being led blindfolded around a room. At the end of the exercise, family members discuss their feelings about trusting and being trusted.	Facilitate family process and self-awareness
Rolling or rocking exercise	Family members form a circle. Turns are taken going into the center of the circle and being rolled from one family member to another. After the exercise, feelings about giving up control to others and being entrusted with another's well-being are discussed.	Facilitate family process and self-awareness
Shadowboxing and fight games	Family members punch at their own shadows or fight nonphysically by yelling and screaming. Purpose is to vent aggression and hostility and relieve tension. At the end of	Facilitate family process and self-awareness

Sources consulted include Madanes (1984), Van Servellen (1984), and Sturkie (1986).

TABLE 14-4   Family therapy techniques—cont'd

Technique	Explanation	Purpose
	the exercise, methods of fighting and feelings during the "fight" are discussed.	
Visualization and imagery	Family members are asked to imagine the issues or feelings that would arise in given hypothetical situations.	Facilitate family process and self-awareness
Video feedback	A family therapy session is videotaped. Video feedback is used to confront family members about their communication behaviors and methods of problem solving.	Improve communication and self-awareness
Locking-unlocking exercise	Family members are directed to physically "unlock" their bodies (e.g., uncross extremities, swing arms). Discussion follows about the ways their bodies contribute to and/or reflect openness in communication.	Improve communication and self-awareness
Role play	Family members are directed to reverse roles in simulations of actual situations.	Improve interpersonal and self-awareness
Cognitive clarification	Therapist describes what just happened: "When you and your wife started to fight, your daughter began to cry."	Facilitate family process and interpersonal awareness
Interpretation	Therapist explains the meaning of what just transpired: "Your son is afraid you will get a divorce, and he wants to keep you together."	Facilitate family process and interpersonal awareness
Affective clarification	Family member is asked what he or she is feeling: "What were you feeling when your parents were arguing?"	Improve communication and self-awareness
Experiential sharing	Therapist shares own feelings about what has just transpired: "I feel like crying too when I see family members who love each other verbally abusing each other."	Facilitate family process and interpersonal awareness
Reframing (paradoxical intent and symptom prescription)	Family members are directed to take a new, exaggerated approach to a situation: "I want you to spend 10 minutes every day arguing with your wife about your mother-in-law and I want Elizabeth to cry while you are arguing."	Facilitate family process and interpersonal awareness
Sorting	Family member is asked to use a different pattern for selecting information: "You keep tellling me how your wife makes all the decisions. Tell me one time that you and your wife made a decision together."	Facilitate family process and communication

Assessment
1. Somatising evidenced by Elizabeth's stomachaches
2. Problems with expression of feelings evidenced by somatising and blocked communication
3. Problems with decision making evidenced by marital discord
4. Change in family membership evidenced by mother-in-law moving in with the family four weeks ago

Nursing diagnosis
Altered family processes related to situational crisis (NANDA 3.2.2; DSM-III-R V61.80).

Outcomes (long-term): family will
1. Recognize the factors that interfere with shared decision making
2. Express feelings openly
3. Renegotiate roles
4. Meet the security needs of its members

Outcomes (short-term): family will
1. Examine the process of decision making in the family
2. Identify feelings related to decision making
3. Examine the effects of decisions on individual family members and the family as a unit
4. Learn new approaches to decision making
5. Identify effects of change in family membership on individual family members and the family as a unit
6. Express feelings related to change in family membership
7. Learn new approaches to role enactment
8. Evaluate effectiveness of current coping behaviors
9. Learn more effective coping behaviors

Nursing strategies
1. Create an atmosphere where family members feel comfortable expressing themselves
2. Include mother-in-law in therapy sessions
3. Explore process of decision making that is being used by the family (e.g., use cognitive clarification, sorting, sculpting)
4. Help family members express feelings (e.g., use affective clarification, experiential sharing, visualization, fight games)
5. Model decision making and conflict resolution within therapy sessions to show that mak-

ing decisions need not elicit recrimination, anxiety, anger, or fear of abandonment (e.g., use role play, video feedback, cognitive and affective clarification)
6. Explore family members' beliefs, rules, fears, and rights concerning role relationships (e.g., use affective clarification, visualization, interpretation, role play)
7. Help family members identify roles that have currently changed with the change in family membership (e.g., use affective clarification, cognitive clarification, role play)
8. Help family members identify ways that roles may be altered or shared in the future to increase role satisfaction (e.g., use cognitive clarification, affective clarification, interpretation, role play)
8. Point out and clarify incongruent, vague or double-bind messages (e.g., use cognitive clarification, affective clarification)
9. Facilitate ownership of feelings and communication by encouraging "I" statements and speaking only for one's self (e.g., use affective clarification, projective drawings)

Evaluation. The family should be included in estimating the degree of achievement of long-term and short-term outcomes. The family needs to feel satisfied with changes in the family situation concerning decision making, role relationships, and expression of feelings.

▶ Techniques of native healers
Native healers also use techniques to resolve family conflict and reduce family tension. These techniques usually (a) identify the source of the problem as supernatural vengeance for a transgression that may have been committed by any one in the extended family and/or (b) enlist the entire family in the implementation of the technique. Healing techniques thereby serve to reincorporate the troubled person into the extended family network. Because the cause of problems is viewed as spiritual rather than emotional, treatment enlists supernatural forces. Healing techniques may facilitate resolution of family schism, promote socially acceptable behavior, and/or reinforce interpersonal bonds. Table 14-5 gives examples of healing techniques that

TABLE 14-5 Native healing techniques

Technique	Explanation	Purpose
Divination	Native healer reaches a judgment about the future or about a problem through the interpretation of signs from a deity or protective spirit. Various techniques may be used, such as the reading of cowrie shells or coconut rinds.	Reinforce interpersonal bonds and resolve family schism
Blessings and prayers	Family member(s) are directed to pray, or the native healer prays or blesses family member(s)	Promote socially acceptable behavior and resolve family schism
Directives and advice	Family member(s) are told to carry out specific rituals, cleansings, repetitive prayers, routines of daily living, or other courses of action	Promote socially acceptable behavior and resolve family schism
Rituals	Native healer and family member(s) participate in activities dependent for success on contact with supernatural forces. Rites may involve plants and herbs, trance, animal sacrifice, and/or exorcism.	Resolve family schism and reinforce interpersonal bonds

Sources consulted include McGoldrick et al. (1982) and Kakar (1982).

facilitate these aims. The way that the techniques are carried out varies from culture to culture.

Maria Sanchez appeared apathetic, listless, depressed, and withdrawn. She had no appetite and she ate little food. When she slept, she was restless and she had nightmares. The Sanchez family believed that Maria's tonalli (soul) had been claimed by an evil spirit and that she was suffering from susto *(magical fright). They brought Maria to a* curandero *who would perform the culturally prescribed* limpia *ritual.*

The purpose of the limpia *was to reclaim Maria's soul. Maria and her extended family members participated in the* limpia. *Spirit forms were cut from bark paper. These bark paper forms were used both to absorb evil spirits and to protect the participants at the* limpia *from evil spirits. A chicken was sacrificed. After the* limpia, *Maria's behavior improved and she once again became a functioning member of her family.*

The ritual techniques of a *curandero* accomplish the same ends as the techniques of the family ther-

apist. A *curandero* acknowledges that a person is suffering from *susto* (also known as *espanto*, a culture-bound syndrome found among Central Americans). *Susto* is related to stress engendered by a self-perceived failure to fulfill sex-role expectations. Once a person is identified as suffering from *susto*, he or she is relieved of normal sex-role expectations and is made the focus of extended family attention. Although the *susto* sufferer is the identified client, *susto* indicates that there is a schism in the extended family. The culturally prescribed *limpia* ritual is a process for resolving the schism (all family members participate) and reincorporating the *susto* sufferer into the extended family (Hernandez et al., 1976). Thus, like the techniques of family therapists, the techniques that native healers use may serve to ease family tension and to resolve family conflicts.

• • •

It is important that nurses recognize that family dysfunction must be understood and treated within its cultural contex. Family therapists and native healers share many similarities. Native healers should not be viewed as charlatans. In fact, the World Health Organization has recommended that Third World nations revive and expand their traditional health care systems. It has also been suggested that native healers and psychotherapists coexist and, whenever possible, work together so that the problems of families may be understood and treated within their cultural contexts.

Nursing Intervention
PRIMARY PREVENTION

The focus of primary prevention is on the promotion and maintenance of healthy patterns of family interaction and functioning—on what family members say, on what they do, and on how they interact with one another in various situations. Nurses engaged in family-centered nursing function as teachers. They educate families, both family units and individual family members, about the following:

1. Potential sources of family stress
2. Effective coping patterns for dealing with stress
3. Life-style changes that may decrease family vulnerability to stress
4. Revision of family roles to accommodate maturational and situational changes in life-style
5. Family strengths that may support family functioning
6. Family weaknesses that may jeopardize family functioning (Jones and Dimond, 1982)

To engage in primary prevention activities with families, nurses need to understand the theories* that explain family functioning. Structural theory will help nurses understand the basic functions of a family. Interactional theory will help nurses identify dynamics of interaction among family members. Multigenerational theory will aid nurses in recognizing family needs and tasks over time. Ecosystem theory will help nurses understand the family in its holistic, multilevel context.

In addition to understanding family theory, nurses should be knowledgeable about stressors and their potential impact on family functioning. Nurses can then assist families in anticipating, preparing for, and ameliorating the effects of stressors on the functioning of the family.* For example, parent-child nurses and community health nurses may help parents anticipate the effect that the birth of a baby or the incorporation of a grandparent into the household may have on their marital relationship and on the needs, tasks, and interactions of other members. Strengths on which the family may rely and weaknesses from which the family needs protection may also be identified.

When a family has experienced a stressor, the nurse's role in primary prevention is to ameliorate the impact of the event so that it does not precipitate family dysfunction. For example, if the mother of a family has a mastectomy, the nurse may refer her to Reach to Recovery or to other mastectomy support groups. If a family member dies, the nurse may refer other family members to such grief support groups as widows and widowers groups (for bereaved mates) and The Compassionate Friends (for bereaved parents). Referrals to such self-help groups assist family members in coping with family stressors. Families are thereby helped to maintain equilibrium and to avoid dysfunction.

Moreover, knowledge about the influences of culture on family form and family dynamics is vital if nurses are to promote culturally acceptable patterns of family functioning. Should the cultural context not be considered, nurses might mistake culturally acceptable family functioning for family dysfunction.

Nurses in the labor and delivery suite of a hospital whose catchment area included Chinese and Japanese enclaves observed that American and Asian fathers-to-be behaved very differently. Most of the American men either coached their wives through labor and delivery or waited in the solarium until their wives had delivered. In contrast, most of the Asian men brought their wives to the hospital and then returned home to await the birth of their children. The

---

*Refer to Chapter 5 for a discussion of family theory.

*See Chapter 15 for a discussion of the nurse's role in anticipatory guidance and crisis intervention.

nurses thought the Asian parents-to-be were "emotionally divorced," and they began to regard the Asian families as dysfunctional.

Only after conferring with a nurse-anthropologist were these nurses able to understand that in the Chinese and Japanese cultures, women have traditionally assisted women during childbirth. Men traditionally have been uninvolved. The reasons for this sex-role behavior include: (1) Chinese and Japanese men and women usually do not openly express emotion in public; (2) traditionally, Chinese and Japanese men view childbirth as women's work; (3) Chinese and Japanese women usually would be embarrassed to have their husbands present during the functioning of the female body.

Instead of promoting the culturally approved patterns of family functioning, the nurses had viewed the noninvolvement of Asian fathers-to-be and the absence of the expression of emotion between Asian spouses as evidence of emotional divorce. The nurses had identified family dysfunction where there was none. Their lack of knowledge about the cultural context of client-families had led them to inaccurately assess family functioning.

Understanding of family theory, family stressors, and cultural influences on the family system is therefore essential if nurses are going to promote and maintain healthy patterns of family interaction and functioning.

In addition, because overcrowding, poverty, and scarcity of resources may act as sociocultural stressors on the family system, nurses need to be aware of changes in local and national social programs. Nurses, as informed citizens and as client advocates, need to militate for social change. When budgets are streamlined, money for social services is usually cut. Yet this type of economizing often contributes to family stress. Promoting social changes that prevent socioeconomic stress or improve living conditions for families is an essential component of primary prevention of family dysfunction. Toward this end, Friedmann (1987) suggests that nurse clinicians and nurse researchers work together on applied research projects that are aimed at preventing family dysfunction in vulnerable families.

SECONDARY PREVENTION

The focus of secondary prevention is on intervention into family dysfunction and restoration of functional patterns of family behavior. Knowledge about principles of family therapy helps nurses understand the dynamics that contribute to family dysfunction. The symptoms of individuals are seen as developing from and feeding back into relational struggles and conflicts within the family system. The goal of nursing care is to help family members function more effectively in their role relationships and interactions.

Nursing process

The nursing process provides the framework for intervention with client-families. (See Table 14-6.)

ASSESSMENT

When nurses assess families, they need to consider the multifaceted contexts in which families exist. Family functioning and mental health are outcomes of many levels of interrelatedness: individual family members with each other and with the family as a unit, the family with other social systems, and individual family members with other social systems. Table 14-8 illustrates some of the factors that Van Servellen (1984) believes may lead to family dysfunction.

The following family process assessment guide has a threefold purpose: It has been designed to assist nurses in assessing a family's functioning, in establishing goals, and in developing nursing strategies consistent with the family's cultural orientation.

    1. Demographic data*
       a. Names of family members
       b. Ages of members
       c. Sexes of members
       d. Relationship between members: affinal; consanguinal
       e. Educational levels of members
       f. Occupations of members

---

*When time for assessment is limited these factors should be assessed first. Other factors can be assessed as the nurse is working with the family.

TABLE 14-6   Use of nursing process with families

Step of nursing process	Aim	Nursing activities
Assessment	Obtain information from verbal and nonverbal family communication	Gather information about the family's • perception of the problem • interaction patterns • role relationships • strengths and limitations • present environment (physical and social) • holistic health status of family members • factors that precipitated the problem • interaction patterns between the nurse and individual family members and the family as a unit
	Verify the data	Confirm observations and perceptions through consensual validation or by obtaining additional information from family members or other sources (e.g., family photograph album, genogram) Chart family assessment data
Analysis of data	Understand the nature of the family's dysfunction	Identify family dynamics, family role relationships, and family stressors Identify the interrelationship between family dynamics, family role relationships, predisposing and precipitating factors, holistic health status of family members, and the family's perception of the problem Formulate a nursing diagnosis that states both the family's dysfunction and the contributing cr related factor (see Table 14-7: NANDA diagnoses that apply to family therapy)
Planning	Develop a plan of action for initiating family change or for enabling a family to better cope with a problem	Refer the family to a family therapist. Nurses who work with families in community or institutional settings but who are not family therapists should not attempt to provide family therapy. After assessing a family, analyzing the data, and making a nursing diagnosis concerning family functioning, these nurses should refer the family for counseling. Nurses who are family therapists should: • determine the family's locus of decision making • in accordance with the locus of decision making, (1) assist or support the family in establishng outcomes (e.g., husband and wife will renegotiate roles; parents will utilize existing support systems) (2) assist or support the family in establishing priorities among outcomes (3) assist the family to differentiate between long-term and short-term outcomes
	Design and modify a care plan that is consistent with the family's beliefs and orientations	Anticipate family needs on the basis of its outcome priorities and the life stages of family members Include all family members in the development of intervention strategies. It is important that all persons who are defined as family members be included (e.g., extended kin, fictive kin)

TABLE 14-6   Use of nursing process with families—cont'd

Step of nursing process	Aim	Nursing activities
Implementation	Counsel the family	Plan strategies that are congruent with the life stages of family members, the life-cycle stage of the family, and the cultural orientation of the family
		Identify family therapy approaches to be used for specific types of family dysfunction (e.g., teach the family new scripts for family relationships; help the family clarify rules that govern family interaction)
		Provide an environment where the family can express their concerns and engage in problem solving
		Facilitate trust among family members
		Help the family identify stressors
		Help the family evaluate current patterns of coping and communication
		Support effective patterns of coping and communication and/or teach new coping and communication behaviors
		Facilitate self-expression among family members if this is consistent with their cultural orientation
		Provide information or clarify misconceptions (e.g., a child may feel responsible for her father's incestuous behavior; a wife may feel she is the cause of her husband's abusiveness. These misconceptions should be clarified. Information about protective services and shelters should be given)
		Refer the family as a unit or refer individual family members to appropriate community resources (e.g., legal services, social services, support groups)
		Support family members in their decision making
Evaluation	Include family members in estimating the family's progress in achieving outcomes	Family members are able to listen to feedback without becoming defensive
		Family members are able to ask each other for clarification of vague or ambiguous communication
		Family members are able to offer feedback to each other instead of being resentful, blaming, or derogating
		Family members are able to state expectations of each other, ways that these expectations may be met, and any unmet expectations
		Family members are able to differentiate between their intentions and the ways that others perceive their behavior.
		Identify outcomes that need to be modified or revised
		Evaluate the effectiveness of family therapy approaches
		Identify aspects of family therapy approaches that need to be modified or revised
		Bridge the family to support systems other than the family therapy relationship such as
		• people in the social environment (e.g., friends, clergy, relatives, native healers) who are willing to serve as support systems for the family
		• community agencies that offer help with problems that the family may encounter in the future (e.g., agencies that offer services to families experiencing maturational or situational crises)

TABLE 14-7 Examples of primary NANDA diagnoses that apply to family therapy

Primary NANDA diagnosis	Definition
Altered parenting	Inability of nurturer(s) to provide an environment that will facilitate the optimal growth and development of a child
Potential altered parenting	Possibility of disruption of ability of nurturer(s) to provide an environment that will facilitate the optimal growth and development of a child
Altered family processes	Dysfunction in a normally functioning family system as a response to situational or maturational crisis
Ineffective family coping: disabling; ineffective family coping: compromised	Patterns of family coping characterized by inadequate, ineffective, or compromised support behaviors (psychosocial, physical, cognitive, or spiritual) in response to internal or external stressors
Family coping: potential for growth	A state of effective coping characterized by desire and readiness for a higher level of wellness and functioning

g. Ethnicity (optional)†
h. Religion (optional)†
i. Other (describe)
2. Family organization*
a. Type of family: nuclear; extended; blended; single-parent
b. Type of system: open; closed; boundary-maintaining mechanisms (describe); norms; rules
c. Members involved in child rearing
d. Members vested with authority
e. Sense of obligation among family members
f. Family roles: peacemaker; protector; attacker; provider; interpreter; rescuer; other
g. Sex-defined roles: stereotyped male-female relationships; amount of independence permitted men and women
h. Other (describe)
3. Family world view
a. Relationship to people: individualistic; group oriented; egalitarian; authoritarian
b. Relationship to time: past oriented; present oriented; future oriented

c. Relationship to the world: personal control; goal directed; fatalistic
d. Other (describe)
4. Family spiritual orientation
a. Ideology
(1) Nature of belief in a supernatural being or supernormal energy
(2) Nature of belief in communion between a supernatural being or supernormal energy and people alive or dead
(3) Conceptualizations about the quality of life and the quality of death
(4) Nature of belief in life after death
b. Inner life
(1) Frequency and type of inner-life activity (meditation, yoga, prayer)
(2) Interrelationship between family members' spiritual life and the other parts of their life (for example, family meditates when under stress; family prays when in trouble)
c. Other (describe)
5. Family perceptions and definitions
a. Family
b. Privacy
c. Intimacy
d. Health (mental and physical)
e. Illness (mental and physical)
f. Presenting family problem (for example, which family members identify a prob-

*When time for assessment is limited these factors should be assessed first. Other factors can be assessed as the nurse is working with the family.
†Legislation protects people from being required to reveal ethnicity and religion.

TABLE 14-8 Factors contributing to family dysfunction

Factor	Example
Psychophysiological alteration in an individual family member	Parents have recently learned that their 5-year-old son has leukemia
Alteration in family group process	Wife criticizes her husband for not earning enough money to support the family; husband responds by blaming the family's financial problems on his wife's spending habits
Disjunction in interrelatedness between the family and other social systems	A family uses a folk medical system and brings their son, who has cancer, to a native healer instead of to a medical doctor
Alteration in family communication evidenced by failure to transmit and/or reinforce cultural values	Parents experience role overburdening and do not inculcate in their children such values as respect for elders and responsibility to and for the family
Disjunction between the family and specific characteristics of the community in which they live	An immigrant family is accustomed to the practice of unmarried women being chaperoned on dates. They continue this custom with their adolescent daughter even after moving to the United States.

lem; clarification of discrepant views of the problem)

    g. Other (describe)

6. Family health care patterns

    a. Ideas concerning causes of illness (mental and physical)

    b. Ideas concerning treatment of illness (mental and physical)

    c. People consulted in times of crisis or for treatment of mental and physical illnesses (family member; native healer; mental health therapist; clergyman; pharmacist; physician; other)

    d. Other (describe)

7. Family living arrangements

    a. Type of residence: multifamily dwelling; single-family dwelling; one-room dwelling; other

    b. Environment of residence: urban; suburban; rural; inter-ethnic neighborhood; ethnic enclave

    c. Time in residence: length of time in present residence; length of time in previous residences

    d. Family members living in another household (describe relationship)

    e. Persons other than family members living in the household (describe living arrangements).

    f. Sleeping arrangements: number of rooms serving as bedrooms (differentiate between rooms functioning solely as bedrooms and those that have other functions); family members sharing bedrooms; family members not sharing bedrooms

    g. Eating arrangements: family members eat together; eat alone; eat in shifts

    h. Privacy arrangements: rooms or sections of rooms reserved for specific family members; furniture (for example, chairs) reserved for specific family members

    i. Other (describe)

8. Family interaction patterns*

    a. Communication patterns

      (1) Verbal

        (a) Language spoken at home

        (b) Language spoken outside home

      (2) Kinesic

        (a) Touching

        (b) Gesturing

      (3) Proxemic

        (a) Interpersonal spacing

        (b) Fixed and/or built space

---

*When time for assessment is limited these factors should be assessed first. Other factors can be assessed as the nurse is working with the family.

(4) Themes
  (a) Double-bind messages
  (b) Manipulation
  (c) Scapegoating
  (d) Intellectualization
  (e) Blame placing
  (f) Validation
  (g) Other (describe)
b. Behavior patterns
  (1) Physical acting out
  (2) Isolation
  (3) Differentiation
  (4) Cooperation
  (5) Competition
  (6) Overdependence
  (7) Other (describe)
c. Social patterns
  (1) Alliances
    (a) Among family members
    (b) Between family members and members of social network
    (c) Conflict between alliances
    (d) Resolution of conflict between alliances
  (2) Dissemination of information
    (a) Sources of information
    (b) Patterns of communicating information
  (3) Social interaction
    (a) Social network: relatives; friends; employers; coworkers; neighbors; clergy; other (describe)
    (b) Community involvement: school; church; labor union; neighborhood; other (describe)
    (c) Patterns of recreation
    (d) Patterns of intimacy
  (4) Other (describe)
9. Family role relationships*
  a. Authority
    (1) Nominal authority figure(s)
    (2) Actual authority figure(s)
    (3) Patterns of authority
    (4) Implementation of authority: direct; delegated

b. Decision making
  (1) Nominal decision-making figure(s)
  (2) Actual decision-making figure(s)
  (3) Patterns of decision making
  (4) Implementation of decisions
c. Regulatory
  (1) Peacemaker figure(s)
  (2) Protector figure(s)
  (3) Interpreter figure(s)
  (4) Attacker figure(s)
  (5) Domineering figure(s)
  (6) Submissive figure(s)
d. Other (describe)
10. Family stressors*
  a. Changes in family membership: loss of a member through divorce, separation, death, or hospitalization or addition of a member through birth, adoption, or incorporation (for example, grandparents move into the household)
  b. Sociocultural strains: environmental pressures such as inadquate support systems, community disorganization, discrimination, inadequate housing, culture shock, and poverty
  c. Maturational events: transitions between developmental stages, such as marriage, entrance of a child into school, and retirement
  d. Disordered family relationships: imbalance in the internal structure of the family; related to such factors as double-bind communication, parental overburdening, overbonding to the family, and psychosomatogenesis
  e. Other (describe)
  f. No significant stress
11. Family coping mechanisms*
  a. Coping mechanisms used (indicate whether mechanisms are used only by specific family members)
  b. Effectiveness of coping mechanisms
  c. Family's perception of mechanisms that are effective in reducing stress
  d. Other (describe)

---

*When time for assessment is limited these factors should be assessed first. Other factors can be assessed as the nurse is working with the family.

*When time for assessment is limited these factors should be assessed first. Other factors can be assessed as the nurse is working with the family.

12. Family resources*
    a. Familial: interests; leisure time activities; physical and mental abilities; other
    b. Socioeconomic: interpersonal support systems; economic support systems (health insurance, sick leave, union benefits); food, shelter, clothing; other

TERTIARY PREVENTION

Families may have to continue to exist in environments that contributed to the development of family dysfunction. After the termination of family therapy, ongoing support in the form of *rehabilitative* services may be needed. Tertiary prevention programs are available in the following areas:

1. Educational training. Depending on the ages, interests, and abilities of family members, continued education, including college and vocational training (or retraining), may be indicated. Education increases self-esteem and prepares family members to be as financially self-reliant as their potential permits. This may help to reduce the impact of chronic sociocultural stressors on family functioning and to limit the degree of family dysfunction.

2. Self-help groups. Some self-help groups function to limit the degree of dysfunction in already dysfunctional families. Such groups are composed of people who have learned or who are learning to cope with chronic stressors and with family dysfunction. For example, after divorce (a type of family dysfunction), Parents Without Partners helps single parents to cope with the social and emotional demands of parenting and to avoid parental overburdening, thereby preventing the development of further family dysfunction. Spouse support groups and Parents Anonymous offer help to abusive family members. Support groups are also available for the victims of family abuse and for families with mentally ill members.

3. Voluntary rehabilitation groups. The purpose of voluntary rehabilitation groups is similar to that of self-help groups. What differentiates them from self-help groups is that their members may not have experienced the same stressors that the client families have experienced. The Salvation Army and the St. Vincent de Paul Society are examples of voluntary rehabilitation groups. Emergency aid in the form of financial assistance, housing, and food is usually available. In addition, counseling, assistance in finding employment and housing, work projects, and leisure time activities may be offered. Family abuse shelters may be operated by religious, quasi-religious, or secular groups. Such shelters not only offer temporary assistance for battered family members, but often also bridge family members to agencies that provide economic assistance, legal services, support groups and assertiveness training programs. Thus, voluntary rehabilitation groups help to reduce the impact of chronic life-style stressors on family functioning and to limit the degree of family dysfunction.

CHAPTER SUMMARY

Throughout the United States, there is a growing tendency to view the family rather than the individual as the client of choice for the delivery of health care. To effectively work with families, nurses need to become knowledgeable about family organization and family process.

The family is a system and has the properties of any social system. As the family interacts with other social systems in its context, it may become vulnerable to stressors that affect family structure and function. Chief among these stressors are changes in family membership, sociocultural strains, maturational events, and disordered family relationships. Combinations of these stressors may interrelate as they influence family functioning.

Several models of family therapy may be used with dysfunctional families. These models are the structural model, the interactional model, the multigenerational model, and the ecosystem model. However, nurses should be aware that cultural presuppositions may be inherent in some aspects of these models. It is important for nurses to be mind-

---

*When time for assessment is limited these factors should be assessed first. Other factors can be assessed as the nurse is working with the family.

ful of the culture-bound aspects of family therapy models so that their assessments, interpretations, and goals will not be value laden. Whenever possible, family therapists and native healers not only should coexist but also should collaborate to ensure that family dysfunction will be understood and treated within its sociocultural context.

Nurses who work with families may engage in activities of primary, secondary, and/or tertiary prevention of family dysfunction. Primary preven-

tion focuses on the promotion and maintenance of healthy patterns of family interaction and functioning. The focus of secondary prevention is intervention into family dysfunction and restoration of functional patterns of family behavior. The nursing process provides the framework for intervention with client-families. Tertiary prevention focuses on limiting the degree of family dysfunction and providing rehabilitative services.

SELF-DIRECTED LEARNING

Sensitivity-Awareness Exercises

The purpose of these exercises are to:
- Develop awareness about the vulnerability of your own family and of client-families to stress
- Develop awareness about the interrelationship between families and their context (physical, emotional, cultural, and social)
- Develop awareness about your own feelings and attitudes when working with dysfunctional families

1. Using the family process assessment guide in this chapter, assess the dynamics, strengths, limitations, stressors, coping patterns, health care patterns, and sociocultural orientations (toward family, privacy, intimacy, health, illness, and spirituality) of your own family. On the basis of this assessment, discuss your evaluation of your family's functioning. What level(s) of prevention (primary, secondary, and/or tertiary) are indicated? Repeat this exercise, this time assessing a client-family.

2. Look at the nature of stressors that have impaired or that are presently impairing the structure and functioning of your own family system. How did your family cope with each stress situation? How did the stress affect the ability of individual family members, including yourself, to accomplish their developmental tasks? How did the responses of each family member to the stress situation affect the responses of other family members?

3. Use one or more of the following techniques to describe the conflicts and alliances in your family system: sculpting (constructing a live family portrait), drawing a family picture, role playing.

4. Use the following self-assessment tool to become more aware of your own feelings and attitudes about working with dysfunctional families:
   a. What personal needs of my own do I try to meet when I work with dysfunctional families?
   b. When I work with dysfunctional families, to what extent do I feel helpless? Frustrated? Angry? Pity? Overwhelmed?
   c. How do my feelings vary according to the stressors the family is encountering? According to the family's coping patterns?
   d. To what extent do I try to cope with my feelings by avoiding the client-family? Blaming the client-family? Pushing the client-family to make a decision or to implement a decision?
   e. To what extent do I focus on the problems and limitations of the client-family?
   f. To what extent do I focus on the strengths and resources of the client-family?

Questions to Consider

1. Families may experience stressors that impair family functioning and structure. Retirement of a family member is an example of which type of stressor?
   a. Change in family membership
   b. Maturational event
   c. Emotional divorce
   d. Situational event
2. In assessing a family's functioning, a nurse determined that the parents often conveyed one message verbally and a conflicting message nonverbally. This pattern of communication is referred to as

SELF-DIRECTED LEARNING—cont'd

a. Pseudomutuality
b. Tangentiality
c. Vagueness
d. Double-bind communication

3. A clinical nurse specialist was working with a dysfunctional family. The nurse's goal was to help the family clarify the rules that governed their family relationships. The nurse was following which model of family therapy?
a. Interactional model
b. Multigenerational model
c. Structural model
d. Ecosystem model

4. Mr. and Mrs. Foster have little emotional involvement with one another, but they are "staying together for the sake of the children." Their pathological pattern of relating is referred to as
a. Pseudomutuality
b. Emotional divorce
c. Scapegoating
d. Mystification

5. A community health nurse conducts family life classes for young adults. These classes cover potential sources of family stress, life-style changes that may decrease family vulnerability to stress, and effective coping patterns for dealing with stress. The community health nurse is engaging in which level of preventive intervention?
a. Primary
b. Secondary
c. Tertiary

Match each of the following terms with the statement that is associated with it:

6. Pseudomutuality
7. Structural model of family therapy
8. Ecosystem model of family therapy
9. Sculpting
10. Scripting

a. Constructing a live family portrait that depicts family alliances and conflicts
b. Ecological orientation, layering of contexts, network relationships
c. Developing new family transaction patterns
d. Surface harmony and agreement cover family conflicts and confusing family communication
e. Scripts, generic constraints, idiosyncratic constraints

Answer key

1. b	6. d
2. d	7. e
3. a	8. b
4. b	9. a
5. a	10. c

REFERENCES

Aguilera DC and Messick JM: Crisis intervention: theory and methodology, ed 5, St. Louis, 1989, The CV Mosby Co.

Arnold J and Gemma PG: A child dies: a portrait of family grief, Rockville, Md, 1983, Aspen.

Auerswald EH: Interdisciplinary versus ecological approach, Family Process 7:205-215, 1968.

Bowen M: Family therapy in clinical practice, New York, 1978, Jason Aronson, Inc.

Cooney TM et al: Parental divorce in young adulthood: some preliminary findings, Am J Orthopsychiatr 56(3):470-477, 1986.

Critchley DL: The child as patient: assessing the effects of family stress and disruption on the mental health of the child, Persp Psychiatr Care 11(5 and 6):144-155, 1981.

Friedemann ML: Families of unemployed workers: need for nursing intervention and prevention, Arch Psychiatr Nurs 1(2):81-89, 1987.

Haley J: Problem-solving therapy: new strategies for effective family therapy, San Francisco, 1976, Jossey-Bass.

Hernandez, CA, Haug MJ, and Wagner NN, editors: Chicanos: social and psychological perspectives, St. Louis, 1976, The CV Mosby Co.

Hoffman L: Foundations of family therapy, New York, 1981, Basic Books.

Johnson SL, Klee L, and Schmidt C: Conceptions of parentage

and kinship among children of divorce, Am Anthropol 90(1):136-144, 1988.

Jones SL and Dimond M: Family theory and family therapy models: comparative review with implications for nursing practice, J Psychiatr Nurs Mental Health Services 20(10):12-19, 1982.

Kakar S: Shamans, mystics and doctors, New York, 1982, Alfred A. Knopf.

Keeney B: Ecosystemic epistemology: an alternative paradigm for diagnosis, Family Process 18:117-129, 1979.

Klein DC and Ross AR: Kindergarten entry: a study of role transition. In Pared H, editor: Crisis intervention: selected readings, New York, 1965, Family Service Association of America.

Lee E: A social systems approach to assessment and treatment for Chinese American families, In McGoldrick M et al, editors: Ethnicity and family therapy, New York, 1982, The Guilford Press.

Madanes C: Strategic family therapy, San Francisco, Calif, 1984, Jossey-Bass.

McGoldrick M: Irish families, In McGoldrick M, Pearce JK, and Giordano J, editors: Ethnicity and family therapy, New York, 1982, The Guilford Press.

McGoldrick M, Pearce JK, and Giordano J, editors: Ethnicity and family therapy, New York, 1982, The Guilford Press.

Miller J: Cultural and class values in family process, J Marital Family Ther 7(4):467-473, 1981.

Minuchin S: Families and family therapy, Cambridge, Mass, 1974, Harvard University Press.

Minuchin S, Rosman B, and Baker L: Psychosomatic families, Cambridge, Mass, 1978, Harvard University Press.

Pasquali EA: Assimilation and acculturation of Cubans on Long Island, Ph.D. Dissertation, State University of New York at Stony Brook, 1982.

Rotunno M and McGoldrick M: Italian families, In McGoldrick M, Pearce JK, and Giordano J, editors: Ethnicity and family therapy, New York, 1982, The Guilford Press.

Satir V: Family systems and approaches to family therapy, In Erickson GD, and Hogan TP, editors: Family therapy: an introduction to theory and technique, Monterey, Calif, 1972, Brooks/Cole Publishing Co.

Scheflen AE and Scheflen A: Body language and social order, Englewood Cliffs, NJ, 1972, Prentice-Hall, Inc.

Searles, HF: Collected papers on schizophrenia and related subjects, New York, 1965, International Universities Press.

Sturkie K: Framework for comparing approaches to family therapy, Soc Casework 67(10):613-621, 1986.

Van Servellen GM: Group and family therapy: a model for psychotherapeutic nursing practice, St. Louis, 1984, The CV Mosby Co.

Wallerstein JS: Children of divorce: the psychological tasks of the child, Am J Orthopsychiatr 53(2):230-243, 1983.

Wallerstein JS and Kelly J: Surviving the breakup: how children and parents cope with divorce, New York, 1980, Basic Books.

ANNOTATED SUGGESTED READINGS

Friedemann ML: Families of unemployed workers: need for nursing intervention and prevention, Arch Psychiatr Nurs 1(2):81-89, 1987.

This study found that paternal unemployment in combination with other types of persistent family stress may contribute to children being more withdrawn or more assertive in their peer relationships. Implications for nursing such as assessment of children's behavior with peers and recognition of the influence of unemployment on parental emotional status, the marital relationship, and the total family stress experience are discussed. Recommendations are made for prevention of family dysfunction in vulnerable families.

van Servellen GM: Group and family therapy: a model for psychotherapeutic nursing practice, St. Louis, 1984, The CV Mosby Co.

This book presents a contextual framework of nursing practice that can be used with both groups and families. The book is divided into four units: Unit 1 presents a conceptual framework for nursing practice in group and family work, Unit 2 explores the scope of nursing practice in group and family work, Unit 3 discusses basic interventions in group and family work, and Unit 4 presents special considerations for group and family work.

FURTHER READINGS

Byng-Halc J: Scripts and legends in families and family therapy, Family Process 27(2):167-179, 1988.

Fife BL: Model for predicting the adaptation of families to medical crisis: an analysis of role integration, Image 27(4):108-112, 1985.

Johnson, HC: Emerging concerns in family therapy, Social Work 31(4):299-306, 1986.

Morofka V: Marital therapy from a systems approach, Persp Psychiatr Care 22(4):145-148, 1984.

Resnikoff RO: Teaching family therapy: ten key questions for understanding the family as patient, J Marital Family Ther 7(2):135-142, 1981.

Stierlin H: Systemic optionism—systemic pessimism: two perspectives on change, Family Process 27(2):121-127, 1988.

Thiederman SB: Workshops in cross-cultural health care: the challenge of ethnographic dynamite, J Cont Ed Nurs 19(1):25-27, 1988.

Tomm K: Interventive interviewing, part III: intending to ask lineal, circular, strategic, or reflexine questions? Family Process, 27(1):1-15, 1988.

Zaslow MJ: Sex differences in children's responses to parental divorce, part I: research methodology and postdivorce family forums, Am J Orthopsychiatr 58(3):355-378, 1988.

CHAPTER 15

Crisis intervention

CHAPTER FOCUS

Crisis can be viewed as an integral component of everyday life situations. Crisis may be growth promoting and has the capacity to enhance one's self-esteem through the use of effective problem solving. A crisis may be situational, maturational, or social. One type of crisis may be compounded by another at any given time. Response to crisis depends on many factors: perception of the precipitating event and its impact on the future, available support systems, repertoire of effective coping strategies, personal vulnerabilities and emotional support.

Crisis theory provides a conceptual framework from which to provide active intervention. The methodology of crisis intervention follows a sequence of steps similar to the nursing process. Assessment of the presenting issues is made through data collection, and a plan is determined. Strategies are implemented, and evaluation is an ongoing process. Ego defenses are supported while more adaptive strategies are explored.

Nurses function as part of the interdisciplinary team in the use of crisis intervention as a therapeutic modality. Nurses may employ crisis techniques in their work with high-risk groups such as clients with chronic diseases, new parents, and bereaved persons. Crisis intervention techniques are not restricted to outpatient settings. They are effective in all units of general hospitals as well as in community settings. Nurses may also use crisis intervention in dealing with intragroup staff issues and client management issues.

CRISIS THEORY AND INTERVENTION
History

The philosophical base of crisis theory can be found in the works of Freud and others in the psychoanalytic movement. Freud noted that individuals' current behaviors are influenced by their genetic past. Early life experiences have a profound effect on later development. He also noted that individuals who were able to identify and mobilize coping strategies to resolve their conflicts were more likely to experience satisfaction in their lives. The psychoanalytic model, with its individualized approach, was helpful in assisting clients in their adaptation to stressful situations. The process of analysis was very costly, lengthy, and available to only a limited number of individuals.

The early 1940s saw the emergence of preventive psychiatry with its focus on maintenance of mental health and the prevention of mental illness. It was at this time that therapists in the field began to use certain psychoanalytic techniques such as catharsis and empathic listening to facilitate individuals' healthy resolution of stressful experiences.

One of the leaders in the development of crisis theory was Eric Lindemann. His comprehensive study (1944) of bereavement following the Coconut Grove fire in Boston in 1943 laid the groundwork for our current understanding of the grieving process. He determined that there was a well-defined sequence of responses that bereaved individuals experienced following that catastrophic event. His observations revealed both physiological and psychological symptomatology. Lindemann's study further revealed that morbid grief reactions might also occur under certain circumstances. The morbid grief response represents a distortion of the acute grief response. He suggested that the most frequent distortion was that of a delayed reaction, which occurs, for example, sometime after the individual is confronted with a significant loss and at a time when he or she is facing other, more significant tasks. Lindemann (1944) presents the example of a young girl who lost her parents and her boyfriend in the fire and was seriously burned herself. During the course of her hospitalization she showed no signs of distress until approximately the tenth week, when she began experiencing tightness in her chest, feelings of emptiness, and a preoccupation with her deceased parents. Individuals may also attempt to hurry their way through the grieving process or to deny their grief by becoming engrossed in other activities or disposing of possessions of the deceased individuals. Lack of acknowledgement of the sense of loss and the accompanying feelings serves only to distort the grief response and delay reinvolvement with others.

Lindemann's observations defined a sequence of responses to loss that can be applied to any situation where individuals experience loss—whether it be loss of self-worth, of independence, of function, of status, or of a significant person or love object. Individuals throughout the life cycle experience loss at many different points. The significance of Lindemann's work lies in the fact that the knowledge of these stages can enable nursing and other helping professions to facilitate individuals' adaptation to potentially stressful events. Crisis intervention, as Lindemann envisioned it, would provide brief, active, collaborative therapy to mobilize clients' own resources within their own communities. The Wellesley Project was set up by Lindemann and Caplan as a community-wide program designed to provide crisis intervention services.

Concurrently, during World War II soldiers who were experiencing stress-induced reactions were treated immediately at the front rather than being sent back home. These men were able to return to combat and did not need further treatment in an inpatient setting. Glass (1957) substantiated these findings in his observations of troops in the Korean War.

Gerald Caplan (1964) developed a theory of individuals in crisis and defined crisis intervention as a modality of treatment. His major emphasis was on the role that the community and its members play in the prevention of mental illness and maintenance of mental health. Caplan presented the concept of primary, secondary, and tertiary levels of prevention as essential factors in community mental health practice. Primary prevention may be viewed as a two-pronged focus involving social and interpersonal action. Social action directs its attention to social and political groups to generate necessary community reform. Large social issues, such as poverty, inadequate housing, poor educational services, and fragmented or nonexistent health services, are the target of social action intervention. Interpersonal action focuses on individuals and assists them in using effective problem-solving strategies.

Primary preventive techniques include educating individuals and providing consultation and crisis intervention. Education about stressors—physiological, environmental, emotional—assists individuals to modify their lives to reduce or eliminate the effects of those stressors. This concept applies to communities, families, and individuals. For example, recent warnings about dioxin helped public health officials to alert affected communities and to institute screening measures to prevent possible physiological effects in the future. Consultation and crisis intervention can be used with clients and families in the general hospital setting to facilitate their adaptation to the crisis of illness with its concurrent role changes and alterations in body image and independence levels. Individuals are encouraged to identify their own stressors (see the Holmes and Rahe scale in Chapter 8) and pursue strategies to reduce their vulnerability. As individuals' coping strategies increase, their sense of vulnerability decreases. Being aware of potential stressors increases a feeling of control and allows individuals to be managers of their own lives. Other examples of primary preventive strategies include parenting classes for new parents, couples groups for those considering marriage, support groups for women in their middle years, and groups for divorced individuals. Counseling in the form of individual support may also be provided for the above-mentioned groups, as well as for those who are retiring and for those individuals and families who are transferred frequently by employers. Situations that present *potential* crises can be identified and worked through to prevent increased vulnerability. Success, however, depends mainly on the individuals' ability to be responsive by modifying their situations, on their previous coping skills and levels of success, and on their support systems.

Secondary prevention includes actions designed to reduce the number of existing cases by early diagnosis and treatment. In this level, the goal is to provide services that prevent lengthy periods of disability. The assumption can be made that either primary preventive services were unavailable or that the affected individual was unable to benefit from these services. From a nursing perspective, it is important that individuals be assessed accurately and be referred to appropriate resources immediately. Short-term therapy as opposed to prolonged hospitalization focuses on the return of individuals to their communities. Crisis intervention may be viewed as part of secondary prevention in that its goal is the healthy resolution of crisis and the return to at least a precrisis level of functioning.

Tertiary prevention involves techniques to reduce the long-term effects of mental disability. Rehabilitation programs are a way to assist individuals to return to their previous occupations and social roles or to enable them to learn new skills. Crisis intervention is an integral component of tertiary prevention—individuals are assisted in developing new methods of coping with stress and reaching their maximum rehabilitative states.

The evolution of community psychiatry and crisis theory was further influenced by the Report of the Joint Commission on Mental Health and Mental Illness (1961). The book *Action for Mental Health* documented the need for short-term crisis-oriented services based in the community. It noted a dearth of services, long waiting lists, and inappropriate, expensive therapies. The report further stated that 42% of people in crisis went to their clergymen or their family physicians rather than seeking mental health professionals. Large numbers of people were not receiving services when or where they needed them. The entire mechanism of providing psychiatric services needed revision. Through federal funding in 1963 and 1965, community mental health centers were developed to provide the comprehensive services necessary to meet the needs of large communities within their own community environments. Paraprofessionals or "indigenous workers" were identified as valuable resource persons who could be of great support in crisis situations. Crisis intervention techniques as a short-term problem-solving modality were found to be the appropriate method of treatment. Inpatient and outpatient crisis programs have demonstrated their effectiveness in meeting the needs of the masses and have reduced the need for long-term hospitalization. Crisis intervention as a valid modality of treatment has earned its place in community psychiatry.

Last, the suicide prevention movement, begun in the late 1950s, was spearheaded by the efforts of Norman Farberow and Edwin Schneidman at the Los Angeles Suicide Prevention Center. Their work added to the development of crisis intervention techniques as appropriate strategies for meeting the needs of suicidal clients. As a result of their efforts, the suicide prevention movement grew, as did the number of centers providing crisis intervention services.

Definition of crisis

A crisis is a situation that cannot be readily resolved by an individual's normal repertoire of coping strategies. Anxiety increases, the individual becomes more immobilized, and a sense of disequilibrium results. Crises are time limited in the sense that either positive or negative outcomes result within a 4- to 6-week period. Crises are perceived as threatening and arise from precipitating events usually related to loss (or the *threat* of loss), illness, a change in status such as new responsibilities at work or birth of a child. The event may have occurred recently or within the last few weeks or months, and the individual may not connect the event to the actual crisis situation. It is important to note that crisis is defined by the individual—not all stressful situations are crises. If an individual views a situation as being overwhelmingly stressful, the individual may be unable to resolve the situation, and a crisis results. A state of crisis has growth-promoting potential. It may act as a catalyst to jar old habits and evoke new responses. Crisis has the potential to strengthen an individual's adaptive capacity and sense of self-worth. Crisis intervention as a short-term modality focuses on the resolution of the immediate issue through the mobilization of social, environmental, and intrapersonal resources. All individuals experience crisis throughout life. Reaching out for help in a time of crisis and effecting resolution serves to promote an overall sense of control and well-being. Through this process individuals emerge at an even higher level of functioning than in the precrisis state.

TABLE 15-1 Phases of crisis

Phase	Description
1	Perceived threat acts as a precipitant that generates increased anxiety. Normal coping strategies are activated; if unsuccessful, individual moves into phase 2.
2	Increased disorganization with resulting vulnerability and lack of control. Immobilization or random attempts to control anxiety occur. Unresolved anxiety leads to phase 3.
3	Redefinition of the crisis is attempted. Individual is most amenable to assistance in this phase. New problem-solving measures may also effect a resolution. Return to precrisis level of functioning may occur. If problem solving is unsuccessful, further disorganization occurs in phase 4.
4	Severe to panic levels of anxiety with profound cognitive, emotional, and physiological changes may occur. Referral to further treatment resources is necessary.

Phases of crisis

As a result of his work, Caplan (1964) has delineated four phases of crisis described in Table 15-1.

Factors influencing the perception of crisis

As noted above, a crisis is defined by the individual. Aguilera and Messick (1986) have developed a paradigm that explores several balancing factors that can affect the manner in which a crisis is resolved (see Fig. 15-1). A healthy resolution depends upon the following three factors:

1. Realistic appraisal of the precipitating event. Recognition of the relationship between the event and feelings of anxiety is necessary for

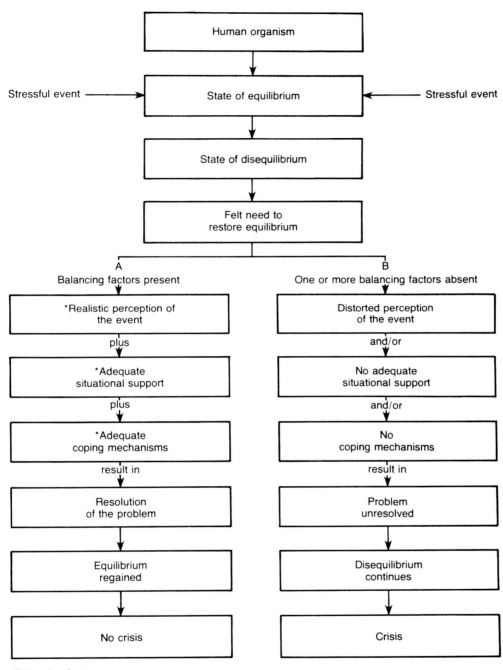

*Balancing factors.

Fig. 15-1 Paradigm: the effect of balancing factors in a stressful event. (From Aguilera DC and Messick JM: Crisis intervention: theory and methodology, ed 5, St. Louis, 1986, The CV Mosby Co.)

effective problem solving to occur. Distortions in perception impair problem solving, thus increasing already high levels of stress.

2. Availability of support systems. It is critical to mobilize existing support systems to prevent feelings of isolation and vulnerability.

3. Availability of coping measures. Over a lifetime, a person develops a repertoire of successful coping strategies that enable him or her to identify and resolve stressful situations. Although these coping strategies may not be successful immediately in new stress-producing situations, the person recognizes that they have succeeded in the past and will do so again.

Crisis proneness

Hendricks (1985) suggests that certain individuals are more prone to crisis than others. The following are characteristics often found in those identified as susceptible to crisis:

1. Dissatisfaction with employment or lack of employment
2. History of unresolved crises
3. History of substance abuse
4. Poor self-esteem; unworthiness
5. Superficial relationships with others
6. Difficulty coping with everyday situations
7. Underuse of available resources and support systems
8. Projection of aloofness and lack of caring and impulsive acts

Increased incidence of crisis may be related to one or more of the characteristics listed above. It is important to note that individual personality traits must also be considered in conjunction with those characteristics. Crisis is defined by the individual; thus, what is a crisis for one is merely an occurrence for another. This factor is a critical component that must be evaluated in relation to crisis-prone characteristics as well as personality traits.

Types of crisis

Initially crisis had been defined as either maturational or situational. Chamberlin (1980) suggested a third category, "unanticipated social crisis,"

which includes catastrophic events involving multiple simultaneous losses. A person may experience more than one crisis at a time. Often a maturational crisis is compounded by a situational crisis. An adolescent who is struggling with his or her changing body image is confronted with the diagnosis of leukemia. The stressors of both crises may be so overwhelming that the individual may find it necessary to seek help.

MATURATIONAL CRISES

Maturational crises can be defined as the predictable processes of growth and development that evolve over a period of time. The ultimate goal of these processes is maturity. Erikson (1963) describes the developmental sequence of the eight stages of man—each of which is characterized by a major task that is resolved on a continuum. The transition points—or those junctures where individuals move into successive stages—often generate disequilibrium. Individuals are required to make cognitive and behavioral changes and to integrate those physical changes that accompany development. The extent to which individuals experience success in the mastery of these tasks depends on previous successes, availability of support systems, influence of role models, and acceptability of the new role by others. Williams (1971) suggests that success in previous transition periods lays the foundation for successes in stages that follow. Unresolved issues cause susceptibility to crisis and influence the ability to cope with the disequilibrium that can accompany transition points. In fact, unresolved dependency issues, for example, may be found as an underlying factor in individuals experiencing depression and gastrointestinal disorders.

Gender-identity confusion may result in an unclear concept of oneself as a sexual being. A person may then have difficulty in establishing intimate relationships with members of the same sex or with members of the opposite sex. Conflict with authority figures may begin in adolescence and later have a profound impact in the young adulthood phase in the form of abusive or acting-out behavior. Any form of conflict, whether it be around the issue of values, sexuality, or dependency, generates anxiety and has the potential for creating a crisis for the individual involved (Baldwin, 1978). Appropriate intervention depends on the determination of the presence of unresolved issues so that further disequilibrium and personality disorganization can be prevented.

Role models who act as mentors function as available support systems as well as examples of the appropriate manner in which to behave as one moves along in the maturational process. Support systems are a crucial factor in responding successfully to the stress associated with transition points. (Each phase requires new, more sophisticated modes of responding that often generate much anxiety.) Individuals need a safe, trusting environment where new roles can be tried out without fear of repercussion or embarrassment.

The transitional periods or events that are most commonly identified as having increased crisis potential are adolescence, marriage, parenthood, midlife, and retirement. This is not to say, however, that crises cannot occur at other transition periods. The following is a case study of a maturational crisis—a crisis of parenthood:

Marian J., a 34-year-old white, single woman presented herself at the mental health clinic two months after the birth of her daughter, Rebecca. Marian stated that she felt depressed most of the time. She described sleeping difficulties, poor appetite, lack of energy, increasing frustration with the baby, and feelings of hopelessness and helplessness. Marian had previously been employed as a fashion designer for a large dress firm in New York City. She was college educated, came from an upper-middle-class Catholic family, and had no siblings. Her parents were currently living in a retirement community in Florida. Further exploration of Marian's situation revealed that she had planned the pregnancy, had no desire to marry the father, and planned to return to work when the infant was 6 months old. Day care facilities were provided by her place of employment. Marian stated tearfully that she had not realized taking care of a baby would require so much time and attention. She felt frustrated when the baby did not adhere to any schedule and seemed to cry a great deal. When asked about support systems, Marian said that her friends and co-workers were supportive of her decision to have the child; however, she felt out of the mainstream of activities. As Marian described it, she "could no longer just pick up and go." Although she had been aware that there would be changes in her routine after the birth of

the baby, she clearly had been unaware of the extent of the impact of the arrival of the child. Marian also stated that her parents were of little support; her father could not understand her decision and refused to talk to her, while her mother expressed a desire to offer assistance. However, her mother felt caught between her father and Marian and therefore decided to remain in Florida "to keep peace."

Assessment. Assessment of Marian's crisis situation revealed difficulty in adjustment to the new role of parent (including unrealistic expectations of self), loss of previous status as an employed person, lack of available support systems, and lack of a role model as possible precipitants of the crisis. Biochemical changes related to the pregnancy also merited exploration as a basis for her responses.

Potential nursing diagnoses. They include the following:

- Social isolation related to lack of direct contact with friends and her parents living in another state. (NANDA 3.1.2.; DSM-III-R 309.90)
- Altered parenting related to feelings of inadequacy as a new mother (NANDA 3.2.1.1.1; DSM-III-R 309.00)
- Altered role performance related to role changes resulting from loss of employment (NANDA 3.2.1; DSM-III-R 309.00, 309.82)

Planning

Long-term outcomes
1. Development of social support systems
2. Development of positive sense of self within the context of the new parenting role

Short-term outcomes
1. Identification of existing social supports
2. Identification of areas of strength as a parent
3. Exploration of methods to increase competence in the parenting role

Implementation

Generic intervention
- Facilitate Marian's movement through the phases of grieving as a healthy response to loss of employment status and change of role.

Individual intervention
- Incorporate *environmental manipulation* by as-

sisting Marian to locate appropriate day-care facilities so that she has time for herself.
- Encourage Marian to reconnect to old friends.
- Identify and support Marian's involvement in a support group for new parents.
- Provide *anticipatory guidance* relative to expected feelings and behaviors that occur within the context of the mothering role.
- Reinforce sense of self-esteem by giving positive feedback regarding mothering behaviors and attempts to reconnect with friends.
- Explore the possibility of communicating with parents.
- Assist Marian to develop more effective methods of coping with stress.
- Discuss options of returning to work on a part-time basis.

Evaluation
- Determine degree of Marian's accomplishment of long-term and short-term outcomes and her need for further intervention.

SITUATIONAL CRISES

A situational crisis is one that is precipitated by an *unanticipated* stressful event that creates disequilibrium by threatening one's sense of biological, social, or psychological integrity (Aguilera and Messick, 1986). The severity of the crisis is, however, determined by the individual's own perception of the situation and the impact of the balancing factors previously discussed. A situational crisis poses the threat of loss—whether it be loss of health, loss of a loved one, or loss of job status through either a promotion or a demotion. Role change occurs that influences not only the individual but also family and significant others. It is interesting to note that an individual's perception of crisis may change from moment to moment or from situation to situation. Each stressful event has the potential to create a crisis; the impact of the stressor depends on the effectiveness of coping strategies, previous experience with the stressor, availability of support systems, and flexibility of individuals in their current situation. Examples of events that can precipitate situational crises are premature birth, status and role changes, death of a loved one, physical or mental illness, divorce, change in geograph-

ic location, and poor performance in school.

Caplan (1964) suggests that a critical factor in the definition of a situational crisis lies in the concept of hazardous event. Because of its unpredictable nature, the presence of a hazard enhances the possibility of individual, family, or group disorganization. Situational crises have the potential to promote positive growth and change or to create multiple disruptions. The following is a case study of a situational crisis—a crisis of physical illness:

Mr. W., a 58-year-old white, single male, was admitted to the local general hospital with dizziness, syncopal episodes, shortness of breath, and feelings of pressure in his chest. After several days in the CCU, he was transferred 60 miles by ambulance to a large urban teaching hospital for further diagnostic studies. His preliminary diagnosis was ventricular tachycardia, a lethal arrhythmia initiated by an electrical deficit in the heart. During his first two days in the unit, he was quiet and remained in his room most of the time. After he had completed the first set of diagnostic studies. Mr. W. seemed more agitated. He frequently paced the hallways and snapped at the nurses. Concurrently his physicians told him that he would need further studies (which were quite painful and frightening). He was also told that the medications used thus far to control the arrhythmia had not been successful. One evening he was sitting on the edge of the bed crying when the nurse entered to give him his medications. He snapped, "Why should I take these—they aren't helping anyway" and threw them to the floor. Exploration with Mr. W. of his current state revealed the following data: his insurance was running out in ten days; he lived alone and bills were going unpaid; his current job status was uncertain because he was no longer going to be able to work with heavy machinery (he was too young to retire, yet too old to find other employment); he feared he would be unable to receive Social Security disability payments. Mr. W. described his brother and sister-in-law as support systems. When asked whether they would be interested in learning cardiopulmonary resuscitation. Mr. W. stated that he didn't want them to "assume that kind of responsibility."

Assessment. Assessment of Mr. W.'s situational crisis precipitated by his hospitalization revealed difficulty in adjusting to potential change in role and possible loss of life and inability to mobilize support systems. Physiological changes related to medications were also considered.

Potential nursing diagnoses. They include the following:

- Altered role performance related to diagnosis of chronic cardiac disease. (NANDA 3.2.1; DSM-III-R 309.28; 309.90).
- Social isolation related to inability to request help from family members. (NANDA 3.1.2; DSM-III-R 309.90).

Planning

Long-term outcomes

1. Development of social support systems
2. Development of adaptive measures to cope with change in role
3. Development of a positive sense of self-esteem

Short-term outcomes

1. Identification and mobilization of existing support systems
2. Exploration of options regarding further diagnostic studies
3. Identification of options regarding insurance coverage and other social and economic issues

Implementation

Generic intervention

- Facilitate Mr. W.'s resolution of the grieving process in relation to his potential change in role and acceptance of life-threatening illness.

Individual intervention

- Facilitate *environmental manipulation* by assisting Mr. W. to become involved in a support group for clients with chronic cardiac disease.
- Identify community resources such as the American Heart Association that can provide information and other resources as necessary.
- Connect Mr. W. with a social worker who can provide assistance with insurance as well as other financial issues.
- Encourage client to communicate with relatives regarding learning of CPR.
- Reinforce Mr. W.'s attempts to modify his life style, i.e., stopping smoking, walking daily, and following a low-cholesterol diet.
- Support Mr. W.'s decision to withdraw from further diagnostic studies.

- Provide alternative options to diagnostic studies as appropriate.
- Identify more effective methods of coping with stress.
- Discuss options for activities that would enhance positive sense of worth as a productive person.

Evaluation

- Determine the degree of Mr. W.'s accomplishment of long-term and short-term outcomes and his need for further intervention.

SOCIAL CRISES

A relatively recent addition to the discussion of crisis is the concept of "social crisis." Chamberlin (1980) describes social crises as accidental, uncommon, and unanticipated crises that result in multiple losses and radical environmental changes. Social crises include natural disasters that impact on large numbers of people—floods, earthquakes, major fires. Violence and large-scale tragedies resulting from man's actions are also considered social crises—for example, group hostage taking and riots, nuclear accidents, mass killings (as in the Tate-LaBianca murders), contamination of large areas by toxic wastes, wars, rape, and persecution of large groups of people because of ethnicity or race. This type of crisis is unlike maturational and situational crises because it does not occur in the lives of all people.

Because of the severity of the effects of social crises, coping strategies may not be effective. Individuals confronted with social crises usually do not have previous experiences from which to draw. Support systems may be unavailable because they may also be involved in similar situations. Mental health professionals are called on to act quickly and provide services to large numbers of people and in some cases whole communities.

DSM-III-R defines posttraumatic stress disorder as a disorder characterized by the development of symptoms following a psychological event that is outside the range of human experiences. The stressor, which could involve a serious threat to one's self, one's children, or one's spouse; sudden destruction of one's home or community; seeing another individual being seriously injured or killed; or learning about serious threat or harm to close friends or relatives, would be perceived as distressing to almost anyone. It is experienced with intense fear, terror, and helplessness. Major characteristic symptoms include reexperiencing the event, avoidance of stimuli related to the event, and blunted responsiveness. The diagnosis is applicable only when the symptomatology occurs for longer than 1 month.

Trauma related to this disorder may be experienced singly or within the context of a group or community. DSM-III-R notes that the duration and intensity of the disorder are apparently more severe and longer lasting if the stressor is of human design.

The primary characteristic—reexperiencing the event—can occur in several ways:

1. Recurrent intrusive recollections or dreams
2. Dissociative state in which components of the event are relived
3. Exposure to similar stimuli or stimuli that symbolize the event such as an anniversary

Individuals may also make a conscious effort to avoid thoughts or feelings related to the trauma or may avoid activities that resemble the event. Feelings of social isolation and alienation may arise; isolation of affect may be present; and lack of spontaneous relationships is apparent. In some cases, violent behaviors may erupt.

Figley (1978) describes a model of posttraumatic stress reaction that can be applied to those veterans returning from the Vietnam conflict. He outlined four phases of emotional adjustment and explored their implications for the Vietnam veteran.

The first phase, recovery, is that period immediately following the war. Vietnam veterans had little if any time to readjust to being home before being expected to return and participate in life as they had prior to their leaving. There was no sense of support from comrades or Americans in general as there had been in previous wars. They also experienced guilt about their participation in the conflict as well as about leaving friends who were still in combat.

The second phase, avoidance, is an attempt by survivors to avoid any reminders of what has occurred. Individuals who are exposed to situations that trigger off a recurrence of the traumatic event may be subject to a posttraumatic stress response.

Crisis intervention skills are most effective in facilitating the confrontation and resolution of this occurrence. If an adaptive resolution results, the veteran is able to enter the reconsideration phase.

Figley describes the third phase as that of the "healing," or reconsideration, phase. During this phase, the veteran seeks to understand what has happened to him during the war and why. Last, the final phase, that of adjustment, incorporates the reentry of the veteran into the mainstream of society as a viable, productive, emotionally healthy individual. The veteran has come to grips with his participation in the war and is able to accept his role and his actions.

However, Figley notes that Vietnam veterans may be more prone to posttraumatic stress due to the nature of the war itself. He describes five characteristics that may affect the process of readjustment:

1. Lack of sense of camaraderie and support. Soldiers did not share a circumscribed period of time together as soldiers in other wars did.
2. Nature of the war itself. Vietnam was not a war declared by Congress but a "conflict." Soldiers were young, ill prepared, and forced to fight using guerilla warfare in a country that was not totally supportive of the conflict.
3. Inappropriate diagnosis of psychological casualty rates due in part to the long-term effects left by the war itself.
4. Lack of an appropriate transition period from combat to former roles in society.
5. Lack of support for the war itself. Many veterans returned to the United States to be confronted by antiwar rallies and peace marches. Often they were left with the impression that their efforts and those efforts of individuals who had lost their lives were not recognized by their fellow countrymen.

In conclusion, the Vietnam War can be considered a primary example of a social crisis or Class 3 crisis, having the potential to precipitate a posttraumatic stress response. The nature of the war itself may provide obstacles for the healthy resolution of this crisis; this must be considered by those health professionals who work with Vietnam veterans, their families, and their significant others.

Typology of crisis

Burgess and Baldwin (1981) have described crisis situations as "critical points of attention in health care delivery." Secondary prevention can be practiced as a part of crisis intervention through the detection of emotional illness and the referral of clients to appropriate agencies. Burgess and Baldwin stress the importance of establishing structure in crisis intervention, placing emphasis on the development of contracts with clients that facilitate crisis resolution. These authors also place emphasis on the working through of maladaptive responses, the support for those responses, and the development of strategies that are more effective. Burgess and Baldwin suggest that a "typology of crisis" seeks to understand and present interventions for client populations that have previously been neglected in the literature and in practice.

Assessment of a crisis is focused on identifying its effects on individuals, the community, the state, the nation, and perhaps the world. Intervention occurs in two phases: the first phase deals with the immediate effects, while the second phase is more concerned with the posttraumatic issues, as noted in the diagnostic criteria for posttraumatic stress disorder.

Baldwin (1978) originally developed the following classification system, which is based on severity of crisis. As one moves from class 1 to class 6, the crisis becomes more severe, and the locus of the stressor moves from external to internal.

CLASS 1—DISPOSITIONAL CRISIS

Butcher and Mandel (1976) define a dispositional crisis as a problematic situation that presents a sense of immediacy. The clinician's role may be to provide information, make a referral to an appropriate agency or discipline, or provide administrative leverage. Examples of dispositional crises include meeting the parenting needs of one's children, experiencing stress resulting from the behavior of a substance abuser in the family, and being unable to study properly because of a roommate's lack of concern for study hours.

Strategies for intervention involve clarification of the issues and providing the necessary services and support.

CLASS 2—CRISES OF ANTICIPATED LIFE TRANSITIONS

There are normal life crises that are anticipated to some degree by clients and over which they may or may not have control. In some cases clients request help prior to the actual onset of the transition, while in other cases clients seek help during or following the transition. Examples of such transitions include going away from home for the first time, midlife career changes (going back to work or school or changing jobs), retirement, and separation and divorce.

The emphasis in strategies of intervention is on assisting clients in developing an understanding of the changes that will occur or are occurring and exploring what those changes mean. Effects on current life-style and family systems are assessed, and more adaptive coping strategies are developed. Group approaches have been useful in providing support to these client populations.

CLASS 3—CRISES RESULTING FROM SUDDEN TRAUMATIC STRESS

Crises of this nature are precipitated by powerful external stressors that are unexpected and over which the client has little control. Clients feel overwhelmed, and coping strategies are immobilized. Examples are sudden death of a spouse, family member, or significant other; rape; natural disasters such as floods; and war combat stress.

Providing or mobilizing support following the impact of the stressor is the initial goal of intervention. Clients are encouraged to acknowledge both positive and negative emotions resulting from a situation that has not been encountered previously. Clients are assisted in exploring other methods of coping that will be effective in meeting the changes that result from the stressor.

CLASS 4—MATURATIONAL / DEVELOPMENTAL CRISES

These crises result not from an external source of stress but rather from one that is more internal and that is based on the psychodynamics of the individual client. These crises result from ineffective attempts to resolve interpersonal situations that are related to more deep-rooted developmental issues such as dependency, power, value conflicts, intimacy, and sexual identity. Attempts to attain emotional maturity are unsuccessful, and repeated patterns of relational difficulties are often noted. Examples of crises reflecting power, intimacy, and sexual-identity issues in particular are child abuse and incest.

Strategies of intervention focus on assisting the client to identify and understand the nature of the developmental issue that is the underlying precipitant. Clients are encouraged to respond to the manifest problem while concurrently developing coping strategies to resolve the developmental conflict.

CLASS 5—CRISES RESULTING FROM PSYCHOPATHOLOGY

Preexisting psychopathology may act to precipitate a crisis or may be instrumental in impairing or complicating crisis resolution. Such a crisis is precipitated by unresolved internal issues that are triggered by events within a relational context. Individuals in this class present with multiple problems that impact on several areas of functioning. Crises of this nature are frequently seen in people with borderline personalities, severe neuroses, characterological disorders, and nonorganic psychoses.

Intervention is directed toward resolving the presenting issue by developing problem-solving skills and manipulating the environment to effect changes in behavior. Stabilization of function to its maximal level is the primary goal. Referral to appropriate long-term therapy is made once the immediate crisis has been resolved.

CLASS 6—PSYCHIATRIC EMERGENCIES

In these crises overall functioning is impaired and clients are no longer responsible for their actions. Crises of this type include acute psychoses, drug or alcohol intoxication, and impulse-control problems such as suicidal or homicidal behavior and uncontrollable anger and aggression.

Intervention with this type of crisis may be difficult in that the client can only provide limited information while service must often be instituted immediately. The goals are to work quickly and effectively to assess the medical and psychological condition, to assess the precipitant, and to pro-

vide intervention as rapidly as possible, particularly in life-threatening situations.

• • •

The importance of Baldwin's "typology of crisis" lies in the fact that it enables mental health professionals to understand more thoroughly the nature of a particular crisis. Strategies of intervention can therefore be made more appropriate to the crisis situation, and they can be more effective in resolving the particular issues of the situation.

CRISIS THEORY AS A TREATMENT MODALITY

Individuals are most amenable to the helping efforts of health professionals and are more likely to respond positively to the efforts of others to change ineffective methods of coping during crisis periods. Previously utilized methods may have maintained some form of equilibrium; therefore, change and growth tended to be limited. Initially, individuals do not consider crisis situations to have growth-promoting potential. Anxiety is increased; problem-solving strategies that were successful in past situations no longer are effective. The crisis intervention process provides the opportunity for clients to confront the identified precipitating event. Through a short-term, goal-directed therapeutic process the client develops more effective coping measures and returns to at least a precrisis level of functioning. Individual crisis therapy has historically been the focus of crisis intervention. However, the concepts of crisis theory are universal in nature and can be utilized appropriately within the context of family, group, and community interventions.

Family intervention

Within the context of family intervention, crisis theory addresses the family as the client. Symptomatology may be reflected in the behaviors of one individual; however, intricate family dynamics are a contributory factor in the expression of these symptomatic behaviors. The assessment of the crisis follows a similar format to that of assessment of individual crisis response. For example, when an aging parent moves into the home of his adult daughter and son-in-law, the son-in-law begins to spend more and more time away from home. Concurrently, the adult daughter is caring for her two young daughters as well as providing emotional and physical attention to meet her aging father's needs. The daughter begins to experience periods of overwhelming anxiety and finally seeks help from the community mental health center near her home. Although she is the primary symptom-bearer, role change and conflict within the family system are indicative of a family crisis. Assessment reveals that the precipitating event is the demand made by her father that she spend more time with him. The nurse assesses the family's methods of coping with previous situations and their effectiveness at this time. She observes family communication style and the manner in which roles are assumed and acted out. During the second and third sessions, it is apparent that the family is having difficulty meeting needs as they were met traditionally. No one feels that he or she is being heard or that he or she matters as an important person. The nurse assists in the clarification of relevant issues and in understanding the emotional impact that a crisis has. Each family member is encouraged to share feelings—to bring them into the open to reduce the tension that is being generated. In the fourth and fifth sessions, family strengths are reviewed and alternative methods of coping are identified and tested out. In this case, specific tasks are assigned and roles are redefined to include the new member of the family. The burden of responsibility of meeting all emotional needs of the family is shifted from the mother/wife/daughter to all members of the family system. These tasks are tested in the home environment, evaluated, and discussed in the therapy sessions. The goal of crisis intervention with this family was to facilitate the development of more adaptive coping measures, to reduce tension, and to return to a precrisis level of functioning.

Crisis intervention with families can be utilized in a variety of settings. Nurses may work with families of clients who are in intensive care settings, who enter emergency rooms, and who are in general hospital or ambulatory care settings. Clients and families are assisted to cope with changes in body image, loss of function, change in life-style, and the potential or actual loss of life. Particular populations at risk include families of clients with cardiac disease; dialysis and transplant clients; clients with cancer; clients with chronic, debilitating illness; families with a premature infant; families who are survivors of a suicide victim; and families of chronically mentally ill clients. Crisis intervention is a most effective method to assist families to mobilize resources and develop more adaptive measures to cope with those situations which created disequilibrium in the family system. Anticipatory guidance, as a component of crisis intervention, can be useful in providing information to families regarding the parameters of expected feelings, thoughts, and behaviors relative to maturational crises, such as pregnancy or adolescence, and situational crises, such as loss or change in function or role. The knowledge of what is to be expected and the feelings of "normalcy"—that others feel and act as they do in similar situations—provide a sense of control and decrease anxiety levels.

Group intervention

Aguilera and Messick (1986) describe a crisis group as a "collection of individuals who are unknown and unrelated to each other who meet as a group with a therapist to work together toward resolution of their individual crises through group interaction" (p. 36). The purpose of the crisis group is similar to that of crisis intervention with individuals: the restoration of members to at least a precrisis level of functioning and potentially to a higher level of problem-solving capability. Sessions are limited to six; the role of the therapist is active and direct with the exploration of precipitating events and past coping measures, the development of an understanding of the relationship between the crisis and feelings experienced, and the tapping of support systems as the primary foci. Groups may be composed of individuals experiencing similar problems, for example, those who have recently experienced the loss of a spouse. Composition of groups may also be mixed, including individuals who are experiencing different types of crisis. The decision as to the composition is often left to the discretion of the group leader and is based on level of expertise and comfort with a particular format.

Aguilera and Messick note that there are several advantages and disadvantages to group crisis intervention. Advantages of this format include willingness of individuals to participate in short-term versus long-term therapy; basic format of crisis intervention, which is understandable and less threatening than other forms of traditional therapy; and less social stigma attached to this type of therapy as opposed to more traditional therapies. Disadvantages of group crisis intervention must also be considered. Due to its short-term nature, process analysis is limited, thus reducing the potential effect of the group on each individual. There seems to be a decided lack of spontaneity in the sense that the therapist must focus on the "telling of each individual story" by group members. Aguilera and Messick also note that the group composition may change frequently, thus necessitating the need to repeat information to maintain any sense of continuity. Last, they note the inability to utilize the transference phenomenon due to the lack of time for development of adequate support relationships between and among group members and therapist.

The process of group crisis intervention can be useful in selected situations. Anticipatory guidance measures, as noted above in the discussion of family intervention, are effective for presenting parameters of expected behaviors, cognitions, and feelings within the context of the group setting. These measures can be utilized with groups of clients, parents, educators, health professionals, or those who may be confronted with a particular social, maturational, or situational crisis as a primary preventive intervention. Hendricks (1985) suggests that crisis theory is a useful model for conflict resolution. It is goal directed; expression of feelings is encouraged; new ideas emerge as a result of active problem solving; and it is a time-limited process. For example, a psychiatric liaison nurse conducts a group with the staff on a very active cardiac surgery unit for the purpose of resolving client management problems as well as developing more effective coping methods for handling intrastaff issues relative to professional stress and vulnerability.

Community intervention

The community also has potential for the utilization of crisis intervention skills. Social or "adventitious" crises (Stuart and Sundeen, 1987) are those crises which are of catastrophic nature and impact on large numbers of individuals. As noted in the previous discussion on social crises, such events as floods, earthquakes, or major fires as well as mass killings, hostage taking, or persecution of large groups of ethnic minorities present a situation not encountered previously in the lives of a majority of the people it affects. The need for appropriate problem-solving skills and the mobilizing of support systems becomes a critical imperative in these incidences. For example, on May 20, 1988, in the quiet suburban North Shore area of Winnetka, Illinois, a young woman initiated a violent rampage that began in the home of her former employer and ended in the elementary school where one child was murdered and several others were critically wounded. Immediately after the event occurred, a team of psychologists, social workers, and other mental health professionals was sent to the school to begin talking with the children and teachers—facilitating the expression of their feelings, helping them to understand what had happened, and mobilizing their support systems. In the weeks that followed, the team worked within the community conducting groups for parents and children alike to facilitate a healthy resolution of this crisis that would impact on their lives forever. Anticipatory guidance was provided to parents to alert them to signs that their children might be experiencing residual effects from the event; information was provided as to what they might expect in terms of the responses their children might have and for what duration; and parents and children alike were encouraged to share their feelings together, to express their feelings of vulnerability and anger—that their lives would not ever be the same from that point on—and to support one another in this difficult period. Although the crisis intervention itself is of short duration, the identification of further resources for future assistance is of importance due to the fact that psychological ramifications may occur months after the event.

Within the community itself, nurses can also

identify those populations at risk for crises such as adolescents, individuals who have recently relocated, older individuals who are planning to retire, pregnant couples, and women whose children have left home. Individuals can be educated to identify potential crises in their own lives as well as in the lives of those around them. They are then able to develop more adaptive coping strategies and mobilize support resources prior to the actual onset of the crisis and the resulting increased anxiety.

For crisis theory to exist as a valid framework of therapy, Burgess and Baldwin (1981) state that mental health professionals who utilize crisis intervention techniques must develop skills at the following levels:

1. Conceptual—theoretical knowledge that provides a framework for understanding client problems and for problem resolution
2. Clinical—Gestalt model techniques that effect change; they evolve from the conceptual framework
3. Communication—therapeutic skills that create a nonthreatening atmosphere where clients can explore the impact of crisis on their lives

The authors believe that once the above skills have been developed, crisis intervention will no longer be considered a "one-shot" type of therapy—a holding action practiced by paraprofessionals—but will assume its place as a valid form of therapy. Brownell (1984) suggests, however, that the concept of crisis must be reconceptualized and more clearly defined. A clear-cut definition of crisis will then be the basis for the methodology of crisis intervention as a form of therapeutic approach.

Pitfalls in the crisis approach

Gordon and Partridge (1982) identified several factors that may compromise crisis intervention. They are as follows:

1. Failure to gather information from as many sources as possible
2. Incomplete or premature diagnosis made prior to the analysis of all pertinent data
3. "Rescue syndrome"—need of the therapist to

"save" the client, do too much for the client, and set unrealistic goals
4. Hasty identification of the precipitating event without further assessment
5. Failure to recognize that clients with preexisting psychopathology can have crises

Crisis intervention can be a useful tool for the confrontation and resolution of immediate issues; however, nurses must realize that this methodology has its drawbacks as do other treatment modalities.

PHASES OF CRISIS INTERVENTION

The phases of crisis intervention as a therapeutic tool parallel the steps of the nursing process.

Assessment

Accurate assessment is a key factor in the appropriate use of crisis intervention techniques. Data are collected regarding the presenting problem and precipitating event. An exploration of the precipitating event is necessary to facilitate the development of effective coping strategies. Burgess and Baldwin (1981) present the following model for assessment:

1. Assessment of the precipitating event
   a. Time and place. It is often difficult for client and therapist to define the event within the client's recent past. Usually the event is clarified through the coping process of crisis intervention.
   b. Interpersonal dimensions. Crisis is related to the context of the client's relationships, whether they be those of the past or the present.
   c. Affective reactions. Emotional responses to crisis are expected and should be explored and *affirmed*. Clients have the *right* to experience emotional disequilibrium. The nature of the responses must be accurately and quickly determined to protect clients from their own impulses (suicidal, homicidal, or other aggressive acting-out behaviors). Feelings commonly experienced are: +3 and/or +4 anxiety,

fear, embarrassment, anger, guilt (see Chapter 8).

d. Client's request for help. A request for help may be directly or indirectly conveyed and may be adaptive or maladaptive. Requests for help enable the therapist to understand in some measure how the client has problem solved in previous situations. Clients may wish support, therapy, an authority figure, or nothing (Lazare et al., 1972). Lazare further suggests that response to the request is critical in that a lack of response may lead to progressive deterioration of client behavior.

2. Assessment of psychodynamic issues. Assessment involves the exploration of the crisis precipitant within the context of current experiences. However, it is the role of the therapist to identify past traumatic experiences that may be analogous to current ones and to identify any events that may cause anticipatory fear of reexperiencing an old trauma. An event occurring in the present environment may recall similar affect and behavior from past traumatic experiences. For example, a Vietnam veteran might experience a crisis response when confronting a situation in his present life that triggered feelings of inadequacy and helplessness similar to those experienced during his tour of duty in Vietnam.

3. Assessment of present coping strategies. When individuals experience a crisis, coping strategies that are a part of their normal repertoire are no longer effective. Assessment of these strategies offers information regarding the crisis and the client's understanding of the need for the use of particular coping strategies within the context of various relationships.

a. Maladaptive coping responses. What would happen if the client were to modify behaviors and resolve the presenting problem? The assessment must evaluate the gains experienced through the use of maladaptive responses: security may be maintained at the cost of healthy equilibrium, and uncomfortable feelings such as

anger, guilt, loss, and shame may not need to be confronted. Exploration of the need for maladaptive coping strategies leads to a more in-depth understanding of the crisis itself.

b. Definition of alternative strategies. Once clients understand their use of maladaptive coping strategies, they are able to conceptualize and define more effective coping strategies. Nurses can present possible alternatives that can be tested by clients as a means of educating clients in relation to their own levels of emotional maturity.

4. Assessment of precrisis functioning
a. Client's usual repertoire of coping strategies. Exploration of coping strategies employed prior to the onset of the crisis will reveal the range of responses called on in various situations. It may be determined that the client has a limited scope of coping measures when confronted with a situation that produces feelings of inadequacy or helplessness but that coping strategies used to resolve anger are quite effective. The process of exploration allows the client to gain insight into usual responses to situations that require adaptation and change.

b. Emotional style and communication skills. Assessment of emotional style reveals a client's capability to respond fully to events in his or her life. For example, does the client experience emotions such as anger or affection, or does he or she keep them in check so as not to lose control? Clients may not even be aware of feelings they are experiencing until the feelings are pointed out to them. The more open clients are to the expression of their emotions, the more able they will be to recognize relationships between emotions and particular events.

c. Social support system. A person exists within the context of many relationships; in fact, a person cannot exist without some type of relatedness to others. Assessment of support systems indicates the number and depth of relationships. A client may have many superficial relationships but no one to actually count on. Through an exploration of relationships, the nurse may note the circumstances in which relationships are initiated and how much energy is expended by the client in maintaining the relationship. Solitary time is important to most individuals; it must be determined whether the client spends time alone because the client wants to or because no one wants to spend time with him or her. Often individuals in the client's community may be called upon to provide support, such as the corner grocer, the postman, or a clergyman, or the client may be invited to join a group of similar individuals as part of a support system.

    d. Personal vulnerabilities. All individuals feel vulnerable at some time in life; however, vulnerability is not characteristic of life in general. Vulnerable areas are often at the base of crisis experiences where coping strategies have not been developed. An assessment of these areas may reveal issues that were in part responsible for the onset of the crisis itself.

    e. Self-report of personality. It is important to listen and *hear* clients' descriptions of themselves. How balanced are their lists of strengths and weaknesses? Do they describe themselves as basically good, or do they constantly put themselves down? Adjectives used to describe self are also important. Perceptions of self prior to the crisis can be compared to current perceptions. The client's sense of self and personal strengths can be used in crisis resolution.

5. Related areas of assessment. The following areas are integral parts of a comprehensive psychosocial assessment: suicidal behavior, substance use and abuse, recent medical history, and recent psychiatric history.

Following a comprehensive assessment, nursing diagnoses are determined that reflect the major issues occurring within the immediate context of the client's life.

Planning

Following data collection and analysis, client and nurse must collaborate on defining goals and interventions to resolve the identified issues. The locus of decision making in the crisis intervention process is shared for the most part. The assessment plan is primarily nurse directed. However, in the planning and implementation phases the relationship assumes a more collaborative nature; in fact, a well-skilled clinician will facilitate the client's development of adaptive strategies rather than solve the problems himself or herself. Through the assessment process the nurse gains a clearer understanding of how to maximize client strengths and provide appropriate client support.

Implementation

The third phase is implementation of the plan designed by client and nurse. In this phase the nurse maintains a goal-directed focus to facilitate the client's resolution of the presenting issue within a limited time frame (six to eight sessions).

During the intervention phase the nurse uses already developed communication skills to help the client understand the impact of the crisis and resolve presenting issues. The nurse encourages the open expression of feelings by affirming the client's right to experience those feelings. The nurse may also protect the client from harmful impulses resulting from an overwhelming sense of helplessness and depression. Clarification of issues facilitates client perception of contributory relationships and an understanding of the emotional effect generated by the crisis develops. Because of the client's feelings of vulnerability, efforts by the nurse are directed toward ego support and acknowledgment of effective coping strategies. Mobilization of support systems is initiated, and the client is encouraged to employ those resources appropriately. See the box on p. 434.

Jacobsen, Strickler, and Morely (1968) suggest that crisis intervention may occur at a generic level

---

Crisis intervention communication skills

- **Clarification of issues**
  Nurse: "From what you've described, it seems that each time the baby cries, you feel you're not a good enough mother and your anxiety increases."
- **Validation of normalcy**
  Nurse: "Many new parents have described their frustrations with the changes that occur when a baby arrives. It's important for you both to know that what you are feeling is expected."
- **Support for new coping measures**
  Nurse: "Since you have started participating in the group for single mothers, you seem to be less anxious when you describe the baby's crying episodes."
- **Exploration of alternatives**
  Nurse: "Several of your friends have toddlers in day care. Have you thought of contacting them for information about cost and time?"
- **Ventilation**
  Nurse: "Can you tell me how you felt when you first came home from Vietnam?"
- **Positive reinforcement**
  Nurse: "I know you have been able to cope successfully with several relocations in the past. I think you'll be able to do it again, although it may not seem that way right now."
- **Mobilizing available support systems**
  Nurse: "Have you contacted the Newcomers group or the Welcome Wagon organization? They often have helpful information about services and activities in the area."

---

or at an individual level. The *generic* approach assumes that there are generalized patterns of behavior in any crisis. The working through of grief is an example of a defined sequence of responses to loss. This pattern of response is not only applicable to loss through death but also to loss of function, loss of role status, or loss of independence. Intervention at the generic level focuses on facilitating the client's movement through the prescribed phases to reach resolution. Individual psychodynamics are not emphasized. *General support* is provided, giving clients a sense that they are not alone and that problem resolution can be effected. *Environmental manipulation* seeks to alter the current situation that may be potentiating the effects of the crisis. For example, assume that a young doctoral student has been feeling overwhelmed by her studies and her full-time job. With support from a nurse, the student seeks to reduce her stress by temporarily reducing her job to part-time status during the semester in which she has the heaviest course load. Feelings of helplessness are alleviated, and she is able to resolve the crisis successfully. *Anticipatory guidance* assists clients in responding to the crises of life that most individuals experience, such as death of a loved one, birth of a child, and the transition from one developmental phase to the next. Nurses can present parameters of expected cognitions, emotions, and actions based on what is known to be the experience of the majority of individuals in similar situations. A sense of control is reestablished when clients feel that what they are experiencing is similar to the experiences of others. The universal statement "Many times clients have expressed . . ." indicates to the client that these feelings and perceptions are shared and understood. This does not deny, however, the uniqueness of the individual. Further exploration of feelings can be pursued. Through anticipatory guidance, clients can be prepared to cope with anticipated events and transition periods and reduce the potential of another crisis response in the future.

The *individual approach* differs from the generic in that there is an emphasis on individual psychodynamics as they exist within the context of relationships. The individual approach focuses on specific needs of a client and on the resolution of a situation peculiar to that client. This approach can be effective in situational and maturational crises. It is often employed when the generic approach has not effected crisis resolution. The individual approach reflects an understanding of unresolved emotional issues of the past, such as dependency and value conflicts, and their connection with the occurrence of behaviors in the present. The intent, however, is not to restructure the personality. Crises that involve impulsive, acting-out behavior, such as aggression directed toward self or others, need to be addressed by an individual approach rather than the generic in order to protect clients from themselves and to protect others from the impulsive behavior. The individual approach does in fact include the generic approach, general support, and environmental manipulation.

Evaluation

Evaluation, the fourth and final step in crisis intervention, involves a review of the effectiveness of the strategies. Has crisis resolution occurred? Have goals been met, and has positive behavioral change been effected? Have adaptive coping strategies been developed and used? What have clients learned about themselves, their responses, and their potential for healthy adaptation in the future? The evaluation phase acts as a period of summation, during which clients can review events of crisis situations, their responses, and the ways in which they were able to resolve the issues. Other areas that need further exploration are identified, and measures to meet those needs are discussed. Nurse and client share the decision making in this phase and determine whether referral to another agency or health professional is appropriate.

SAMPLE INTERACTION

This sample interaction will illustrate the four phases of crisis intervention utilizing selected communication techniques.

Initial assessment

Jack H., a 36-year-old white male, presented at the local mental health center complaining of feeling depressed and highly anxious. Upon arrival, he was assigned to Ms. D., the nurse-therapist.

Ms. D. *Can you tell me what brought you here today at this time?*

Jack *The lawyer called me to set up an appointment to review the divorce and custody arrangements about two hours ago.*

Ms. D. *What did that mean to you?*

Jack *I guess I thought it would never really happen—I mean the divorce and losing the kids.*

Ms. D. *What did you think would happen?*

Jack *I don't know—we had been having problems for a while and saw a counselor, but my wife wants to lead her own life.*

Ms. D. *Do you have anyone to talk to when you're having problems?*

Jack *Not really—we just moved to this area six months ago. I know some people where I work, but I wouldn't talk to them. My parents live about 1200 miles away, and I don't want to bother them.*

Ms. D. *What do you usually do when you have a problem— how do you handle it?*

Jack *I used to play a lot of racquetball, but I haven't done that recently—it helps me wind down.*

Ms. D. *Have you thought of hurting yourself?*

Jack *No—I don't want to die; I just want to feel better.*

Analysis of data. Following the initial session, analysis of the data reflected these nursing diagnoses:

- Dysfunctional grieving related to the failure of the marriage. (NANDA 9.2.1.1; DSM-III-R 309.00)
- Situational low self-esteem related to feelings of inadequacy and loss. (NANDA 7.1.2.2; DSM-III-R 309.28)

Planning. Long and short-term outcomes were developed to assist Jack in resolving feelings of guilt and to reestablish a positive sense of self-worth. Specific long-term outcomes include return to precrisis level of functioning, develop positive sense of self, and develop more effective coping strategies. Short-term outcomes include identify the relationship between the crisis and the feelings experienced, develop social support systems either within the work environment or within his condominium complex, actively participate in the divorce proceedings and child-custody action, and take a two-week leave of absence from work.

Implementation. Nursing intervention includes the use of a generic approach based on Jack's response to the loss of his marriage and loss of his role as a father. An individual approach focused on the impact of Jack's parents' divorce and its relationship to his current situation.

Support provided by the nurse enables the client to explore feelings and test out new measures of coping in a nonjudgmental, unbiased, empathic environment. Jack's level of anxiety was reduced, and his feelings of worthlessness were challenged as he and the nurse identified his strengths. Reduction of anxiety made more energy available to actively participate in the divorce proceedings rather than be a passive recipient of the event's effects. Jack came to recognize that both he and his wife had responsibility for the failure of the marriage; it was not his alone. He also began to recognize the feelings that he had experienced during his parents' divorce and the effects of those feelings on his current behavior.

By the completion of the sixth session, Jack was experiencing less anxiety and had a clearer perception of his role in the marriage and impending divorce. He was able to make decisions regarding his job, the custody of his children, and his future relationships with his wife and other women. Jack's support systems were still somewhat limited. He made plans to join an exercise club in his condominium complex.

Evaluation. As a result of Jack's more active involvement in directing the events of his life, he felt an increased sense of competence, self-worth, and control. His inability to concentrate, lack of appetite, and insomnia were decreasing, as was his anxiety level. Those coping measures which had been effective prior to the crisis were so once again. He had also developed new coping strategies that added to his repertoire for future use. Jack and the nurse reviewed the experience and the manner in which Jack had successfully used problem-solving techniques. The defined goals had been achieved.

CHAPTER SUMMARY

A crisis can be defined as a situation that cannot readily be resolved by an individual's normal or available repertoire of coping strategies. Events that precipitate crises may be anticipated, as in the case of the transition from one developmental phase to another. Situations of an external nature that threaten one's sense of biological, psychological, or social integrity may also precipitate crises.

Crisis theory provides a conceptual framework for active intervention. Contracts are time limited to six to eight sessions in which presenting issues are explored, interventive strategies are implemented, and clients learn to modify behavior as necessary. Further referral is made if it is appropriate. Crisis intervention is no longer considered a "band-aid" approach or "one-shot" therapy. It is a valid modality of treatment practiced by clinicians who are skilled in the use of crisis strategies.

The methodology of crisis intervention involves a sequence of steps similar to those of the nursing process. An assessment of the presenting issue is made through data collection and analysis. A plan is determined through a collaborative effort with the client. Strategies of action to enhance coping measures are implemented. Finally, the effectiveness of the plan is reviewed, and a determination is made in regard to further action. Steps are followed sequentially and may be returned to as appropriate.

Nursing intervention is based on sound therapeutic communication skills. Ego defenses are supported while more adaptive strategies are explored. Manipulation of the environment alters stressful situations so that individuals are able to explore more effective resolutions.

Crisis intervention can be used in many settings and formats. Group crisis intervention reaches larger numbers of individuals. Examples include parenting groups, groups of at-risk clients such as those with cardiac disease, and families of clients in intensive care settings. Crisis techniques can be used in all general hospital units, as well as in community settings, including schools and industries. Nurses may also employ crisis strategies in dealing with intragroup issues concerning a nursing staff and in dealing with client management issues.

SELF-DIRECTED LEARNING

Sensitivity-Awareness Exercises

The purposes of these exercises are to:
- Develop an awareness of the impact of maturational, situational, and social crises on individuals
- Develop an awareness of your own responses to clients who are in crisis

1. Read accounts in your local newspaper of crisis situations such as mass murders, major earthquakes, contamination of large areas of natural resources.
   a. What type of messages are conveyed about the crisis itself? How are the victims of the crisis portrayed? Is there any mention of emotional ramifications either short or long-term? How is the management of the crisis depicted?
2. Try to imagine yourself as a victim of one of the following:
   a. Major earthquake
   b. Hostage situation with a known murderer
   c. A Vietnam veteran
   d. A parent whose child was wounded in a random shooting
3. Describe the feelings you might have if you were to:
   a. Lose the job you love
   b. Fail your first nursing examination
   c. Separate from your spouse
   d. Contract a terminal physical illness
4. Develop a plan of crisis intervention for the following: families of dialysis clients; new parents; recently widowed individuals; parents of children who were exposed to a shooting rampage.

Questions to Consider

Bill, a 17-year-old high school senior, called the mental health hot line. He blurted out that he was experiencing overwhelming stress, had too many things in his life to handle, and had reached the breaking point. He was sure he wouldn't get into the college he wanted. He didn't know what to do or who to talk to. He had never felt this way before. He didn't want to worry his parents, but he needed to do "something."

1. The nurse's initial response should be
   a. "What caused you to call the center today—right now?"
   b. "Tell me what your parents know about your situation."
   c. "I think we can help you feel better."
   d. "Have you ever visited a psychiatrist before?"
2. Short-term outcomes for Bill might include
   a. Identification of unresolved conflicts with parents
   b. Exploration of realistic options for college
   c. Consideration of a preparatory school for one year prior to college
   d. Reduction of all outside activities for 6 months
3. During the fourth session the nurse assists Bill in determining how the current situation can be altered to reduce his feelings of stress. This method of intervention is termed
   a. Anticipatory guidance
   b. General support
   c. Values clarification
   d. Environment manipulation
4. The primary characteristic of phase three of Caplan's model of crisis is
   a. Redefinition of the crisis
   b. General increase in anxiety
   c. Profound cognitive, emotional and physiological changes
   d. Increasing disorganization and vulnerability

Continued.

SELF-DIRECTED LEARNING—cont'd

Questions to Consider—cont'd

Select the statement from Column B that best matches the class of crises in Column A.

Column A

5. Problematic situations such as meeting the parenting needs of an adolescent that present a sense of immediacy

6. Situations, such as retirement, midlife career changes, or leaving home for the first time, over which the client may or may not have control

7. Situations precipitated by powerful exterior stressors that are unexpected and over which client has little control

8. Situations that result from ineffective attempts to resolve such issues as dependency, power, value conflicts, and intimacy

9. Situations that are precipitated by such acute problems as homicidal behavior and acute psychoses

10. Situations precipitated by unresolved internal issues that are triggered by events within a relational contest

Column B

a. Sudden traumatic stress crises

b. Maturational crises

c. Crises resulting from psychopathology

d. Dispositional crises

e. Anticipated life transition

f. Psychiatric emergencies

Answer key

1. a	6. e
2. b	7. a
3. d	8. b
4. a	9. f
5. d	10. c

REFERENCES

Aguilera D and Messick J: Crisis intervention: theory and methodology, ed 5, St. Louis, 1986, The CV Mosby Co.

American Psychiatric Association: Diagnostic and statistical manual III-R, Washington, DC, 1987.

Baldwin B: A paradigm for the classification of emotional crises: indications for crisis intervention, Am J Psychiatr 4:538, 1978.

Brownell MJ: The concept of crisis: its utility for nursing, Adv Nurs Sci 7:10-20, 1984.

Burgess A and Baldwin B: Crisis intervention theory and practice: a clinical handbook, Englewood Cliffs, NJ, 1981, Prentice-Hall, Inc.

Butcher JM and Mandel G: Crisis intervention, In We I, editor: Clinical methods in psychology, New York, 1976, John Wiley & Sons, Inc.

Caplan G: Principles of preventive psychiatry, New York, 1964, Basic Books, Inc.

Chamberlin BC: The psychological aftermath of disasters, J Clin Psychol 41:238-243, 1980.

Erikson E: Childhood and society, New York, 1963, WW Norton & Co.

Figley C, editor: Stress disorders among Vietnam veterans: theory, research & treatment, New York, 1978, Bruner/Mazel, Inc.

Glass A: Observations upon the epidemiology of mental illness in troops during warfare, In National Research Councel, editor: Symposium on preventive and social psychiatry, Washington, DC, 1957, Walter Reed Army Institute.

Gordon J and Partridge R, editors: Practice and management of psychiatric emergencies, St. Louis, 1982, The CV Mosby Co.

Hendricks J: Crisis intervention, Springfield, Ill, 1985, Charles C. Thomas Publishers.

Hradek E: Crisis intervention and suicide, J Psychosoc Nurs Mental Health Serv 26(5):24-28, 1988.

Jacobsen G, Strickler N, and Morely W: Generic and individual approaches to crisis intervention, Am J Public Health 47:339-345, 1968.

Joint Commission on Mental Health and Mental Illness: Action or mental health, New York, 1961, Basic Books Inc.

Lazare A et al: The walk-in patient as a customer: A key dimension in evaluation and treatment, Am J Orthopsychiatr 23:872-875, 1972.

Lindemann E: Symptomatology and management of acute grief, Am J Psychiatr 32:141-151, 1944.

McLane A, editor: Classification of nursing diagnoses, St. Louis, 1987, The CV Mosby Co.

Stuart G and Sundeen S: Principles and practices of psychiatric nursing, St. Louis, 1987, The CV Mosby Co.

Williams F: Intervention in maturational crises, Persp Psychiatr Care 17:240-245, 1971.

ANNOTATED SUGGESTED READINGS

Baldwin B: A paradigm for the classification of emotional crises: implications for crisis intervention, Am J Orthopsychiatr 48(3):538, 1978.

This article presents an integrated crisis theory based on the author's development of six classes of crisis. Formats of intervention are well defined for each class. The comprehensive and pragmatic nature of this work serves to fill the gap left by other crisis theories.

Britton J and Mattson-Melcher D: The crisis home: sheltering patients in emotional crisis, J Psychiatr Mental Health Services 23(12):18-23, 1985.

The authors describe a unique program that provides cost-effective alternative care for the chronically mentally ill. The program is run solely by nurses and utilizes a home environment rather than placing the client back in a chronic institution. The program enjoys continued success and can be utilized as a model for similar programs in other areas of the country.

Brownell MJ: The concept of crisis: its utility for nursing, Adv Nurs Sci 7:10-20, 1984.

Brownell notes the importance of the concept of crisis to nursing yet suggests that discrepancies exist in the manner in which the concept is utilized conceptually and clinically. She reviews the more recent definitions of crisis using related theories of stress and threat. The utility of crisis is discussed within the context of a continuum rather than as a dichotomous entity. Implications for further research and clinical practice are presented.

Geisler E: Crisis: what it is and is not, Adv Nurs Sci 7:1-5, 1984.

Geisler utilizes the technique of concept analysis to develop four critera for the diagnosis of a client as having attributes congruent with the concept of crisis. She differentiates the concept of crisis from related concepts such as stress and emergency. Variations of the model were presented to demonstrate what crisis is and is not. The author also identified antecedents, consequences, and empirical referents for crisis that are necessary for a more comprehensive understanding of the concept of crisis.

Lindemann E: Symptomatology and management of acute grief, Am J Psychiatr 101:141, 1944.

This classic study of the grief response evolved out of the author's work with the survivors of the Coconut Grove fire in Boston. The article played a significant role in the emergence of crisis intervention as a valid method of coping with the grief response.

Taylor L: Policemen and students: a crisis intervention team, J Psychiatr Mental Health Serv 23(9):26-30, 1985.

Taylor presents a discussion of a course that teams nursing students with police officers to provide a unique method of teaching crisis intervention skills. Theory is taught in the first week of the course by an interdisciplinary team, and the remaining clinical experience is spent with the police officers on duty. Students found the experience very positive. They gained a greater appreciation for police officers and their work. Students also noted that the exposure to people in the community in all walks of life facilitated a greater understanding of the mentality, values, and pressures that individuals of diverse cultures experience daily.

FURTHER READINGS

Dixon S: Working with people in crisis: theory and practice, St. Louis, 1979, The CV Mosby Co.

Donovan J, Bennet M, and McElroy C: The crisis 'group'—an outcome study, Am J Psychiatr 13:906, 1979.

Goldstein D: Crisis intervention: a brief therapy model, Nurs Clinics N Am 13(4):657, 1978.

Hanke N: Handbook of emergency psychiatry, Lexington, Mass, 1984, The Collamore Press.

Harrison D: Nurses and disasters, J Psychosoc Nurs Mental Health Serv 19(2):34, 1981.

Hoff LA: People in crisis: understanding and helping, Menlo Park, Ca, 1978, Addison-Wesley Publishing Co.

Lancaster J and Berkovsky D: An ecological framework for crisis intervention, J Psychiatr Nurs 16:17, 1978.

Merker M: A psychiatric emergency evaluation, Nurs Clinics N Am 21(3):387-395, 1986.

Puryear D: Helping people in crisis, San Francisco, 1979, Jossey-Bass, Inc.

Rickel L: Making mountains manageable: maximizing quality of life through crisis intervention, Oncol Nurs Forum 14(4):29-34, 1987.

CHAPTER 16

Community mental health

CHAPTER FOCUS

Mental health care has been undergoing an evolutionary, some even say a revolutionary, process for more than a quarter of a century. The community mental health movement has been an important part of this process since its implementation on a nationwide basis in the 1960s.

The Comprehensive Mental Health Centers Act, passed by the United States Congress in 1963, along with subsequent legislation, has changed the mental health care delivery system. The 1963 legislation was unique in that it increased the involvement of the federal government in mental health care. Prior to the passage of the community mental health legislation, major responsibility for mental health care was a function of state and local governments and the private sector. The federal government has been involved only in funding research, education, and a few other aspects of mental health care and in providing health services to special groups such as the armed forces and veterans. The legislation established national guidelines for mental health services and provided some funding in the form of grants for construction and staffing of mental health centers. The guidelines were broad enough to allow programs to meet local and regional mental health needs.

Community mental health care involves a complex, multifaceted approach to meeting one of the nation's major health problems. Concepts of community mental health place emphasis upon reducing the incidence of mental disorders through locally available and comprehensive services for prevention, early treatment, and rehabilitation. As a means of achieving these objectives and of bringing mental health care into the mainstream of modern health practices, an integrated system of health, social welfare, and other human services was conceived.

Implementation of the goals of the community mental health movement is an evolving process in which communities; governmental, health, and social agencies; professional practitioners; and consumers develop collaborative, cooperative programs to promote mental health. Because of variations in population density and the multiplicity of ethnic and sociocultural groups in the United States, the mental health needs and the organization of mental health services to meet those needs vary considerably from one community to another. Certain concepts, however, are characteristic of all community mental health programs. Among these concepts are the following:

1. Emphasis on preventive psychiatry and the availability of comprehensive services for the prevention, treatment, and rehabilitation of mental disorders
2. Provision of mental health services in a setting in which there is the least possible disruption of social and kinship support systems and the least possible interference with personal and civil liberties
3. Responsiveness to consumer needs through community involvement in the planning and evaluation of programs to meet mental health needs
4. Provision of mental health services by interdisciplinary mental health teams

The community mental health movement has had a major impact upon the treatment of persons with psychiatric disorders. There has also been an influence upon the roles and functions of health professionals involved in providing health services. As a basis for understanding current mental health practices, this chapter will focus on major aspects of community mental health including the provision of culturally relevant care. The present status of community mental health care and some of the factors that have influenced the realization of the goals of the movement will be discussed.

CONCEPTS UNDERLYING COMMUNITY MENTAL HEALTH CARE

The community mental health movement embraces a broad-spectrum approach to meeting mental health needs. Theoretical concepts place emphasis on the interrelationship of biological, psychological, intellectual, spiritual, and sociocultural forces inherent in a *holistic view* of the individual interacting with the environment (see Chapter 1). Developments in psychopharmacology and biochemical research and advancements in the knowledge of the effects on mental health of such sociocultural stressors as poverty, racism, and unemployment have emphasized the importance of a holistic approach to mental health promotion.

The community mental health concept uses *systems theory*,* taking an *ecosystem approach* to the organization of services to meet the mental health needs of communities (See Fig. 16-1). A human ecosystem is the environment, physical and social, of which the individual is a part and with which he or she interacts. The unit of analysis is the community. An ecosystem approach to community mental health is based on the following assumptions:

1. Alteration in the number of admissions to a local community mental health agency will not only affect the operation of other local mental health agencies but also the resources, economy, and composition of the community (for example, there will be a change in the number of people employed and the amount of income earned).
2. There is a relationship between the environment and behavior. For example, overcrowding, inadequate housing, urban renewal, and migration influence behavior.
3. There is a relationship between human behavior and such elements of the immediate social environment as the family, school, and place of employment.
4. Social structure and the physical environment interrelate and influence the well-being of community members (both individuals and families) and communities.

---

*Refer to Chapter 1 for discussion of systems theory.

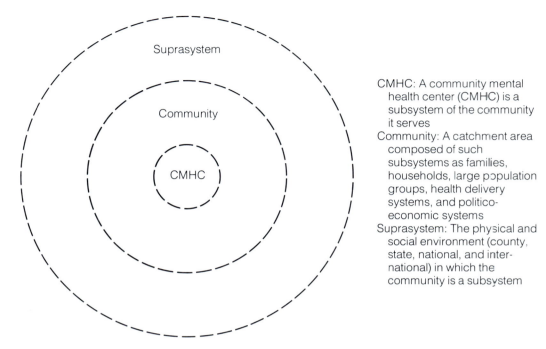

Fig. 16-1   Community as client system.

5. Community mental health professionals will have an inadequate data base if they assess only one aspect of the ecosystem. This may lead to ineffective intervention (Lancaster, 1980; Shamansky and Peznecker, 1982).

Therefore, from an ecosystem perspective, mental illness occurs when communities are unable to obtain adequate resources or to equitably distribute resources to their members. The origin of psychopathology is not located solely in the individual but within the entire ecosystem, of which the individual is one interdependent part.

Community mental health nurses facilitate the effective functioning of human ecosystems by engaging in primary (anticipatory), secondary (corrective), or tertiary (rehabilitative) preventive intervention.* Because human behavior is both affected by and affects the family and the community, all three levels of intervention may be engaged in seri-

---

*Levels of preventive intervention will be discussed later in this chapter and have been discussed in depth in Chapter 1.

ally or simultaneously (Lancaster, 1980). For example, secondary and tertiary activities may be aimed at treating and rehabilitating both the perpetrators and victims of violence (a symptom of system dysfunction), while primary activities may be aimed at preventing a recurrence of the overcrowding, inadequate housing, and parental overburdening that may contribute to future dysfunction in the ecosystem. In addition to an ecosystem approach, any of the conceptual models summarized in Table 16-1 may be used in community psychiatry.

FACTORS INFLUENCING THE COMMUNITY MENTAL HEALTH MOVEMENT
Scope of the mental health problem

World War II, which brought universal conscription of young men for military service in the United States, focused national attention on the extent of the nation's mental health problems. Neuropsychiatric disturbances were responsible for the greatest

TABLE 16-1 Conceptual models

Model	Focus	Goal
Medical	Individual psychopathology	Treat an individual's psychiatric symptoms and pathology
Public health	Incidence of mental illness in a catchment area (geographically defined area with a population of 75,000–200,000)	Decrease or eliminate the incidence of mental disorders in a catchment area through primary, secondary, and tertiary preventive intervention (see Table 16-2)
Social	Problems of daily living that generate mental illness in specific populations (target populations)	Improve the social milieu through social and political action; mobilize the resources and strengths of the community to help individuals and families cope with crises and problems of daily living
Holistic	People as biological, psychological, sociocultural, and spiritual beings	Engage the client as a partner in attaining a high level of wellness that reflects balance and integration of mind, body, and spirit (see Chapter 1 for an in-depth discussion of the holistic health model)

TABLE 16-2 Levels of preventive intervention*

Level of prevention	Objective	Example of a nursing activity
Primary	Identify potential mental health problems and plan and implement preventive programs	Developing a program to prevent drug abuse in a population of high school students
Secondary	Identify and effectively treat mental disorders	Recognizing the symptoms of depression in an elderly man living alone and referring him for treatment
Tertiary	Provide treatment or rehabilitation services, in the least restrictive setting possible, to people with chronic psychiatric disorders	Implementing a program to remotivate and resocialize chronically mentally ill clients

*See Chapter 1 for further discussion of levels of preventive intervention.

number of medical discharges from the armed services during the war. The impact on the state budgets, which had to be increased to provide essential services, and on capital spending, to expand the institutions to meet the mental health needs of the steadily increasing institutional populations, was profound. In many states, the cost of mental health services became a major budgetary expense—and therefore a sociopolitical concern that served to focus attention upon the mental health problem.

The ever-rising costs of services gave impetus to the use of newer therapeutic modalities, particularly chemotherapy, and focused the attention of the federal government upon the nation's mental health needs.

Legislative action

In 1955 the United States Congress passed the Mental Health Studies Act, which directed that a Joint Commission on Mental Health and Mental Illness be appointed to study "the needs and resources of the mentally ill in the United States and to make recommendations for a National Mental Health program" (Joint Commission on Mental Health and Mental Illness, 1961). The Joint Commission, appointed by the National Institute for Mental Health, was an interdisciplinary group drawn from 28 national organizations concerned with mental health. The American Nurses' Association and the National League for Nursing were among the professional organizations supporting the study.

In 1961 the Joint Commission issued its final report in the form of a book entitled *Action for Mental Health: A Program for Meeting the National Emergency*. The report included the following recommendations:

1. To promote publicly supported research and the development of research centers. The report noted that education and scientific knowledge should be regarded as national resources.
2. To achieve better use of present knowledge and experience. The report recommended that "psychiatry and the mental health professions should adopt and practice a liberal philosophy of what constitutes and who can do treatment. . . ." The report noted that certain examinations and treatments should be done by physicians and that psychoanalysis and related forms of insight therapy must be conducted by persons with special training. It recommended, however, that nonmedical mental health workers "with aptitude, sound training, practical experience and demonstrated competence should be permitted to do short-term psychotherapy."
3. To increase the number of mental health professionals. The report recommended federal support of education in the mental health professions. The report also recommended that the mental health professions conduct national recruitment drives and training programs for all categories of mental health workers and that professional leaders become actively engaged in supporting constructive legislation for general and professional education.
4. To increase federal funding for mental health care and improvement in mental health services.

5. To improve services provided to people with emotional disturbances. Among the recommendations were increases in the number of community mental health clinics and psychiatric units in general hospitals, provision of counseling services in the community as secondary prevention measures, improvement in facilities for the chronically ill as tertiary prevention measures, and dissemination of information aimed at increasing public understanding and attitudes about mental illness.

President Kennedy's interest in mental health gave further impetus to the community mental health movement. In 1963 he spoke about the crisis in mental health. Congress responded by passing the Community Mental Health Centers Act, which allocated monies for mental health care and developed guidelines for mental health services.

The Community Mental Health Centers Act incorporated many of the recommendations of the Joint Commission. The basic principles of the act included the following:

1. Providing services for mental health care that are readily available to community residents
2. Providing comprehensive services to meet the varying needs of community residents
3. Providing services appropriate to the individual's problems

The original intent of the act was to establish community mental health centers to treat and rehabilitate the mentally ill within the community (Jerrell and Larsen, 1986).

A major effect of the Mental Health Studies Act and subsequent legislation on nursing and other, nonmedical health professions was a resolution of the problem of who was qualified to do short-term psychotherapy. The practice of short-term psychotherapy by qualified nurses, social workers, and other professionals became accepted.

CHARACTERISTICS OF COMMUNITY MENTAL HEALTH SERVICES
Essential services

The Community Mental Health Centers Act of 1963 established guidelines for mental health care and defined five essential services that a health cen-

TABLE 16-3 Comparison of target groups being served by community mental health centers (CMHC)

Target group	Demographic trend	CMHC service shifts
Chronically mentally ill	Increase in 18–35-year-olds	Increased services for older clients who have received long-term care and for younger clients who have not received long-term care; beginning focus on psychosocial and vocational rehabilitation; improved case management (e.g., needs assessments, coordination of services); increased residential programs
Children and adolescents	Maintenance of previous pattern	Increased preventive services in the areas of child abuse, sexual abuse, maternal-infant relations, and family problems (especially those associated with unemployment); increased services for autistic and hyperactive children
Elderly	Increase (population will double by year 2020)	Some increased consultation services to nursing homes; decreased outreach programs

Sources consulted include Pepper, Kirshmer, and Ryglewicz (1981), Talbott (1981), Jerrell and Larsen (1986).

ter must provide to be eligible to receive federal funds. The five essential services were (1) around-the-clock inpatient care, (2) outpatient clinic services, (3) facilities for partial hospitalization (for example, day or night hospitals), (4) walk-in facilities for emergency services, and (5) community consultation and education services for prevention of mental illness and promotion of mental health.

The 1963 legislation listed additional services that could be provided but that were not mandatory: diagnostic services, rehabilitation services, research, and evaluation and training of mental health workers.

Between 1963 and 1979, the Community Mental Health Centers Act was amended several times. Each time, the scope of the program was expanded (Jerrell and Larsen, 1986). For example, such originally optional services as diagnosis, rehabilitation, research, evaluation, and training of mental health workers became required. In addition, amended legislation required services for special groups—

particularly children, the aged, ethnic minorities, and persons with special problems such as drug or alcohol addiction—and recommended coordination of health and human services systems to meet mental health needs.

Delivery of services

The manner in which community mental health services are organized and the programs that are developed to provide comprehensive services may vary from one community to another. Many factors can influence the way in which community mental health programs are implemented. Variations in geographic distribution of population, population density, and mental health needs necessitate variations in the organization of mental health services. Socioeconomic and demographic factors and the availability of already existing mental health and human services systems may also affect the ways in which programs are plannd to meet mental health needs. Table 16-3 compares target groups that are being served by community mental health services.

The ideal toward which the community mental health movement strives is a system characterized by collaborative endeavors of all agencies and personnel providing human services. However, Aiken (1987) believes that services are fragmented and that mental health professionals, while striving for effective case management, are finding it difficult to coordinate services. For instance, in many states nursing homes are being used as alternatives to hospitalization of the elderly in state hospitals. Moreover, the treatment of acute mental illness is primarily shifting to general hospital psychiatric services. Also, although the duration of stay in state mental hospitals has decreased, the number of readmissions has increased.

Unmet need for services: The homeless mentally ill

Freeman (1986) estimates that the mentally ill have a 20 times greater likelihood of being homeless than the general population. Some of the homeless mentally ill are chronically mentally ill people who have been deinstitutionalized or have been repeatedly treated in ambulatory mental health programs. Many "young chronics" are in this category. Others are "bag ladies" or "grate men" who live relatively isolated lives, evidence bizarre behavior, and have some degree of mental illness. Still others are chronic alcoholics who live on the streets (Fisher and Breakey, 1986).

Such factors as deinstitutionalization, shortage of low-cost housing, and decreases in social service funding have contributed to the problem of homelessness. Hopper (1988) sees the problem of homelessness as an indication that the fundamental needs-meeting mechanisms of society are failing and looks at system-wide developments in society that have generated this problem. Nation-wide unemployment and recession, curtailment of federal housing-assistance programs for the poor, gentrification (reclaiming of rundown but inhabited neighborhoods for high-income dwellings), abandoned dwellings, and conversion of vacated dwellings to cooperatives or condominiums (usually preceded by buying tenants out or displacing them by allow-

ing services to deteriorate until tenants move) all have contributed to the crisis of homelessness. Hopper suggests that it is under such circumstances that psychiatric impairment converts into social handicap. Within a socioeconomic context of competition for increasingly scarce and expensive housing, the mentally ill, who have impaired coping abilities, are at a decided disadvantage, and they succumb to homelessness. Public shelters have not been a solution, for many homeless people find shelter environments menacing. Shelters are usually located in the most unkempt and marginal areas of cities, where there is a high incidence of crime and violence. Homeless mentally ill people often are victimized in such environments.

Some community mental health centers have street rescue teams that hospitalize homeless mentally ill people on a short-term, involuntary emergency treatment basis. This approach has received criticism for infringing on the civil rights of homeless people. Sometimes criminal charges may be brought against the homeless mentally ill, and they may be jailed. French (1987) emphasizes that jail is not an acceptable alternative to clinical treatment. Moreover, the stress associated with the experience of incarceration may exacerbate the mental disorders of the homeless mentally ill and further increase their chances of being victimized (French, 1987).

To deal effectively with the needs of the homeless mentally ill, French (1987) believes that the criterion for treatment and placement should be changed from "least restrictive" to "most therapeutic." In addition, he would like the definition of legal incompetency to be broadened to include all clinical conditions that impede judgment. Such changes would encourage accountability of treatment staff and case managers for therapeutic treatment of clients whether they are in an institutional or community setting. Table 16-4 outlines some strategies that have been suggested for serving the homeless mentally ill in community settings.

CURRENT STATUS OF COMMUNITY MENTAL HEALTH

During the past two decades there has been remarkable progress in the implementation of the

TABLE 16-4   Suggested community mental health center services for the homeless mentally ill

Service	Description
Crisis intervention	Information and referral to shelters, food pantries, food-stamp offices, thrift shops, and loan closets (for clothing and furniture); job counseling (e.g., job retraining, job leads, coaching about presentation of self to prospective employers); relational services
Relocation assistance	Housing leads (e.g., available private housing, available structured group housing); counseling about how to follow up on housing leads (e.g., presentation of self to prospective landlords, securing financial assistance with rent); collaboration with local public housing authorities; provision of transportation to housing leads
Outreach mental health services	Mobile mental health diagnostic and treatment services administered in such settings as group homes, homeless shelters, and city streets
Drop-in centers	Located in geographic areas where the homeless congregate; loosely structured; make few demands on clients; no appointment necessary; offer crisis intervention and information and referal services

Sources consulted include Hutchison, Searight, and Stretch (1986), Hagen (1986), Appleby and Desai (1987), and Aiken (1987).

community mental health concept. This progress is reflected in major changes in services for the treatment of persons with psychiatric disorders and developmental disabilities.

Long-term hospitalization in institutions has largely given way to brief hospitalization in times of crisis and the development of treatment and prevention services in local communities throughout the country. State hospital populations have declined, despite a relatively stable number of admissions or, in some institutions, even a slight increase in admissions. For many persons with chronic disabilities, forms of supervised housing in the community have replaced the institution as a home. This pattern has become increasingly prevalent as the constitutional rights of persons with mental health problems have been affirmed by the courts.

Progress has also been made in primary prevention, including public education about mental disorders and promotion of collaborative efforts between health and social service systems for the improvement of mental health care.

Despite the progress that has been made, many problems and difficulties lie ahead. Much criticism has been leveled against the community mental health movement in recent years by health professionals and the public at large. Community mental health has been accused by many authors of moving too far too fast, of failing to live up to early expectations and promises, and of moving people out of the back wards into the back alleys. That problems would be encountered and criticisms would arise as a result of a change in health care of the magnitude of that brought about by the community mental health movement was to be expected. Challenges to long-standing beliefs, attitudes, and practices and to areas of vested interest were threatening to many people.

In many communities, for example, there has been public resistance to the presence of mental health treatment and rehabilitation facilities. This problem has been exacerbated in some areas because of the large numbers of people with chronic disorders who have been housed or "dumped" in some communities. The problem, to some extent, reflects a lack of funding by state, local, and federal governments, which could have made possible the wider distribution of the mental health facilities necessary to provide care and treatment for persons with chronic disorders.

The maldistribution of health professionals is another major concern, particularly since the persons most in need of mental health services often reside in poor neighborhoods or in rural areas, where few health professionals practice and where the services that are available are often provided by local residents or self-help groups with inadequate preparation. There has also been a decrease in staff in alcohol and drug abuse services (Jerrell and Larsen, 1986).

Deinstitutionalization

In the past 20 years, state mental hospitals have experienced a decline of almost 80% in the number of residents. The total of all client populations has decreased from approximately 559,000 to fewer than 120,000 people (Aiken, 1987). The practice of discharging chronically mentally ill clients into the community is known as deinstitutionalization. Because the ability to cope with the stress of living in the community without decompensating and developing psychiatric symptoms is different for each chronically mentally ill person, the population of deinstitutionalized clients ranges from those who can tolerate very little stress to those who, with assistance, can cope with the stressors of community living (Lamb, 1981).

However, planning for deinstitutionalization is often inadequate. The desire to shift the cost of care for chronically mentally ill clients from the state to the federal government often results in discharging clients into the community without ascertaining whether community service facilities exist. There is usually little assessment of client needs and level of functioning and little consideration of whether hospital or community is the best treatment setting for a particular client. Clients are frequently discharged from a state institution into a hostile community. The lack of aftercare and support services to facilitate the transition from a highly structured hospital setting to a less structured community setting may have devastating effects on a client. One effect is the social breakdown syndrome.

The community mental health movement is oriented toward preventing or reversing the social breakdown syndrome. The social breakdown syndrome begins when individuals who are experiencing psychiatric symptoms become unable to meet the behavioral expectations of their culture and develop feelings of isolation and detachment. Brief hospitalization for treatment of acute psychotic states, in a therapeutic milieu, with follow-up care in outpatient departments of community mental health centers is one strategy used to prevent or reverse this syndrome. Although the family is often the most important part of a person's social network, a major psychiatric disorder may cause a breakdown in a person's relationship with the family. A family member who is regarded as mentally ill may become alienated from the family. Nurses may ameliorate or prevent such alienation of psychiatric clients by working with family members as part of the treatment and rehabilitation process and by facilitating communication between clients and their families and other social networks. Treatment in community settings, with minimal restrictions on client freedom and maximum opportunity for the maintenance of social contacts, is another important measure in preventing the social breakdown syndrome.

For some clients with chronic mental illness and especially for those deinstitutionalized clients who have experienced long-term isolation from their social support systems, efforts to develop new social networks may be necessary. Ethnic and religious groups and community mental health services may provide such networks. For example, Alcoholics Anonymous often serves as a major social support system for persons with disorders related to alcoholism.

ORGANIZATIONAL STRESSORS

Factors inherent in providing care to chronically mentally ill clients in the community may produce organizational stress and ineffective and inefficient delivery of care. Table 16-5 summarizes some of these stressors.

According to Scheper-Hughes (1982), because the cost of many programs for deinstitutionalized clients are financed by Medicaid monies, the focus of these programs is usually on medical and psychiatric treatment and sheltered-workshop types of employment. Yet what is most often needed by deinstitutionalized clients are such supportive services as adequate housing, provision of nutritious food, and a place to "hang out." Deinstitutionalized clients who spend their days in libraries, public parks, diners, and donut shops are usually viewed either with suspicion or as public nuisances.

The need for a place to spend free time and the desire to socialize with people like oneself are common human needs and are found among many

TABLE 16-5 Organizational stressors associated with community care of chronically mentally ill clients

Organizational stressor	Description
Rehabilitation goal	The goal of the community mental health movement—to reintegrate clients into the community as independent, gainfully employed, well-functioning individuals—may be unrealistic for many deinstitutionalized clients. Many chronically mentally ill clients do not have access to social networks, community support, or aftercare services. For them, the goal of rehabilitation may be to live with comfort and with dignity in the community. Board-and-care homes, which offer varying degrees of supervision and structure, may meet their needs. Nurses and other mental health professionals who are unable to modify their goals to meet the different needs and coping abilities of clients may experience stress when total reintegration into the community is unrealistic. Mental health professionals may try to deal with their stress by engaging in blame placing (blaming clients or the community) and by rejecting deinstitutionalized clients.
Service ideal	The ideal of community mental health centers is to serve the entire community. Treating deinstitutionalized clients is time-consuming. If community mental health professionals work with deinstitutionalized clients, they have less time to serve the rest of the community. This dilemma may cause conflict and stress. Many nurses and other mental health professionals resolve the conflict by concentrating on primary and secondary prevention to the exclusion of tertiary prevention. This approach results in the abandonment of deinstitutionalized clients.
Threat to professional esteem	Among nurses and other mental health professionals, status and professional recognition tend to be associated with the care of acutely ill, rather than chronically ill, clients. Acutely ill clients may be viewed as more challenging and more satisfying to work with than chronically ill clients. In addition, the education of most mental health professionals does not provide the special skills needed to work with chronically mentally ill clients. These factors tend to threaten professional esteem.
Threat to professional ability	When nurses and other mental health professionals work with deinstitutionalized clients, they may experience frustration, helplessness and hopelessness, and, eventually, burnout. For this reason, mental health professionals often try to avoid treating deinstitutionalized clients and may delegate this responsibility to nonprofessionals.
Reality of chronicity	Chronic mental illness is rarely cured. Many nurses and other mental health professionals judge their effectiveness by their ability to cure clients. To satisfy their need for client progress, many mental health professionals may pressure deinstitutionalized clients to alter their behavior, may establish short-term goals that deal only with dysfunction, and may ignore long-term goals that would deal with problems related to chronicity. A power struggle between client and therapist may develop overcontrol or definition of the therapeutic relationship.
Reality of deinstitutionalization	The discharge of chronically mentally ill clients into the community may present many problems. Communities may be hostile and resistant. Families may feel overwhelmed. Clients may feel isolated and insecure in their new community surroundings and may wish for the security associated with hospital routine. Aftercare facilities for deinstitutionalized clients may be inadequate.

Sources consulted include Stern and Minkoff (1979), Lamb (1981), White and Bennett (1981), Harris and Bergman (1986), Plum (1987), Swearingen (1987).

deinstitutionalized clients. The despair and isolation experienced by deinstitutionalized clients who have been "dumped" into a community without any support systems contribute to a high suicide rate among deinstitutionalized clients. However, some deinstitutionalized clients who live in single room occupancy hotels, rooming houses, or apartments with other deinstitutionalized clients have been able to establish and maintain social support systems among themselves (Scheper-Hughes, 1981). It is vitally important that community mental health workers facilitate the formation and maintenance of such client support systems.

IMPLICATIONS FOR THE FUTURE

The gestalt of the community mental health movement may need to be altered to include the hospital as an integral part of the community. The hospital and the community mental health agency will need to cooperate with and complement each other. The hospital may need to introduce creative approaches to chronicity and to increase the type and number of services for chronically mentally ill clients. To prevent duplication of services, hospitals and community mental health agencies may need to cooperate in planning programs aimed at problems associated with chronicity. This approach necessitates a recognition of such unique service needs of chronically mentally ill individuals as resocialization, housing, vocational rehabilitation, and employment opportunities.

The goal of reintegrating all mentally ill clients into the community may need to be reexamined. Long-term institutionalization may be indicated for people who are so severely chronically ill that the structure and nursing care available in hospitals are necessary. For people who are mildly or moderately chronically ill, reintegration into the community may be a viable alternative to institutionalization. However, it will be necessary to provide adequate aftercare and supportive services and to involve communities in planning and delivering services. In addition, to obtain continuous information about the needs of chronically mentally ill individuals, outreach programs for deinstitutionalized clients may need to be developed (Plum, 1987; Swearingen, 1987).

The education of nurses and other mental health professionals may also need to be reexamined. Clinical specialization and in-service education programs for the care of chronically mentally ill individuals will need to be encouraged. Development of skills that are effective in the treatment of chronically mentally ill clients may lessen the threat to professional esteem that many nurses and other mental health professionals often experience and may help to keep professionals involved in the care of chronically mentally ill clients (Stern and Minkoff, 1979).

Impact of decreased funding

The Community Mental Health Centers Act of 1963 allocated monies, using a "seed money" concept, for community mental health centers. The concept of seed money was based on the belief that community mental health centers should gradually become less dependent on National Institute of Mental Health (NIMH) funding. Federal regulations for nonpoverty areas stipulated the following funding formula to finance community mental health centers' operational costs: 80% NIMH funding during the first year of a center's operation; 65% funding during the second year; 40% during the third and fourth years; 35% during the fifth and sixth years; and 25% during the seventh and eighth years. In some instances, NIMH funding was continued through the twelfth year of a community mental health center's operation. Poverty areas received 90% NIMH funding for the first two years of operation, and then the funding was gradually decreased to 30% in the eighth year. NIMH money was to be "matched" by gradually increasing amounts of nonfederal monies. Thus, community mental health centers would progressively become financially independent of Federal grant money and would find other sources of revenue (Weiner et al., 1979; Kenig, 1986).

Medicare, Medicaid, and other third-party payments have not replaced NIMH funding, but they have been a source of some revenue. Client fees for direct services and local grants augment third-party reimbursements (Jerrell and Larsen, 1986).

In 1981, the Omnibus Budget Reconciliation Act incorporated the mental health services support programs formerly administered by NIMH into an alcohol, drug abuse, and mental health (ADM) services block grant. Because states have the option of transferring grant monies among alcohol, drug abuse, and mental health categories, it is advantageous for community mental health centers to refer clients to existing local and state drug and alcohol treatment services instead of developing such programs themselves (Jerrell and Larsen, 1986).

The impact of decreased federal funding for community mental health centers is reflected in (1) fragmentation of services and (2) development of specialized service programs aimed at those target populations that are sources of revenue. For example, services for the severely acutely mentally ill are increasing as a result of state directives giving high priority as well as money to support programs for these clients. In addition, staff lay-offs and hiring freezes that were so common in the early 1980s seem to have come to an end. Many administrators are recognizing that they need credentialed mental health professionals to qualify for third-party reimbursement (Jerrell and Larsen, 1986; Kenig, 1986).

IMPLICATIONS FOR THE FUTURE

Some questions facing the community mental health movement are (1) Will future policy changes focus on different client groups? (2) What will be the quality and effectiveness of service changes? and (3) Will public funding be able to expand the scope of mental health services for those in need or even be able to maintain the current range of services? (Jerrell and Larsen, 1986).

Several factors favor the continuation and possibly the expansion of the community mental health movement, even during a period of economic uncertainty. One factor is economic. Providing services which treat people with psychiatric disorders and disabilities in the community is less costly—in both human and economic terms—than maintaining large inpatient populations in public hospitals. Although it is necessary in times of fiscal restraint to establish priorities in relation to mental health programs, economic considerations favor the community mental health approach. Prevention of disorders is also far less costly in human and economic terms than secondary and tertiary programs.

Another factor that augurs well for community mental health programs is the court actions that have upheld the constitutional rights of persons with psychiatric problems. Our legal system is based on precedents established by decisions of the courts. The many lawsuits adjudicated in state courts across the nation and in the United States Supreme Court during the past two decades have established precedents and upheld clients' constitutional rights concerning mental health care, including the right to such care in the least restrictive setting.

The strong commitment to the community mental health movement that has been demonstrated by many mental health professionals and many consumers of health care holds promise for the development of the movement in the future. Participation in social, political, and community action to promote mental health programs and facilities is an important function of nurses and members of the other health professions.

CULTURE AND COMMUNITY MENTAL HEALTH
Cultural background of the community

For health care givers to effectively meet the mental health needs of a given community, they must understand the cultural background of that community. The cultural background of community residents affects their conceptualization of and response to mental health and mental illness. Some major conceptual differences between traditional non-Western ethnomedical systems and modern Western medicine are summarized in Table 16-6.

Sometimes, ethnomedical and modern Western medical systems coexist in a community. People recognize the effectiveness of using modern Western medicine to treat biophysical conditions while also recognizing and using ethnomedicine to explain and remedy "why" (the disharmonic conditions) they have fallen victim to illness. Other times, ethnomedical and modern Western medical systems operate in a community as mutually exclusive systems. Traditional health or religious groups may have very highly developed healing ministries,

TABLE 16-6   Conceptual differences between traditional and modern health care systems

Health-related concept	View of health care system
Body	*Ethnomedicine:* body is a microcosm of the universe and/or an integration of self and social relationships *Western medicine:* body is a complex machine; behavior is motivated by habit, instinct, and/or searches for meaning, self-actualization, and altruism
Mind-body relationship	*Ethnomedicine:* mind, body and spirit are interrelated; illness cannot be located in only the mind or only the body *Western medicine:* mind and body are distinct entities; locus of illness may be in the mind or in the body
Social relationships	*Ethnomedicine:* labeling, causation, and treatment of illness usually involve the entire family (including extended family and/or ancestors) *Western medicine:* labeling, causation, and treatment of illness may involve only the individual (except in such areas as family therapy or holistic health practice)
Health	*Ethnomedicine:* health is a balanced state of being in harmony with self (mind, body, and spirit) and with nature *Western medicine:* physical and mental health may be viewed as two different states of well-being or absence of disease

Sources include Rappaport and Rappaport (1981), Scheper-Hughes and Lock (1987), and Williams (1988).

and their practitioners and followers may view modern Western medicine as useless or meaningless. At the same time, modern Western medical practitioners may make little attempt to accommodate ethnomedical beliefs and practices. There are also times when ethnomedical and modern Western medical systems have a complementary relationship. Practitioners and followers of each system recognize the strengths and weaknesses of both systems, and practitioners work together to fill voids created by deficits inherent in each system (Milner, 1983).

Because there is an interrelationship between the medical and social realms in society, traditional ethnomedical systems are able to meet many of the special needs of ethnic group members and to make significant contributions to the health of communities (Clinton, 1987).

A community may comprise various minority groups, which display different and distinct orientations and responses to health and illness. A cluster of characteristics that many minority groups share is summarized in Table 16-7.

Because ethnic group members may come from different geographic locales, differ in age and ethnic generation (e.g., immigrant vs. second-generation ethnic American), follow different religious

beliefs and practices, come from different educational and socioeconomic backgrounds, speak different languages, and have different personalities, there tends to be great variation within ethnic groups, and stereotyping and generalizing should be avoided. For example, Asian Indians may practice the Hindu, Moslem, or Christian faith. Chinese immigrants may speak one of three major Chinese dialects: Mandarin, Shanhainesse, or Cantonese. Southeast Asian refugees may come from Cambodia, Vietnam, or Laos; speak different languages; and have different beliefs and practices. Hispanics may come from South America or Central America and have different ethnomedical systems.

Utilization of community mental health services

Among the various cultural groups in American society, there are differences in attitudes toward accepting mental health care and using community mental health centers. Community residents who are members of the lower socioeconomic class or who are members of minority racial or ethnic groups may be apprehensive or suspicious of a community mental health staff that is predominantly

TABLE 16-7   Characteristics common to minority groups

Characteristic	Description
Victim orientation	Some minority groups may be the victims of institutionalized racism or discrimination, or they may experience social stigma attached to illegal alien status or poverty. Many minority groups are segregated in ghettos or on reservations.
Communication problems	A language barrier (both verbal and nonverbal) may exist between minority group members and members of mainstream America. Differences in cultural orientation and lifestyle may result in differences in perception, interpretation, and response to events and situations (refer to Chapter 10 for a discussion of culture and communication).
Definition of family	Members of many minority group cultures have an extended family orientation that encompasses many households and several generations. There usually is a sense of responsibility for one's extended family and an inclusion of extended kin, both actual and fictive, in problem solving. This orientation is different from that of mainstream Americans, who tend to engage in problem solving on a nuclear family level or on an individual level (refer to Chapter 5 for a discussion of culturally influenced family forms).
Respect for elders	In various minority groups, elderly family members may be looked to for advice, and their advice is usually followed. Elderly family members may also be the authority figures in the family. This is different from the situation in many mainstream American families, which tend to be egalitarian or to devalue elderly family members.
Fatalistic orientation	Many minority groups tend to be fatalistic and to believe that their existence and health are at the mercy of the environment and/or God. They may feel that they have little personal control over their fate except to remain in harmony with the environment and/or God. On the other hand, mainstream Americans usually believe that they can control what happens to them—that they are "masters of their fate."
Holistic health orientation	Many minority groups view health and illness as complex physical, psychological, and spiritual conditions. When they become ill, this holistic orientation is usually reflected in a mixture of somatic, spiritual, and emotional complaints. Ethnic healers, rather than traditional community mental health professionals, can relate to this admixture of complaints, conceptualize health and illness in the same way as do minority group clients, and involve extended family members in the therapeutic plan.

Sources consulted include Weaver and Sklar (1980), Flaskerud (1982), McGoldrick, Pearce, and Giordano (1982), and Scheper-Hughes and Lock (1987).

white and middle class. These minority group community members may associate community mental health centers with other mainstream American–controlled institutions, such as the police and the courts, that they have found repressive. Also, the previously discussed cluster of shared differences between many minorities and mainstream Americans may contribute to a sense of alienation of minority group residents from community mental health centers. For example, Mexican-Americans, Puerto Ricans, and Native Americans who are on the lower end of the socioeconomic class system tend to underutilize community mental health centers. Primary reasons for this underutilization include (1) different values, different expectations, and different world views than those held by mental health professionals; (2) lack of culturally appropriate services; (3) self-perceived stigma attached to mental health services; and/or (4) financial constraints (Rappaport and Rappaport, 1981; Hough et al., 1987).

Even within the same cultural group, attitudinal differences based on sex may exist. In many cultures it is more acceptable for women than for men to express emotional distress and to seek help for their problems. This is a major factor in explaining why, throughout the United States, women not only use community mental health facilities more often than do men but also seek help earlier in the course of their problems than do men (Kerson, 1981).

In addition, a lack of knowledge about the services offered by the community mental health center and the fees it charges may contribute to underuse of the facility. The existence of a sliding scale, based on income, is often unknown to community residents.

Implications for transcultural nursing

To better meet the mental health needs of minority group community residents, community mental health nurses need to be knowledgeable about the cultural backgrounds of clients and potential clients and adapt nursing-care approaches to clients' cultural orientations. Clinton (1987) suggests that nurses broaden their perspective of health so that it (1) encompasses cultural diversity, (2) understands the role of culturally derived beliefs and practices in health promotion, (3) recognizes biases engendered by professional socialization, (4) promotes complementary and egalitarian interaction between traditional ethnomedical and Western medical systems, and (5) uses politicoeconomic influence to remedy social inequalities. Nursing psychotherapy is ideal for providing culturally relevant nursing therapy because it focuses on clients as biopsychosocial beings, integrates mental and physical health care, encompasses a multifaceted approach that includes a spectrum of support services to meet clients' socioeconomic needs, and delivers nursing psychotherapy in a multiplicity of settings and with emphasis on family-centered care (Flaskerud, 1987). Table 16-8 illustrates some nursing approaches that may increase the use and effectiveness of community mental health services.

In addition to the nursing approaches and activities described in Table 16-8, community mental health nurses need to use culturally acceptable interactional approaches to establish rapport with ethnic clients. Provision of culturally relevant psychotherapy is predicated on an understanding of clients' perceptions, values, beliefs, and attitudes about maintenance of health and prevention and treatment of illness. To accomplish this, nurses should shift from relying on cultural stereotypes in delivering nursing psychotherapy and shift toward utilization of knowledge about cultural differences. Nurses should also stop interpreting behavior as a predominantly psychological phenomenon and start understanding it from the cultural perspectives of clients. Therefore, the traditional world views, or cultural perspectives, of several cultural groupings will now be discussed. It is important to remember that great variation exists among ethnic groups within each cultural grouping as well as within each ethnic group.

NATIVE AMERICAN WORLD VIEW

Traditionally, Native Americans view the world as a dynamic system of interrelated parts, with each part governed by a supernatural force or spirit being. For instance, Cheyenne spirits include the Spirit who Gives Good Health, the Spirit who Rules the Universe, and the Spirit who Rules the Summer. The power of spirits, including ancestors, is derived not from their ability to create and rule domains of the universe but from their wisdom and knowledge about the workings of the universe. The energy of the world and any of the objects in it is finite. Because people expend energy through activity, they must regenerate it if they are to survive. Ceremonials are one way of renewing energy and therefore are critically important in the life-styles of Native Americans.

Although nature/environment (comprised of such elements as weather, plants, animals, people, and supernatural forces) tends to be beneficent, human beings cannot control it. It is therefore important for people to keep themselves in harmony with nature.

The kin group rather than the individual is emphasized. Kinship is the basis for personal identity, and all aspects of life tend to be group oriented. The extended family system continues to prevail among a majority of Native Americans.

Health reflects a harmonious relationship with nature that includes not only balance with the physical environment but also accord with supernatural forces, respect for taboos and ancestors, responsibility for one's actions and decisions, and family unity. Health and religion are intertwined and are considered inseparable. The medicine man (or shaman) possesses supernatural power and is

TABLE 16-8 Community mental health nursing approaches and activities

Nursing approach	Nursing activity
Collaboration	Work with other community mental health workers and with community leaders and community residents in planning comprehensive services that address such problems as poverty, housing, unemployment, discrimination, and social and medical concerns. Include community leaders and community residents in evaluating community mental health services. Encourage community members to use the physical facilities of the local community mental health center for community meetings and activities. Work with clergy and pastoral counselors to help clients with the spiritual components of their problems.
Advocacy	Assist clients to navigate the community mental health system and/or other social systems. This involves supporting, guiding, and interceding for clients, as well as helping clients learn to navigate the system(s) for themselves (refer to Chapter 3 for a discussion of client advocacy).
Availability	Make community mental health services readily available to *all* community residents. This may mean locating a community mental health center in an ethnic area, lobbying for adequate public transportation, and making home visits to clients who are homebound or who do not have babysitters. It may also mean the scheduling of ample evening and weekend hours and walk-in appointments so that clients will not have to take off from work to utilize community mental health services.
Family-centered nursing	Utilize family therapy in nursing psychotherapy and encourage other professional team members to use family therapy. When culturally appropriate, include extended kin in the family grouping.
Holistic orientation	View clients as biopsychosocial beings with complex problems. Use crisis-oriented therapy that focuses on clients' presenting problems and that offers concrete goals and results.
Communication	Whenever possible, converse with ethnic clients in their native languages. Otherwise, nurses should urge that indigenous workers be hired to act as culture brokers and translators of behavioral expectations and codes of conduct.
Complementarity	Facilitate the incorporation of ethnic healers into community mental health centers. Ethnomedical healing may be used in conjunction with traditional Western therapies, or a system of mutual referrals may be set up between ethnic healers and community mental health workers.
Acculturative assessment	Assess the level of acculturation of clients. Nurses should be aware that, because children often acculturate more rapidly than their parents, intergenerational problems may develop and role relationships may be reversed (refer to Chapter 4 for a discussion of acculturation and its assessment).

Sources consulted include Weaver and Sklar (1980), Pasquali (1982), Flaskerud (1982), Milner (1983), and Flaskerud and van Servellen (1985).

wise in the ways of both nature and people. This wisdom embraces the interrelationship among people, the earth, and the universe as well as the workings of plants, animals, and the galaxy. The shaman treats by trying to correct the cause of illness. Treatment may include confession, making amends to family or tribe, therapeutic agents, and negotiation with the spirit world (Attneave, 1982; Scheper-Hughes and Lock, 1987; Rogers and Evernham, 1983; Herrick, 1983).

ASIAN-AMERICAN WORLD VIEW

Asian-Americans encompass such ethnic groups as Chinese, Koreans, Japanese, Cambodians, Laotians, Vietnamese, and Filipinos. While each ethnic group has unique beliefs and customs, a core of beliefs is shared. The universe is viewed as indivisible. Each part, or element, has a definite function, and all parts interrelate in harmonious balance. The aim of life is to achieve harmony with nature. Each person is a reflection of the forces that govern the universe. Meditation and ceremonials free a person from distractions so that there is freedom for inter-action of cosmic forces within the self. Filial piety, reverence for family and ancestors, moral behavior, evenness of feeling, cooperation, tolerance, and saving face are necessary to achieve harmony and balance. Saving face (the avoidance of shame and humiliation) refers to a person's moral reputation. The self is supposed to remain inconspicuous and unexpressed. Calling attention to one's self, whether through violation of norms, public failure, or excelling, may result in shame and the loss of face. If attention is focused on one's self, it is culturally prescribed to act embarrassed or shy. Shame and the loss of face are associated with the withdrawal of family and community support. In a society that is socially group-minded and stresses interdependence, the threats of losing face and having social support systems withdrawn help to reinforce conformity to family and societal norms and expectations.

Polytheism is reflected in a pantheon of gods and sacred places or shrines. Spiritual emphasis is on protection from the caprices of gods and nature and living a good life. Among many Asians, deceased parents and grandparents are believed to influence the well-being of their living descendants, and they therefore must be honored. Household shrines often are the locus of ancestor honoring.

The kin group, rather than the individual, is emphasized. Identity is derived from one's place in the extended family, which may include ancestors as well as living relatives. Families tend to be parent, rather than child, oriented. Parents and elders are honored and respected, and parental advice must be followed. Obligations to one's parents often supersede those to one's spouse or children. To maintain family harmony, expression of negative feelings, emotional states, and conflict tends to be avoided.

Health is viewed as a balanced state. Moderation in all things is seen as a means of maintaining balance and staying healthy. Balance should be maintained through a disciplined life, control of emotions and desires, healthy diet, and adaptation to environmental changes. Illness is a state of imbalance. The goal of treatment is to reinstate balance and harmony. Reinstatement of balance may be

achieved through regulation (e.g., following specific dietary patterns or manifesting culturally prescribed "correct" behavior) and replacement (e.g., supplementing with foods and herbs prescribed according to symptoms, age, season, etc.) (Shon and Ja, 1982; Lebra, 1983; Kakar, 1982; Roberts, Morita, and Brown, 1986; Manio and Hall, 1987; Flaskerud, 1987).

AFRO-AMERICAN WORLD VIEW

Traditionally, Afro-Americans view life as a process. Everything, whether it is alive or dead, is interrelated and interdependent, exerting influence one on the other. This extends to the interrelationship of mind, body, and spirit. God is seen as the source of all good things, including health. People should have faith, trust, and belief in God, who is omnipotent and beneficent. God has a plan for each person. While God's plan may not always be understandable to people, neither should people try to judge that plan. Because Satan is always trying to tempt people and gain mastery over their souls, people fall into sin. However, through prayer and repentence, people can save their souls and live for eternity in the afterworld.

The collateral and affiliation orientations valued in African culture are reflected in the Afro-American extended family. Lateral relations are very important, and loyalty to, interdependence with, and responsibility for the extended family of real and fictive kin are stressed (see Chapter 4 for a discussion of collateral orientation). In addition, children are highly valued, and elders are respected.

Health is viewed as a state of balance. Health maintenance and illness prevention are strongly influenced by religious beliefs. Christian living offers protection from evil behavior and evil spirits and is essential to one's spiritual, physical, and emotional well-being. However, being a good Christian does not ensure health. Behavior that disrupts the balance between one's self and the environment (social and physical) can result in illness. Potential causes of illness may be either supernatural (e.g., punishment from God or the result of demons, spirits, spells, or hexes) or natural (e.g., stress, negative mental attitudes, personal actions that disrupt self-nature harmony). Therefore, daily examination of one's behavior is necessary to maintain health and to explain illness. The restoration of balance to regain health is achieved by trying to remedy the cause of illness, whether it is naturally caused or supernaturally caused. Illness due to supernatural cause is treated by root doctors or voodoo doctors who use magico-religious interventions that include potions, prayers, laying-on-of-hands, and recitation of psalms. Illness due to natural cause is treated by "granny healers" who use home remedies and herbal medicines (Hill and Mathews, 1981; Pinderhughes, 1982; Powers, 1982; Roberson, 1985).

HISPANIC-AMERICAN WORLD VIEW

Traditional Hispanic-American world view has been shaped by Spanish, African, and Amerindian beliefs. Spanish influence is reflected in the belief that fortune and misfortune are God given. Living according to God's laws and praying to saints, who serve as intermediaries to God, are "precautions" that one may take against misfortune. However, such precautions do not guarantee good fortune, and hardship is accepted as part of life. Amerindian influence is reflected in beliefs about supernatural forces and predestination. Supernatural forces, in the form of gods, ghosts, and demons, victimize people from birth to death. The soul, or vital breath of a person, may be lost if a person is subjected to such strong emotions as anger and fear. Although there is a divine design to life, destiny can be altered through self-discipline, prayers, potions, and incantations. African belief about a pantheon of powerful gods or supernatural forces shaping one's destiny, a destiny that can be altered through behavior and knowledge about people and the world, also contributes to acceptance of predestination. The synthesis of Spanish, Amerindian, and African beliefs results in (1) viewing the natural world and the supernatural world as interrelated, (2) having a fatalistic attitude: what happens is predestined or God's will, (3) holding belief systems such as Santeria or the Cult of Chango, in which African gods are syncretized with Catholic saints.

Family form and attitudes about the family have also been influenced by Spanish and African culture contacts. The traditional Hispanic family is an extended family of real and fictive kin. Children are reared to have a sense of responsibility to and for extended family members. Identity is derived from one's position in and relationship with the extended family. Patriarchal authority in the family reflects traditional sex roles of male dominance and female submissiveness.

Health is viewed as a state of harmony or balance: (1) balance between four humors (blood, phlegm, black bile, and yellow bile) and (2) balance and oneness of mind, body, and spirit. Illness, which results from a state of imbalance, is God given and cannot be prevented. However, certain "precautions" (e.g., living a "good" life, having proper eating and sleeping habits) can be taken. Agents that may provoke illness include strong emotions, excesses of food and drink, certain people (e.g., witches and givers of the evil eye), and natural elements (e.g., spoiled food, night air, drafts). All foods, animals, people, beverages, and medicines may be classified as either hot or cold. This is a colloquial application of the Hippocratic humoral theory that was brought to Latin America by Spain and superimposed on the Amerindian lifestyle. This hot-cold system provides a way of classifying and treating illness. Hot illnesses are treated with cold remedies, and cold illnesses are treated with hot remedies. Thus, balance is restored. However, there tends to be much individual variation as to what is considered "hot" or "cold." If home remedies and the advice of family and friends fail to restore health, ethnic healing specialists (e.g., Mexican *curanderos*, Puerto Rican *espiritistas*, Cuban *santeras*) may be sought. In a world view where natural and supernatural worlds interrelate, ethnic healers act as liaisons between the two worlds (Martinez, 1978; Delgado, 1981; Pasquali, 1982; Foster, 1987; Scheper-Hughes and Lock, 1987).

Common to the four world views just discussed are beliefs that (1) the natural and supernatural worlds are interrelated, (2) body, mind, and spirit are inseparable, (3) health is a state of balance, and (4) illness is a state of imbalance. While mindful that there is a wide range of cultural diversity among different ethnic groups (even those within the same cultural grouping) as well as within ethnic groups, community mental health nurses should develop culturally relevant interactional approaches for establishing rapport with ethnic cli-

TABLE 16-9 Culturally relevant interactional approaches

Approach	Rationale
Assess cultural orientation	Diversity in cultural beliefs, attitudes, and/or behaviors may exist among members of the same ethnic group and sometimes among different generations of the same family (see Chapter 4 for a cultural assessment guide)
Be supportive rather than confrontive	Overt conflict and/or strong emotions such as anger may be believed to disrupt balance and harmony
Ask about client's physical health	Emotional distress may be expressed somatically in clients whose cultural orientation prescribes against verbal expression of feelings or emotional states; world view may hold mind, body, and spirit as inseparable and interrelated
Monitor own eye contact	Maintaining eye contact may be considered rude behavior or an indication of hostility
Utilize strategies other than verbalization of feelings or problems	Verbal expression of feelings, conflicts, and/or emotional states may be culturally unacceptable; fear of incurring shame may keep client from talking about problems; culture may prescribe that problems be resolved on one's own or within the family and not expressed outside the family
Listen to recountings of daily events	Telling about daily life events may be client's way of trying to identify factors that contributed to illness; client may be used to the interest of ethnic healers in daily events as a means of understanding the cause of illness
Ask about healing systems being used	Mental health professionals and ethnic healers may be simultaneously consulted; ethnic healers may serve as a natural support system and look at problems from the client's cultural perspective
Seek client's opinion of the problem	Emotional problems may be categorized as having spiritual (supernatural) causes
Take a holistic approach	Mind, body, and spirit may be viewed as inseparable and interrelated; emotional distress may be expressed somatically
Include the family in the treatment plan	Family ties may be strong; personal identity may be related to one's place in the extended family; extended family may be an important natural support system; culture may prescribe that problems be resolved within the family
Deal with hostility or suspiciousness, but do not take it personally	Expressions of hostility or suspiciousness may evidence social anxiety and be adaptive responses to encounters with prejudice and discrimination against ethnic minorities

Sources consulted include McGoldrick, Pearce, and Giordano (1982); Orque, Bloch, and Monroy (1983); Delgado (1983); Flaskerud (1987).

ents. Table 16-9 illustrates some of these approaches.

COMMUNITY MENTAL HEALTH NURSING

A community approach to mental health may require an adjustment in the tasks of mental health nurses. Community mental health nurses need to focus on activities in primary mental health care for the community in general and for subcultures within the community. This means that nurses should participate in programs that promote or reinforce the strengths and effective coping behaviors of members of a particular community. Community mental health nurses also should identify high-risk populations and provide services that reduce stress

Community mental health **459**

and deal with other psychosocial factors before healthy emotional functioning is disrupted.

Levels of practice

Community mental health nurses engage in a variety of levels of practice that involve assessing, planning, implementing, and evaluating mental health services for communities of people. Nurses function in organizational, advisory, advocacy, direct service, and consultative positions in community mental health agencies. The American Nurses' Association Division on Psychiatric and Mental Health Nursing Practice (1982) has identified *process criteria* (criteria focusing on nursing activities) and *outcome criteria* (criteria focusing on observable or measurable end results) for the practice of community mental health nursing. Process criteria specify that:

1. Nurses use their knowledge of systems theory and community and group dynamics in the analysis of community systems.
2. Nurses are cognizant of the influence of sociopolitical issues on community mental health problems.
3. Nurses encourage the participation of community members in the assessment and development of programs to address the mental health needs of the community.
4. Nurses are activists in articulating community health needs to such appropriate individuals and groups as legislators and regional and state planning boards.
5. Nurses engage in didactic and experiential teaching programs that meet the community's mental health needs.
6. Nurses serve as consultants in designing and implementing community mental health programs.
7. Nurses explain available mental health programs to members of the community.
8. Nurses collaborate with health team professionals and with community members in developing, implementing, and evaluating mental health programs.
9. Nurses identify populations at risk in the community and delineate areas of scarcity in community services.

10. Nurses assess the strengths and coping behaviors of individuals, families, and the community in order to promote, maintain, and improve their levels of mental health.
11. Nurses are knowledgeable about, refer clients to, and facilitate the use of appropriate community resources.
12. Nurses collaborate with inter-agency personnel to facilitate continuity of care for consumers of agency services.

Outcome criteria specify that:

1. The activities of nurses in primary, secondary, and tertiary mental health care are documented.
2. Mental health services that address the needs of the community are provided.
3. Nurses assume leadership roles in voluntary and governmental community health groups.

Qualities of community mental health nurses

Whether nurses in community mental health agencies are functioning as staff nurses prepared at the baccalaureate degree level or as clinical specialists prepared at the master's or doctoral degree level, they need to have a sound understanding of the unique contributions of nurses to the community mental health team. They also need high degrees of assertiveness and flexibility. Without these qualities, community mental health nurses may find that they are losing their identities in the role blurring that is common among community mental health professionals or that they are jeopardizing their effectiveness by being nonassertive in interdisciplinary altercations and exploration of roles.

Community mental health nurses also need to be clinically competent; knowledgeable about change theory, community organization, and the politics of institutions; and innovative, so that they can define their roles, demonstrate to colleagues the contributions nurses can make to community mental health programs, develop their own case loads, and engage in community outreach and consumer advocacy programs.[*] In addition, community mental

---

[*]Refer to Chapters 1 and 12 for further discussion of the role of the nurse and the mental health team.

TABLE 16-10   Knowledge about the community

Data	Description
Community attitudes	The attitudes of health professionals, special interest groups (e.g., neighborhood associations or parents of emotionally disturbed children), and community residents toward mental health needs and services should be elicited. This process necessitates ongoing dialogue among consumers, other health care providers in the community, and community mental health nurses.
Community strengths and limitations	The availability of trained mental health workers, such as psychiatric nurses, social workers, and psychologists, and of nonpsychiatric health professionals, such as community health nurses, physicians, clergymen, and teachers, should be determined. In addition, such physical resources as already functioning mental health clinics, halfway houses, hospitals, and nursing homes should be identified and their accessibility to and use by the community evaluated. Finally, any overlapping of services or fragmentation of services that are already available to the community should be identified.
Target population	The geographic catchment area should be delineated. The size of the population in need of mental health services (currently and potentially needy clients) should also be determined, and then this population should be segmented according to specific characteristics (e.g., ethnicity, social class, religious beliefs). Finally, the needs, problems, attitudes, and perceptions of the target population, as well as their desire for change and the direction in which they want that change to occur, should be determined.

Sources consulted include Clark (1978), Lancaster (1980), Flaskerud and van Servellen (1985).

health nurses often are responsible for training community paraprofessionals or indigenous community workers. During these training sessions, nurses sometimes find that they must reexamine their own perceptions, value systems, purposes, and functions (Lancaster, 1980; Koldjeski, 1984).

Thus, community mental health nurses need to be knowledgeable, assertive, flexible, and innovative to achieve their goals and to maximize their effectiveness in planning and delivering mental health care to communities.

Community assessment

To effectively function as community mental health nurses, nurses need to be aware of the strengths, deficits, and needs of the community they are serving. Table 16-10 describes three types of information that nurses need to know about the community.

The following community assessment guide* has

*Sources consulted in the preparation of this assessment guide include Clark (1978), Lancaster (1980), and Flaskerud and van Servellen (1985).

been designed to help nurses assess communities and to identify areas for community intervention:

1. Physical description of the community: Geographic parameters of the community; territorial distribution patterns (zones of business and residence; shopping, cultural, recreational, and health facilities; areas of overpopulation and underpopulation; multiple-family dwellings and single-family dwellings; interethnic neighborhoods or ethnic enclaves)

2. Target population: Age, sex, and types of family and/or household groupings; ethnic composition of the community (ethnic groups represented; degree of acculturation and assimilation; degree of interaction among ethnic groups); socioeconomic levels of the population (income levels represented; proportion of population in each income level; occupational groups represented; educational levels represented); spiritual orientations of the population (beliefs and rituals concerning birth, illness, and death; nature of belief in a supernatural being and/or supernormal energy; conceptualization about the quality of life and quality of death); health status of the population (support systems; strengths; prev-

alence of physical and mental disorders; acculturative pressures; minority status stressors)

3. Community resources: Existence of schools, health facilities, shopping areas, recreational facilities, self-help or support groups, and neighborhood action groups; availability of these resources (accessible by public transportation or by walking; open on weekends and in the evening); degree of satisfaction of community residents with community resources (perceived fit between community needs and services; overlap of services; fragmentation of services; cultural barriers or facilitators to use of community resources such as personnel who speak the language of minority group consumers)

4. Community attitudes about deviance: Attitudes about mental illness (fear mentally ill people; include mentally ill relatives and friends in their social networks); attitudes about social deviance* (reject people who have a history of social deviance; try to emulate social deviants); attitudes about treatment facilities for deviants (feelings about locating treatment facilities within the community; prevailing view that deviants should be treated/should be punished)

5. Community functioning: Decision-making patterns (decisions are based on adequate/inadequate information; are made by default; are arrived at by community consensus); communication patterns (patterns reflect stereotyping of or distance maneuvers between groups; nature of formal and informal communication channels; efficiency or fragmentation of communication patterns); leadership patterns (identifiable community leaders; leadership shifts according to the situation at hand; leadership is concentrated among a few groups; leadership is distributed throughout the community; degree of trust between community leaders and community residents); power patterns (location of power in the community; perception of how power is used)

6. Community integration: Incidence of "broken" homes (for example, dysfunctional families); incidence of violent, criminal, or delinquent behavior; adequacy and use of recreational facilities; adequacy of associations (degree to which people group around such common interests as religion, work, or recreation; cohesiveness of existing groups); presence of isolation factors (poor transportation systems; absence of telephones; poor interpersonal relationships)

7. Community attitudes toward change: Perception of change (views about how customs, lifestyles, and institutions will be affected by change; past experiences with change); forces facilitating or inhibiting change (relationship between change agents and the community; degree of awareness of need for change; degree of anticipated personal suffering or personal benefit from change; degree of involvement of community residents in planning for change; previous degree of openness of the community to change)

8. Community health care patterns: Prevalent definition(s) associated with specific community groups of health and illness; ideas concerning causes of illness (for example, evil spirits; punishment for sins; stress); ideas concerning treatment of illness; people consulted when ill (family member; native healing specialist; physician; pharmacist) and the order in which they are consulted

A comprehensive community assessment will provide community mental health nurses with the information necessary for identifying community mental health problems and for planning community mental health services that will address those problems. Lancaster (1980) lists five essential aspects of effective community mental health planning: (1) awareness that uncoordinated inter-agency planning tends to produce fragmented services or duplication of services; (2) recognition of the importance of involving the community in or obtaining community support for plans; (3) ability to define the range of essential services that will be provided to the community; (4) collaboration between mental health professionals and community residents; and (5) awareness of the importance of a systems approach to planning.

*Refer to Chapter 20 for a discussion of social deviance.

CHAPTER SUMMARY

The community mental health concept embraces an interacting system of health, welfare, and social services oriented toward meeting the mental health needs of a community. Programs are organized to provide mental health services for populations in geographically defined communities termed catchment areas. Each catchment area may have a population of from 75,000 to 200,000 people. Programs to meet community needs are, ideally, developed through a cooperative effort between health and social agencies, community organizations, and residents of the community served.

Although many factors influenced the development of the community mental health movement, the Community Mental Health Centers Act, passed by Congress in 1963, was a major factor in the implementation of mental health programs on a national basis. The act provided some federal funding for mental health care and established principles and guidelines to meet comprehensive mental health needs of residents in their local communities. Subsequent legislative actions further defined mental health care and upheld the constitutional rights of persons who have psychiatric disorders.

Although it continues to be an evolving process, the community mental health movement has significantly changed the treatment of persons with psychiatric disorders. Before the community mental health movement, mental health care had usually been available only in public hospitals, where long-term hospitalization was often a major form of treatment.

The community mental health concept uses a public health approach to meeting mental health needs of culturally diverse populations. This approach involves primary, secondary, and tertiary prevention. Primary prevention seeks to reduce the incidence of psychiatric disorders, secondary prevention seeks to reduce the disability rate through early and effective intervention, and tertiary prevention seeks to prevent or reduce the severity or duration of long-term disability.

The characteristics of agencies providing mental health services and the ways in which mental health teams function vary from one agency to another and according to the philosophies and professional orientations of health team members. The mental health services offered also vary according to the priorities established by a particular community.

SELF-DIRECTED LEARNING

Sensitivity-Awareness Exercises

The purposes of the following exercises are to:
- Develop awareness about your own attitudes and the attitudes of others toward mental health care and community mental health facilities
- Develop knowledge about the functioning and use of a local community mental health center
- Develop insight into the strengths, deficits, and needs of your community and/or your client's community
- Develop an ecosystem perspective to community mental health

1. Using the community assessment guide in this chapter, assess your community and/or your client's community. From the data obtained from your assessment, identify and describe:

a. Community attitudes about community health needs and services
b. Community strengths and limitations (physical, cultural, technological, and social)
c. Size and composition of the target population; be sure to include the ethnic and socioeconomic characteristics of the target population, as well as health status and attitudes and perceptions about mental health and mental health care
d. Implications for primary, secondary and tertiary intervention
2. Using the community assessment guide in this chapter, assess the functioning and integration of your community and/or your client's community. Identify and describe:
a. Decision-making patterns

SELF-DIRECTED LEARNING—cont'd

b. Communication patterns
c. Leadership patterns
d. Power patterns
e. Incidence of "broken" homes
f. Incidence of violent, criminal, and/or delinquent behavior
g. Adequacy and use of recreational facilities
h. Adequacy of associations
i. Isolation factors

3. Interview neighbors, health professionals, other professionals (for example, teachers, clergy) and small business owners. What are their attitudes about mental illness? About social deviance? About types of treatment and aftercare services that should be offered? About the location of treatment and/or aftercare facilities in their own community?

4. Visit a community mental health center and assess the following:
   a. Availability to clients (for example, intake procedures, hours open, length of waiting list, accessibility by public transportation or walking, fee scale)
   b. Staff-client interaction (for example, degree of rapport between staff and clients, incorporation of native healers or indigenous workers into the health team, use of client's native language)
   c. Treatment services (for example, "fit" between clients' cultural orientations and therapeutic modalities, types of essential and recommended services, relationship (if any) between ethnomedical system and modern Western medical system)

Questions to Consider

1. A nurse who has an ecosystem perspective to community mental health would
   a. Look for the origin of psychopathology in the individual
   b. Assess one aspect of the ecosystem as a data base on which to develop intervention
   c. Recognize an interrelationship between the environment and human behavior
   d. Recognize that social structure and human behavior are unrelated

2. A nurse assessed that the feelings of isolation and estrangement experienced by a client who had been institutionalized for 10 years were related to an inability to meet the behavioral expectations of society. This syndrome is referred to as the
   a. Social breakdown syndrome
   b. Deinstitutionalization syndrome
   c. Dumping syndrome
   d. Homeless syndrome

3. A nurse is involved in designing mental health services for homeless mentally ill people in the community. The nurse should recognize that all *except* which of the following services would be appropriate?
   a. Crisis intervention
   b. Relocation assistance
   c. Drop-in centers
   d. Long-term treatment

4. Culturally relevant interactional approaches for ethnic clients who have an extended family orientation and cultural prescriptions against expression of conflict and emotional states would include all *but* which of the following?
   a. Inclusion of the family in the treatment plan
   b. Encouragement to verbalize feelings
   c. Attention to somatic complaints
   d. Supportive rather than confrontive interventions

5. According to the American Nurses' Association Division on Psychiatric–Mental Health Nursing Practice, which of the following is a *process* criterion for the practice of community mental health nursing?
   a. The activities of nurses in primary, secondary, and tertiary mental health care are documented.
   b. Mental health services that address the needs of the community are provided.
   c. Nurses assume leadership roles in voluntary and governmental community health groups.
   d. Nurses explain available mental health programs to members of the community.

Continued.

SELF-DIRECTED LEARNING—cont'd

Match each of the following terms with the statement that is associated with it.

6. Target population
7. Community integration
8. Block grants
9. Essential service

a. Outpatient clinic service
b. Federal monies allocated by the Omnibus Budget Reconciliation Act of 1981 for alcohol, drug abuse, and mental health services
c. Group of people designated for community mental health services
d. Practice of discharging chronically men-

10. Deinstitutionalization

tally ill clients into the community
e. Measured by incidence of violence and "broken" homes, adequacy of recreational facilities and associations, and presence or absence of isolation factors

Answer key

1. c   6. c
2. a   7. e
3. d   8. b
4. b   9. a
5. d   10. d

REFERENCES

Aiken LH: Unmet needs of the chronically mentally ill: will nursing respond? Image 19(3):121-125, 1987.

American Nurses' Association Division on Psychiatric–Mental Health Nursing: Standards of Psychiatric and Mental Health Nursing Practice, Kansas City, 1982, The Association.

Appleby L and Desai P: Residential instability: a perspective on system imbalance, Am J Orthopsychiatr 57(4):515-524, 1987.

Atteneave C: American Indians and Alaska native families: emigrants in their own homeland, In McGoldrick M, Pearce JK, and Giordano J, editors: Ethnicity and family therapy, New York, 1982, The Guilford Press.

Clark CC: Mental health aspects of community health nursing, New York, 1978, McGraw-Hill Book Company.

Clinton J: Sociocultural issues relevant to health, Cultural Connections 7(1):1-2, 1987.

Delgado M: Hispanic cultural values: implications for groups, Small Group Behavior 12:69-80, 1981.

Delgado M: Hispanic natural support systems: implications for mental health services, J Psychiatr Nurs Mental Health Serv 21(4):19-24, 1983.

Fisher P and Breakey W: Homelessness and mental health, Int J Mental Health 14:11-12, 1986.

Flaskerud JH: Community mental health nursing: its unique role in the delivery of services to ethnic minorities, Persp Psychiatr Care 20(1):37-43, 1982.

Flaskerud JH: A proposed protocol for culturally relevant nursing psychotherapy, Clin Nurse Specialist 1(4):150-157, 1987.

Flaskerud JH and van Servellen GM: Community mental health nursing: theories and methods, Norwalk, Conn, 1985, Appleton-Century-Crofts.

Foster GM: On the origin of humoral medicine in Latin America, Med Anthropol Q 1(4):355-393, 1987.

Freeman RB: Permanent homelessness in America? Stanford, Calif, 1986, National Bureau of Economic Research.

French L: Victimization of the mentally ill: an unintended consequence of deinstitutionalization, Social Work 32(6):502-505, 1987.

Hagen JL: Gender and homelessness, Social Work 32(4):312-316, 1986.

Harris M and Bergman HC: Case management with the chronically mentally ill: a clinical perspective, Am J Orthopsychiatr 57(2):296-302, 1986.

Herrick, JW: The symbolic roots of three potent Iroquois medicinal plants, In Romanucci-Ross L, Moerman DE, and Tancredi LR, editors: The anthropology of medicine: from culture to method, South Hadley, Mass, 1983, Bergin and Garvey Publishers, Inc.

Hill CE and Mathews H: Traditional health beliefs and practices among southern rural blacks, In Black M and Reed J, editors: Social science perspectives on the south, New York, 1981, Breech Science.

Hopper K: More than passing strange: homelessness and mental illness in New York City, Am Ethnol 15(1):155-167, 1988.

Hough RL et al: Utilization of health and mental health services by Los Angeles Mexican Americans and nonhispanic whites, Arch Gen Psychiatr 44(8):702-709, 1987.

Hutchison WJ, Searight P, and Stretch JJ: Multidimensional networking: a response to the needs of homeless families, Social Work 31(6):427-430, 1986.

Jerrell JM and Larsen JK: Community mental health services in transition: who is benefitting? Am J Orthopsychiatr 56(1):78-88, 1986.

Joint Commission on Mental Health and Mental Illness: Action for mental health, New York, 1961, Basic Books, Inc.

Kakar S: Shamans, mystics and doctors, New York, 1982, Alfred Knopf.

Kenig S: The political economy of community health, Med Anthropol Q 17(5):132-134, 1986.

Kerson TS: The impact of ethnicity on community mental health, J Nurs Educ 20(3):32-38, 1981.

Koldjeski D: Community mental health nursing: new directions in theory and practice, New York, 1984, John Wiley & Sons.

Lamb HR: What did we expect from deinstitutionalization? Hosp Commun Psychiatr 32(2):105-109, 1981.

Lancaster J: Community mental health nursing: an ecological perspective, St. Louis, 1980, The CV Mosby Co.

Lebra TS: Shame and guilt: a psychocultural view of the Japanese self, Ethos 2(3):192-209, 1983.

McGoldrick M, Pearce JK, and Giordano J, editors: Ethnicity and family therapy, New York, 1982, The Guilford Press.

Manio EB and Hall RR: Asian family traditions and their influence in transcultural health care delivery, J Assoc Care Children's Health 15(3):172-177, 1987.

Martinez RA, editor: Hispanic culture and health care: fact, fiction and folklore, St. Louis, 1978, The CV Mosby Co.

Milner C: Filling the void: an analysis of complementarity between folk and contemporary health-care systems in urban Brazil, Paper presented at the International Health Conference, Washington, DC, June 13, 1983.

Orque MS, Bloch B, and Monroy LSA: Ethnic nursing care: a multicultural approach, St. Louis, 1983, The CV Mosby Co.

Pasquali EA: Assimilation and acculturation of Cubans on Long Island, PhD dissertation, State University of New York at Stony Brook, 1982.

Pepper B, Kirshmer MC, and Ryglewicz H: The young adult chronic patient: overview of a population, Hosp Commun Psychiatr 32(7):463-469, 1981.

Pinderhughes E: Afro-American families and the victim system. In McGoldrick M, Pearce JK, and Giordano J, editors: Ethnicity and family therapy, New York, 1982, The Guilford Press.

Plum KC: Moving forward with deinstitutionalization: lessons of an ethical policy analysis, Am J Orthopsychiatr 57(4):508-514, 1987.

Powers BA: The use of orthodox and black American folk medicine, Adv Nurs Sci 4(3):35-47, 1982.

Rappaport H and Rappaport M: The integration of scientific and traditional healing: a proposed model, Am Psychol 36(7):774-781, 1981.

Roberson MHB: The influence of religious beliefs on health choices of Afro-Americans, Topics Clin Nurs 7(3):57-63, 1985.

Roberts JM, Morita S, and Brown LK: Personal categories for Japanese sacred places and gods: views elicited from a conjugal pair, Am Anthropol 88:807-824, 1986.

Rogers SL and Evernham L: Shamanistic healing among the Digueno Indians of southern California, In Romanucci-Ross L, Moerman DE, and Tancredi LR, editors: The anthropology of medicine: from culture to method, South Hadley, Mass, 1983, Bergin and Garvey Publishers, Inc.

Scheper-Hughes N: Dilemmas in deinstitutionalization, J Operational Psychiatr 12(2):90-99, 1981.

Scheper-Hughes N: A proposal for the aftercare of chronic psychiatric patients, Med Anthropol Q 14(2):3-15, 1982.

Scheper-Hughes N and Lock MM: The mindful body: a prolegomenon to future work in medical anthropology, Med Anthropol Q 1(1):6-33, 1987.

Shamansky SL and Peznecker B: A community is . . ., In Spradley BW, editor: Readings in community health nursing, Boston, 1982, Little, Brown and Company.

Shon SP and Ja DY: Asian families, In McGoldrick M, Pearce JK, and Giordano J, editors: Ethnicity and family therapy, New York, 1982, The Guilford Press.

Stern R and Minkoff K: Paradoxes in programming for chronic patients in a community clinic, Hosp Commun Psychiatr 30(9):613-617, 1979.

Swearingen L: Transitional day treatment: an individualized goal-oriented approach, Arch Psychiatr Nurs 1(2):104-110, 1987.

Talbott JA: The emerging crisis in chronic care, Hosp Commun Psychiatr 32(4):447, 1981.

Weaver C and Sklar D: Diagnostic dilemmas and cultural diversity in emergency rooms, Western J Med 133(4):356-366, 1980.

Weiner RS et al: Community mental health centers and the "seed money" concept: effects of terminating federal funds, Commun Mental Health J 15(2):129-138, 1979.

White HS and Bennett MB: Training psychiatric residents in chronic care, Hosp Commun Psychiatr 32(5):339-343, 1981.

Williams K: World view and the facilitation of wholeness, Holistic Nurs Prac 2(3):1-8, 1988.

ANNOTATED SUGGESTED READINGS

Capers CF: Cultural diversity and nursing practice, Topics Clinical Nurs (entire issue) 7(3):1-88, 1985.
This journal issue assists nurses in recognizing the uniqueness of ethnic and cultural factors and in accepting and using these factors in nursing intervention. The journal includes articles on health care of Afro-Americans, Chinese-Americans, Navajo Indians, and Cuban refugees.

Plum KC: Moving forward with deinstitutionalization: lessons of an ethical policy analysis, Am J Orthopsychiatr 57(4):508-514, 1987.
The author, a nurse, takes an ethical approach in reconceptualizing historical and contemporary dilemmas associated

with deinstitutionalization and the community mental health movement.

Swearingen L: Transitional day treatment: an individualized goal-oriented approach, Arch Psychiatr Nurs 1(2):104-110, 1987.

The article discusses the importance of transitional day treatment programs in facilitating the return of chronically mentally ill clients to the community. A transitional treatment program that utilized an individualized goal-oriented treatment model that allowed clients to proceed at their own pace is described.

FURTHER READINGS

Elpers JR: Are we legislating reinstitutionalization? Am J Orthopsychiatr 57(3):441-446, 1987.

Gary LE: Attitudes of black adults toward community mental health centers, Hosp Commun Psychiatr 38(10):1100-1105, 1987.

Gibbs JT: Identity and marginality: issues in the treatment of biracial adolescents, Am J Orthopsychiatr 57(2):265-278, 1987.

Humm-Delgado D and Delgado M: Gaining community entree to assess service needs of Hispanics, Social Casework 67(2):80-89, 1986.

James JF: Does the community mental health movement have the momentum needed to survive? Am J Orthopsychiatr 57(3):447-451, 1987.

Lipton FR, Nutt S, and Sabatini A: Housing the homeless mentally ill: a longitudinal study of a treatment approach, Hosp Commun Psychiatr 39(1):40-45, 1988.

Moffett MJ: Evolution of psychiatric community care, J Psychosoc Nurs 26(7):17-21, 1988.

Pepper B: A public policy for the long-term mentally ill: a positive alternative to reinstitutionalization, Am J Orthopsychiatr 57(3):452-457, 1987.

Sallinger N: Relapse, J Psychosoc Nurs 26(6):20-23, 1988.

Walfish S and Janzen L: Financing outpatient mental health care: how much does insurance actually help? Am J Orthopsychiatr 58(3):470-472, 1988.

Weltman K et al: Impact of community based psychosocial treatment on clients' level of functioning, Hosp Commun Psychiatr 39:550-553, 1988.

Worley NK and Lowery BJ: Deinstitutionalization: could the process have been better for patients? Arch Psychiatr Nurs 2(3):126-133, 1988.

UNIT 4

Client behavior and nursing practice

The fourth section of this book focuses on major psychogenic and psychiatric conditions of children, adolescents, and adults. Although each chapter looks at the development and/or implications of particular disorders throughout the life cycle, two chapters focus on patterns of conflict and stress specific to age groups: children and adolescents (Chapter 17) and the elderly (Chapter 18).

A client system—whether it is an individual, a family, a small group, or a community—has permeable boundaries. During the process of self-regulation (a characteristic of all living systems), matter energy and information are both taken into the system (input) and given out to the environment (output). When self-regulatory processes are successful, a client system maintains itself in dynamic equilibrium. More energy is produced or stored than is expended, and growth and holistic wellness (negentropy) evolve. When self-regulatory processes fail, more energy is expended than is produced or stored. Disharmony develops and contributes to various degrees of pathology (entropy).

Client systems are open systems, constantly interacting with the environment. This interaction contributes to states of mental health (negentropy) or mental illness (entropy). A critical understanding of the dynamic quality of interrelatedness between a client system and its environment (both internal and external) is necessary. Internal factors—such as genetics, temperament, and physiology—as well as such external factors—such as pollution, socioeconomic status, and nature of support systems—are intrinsic to the relationship of any given client system with its environment. Coping behaviors are one way that a client system interacts with the environment. Coping behaviors serve either as positive or negative feedback. The notion of linear causality should be discarded, and in its place multifactorial interrelationships should be examined. For example, if a client system is malfunctioning (inappropriate behavior is displayed), stress and malfunction may be generated by a problem with relationships.

The patterns of behavior that are discussed in these chapters range across the mental health continuum. The earlier chapters deal with conditions that involve relatively little interference with psychosocial functioning, and the later chapters deal with conditions in which there may be great interference with psychosocial functioning. The DSM-III-R categories associated with specific behavior patterns are given.

The framework of systems theory provides a foundation for understanding a client system. Systems theory structures nursing assessment, planning, intervention, and evaluation in such a way that the interrelationship of parts or factors is considered and given validity. For example, a nursing assessment reflects the interrelatedness of biophysical, psychosocial, and spiritual factors. Due to the complexity of these multifactorial relationships, the nurse should determine, ideally in consultation with the client, what relationships are meaningful at the time and in light of the problem under consideration. Planning and intervention should begin at that point. Intervention, which involves entering a particular part of a client system, will generate change throughout the system through a process of mutual interaction.

Each chapter in this unit utilizes the nursing process. Primary NANDA nursing diagnoses are used in developing nursing care plans. Treatment modalities are discussed in relation to particular patterns of behavior. In addition, each behavior pattern is explored in terms of primary, secondary, and tertiary prevention.

Patterns of conflict and stress in childhood and adolescence

CHAPTER FOCUS

The Report of the Joint Commission on Mental Health of Children (1969) identified several factors that act as precipitants for the development of emotional disorders; these factors include faulty life experiences, relational difficulties between parent and child; adjustment reactions to school and social experiences; internalized conflicts; and adjustment difficulties related to physical handicaps and severe ego dysfunction. More than 80% of emotionally disturbed children fall into the first two categories— life experiences and relational difficulties. Nurses in school health, community health, family practice, and camp settings, in addition to nurses in well-child clinics, should be able to identify these potential factors and intervene at a primary level. Nurses can act as educators and as support and resource systems for the family within which a child exists. Thus, the focal point of nursing assessment and intervention is twofold: assisting the child to modify unhealthy behaviors and enabling the family to develop more effective means of communication and more effective parenting skills.

This chapter begins with descriptions of selected disorders of childhood and adolescence; primary characteristics of each are discussed to provide guidelines for nursing assessment. Specific underlying etiologies are also discussed. Emphasis is placed on a systems approach to the understanding of childhood and adolescent disorders and subsequent interventions. The authors stress the importance of an assessment that reflects a multifactorial approach to the development of these disorders.

Modalities of treatment reflect a varied approach as well. Individual therapy, milieu therapy, groups for both parents and children, and family therapy are explored in depth. Somatic therapy, including psychopharmacology and electroconvulsive therapy, is presented as it relates specifically to children and adolescents.

The final section of the chapter covers the nursing process. Primary prevention focuses on screening for risk—identifying children and families who may be in potential difficulty as a result of poor environmental factors, a lack of knowledge regarding parenting, or a lack of appropriate problem-solving skills. Secondary prevention is explored in light of the increased emphasis on case finding and early diagnosis. Specific diagnoses are presented relative to the disorders of childhood and adolescence discussed in the earlier section. Family diagnoses are also discussed. Long- and short-term goals and nursing strategies are specifically delineated for each diagnosis. General outcome criteria are included at the conclusion of the discussion of secondary prevention. Tertiary prevention involves the use of therapeutic measures directed toward ensuring the optimum level of functioning in cases where there is chronic dysfunction. Residential placement is included in the discussion of tertiary prevention.

The purpose of this chapter is to give nurses a greater understanding of emotional disorders of childhood and adolescence, as well as of specific interventive techniques. The emphasis on a systems approach provides guidelines that facilitate nurses' comprehensive assessment and intervention with children and adolescents and with their families.

HISTORICAL PERSPECTIVES

In 1972, Fagin cited the findings of the Report of the Joint Commission on the Mental Health of Children (1969) that 1,400,000 persons under the age of 18 needed professional psychiatric help. At that time a third were receiving some form of assistance from mental health facilities, while 3% were being treated in residential living centers. In 1978, the President's Commission on Mental Health sup-

ported the findings noted by Fagin. The Joint Commission further delineated the problems that seemed to act as precipitants for the development of emotional disorders. These are:

1. Faulty life experiences and training
2. Surface conflicts between children and parents, such as relational difficulties among siblings and adjustment difficulties in the areas of school, social relations, and sexuality
3. Internalized conflicts of a deeper nature that lead to neurotic responses
4. Adjustment difficulties related to physical disorders and handicaps
5. Adjustment difficulties related to severe mental disorders such as psychotic behaviors and mental retardation.

The Joint Commission noted that approximately 80% of the children who need treatment fall into the first two problem areas. These children are able to live within the context of their families and the larger environment. Treatment, when appropriate, can be provided for both child and family on an outpatient basis. Often school nurses, community health nurses, or family nurse practitioners are able to identify troublesome areas and provide education, support, or referral to mental health professionals when it is necessary. Tertiary care is most appropriate for the remaining 20% of the identified population. In some instances, as with severe psychosis, institutionalization and close supervision are necessary.

Since a child exists within the context of his or her family, the provision of services has been influenced by the family system. Children, particularly young children, are not often encouraged to seek out mental health services, nor are they often able to seek out such services. Parental attitudes toward mental health professionals and their practice are often negative. Yet parental expectations, previous experiences within parents' own families of origin, and parents' lack of clear communication patterns serve as the basis for the development of emotional and mental disorders. It is important to identify high-risk families, to connect members of these families with appropriate resources, and to assist parents in becoming more effective.

One difficulty in the provision of services relates to family members' lack of awareness of their own problems. Often parents themselves do not realize that they have questions regarding parenting. For example, parents may not be aware that consistency is important in a relationship with a child. It must be emphasized also that children under the age of 3 do not often come to the attention of those who provide mental health services. It becomes critical for nurses in well-baby clinics and other health facilities, such as health maintenance organizations (HMOs) and hospital emergency rooms, to be able to assess accurately the developmental status and emotional response of a child, as well as the parent-child interaction. If undetected, emotional difficulties may establish maladaptive patterns of behavior, leading in turn to future adjustment difficulties. It was noted by the Joint Commission that in childhood the foundations in all areas of development, including physical, social, emotional, and intellectual, are laid for the ensuing years. Negative experiences learned in the parents' families of origin can be played out in the current family system, leaving open the possibility of generating similar maladaptive methods of coping. Supportive-educative services are not uniformly offered to parents and families; it is only when children begin to display inappropriate behaviors that resources are made available.

Other factors that impact on provision of services include socioeconomic background, cultural and religious values, and attitudes toward mental health services (see Chapter 16 for further discussion of attitudes toward mental health services). Socioeconomic status has a profound influence on families' abilities to use mental health services. There are too few programs in which fees are based on a sliding scale or in which reduced fees are available for parents in lower economic brackets. Often it is this population that is most in need of services, yet services are too costly or federally sponsored programs such as Medicaid do not cover psychiatric expenses.

Cultural and religious values not only may influence familial child-rearing practices but also may dictate certain norms, values, and expectations that may conflict with societal norms and expectations. Mental health services and the providers of services may be viewed with apprehension. The family may draw together to protect a child who is experiencing difficulty rather than expose the family to the scrutiny and intervention of outsiders. Cultural and religious values do have a significant influence on children, yet one needs to remember that each child is unique and needs an environment in which expectations of behavior and communication are clear.

Role of the nurse

Statistics indicate that a large number of children and youth are in need of some level of psychosocial intervention. Nurses, as the largest group of health care providers, potentially possess assessment skills and the ability to design and implement relevant plans of care for this population. The ANA (1985) has emphasized the need for skilled practitioners in the area of child and adolescent mental health by setting standards for generalists and specialists (see Appendix D). Furthermore, nurses have limitless opportunities for contact with children and families. However, Fagin (1972) states that few nursing students are exposed to child psychiatric concepts in their undergraduate curricula. Some mental health concepts relating to childhood and adolescence may be incorporated into the pediatrics component, yet insufficient attention is directed toward this area because of the large amount of biophysiological information currently taught relative to health care of children. Therefore it can be said that nurses currently complete their undergraduate studies with little or no knowledge of child and adolescent psychiatric problems and interventions. With the current focus of nursing assessment and intervention directed toward the concept of family, it would seem logical to discuss issues of the child and adolescent within the context of the family system.

Intervention with children who are experiencing difficulty coping with life situations or with those who display psychotic behaviors can be an emotionally upsetting experience for nurses. Feelings of vulnerability are aroused in the nurse. A sense of overwhelming inadequacy may also be felt by the nurse when confronted with the extensive patterns of behavior and the wide variety of developmental tasks to be accomplished throughout childhood and adolescence. These factors often seem incomprehensible to health practitioners, as well as to families who are moving through those phases.

The primary role of the nurse is to understand the child within the context of the family. Before they can accomplish this, nurses must be aware of their own values and beliefs regarding family: their roles within their own families, expectations of behavior, how feelings are expressed, what the lines of communication are. Nurses may perceive other families as behaving inappropriately in terms of the nurses' own values and experiences within their own family systems. A family that is already experiencing distress can detect feelings of ambivalence or a blaming attitude on the part of a nurse, which immediately places a barrier between nurse and family. The family then takes a defensive position that does not allow open communication to occur. The child's maladaptive behavior may then escalate as he or she responds to the increased anxiety level within the family system. Nurses should be aware that feelings of guilt and failure in the parental dyad can be quickly reinforced by nurses' thoughtless comments.

Nurses may become easily frustrated with parents who do not promptly change their patterns of child-rearing when it has been demonstrated that these behaviors may be less effective than others. It is difficult to change lifelong patterns—even more so when disequilibrium in the family is already occurring. Individuals tend to revert back to old behavior patterns or become immobilized in the face of escalating anxiety. Even though parents may understand intellectually the need for more open communication or for changing a maladaptive manner of responding, it is much more difficult to operationalize those changes and to become emotionally committed to them. Parents bring their own experiences from childhood, which influence their behaviors as parents as well as their expectations of their children. In some situations parents do not communicate their expectations to one another, creating an ambiguous situation for the child.

Nurses need to feel comfortable with their own feelings and with their expectations in regard to roles in the family system. After accomplishing these objectives, a nurse can create an atmosphere within which the members of a family can discuss alternative coping strategies and can explore their feelings and gain support from one another and from the nurse, thus emerging as a more healthy unit in a holistic sense.

It must be noted that adults are prepared for the jobs or careers they intend to pursue; however, they undergo little or no preparation for their most critical task—parenting the next generation. With that thought in mind, nurses should believe that parents are most likely doing the best they know how, based on their own experiences and their current physical, social, economic, emotional, educational, and religious resources. It is part of nursing to support the parental role when appropriate—to be empathic and to set realistic goals for the family as a whole unit and for the child who is demonstrating maladaptive methods of coping.

DISORDERS OF CHILDHOOD

Long (1985) notes that the diagnosis and acceptance of mental illness in children and adolescents is difficult. She states that historically society has ignored and mislabeled those children who were actually experiencing mental health problems. Often health care professionals reassure parents falsely that problems are "developmental" and will be "outgrown." Long cites National Academy of Science statistics that indicate the growing number of children who require immediate care for mental health problems. Significantly small numbers of children and adolescents, however, will receive the treatment that they need.

Talan (1988) states that the number of children, particularly adolescents, who are institutionalized has increased 400% from more than a decade ago. Studies demonstrate no significant increase in the diagnosis of schizophrenia and manic depression; however, parents seem to be hospitalizing children and adolescents when they are unable or unwilling to cope with problems that in the past have been handled within the context of the home environment. Talan cites several possible reasons for the increase:

1. Insurance coverage of inpatient stays but little or no coverage for outpatient therapy
2. Increase in the number of private psychiatric hospitals offering programs that purport to

offer "cures" for everything from running away to poor grades

3. Rapid increase in the number of teen suicides that causes parents to seek inpatient treatment rather than outpatient therapy
4. Psychiatric coverage is not as limited to number of days covered in an inpatient setting; therefore, there is an increasing number of psychiatric beds available
5. There is a shift away from sending delinquent children and adolescents to jail. Professionals hope that psychiatric treatment will be successful in changing criminal behavior before it becomes ingrained

Talan supports Long's belief that there is an inherent difficulty in diagnosing mental illness in children and adolescents due to the developmental turmoil that is part of the changes the individual experiences. The controversy surrounding the decision to admit a young person to inpatient care has become a critical one. Those who are invested in the notion of private, inpatient care state vehemently that such behaviors as running away, truancy, or stealing are signs of serious mental illness. Ad campaigns for private hospitals ask parents to wonder, "Do you know where your children are?" They highlight a portrait of a troubled child with a gun pointed to his temple and then flash the name of a psychiatric hospital on the screen. Parents are then willing to hospitalize their children for problems that historically have been dealt with successfully in other less restrictive ways. Those professionals who believe that parents are being coerced to hospitalize and stigmatize their children note the lack of convincing statistics to demonstrate the success of hospitalization. Adolescents are being hospitalized, unlike adults, for the extremeness of their behavior as a sole factor rather than for the severity of their illness. Talan quotes research from several sources including Knitzer, whose study with adolescent and child admissions found that 40% of these admissions were inappropriate, as well as a study conducted by Schwartz, which concluded that young people were admitted to hospitals for far less serious problems than adults and were hospitalized for longer periods of time than adults. Schwartz also noted that more than half the admissions were inappropriate.

The concern of health professionals, including nurses, who care for children and adolescents must be the accurate assessment and determination of a program of care that meets that individual's needs. Hospitalization may not be the panacea as it is portrayed by convincing media advertisements. The stigma attached to mental illness continues to exist in our society. What effect will a hospitalization in childhood or adolescence have on that individual in later life in terms of college, employment, or other facets of life? Yet some health professionals suggest that there are few outpatient programs available to assist troubled parents and children. Often, as Talan notes, the exhausted family has little energy left, the child is considered dysfunctional, and the only viable option is hospitalization.

DSM-III-R has attempted to categorize behaviors by specific disorders rather than cluster behaviors; this clouds assessment and diagnosis. DSM-III-R delineates disorders in the following manner: developmental disorders, disruptive behavior disorders, anxiety disorders, eating disorders, gender-identity disorders, tic disorders, elimination disorders, speech disorders, and other disorders of infancy, childhood, or adolescence. (See Appendix A).

Disruptive behavior disorders
ATTENTION DEFICIT HYPERACTIVITY DISORDER

Popper (1988) describes the hyperactive child as one who is impulsive, wriggling, fidgets, is easily distractible, and has a short concentration span. Statistics demonstrate a higher incidence among boys (10%) than girls (2%), and attention deficit disorders are frequently found in conjunction with other disorders such as conduct and mood disorders as well as autistic and pervasive developmental disorders.

Popper (1988) states that the behaviors associated with attention deficit disorder may be worse at the end of the day, perhaps resulting from anxiety. Further signs of attention deficit disorders include clumsiness, confusion of right and left and front and back, lack of symmetry of five finger-hand movements, and intellectual and memory faults. Children who are hyperactive are described as restless, impulsive, and quarrelsome. Their behavior often distracts others in the same environment and makes it impossible for themselves or others to maintain task orientation and to complete objectives. The inability to complete assignments or follow directions may lead a child to cope in a maladaptive manner by withdrawing, being negativistic, playing the class clown, or denying any difficulty exists. It is important for nurses to recognize that whatever the behavior, children are labeled in a negative or derisive manner, which then acts as a feedback mechanism to generate further socially unacceptable behavior.

CONDUCT DISORDERS

Popper (1988) describes conduct disorder as the most common diagnosis found in child and adolescent patients. Children who have assaultive tendencies, who start fights for no apparent reason, who are cruel to animals and others, and who are malicious with intent are characteristic of disturbances of conduct. The syndrome is composed of alterations of attention and learning disorders, cheating, lying, manipulation, lack of a sense of consequences of events, impaired interpersonal relationships, lack of understanding of the relationship of behavior to events, lack of conscience, and lack of empathy toward others. Kalb (1979) notes that there may be evidence of superego defects or lacunae that are related to the lack of a development of a sense of conscience or right or wrong. Popper also indicates that traditionally conduct disorders were found to a greater extent among the male population; however, the prevalence among females is increasing. The epidemiology of conduct disorders will continue to change in relation to societal changes, family structure, and socioeconomic conditions.

Although there is some support for the psychoanalytic basis of conduct disorders, it seems that sociologic theories and family history impact most on the development of this syndrome. Elliott et al. (1985) note that social deprivation, status-seeking behavior, and the need to escape from a feeling of entrapment are critical in the etiology of conduct disorders. Family history often reveals inconsistent parenting, alcohol and drug abuse, parental rejection, cruel discipline, and general family discord.

The child is unable to develop a strong sense of identity in an environment where positive reinforcement is unknown, and he or she is unable to engage in intimate, caring relationships. Adolescents may find the necessary support and encouragement to develop a sense of self-worth from a peer group that, in many cases, is delinquent. The conduct disturbance in and of itself may serve to enhance self-worth and provide courage and independence in the face of anxiety-provoking situations. Popper states that involvement with peers often increases socialization skills, which serves as a positive outcome predictor relative to long-term behavior. Further studies are being conducted by Elliott to determine the role of socialization in the development of delinquency and drug abuse. Frequently children and adolescents who have conduct disorders also have difficulties in school; become involved with the law; have higher rates of teenage pregnancy and venereal disease; are more likely to commit suicide or be murdered; and are more likely to abandon their families when in the adult parenting role. Thus, as these individuals become adults, there is an increased risk for more serious crimes and incarceration. However, Popper does point out that children with a conduct disturbance can achieve a positive outcome in adulthood. The variables that may predict this outcome are not clear, although he does suggest that socialization skills are at least a partial predictor of a positive outcome. Nursing assessment and intervention can then be directed toward assisting these children in developing positive relationships with others through the use of effective socialization skills.

DSM-III-R does differentiate between conduct disorder and the less disruptive behaviors that make up the syndrome of oppositional defiant disorder. Briefly, these children exhibit argumentative, disobedient behavior but do not infringe upon the rights of others. They do not experience the severity of symptoms as those diagnosed with conduct disorders and frequently have attention deficit problems or other psychiatric problems. As Popper describes, the most characteristic behavior of this disorder is the need to win a struggle at any cost. Children will assume a self-defeating stance, which often causes them to lose the actual item or privilege, yet they will "hold on" to the struggle until their point is won. Behaviors noted in this disorder may also be found in normal development; however, nurses must be cognizant of the fact that these behaviors must occur for a period of 6 months or more to be considered an oppositional defiant disorder.

ANXIETY DISORDERS

Rutter et al. (1986) found in their study that approximately 1% of children experienced some form of anxiety disorder, although other research suggests that this estimate is far too low. Anxiety is frequently mislabeled or missed completely by pediatricians and parents. This phenomenon is due in part to the fact that anxiety is commonly experienced to some degree in childhood: fear of snakes under the bed at night; fear of thunderstorms and lightning; and anxiety related to peers and school performance. It becomes imperative for nurses and other health professionals to assess normal developmental anxiety as well as to recognize anxiety that is disruptive. Anxiety disorders cause much distress to the child himself, whereas conduct disorders cause distress to those around the child; thus, anxiety disorders impact on the child's ability to interact with others, to achieve in school, and to develop some sense of identity.

DSM-III-R delineates two categories of anxiety disorders—separation anxiety disorder and overanxious disorder. Separation anxiety as a normal developmental process occurs between the ages of 18 months and 30 months. (For further discussion, see Chapter 9). Popper suggests that school phobia or school absenteeism may be due to separation anxiety disorder, but they are not synonymous. Last and Hersen (1987) note that not all children with school absenteeism are experiencing separation anxiety. They note that school phobia may actually be a form of truancy without any implication of "phobia." Last indicates that refusing to go to school may be one of a cluster of symptoms of separation anxiety in conjunction with feelings of dread and apprehension that something will happen to self or to others such as parents or siblings: refusing to sleep or be alone, disruption in cognitive processes, and somatization. Frequently separation anxiety is seen in children who are also experiencing mood disorders or other developmental difficulties; however, they may not be experiencing school absenteeism. School absenteeism may be seen in children who are depressed or who are experiencing panic levels of anxiety. The major point of assessment is recognizing that separation anxiety and school absenteeism are separate entities, yet separation anxiety may be a prominent characteristic of school absenteeism. This factor is supported by studies that demonstrate familial psychodynamics based on fears of separation. Parents may fear separation; this fear is then transferred unconsciously to the child. An examination of family dynamics may reveal ambivalence or a lack of clarity of parenting roles. Parents may also feel a strong sense of protectiveness toward the child while at the same time resenting the dependent relationship that has developed. Popper notes the influence of family values and behaviors in the development of anxiety disorders and school truancy. More than half the children studied who had some form of anxiety disorder had parents who had a history of anxiety and mood disorders. Family values regarding the importance of school were also reflected in school absenteeism behaviors. In some cases, children were kept home from school to go shopping with a parent or to babysit other children at home. An increased incidence of school absenteeism is also noted in cultures where poverty is prevalent and where there is little value place on obtaining an education.

Differentiation between normal separation anxiety, separation disorders, and school absenteeism is critical. Intervention must be directed toward assisting children and parents to develop more effective methods of coping with anxiety and to develop a positive sense of self as an individual. Sociocultural factors as they impact on the family and the child must also be considered within the broad context of society if treatment is to be successful.

Other disorders of infancy, childhood, or adolescence
REACTIVE ATTACHMENT AND WITHDRAWAL

Popper suggests that physical and/or emotional abuse, which may include sexual abuse, inconsistent or inappropriate parenting, neglect, unstable home environment, and lack of consistent bonding behaviors within the context of the family system, incorporates both decreased and increased social interactiveness following trauma in infancy or early childhood. Often these children are diagnosed with "failure-to-thrive" syndrome, which encompasses physical manifestations of malnutrition as well as the emotional factors that disrupt the maternal-child relationship.

Shyness, withdrawal, inability to relate socially to peers, and oversensitivity characterize children who are experiencing disorders in social relatedness. These children often demonstrate excessive worrying and submissive behaviors. Within the family system, activity is not tolerated well and is often punished. Because these children do not form intimate relationships with peers, they engage in daydreaming to provide the support they are not receiving from significant others. If withdrawal continues, it is likely that impairment of reality will increase. Affective impoverishment becomes more apparent as the child seeks to create a world that is less punitive.

Reactive disorders bear discussion because they occur frequently—individuals cannot progress from infancy through adolescence without some level of stress occurring as a result of life events. Individuals who do not experience stress and are not confronted with the need to change to progress in their development might be considered a poor risk for adjustment in future life situations. Through confrontations with situations that require individuals to adopt alternative behaviors, they learn that change can be effected and that they can be in control of their lives. They may also learn that in failing, learning can occur. However, as Kessler (1979) points out, there is a fine line between normal adaptive responses and pathology. There is a complex interrelationship among the nature and impact of the stressor, current and past experiences with stressors, the level of support from significant others, and the current emotional and physical health of the child. Particularly with younger children, it becomes difficult to predict how a child will adapt to stressful situations. It is important to note here that infants and preschool children are more vulnerable to the impact of stressors for those reasons noted above. Children at this age have limited coping strategies; at the same time, however, they may be more flexible in their coping if they have the appropriate support systems. The critical factor in reactive disorders is the identification and amelioration of traumatic stressors. This will reduce the risk of lasting alterations in the child's personality.

Reactive responses may be subtle; therefore, assessment must be directed toward identifying changes in behavior—for example, increased withdrawal, night terrors, bedwetting, eating problems, and hyperactivity—as well as identifying the stressor causing those changes. Intervention requires parental involvement and the willingness to consider the behavioral response of the child within the context of the family rather than as a singular event solely involving the child. Parents who are able to consider their own reactions and expectations and their influence on their children are more able to respond clearly and consistently to their children's needs. When there is little role confusion and ambiguity between parent and child and when needs of parents are not confused with needs of the children, there is decreased risk of development of maladaptive coping responses.

Developmental disorders

DSM-III-R has coded developmental disorders on Axis II as opposed to their inclusion as clinical syndromes. Mental retardation, pervasive developmental disorders, specific developmental disorders, and other developmental disorders not otherwise specified are included in this category. The following discussion will address autistic disorder and childhood onset pervasive developmental disorders as categories of pervasive developmental disorders. Popper notes that these disorders are characterized by deficits across multiple areas of functioning: thus the connotation "pervasive" disorders.

Disorders first diagnosed in infancy or childhood reflect alterations in thinking, affect, speech, and perceptions. These children display an inability to relate to others, clinging behavior with the parenting figure, body image distortion, and difficulty with speech or no speech at all. There may also be poor development of locomotor, fine motor, and visual-motor skills, which results in erratic and peculiar patterns of functioning (Fish and Ritvo,

1979). It is important to note that the degree of personality disorganization varies from time to time within the same child, as well as among children having the same disturbance.

AUTISTIC DISORDER

Freeman and Ritvo (1982) describe the following characteristics as significant diagnostic criteria: onset before the age of 30 months; delayed or deviant developmental progression, particularly in the area of language development; disturbed responses to stimuli; and a marked lack of social relatedness. The latter is of particular importance in the diagnosis of autistic disorder. Characteristic changes occur in relation to speech, language, perceptual and motor response, affect and mood, and interactions with others. To accurately assess a child, these areas must be comprehensively evaluated.

▶ Speech, language, and thought disturbances

Autistic children exhibit all levels of speech retardation. Some remain mute, whereas others may speak only in the present tense even when referring to past occurrences. Fish and Ritvo (1979) state that a critical characteristic is the coexistence of jargon and unintelligible speech with mature speech. As the percentage of unintelligible speech increases, the prognosis for these children worsens. Comprehension of speech may vary: some children are oblivious to meaning, whereas others may be unable to understand subtle or abstract meanings.

Kanner (1955) suggests that rigid echolalic speech can be identified in children whose speech has progressed beyond jargon and simple words. Literal repetition of statements and questions indicates that there is no change in the use of pronouns nor in the inflection of voice.

Formal thought disturbance is reflected in conceptualization and logic of thought. There may be a lack of connectedness between sentences, distorted grammar, pronoun reversal, and sudden irrelevancies. Kanner (1955) further notes that words can be condensed or distorted to create neologisms. These children have been observed to create worlds characterized by endless illogical connections and juxtapositions that hold little if any meaning for themselves and those around them.

▶ Perceptual and motor disturbances

Many children demonstrate unpredictable and disorganized responses to environmental stimuli. Inappropriately exaggerated responses to insignificant stimuli, with inattention or shortened attention to new or obvious stimuli, have been noted. These children do not use visual cues to learn about their environment but rather manipulate their environment through their mobility. Those objects in the environment that move can be readily discerned. Autistic children have difficulty separating an object figure from its background, creating the need to move objects while inspecting them. During assessment, lack of response to voices or loud noises is often seen. Kanner (1955) states that autistic children do not adapt to a wide variety of activities or use of different objects. There is attention to specific details of objects without regard for the object as a whole. There is little creative or imaginative play as is found in age-appropriate children. Brightly colored toys and objects attract the attention of autistic children.

Motor development is characterized by simple, repetitive movements such as hand flapping, finger twiddling, rocking, and whirling. Infants are fascinated by movement of any kind, yet autistic infants demonstrate this interest to excess. This need for motion is carried further into forms of self-stimulation such as banging of the head and rocking.

▶ Affect and mood

Kanner (1955) observed that the "blank expression" of autistic children reflects the indifference of these children to those around them. Temper tantrums and outbursts of tears, rage, and other aggressive responses are initiated when the child's routine or need for "sameness" is interrupted. Bender (1947) describes excessive anxiety that tends to be precipitated by change in the environment or disruption of normal activities. The flat affect may be incongruent with thought processes, and it does not necessarily correlate with changes in the environment; in fact, it may occur in the absence of stimuli. Although anxiety is common in many childhood disorders, the illogical eruptions demonstrated by autistic children are a distinguishing feature.

▶ Social relatedness

Autistic children are often viewed as aloof and distant. The avoidance of eye contact has been noted as early as six months. Kanner (1955) differentiates this inability to relate to others from withdrawal from relationships in that the latter requires a previously existing relationship. Autistic children are unable to relate to others from the very beginning of life. Although clinging and symbiotic behavior may also be observed, there is little if any emotional attachment to other persons. Less severely autistic children may interact periodically but are unable to sustain a lasting relationship. These children infrequently initiate social relationships and are often observed as being isolated and preoccupied.

Numerous theories have been postulated as the cause for autistic disorder; however, a more plausible explanation may be derived from a systems perspective. Multiple factors—biological, developmental, sociocultural, and psychodynamic interact in a mutual and simultaneous manner. However, successful intervention with these children is limited; caring for them is often difficult and frustrating. Vessey (1988) suggests that maintaining an "en face" position, gently holding the child's hand and maintaining continuous eye contact assists in establishing an initial relationship. Simple, short sentences are useful; do not use words that can be misconstrued or taken literally. Vessey uses the example of "taking your blood pressure," which to the autistic child literally might mean taking the blood pressure away from the child. Vessey also notes that utilizing parents is an invaluable resource for the nurse in planning and implementing nursing strategies. The following sample interaction involves a 2-year-old autistic child who has been admitted to the hospital for a tonsillectomy. The nurse is establishing contact with this child for the first time.

Nurse	*Hi, Samantha—I'm Mrs. D. and I will be here with you for the next hour.*
Samantha	*(Rocks back and forth; does not look at the nurse.)*
Nurse	*(Holds the child's hand and looks at her face.) I will be putting a hospital gown on you and giving your clothes to your mother for now. Can I get you a drink of water?*
Samantha	*(Rocking more rapidly; bangs her head on the side rail in a repetitive manner; does not look at the nurse.) Can I get you a drink; can I get you a drink; can I get you a drink.*
Nurse	*Samantha (takes hand again and looks into her eyes), I'll get you a drink of water; you can stay here in your crib.*
Samantha	*(Continues head banging and rocking with no eye contact—takes the water from the nurse when she returns; then throws the water on the floor.)*
Nurse	*You won't hurt anyone by throwing the water— that's all right. (Looks directly at child; speaks gently.)*
Samantha	*(Continues to rock back and forth; no eye contact.)*

The nurse in this situation attempts to define the environment for the child without imposing herself on the child. She maintains contact through touch and visual means. The nurse permits the child to continue self-stimulating behavior as long as it remains within reasonable limits. Vessey notes that this type of behavior may serve to reduce anxiety for the child while she is in a strange environment. If the child is in no apparent physical danger, Vessey indicates that allowing a temper tantrum to run its course is permissible. Restraint should be utilized only if the child is in danger of hurting self or others.

CHILDHOOD ONSET PERVASIVE DEVELOPMENTAL DISORDERS

Disturbances in thought, affect, social relatedness, and behavior emerge in children between ages 30 months and 12 years. Children in this category may have experienced a relatively symptom-free relationship within the family system. Precipitating factors of a severe nature such as loss of a parent through death or separation, repeated separating, sexual abuse, or violence often initiate high levels of anxiety, resulting in ego fragmentation. It is important to note that no one factor leads to the onset of symptoms. There is a complex interrelationship of factors that must be considered during the assessment process.

Children who develop symptoms after the first three years of life seem to have a more favorable prognosis than children diagnosed as autistic in the infancy period. Areas similar to those in infantile autism are affected: thought processes, behavior, affect, and relatedness. Those areas are assessed in relation to continuing age-appropriate characteristics. Thus, characteristics noted in the infantile autistic disorder group will be observed in varying degrees in this group. The following behaviors are characteristic of childhood-onset developmental disorders.

▶ Speech, language, and thought disturbances

Speech may have developed appropriately up to the point of diagnosis. Elective mutism may be present, as well as impairment of nonverbal communication. Cognitive function is impaired, including insight and judgment. Bizarre fantasies and preoccupation with unusual thoughts may also be observed. Echolalic repetition characterizes speech; distorted syntax and fragmented speech patterns result. Although delusions and hallucinations occur in later years, they are not apparent in childhood disorders. Looseness of association and lack of logical connections also characterize this group of children.

▶ Perceptual and motor disturbances

Extreme hypoactivity or hyperactivity may occur, as well as ritualistic movements such as rocking, turning, and whirling. Perception of body boundaries is also impaired. Bender (1947) noted that drawings of the human body are often distorted, with an emphasis on peripheral details such as hair, extremities, and fingers. There is also a distortion in the perception of the relationship of one's own body to other objects in the environment.

▶ Affect and mood

These children display inappropriate affect with mood swings that range from rage to passivity and apathy. Their responses to dangerous situations do not approximate the normal response. As noted previously, illogical anxiety that has no apparent relationship to external events is also exhibited by these children.

▶ Social relatedness

A striking characteristic is the lack of attachment to and hence the withdrawal from peers and peer groups. There is a social distance that is maintained throughout relationships. A lack of response to the feelings of others as human beings and little sense of cooperative interaction can be observed. These children experience much anxiety when changes occur in their environment, and they lack flexibility in adaptation to new persons or events in their surrounding territory. Distorted perception of body boundaries is reflected in these children's inappropriate touching of others and taking of objects belonging to others as if they were their own.

Depression in children

DSM-III-R does not identify a specific category for depression in children and adolescence. Cytryn and McKnew (1979) suggest that this omission perpetuates the myth that children do not experience depressive reactions when in fact they do. Rhyne et al. (1986) note that as many as 20% of school-aged children suffer from depression. The authors indicate that perhaps the stressors of society increase the likelihood that children do not have the support that is necessary to cope effectively with these situations, thus leading to a depressive response. Rhyne et al. discuss several factors that increase the incidence of depression in children:

1. Divorce with accompanying feelings of abandonment or responsibility for the divorce
2. Death of a parent—surviving parent has little energy to cope with the grief of the child
3. Abandonment/separation—parents are jailed or hospitalized, causing children to be placed in one or several foster homes
4. Distancing by parents—events such as a new baby, mother returning to work full-time, or preoccupation by other stressful situations may cause children to feel emotionally distanced from their parents
5. Parental psychopathology—parents who are emotionally unstable themselves are less able to communicate effectively, to offer affection and recognition, and are more likely to provide a chaotic home environment
6. Loss of self-esteem, which results from lack of

consistent positive feedback, leads to feelings of vulnerability

7. Physical disabilities can influence perceptions of self, particularly if illness is life-threatening

Accurate diagnosis of childhood depression is made difficult by the widely divergent symptoms found in this category. Clinical symptoms are age related and often are quite different from the clinical picture of depressed adults. Cytryn and McKnew (1979) state that the depressive process manifests itself in three ways:

1. Fantasy. Depressive themes are demonstrated in dreams of spontaneous play or are elicited through projective testing. Fantasy is present in almost all children who are diagnosed as experiencing a depressive reaction.
2. Verbal expression. Depression is evident through talk of hopelessness, suicide, and being worthless, unloved, and unattractive.
3. Mood and behavior. Observable signs include psychomotor retardation, sadness, crying, anorexia, and sleep disturbances. Masked depression evidences itself in hyperactivity, aggressiveness, school failure, delinquency, and psychosomatic symptoms.

This last category is characterized by the least stability on the part of the child. The authors note that the first line of defense is the development of depressive fantasy, which enables the child to project or deny through fantasy life. Acute depressive reactions are marked by verbal expression of depression, whereas mood and behavior changes are more frequently noted in chronic depressive reactions. At this last level, the preceding defenses against depression have failed, thus permitting mood and behavior changes to surface.

It is important to note that in childhood several factors enhance the ability to defend against depression. During infancy, the maturational process, which promotes a sense of hope and fulfillment and the ability to substitute love objects (since object constancy has not yet been attained), serves to counteract the depressive process. During preschool and latency, the still-rich fantasy life, immature reality testing, and ability to substitute love objects allow for the containment of depressive symptoms at the fantasy level. As the child moves

into adolescence and young adulthood, depressive symptoms are expressed through verbal means, and mood and behavior changes are noted. More mature reality testing and verbalization of feelings counteract the use of fantasy life and other more primitive defenses used in earlier life. Thus, the frequency of overt depression in adult life is greater than in earlier stages of life. (Even in adult life, overt depression does not occur in situations where denial and other primitive mechanisms are in operation.)

Several variables influence the development of a depressive response in children. Toolan (1978) notes that the younger the child at the time of a significant loss, the more serious the consequences of that loss. Other studies support the notion that parental loss before the child reaches the age of 7 increases the incidence of depression. However, Wallerstein (1984) found that preschool children at the time of divorce were troubled; ten years postdivorce, these same children were experiencing less difficulty than those children who were older at the time of the divorce. Stress is seen as a significant variable whether it is related to family disequilibrium, financial difficulties, or frequent relocations. Yet it must be pointed out that stress may be mediated in any of these cases by the presence of a stable support system, which may come from outside the family system.

Early detection requires an assessment of multiple factors that may interact in a mutual relationship to cause a depressive response. Nodal events such as the loss of a parent or the hospitalization of a parent may place a child at risk; changes in school performance and behavior may also increase risk. Trad (1986) notes that the critical developmental milestones must serve as a baseline measurement from which to analyze data. Factors to be assessed include temperament, attachment behaviors, object permanence and constancy, empathy, self-concept, neuroendocrinology, and learned-helplessness phenomena. One must also consider the child's perception of the stressor and the attendant coping strategies. What may be stressful for one child may not be perceived as stressful for another. This model repudiates the use of an adult model of depression and considers in its stead both normal and abnormal maturation as the context of assessment. Once diagnosis of depression has been made, treatment is instituted based on age of the child, severity of behavioral symptoms, length of depression, family resources and support, and other available resources.

The following sample interaction involves a depressed 6-year-old Peter, his mother, and the nurse-psychotherapist at the community mental health center. They were referred by the school nurse and Peter's teacher.

Mother	*I don't know what to do; he won't go to school anymore.*
Nurse	*Can you tell me when this behavior started—was there a specific event?*
Mother	*No, not that I can think of—my husband and I separated several months ago, but he seemed all right after that.*
Nurse	*Does he seem different in other ways?*
Mother	*He doesn't eat as much; he starts fights with other children, and he doesn't seem to enjoy anything any more.*
Nurse	*Peter, can you tell me what might be bothering you?*
Peter	*I feel sad since my daddy left (starts to weep uncontrollably).*
Nurse	*(Puts her arm around Peter to comfort him.) It must be hard for you not to have your daddy around, too.*
Peter	*(Through his tears) It must have been my fault—I know I can be good if he just comes back.*
Mother	*Peter, I've told you that it wasn't your fault (seems to be emotionally distanced—doesn't reach to touch or comfort Peter).*
Nurse	*It must be a difficult time for both of you—I think it would be helpful for me to see Peter individually for a period of time, but I would like to see you as well.*
Mother	*I think it would be helpful—I don't know what to do to make either one of us feel better.*

This vignette illustrates Peter's perception of a stressor—the loss of his father—as being his responsibility. The inability to cope with this loss effectively leads to a depressive response. This depressive response was evidenced by major changes in behavior that were not spontaneously getting better over time. Both Peter and his mother would be able to benefit from individual therapy to alter ineffective coping measures.

DISORDERS OF ADOLESCENCE

Adolescence has been described as one of the major developmental periods. Erikson views adolescence as a period of great physical and emotional change, the goal being a beginning sense of identity—a separation from parents as the primary support system. Self is the focus of development in adolescence. Peer groups guide identity in such areas as dress, activities, academic excellence, and college selection. It has also been called a period of "turmoil" and "adjustment." Adolescents themselves find this time one of ambivalence—the exhilaration of the adult life ahead mingled with the desire to run back to the "nest" and be taken care of. It is maintaining this delicate balance within the family system that contributes to the successful mastery of this period.

Physical changes are apparent in this period. Early in adolescence, secondary sex characteristics emerge with the attendant biological changes. Penis size increases, and breasts develop; the female begins to display the rounded figure; and pubic hair appears in both sexes. Menses may begin as early as age eleven. Voice changes in the male occur. As adolescence progresses, hormonal and growth activity lead to further changes. Males begin to lose their gawkiness; muscle mass increases to fill out the body. Females experience an increase in estrogen as the body prepares for ovulation and pregnancy becomes a possibility. Females experience continued growth and fullness in the breasts and hips. A primary physical change throughout adolescence is the occurrence of acne. Endocrine activity experiences an upsurge in this period, leading to increased production of the sebaceous glands. Adolescents find these varied physical changes difficult to adjust to, and their adjustment is compounded by the emotional swings common to this period.

Emotional changes are wide and varied. Adolescents are noted for their heightened sensitivity to events around them, as well as to their own bodies. Initially, adolescents are uncomfortable discussing the changes they are experiencing.

Elizabeth had just begun her menses. Her mother noticed some pink-tinged tissues in the bathroom. When she openly brought the issue to Elizabeth's attention, Elizabeth promptly turned red and began to deny the occurrence. The mother continued to gently acknowledge the naturalness of this phenomenon and provided support until Elizabeth seemed to be less threatened by the situation.

Often adolescents feel a lack of control over their own bodies and over external events, as is demonstrated by this vignette.

Abrupt changes in mood, impulsive behavior, fluctuations between responsibleness and "flakiness," dress styles, and overt rebellion against parental values are often at the core of adolescent-parent struggles. As noted earlier, beginning at early adolescence peer groups become the major shaping forces, which is frequently frightening to parents. Adolescents' need to control often drives parents and adolescents into struggles that result in benefits to no one. Jay Haley (1980) noted in his book *Leaving Home* that some struggle must occur for the adolescent to separate and develop as an individual; however, the essence of the struggle is critical. Those "minor" struggles, over issues such as curfews and styles of clothing and hair, have less serious consequences than those that involve major value conflicts. Haley's point, which is a valid one, is that separation cannot occur unless there is some force that activates the separation.

Critical to the parent-adolescent relationship is the maintenance of a delicate balance of control. Although adolescents struggle for independence, parental limit setting and expectations are necessary, particularly in early adolescence. Those parents who want to be "friends" to their children promote further role confusion at a time when the adolescent needs clarity. The major focus of parenting is on the provision of support and guidance as the adolescent moves toward independence. To actualize this support, parents must have a clear definition of their own roles and expectations, must be able to tolerate the mood swings and other behaviors that are a part of the emerging individual, and, last, must be able to separate out their own goals, desires, *and* unresolved conflicts.

Adolescent depression and suicide

Studies by Rutter et al. (1986) and others indicate that depression in adolescence is rising at a significant rate. Often depression in adolescence is mislabeled or dismissed as part of the "normal" adolescent turmoil. However, it is clear that adolescents who are depressed often turn to suicide as a means of coping with their situation. Rutter et al. note that postpubertal depression increases more than twofold; the sex ratio also changes, with depression seen more frequently in girls in the postpubertal period. Mania is rarely seen in childhood; however, there seems to be a more frequent appearance in the adolescent period. Rutter et al. indicate that bipolar disorders may begin in childhood but that the manic phase does not appear until adolescence. There is evidence of these changes; however, there is little empirical data to support a rationale for why sex ratio and age changes occur as they do.

What places an adolescent at risk for depression? Why do some adolescents become depressed while others do not? As has been discussed in Chapter 8, stress is perceived differently by individuals who may be in similar situations. What is perceived as stressful for one may not be for another. An individual may also be more vulnerable to stress at certain points in the life-cycle. Rutter delineates the following risk factors:

1. Frequent changes in care takers
2. Changes in family roles due to physical or emotional illness; other circumstances
3. Financial and social strain, i.e., loss of parental employment
4. Death of a parent and impact on surviving parent
5. Break-up of family system
6. Blending of stepfamilies
7. Emotional and/or physical abuse within family system
8. History of alcohol/drug abuse within family system
9. Physical disability or handicap of adolescent

Assessment of depression in adolescents is difficult due to the very nature of the adolescent phase of development. Often parents, teachers, and mental health professionals are hesitant to identify signs of depression—either assuming that the behaviors are normal or fearing that the adolescent and the family will be labeled as "mentally ill." Often there is no specific event that initiates a depressive response; a chronic sense of poor self-worth and feelings of failure characterize the depressive response in the adolescent. Other significant signs of adolescent depression include:

1. Lack of concern for physical appearance
2. Withdrawal from others and usual activities
3. Negative attitude toward self and others
4. Physical complaints such as chronic fatigue, alteration in sleep and eating patterns
5. Difficulties in school—decrease in grades; acting out behaviors toward teachers, peers, others
6. Decrease in attention and concentration
7. Persistent feelings of hopelessness and powerlessness
8. Flat or blunted affect
9. Sexual difficulties
10. Pervasive unhappy mood

Although the assessment of depression in adolescents may be complicated by the nature of the developmental phase itself, nurses can be alert to these behavioral cues and utilize them to determine an appropriate plan of intervention.

ADOLESCENT SUICIDE

Valente and Saunders (1987) cite the rising trend of adolescent suicides, which has reached the national mean, and the fear that adolescent suicide will become epidemic. Maris (1985) notes a 273% rise in adolescent suicide during the period 1960–1980; further studies are being conducted to determine the validity of these statistics as well as to determine the predictor behaviors of adolescent suicide.

Adolescent suicide is not the result of a single causative factor but rather emerges as a response to the interaction of multiple factors. Hendin (1987) discusses adolescent suicide within the context of the sociocultural environment. He suggests that to gain a comprehensive psychosocial perspective, one must understand the social context in which suicide occurs as well as the factors that have affected the adolescent and his or her perceptions of those factors. Hendin describes the following factors that must be considered within the framework of a psychosocial perspective: the concurrent rise in drug abuse, alcohol abuse, delinquency, and crime among adolescents; the emergence of significant biological correlates of suicide; increased stress resulting from an increased number of youth in the population with an accompanying increase in competition for desired options in society, i.e., employment, college, etc. These young people will have more difficulty fulfilling their aspirations; may encounter more marital stress; and divorce rates among this group as they move through young adulthood will be higher. Hendin also notes the importance of family dynamics in relation to suicidal behavior. He found that the family situation of suicidal adolescents revealed disturbances in the parent-child relationship beginning in the early life experience. The parents were perceived as rejecting, unkind, emotionally distanced, and unable to establish intimate relationships with their children. Hendin suggests that adolescent suicide may be conceptualized as the adolescent's response to loss, separation, or abandonment. Support for the sociocultural perspective of suicidal behavior can be found in Berlin's (1987) study of suicide among American Indian adolescents. He notes that the rate of suicide has dramatically increased in the American Indian population over the last decade. Postmortem interviews with families and significant others reveal the following etiological factors: early loss of care takers; increased incidence of arrest and incarceration of both care taker and adolescent; emotional instability in the family; alcoholism and drug abuse; increased number of both parents involved in employment out of the home; and severe environmental changes. Berlin cites a study conducted with a black and Hispanic population that delineates a three-phase process that leads to suicide: (1) chronic history of childhood problems; (2) escalation of these problems which causes strained and distant relationships with parents and struggle for independence creates feelings of misunderstanding between parents and adolescent; (3) final period of days or weeks prior to the attempt is characterized by breakdown of social relationships with peers and family.

Within the sociocultural context, one must consider the issue of "cluster" suicides as defined by

Valente and Saunders. The authors note that there is not a clear-cut definition of "cluster" suicide, although some indicate that the term should be utilized only if the individuals have discussed their suicidal ideations. Most recent statistics as presented by Valente and Saunders indicate that there has been an increase in the incidence of cluster suicide as evidenced by the deaths of five adolescents in Westchester County, New York; four adolescents in Bergen County, New Jersey; nine adolescents on the Wind River Indian Reservation, Wyoming; and six adolescents in Clear Lake City, Texas. There is added concern that media coverage increases the romantic notion of suicide, thus increasing the number of imitative responses. Phillips and Carstensen (1988) note in their demographic study of the effects of suicide stories that these stories do in fact impact on the population at large. However, the authors point out that adolescents tend to be most affected.

The etiology of adolescent suicide also reflects biochemical changes that lead to a depressive response. Suicide may be a learned behavior within the context of a family system where other members have coped with stress through the suicidal act. A sense of learned helplessness wherein the adolescent believes that he has no control over his environment, feels hopeless, and ultimately turns to suicide may also be noted. As previously discussed, suicide must be assessed and understood within the context of the interaction of multiple factors.

Who is at risk for adolescent suicide? Valente and Saunders state that young males commit suicide four times more often than young females, while young females make four times more attempts than young males. This is consistent with statistics for the adult population in general. What are specific risk factors for suicide? Smith and Crawford (1984) identify high-risk groups that include teens with such characteristics as depression, particularly related to the loss of a loved one or a valued object or possession; alcohol and drug problems; schizophrenia; past suicide attempts; alienation or stigmatization related to one's behavior (homosexuality) or to one's appearance (physical disability or illness); previous exposure to child abuse, family suicide, and incest; and marital and/or family instability and

conflict. Hart and Keidel (1979) suggest that adolescents who do not demonstrate the characteristic signs of turmoil yet are subject to the above-mentioned risk factors are candidates for suicidal behavior. However, this premise does not account for the large population of adolescents who, during the adolescent phase, are subjected to these risk factors but do not utilize suicidal behaviors.

The impact of adolescent suicide is far reaching. Parents and siblings, teachers and coaches, best friends and acquaintances are left with feelings of depression, anger, guilt, and, in some cases, a sense of relief. Ojanlatva, Hammer, and Mohr (1987) state that each year teens leave behind more than 25,000 survivors who must cope with the social stigma that surrounds the issue of suicide. They note that sadness is the most obvious reaction, yet the most enduring is anger and guilt. Anger may be directed toward friends of the adolescent; toward teachers, clergy, psychiatrists, or other health professionals; toward God for allowing this to happen; and toward the adolescent for dying. Survivors view suicide as a rejection and feel that they must have done something to cause the victim to choose death rather than life. Guilt is generated by this perspective, which is further perpetuated by feelings of anger toward the victim and then by feelings of relief that the victim no longer must suffer. Although feelings of anger and relief may be viewed as part of the normal grieving process, the ensuing feelings of guilt may be long-lasting. To facilitate healthy adaptation of survivors and to prevent the incidence of further suicidal behavior, programs of postvention and prevention have been identified. Ojanlatva et al. (1987) suggest that supportive programs be instituted that incorporate the use of school administration and teachers. They note the need for crisis intervention with students, which may then refer students needing further assistance to ongoing support groups. Last, the authors suggest that parents of the victim be referred to community programs that provide supportive therapy. Valente and Saunders (1987) describe school suicide prevention programs directed at reducing adolescent suicide through education about suicidal behavior, choice of alternatives to suicide, and referral to counseling when necessary. They note that these programs seemed to increase awareness of suicidal clues, triggered increased community involvement with adolescents, and encouraged adolescents to become active suicide prevention advocates. However, critics indicate that there are no empirical data to support the notion that these programs do reduce suicidal behavior. They also believe that programs of this type may dramatize suicide and instigate suicidal behavior in those adolescents who may not ordinarily consider suicide as an option. However, studies by Nelson (1986) reveal that over 65% of students reported some degree of suicidal ideation or suicidal activity. Thus, it would seem that programs of this nature do not put thoughts into the heads of adolescents but rather may make them aware of options that are more adaptive than suicide.

In summary, adolescent suicide is emerging as a leading cause of death in that age group. Accurate assessment is dependent upon the understanding of potential stressors and risk factors as well as having a knowledge of the underlying dynamics of suicidal behavior. Nurses are in key positions in schools and communities to identify at-risk individuals, to implement programs of prevention and community awareness, and to facilitate support groups for survivors. The following is a sample interaction with a 14-year-old female, Cathy, who has been admitted to the psychiatric unit for attempted suicidal behavior.

Nurse	*Cathy, I'd like you to tell me what happened in your own words.*
Cathy	*I was upset; I took a bottle of aspirin, but then I called my mother at work.*
Nurse	*Can you tell me what was upsetting you right at that point in time?*
Cathy	*Everything—nothing was going well. I broke up with my boyfriend and then he told me he didn't care about me anyway.*
Nurse	*How did that make you feel?*
Cathy	*It was just one more thing to make me feel bad.*
Nurse	*I'm not sure what you mean.*
Cathy	*I can't do anything well—my grades aren't that good, and my parents keep telling me I won't go to college.*
Nurse	*Is there something that makes you feel good about yourself?*
Cathy	*I don't know—I can't think of anything.*

Nurse	*It sounds as though it feels pretty awful right now being you.*
Cathy	*I just didn't want to feel that way any more. I thought the pills would take care of that.*
Nurse	*I think we can work on some things to help you begin to feel more positive about who you are. Since you have been here, have you felt like hurting yourself?*
Cathy	*No, not right at the moment.*
Nurse	*Before I leave you for today, I'd like to contract with you that you'll talk to me if you have feelings of wanting to hurt yourself again. I care about what happens to you.*
Cathy	*I think I can do that—but nobody has said that they care about me in a long time.*

In the initial interaction, the nurse begins to establish a trusting relationship with the client. She attempts to determine precipitating factors, feelings associated with suicidal behavior, and sets the tone for a positive, goal-directed relationship.

Impulsive behaviors*

In an attempt to separate and individuate, the adolescent may use inappropriate measures to achieve independence; antisocial behavior such as stealing, truancy, and running away may represent attempts to escape from tension-producing family situations, as well as being a method to achieve some measure of independence. Often parent-child relationships are characterized by rejection and ambivalence over the parenting role. Open communication between parent and child is not encouraged; the adolescent is not given the opportunity to work through the emotional conflicts that are experienced as part of adolescence. An adolescent's anger toward parents or caregivers is expressed through stealing and running away—the motivation being to punish the parents for their lack of attention and love. In the case of stealing, the parents are often the focus of the punishment from the police or other authorities. Adolescents may feel that outside authorities will have an effect on parents when they themselves do not have any impact. Adolescents who run away may also feel

---

*Eating disorders and substance abuse will be covered in Chapters 23 and 21 respectively.

that they are punishing their parents; unfortunately in some cases, parents may feel relief at having the responsibility removed. Impulsive behaviors such as those noted are used by adolescents to exert some measure of control, to separate from an untenable family situation, to express anger and frustration at parents, and to develop a sense of self-worth through their acts.

EXPLANATORY THEORIES

The following section will present theories of child and adolescent mental health from a variety of perspectives. Each theory is recognized for its individual contributions; however, it is an underlying premise of this book that a systems perspective should be considered to provide effective nursing intervention at all levels—primary, secondary, and tertiary.

Psychodynamic theory

Psychodynamic theory incorporates both the analytic viewpoint and those theories which are extensions or derivations of Freudian theory.

A primary characteristic of childhood disorders is the lack of appropriate ego functioning. Ego deficits may occur as a result of organic changes or faulty development in childhood. Freud states that fixation during a particular period of childhood will then determine the future level of functioning. Children with ego deficits are unable to control their impulses. Berman (1979) notes that their levels of tolerance of frustration are minimal. Immediate gratification of desires is necessary; aggressive acting-out behavior results when these children are placed in situations that create anxiety and frustration.

The lack of a sound ego prevents these children from forming relationships with others. Lack of ego boundaries causes them to fear engulfment from others while also desiring a warm, caring relationship. These children have few problem-solving skills; thus they are unable to adapt to situations around them. They are unable to learn from their mistakes and move on to new experiences. Multiple stimuli generate panic rather than provide an opportunity for learning. These children may be insensitive to others and are unable to function within the accepted social norms. This behavior causes others to avoid and castigate them, which further forces them into a fantasy world and social isolation.

Popper notes in the case of conduct disorders that there may be superego defects, which in turn impact on the development of a sound conscience. He also suggests that conduct disorders may be a reflection of the parents' acting out of their own unverbalized antisocial wishes and/or impulses. Separation anxiety disorders may result from unconscious internal conflicts regarding aggressive and sexual impulses as well as uncertainty regarding the caretaker's presence following the toddler's initial step-taking and anxiety induced by the parents themselves.

Blos (1962) describes the dynamics of adolescence as being crucial in the individuation of the self. The adolescent returns to former modes of adaptation in an attempt to renegotiate his or her role as an independent self—separate from the adult parents. Again, sound foundation in the early phases of life must be present for adolescents to successfully individuate from the parental system. As Blos further describes, adolescent behavior such as anger, argumentative behavior, and resistance to authority serve as ways to facilitate separation. The importance of sound ego functioning is also supported by Erikson in his delineation of the eight stages of development. His description of the task of adolescence focuses on the need of the adolescent to define self in relation to environment, peers, parents, and life goals. For an adolescent to move along and complete further tasks, he or she must develop a sound sense of self.

Constitutional-biological theory

Temperament characteristics—characteristics that exist at birth—may influence a child's level of stress tolerance and shape the child's future life experiences. Thus the situations children find themselves in are influenced by their very temperaments. A quiet, shy child will select experiences that reflect a quality of interaction that is quite different from that of a child who is extremely active.

Temperament in an indirect manner directs choice of peers, quality of interaction, and roles a child will play. These factors in turn have a relationship to the development of psychopathology.

The New York Longitudinal Studies (Chess et al., 1970) have demonstrated that certain temperamental characteristics were connected to the development of psychiatric disorders. Nine assessment categories were identified as a result of the study: activity level, rhythmicity, approach-withdrawal, adaptability, threshold of responsiveness, intensity of reaction, quality of mood, distractibility, and attention span and persistence. It was determined that there was not a direct correlation between temperamental characteristics and psychopathology; however, it was also determined that a child with vulnerabilities in one or more categories can become the target of parental frustration and irritability. Thus, one must consider not only the temperament of the child but also the attitude and response of the parents. Chess et al. (1970) suggest that normal development results from a "goodness of fit" between the child's individual characteristics and the expectations of the family environment.

Individual differences in infants have been reported by Schaffer (1974) and Bridger and Birns (1968). Sucking behaviors in infants showed marked differences, as did startle responses. Consistent individual variation in heart rates in response to being touched was also noted. Bridger and Birns noted that an NIMH study provided empirical data that supported evidence that identical (monozygotic) twins are born with very different temperaments. Major differences were noted in the areas of attention span, physiologic adaptation, and level of calmness. The authors concluded that there was a strong indication of nongenetic factors affecting early congenital differences in temperament.

Bell (1971) in his research supports the aforementioned findings. He notes that there are congenital determinants of such childhood traits as assertiveness, sensorimotor capabilities, and sociability. Individual variations in these traits will affect the manner in which the parent responds. He concludes that these behaviors arouse a particular level of parental response that occurs within a response hierarchy and that reinforces certain parental behaviors once they have been elicited.

Chess et al. (1970) present data that support the genetic component in a longitudinal study of eight pairs of twins. Those characteristics that reflected the strongest genetic evidence were activity, approach-withdrawal, and adaptability. During the first year of study, the genetic influence seemed stronger than during the subsequent two years.

Further studies have been conducted that examine correlations between temperament and children's coping responses. Dunn and Kendrick (1980) report that there are specific changes in children's behavior after the birth of a sibling that seem to be correlated with the temperament of the child. Rutter et al. (1983) found the child's temperamental features increased the liability to behavioral changes after the birth of a sibling. These individual differences also interacted with the mother's emotional state and the nature and quality of the mother-child relationship. Wertlieb et al. (1987) conclude from their preliminary research that there is strong evidence for a relationship between stress and temperament and their effect on behavior, thus supporting the notion that temperament is relevant to socioemotional functioning and the outcome of stress reactions in children of school age.

Popper indicates that there is a definitive genetic etiological component in the development of attention deficit disorders, conduct disorders, and autistic disorders. In the latter, research indicates that autosomal recessive inheritance may be instrumental in the development of certain cases of autistic disorder. Vandenberg, Singer, and Pauls (1986) state that although genetic studies on attention deficit disorders are in the preliminary phase, it seems that at least some children have a genetic contribution.

Neurological studies indicate that there is support for a neurochemical basis of disorders in childhood and adolescence. Bellinger et al. (1987) note that pre- and postnatal exposure to toxic levels of lead can precede attention deficit and cognitive disorders. Popper suggests a correlation between prenatal factors as opposed to birth complications and attention deficit disorders. Herskowitz (1987) concludes that intrauterine exposure to alcohol may also be instrumental in the development of hyperactivity, impulsive behavior, and attention deficits. Popper notes a significant correlation of history of physical abuse with head and face injuries with conduct disorders in youth in conjunction with a history of seizure disorders. Last, Popper notes that there are autoantibodies to serotonin-A in the cerebrospinal fluid and in the blood of 40% of autistic children that are not found in other clients. He indicates that it is unlikely that one single neurological deficit is responsible for the development of autistic behavior.

Effects of sex differences on the development of childhood psychopathology were studied by Hutt (1974). She noted three aspects of male development: males experience an increased risk of and are more vulnerable to various dysfunctions; males are subject to greater phenotype variability; and males are slower in their development. Male infants seem to be more susceptible to postnatal complications. Cantwell and Tarjan (1979) support Hutt and suggest that dysfunctions such as childhood psychosis, learning disabilities, language disturbances, and behavioral disturbances occur to a greater degree in males than in females. Hutt (1974) suggests that increased susceptibility may result in part from the extended developmental period experienced by males. Extended developmental periods would provide longer critical periods, increasing the amount of time stressors have to operate. Rutter (1970, 1986) further supports the premise of vulnerability in males. In his study of high-risk families (those having one parent with mental illness), he found that male children were more stressed by family dysfunction than females. A study of stresses experienced as a result of short-term admissions of a parent into an institution also indicated a greater incidence of behavioral dysfunction in boys.

Sameroff and Chandler (1975) have developed three models to describe the relationship between constitutional-organic factors and the environment. The first model, the main effects model, states that an organic deficit will result in deviant behavior regardless of environmental influences. The interaction model suggests that deviant behavior is a result of the interaction between the child's constitutional-organic factors and psychosocial factors in the environment. However, this model does not emphasize the reciprocity of influence. Sameroff and Chandler suggest that a third model, the transactional model, considers the mutual influence child and environment have on one another. Neither factor exerts greater influence; each must be considered in concert. Thus, in the next section, the sociocultural and familial influences on the development of behavioral and emotional dysfunctions will be considered.

Sociocultural theory

Children exist within the context of their families; however, the influence of the larger society also impacts on their development and their behavioral responses. Thus, the community or cultural context within which the child grows up will define various behaviors as abnormal. That definition of abnormal may vary depending on the age of the child. For example, crying, temper tantrums, and clinging behaviors may be age appropriate until the age of five or six. These are unacceptable behaviors for the twelve-year-old and are likely to be indicative of a behavioral disorder. The people within the culture interpret behaviors and determine whether they are acceptable within the framework of that particular culture. As Looff (1979) notes, children are referred to mental health resources by those in the community such as nurses, teachers, local physicians, and guidance counselors, whose determinations are made by comparing presenting behaviors with culturally defined behaviors based on peer norms. A study of the Hutterites (Eaton and Weill, 1955) revealed that neurotic symptoms (for example, psychophysiological and depressive responses) were socially acceptable methods of tension relief in that culture. In another example of regional cultural influence, Looff (1979) indicates that in Southern Appalachia certain behavior patterns do occur with reasonable frequency while others do not. The children of Southern Appalachia rarely display symptoms of primary behavior disorders or impulse disorders. However, this population seems to reflect an increased occurrence of disorders based on sexual conflict, indicative perhaps of exaggerated sexual attitudes in this particular area. Loof further notes that verbal communication is a problem among these families, thus severely restricting their ability to discuss problems and solutions. He suggests that children from these families often have emotional problems that reflect nonverbal themes, a situation resulting from a lack of experience in verbally expressing difficulties.

It is also important to consider sociocultural influences on the development of strengths. The culture impacts on the shaping of the healthy aspects of the personality—in terms of developing effective methods of coping and basic ego strengths. Looff notes the strengths of the Southern Appalachian culture: the family is basically stable and organized; there is a remarkable sense of relatedness and trust with little sense of personal isolation, and there is an impressive capacity to deeply experience and differentiate feelings related to one's own experiences.

As has been stated throughout, the child exists within the context of the larger society and within the context of the family. In the last section, the family will be discussed in relation to its impact on the developing child. (For further reference to the family, see Chapters 5 and 14.)

Lidz (1963) indicates that familial influences are the first imprint on the newborn child. These influences are so pervasive and consistent that they shape the child's life in such a way that they can be modified in later life but never truly altered.

Because every aspect of the child reflects the familial influence, certain family factors contribute to disturbances in childhood and adolescence. The ability to communicate in an open, honest manner, the ability to develop trusting relationships, and the ability to resolve conflict through effective coping strategies emerge out of early familial interaction.

Spitz (1951) noted that lack of human contact in the form of maternal deprivation and lack of stimulation were central factors in the development of disturbed behavior in the early stages of life, resulting in the "failure to thrive" syndrome. Kanner's early work (1955) suggests that infantile autism results from a disturbed parent-child relationship. According to Kanner, mothers of autistic children tend to be aloof and distant and to have little emotional attachment to their children; the relationship between mother and child exists primarily on an intellectual level.

Several family theorists suggest a strong reciprocal relationship among family members in the development of behavioral and emotional disorders in children and adolescents. For example, Laing (1964) notes that deficiencies in communication and parenting skills and disturbed family behavior patterns occur early in the family life-cycle. In his work he described the distorted patterns of communication that characterize these families. He also described the concept of mystification, whereby family members have little, if any, specific identity. There is no sense of individual personality or spontaneity. The process of mystification includes many contradictions and inconsistencies, so much so that members are unable to determine what is actually so and what is not.

Bowen (1978) describes family relationships in regard to the degree of differentiation between the two members of the parental dyad. Parents who are unable to define self clearly experience a fusion that influences their ability to relate to the child as well as to one another. Bowen suggests that for these parents to control tension and resolve conflict, two actions must take place: (1) the child is triangled into the parental dyad and (2) the projection process occurs whereby the focus of the disturbance is placed on the child, taking the pressure off the parental dyad. Eventually, Bowen suggests, the child lives up to the distorted projections placed on him by the parents and dysfunctional behavior does occur.

Minuchin (1974) and his colleagues at the Child Guidance Clinic support the belief that family dynamics influence the development of psychosomatic illness. He notes that behavioral events and stressful interactions that occur among family members can be measured in terms of increases in the levels of hormones and other substances in the bloodstreams of family members as the events occur. Minuchin describes these families as being characterized by enmeshment, rigidity, and inability to effectively problem solve. For example, clients with eating disorders such as anorexia and bulimia experience difficulty in gaining control over and individuating self. Families of these clients are often characterized by a facade of "normalcy," whereas beneath the facade exists little room for the development of a personal identity. Control over one's own body is perceived by the anorectic/bulimic as perhaps the singular form of control he or she has. Often the mother is viewed as controlling and chronically depressed, while the father is seen as passive. Feelings and differences of opinion are not commonly expressed in this enmeshed family system. Thus one can begin to understand the complex relationship between parent and child and its effect on developing behavior patterns.

Elliott et al. (1985) report that sociocultural theories focus on the effects of poverty and cultural disadvantage, variations in local mores and norms, including the importance of street gangs, and the escape from social entrapment. These factors impact on the development of conduct disorders as well as oppositional defiant dysfunctions. Family history research demonstrates a preponderance of antisocial behavior, alcohol and drug abuse, mood disorders, schizophrenia, and other behavioral disorders in families of children with conduct and attention deficit disorders. It has been reported that over half the parents of children with anxiety disorders suffer from some form of mood disorder as well. Although the role of family dysfunction is apparent in the etiology of such illnesses as conduct disorder, separation anxiety, and attention deficit, one must be cautious in making assumptions about the direct correlation of family and disorder. Certain factors can act as a protective mechanism, for example, consistent caretaking when parents are unable to be in the home and other support systems such as extended family and friends. In light of the number of factors that operate within the context of the family system, it is difficult to develop a foundation of predictive knowledge relative to the etiology of childhood and adolescent disorders.

Family dynamics—relationships between parents, relationships between parent and child, inconsistent parenting skills, inappropriate expectations of child and adolescent behavior, lack of adequate support systems for parenting role, lack of effective problem-solving skills, inability to express feelings directly, lack of knowledge regarding normal growth and development, undifferentiated self with a poor sense of worth, residual unmet dependency needs, isolation, and alienation as a family unit—are factors that may operate at critical points throughout the family life-cycle and exert a pro-

found impact on the growth and development of children within the family system. To fully understand family dynamics, these factors must be considered in the assessment and implementation phases of the nursing process.

Systems theory

Each theory presented suggests a distinct etiological underpinning for the development of disorders in children and adolescents. Research has demonstrated that a particular temperament may be present at birth as well as a preexisting vulnerability that influences the manner in which the newborn later utilizes those capacities to interact within the context of the environment. Severe ego dysfunction in children may have a neurologic as well as a biochemical base. Profoundly disturbed behavior in children may elicit disorganized and dysfunctional responses from a parenting system that does not have the knowledge or capacity to cope with disturbed behavior. In some instances, there is evidence of emotional disturbance in one or both parents that then reinforces inappropriate behavior in the child or adolescent. There is a mutual, simultaneous interaction between child and environment where each impacts upon the other. The degree to which the child can affect the environment is dependent in part upon constitutional make-up, neurological and biochemical factors, sociocultural influences, societal expectations, and family relationships. Thus, the development of disorders in children and adolescents is reflective of the mutual interaction of multiple factors—both internal and external.

TREATMENT MODALITIES
Emergency intervention

Crisis intervention theory provides the framework for short-term measures that can assist children, adolescents, and their parents to cope with depressive and/or suicidal feelings. Crisis services may be offered through community mental health centers, hot lines, and emergency room settings. School nurses are in a critical position to identify signs of depression, as adolescents often utilize the school nurse as a sounding board for expressing their feelings of discouragement, their disappointments, and their feelings that life may not be worth living. Acute listening skills, an understanding of the dynamics of adolescent behavior, awareness of the signs of emotional distress, and the ability to form genuine empathic relationships are necessary tools for the school nurse. School nurses, as well as those nurses working on a pediatric unit, may be in a position to identify signs of developmental delays as well as overt and subtle signs of anxiety disorders, disruptive behaviors, eating disorders, and gender disturbances. Pediatric nurses may also provide short-term measures that assist parents in coping with the hospitalization of their children as well as assisting them to cope with the needs of other children at home. Nurses in the general hospital setting who care for adults can also assess how children in the family are coping with the illness of the parent and adapting to changing roles and expectations that may result from the illness of a parent.

Emergency outpatient care for suicidal teens is described by Talan as an alternative to inpatient hospitalization. Talan notes that the care at these emergency outpatient centers involves not only the adolescent but also family members and significant others. Statistics indicate that approximately 75% of the adolescents treated in the emergency outpatient centers show significant improvement, which is somewhat better than inpatient programs. This alternative to inpatient hospitalization shows promise; however, the scarcity of such programs remains a major issue at this time. (For further discussion of crisis intervention, see Chapters 15 and 22).

Family therapy

As has been noted earlier in this chapter, children and adolescents exist within the context of a family system. Thus, regardless of whether a child is in residential treatment or outpatient therapy, the family should be considered as part of the treatment process. Goren (1984) notes that the family enters treatment because the child is ill, but the remaining family members consider themselves healthy. Family function will improve, it is thought, if the child's behavior is altered. The goal

of family therapy, then, is to reframe the problem as reflective of the dynamics of the family system. Goren suggests that the focus of intervention is to enable family members to understand that symptomatic behavior of the child continues because it is supported in many ways by other members of the family. For example, a sibling of a "good" child may find that a satisfactory method of gaining parental attention is through acting-out behavior. Goren adds that altering the acting-out behavior will influence the "good" behavior of the other child because both participants are necessary for the interaction to occur. Identifying the process of interactional effects within the system will assist family members in understanding their influences on others' roles. Improved communication with clearly stated expectations and increased expression of feelings are also critical outcomes of family therapy. Within the therapy setting, the nurse acts as a role model in the direct expression of feelings as they relate to specific situations. Parents learn that rules, regulations, and consequences can be determined and maintained. Positive reinforcement is offered to support appropriate parenting behaviors. Smith and Murphy (1984) state that parents can learn how to *listen* to one another and their children, as well as how to spend more productive interactional time with their children. The family therapy setting provides an arena where aspects of normal growth and development can be identified and explored, providing anticipatory guidance for both parents and children by increasing their awareness of developmental tasks and behavioral changes. Finally, through treatment, family members learn to use their own strengths and capabilities to develop more effective problem-solving methods (Goren, 1984). (For further discussion of family therapy see Chapter 14.)

Individual therapy

Individual therapy can be done on a verbal or play level; the choice depends on the ability of the child to verbally express feelings and on the child's cognitive level. Axline (1969) states that play therapy as a treatment modality uses the child's natural medium of self-expression. Hostility toward a doll, for example, can be more readily expressed with no repercussions than can hostility toward a newborn sibling. The manner in which children respond to various games, the roles they choose to play (mother, father), and the media they use (clay, water, paints) are critical assessment data. Through play therapy children are permitted to experience and explore their feelings in a trusting, stable environment where they can begin to define their own senses of individuality. Thus, the individual setting—whether on a verbal level or a play level—can be used to explore relationships with peers and with family members.

Smith and Murphy (1984) support Axline's premises and suggest that play therapy is appropriate for children from preschool age through latency, particularly in cases in which behavior has regressed from a higher level of functioning. Adolescent individual therapy may be used as a means to explore developmental issues such as achieving independence and coping with emerging sexuality.

Milieu therapy

Jones (1953), who initiated the concept of therapeutic community, believes that mental illness results from an individual's inability to function effectively within the context of interpersonal relationships. Thus, relationships with staff members and other clients have an influence on an individual client, and that influence is reciprocal. Clients mature and learn through their experiences within the milieu. Community meetings are an integral part of milieu therapy. Issues of daily living are raised and problem-solving is explored. Milieu therapy within the context of residential treatment provides a structured environment where new coping skills can be tested and more effective communication skills can be developed. Smith and Murphy (1984) state that milieu therapy for children must provide basic rules to follow and consistent consequences for noncompliant behaviors. Inconsistencies may result in confusion for the child and regressive behaviors. Principles of behavior modification may be used to reinforce positive behaviors. Smith and Murphy add that development of rewards and consequences must be determined in relation to age and comprehension level of the client popula-

tion. Consideration also must be given to the frequency and duration of the consequences and rewards.

Group therapy

Moss (1984) notes that some current literature supports the validity of child group therapy for a variety of clients and using different approaches. An open, unstructured group may be used for school-age and latency-age children; topics can be decided on by group members themselves. Younger children may use the group setting as a means to learn cooperative play and to view their behaviors as they relate to their peers (Smith and Murphy, 1984). Smith and Murphy also suggest that staff-directed, structured groups can be useful in assisting children in learning and practicing more effective methods of handling feelings and difficult situations. Staff members select a particular topic and develop a role play, puppet, or story-telling activity to deal with the identified issue.

Group therapy may be used for a variety of purposes: to increase object development, to correct family experiences, to improve interaction with peers, and to reduce ego dysfunction. Moss (1984) supports the belief that group therapy can be a productive treatment modality for children and adolescents with many different types of problems: psychoses, physical handicaps, victims of abuse, school behavior problems, and mental retardation. Consistency and structure are critical elements in the success of group therapy. Moss further notes that a diverse group enhances the potential therapeutic effect. For example, a withdrawn child gains when he or she reaches out to help a child who is hyperactive. The hyperactive child, on the other hand, profits from focusing attention on the interaction. The strengths of one child can be used to support another child, within the context of that child's limitations.

Child group therapy can be a useful means to reduce psychological and emotional dysfunction. Various techniques can be utilized by the therapist, such as role-playing, behavior modification, and activities to facilitate development of interpersonal skills and more appropriate behavioral responses.

It is important to note that the success of child group therapy depend on parental support. Moss (1984) and Kaplan and Sadock (1985) identify the need for concurrent parent support groups. Through such a group, parents gain a better understanding of their child's problems and strengths. The group setting provides an opportunity to discuss their own feelings and to explore more effective methods of coping.

Somatic therapies

Pharmacological treatment is used with caution. Major tranquilizers may be given to reduce severe personality disorganization. Baer and Williams (1988) suggest that the drug of first choice should be a common one so that side effects and dosage level are more well known. Behaviors should be specifically targeted so that effects can be monitored accurately. Lowest dosages possible should be used, and their dosages should be increased gradually until target symptoms are reduced or side effects result.

Tricyclic antidepressants may be used for childhood and adolescent depressions, although DSM-III-R does not list these as separate disorders. Judicious use of imipramine (Tofranil) has demonstrated success in the treatment of separation anxiety disorder. Lithium is not currently approved for use with children under 12 years of age. As yet its efficacy in the treatment of major affective disorders in childhood has not been proved (Kaplan and Sadock, 1985).

Methylphenidate (Ritalin) and dextroamphetamine (Dexedrine) have been used with reasonable success in the treatment of attention deficit disorders. Side effects are for the most part transient and decrease as the dose is adjusted. Tofranil has also been used, yet Kaplan and Sadock note that there tends to be a higher incidence of side effects.

There is a controversy over the use of electroconvulsive therapy (ECT). Bender (1947) states that children can significantly improve following electroconvulsive therapy and are then more amenable to concurrent therapies. Kaplan and Sadock (1985), however, believe that there is no justification for the use of ECT in childhood disorders.

Nursing Intervention
PRIMARY PREVENTION

Primary prevention in the area of child and adolescent mental health focuses on assessment or screening for risk. To provide a comprehensive assessment, nurses must be aware of the criteria for mental health and of those factors that influence the child's ability to respond and adjust appropriately to environmental and internal stimuli. Bumbalo and Siemon (1983) suggest that there are three areas to consider when screening for risk: (1) environmental factors, (2) parental characteristics, and (3) characteristics indicative of increased vulnerability. Based on an expansion of these factors, principles can be derived to act as guidelines for the development of goals in primary prevention. These are:

1. Emotional difficulties in children and adolescents often arise from faulty or inconsistent child-rearing practices.
2. Surface conflicts may emerge from developmental transitions such as entry into school and development of sex characteristics.
3. Environmental factors such as poverty, lack of adequate support systems, major cumulative life stresses, and maternal employment influence coping abilities of children and adolescents.
4. Constitutional factors, or those characteristics within the child or adolescent, affect level of individual vulnerability.
5. Children and adolescents who have a secure sense of self are able to engage in satisfying relationships, learn new skills, and perceive the world without distortion.
6. Cultural factors influence each family's perception of child-rearing practices.

The goals for primary prevention of emotional disorders in children and adolescents include:

1. Providing knowledge of normal growth and development to parents
2. Minimizing the effects of factors that predispose children and adolescents to emotional disorders
3. Screening groups that represent high-risk parental systems—that is, abusive families, indulgent families, families with chronic illnesses, and families that engage in drug or alcohol abuse.

Nurses in schools and in community agencies are in key positions to observe children in their school environments and in family interactions. Children may not be symptomatic yet exist within the context of a family environment that presents a potential risk. An assessment should address the following areas:*

1. Environmental factors
   a. Socioeconomic level
   b. Maternal employment
   c. Adequacy of housing, food, and clothing
2. Social support, resources, functioning
   a. Adequacy and availability of support systems
   b. Stability of family system (including number of major life changes)
   c. Characteristics of parental system
      (1) Abusive behaviors
      (2) Alcohol or drug abuse
      (3) Chronic illness (either physical or emotional)
      (4) Overindulgent, immature
      (5) Rejecting
   d. Cultural and spiritual factors influencing child-rearing practices
   e. Relationships existing among family members
      (1) Discipline practices
      (2) Consistency of approach to children or adolescents
      (3) Presence of maladaptive coping measures
3. Developmental level of child or adolescent
   a. Age-appropriate behaviors and intellectual functioning
   b. Sense of body image and personal identity (including major changes due to trauma or illness)
4. Level of vulnerability
   a. Primary vulnerability (congenital deficits or those acquired during the first six months of life, such as sensory deficits, developmental disabilities, or difficult temperament)
   b. Secondary vulnerability (which results from the individual's reaction to environmental stressors previously noted).
5. Knowledge of normal growth and development
   a. Awareness of transition periods as stressors (for example, entry into school, going away to college)
   b. Awareness of situational crises (for example, illness in the family, loss of employment)

This assessment considers the child within the context of the family, with an emphasis on the three primary factors as noted by Bumbalo and Siemon (1983). Further data may be included for each individual situation. Bumbalo and Siemon also state that specific techniques such as children's drawings are good projective sources of information. Nurses may also use peer ratings and teacher ratings to assist in identifying children and adolescents at risk.

Primary prevention actually begins within the context of the family environment. Many theorists suggest that children learn behaviors through early parent-child interactions. Child-rearing practices are carried from one generation to the next. For example, there is literature to support the fact that parents who are abusive to their children were abused themselves. Methods of coping and problem solving are learned through family interaction, which suggests that unhealthy methods of coping are also transferred to children.

Parenting is perhaps the most important task an individual will confront in his or her lifetime—yet little has been done to help people to be more effective parents. Parent effectiveness programs such as P.E.T. are addressing this issue; however, parents who are struggling with such problems as low income, inadequate housing, and lack of support systems are not likely to be able to afford the time and money to take part in these programs. Active attention needs to be directed toward these at-risk populations to assist them in identifying the stressors they are experiencing in parenting and to actively explore problem-solving measures that are effective (for example, how to negotiate with large government agencies, such as departments of social services, in order to meet their needs).

Families need to learn appropriate means of

*Adapted from Murphy and Moriarity (1976).

communicating directly and honestly—to express feelings rather than to channel them in unhealthy directions such as abusive or psychosomatic behaviors. Through authentic expression of feelings, family members will develop sound feelings of self-worth—a key factor in healthy growth and development. Stress-reduction techniques can be taught to individuals so they can be active managers of their lives rather than passive victims. Parents need to recognize that they too have feelings and needs that require attention and expression. When these needs are thwarted, the frustration is often directed toward other members of the family. Parents and prospective parents can be assisted in recognizing their own needs and the importance of meeting those needs through effective problem solving.

Nurses as health care providers are active in this area of promoting physical and mental health. Health education, family life curricula in school systems, anticipatory guidance in the prenatal and perinatal periods, and support groups for parents are necessary elements in effective primary prevention. It seems that how children feel about themselves as they develop into adults is the foundation for their behavior as prospective parents. The development of a healthy self-concept as a child and an adolescent is an essential component of a sound foundation for parenting.

SECONDARY PREVENTION

It is increasingly apparent that the role of nurses in hospitals, clinics, schools, and community agencies is being directed toward case finding and early diagnosis. Through observation of children and adolescents in activities at school, church, or elsewhere in the community, as well as within the context of the family environment, nurses have the opportunity to detect early signs of stress, such as extended clinging behavior following the birth of a sibling or possible behavioral problems such as attention or conduct disorders. Secondary prevention is involved in addressing the following objectives:

1. Early identification of disorders of childhood and adolescence
2. Seeking prompt and effective treatment to re-

store individuals and their families to optimum levels of functioning
3. Assessment of community resources available (for example, for abuse victims and their families)
4. Expansion of community resources as is appropriate

Case finding is most critical in the area of child and adolescent mental health. Nurses as members of the primary health care team are in contact with children and their families throughout the life cycle. A community health nurse, while providing health services to a person newly diagnosed as a diabetic, might observe that one of the person's children is experiencing difficulty relating to strangers. If this behavior occurs over an extended period of time, it may be an early sign of overwhelming stress. Nursery school, elementary school, and secondary school settings are fertile ground for observation of behaviors that may be indicative of problems. Settings where children and adolescents gather to participate in activities are also prime target areas for early case finding. Although nurses may not always function directly with children and adolescents, they may act as consultants to those individuals, such as teachers, who are in positions of direct-line activity.

Early assessments may be tentative and are subject to validation with the family, including the child (when age appropriate), and other health team members. The nature of the relationship between the nurse who has identified the early signs and the child or adolescent is a critical factor. A comfortable, accepting atmosphere permits the individual child or adolescent to explore his or her potential difficulty within the context of an environment that is supportive and trusting. Parents may be resistant to others entering the family system and identifying difficulties that their children may be experiencing. Again, the circumstances under which the client system (the family) and the nurse come together will set the tone for the relationship in the future. Often nurses who first identify early warning behaviors do not feel prepared to resolve presenting behavioral disorders. Nurses may then refer the family to mental health resources such as child guidance clinics, school psychologists, or independent nurse psychotherapists, depending on availability, financial status, and preference of the family. In any case, the goal of early identification is referral to mental health resources for appropriate intervention.

The focus of secondary prevention is best stated by the Report of the Joint Commission of Mental Health of Children (1969). The goals of secondary prevention are to improve the actual conditions or behavior and to prevent the possibility of its deterioration. Goals for the family include restoration of family system functioning by increasing effective parenting and prevention of deterioration in the future. The following principles of secondary prevention apply to family systems regardless of symptom picture:

1. The focus should be on the individual child or adolescent as he or she exists within the context of the family system.
2. Family system behavior represents the most effective level of functioning at that given point in time.
3. Individual symptoms and behaviors are defense mechanisms designed to maintain ego integrity and reduce anxiety.
4. Support and empathy are necessary to establish a relationship that provides for effective problem resolution.
5. Behavior of one individual within the family system affects all other members, and there is a reciprocal response.
6. Nursing interventions should be directed toward alleviating symptomatic behavior and assisting parents in developing more effective strategies of parenting.
7. Nurses must recognize their own emotional responses to parents and children (for example, their own frustration with parental responses and child-rearing practices).

Knowledge of these basic principles will facilitate nursing intervention with children, adolescents, and parents who are experiencing emotional or behavioral disorders.

Nursing process

The nursing process acts as a framework for therapeutic intervention.

ASSESSMENT

Bumbalo and Siemons (1983) suggest that there are three primary means to collect data: (1) use of self, (2) use of data from the child and family, and (3) other assessment techniques. As these authors note, assessment data are basically invalid unless a therapeutic climate has been established. Meaning can be attached to data that signifies the "who, what, and how" of the problem. Without this significance of meaning, there is little rationale for doing the assessment.

The family and the child or adolescent are major sources of data. Questions will depend on the nature of the problem and the age of the child. The information gathered should provide a profile of the course of development—where difficulties lie, as well as strengths, duration of problem, effectiveness of coping strategies, problematic family behavior, and family relationships. The third area of assessment may be the use of specific tools as adjuncts to the sources of information previously noted.

The assessment should include the following*:

I. Child or adolescent interview
   A. Developmental screening (Denver Developmental); used for infants through preschoolers
   B. Major areas to be considered for all age groups
      1. Gross motor skills
      2. Fine motor skills
      3. Communication skills
      4. Social interaction (self-concept)
   C. Relationships with peers, authority figures, parents, and other family members
   D. Play behavior (solitary, fantasy)
   E. Emotional state (including affect and mood)
   F. Perception of world and his or her place in it
   G. Perception of presenting problem (if age appropriate)
   H. Coping measures and effectiveness
II. Parent system interview

---

*This assessment guide draws on concepts from Critchley (1979), Bumbalo and Siemons (1983), and Lourie and Reiger (1974).

A. Perception of presenting problem
B. Perception of developmental functioning (including knowledge of normal growth and development)
C. Duration and frequency of behavior.
D. Effectiveness of relief measures
E. Responses of other family members to current functioning
F. Previous developmental or behavioral difficulties of this child
G. Situational crises occurring with or prior to present difficulty
   1. Trauma
   2. Separation from significant others
III. Family assessment (see Chapter 14 for comprehensive assessment tool)

The family assessment considers the family unit in light of current stressors, availability of support systems, previous successful coping strategies, significant nodal events in the family life cycle, family constellation, differentiation of roles, maladaptive coping styles (for example, history of alcoholism, drug abuse, or physical abuse), knowledge and experience relative to successful parenting (including parental expectations), and cultural and religious factors influencing child-rearing practices.

Bumbalo and Siemons (1983) note the importance of validating information collected through the assessment process. They suggest that practitioners may use one or more of the following measures to validate the data:

1. Observations of the child or adolescent in more than one setting
2. Input from a second observer (determine interrater reliability)
3. Videotaping in school, play, or other appropriate settings
4. Review of previous health records
5. Consultation with other health team members
6. Sharing observations with parents and child when appropriate
7. Use of specific tools, such as Achenbach Child Behavior Profile and Coopersmith Self-Esteem Inventories, that have established reliability and validity

Through the process of validation of information, nurses can determine whether enough data have been collected to make inferences or whether further assessment is necessary.

ANALYSIS OF DATA

As nurses assess the child or adolescent within the context of the family, they may begin to understand not only the presenting problem(s) but also the complex interrelationship between family dynamics, vulnerability, precipitating factors, and problem-solving measures. The analysis of data leads to the formulation of nursing diagnoses. The next two sections will present nursing diagnoses that are frequently made—first those related to the parenting system and then those specifically related to the child or adolescent.

▶ Family nursing diagnoses

Children and adolescents exist within the context of their family environments—whether the environment be a single-parent family, a reconstituted family, a nuclear family, or an extended family. Behaviors of children and adolescents reflect the mood and dynamics of the family in the sense that what occurs within the family setting may be exhibited in symptoms displayed by the child or adolescent. For example, a member of a dysfunctional marital dyad may displace frustrations with his or her spouse onto a particular child, who in turn displays disruptive behavior in school. It is critical that nurses understand the interrelationships of parent and child within the context of the system as a whole. Families who have autistic children or children with childhood-onset developmental disorders may experience a mixture of ambivalence, guilt, anger, and frustration. These feelings may be projected onto others in the environment, such as other children, friends outside the family, or the health care professional. Conflict may exist within the family as to which is the best method of working with the child. One or both parents may attempt to deny that a problem exists, stating that the child will "outgrow" the disruptive behavior. In an attempt to protect the child from outside stressors, the parents may refuse assistance from other family members and friends, thereby eliminating any possible relief from the daily care of the child. This may result in a further escalation of anger, guilt, and frustration in the parental system. The effect of these feelings may be felt in the husband's or wife's job performance, other siblings' school participation, the family's social activities, and other areas of the family system.

Parents may lack appropriate parenting skills or knowledge of developmental phases, which may then cause the imposition of unrealistic expectations on the child or adolescent. For example, it is important that parents of an adolescent recognize the ambivalence of that phase—of the desire to be independent yet still be taken care of. Undue pressure, whether verbal or nonverbal, from the parental system can increase feelings of helplessness, hopelessness, and lack of a secure identity. Lack of knowledge of age-appropriate behaviors may result in parental frustration and anger, which can then be projected onto the child and increase the probability of inappropriate behaviors. This process, in turn, becomes a vicious cycle in which both parent and child experience frustration and a loss of control. Further family system disruption may occur when parents do not share similar perceptions and expectations regarding child care. Inconsistent messages are transmitted to the child that may immobilize the child or may potentiate present disruptive behaviors. Children may learn to manipulate the dysfunctional parental system, which may further increase disruptive behavior.

Thus, family diagnoses may reflect various dysfunctional dynamics within the family system. Examples of family diagnoses include
- knowledge deficit related to age-appropriate behaviors and tasks (NANDA 8.1.1, DSM-III-R V61.20 or V61.80)
- altered family processes secondary to inconsistent parenting/inability to manage disruptive behaviors (NANDA 3.2.2; DSM-III-R V61.20; V61.80)
- altered parenting role secondary to feelings of guilt regarding perceived inability to care for developmentally delayed child (NANDA 3.2.1.1.1; DSM-III-R V61.20).

PLANNING AND IMPLEMENTATION

Long-term outcomes include increasing healthy communication among family members; increasing individual sense of positive self-esteem within the family system; decreasing power struggles among

family members. *Short-term outcomes* are defined for each diagnosis as is appropriate.

The following general nursing strategies can be utilized within the context of the family system:
1. Facilitate open lines of communication and effective problem-solving techniques
   a. Identify unrealistic parental expectations
   b. Help parents to explore personal feelings regarding parenthood and their childhood experiences with their own parents
   c. Explore effective means of resolving inconsistent parenting approaches
   d. Support ego strengths of parental dyad
   e. Reinforce effective parenting behaviors as appropriate (for example, for promoting progressively more independent behavior on the part of an adolescent)
   f. Encourage parental verbalization of feelings of guilt, anger, and frustration (for example, the frustration involved in caring for a mentally retarded child on a day-to-day basis or the guilt of a working mother who is leaving her child in a day care center for the first time)
      (1) Validate those feelings as expected and situation-appropriate
      (2) Explore more effective methods of resolving these feelings
2. Act as a resource person
   a. Provide information on parent effectiveness programs, normal growth and development, and age-appropriate behaviors
   b. Facilitate access to further mental health treatment (for example, psychotherapy, family therapy)
   c. Mobilize support systems (other extended family members; clergy; close friends; church groups) and stress importance of support for one another in parental dyad
   d. Suggest "relief" options for parents of severely disturbed children (for example, periodic babysitting; special schools; day camps)
   e. Explore residential treatment as is appropriate and support parental decision regarding residential placement

Again, one must recognize that children exist within the context of the family—each member influences the others. Parents' behaviors are molded by their current situation and experiences as well as their experiences with their own parents—each factor contributing to the perception and actualization of parenting behaviors. We have noted specific disruptive or dysfunctional behaviors of children and adolescents that merit specific interventions. However, we must conclude that those specific interventions must exist within the context of the family as a whole system. (For further discussion of family therapy, see Chapter 14.)

The next section presents selected nursing diagnosis as well as long-term and short-term outcomes that are specifically related to children and adolescents.

NURSING CARE PLAN

Children and Adolescents

Long-term Outcomes	Short-term Outcomes	Nursing Strategies
Nursing diagnosis: (NANDA 5.1.1.1.1)	Impaired adolescent adjustment related to impending separation due to college enrollment	
Integrate life experiences as an independent person into a holistic sense of self.	Identify separations as potentially anxiety-producing situations Verbalize feelings of ambivalence regarding independent status Develop effective modes of coping that will facilitate current and future individuation Realistically perceive self as multidimensional (biological, intellectual, phychological, sociocultural, spiritual)	Support current ego strengths—what the client has accomplished in his or her life Positively reinforce decisions client has made regarding separation (going away to college, finding own apartment) Assist client in viewing self within the context of family as an independent person Explore potential changes in family relationships as a result of separation Explore family's role in individuation process of the client Support effective methods of coping with separation (verbalization of feelings honestly, recognition of process of separation as a form of grieving) Share with client the maturational tasks of this period
Nursing diagnosis: 5.1.1.1; DSM-III-R V 71.02)	Ineffective individual coping related to inability to control acting-out behaviors (NANDA	
Decrease use of socially unacceptable behavior Increase adaptive behavior within the family as a whole	Recognize situations that arouse anxiety, anger, frustration Relate current stressful situations to past situations that generated similar feelings Develop more effective interpersonal coping skills Recognize influence of maturational task on current behavior Identify behavioral responses as occurring within the context of the family	Assist adolescent in identifying situations that generate anger and anxiety Explore other means of expressing angry feelings (for example, jogging, racquetball) Intervene in situations before anxiety levels become overwhelming Reinforce verbalization as a healthy, adaptive mode Support ego strengths of adolescent as a competent human being Assist adolescent in managing life situations in a manner that is positively directed toward achieving developmental goals

Continued.

NURSING CARE PLAN—cont'd

Children and Adolescents

Long-term Outcomes	Short-term Outcomes	Nursing Strategies

Nursing diagnosis: Potential for self-directed violence related to lack of ego differentiation (NANDA 9.2.2; DSM-III-R 299.0)

Long-term Outcomes	Short-term Outcomes	Nursing Strategies
Reduce self-mutilating behaviors Develop more effective methods of controlling anxiety	Recognize situations that precipitate head-banging, picking behaviors Verbalize anxiety, anger, other feelings Use other effective methods of expressing needs (for example, punching bag)	Point out situations that stimulate self-mutilating behavior Protect child while head-banging occurs, through use of helmet or other devices as necessary Encourage the use of other body gestures that enable the child to explore the environment Recognize increased levels of anxiety and prevent use of self-destructive behaviors

Nursing diagnosis: Impaired social interaction related to poor sense of self-esteem (NANDA 3.1.1; DSM-III-R 299.0)

Long-term Outcomes	Short-term Outcomes	Nursing Strategies
Increase ability to establish a trusting relationship	Respond to touch and eye contact in an appropriate manner Communicate in simple sentences to express needs	Work on a one-to-one basis with child Provide an accepting, warm environment Encourage interaction with child through use of favorite toy or other object Initially use eye contact as means of interaction, with reinforcement for appropriate responses to nurse Use other modes of relating, such as touching, smiling, hugging Reinforce child's attempts to relate to others as he or she feels comfortable Accept child's need for physical distance at times

Nursing diagnosis: Disturbed perception of personal identity related to inability to differentiate self from environment (NANDA 7.1.3; DSM-III-R 299.0)

Long-term Outcomes	Short-term Outcomes	Nursing Strategies
Develop ability to recognize physiological and emotional needs as separate from those of other people Increase level of trust	Learn ways to increase sense of self as separate from others Experience reduced anxiety levels generated by contact with others	Work on a one-to-one basis with child Use touching and physical contact cautiously Assist child in identifying own parts of body correctly Point out differences between self and nurse through touch and other appropriate measures Use photographs of child, drawings, and mirrors to reinforce own boundaries Use self-directed activities such as dressing and feeding to reinforce self as separate from others

Long-term Outcomes	Short-term Outcomes	Nursing Strategies
Nursing diagnosis: DSM-III-R 309.00)	Potential for violence (suicidal behavior) related to feelings of poor self-esteem (NANDA 9.2.2;	
Increase feelings of self-worth as a competent and functioning individual Decrease use of self-destructive behaviors	Identify feelings of anger, loneliness, rage Identify situations that precipitate use of self-destructive behaviors Use non-self-destructive methods of coping with feelings	Provide an atmosphere where the client can begin to develop a trusting relationship Observe for signs of self-destructive behaviors Complete a suicidal risk assessment (see Chapter 22) Provide suicidal precautions (if on an inpatient unit, see Chapter 22) Reinforce appropriate coping measures Explore with client the effects of self-destructive behavior on his or her parents Facilitate open lines of communication between parents and client. • Assist parents in recognizing seriousness of self-destructive behaviors • Help client to note contagious effects of suicide and to be alert to such acts in the local community • Educate parents regarding developmental tasks of adolescence and age-appropriate behaviors • Assist parents in differentiating age-appropriate behaviors from age-inappropriate behaviors (withdrawal, change in peer relationships, poor school performance, change in regular activities) Administer medication judiciously
Nursing diagnosis: 313.21)	Increased anxiety level related to inability to manage separations (NANDA 9.3.1; DSM-III-R	
Resolve conflict that generates ambivalent feelings regarding separation (parents) Return to school setting (child) Experience decreased level of anxiety	Verbalize feelings of anxiety and ambivalence Identify situations in the past which generated similar feelings Develop more effective interpersonal coping skills	Do a physical assessment to rule out any physical problems Encourage the child's return to school on a day-to-day basis Explore the child's fears of leaving home Recognize parents' and child's anxiety as real Assist parents in recognizing the effect of their ambivalent feelings on the child Reinforce positive attempts by parents and child to manage the separation Mobilize other support systems in the environment that parents can use Incorporate school nurse, teacher, and other school officials in the treatment plan

Continued.

NURSING CARE PLAN—cont'd

Children and Adolescents

Long-term Outcomes	Short-term Outcomes	Nursing Strategies
Nursing diagnosis: Sensory alteration resulting in disruptive behavior secondary to inability to attend to appropriate stimuli (NANDA 7.2; DSM-III-R 314.0)		
Modify inappropriate responses to environmental stimuli	Finish one project to completion Organize school work in a manner that is meaningful Increase length of time that is spent sitting appropriately	Evaluate neurologically; use appropriate psychological testing to determine accurate diagnosis Administer medication judiciously and monitor target symptoms Structure the environment to minimize stimuli, in school as well as home • Provide a predictable environment and experiences that can be managed with little frustration • Encourage participation of the child in setting the structure Educate parents to set limits and to recognize that permissiveness can be destructive Encourage open lines of communication between parents and child Use behavior modification to control impulsive and inattentive behaviors and to reinforce appropriate behaviors Provide physical outlets for motor restlessness

EVALUATION

Evaluation of child and adolescent behavioral and emotional dysfunctions occurs within the context of the family system. It reflects client and family participation in the achievement of goals. In cases where individual client behaviors are targeted, evaluation should reveal a positive change in behavioral symptomatology—for example, reduction in autoerotic activity, increased attention span, and reduction in impulsive behaviors. Outcome evaluation of the family system should reflect improved communication among members, more effective parenting skills, increased level of knowledge regarding normal growth and development and age-appropriate behaviors, and, finally, more effective coping strategies.

During the evaluation process, the nurse identifies goals that may need to be modified and goals that are to be met in the future. Referral sources outside the nurse-client relationship, such as community agencies and significant others in the network of the client and family, are important factors in the ongoing success of the therapeutic process. Reinforcement of behavioral change and of learning to identify and cope with potentially troublesome issues will enable clients to assume increased control over their situations. The ability to recognize the need for outside assistance also needs to be reinforced as part of the evaluation process.

Finally, evaluation must reflect an assessment of the nurse's own self. Intervention with the family may generate feelings of anger, protectiveness, and disgust. The nurse's careful assessment of his or her own responses throughout the nurse-client relationship and during the evaluation phase is critical to the success of therapeutic intervention.

TERTIARY PREVENTION

Tertiary prevention should include provision of ongoing services for those children and adolescents who do not show improvement as a result of secondary interventions. The chronicity of the behavioral dysfunction may require referral to other specialized agencies for further treatment. Children who display severe ego impairment may need residential treatment or perhaps a day treatment center. Adolescents may also need to be placed in residential treatment if impulsive, acting-out behaviors continue to disrupt the family system. In some cases where truancy or juvenile delinquent behavior occurs, adolescents come in contact with the police and court systems. Residential treatment may then be offered as an alternative to a sentence of confinement.

The role of the nurse in tertiary prevention is varied. Nurses may provide ongoing group, individual, and family therapy for clients who present chronic behavioral and/or physical dysfunction. In addition, nurses may identify children, adolescents, and their families who exhibit chronically disturbed patterns of functioning, yet have not received any form of treatment. Finally, nurses may act as resource persons who can provide referrals for various treatment modalities and act as a link between client and resource facility.

The goals of tertiary prevention are to prevent or reduce the residual effects of long-term impairment. Interventive techniques are designed to restore the client and the family system to their optimum level of functioning.

CHAPTER SUMMARY

The field of child and adolescent mental health has historically received little attention in undergraduate curricula. However, nurses are in key positions to assess and intervene with new parents and children in school, camp, and clinic settings. Nurses are able to observe families as they interact in the community health setting. Identification of behavioral disturbances can be made earlier and intervention initiated to reduce the incidence of major pathological disturbances.

Child and adolescent behavioral dysfunctions may be viewed within the context of the family system. Underlying dynamics reflect a holistic interrelationship of factors: biological, psychodynamic, familial, and sociocultural. Nursing assessment is directed toward collecting data relative to the above-noted factors and making a nursing diagnosis. The diagnosis may specifically target a behavior, such as autoerotic activity or adolescent impulsive, acting-out behavior. Intervention is designed to reduce the target symptoms of the individual. However, particularly with children and adolescents, the parenting system needs to be addressed as well. The nurse may use behavior modification techniques with the child or adolescent client. At the same time the nurse may act as an educative-supportive person for the parents, providing information on normal growth and development and age-appropriate behaviors. Nurses may provide ongoing group, individual, and family therapy. They may also function as a vital link between client and other appropriate resources in the community.

Thus, nurses play a valuable role in the promotion of the mental health of children and adolescents, as well as assist in the maintenance of optimum levels of functioning in children, adolescents, and their families.

SELF-DIRECTED LEARNING

Sensitivity-Awareness Exercises

The purposes of the following exercises are to:

- Develop awareness of the vulnerability of families to the development of childhood or adolescent emotional or behavioral disorders
- Develop awareness about the interrelationship of factors in the etiology of childhood and adolescent disorders
- Develop awareness about the subjective experiences of clients who are suffering from these disorders and of the experiences of clients' families
- Develop awareness about your own feelings and attitudes when working with clients who are suffering

1. Try to imagine that you are a child or adolescent who is experiencing one of the following disorders, and explain why you selected that particular disorder. Then describe what you think it would be like to suffer from that disorder.
   a. Attention deficit with hyperactivity
   b. Anorexia nervosa
   c. Autistic disorder
   d. Withdrawal and depression
   e. Impulsive behaviors
2. Describe what you think it would be like to have a family member suffering from one of the disorders listed in exercise 1. Which disorder do you think would be easiest to tolerate in a family member? Why? Which disorder do you think would be hardest to tolerate? Why?
3. What might be some of your feelings and reactions as a nurse caring for clients and families who are suffering from emotional disorders of childhood and adolescence? Would your feelings and reac-

tions vary with the disorders experienced by clients? Explain why.

4. Imagine that you are a community health nurse engaged in health supervision activities with new parents. What high-risk factors (biological, psychological, intellectual, sociocultural, spiritual) would you look for that might predispose children to the development of emotional and behavioral disorders?
5. Develop a plan for counseling parents about child-rearing that incorporates principles and goals for the primary prevention of disorders of childhood and adolescence.

Questions to Consider

1. Strategies of a primary preventive nature include all of the following except
   a. Stress management techniques
   b. Parent effectiveness programs
   c. Case finding
   d. Provision of knowledge about normal growth and development
2. Principle elements of group therapy with children to ensure its effectiveness are
   a. Consistency and structure
   b. Role modeling and rewards
   c. Positive reinforcement and behavioral modification
   d. Homogeneity and definitive guidelines
3. Significant factors in the etiology of suicide in the American Indian adolescent include
   a. Native healers view suicide as honorable
   b. Early loss of caretakers
   c. Unstable tribal leadership
   d. Lack of homogeneous reservation populations

SELF-DIRECTED LEARNING—cont'd

Theresa, aged 8, has been diagnosed as having an attention deficit disorder. During class, she is unable to sit still, has a short attention span, and is unable to complete her school work on a regular basis. Questions 4 through 6 relate to this situation.

4. Which of the following short-term outcomes would be most appropriate?
   a. Sit through the day with two prescribed break periods
   b. Express emotions as she experiences them
   c. Complete one homework assignment fully each day
   d. Work on a project with two other children

5. Nursing strategies to assist the teacher in working with Theresa in the classroom would include
   a. Encouraging the teacher to use negative reinforcement to reduce disruptive behavior
   b. Assisting the teacher to define specific activities that can be completed in a short period of time
   c. Providing an assistant to work in the classroom
   d. Supporting the teacher's desire to permit Theresa to express her emotions freely

6. To assist Theresa in meeting the above short-term outcome, which nursing strategy would be most effective?
   a. Providing a safe but unstructured environment
   b. Designing special projects for Theresa that limit her interaction with others
   c. Defining reasonable boundaries within which Theresa can function

   d. Assigning a teacher's assistant to monitor her classwork

7. A nursing strategy that can be effectively utilized with children experiencing separation anxiety is
   a. Completing a comprehensive physical assessment to rule out physical problems
   b. Encouraging parents to permit the child to stay at home until he feels comfortable
   c. Inviting the teacher to come to the home to decrease the child's fear
   d. Reassure the child that there is nothing to be afraid of in school

8. The primary role of the nurse in working with children and adolescents is to
   a. Recognize that alterations in behavior exist within the context of the family
   b. Determine the frequency and degree of behavioral dysfunction
   c. Refer families to the appropriate resources
   d. Maintain family boundaries and decrease differentiation

Answer key

1. c
2. a
3. b
4. c
5. b
6. c
7. a
8. a

REFERENCES

American Nurses' Association: Standards of child and adolescent mental health nursing practice, New York, 1985, Pergamon Press.

American Psychiatric Association: Diagnostic and statistical manual III-R, Washington, DC, 1987.

Axline V: Play therapy, New York, 1969, Ballantine Books.

Baer C and Williams B: Clinical pharmacology and nursing, Springhouse, Pa, 1988, Springhouse Publishing Co.

Bell R: Stimulus control of parent or caregiver behavior by offspring, Developmental Psychol 7(1):41-44, 1971.

Bellinger D et al: Longitudinal analyses of prenatal and postnatal lead exposure and early cognitive development, N Engl J Med 316:1037-1043, 1987.

Bender L: Childhood schizophrenia: clinical study of one hundred schizophrenic children, Am J Orthopsychiatr 17(1):40-45, 1947.

Berlin I: Suicide among American Indian adolescents: an overview, Suicide Life-Threatening Behav 17(3):218-232, 1987.

Berman R: Ego differentiation, In Noshpitz J, editor: Basic handbook of child psychiatry, vol 2, 1979, Basic Books.

Blos P: On adolesence, New York, 1962, The Free Press.

Bollen K and Phillips D: Imitative suicides: a national study of the effects of television news stories, Am Sociol Rev 47:802-809, 1982.

Bowen M: Family therapy in clinical practice, New York, 1978, Jason Aronson, Inc.

Bridger W and Birns B: Experience and temperament in human neonates, In Newton R and Levine S, editors: Early experience and behavior, Springfield, Ill, 1968, Charles C Thomas, Publisher.

Bumbalo J and Siemon M: Nursing assessment and diagnosis: mental health problems of children, Topics Clin Nurs 5:41-45, 1983.

Cantwell D and Tarjan G: Constitutional-organic factors in etiology, In Noshpitz J, editor: Basic handbook of child psychiatry, vol 2, New York, 1979, Basic Books.

Chess S et al: The origins of personality, Sci Am 223:102-110, 1970.

Critchley D: Mental status examinations with children and adolescents: a developmental approach, In Nursing clinics of North America, Philadelphia, 1979, WB Saunders.

Cytryn D and McKnew R: Depressive disorders, In Noshpitz J, editor: Basic handbook of child psychiatry, vol 2, New York, 1979, Basic Books.

Dunn J and Kendrick C: Studying temperament and parent-child interactions: comparisons of interview and direct observation, Dev Med Child Neurol 22:494-496, 1980.

Eaton J and Weill R: Culture and mental disorders: a comparative study of the Hutterites and other populations, Glencoe, NY, 1955, The Free Press.

Elliott D et al: Explaining delinquency and drug use, Beverly Hills, Cal, 1985, Sage Publications.

Fagin C, editor: Nursing in child psychiatry, St. Louis, 1972, The CV Mosby Co.

Freeman B and Ritvo E: The syndrome of autism: a critical review of diagnostic systems, follow-up studies, and the theoretical background of the Behavioral Observation Scale, In Staffen J and Karoley P, editors: Autism and severe psychopathology: advances in child behavioral analysis and therapy, Lexington, Mass, 1982, Lexington Books.

Fish B and Ritvo O: Psychoses of childhood, In Noshpitz J, editor: Basic handbook of child psychiatry, vol 2, New York, 1979, Basic Books.

Goren S: Points of view, J Psychosoc Nurs Mental Health Serv 22(1):51-55, 1984.

Haley J: Leaving home: the therapy of disturbed young people, New York, 1980, McGraw-Hill.

Hart N and Keidel G: The suicidal adolescent, Am J Nurs 79(1):80-83, 1979.

Hendin H: Youth suicide: a psychosocial perspective, Suicide Life-Threatening Behav 17(21):151-164, 1987.

Herskowitz J: Developmental neurotoxicology, In Popper C, editor: Psychiatric pharmacosciences of children and adolescents, Washington DC, 1987, American Psychiatric Press.

Hutt C: Sex: what's the difference? New Scientist 62:405, 1974.

Jones M: The therapeutic community, New York, 1953, Basic Books.

Kanner L: To what extent is early infantile autism determined by constitutional inadequacies? Proc Assoc Res Nervous Mental Dis 33:378-385, 1955.

Kaplan H and Sadock B: Comprehensive textbook of psychiatry, ed 4, Baltimore, 1985, The Williams & Wilkins Co.

Kalb C: Conduct disorder, In Noshpitz J, editor: Basic handbook of child psychiatry, vol 2, New York, 1979, Basic Books.

Kessler J: Reactive disorders, In Noshpitz J, editor: Basic handbook of child psychiatry, vol 2, New York, 1979, Basic Books.

Laing R: Mystification, confusion and conflict, In Boszormenyi-Nagy I, and Framo J, editors: Intensive family therapy: theoretical and practical aspects, New York, 1964, Harper & Row.

Last C and Hersen M: Separation anxiety and school phobia—a comparison using DSM III criteria, Am J Psychiatr 144:653-657, 1987.

Lidz T: The family and human adaptation, New York, 1963, International Universities Press.

Long K: Are children too young for mental disorders? Am J Nurs 3(1):1254-1257, 1985.

Looff D: Sociocultural factors in etiology, In Noshpitz J, editor: Basic handbook of child psychiatry, vol 2, New York, 1979, Basic Books.

Lourie R and Reiger R: Psychiatric and psychological examination of children, In Arieti S, editor: American handbook of psychiatry, ed 2, New York, 1974, Basic Books.

McLane A, editor: Classification of nursing diagnosis, St. Louis, 1987, The CV Mosby Co.

Maris R: The adolescent suicide problem, Suicide and Life Threatening Behav 15(2):91-110, 1985.

Minuchin S: Families and family therapy, Cambridge, Mass, 1974, Harvard University Press.

Moss N: Child therapy groups in the real world, J Psychosoc Nurs Mental Health Serv 22:43-48, 1984.

Murphy L and Moriarity A: Vulnerability, coping, and growth, New Haven, 1976, Yale University Press.

National Society for Autistic Children: Definition of the syndrome of autism, J Autism Childhood Schizophren 8:162-169, 1978.

Nelson F: A research note on knowledge of youth suicide among high school students, J Commun Psychol, in press.

Ojantlatva A, Hammer A, and Mohr M: The ultimate rejection: helping the survivors of teen suicide victims, J School Health 57(5):181-182, 1987.

Phillips D and Carstensen L: Effect of suicide stories on various demographic groups, Suicide Life Threatening Behav 18(1):100-114, 1988.

Popper C: Disorders usually first evident in infancy, childhood, or adolescence, In Talbott J, Hales R, and Yudofsky S, editors: Textbook of psychiatry, Washington DC, 1988, The American Psychiatric Press.

Report of the Joint Commission on Mental Health of Children: Challenge for the 1970's, New York, 1969, Harper & Row.

Rhyne M et al: Children at risk for depression, Am J Nurs 12(1):1379-1382, 1986.

Rutter M et al: Depression in young people, New York, 1986, Guilford Press.

Rutter M: Sex differences in children's responses to family stress, In Anthony E and Koupernick C, editors: The child and his family, London, 1970, John Wiley.

Rutter M: Stress, coping, and development: some issues and some questions, In Garmezy N and Rutter M, editors: Stress, coping and development in children, New York, 1983, McGraw-Hill.

Sameroff A and Chandler M: Reproductive risk and the continuum of caretaking causality, In Horowitz F, editor: Review of child development research, vol 4, Chicago, 1975, The University of Chicago Press.

Sanger E and Cassino T: Avoiding the power struggle, Am J Nurs 84:30-35, 1984.

Schaffer D: Psychiatric aspects of brain injury in childhood: a review, Development Med Child Neurol 15:211-225, 1974.

Smith C and Crawford S: Suicidal behavior among normal high school students, Paper presented at the Fourth Annual Conference on Suicide of Adults and Youth, Topeka, Kan, 1984.

Smith C and Murphy K: Developing a children's inpatient psychiatric unit, J Psychosoc Nurs Mental Health Serv 22:31-36, 1984.

Spitz R: The psychogenic diseases in infancy, In Eissler R, editor: Psychoanalytic study of the child, vol 6, New York, 1951, International Universities Press.

Talan J: The hospitalization of America's troubled teenagers, Newsday, January 5, 1988.

Teicher J and Jacobs J: Adolescents who attempt suicide, Am J Psychiatr 122:1248-1256, 1966.

Toolan J: Therapy of depressed and suicidal children, Am J Psychother 32:244-248, 1978.

Trad P: Infant depression: paradigms and paradoxes, New York, 1986, Springer-Verlag.

Valente S and Saunders J: High school suicide prevention programs, Pediatr Nurs 13(2):108-112, 1987.

Vandenberg S, Singer S, and Pauls D: The heredity of behavior disorders in adults and children, New York, 1986, Plenum Publishing Co.

Vessey J: Care of the hospitalized child with a cognitive developmental delay, Holistic Nurs Prac 2(2):48-54, 1988.

Wallerstein J: Children of divorce: preliminary report of a ten-year follow-up of young children, Am J Orthopsychiatr 54:444-458, 1984.

Watzlawick P et al: Pragmatics of human communication, New York, 1967, WW Norton.

Wertlieb D et al: Temperament as a moderator of children's stressful experiences, Am J Orthopsychiatr 57(2):234-245, 1987.

Zoltak B: Autism: recognition and management, Ped Nurs 12(2):90-95, 1986.

ANNOTATED SUGGESTED READINGS

Hendin H: Youth suicide: a psychosocial perspective, Suicide and Life-Threatening Behav 17(2):151-164, 1987.
This article presents a comprehensive discussion of the author's study of different cultures and subcultures as well as different age groups for the purpose of understanding the nature of adolescent suicide. His perspective utilizes disciplines ranging from demography to psychodynamics to explore the relationship of multiple factors such as violence and the role of families to suicidal behavior. The author also identifies goals for future research in this area.

Valente S and Saunders J: High school suicide prevention programs, Pediatr Nurs 13(2):108-112, 137, 1987.
The authors describe the development of high school suicide prevention programs as a means of addressing the rising rate of adolescent suicide. Goals of this type of program as well as criticisms were discussed in an unbiased and clear-cut manner. A significant contribution of this article is the authors' delineation of the role of the nurse in various settings for the development, implementation, and evaluation of these programs and the highlighting of the significance of such a role.

Vessey J: Care of the hospitalized child with a cognitive developmental delay, Holistic Nurs Prac 2(2):48-54, 1988.
The author notes that research has impacted positively on the care of hospitalized children in general; however, there has been little written relative to the care of hospitalized developmentally delayed children. Vessey discusses specific diagnoses concerned with cognitive capabilities and the role of the nurse. She identifies intervention strategies including behavior management and the use of medication that can be useful in the care of this special group of children.

Wertlieb D et al: Temperament as a moderator of children's stressful experiences, Am J Orthopsychiatr 57(2):234-245, 1987.
The authors present the findings of their research on temperament and stressful experiences. They note that undesirable life events and intense "hassles" were correlated with behavioral symptoms. Temperament was found to moderate this influence, but there was little appreciable variance of symptoms. Consideration was given to the fact that there is much

controversy over the definition of stress and temperament predictor variables. The authors describe the data as pioneering efforts to examine the relationship among stress, temperament, and behavioral symptoms in middle childhood. They note the need for further research to determine the role of key contextual moderators such as social support in the development of effective coping strategies.

FURTHER READINGS

Blom S, Lininger R, and Charlesworth W: Ecological observation of emotionally and behaviorally disordered students: an alternative method, Am J Orthopsychiatr 57(1):49-59, 1987.

Dalton R et al: Short-term psychiatric hospitalization of children, Hosp Commun Psychiatr 38(9):973-976, 1987.

Gentilin J: Room restriction: a therapeutic prescription, J Psychosoc Nurs Mental Health Serv 25(7):12-16, 1987.

Greydamus D et al: The behavioral medicine unit: a community hospital model for in-patient treatment of adolescent depression, Sem Adolescent Med 2(4):311-319, 1986.

Katz-Leavy J et al: Meeting the mental health needs of severely emotionally disturbed minority children and adolescents: a national perspective, Child Today 16(5):10-14, 1987.

Pothier P: Psychiatric skills: preventive measures...children in need of mental health services, Nurs Times 83(4):42-43, 1987.

Rauch S et al: School-based, short-term group treatment for behaviorally disturbed young adolescent males: a pilot intervention, J School Health 57(1):19-22, 1987.

Valente S: Assessing suicide risk in the school-aged child, J Pediatr Health Care 1(1):14-20, 1987.

Wiack M: Family therapy and the out-of-control teenager, Michigan Nurse 60(5):8-9, 1987.

Yarcheski A et al: Perceived stress and symptom patterns in early adolescents: the role of mediating variables, Res Nurs Health 9(4):289-297, 1986.

Zaozirny J: Separation in the adolescent therapeutic community...losses produce a crisis for many patients, J Psychosoc Nurs and Mental Health Serv 26(1):20-23, 1988.

Patterns of conflict and stress in the elderly

CHAPTER FOCUS

The profession of nursing has a long tradition of caring for elderly clients in institutions such as nursing homes and through visiting nurse services in the community. As the population of elderly American people continues to increase and as the demand for optimum, client-collaborative health care services also increases, the need for informed and empathetic psychosocial nursing intervention becomes more and more urgent.

The experience of "aging in America" is a complex one, reflecting our changing society, the heterogeneity of the aging population, and the complexity of the aging experience itself. Aspects covered in this chapter include health care and its economic aspects, financial stressors, women and aging, ethnicity and aging, retirement and adaptation to role changes in the area of work, "ageism" and legislation related to it, and self-help groups for the elderly.

Loss and *change* are major themes as we grow older, but so is *heterogeneity;* an appreciation of the differences among aging people is essential to prevent stereotyping that can lead to misdirected and ineffective interventions.

The treatment modalities that are effective for younger people are also helpful to the elderly. Individual therapy, group and activities therapy, family and marital therapy, and somatic therapies may all at times need to be modified to meet the special needs of older clients, but priniciples remain the same. Some particular types of therapy that have been found useful for elderly clients include *logotherapeutic use of the past, reminiscing* and *the life review,* and *pet therapy.* The importance of response to medication regimens is also discussed.

Because of the evident heterogeneity of the elderly population and the variety of aging experiences that people have, *primary prevention* in the elderly is approached with a dual focus on (1) pathological vs. "normal" and (2) usual vs. successful.

Secondary prevention in the aged is reviewed using the nursing process as a framework. Nursing diagnoses related to some important areas of concern for the elderly—depression, anxiety, and substance abuse are covered in Chapters 8, 20, and 22. Nursing process related to diagnoses of potential for injury, sleep pattern disturbances, altered family processes related to nursing home placement, memory loss, and spiritual distress are highlighted here. Spiritual distress is of particular relevance to this age group, and, in this chapter, it is related to Erickson's epigenetic crisis of integrity vs. despair.

The section on *tertiary prevention* acknowledges an important and growing area in the care of the elderly client and his or her family. *Day care, home care*, and *respite care* are presented as possible alternatives to institutional long-term care.

HISTORICAL PERSPECTIVES: THEORIES AND MYTHS RELATED TO AGING
History

The Mental Health Act of 1946 (Chapter 2), the Mental Health Studies Act of 1955, and the Community Mental Health Centers Act of 1963 (Chapter 16) are all important examples of legislation aimed at improving the delivery of mental health services to the American people. Until quite recently, however, society has tended to exclude the elderly as a group with special needs for psychological care. In 1975, the federal government created the National Institute on Aging to conduct and support biological, behavioral, and sociological research relating to the aging process and the health problems of the aged (Encyclopedia of Social Work, 1977). The establishment of this institute and the extension of the Community Mental Health Centers Act of 1975 helped to improve the situation, as

did the earlier enactment in 1965 of Medicare and Medicaid to help provide for the health care needs of the elderly and indigent (Blazer and Maddox, 1984; Crooks, 1984). The extension of the Community Mental Health Centers Act specified that the elderly constitute a subgroup of the population with special needs. In doing so, it designated specialized inpatient, outpatient, liaison, and referral services for meeting these needs (LeBray, 1984). In 1980, the Mental Health Systems Act was passed to fund broader, better coordinated mental health services for the needy elderly. The act linked mental health services to community nursing homes (Crooks, 1984). Despite all this legislation, there are still many inadequacies in the delivery of mental health care to the elderly (Blazer and Maddox, 1984; Crooks, 1984; LeBray, 1984). Citing recent studies of existing mental health centers, Blazer, Maddox, Crooks, and LeBray all point out that few of them have developed integrated programs specific to the needs of the elderly. But the passage of legislation did reflect a growing awareness of the increasing number of aged people in this country and the need for improved mental health services to help them deal with the stresses of aging. These are related to life's inevitable changes and losses. The ways in which our society deals with the elderly also engender stress. For example, in a youth-oriented culture such as ours, the prevalent stereotyping of the elderly, leading to "ageism," inevitably induces stress. Other stressors are the inadequate support networks and the complex health care system that can foster acute feelings of helplessness—particularly in the frail elderly.

While negative stereotyping, ageism, neglect, and even mistreatment have long been elements in humanity's approach to aging and the aged, there are cultural variations. The elderly were revered in some early cultures (Achenbaum, 1985), and they are respected and well cared for in some present-day societies (Chae, 1987). Societies throughout the world whose values and norms tended to foster altruism and close emotional attachments have typically cared well for children and the very old, while societies that were less developed in these areas tended toward harshness in the treatment of their more vulnerable members (Gutmann, 1977).

The ancient Hebrew culture apparently represented a model of respect for elders. For example, the fifth commandment provided an important guideline:

Honor your father and your mother as the Lord your God commanded you; that your days may be prolonged and that it may go well with you in the land which the Lord your God gave you. (Deuteronomy 5:16)

The early Christians also carried on this tradition of respect and honor for the elders of the community. Early Madhyamika Buddhists and the Chinese Taoists both viewed old age as a very important part of life, a time for the ripening of wisdom and the spirit. It was an opportunity for detachment from worldly preoccupations and for concentration on inner truths. The liabilities of aging were considered just as valuable as the advantages because both enhanced the opportunities for acceptance of self and reality. Indeed, learning to cope with one's troubles fostered a better understanding of the ultimate meaning of existence (Achenbaum, 1985).

In classical antiquity, both negative and positive images of aging were reflected in philosophy, drama, and mythology. These images were often heroic and tragic. Tales of intergenerational hatred and distrust were frequent, and older men and women were sometimes feared or respected because it was believed that they possessed supernatural powers. In Sparta, the "gerusea," a political body empowered to make important decisions, was composed of the richest and oldest men of the society. Like the Buddhists and the Taoists, Cicero's *De Senectute* downplayed the diminished physical strength of old age in comparison to the increased wisdom and spiritual development that natural aging provided. This view is in stark contrast to the primitive practice of drowning disabled senior citizens in the Tiber River. Other famous Roman writers made cruel fun of the aged and the aging process; Seneca concluded that old age is simply a "disease" (Achenbaum, 1985). This view of old age as a disease has continued in present times to color our beliefs in a negative manner (Callahan, 1987; Rowe and Kahn, 1987).

In the Middle Ages, there were a variety of approaches to aging. Stories about Charlemagne and various versions of *Le Mort d' Artur* pay homage to the wisdom and courage of old age. But Chaucer and Boccaccio depicted foolish, lustful older women and older cuckolds. Grimm's fairy tales focused on the ugliness and disgusting behavior of the old people in the stories. Shakespeare, as always, was more complex and presented conflicts and contrasts, as, for example, in *King Lear*, when the assets and liabilities of old age were distilled into powerful symbols of the "isolated and alienating creativity of late life" (Achenbaum, 1985).

A tragic example of extreme negativity that was particularly applied to older women during the Middle Ages was the burning of "witches." While some of this was done to rid society of mentally ill people (see Chapter 25), it was also a way of obtaining the wealth and property of elderly widows. These women were past their childbearing years and were no longer considered useful in a sexist and ageist society (Walker, 1985). Modern aging women are not treated so cruelly, but as a group they do suffer hardships specific to their gender in this society (see discussion below).

In early American times, the society appears to have been quite "age integrated," and age brought neither extra privileges nor special discrimination. Physical or financial problems were considered the responsibility of individuals, not of society. This probably led to a "catch-22" situation for many of those growing in frailty and vulnerability. During the Great Depression of the 1930s, it became quite evident that many elderly Americans were in desperate financial circumstances. This fact helped to define the position of the elderly as a "problem," and some sort of assistance was seen as necessary. The Social Security Act was passed in 1935.

In modern times, our youth-oriented culture determines how the elderly are viewed and, ultimately, how they are treated. A possible explanation for this persistent youth cult is our need to deny death—the elderly are associated with the inevitability of death and are thus "excluded from a world awed by the vitality of youth" (Achenbaum, 1985). There are some signs of change or even a countermovement in this distortion of intergenerational relationships (Achenbaum, 1985; Collins, 1987, Tavris, 1987). Magazine advertisements have changed a little—one does see older models even if they are somewhat sexist in combining an obviously older man and a much younger women. Television shows have "come of age" and feature older men and women in roles of power and attractiveness (Taylor, 1987). Frazer (1975) has pointed out that society's view of aging is an essential part of one's view of oneself. The second assumption on which nursing theorist Martha Rogers builds her nursing science is relevant to our understanding of society's attitudes and the aging process: "The constant interchange of matter and energy between man and environment is at the basis of man's becoming" (Rogers, 1970).

The pattern of an elderly individual's social situation is in constant change as the patterning of the whole society and of the individual person continues to change. The elderly person's achievement of "successful aging" (Rowe and Kahn, 1987) depends on his or her own patterns of coping and on the attitudes of significant others in the environment. It is important for us, as nurses, to remember this. The way we view the aged and the aging process (and our own aging) will affect the care we give and the ways we relate to our elderly clients. This ultimately will have some effect, positive or negative, on the self-view of the client.

Frazer's point about the effect of society's judgment on self-concept is well taken. In light of it and the trite but true saying "you're only as old as you feel," any change in society's attitudes toward aging is a welcome one. The fact remains, however, that the changes are not coming soon enough for most of the elderly today and, for many of them, life is stressful.

Definitions

There are several ways of defining the aging process. For instance, Neugarten (1974) divides the older population into three groups.

1. *The young old*—those who are age 55 to 65. Generally they are still employed and perhaps at their peak as far as income and social prestige are concerned.
2. *The middle old*—people between the ages of 65 and 75. This group includes a large proportion of the retired in our country. There is a drop in income, and they have given up a life-time occupation. But many in this group are still in good health and enjoying the increased time at their disposal.
3. *The old old*—individuals who are over the age of 75. This group contains the most isolated, ill, and impoverished members of our senior citizenry, and it is a group that is designated "the problem population" by Neugarten.

Biological aging refers to changes that occur in the body over time, ending with the death of the individual (Myers, 1984). This term can be further broken down into *primary aging*, or the inevitable decline of all organisms that is independent of disease, trauma, or stress and *secondary aging*, which describes changes that *are* related to these variables. Myers points out that to adequately assess an aging client's status, it is important to understand that individuals (and individual organs and systems within an individual) differ in their rates of natural biological change. Second, trauma or disease can affect various organs or systems, and this varies among individuals.

Citing several groups of gerontological researchers, Birren and Abrahams (1984) conclude that there are three metaphors that define aging. These are *senescing, eldering,* and *geronting*.

senescing   The term used to describe biological processes that render a person vulnerable to physical deterioration over a period of time. It culminates in the death of the person.
eldering   The term is related to senescing, but it is independent of it and refers to a process of moving into age-appropriate roles. Social and family roles change for people throughout the life cycle, and while America has not defined age-related roles as distinctly as some other societies, this process does occur—people retire and become empty-nesters and grandparents.
geronting   This term defines the process of coping with the interaction of senescing and eldering. It is the individual organism repatterning in response to inner forces of biological imperatives and to outer, societal forces and, simultaneously, to how these forces interact with each other.

A definition of aging, holistic in nature, is one that was first proposed by Birren and Renner (1977) in the first edition of the encyclopedic *Handbook of Aging.* Noting the need for continued study of human functioning that includes incremental as well as decremental changes, they conclude that aging is the "regular changes that occur in mature genetically representative organisms living under representative environmental conditions as they advance in chronological age" (p. 4).

Theories related to aging

Sigmund Freud's theory of human development focused on childhood stages of development (Chapter 6). Erik Erikson's theory (1950) goes further—it includes adolescence, adulthood, and aging (see Chapter 6 for a detailed discussion of Erikson's life stages). The developmental stage that encompasses late life is the eighth and is called "the development of a sense of ego integrity versus despair." It is the culminating stage of life and success, and mastering it depends on how a person mastered the preceding seven stages. It requires an acceptance of one's one and only life and the acceptance of death. Despair comes from feeling that life is now too short to "start over" and to make other choices, to try different routes to achieve integrity. Erikson ties his theory of lifestage development to a continual interaction between an individual and society, and the task is to continue growing and adapting in the midst of all of the changes and losses of the aging process (Myers, 1984).

Carl Jung emphasized that the latter half of life prepared one for the inevitability of death (Frazer, 1975). Jung's thoughts on aging also included a belief that the second half of one's life balanced the first half to produce a sense of wholeness for the person. Growth toward *individuation* of the many aspects of the psyche and *integration* of these aspects into the *self* are the two main tasks for the maturing human being. For example, knowledge and understanding of how the collective unconscious and its archetypes (such as the persona, the anima or animus, the shadow, and the self) are manifested in one's particular psyche would be part of the quest for maturity.* Integration of all the

*For an understanding of Jung's psychology and the meanings and significance of the archetypes see: *A primer of Jungian psychology* by C.S. Hall and V.J. Nordley, New York, 1973, New American Library, or *An introduction to Jung's psychology* by F. Fordham, Baltimore, Md, 1966, Penguin Books.

components of the total psyche into a unified *self* is also part of it. Jung sees a dramatic change in development occurring in middle age. There is a transition from adaptation to the outer world to adaptation to one's inner world. Thus, individuation and integration can be the focus of concentration. The second half of life is when new meaning and purpose in life are to be sought, and Jung believed it was best accomplished by attending to whatever had been neglected in the first half (Fordham, 1966). If a person had been mostly concerned with mastery of the environment while neglecting the interpersonal aspects of life, a change in focus to bring about a more balanced synthesis of the two aspects would be best. Because our society has fostered sex roles with differing directions, the emphases for men and women seem to change at midlife. Research has supported that this shift occurs—middle-aged men tend to move away from preoccupation with mastery toward interpersonal commitments and women shift in the opposite direction toward self-assertion (Lowenthal, 1977). This supports Jung's thesis that the task of late life is the balancing of one's earlier life.

There are several specific theories of aging that can help us to understand the process—three will be discussed here; *the disengagement theory, the activity theory,* and *the continuity theory.*

Disengagement theory contends that there is a natural and mutual agreement between an aging person and society that interactions with others will gradually decrease and that the earlier social roles of the person will become less important. It is a mutual withdrawal (Cumming and Henry, 1961; Frazer, 1975; LeBray, 1984). The theory is based on observation and research demonstrating that as people age

1. There is a change from active mastery to a more passive mode
2. Introversion increases
3. Intellectual efficiency declines
4. Activities and interest decline (Birren, 1964; Burrus-Bammel and Bammel, 1985.)

Disengagement is thought to begin in middle life when one begins to become more aware of the inevitability of death (Cumming, 1963). Proponents of the theory believe that barring the intervention of negative social pressures, the disengagement process is desirable. The aged person can more easily maintain high morale because more modest wishes and aspirations become more consistent with a declining biological capacity (Encyclopedia of Social Work, 1977) and energy can be expended on the inner self rather than the outer world (Frazer, 1975), which is consistent with both Jung's and Erikson's theories.

The theory of disengagement has been quite controversial (Burrus-Bammel and Bammel, 1985; Encyclopedia of Social Work, 1977; Lancaster, 1980), and there certainly are dangers inherent in a blind acceptance of all its premises. For example, it could produce a harmful effect when used to justify social policy on programs for the elderly (Burrus-Bammel and Bammel, 1985; Lancaster, 1980) or, on a smaller scale, when it affects the attitudes of staff members caring for the institutionalized elderly. It may be a theory that is more appropriate to societies (like ours) where age is not a venerable state. In societies where the elderly are highly respected, involvement may increase rather than decline (Frazer, 1975). In any case, there is evidence that while voluntary disengagement is not a threat to morale, involuntary disengagement (because of ill health, disability, poverty, bereavement, or retirement) is (Chown, 1977).

Proponents of *activity theory* (Havighurst and Albrecht, 1953) don't think that disengagement is beneficial, although they agree that it occurs in some people. Supporters of activity theory believe the greatest satisfaction comes from continuing activities and social roles into late life. Participation in social or group activities, in physical activities, and in cognitive recreation activities (reading, crossword puzzles, Scrabble) were all strong predictors of life satisfaction for elders in the several studies that looked at these variables. There was difficulty in operationalizing such terms as *happiness, morale,* and *self-esteem,* and this presented som. methodological problems, but like disengagement theory, activity theory covers another aspect of the complexity of aging. In 1977, the Encyclopedia of Social Work stated that most studies of aging support a view that includes and extends beyond both disengagement and activity theory. More recent workers agree that the factor of *heterogeneity* in the elderly is a crucial one (Burrus-Bammel and Bam-

mel, 1985; LeBray, 1984; Rowe and Kahn, 1987).

Continuity theory takes into account the influence of early patterns on latter life adjustment (LeBray, 1984), and research supports this (Burrus-Bammel and Bammel, 1985). In their past history, people have had highly individual personality patterns, family situations, and patterns of coping. Aging in our society is a developmental crisis, and past reaction patterns will continue to be stimulated and used. The following is a case study of how aging can be a crisis situation for the client and family systems and how past coping patterns can be reactivated.

Grace is a 78-year-old woman who was widowed at 36 and who worked hard to support her four small children. The children are all self-sufficient adults now, and she has been quite involved in the family life of her only daughter who lives nearby. An active woman before her latest illness, she drove her car around town, went on senior citizen trips with her friends, and even travelled to various vacation spots in her car.

Grace took care of her aged mother, who died at the age of 98 "without ever having to go in a nursing home" as Grace was proud to proclaim. Grace did have several bouts with severe depression throughout her life, and they seemed to be situationally related to times of bereavement and loss (when her cousin, a woman she felt very close to, died in an automobile accident 20 years ago; when her mother died 15 years ago; and, more recently, when a good friend had to be admitted to a nursing home). Grace had been caring for this friend in her own home and felt defeated by the necessity for placement in a nursing home. This last depression was triggered by the loss of her friend and by the fact that the care Grace provided and from which she derived a good deal of meaning for her life was no longer needed. It was also complicated by her own declining health (diabetes, high blood pressure, and some beginning signs of congestive heart failure) and by her secret fears that she too might have to be "put in a home."

Grace depended a great deal on her daughter, and her joys in life revolved around her daughter's family— the grown children and their children. Her sons lived in distant cities and were not so involved with their mother. Janet, her 55-year-old daughter, felt stressed and "squeezed" in the middle. She was working full time, going to school to complete her master's degree, and actively involved with her own young adult children,

the grandchildren, and all the various lifestage prob-
lems. This situation, along with Grace's depression,
her escalating dependency needs, and deteriorating
physical health, produced a high level of stress for
Janet.

Grace had to be hospitalized after she developed
severe anorexia, stopped taking her antihypertensive
medication, and fainted twice—once in the street. She
seemed very depressed and expressed feelings of
helplessness and hopelessness. In the hospital, sever-
al tests were done and a uterine tumor was detected.
A total hysterectomy was performed, and the patholo-
gy report resulted in a diagnosis of uterine carcinoma.
Her recovery was very slow and at times seemed non-
existent. Grace was too weak, too depressed, and too
physically ill to go back to her own house; Janet was
feeling guilty, conflicted, and stressed about having
her come to live with her; the hospital, following DRG*
guidelines, was pushing for discharge and placement,
and the idea of a nursing home threatened Grace's
feelings of security and her beliefs about "family."
Grace felt like she was losing everything.

It cannot be denied that *loss* is a fact in aging—it
is often thought to be the major theme of the elderly client. Until recently, most research focused on
the losses of aging. As in the case described above,
losses include changes and effects on the physiological subsystem, the physical-environmental subsystem, and the spiritual/philosophical subsystem
(Henthorn, 1980). Currently, researchers in gerontology are questioning many of the accepted views
of aging and the defects associated with loss. Rowe
and Kahn (1987), in their discussion of "usual" and
"successful" aging, emphasize the importance of
the *heterogeneity* of the aged population. Heterogeneity has itself been called a theory of aging (Le-
Bray, 1984). Research points overwhelmingly to
vast differences between aging people in such
things as attitudes, abilities, changes in abilities,
life situations, coping patterns, and present adjustments (Baltes and Willis, 1977; Kastenbaum, 1971;

*DRG—Diagnosis Related Groups—Medicare's prospective
payment system, based on classifications arrived at by comput-
erizing the various circumstances under which Medicare beneficiaries are hospitalized. Hospitals are paid set amounts for particular diagnoses no matter how long the client needs to remain
in the hospital (MacLean, 1987).

Rowe and Kahn, 1987; Ryff, 1982). The practical
implication of this heterogeneity in the elderly is
that there isn't any single theory of aging—all are
useful at times, but highly individualized assessment and treatment approaches are necessary in
the psychosocial care of the elderly client. Stereotyping can lead to unfair and inadequate treatment.
Myths of aging abound and reinforce negative stereotyping. Some of the prevalent myths include:

1. Most elderly people are dissatisfied with
   life.
2. The ability to think intelligently is lost or lessened with age.
3. Older people cannot really contribute to society.
4. The elderly are hypochondriacal.
5. Sexuality is a thing of the past for the aged.
6. The elderly are rigid, unable to change.

Fortunately, myths are being challenged, and
gerontological research is helping to change beliefs
about the elderly and the aging process (Tavris,
1987; Rowe and Kahn, 1987). Rowe and Kahn
stress that in gerontological research, the study of
"normal aging" is really not relevant because it pays
no attention to the vast heterogeneity within the
"normal" concept—it simply separates pathology
from changes related to an aging process in people.
This aging process varies greatly among individuals, and Rowe and Kahn prefer to categorize normal
aging into "usual aging" and "successful aging."
Certainly, the lives of many elderly people defy the
stereotyping of age as inevitable decline. A partial
list (we're sure you can add to it) of people who
have helped dispel some of the myths about aging
includes Arturo Toscanini, Pablo Picasso, George
Bernard Shaw, Bertrand Russell, Georgia
O'Keeffe, Martha Graham, Andres Segovia, Artur
Rubenstein, George Burns, Eubie Blake, Grandma
Moses, Eleanore of Aquitane, Lowell Thomas,
Krishnamurti, Averell Harriman, Lillian Gish,
George Abbot, and Rep. Claud Pepper.

Henry Roth, who published his first book, the
critically acclaimed *Call It Sleep*, in 1934, published his second critically acclaimed book, *Shifting Landscape*, in 1987 at the age of 81 (*New York
Times*, November 29, 1987). The biographies of
many famous people and our own observations confirm that human development and creativity con-

tinue throughout advanced old age (Kastenbaum, 1971).

Not so well known, but also living vigorously into old age, is Luba Kahan, who at the age of 90 "lives alone, walks to the local supermarket, reads all night when it suits her and, continues to be busy and independent" (Tavris, 1987). There is also Lucy Lewis, one of the "venerable old ones"—a pueblo artisan in New Mexico who produces pieces of pottery that are genuine works of art. She is in her 90s (Winter, 1987). Benjamin Rosen is 92 and still runs his sheet-music shop in Hollywood by himself (Tavris, 1987). Other elderly people are not so advanced in the self-actualization process, and some are feeling stressed, vulnerable, and perhaps even helpless. It is because of such heterogeneity in the aged population that Rowe and Kahn (1987) caution us against treating age as if it were in itself a variable.

SOCIOCULTURAL ASPECTS: THE EXPERIENCE OF AGING IN AMERICA
Demographics

Improved sanitation and social conditions along with medical advances have contributed to increased human longevity (Achenbaum, 1977). There are strong indications that the number of older people in this country is rapidly increasing (Horton, 1982). Based on census statistics and predictions, the following points may be of interest:

1. In 1980, people over 65 constituted 11% of the entire population of the United States (Callahan, 1987), or 25 million Americans (Myers, 1984; Soldo, 1980).
2. In 1985, there were 25,000 Americans who were 100 years old or more, and by the year 2050 there could be more than a million (*Modern Maturity*, October/November, 1987).
3. In 1985, the number of Americans over the age of 65 exceeded the entire population of Canada (*Modern Maturity*, October/November 1987).
4. By the year 2000, a 30% increase in the population of Americans over the age of 65 will

increase their ranks to 32 million. The proportion of the "younger aged" will decrease, and the proportion of those over 75 will increase. Of the expected increase of 7 million in the elderly between 1980 and 2000, 75% will be in the 75 or older group (Soldo, 1980).
5. The census bureau predicts that by the year 2030, 20% of all Americans will be over 65 years of age—64 million compared to about 26 million now (Collins, 1987a).
6. The fastest-growing group in the United States is those over the age of 85, and they are increasing by 10% every two years. By 2040 it is predicted they will be 21% of the population, and they will need 45% of all health care expenditures (Callahan, 1987).
7. Another sobering thought is that by the year 2040 most of the readers of this text will be over the age of 70. To paraphrase the cartoon character Pogo—*we have seen the elderly and they is us.*

It seems that no matter how we look at it, there definitely is a "graying of America." Some of the characteristics of this graying population, based on a March 1981 *Current Population Survey* supplied by the Social Security Administration are:

1. Older units* predominated—one half of all aged units were 73 or over; two thirds were over 70.
2. Single persons predominated—nearly 60% of all aged units were single.
3. Single-women units predominated—they constituted 47% of all aged units, and single women accounted for nearly four fifths of all nonmarried persons.
4. The median total income declined with age regardless of marital status.
5. Single women had a lower median income than single men—widows had the lowest among all subgroups by marital status (Chen, 1985). This last statement exemplified a problem related to aging in America and being a woman. This and other problem areas are discussed in the following section.

---

*A "unit" refers to the grouping that is receiving payments—an individual, a couple, or family.

Health problems and the cost of health care

There is a very well-documented relationship between chronological age and the state of one's health. In mid and later life, biological changes gradually result in a diminished ability to function and survive. Life tables and epidemiological reports on the distribution of disease and impairment verify that there is an age-related incidence and prevalence. In this country the major causes of death in later life are the chronic, degenerative diseases of the heart, cancer, and strokes. Health problems in this age group are often multiple and include complex mixtures of physical, psychological, and social factors (Shanas and Maddox, 1985). Chronic, organic mental disorders are the most common psychiatric disorders in the elderly. Epidemiological surveys point to a 4 to 6% prevalence in persons over 65 and a 20% prevalence in those over 85 (Matteson, 1984).

Health status in the elderly is defined in one of two ways:

1. The presence or absence of disease and, alternatively,
2. According to one's ability to function or one's general sense of "well-being."

This latter way of assessing health status was summarized by a World Health Organization advisory group in 1959. It states that the degree of ability or fitness in an elderly individual, rather than the amount of pathology that is present, may be used as a guide for determining the level of services the person will require from the community (Shanas and Maddox, 1985). A report in 1974 by the same organization on the planning and organization of geriatric services also declared that *functional diagnosis* is one of the most important innovations in geriatric care. *Impairment* and *disability* were differentiated in the following ways: *impairment*—a physiological or psychological abnormality that does not interfere with normal life activities in the individual; *disability*—a condition that results in a partial or total limitation of the normal life activities of a person (Shanas and Maddox, 1985; World Health Organization, 1982).

As people age, chronic illness and resulting disability become more common. In this country, since the 1960s, death rates for the elderly have

declined sharply; between 1968 and 1978 there was a decline of 1.5% for males and 2.3% for females (Davis, 1985). People are living longer; there are more elderly people in our society, and they are more susceptible to disease and disability as they reach greater ages. There is a discrepancy between the growing health care needs of the elderly and the health care resources available to them. Our health care system tends to focus more on the specialized, acute care system (secondary care) rather than community-centered primary or tertiary care (Shanas and Maddox, 1985). The cost of health care for the elderly is a major concern for the individual and for society. In 1980, people over the age of 65 (11% of the total population) accounted for 29% of a total expenditure of $450 billion. Medicare costs were projected to rise from $75 billion in 1986 to $114 billion in the year 2000 (Callahan, 1987). It is virtually certain that the health care needs of the elderly will make greater and greater demands on our health care system in the forseeable future. Besides an increase in the number of older persons, their average demand for health care is projected to increase (Shanas and Maddox, 1985).

Medicare and *Medicaid* are the names of pieces of legislation enacted to help the elderly meet the financial crunch of health care. Title XVIII of the Social Security Act, Medicare (also known as the Federal Health Insurance Program for the Elderly), was enacted in 1965. Medicare is a governmental economic system that is financed by a payroll tax and that transfers payments to provide for certain kinds of health care for elderly people. Medicare consists of two parts: Part A is compulsory hospital insurance, and Part B is a subsidized, direct payment system. Part A covers hospital, some nursing home services, and home health services, while Part B covers physician, outpatient hospital, home health, and some ambulatory services. Part A covers all eligible persons who also may voluntarily enroll in Part B by paying a premium. Because of the nature of reimbursement, the system tends to focus on acute, episodic care, and it is inadequate to meet all the health care needs of the elderly. It was designed to *reduce the cost* of health care, not to meet the real needs of older people who suffer from chronic health problems. Long-term institutional care was not covered under either Part A or Part B, and Part A covered only 90 days of inpatient hospitalization for any illness (Clark and Baumer, 1985; Eisdorfer, 1985; Pear, 1987a). In October 1987, a bill to protect America's 31 million Medicare beneficiaries against the costs of catastrophic illness was passed by the House and the Senate (Pear, 1987a). On July 1, 1988, President Reagan signed the Medicare Catastrophic Coverage Act of 1988 into law. It is the most significant expansion of Medicare since the program was created (Deets, 1988). The changes in Medicare are complicated, and they are scheduled to be phased in gradually over a period of years. Some costs to the elderly will increase, but the financial risk of sickness has been eased somewhat for the elderly (Coleman, 1988). The bill still does not provide comprehensive coverage for extended nursing home stays, which, according to John Denning, president of the American Association of Retired Persons, are responsible for the greatest catastrophic costs to the elderly. The catastrophic bill would limit some costs (AARP News Bulletin, December, 1987). Many health care costs must still be paid by the elderly under Medicare; a survey by the AARP showed that prescription drugs are their second-highest expense after nursing home care (Pear, 1987a). The bill provides some help for prescription drug costs. The catastrophic illness bill also seeks to prevent the dispiriting consequence of sickness in which an elderly couple must deplete all their financial resources at the time one spouse enters a nursing home. To be eligible for Medicaid payments for the nursing home stay, the spouse remaining at home must be impoverished and live on $340 or less per month. Under the new law, this will improve in 1989 (Coleman, 1988). Nursing home care costs an average of $22,000 a year (*New York Times*, November 9, 1987), often exceeds $30,000 a year (Pear, 1987b), and can reach $50,000 a year (AARP Bulletin, November, 1987).

Medicaid, Title XIX of the Social Security Act, is a federal-state program for people of low income. It helps to finance health care for the poor and the medically needy. It was not specifically intended for the elderly, but persons over 65 accounted for 37.4% of all of its expenditures according to a 1981 report (Davis, 1985). It is an important means of protection for the elderly poor. In addition, it provides a form of "insurance" for extended nursing home care for some elderly persons. It is the only government program that pays for a substantial amount of the costs of nursing home care. This care, which costs over $38 billion a year, is paid by Medicaid (41%) and directly by the person and/or relatives (51%). The requirement that the aged person (and spouse) must first be impoverished to receive these benefits for needed nursing home care has been a hardship for many elderly people. The new catastrophic illness bill will provide some relief and protect these people from poverty. Financial stress is certainly one problem related to aging in our society, and the high cost of health care combined with our escalating need for health care services make it a fact of life for most elderly Americans.

Financial problems

At this time when health may be declining, income is also declining for many elderly people. Retirement, fixed incomes, and inflation can be very hazardous to a person's life-style and sense of security. Some elderly people have retired without pensions or with inadequate pensions. For example, nonunion workers, women, and minorities are often employed by small firms or in fringe occupations, and they are less apt to be eligible for a pension (Streib, 1985).

The *Social Security Act*, otherwise known as the *Old Age and Survivors Benefit*, component of the Social Security system was enacted in 1935. Medicare and Medicaid are parts of that system through amendments that were enacted in 1965 (Encyclopedia of Social Work, 1977; Schulz, 1980). The retirement benefit part, known as Social Security has six basic principles:
1. Participation is compulsory for certain designated groups
2. Benefits are calculated, based on past earnings
3. It provides a "floor" of protection but is not intended to be a sole source of income
4. Funds come from an earmarked payroll tax
5. Social adequacy is attempted through the use of a progressive benefit formula (i.e., higher income, higher payroll deductions and eventually, higher benefits)
6. A retirement test limits the benefits to people

who have substantially reduced work efforts (there are limits on how much a person can earn and still receive full benefits) (Schulz, 1980)

The significance of Social Security for many elderly people is that it defines retirement not as a degrading financial dependency in old age but as a social position that accrues to one by right. It does not, however, protect the very poor, since adequate benefits are paid to those who have strong work records at relatively high earnings. Since eligibility is tied to employment, it can't reach the poorest of our citizens, those who have not had consistent and traditional work records (Encyclopedia of Social Work, 1977). According to Census Bureau figures, one in four elderly persons is living below or just above the poverty level (Carlson, 1988). Many women among the elderly today have never worked at jobs but followed the traditional cultural norms of the times and devoted their lives to homemaking and raising children. Many lost private pension benefits after their husbands died (Doress and Siegal, 1987; Streib, 1985). Women outlive men by an average of seven years, and most women in this culture married older men to begin with. Of today's group of elderly women, few expect to receive a private pension (Streib, 1985), and they must subsist on reduced Social Security benefits (*New York Times*, November 26, 1987, B12). This group of women makes up a substantial proportion of our elderly poor. One study found that a widow's income was half of what it was before widowhood (LoPata, 1979).

Despite these problems, Social Security has been of immense value to elderly people, and because of its programs, poverty rates for older Americans have been cut in half since 1970 (Carlson, 1988). In fact, in a recent study of Census Bureau data, Social Security was found to be the largest source of income for people over the age of 85 (*New York Times*, November 26, 1987, B12).

The aging of women

In general, women seem to be worse off financially in old age than men. There are more elderly women—three times as many single women over the age of 65 as men (Aizenberg and Treas, 1985). One recent study, based on Census Bureau data, showed that among people 85 and over, men are more apt to be married, living in their own homes, have higher incomes, and be healthier than women. The study also showed that nearly 70% of the people over 85 in this country are women. Average personal income was $10,529 for the elderly men compared to $6,931 for women, and 14% of the women were receiving public assistance compared to 9% of the men. While half the men were married, only one tenth of the women were. The study also indicated that approximately half the women had suffered a long-term disability, compared to 38% of the men (*New York Times*, November 26, 1987, B12). Some other interesting facts concerning women include:

1. Of elderly women, 15.6% are poor compared to 8.5% of elderly men.
2. Of the older women living alone, 26.8% are poor.
3. 34.8% of elderly black women are poor.
4. Of black women over the age of 85, 73% are poor (Beram and Chauncey, 1987).

Cultural norms support the marriage of older men to younger women, but the reverse is not operating in this society (Aizenberg and Treas, 1985). The elderly population is becoming more and more a population of single older women—a ratio of 45 men to 100 women in 1980 is expected to be 39 men to 100 women in the year 2000 (Shanas and Maddox, 1985)—and while among the very wealthy, inheritance has enabled some older women to have greater control of wealth (Streib, 1985), many single older women are experiencing great financial stress. One other stress is the change in status that is often part of a woman's aging. If, for instance, she stays in the home after widowhood, she must cope with the difficulties of home repair and maintenance. The culture dictated in past years that this be left to her husband; in widowhood, it falls to her. If she moves in with her children or other relatives, her position as mistress of her own kitchen is lost, and she often must give up prized possessions from her home. Along with the increasing ratio of women to men in this society, there is the finding of several studies that women are more likely than men to utilize the services of the health care system (Streib, 1985). The probable basis for this trend is the necessity for economically deprived women to seek assistance, and it predicts an increasing strain on an already inadequate system.

Ethnicity and aging

Just as gender modifies patterns of aging in America, so does ethnicity. Generally, a person's experience is influenced by membership in an ethnic group, particularly when the person has suffered from the negative impact of racial prejudice, language barriers, and the lack of accessibility of health care services. Because of various kinds of discrimination, members of minority groups are more apt to be poor, to have inadequate housing, and to be in poorer health. Discrimination based on age places the person in double jeopardy ("Age Page," 1987a). Mental health services are particularly inaccessible to elderly members of minority groups. Cultural traditions and beliefs may not sanction the use of these services, and the elderly often cope through the more acceptable somatization of psychological problems, or they go the route of traditional folk medicine (Solomon, 1984). Gaining access to *any* health service is an acute problem for elderly members of the Native American population. In this group, poor health and a long history of inadequate health care contribute to suffering. Elderly Chinese-Americans, because of traditional beliefs, will often avoid modern medicine and particularly hospitals. Instead, they prefer to rely on herbology and traditional healers. When the interventions of modern medicine are needed, it is often too late. Hispanic elderly people may also prefer to use folk medicine rather than the primary care of mainstream American medicine (Solomon, 1984). For elderly Japanese, institutionalization is viewed as family disgrace, and when younger, westernized family members consider it the best option, the elderly person suffers acutely from a perceived "loss of face" (Chae, 1987). Chae, in discussing the problems of older Asians, makes an important point that is applicable to the elderly of all minority groups. Experiences in hospitals, institutions, or with any aspect of our health care system can be traumatic for these people. Insensitivity, or a misunderstanding of someone's cultural background, can have a devastating effect on that person's well-being and health status. Traditional eating habits of some groups such as Cuban immigrants may be at odds with mainstream American nutritional lore, making favorite foods unavailable. This can result in an important loss of comfort and security (Pasquali, 1985).

The concept of retirement does not really exist for many elderly members of minority groups. They are often excluded from pensions or even Social Security benefits because they were employed in jobs without this coverage or were caught up in the erratic employment patterns of discrimination and poverty (AARP Bulletin, January 1988, 6; Solomon, 1984). An advocacy group for Hispanics, the *National Council of La Raza*, points out that government statistics are bleak for elderly Hispanics in this country. The poverty rate for this group was twice that of whites, and one in four did not even receive Social Security benefits (compared to one in twelve whites). Language barriers were cited as one important reason for not obtaining any aid that was available (AARP Bulletin, January 1988, 6).

There are, of course, some positive effects of ethnicity on aging, and they include feelings of shared particularity, cultural patterns of respect for the aged, and a prevalence of extended family ties. An example of the positive effects of belonging to a minority group is the Mexican-American older person whose subculture permits the principle of passive mastery in aging—that is, old age is viewed as the time when one may rest and give others the benefit of years of accumulated wisdom. This enables the older Mexican-American to freely accept help from children and other family members (Gutmann, 1977, 316-317). Elderly blacks who in earlier years have experienced much distress from discrimination may continue to be deeply affected by this in later life (Solomon, 1984), but they are also apt to belong to a family system that has strong intergenerational ties (Gutmann, 1977).

Retirement

Retirement may be a very positive experience for some people, a devastating one for some, and something in between for many others. It is a mixture of positives and negatives. Charges by some younger people that the elderly are unfairly segregated into "geriatric ghettos" in retirement communities seem to be unfounded. Joining a retirement community is voluntary, and a person can leave at any time. Numerous studies have supported the idea that many elderly people prefer to live with people in their own age group (Streib, 1985). It is more likely to be the poverty ghetto or the racial ghetto that provides harsh treatment to the elderly.

Many retirees enjoy the greater opportunity for leisure and continued education. There exists, for example, the *elderhostel* system, in which older people go to various college campuses in the summer months to learn, discuss, and meet with others who have similar interests. Freedom from having to make a living may enable some to continue the task of self-actualization. Others are choosing to retire and settle in college towns instead of the traditional Sunbelt cities. They take advantage of the rich cultural life these places can offer (*New York Times*, November 29, 1987). Successful retirement is a reality for many, but we should remember that it is still a major life change, and there is a natural stress that accompanies even positive changes.

While some people are enjoying retirement, others feel a painful loss of status and income and perhaps even the meaning of their lives if they leave a job where identification was strong. Poverty and ageism deprive many elderly citizens of access to health care, social services, and the cultural activities that can make retirement a time of self-enrichment.

The status bestowed by education seems to persist after retirement, and people with higher education levels express more satisfaction with retirement. For one thing, they usually have higher incomes, which permit them to become involved in a greater variety of activities (Streib, 1985). Even voluntary work activities require money for wardrobe and transportation expenses. When people retire voluntarily and have the health and financial resources to enjoy their freedom, they do consider this to be a "golden" time of life.

Ageism and legislation

Some other elderly people are choosing to work longer into old age. The Age Discrimination Act (ADA) was passed in 1975, and it addresses "ageism" on a broad scale (Eglit, 1985). *Ageism* is a term

that was coined by Robert Butler; it is defined as follows:

Ageism can be seen as a systematic stereotyping and discrimination against people because they are old, just as racism and sexism accomplish this with skin color and gender (Butler, 1975, 144).

Ageism complicates aging in our society in a negative way that intensifies peoples' fears about growing old.

In addition to the Age Discrimination Act, several other laws deal with the problem. The Age Discrimination in Employment Act (ADEA) of 1967 attacks discrimination in the workplace and in all areas of employment, including hiring, firing, promotion, benefits, and discriminatory advertising (Eglit, 1985). The Equal Credit Opportunity Act (ECOA) prohibits discrimination on the basis of age as well as race, sex, marital status, and religion. Using age as a criterion for deciding individual rights and privileges has been common in the past. Fortunately, the consciousness of legislators, judges, and lawyers has begun to reach a level that acknowledges the inequity of distribution of rights, responsibilities, and resources on the basis of age (Eglit, 1985).* The AARP has been active in supporting older workers who have experienced age discrimination at work. They lobby at state and federal levels for increased worker protection (*Modern Maturity*, October/November 1987). Society is beginning to appreciate the value of older workers, up to now an untapped labor force. People over the age of 55 are being sought out to work in many areas that are chronically short of help. One notable area is in child-care services. Gerontologists and child-development specialists both see an advantage in hooking up these two age groups. This is particularly valuable at a time when population mobility has isolated grandparents and grandchildren from one another (Collins, 1987b).

There is a danger inherent in elderly people being sought out for work; they are often exploited in low-paying jobs. But there is the potential, as in the child-care example, for increased self-esteem when an elderly person works at something mean-

---

*In 1986, virtually all mandatory retirement from the work place was abolished by congress (Brickfield, 1987).

ingful. Many elderly people also need the additional income.

Problems of getting and giving care

The frail or disabled elderly still living in the community make up about 20% of all elderly, and they number about 4.5 million (Carlson, 1987). Of this number, nearly 75% were being cared for by relatives or friends rather than health professionals (Antonucci, 1985; Carlson, 1987). The most typical scenario is one of a frail elderly man cared for by an only slightly less frail and elderly wife (Antonucci, 1985). The family remains the major source of care for the sick elderly (Shanas and Maddox, 1985). While several studies have demonstrated that strong family ties and support reduce mortality in the frail elderly (Antonucci, 1985), the responsibility of continuously providing care can impose a strain on the health of the caregiver. The estimated cost for care of the elderly underestimates the real cost borne by family members. An article in a recent issue of *Modern Maturity* states that the term *caregiver* is a "euphemism for unpaid female relative" (Wood, 1987, 30). Women "in the middle" and "sandwich generation" are terms that describe the stressful position of women caring for elderly parents (or parents-in-law) and also providing support for adult children and grandchildren. Elaine Brody, associate director of research at the Philadelphia Geriatric Center, describes the situation as being "like refilling the empty nest—from both sides" (Wood, 1987, 28). Life for the middle-aged woman is further complicated by the fact that more and more are joining the labor force (Shanas and Maddox, 1985), and job responsibilities are added. Families need assistance in the task of caring for elderly members, and they need relief for the care giver through such mechanisms as *home care*, *day care*, and *respite care*. Home care provides for various health and homemaker services to the elderly person in the community; *day care* centers provide centrally located, 9 to 5 supervision, socialization, and therapy for some elderly people; and *respite care* provides the caregiver with short-term "vacations" from the continuous responsibility of caring for an elderly relative. All three concepts are discussed in this chapter under *Tertiary Care.*

Title XX of the Social Security Act allows each state to offer a variety of services to eligible persons. The problem is that "eligible persons" excludes many of our elderly citizens who are not in a financially eligible group because they are not covered by Social Security.

Provision of care by the children of the very old can be a problem when these "children" are experiencing declining health and aging themselves. The childless elderly may depend on relatives who are of a similar age and in marginally better health. A group that is growing in number but receiving little attention is the elderly parents who must continue as long-term caregivers for their disabled and dependent adult children. Because people are living longer (both the parent and the disabled child), this is becoming a crisis situation for some elderly caregivers (Jennings, 1987). For many reasons the role of caregiver is a stressful one. John Wood has listed several danger signals that indicate to a caregiver when help is needed. They are:

1. The elderly person's condition worsens despite the help you give.
2. No matter what you do to help, it is not enough.
3. You feel completely alone in enduring this.
4. You have no time for yourself, for even a brief time.
5. The occasional help that you gave is now a daily part of your routine.
6. Caregiving is seriously interfering with your work and social life.
7. You go on in a hopeless situation because you can't admit failure.
8. You realize that you've excluded others who have offered help and that you are all alone in caregiving.
9. You don't consider your own needs because to do so would be selfish.
10. Your coping patterns are destructive (e.g., overeating, substance abuse, family scapegoating).
11. Exhaustion and resentment prevent happy and caring times—you no longer feel good about yourself or what you're doing (Wood, 1987, 31).

The feelings of dependency engendered by having to rely on others is a feared role change for the previously independent person who becomes frail or disabled. Self-esteem can be damaged. The concept of *role reversal*, believed to be operating when a parent is cared for by an adult child, is really not adequate to describe the situation. The adult child does not reverse roles, and to foster this idea does harm to the relationship. A better term is *filial maturity*, which is defined as the mature adult child's capacity to be depended upon by the parent (Blazer, 1982; Blenker, 1965; Brody, 1979; Encyclopedia of Social Work, 1977).

Care by family members may engender situations that are problematic. Past relationships of severe family conflict may result in acute situational stress within the family, and *elder abuse* is a term that has joined the concepts of child abuse and spouse abuse. Elder abuse can range from passive neglect to active mistreatment, and it may be a well-hidden problem. In 1985, a House Committee on Aging report estimated that there may be as many as a million elderly victims of abuse in the country (*Modern Maturity*, February-March 1988, 87). For a more comprehensive discussion of elder abuse, see Chapter 21.

There are some hopeful signs of change emerging around the issues of caregiving. A growing number of corporations and businesses see the value of helping workers who must care for elderly relatives (Kahn, 1987; Martin, 1988; Quinn, 1987). Recent studies indicate that 20 to 40% of full-time employees are providing some degree of care for elderly relatives (Kahn, 1987). This concept of employer support for caregivers is termed *eldercare* and it is taking many forms, such as:

1. Information and referral
2. Flexible hours to schedule time to meet care needs
3. Company-sponsored day-care centers
4. Financial support in the form of companies allowing workers to designate part of income to pay for various forms of care; following IRS guidelines, this income will be free of taxation
5. Insurance coverage for long-term care (Quinn, 1987)

When community or home-based care is no longer adequate for the needs of the frail elderly, inpatient care becomes necessary. This may be for a temporary, acute episode, and often Medicare will be the method of payment. The number of older people using hospitals has risen steadily since Medicare was introduced (Shanas and Maddox, 1985). With the introduction of DRGs (diagnosis related groups), the length of these stays has decreased. Many geriatric health care workers are deeply concerned about the potential dangers of a rigid, systematic discharge system. This is particularly relevant for the frail elderly person who lives alone. Shanas and Maddox (1985) point out that the goal of avoiding institutionalization and keeping the frail elderly in the community may include the erroneous assumption that there is a family unit to care for the aged person.

When long-term institutionalization (nursing home care) becomes the best choice for elderly people and their families, other stresses become apparent. Some elderly people do not want to enter a nursing home. They may fear abuse or neglect or isolation from friends and family. Since many nursing homes do not have private rooms, they may foresee a lack of privacy. Other elders welcome the relief from the strain of caring for self and home— the chores of food shopping and meal preparation, for example. They may also welcome the increased security if they have been living in areas where crime is rising. Sometimes an elderly person who wants to be admitted to a nursing home and who can afford the cost cannot be admitted because of governmental regulations requiring a greater degree of disability before admission is allowed. This is because of the government's fears that the individual's care must eventually be financed by Medicaid as personal finances are depleted.

Nursing home placement of an elderly relative can be stressful for family members, who may feel intense guilt—particularly when the elder doesn't want the placement. Guilt feelings and past intergenerational conflicts are reactivated, and the family needs support and education from the involved health professionals. Guilt and resentment strain family ties and may weaken the family's continuing emotional involvement with the elderly person. The older person's reluctance to enter a nursing home may be based on real fears about the kind of care he or she will receive. Nursing homes vary in quality from places where neglect and poor care are the norm (*New York Times*, December 26, 1987 A) to the excellent, caring establishment with sensitive, empathetic workers that was described in the *American Nurse* (November-December, 1987) by Jane Chandler, an ANA certified gerontological nurse. In 1986, the Institute of Medicine Committee on Nursing Home Regulation published a study concluding that there are nursing homes throughout this country that provide a "seriously inadequate quality of care and quality of life" (Walgren, 1987). This was despite a supposedly extensive federal regulation of nursing homes. The General Accounting Office of the federal government also issued a report that found more than a third of nursing homes certified to receive Medicare and Medicaid funds were frequent violators of patient-care rules ranging from bad food and bad plumbing to nurse shortages. Under previous federal regulations, violators could stay in the program if the violations were corrected before expiration of their one-year licenses. Loss of certification was the only penalty, and, with a severe shortage of nursing home beds, it was rarely used. The Nursing Home Quality Reform Act of 1987 makes it harder for any homes so terminated to be readmitted, and it expands the authority of the states and the Department of Health and Human Services to impose fines and bans on admissions of new Medicare and Medicaid patients (*New York Times*, December 26, 1987, 22; Pear, 1988). On December 22, 1987, the Omnibus Budget Reconciliation Act of 1987 was signed into law by President Reagan. It is an extremely detailed law that protects many rights for nursing home residents. Included are the following rights:

1. To choose a personal physician
2. To privacy
3. To be free from mental and physical abuse
4. To receive notice before change of room or roommate
5. To meet with other residents in organized groups
6. To voice grievances about care and to have the grievances addressed promptly by the nursing home

The law also states that there will be federal standards for training the nurses' aides who provide most of the care in nursing homes. They would receive at least 75 hours of training in nursing skills. The nursing home must have licensed nurses on duty around the clock and a registered nurse on duty at least eight hours a day, seven days a week. A full-time social worker must be hired by any home with more than 120 beds. Nursing homes must permit immediate access to any resident by that person's relatives. Federal and state ombudsmen must also be admitted to the home to investigate any claims of abuse. Severe fines and penalties are in place to back up these regulations (Pear, 1988).

The government thus is increasingly empowered to help the frail and disabled elderly and to defend those who cannot defend themselves. Many older people *can* defend themselves, and some are becoming more involved in the self-help organizations that have formed in recent times.

Self-help groups

The American Association of Retired Persons (the AARP) is a nonprofit and nonpartisan organization established in 1958. It began with a handful of members; today they number 26 million. Advocacy efforts in Congress to contain health care costs and to protect the rights of elderly persons in the workplace are some of the issues with which the AARP has become involved (Brickfield, 1987; Denning, 1987; Eglit, 1985).

The Gray Panthers is a national activist group. A cofounder of this group, 83-year-old Maggie Kuhn, was the plenary speaker on "Health Care of Older Americans" at the American Nurses' Association convention in 1988. The Gray Panthers is a more militant group than the AARP, and its approach is intergenerational. One important goal is to fight "ageism" whether in the form of mandatory retirement, discrimination based on age, or negative stereotyping of the aged (MacLean, 1987).

The Older Women's League (O.W.L.) was organized in 1980 as a national activist network. It is concerned with issues and problems of health care, retirement and pay equity, job training for displaced homemakers, housing and, in general, the mid-life and aging problems of women. They seek to improve the quality of life for older women through helping one another as a "sisterhood" MacLean, 1987). These organizations have been very effective in influencing legislators around issues of antidiscrimination for our elderly citizens (Eglit, 1985).

LOSSES, CHANGES, AND INTERVENING VARIABLES

Eighty years old! No eyes left, no ears, no teeth, no legs, no wind! And when all is said and done, how astonishing well one does without them! (French poet Paul Claudel, meditating on old age.)

Intervening variables

Traditionally, human aging has been studied in two categories—*normal aging* vs. *pathological aging*. This approach is too narrow because it ignores the heterogeneity of the *normal aging* group. There are wide differences, and some gerontological workers (e.g., Butler and Lewis, 1973; Rowe and Kahn, 1987) have suggested the term *successful aging*. Rowe and Kahn believe that the *normal aging* group should be subdivided into categories of *usual aging* and *successful aging*. In usual aging, extrinsic factors heighten the effects of aging, while in successful aging, extrinsic factors have a neutral or positive effect on aging. The two broad areas of extrinsic factors or intervening variables are lifestyle factors and psychosocial factors. The former, which either enhance a successful and healthy aging or work to promote a more rapid decline, include diet, amount of exercise, and the individual's personal habits (e.g., substance use and abuse). Psychosocial factors at work in this process include:

1. Autonomy and control of the individual— feeling somewhat in control over one's environment makes life seem more predictable and more secure
2. Social support and networks

There is an important relationship between (1) and (2): In the latter, "support" can enhance the elder's life, but it must be the kind of support that doesn't threaten (1)—autonomy and control. It must be *enabling support*. The authors warn that such things as "constraining," "doing for," and "warning" that go beyond the requirements of the situation may convey caring, but they also teach the person helplessness (Rowe and Kahn, 1987). The belief that the normal aging process can be modified, positively or negatively, is an important one for health professionals to consider. Gerontological researchers are questioning the accepted views of aging and the degree of loss and change associated with the process; many believe that it has been overstated. Still, some degree of *loss* and *change* remains a fact of human aging.

Losses and changes

What are these losses and changes? From an ecological approach, they include a repatterning of the physiological subsystem, the physical-environmental subsystem, the sociocultural subsystem, and the spiritual/philosophical subsystem (Henthorn, 1980). The physiological subsystem undergoes changes in the sensory functions, and this can affect all the other subsystems. In general, a person's ability to cope with the environment is directly related to the capacity to detect, interpret, and respond to sensory information (Kline and Schreiber, 1985). There are age-related perceptual losses in a person's senses; limiting perception can limit that person's possibilities, and self-esteem and motivation for social interaction are affected. Activities of daily living are influenced by any significant degree of visual decline, and anyone who reaches old age is likely to experience some degree of visual decline. The illumination required for efficient functioning increases with age because the pupil is shrinking, the lens is yellowing, and there is a loss in accommodation (Fozard, 1982). The ability to see small details and to differentiate colors decreases with age (Horton, 1982). One inevitable visual change is called *presbyopia*, a term from the Greek for "elderly vision." This usually begins in the early 40s and is a growing inability of the lens to focus on nearby objects because of a loss in elasticity; people find themselves holding reading material further and further from the eyes. Presbyopia is treated with reading glasses or bifocals (Henig, 1985).

Manipulation of levels of illumination can help to compensate for many of the visual difficulties the elderly experience. For example, the elderly may need more focused light in the workplace or on stairs rather than in the entire area. Contrast in visual information can be emphasized on such things as labels or information on control panels of appliances (Fozard, 1982).

Hearing impairment also increases with age, and of those who are 65 to 79 years of age, approximately one third have a significant loss of hearing (Shanas and Maddox, 1985). Men find it particularly difficult to hear tones in the higher frequencies (Tavris, 1987). *Prebycusis* refers to age-related changes in hearing. Unlike the inevitability seen for presbyopia, many physicians believe that while hearing loss is associated with age, it is not caused by it. They believe that the majority of cases of hearing impairment can be traced to specific mechanical or neurological causes (Henig, 1985). Changes are related to such things as degeneration of receptor cells and neural units within the cochlea and metabolic changes occurring within the inner ear (Olsho, Harkins, and Lenhardt, 1985). *Otosclerosis* is a genetic condition that causes conductor loss or reduction in sound level reaching the inner ear. The stapes becomes embedded in a growth of spongy bone. An operation called a stapedectomy has been quite successful in treating this condition—the stapes is replaced by a tiny metal prostheses.

As in the case of declining vision, environmental manipulation becomes important as a way of compensating for hearing loss. This includes such things as choosing a seat that is advantageous for hearing in groups or putting one's best hearing ear forward. Some people are helped immensely by the use of hearing aids.

Other sensibilities are changing as we age—pain sensitivity decreases (Horton, 1982), and our sense of smell may be dulled (Bower and Patterson, 1986; Tavris, 1987). The sense of smell affects taste, and many elderly people complain that food doesn't taste as good as it used to. Secondarily, an elderly person's mobility may be decreased by a primary problem with osteoarthritis or osteoporosis. The loss of bone density that can result from osteoporosis and that can lead to minor or life-threatening fractures can be modified by preventive measures such as exercise, cessation of smoking, limited alcohol intake, and adequate nutrition (Rowe and Kahn, 1987).

Myths surrounding the aging process and sexuality are prevalent. Patterns of sexuality do change in response to physiological changes, but here, too, heterogeneity is the important factor. Just as sexuality is highly individualized in younger people, its experience and expression vary widely among the elderly. All too often, the sexuality of elderly people is misunderstood or stereotyped. Allen (1985) points out that sexuality can carry several connotations for individuals—close companionship, opportunities to touch and be touched, one's body image, sexual intercourse or lovemaking. Societal myths about sexuality and the elderly reinforce the older person's image of his or her own sexuality and can lead to an identification of self as nonsexual (Allen, 1985). Alex Comfort (1984, 169) states: "The folklorist view of old age as being ... uninterested and nonfunctional in sexuality, tends to be the expression of a self-fulfilling prophecy." Elderly people, like younger people, can have sexual difficulties, and they can respond to treatment or new information. (See Chapter 7 for a comprehensive discussion of sexuality.) One major problem with sexuality for the elderly may be dealing with the lack of a sex partner because of bereavement. The cultural norm of older men marrying younger women and the greater longevity of women results in many aging, heterosexual women being left without their partners.

Lack of privacy may be an inhibiting factor for the institutionalized elderly, although there seems to be a growing enlightenment among health professionals about this problem.

Some physiological changes do occur with aging that can affect the experience and expression of sexuality. For example, the aging female's vagina lengthens and thins out, and the addition of lubrication may be required. The elderly male's changes include an increased time to arousal, erection, and ejaculation (Masters and Johnson, 1966). This slower time is successfully incorporated by many older couples into a more leisurely lovemaking.

Another myth of aging concerns a supposed decrease in intellectual ability and in the ability to learn. This issue has received a good deal of attention in recent years. Earlier beliefs about declining intellectual ability were based on tests using standard IQ measurements and designed for young people. They showed a steady decrement from postadolescence onward. When test results were analyzed, it was observed that differences seen in particular areas were age related. *Performance* subtests showed greater susceptibility to aging than *verbal* subtests (Birren and Abrahams, 1984). Response time is a critical dependent variable when examining the registering, storing, and retrieving of information and problem solving. This gives youth the advantage in testing for intellectual ability (Omenn, 1977). An age-intelligence relationship is more indicative of certain specific mental functions than it is of overall intelligence. Vocabulary may be (and very often is) much more extensive in the older person than it is in the young adult. Another way of understanding this incorporates the concepts, first proposed by Cattel (1963), of *fluid intelligence* and *crystallized intelligence*. Fluid intelligence is the processing of information, and it reflects the functioning of neurological structures at their peaks of efficiency in adolescence and in young adulthood (Labouvie-Vief, 1985). Crystallized intelligence is based on learned ability, experience, and stored information. It reflects cultural assimilation, and it is highly influenced by formal and informal education. Fluid intelligence decreases postadolescence, but crystallized intelligence increases throughout life. Growth of crystallized intelligence in each person *is* limited by the capacity of the neurologically based fluid intelligence system, and increments do become smaller with age (Omenn, 1977). But crystallized intelligence continues to increase because of the fact that experience and learning accumulate throughout life.

A common psychosocial loss in later life is the loss of a spouse or partner. In their review of the literature on differences in mortality rates between widowed and married people, Rowe and Kahn (1987) confirmed an excess mortality rate for the widowed group. For some unknown reason, the effect is more pronounced in elderly men than in women. Possible explanations for the greater vulnerability of bereaved men include (1) men's greater reliance on their wives for emotional support and (2) poor nutrition because of the men's reliance on their wives for meal preparation. Warner (1987), in her review of the literature, cites a study by Longino and Lipman (1981) that supports a relationship between gender and perceived support during be-

reavement—they found that women perceived the most support. Warner's comparative study of widows and widowers and their perceived support during bereavement did suggest role-expectation differences based on gender. It appears that men may be more vulnerable during this stressful period. Suggested reasons for the increased risk at bereavement for both men and women were increased stress contributing to maladaptive body changes and an altered social support network contributing to a changed life-style (Blazer, 1982).

Residential relocation and the losses associated with it present problems for elderly people. Relocation may involve moving to another community to live with children or other relatives, or it may happen when the elderly person enters a nursing home. Relocation often means the loss of home, friends, and familiar neighborhoods, and this is stressful for most people. Sometimes it can also be a relief when someone no longer needs to worry about the strain of home maintenance, meal preparation, or the dangers of living alone as a frail and vulnerable elderly person.

The loss of friends or age-mates is accelerated as one grows older—friends die or move away or one moves away from them. Loneliness is a common theme. Interestingly, an unpublished study by Russel and Cutrona (Lear, 1987) found that the loneliness of the elderly was most often caused by a lack of friends, not a lack of kin in their lives. Other gerontologists suggested that contrary to popular belief, concentrating older people in retirement communities is likely to facilitate a more satisfying group life with age-mates (Streib, 1985).

Older people also experience changes in job status. Job status can affect one's self-esteem and one's financial security. Some people embrace retirement enthusiastically, and they enjoy a slower pace or the increased time available for pursuing interests or the freedom from the tyranny of a schedule or from a tyrannical boss. Others feel a great loss when they've been closely identified with the roles of their former work life. Financial security may be unaffected or even enhanced for some who have liberal pensions or accumulated savings. Other elderly people may live close to the poverty level or even below it, if they have not been able to achieve a work record that ensures payment of benefits.

Many must depend on welfare or the help of relatives.

The mandatory retirement age is no longer legal in this country for almost all workers. At the same time, the work force is shrinking. These two factors have led to an increase in available jobs for older people, and some senior citizens are remaining at work or going back to work. Older people, it seems, appreciate the nonmonetary rewards of working the most—such things as the opportunity to expand one's social life or doing meaningful and interesting work that contributes to society (Bird, 1987).

Futurists predict that the tendency for a portion of the elderly population to return to work or stay at jobs they already hold will increase (Bird, 1987). Meanwhile, many older people experience a great deal of stress around the changes and losses that occur in relation to jobs or careers.

It seems that elderly people are vulnerable to stress in many areas of their lives. While some may (as Buddhist philosophy suggests) use adversity for an opportunity to grow in wisdom, others are suffering and coping in less than healthy ways.

UNHEALTHY PATTERNS OF COPING WITH STRESS

Depression is the most common psychiatric disorder in the elderly (Goldenburg, 1984; La Rue, 1985; Louden et al., 1985; Matteson, 1984; Slimmer et al., 1987). Depression is a common disorder but not a simple one, and it seems even more complex as it is manifested in the elderly. The complicating factors include:

1. Physical illness masquerading as depression and the reverse
2. Depression being manifested as physical illness
3. Certain medications prescribed for many elderly people (e.g., antihypertensive drugs and barbiturates) exacerbating or initiating a depression
4. A relationship between chronic degenerative illness (more prevalent in old age) and depression. This can be psychologically associated with the disability, or it may be a biochemical relationship between the physical illness and

depression such as in Parkinson's disease with its decrease in the brain chemical serotonin (Blazer, 1982). Some disorders that seem to precipitate or precede depression include cardiovascular disease, neoplasm, and pancreatitis (La Rue et al., 1985).

5. The symptom similarity between dementia and depression that makes an accurate differential diagnosis so important
6. The complex interplay of social, physical, and psychological losses and changes that can occur with aging and that makes an elderly person vulnerable to depression
7. A tendency in elderly people to resist complaining about feeling depressed because they think it's all part of what is to be expected in aging (Neshkes and Jarvik, 1986)
8. A similar sort of denial on the part of many helping professionals who are working with the elderly population (Louden et al, 1985)
9. Elderly people who are severely depressed may have been practicing maladaptive coping patterns for a longer period of time than younger clients—simply because they are older (Zarit and Zarit, 1984)

As a group, elderly people can and do experience all the varieties of depression—endogenous and exogenous depression, bipolar depression, or adjustment disorder with depressed mood (see Chapter 22 for complete descriptions of the various types of depression). Reactive depression occurs more commonly in late life than at an earlier age (Matteson, 1984). The losses and changes are more frequent, often occurring rapidly with little time for the person to recover. Losses are more apt to be "balanced" by gains in younger age groups than in the elderly.

The elderly are more at risk for suicide (Blazer, 1982; Neshkes and Jarvik, 1986). Older persons make fewer attempts and communicate about the attempts less frequently than younger people, but they commit suicide more frequently. Many clinicians report that the depressive symptoms of elderly clients who commit suicide may not appear severe (Blazer, 1982). The elderly male is particularly vulnerable—this group is at highest risk for suicide (Blazer, 1982; Neshkes and Jarvik, 1986).

A particularly significant aspect of depression in

TABLE 18-1   Depression differentiated from dementia

	Dementia	Depression
Memory loss	Increasing and obvious deficits in memory; specific memory "gaps" or patch memory gaps are unusual; recent memory loss is greater than remote (retrograde memory loss)	More often, temporary forgetfulness; complains of memory loss but does not have an obvious, increasing deficit; specific memory "gaps" are usual; recent and remote memory loss are similar
Mental status on psychological testing	Scores much lower Errors frequent Global, profound impairment Static or progressive loss of one or more intellectual abilities (eg., problem-solving; learning)	Scores higher Errors are rare Subtle intellectual impairment present Progressive losses not usually present
Timing of symptoms	Symptoms worsen as the day goes on—worse in the evening	Better in the evening—more outgoing, more in contact with the world in the evening
Complaints, descriptions, and reactions of clients	Fewer complaints, description tends to be vague; client's distress is variable—unconcerned in later stages	More complaints about symptoms—descriptions of symptoms are more detailed; greater distress for the client
Neurological testing, CT scan	Possible abnormal findings (increased ventricle size and cortical atrophy)	Normal

Based on material from La Rue (1985), Loudon et al. (1985), Wells (1979), Zarit and Zarit (1984).

the elderly is the concept of "pseudodementia." Depression in the elderly may be accompanied by temporary cognitive impairment and can present as dementia, while true dementia is usually accompanied by depression. Dementia, or chronic organic brain syndrome, is a disorder found in some elderly people. This topic is covered in Chapter 26. The necessity for making an accurate differential diagnosis between dementia and depression in the elderly is evident. Variability of client responses is great because of the great heterogeneity of this group we call "The Elderly." However, some guidelines for differentiating dementia from depression are useful and are shown in Table 18-1.

Anxiety and helplessness—while elderly people are at risk for developing depression, another common psychological problem is anxiety. Anxiety in the elderly is often associated with helplessness. Verwoerdt (1980) has termed it "helplessness anxiety," and he relates it to increased vulnerability generated by the physical and psychological losses of later life. Helplessness is also related to depression in that it links losses and changes with depression (Zarit and Zarit, 1984). Seligman (1975) proposed a theory of learned helplessness and depression—when people experience losses and change over which they feel they have no control, they begin to view themselves as helpless and no longer able to manage their lives and may become depressed. Since elderly people experience so many losses, they are at risk for developing feelings of depression, helplessness, and anxiety. The depression of elderly people is often accompanied by anxiety—it is frequently an "agitated depression" (Herman, 1984). Anxiety may also be accompanied by physical illness in older persons—sometimes anxiety is generated by the physical symptom, and sometimes it may be the only obvious symptom of underlying physical illness. Roth and Mountjoy (1980) state that the relationship between anxiety and physical illness in an elderly person is complex and that while anxiety may be . . . "an emotional *response* to illness and the threat it poses, it is at times a harbinger of undetected organic disease."

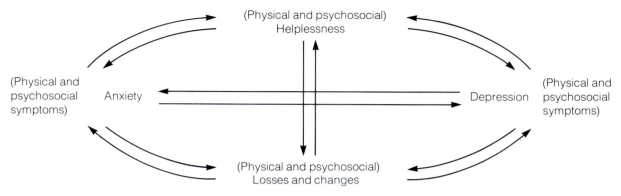

Fig. 18-1   Pathological patterns of coping.

Elderly clients with unexplained anxiety should have a complete medical evaluation.

Anxiety is particularly difficult for an elderly person because of the feelings of helplessness it engenders. This can interfere with functioning that may already be impaired by declining physical health. The physical symptoms of anxiety such as fatigue and insomnia compromise the elderly person who is also dealing with chronic illness. High anxiety can impair cognitive functioning, which, combined with age-related losses and the stress of living, can lead to some degree of confusion in the elderly person. While anxiety is generally thought to be related to unacceptable impulses threatening the person from within, in the elderly, the threat of loss of emotional and social supports seems more relevant.

The problems of anxiety, helplessness, and depression and their relationship to one another are further evidence of the increasing complexity of the elderly person's patterns of coping, as shown in Figure 18-1.

Substance abuse

Elderly people may react to further complicate the patterns illustrated in Figure 18-1 through the various forms of substance abuse. Alcohol is the substance most commonly abused by the elderly (Blazer, 1982). The rate of alcoholism among the elderly is generally the same as that for younger groups—about 2 to 10% of elderly men and 2% of elderly women are believed to experience prob-

lems with alcohol abuse. Rates among elderly widowers are higher (Stern and Kastenbaum, 1984). Because elderly alcoholics tend to be less visible in their drinking behavior, they may not be referred to AA or for other treatment as often as younger people (Mishara and Kastenbaum, 1980). The reasons they are referred less frequently include:

1. Retirement of many, who do not have to report the "morning after" to a job.
2. A reluctance among friends, family, and health workers to separate the person from "one remaining pleasure in life."
3. An unfortunate and widespread attitude that the elderly have a limited life span anyway so that the time and effort of treatment are not warranted.
4. The difficulty in distinguishing alcohol-related physical and mental health problems from those of old age.
5. The failure of some clinicians to take into account the reduced metabolic tolerance for alcohol that occurs with aging. When they use quantity and frequency of drinking as a guideline, it may not be appropriate.

Elderly people generally suffer from more health problems than younger people, and this, in combination with the alcohol abuse, has a profound effect on health status in the elderly alcoholic. Elderly alcoholics are differentiated into two groups: *early onset drinkers*, who have been abusing alcohol since their youth, and *late onset* drinkers, who may have started in middle or late life, often in response to a specific trauma such as bereavement (Rosin and Glatt, 1971; Stern and Kastenbaum, 1984). Some elderly people have started abusing alcohol through using it as an antianxiety agent or as a sedative to induce sleep. The sleep that results is often a fragmented one after alcohol is taken (Blazer, 1982). Elderly alcoholics are at high risk for social isolation and for suicide. There is an increased rate of severe physical illnesses in elderly alcoholics (Stern and Kastenbaum, 1984). Elderly alcoholics and alcohol abusers *must* have adequate, consistent medical care with thorough physical examinations. Alcohol abuse is also dangerous for the elderly because of the large number of prescriptions and over-the-counter medications many of them take. The potential exists for very serious problems in mixing these drugs with alcohol (Stern and Kastenbaum, 1984). While the rate of alcoholism among the elderly is comparable to that of younger age groups, some (e.g., Brody, 1981; Stern and Kastenbaum, 1984) predict that the problem will increase. Brody identifies four factors that can promote alcoholism in the elderly:

1. Retirement that is associated with boredom, loss of job status, and reduced income
2. Bereavement
3. Declining health and physical disability
4. Loneliness

The increased amount of stress that elderly people are susceptible to in daily living puts some of them at increased risk for abusing alcohol. Some researchers have cited possible benefits of moderate use of alcohol for the elderly (e.g., a decreased rate of cardiac disease in moderate drinkers compared to teetotalers). Others in the field of alcoholism research are skeptical, suggesting that the lower rate may be because so many alcoholics die young that fewer remain to be at risk for cardiovascular disease. The studies showing lower rates may not have taken into account the fact that the teetotaler group included many recovering (and abstinent) alcoholics.

For a more detailed description of the development of alcohol abuse in general, the reader should refer to Chapter 20.

Abuse or addiction to illegal drugs, while it occurs in the elderly, does not seem to be a major problem specific to the age group (Whanger, 1984). The problem of *misuse* of drugs is, however, a major one. One possible reason for the small amount of illegal drugs abused by the elderly is the prevalence of abuse and misuse of legal drugs. Some of this occurs because of the large number of medications the elderly are taking. There is a danger of harmful mixtures of medicines and of confusion in dosage and timing of intervals. Drug misuse, the inappropriate use of drugs that were prescribed for therapeutic use, can mean:

1. Overuse
2. Underuse
3. Erratic use
4. Use in unnecessary circumstances
5. Use in contraindicated circumstances (Pascarelli, 1981)

The three most prevalent areas of misuse are:

1. Misuse of prescribed medications
2. Misuse of over-the-counter drugs
3. Physician-related or iatrogenic problems in prescribing drugs (Whanger, 1984)

The elderly population has a much greater risk for experiencing an adverse reaction to drugs than younger people. Some of this risk is due to age-related physiological changes that affect metabolism and excretion and to degenerative illness and poor nutrition, which can affect individual reaction to drugs. Some of it is due to misuse. Among the elderly, noncompliance with a prescribed regimen seems to be the major problem. Several studies report that it is a common occurrence (Whanger, 1984). One study by Schwartz and others (1962) looked at misuse by the elderly and found that the common areas of misuse were:

1. Omission
2. Inaccurate information
3. Erratic self-medication
4. Incorrect dose
5. Incorrect timing

Gollub (1978) identified problems related to *client error* and *health professional error* (see Table 18-2).

Substance abuse and misuse is a particular health problem of the elderly because of their increased physical and emotional vulnerability as they cope with the stress of aging. The self-perpetuating vicious cycle that substance abuse can become represents a trap for many elderly people.

Substance abuse may be a factor in another area

TABLE 18-2 Medical-related problems in the elderly

Client error	Health professional error
Overdose through error	Misdiagnosis
Overdose through emotional disturbance	Inaccuracy in drug treatment (e.g., failure to account for altered reactions of elderly)
Misuse resulting from mental disorder	Polypharmacy—drug interaction
Use of multiple prescriptions without physician's knowledge	Overmedication
Overuse of prescriptions through automatic or telephone refills	Overuse of prescription through automatic or telephone refills
Exchange of prescription medications with others	
Use of outdated medication	

Adapted from Gollub (1978).

of health concern for the elderly—accidents. Other factors include decreased functioning due to osteoarthritis and osteoporosis, declining sensory acuity, and lack of support networks to help with activities of daily living. Older people have a low accident-frequency rate as compared to younger groups, but they have a higher disability and fatality rate from accidents; they are more physiologically vulnerable. With an increased risk for serious injury, accident prevention in the elderly is a major concern for health care professionals. In the over 75 group, falls are the most common cause of accidental injury or death (Sterns et al., 1985). Environmental modification and the installation of protective measures and devices may help to prevent a tragic situation. Such things would include adequate, strategically placed lighting; nonskid rugs; bathtub bars and seats; canes; smoke detectors and antiscald devices; whistling teakettles. Elderly people are also at risk for accidental hypothermia or accidental heatstroke. Our bodies become less able to stand long exposure to heat or cold as we age. With the elderly person who may be suffering from diabetes or heart, circulatory, or lung disease, the problem is magnified. The elderly poor are particularly at risk for accidental hypothermia when they must cope with an inadequate supply of heat in substandard living conditions (Age Page, April, 1987c). This may be compounded by an inadequate support system that does not include people to "look in" on them during severe cold spells.

Malnutrition should be another important concern for those involved with the elderly. Such things as ill-fitting dentures, poor appetite due to

diminishing smell and taste senses, and inadequate finances and difficulty in shopping all complicate the ability to achieve optimal nutrition. Chronic illness, alcoholism, depression, and anxiety further limit intake and can place an individual's nutritional status and health at risk (AARP News Bulletin, October 1987; Barry, 1986). Traditional ethnic ways of cooking and eating provide comfort and solace for many elderly people. Losses and changes occurring with immigration and culture shock have an important effect on the nutrition of elderly people (Pasquali, 1985). Fast foods and highly processed foods take some of the work out of preparation for an elderly person whose energy level has declined, but they also provide too much salt, sugar, cholesterol, and "empty calories." The body has an increasing difficulty in metabolizing and absorbing nutrients efficiently as it ages, and this adds to the older person's susceptibility to nutritional deficiencies (MacLean, 1987).

Sleep disturbance—many elderly people suffer from disturbances in sleep. Sleep patterns do change as we age, and we need fewer hours of sleep per night. Generally speaking, an elderly person may require from 3 to 6 hours a night with a nap during the day. There is, however, a variation in the amount of sleep required among older individuals, and research has indicated that over a third of people over the age of 60 complain of sleeping difficulties. An important concern is the number of awakenings per night and the disruptive effects of these awakenings. Respiratory dysfunction, or sleep apnea, has been documented in the elderly, and it can be exacerbated by sleeping pills (Woodruff, 1985). Considering the normal decline in total sleeping hours required as a person ages, the reliance on sleeping pills with their negative effects on sleep quality seems unwise. Some elderly people get caught in a vicious cycle of sleeping pills and unhealthy sleep patterns. Sleep deprivation studies conducted with the elderly indicate that the quality of subsequent sleep is much better if the individual, instead of taking pills or spending too much time in bed, simply misses a night of sleep (Woodruff, 1985).

One cannot always assume that sleep pattern disturbance in the elderly is simply the need for less sleep. In some individuals it may be something else—depression, for example. Depression in the elderly often goes undiagnosed by clinicians and unrecognized by the client. Sleep disturbance may be an important indicator. Elderly alcoholics, even more than their younger counterparts because of their compromised physiological condition, may also suffer from sleep disturbances. REM sleep seems to be most dependent on CNS structure, and some of that may be damaged or out of synchrony in many elderly alcoholics (Mishara and Kastenbaum, 1980). For nondrug treatment of sleep disturbances in the elderly, any combination of the following measures may be helpful:

1. Back rub
2. Warm tub bath
3. Warm glass of milk (or other L-tryptophan–containing foods)
4. Reading a book
5. Relaxation techniques and visualization of calming scenes
6. Avoidance of stimulants such as coffee or colas
7. Selection of TV programs that are *not* particularly exciting
8. Avoidance of alcohol as a sedative at night
9. Correction of any mattress problems

TREATMENT MODALITIES TAILORED TO THE ELDERLY

Individual treatment—psychotherapeutic treatment for the various difficulties of the elderly do not usually differ from those used at other ages. For example, depression, a commonly occurring psy-

chiatric difficulty in the elderly, is treated as it is at any other age—the same principles apply (see Chapter 22). The therapies and resources for treating substance abuse are similar (see Chapter 20). Some therapeutic techniques are specifically applicable to the elderly client. These are *logotherapeutic use of the past* (or *reminiscing* and *The Life Review*); *memory training* and *pet therapy* to combat loneliness.

Logotherapy, according to existentialist and psychotherapist Viktor Frankl, is "that psychotherapy which centers on the meaning as well as man's search for meaning" (Frankl, 1986, 74). One important aspect of logotherapy pertains to the conception of time. An individual's past is the repository of all that he or she has brought into being. One's future consists of opportunities not yet materialized, but one's past is an invaluable resource for realizing the meaning and satisfaction of accomplishments and experiences in life (Frankl, 1968). Reminiscing helps an elderly person to integrate aspects of a life that has been lived—to gain satisfaction from some accomplishments and events and to let some negative thoughts and feelings go. *The Life Review* is a term coined by Butler (1963)—it is a universal mental process that occurs naturally in individuals and one that is characterized by:

1. A progressive return to consciousness of past experiences
2. The resurgence of unresolved conflicts
3. A simultaneous review and integration of these reviewed experiences and conflicts

Sometimes clinicians, younger than their elderly clients, do not appreciate phenomena such as reminiscing and life review but see it as evidence of regression and living in the past. Often, the pairing of small children (who like to hear stories about the past) with the elderly proves fortuitous. The recent trend of including child day care centers in senior citizen centers or nursing homes helps to facilitate this pairing. The Life Review is recommended as a method for life enhancement and for facilitating the developmental task of late life that both Jung and Erikson have delineated—the integration of the self. Life review therapy can be adapted to group therapy as well as individual therapy.

Memory training—"benign senescent forgetfulness" (Kral, 1978) in the aged implies a change that occurs in most of us as we age; forgetfulness tends to increase (Ferris et al., 1984). It is not to be confused with the massive memory loss associated with such conditions as *Alzheimer's disease* or *multi-infarct dementia* (see Chapter 26). As at any age, anxiety and depression can exacerbate forgetfulness, and forgetfulness can increase anxiety and depression. Memory training for adults can help to increase feelings of security and protect self-esteem.

Remembering requires three steps: encoding, storage, and retrieval. According to research carried out by Smith (Poon, 1985; Smith, 1980), the storage step does not seem to be a problem for the elderly as much as encoding and retrieval. However, the three processes are not independent, and their simultaneous interaction with one another makes them difficult to separate. The end result is that storage is also affected. Mnemonics are memory aids such as those used by most students to memorize sets of facts for upcoming examinations (e.g., Bleuler's 4 A's of schizophrenia or the device used to memorize the cranial nerves: "On Old Olympus's Towering Top a Finn and German Viewed a Hawk"—the first letter of each word represents the first letter of a cranial nerve). Such devices help the elderly to improve memory, and they have been used in programs for this. The principles for using mnemonic devices are:

1. Provide meaning to the material
2. Arrange the information in a systematic way
3. Form meaningful associations
4. Use visualization as an aid
5. Concentrate on the material during the encoding process
6. Provide feedback during the process (Poon, 1984)

Mnemonics are internal aids to memory, and they can be helpful to some elderly people—others prefer to rely on external aids. This would include such things as using calendars, making lists, posting notes to oneself, placing objects in certain places (e.g., the letter to be mailed by the front door), and associating certain chores with dates (e.g., every first of the month, the bills are mailed). Some elderly people are using computers to help memory.

The following learning principles have been helpful for memory training in older adults:

1. Allow self-pacing for the individual
2. Use learning material that is relevant to the person
3. Repeat exposure to the learning material
4. Provide a narrow focus that will enhance concentration
5. Procedures used should be consistent and structural (Birren and Abrahams, 1984)

Birren and Abrahams recommend that the gereclinician who is working in individual therapy with an elderly client should encourage note-taking during therapy sessions by the client and keeping a log between sessions. They believe that this method can help ease the burden on memory, and it can also facilitate between-session work by the client.

Pet therapy—loneliness is often the companion of old age. The scope of the problem of loneliness and the elderly may have been underestimated, particularly in terms of its danger to physical and mental health. Advocates of pet therapy see it as an antidote to loneliness. Pets have been introduced into some institutions and encouraged for community-based elders. Pets can provide companionship, physical contact, affection, and meaning to life through the responsibility required in caring for an "other" (Gatz et al., 1985; MacLean, 1987). The choice of a pet can be matched with the abilities of the elderly person. For example, a self-sufficient indoor cat might be better for a housebound elder than a dog because of the dog's need for "walking."

Family therapy

The same principles that apply to family therapy in general (see Chapter 14) apply to family therapy with an elder. There are some differences, but similarities are far more numerous (Herr and Weakland, 1984). There are some important issues to be aware of in conducting family therapy with an "identified patient" who is an elder:

1. Therapists are apt to give up too soon or set their goals too low when working with an elderly person who is the "identified patient." The possibility of organic impairment is almost always raised either overtly or simply in the therapist's own thoughts.
2. If organic impairment is present, some clini-

cians believe they can have little or no effect on the family system.

3. Therapists may have to be more aggressive in collaborating with the elder's physicians to ensure that any behavioral problems are not the result of chronic diseases, poor nutrition, overmedication, or the interaction of drugs prescribed by different specialists.

4. In family therapy with elders, therapists may have to work harder to get other family members to attend sessions.

5. There may be a need to consider staff members of institutions such as nursing homes as part of an "extended family." Relationships between staff members and the elder's family members may be very important to the person's well-being.

6. The structure of a family is continually changing as its members grow and develop in different ways. When an older client with adult children is the "identified patient," issues of control, autonomy, and dependency are particularly important. For example, filial maturity may be an important goal.

7. Filial maturity, or the ability of an adult child to be depended upon by an aging parent, is an important role change that can have a profound effect on the physical and mental health of an elderly person (adapted from Herr and Weakland, 1984; Wolinsky, 1986).

Marital therapy—marital therapy for people over 60 years of age is becoming increasingly common (Wolinsky, 1986). Techniques and problems are similar to those used with younger couples, but some factors, goals, and tasks are specific to the mature-stage marriage:

1. Intimacy, interactional patterns, and roles need redefining as, after retirement, the couple spends more time together.

2. After retirement, a redefinition of the couple's roles and patterns within the extended family must be accomplished.

3. New goals, appropriate to changing relationships and individual lives, need to be formulated.

4. The mourning of losses related to self, spouse, and marriage will occur as the marital pattern changes through the life cycle.

5. One task may involve the mourning of loss of

a spouse through incapacitation or institutionalization in a nursing home.

6. Another related task would be the acceptance of oneself as an individual and one's life as meaningful, apart from one's spouse (after institutionalization or incapacitation).

7. Validation of all stages of the marriage through such mechanisms as *The Life Review* within the context of the marriage (a marital life review) is a goal (adapted from Wolinsky, 1986).

Group and activity therapies for the elderly

Principles and practices of group and activity therapies outlined and discussed in Chapters 12 and 13 also apply to interventions with elderly clients. One important value of group treatment for elderly people is that it helps to counteract the loneliness, isolation, and withdrawal of a negative disengagement from the world. The negative disengagement is based on low self-esteem and is exacerbated by the losses of aging and the negative stereotyping from society that the elder accepts as inevitable. Feelings of *cohesiveness* within the group and a sense of being *included* by other members can heal these negative feelings. Group leaders working with the elderly use reminiscing or The Life Review to facilitate the task of *integrity* vs. *despair* and the acceptance of one's death as a part of the natural cycle. Guilt over past failures and anxiety over present circumstances are reduced, and self-esteem is increased through the task accomplishment and through the mutual support. Problem solving and reality testing are also enhanced through the structures and process of group treatment (Horton and Linden, 1982; Johnson, 1985; Leszcz et al., 1985; Sorenson, 1986).

There are values to homogeneity and to heterogeneity in structuring the group. A homogeneous age group can work on similar issues and feel understood by one another (Blazer, 1982). A heterogeneous group that mixes age and gender can have the advantage of helping the members to work out specific transferential problems and intergenerational tensions and conflicts. The value of this should be remembered by nurses working on short-term inpatient psychiatric units. Too often, the one or two elderly clients on a unit are excluded from group therapy sessions by staff members who don't understand that differences can provide "grist for the mill" through multiple transference situations.

Various activities are used to facilitate group interaction and to increase self-esteem in the elderly. A person who has no meaningful work or chance to express creativity will experience a lack of balance in life (Hatter and Nelson, 1987). The stereotyping of old age and declining creativity may be the result of an inhibition of our senior citizens. Certainly, as the list of the prominent creative artists earlier in this chapter confirms, older people can be just as creative as their younger counterparts. Encouragement from others can help counteract the inhibition of creativity, and everyone does not have to be Grandma Moses to reap the benefits. There are numerous incidents of elderly people who start to paint or model clay for the first time in senior citizen groups and who then continue to make it a meaningful way of expression. Activity therapies such as art and music and dance groups, besides facilitating expression of creativity, also provide a nonverbal method of interpersonal relating and communicating (Johnson, 1986). The physical exercise of capabilities and creative expression of such groups is also of great value to elderly clients (Hatter and Nelson, 1987). Drama therapy, besides its other values, helps to establish meaningful interpersonal relationships and facilitate insight through transference phenomena occurring among the group members. A form of drama therapy, modified to the needs of clients with impaired cognition, can be particularly helpful in facilitating communication through the supervised "acting out" of feelings, memories, and preconscious thoughts (Johnson, 1985). One might not be able to express, in words, feelings of isolation and powerlessness, but a short "scene" of symbolic acting out of these feelings in a protected atmosphere can help. Material that is too conflictual can be disowned, if necessary, through the medium of a playful and metaphorical atmosphere. Role playing and physical involvement simplify complex feelings, making it easier for group members to focus on problems (Johnson, 1985). The value of activities therapy for the elderly client is an accepted part of treatment rationale and planning in senior citizen groups, nursing homes, and geriatric psychiatric facilities.

Somatic therapies

Somatic therapy for the elderly includes electroconvulsive treatment, nutritional therapy, exercise, and pharmacological treatment. Nutritional problems are common in elderly clients because of cultural conflicts and incompatibilities (Blazer, 1982; Pasquali, 1985), decreased income, and social isolation. Physical factors include dental and denture problems, poor gustatory sensations, and medical problems that interfere with food intake and absorption. Poor nutrition can have a profound effect on the psyche of the elderly client and is of particular importance through its interaction with depression. Depression leads to poor nutrition, which feeds back to depressive symptoms (Blazer, 1982). Blazer believes that clinicians treating depression in the elderly should obtain a dietary history (Natow and Heslin, 1980) from the client.

Exercise as therapy can have a positive effect on the physical and emotional status of the individual. Much attention has been paid to the role of exercise in alleviating the symptoms of depression (Blazer, 1982). Exercise can be a relaxation technique for the elderly and can include deep breathing exercises, mobility and flexibility exercises (stretching), swimming, and walking. Some elders enjoy a modified form of yoga.

Electroconvulsive treatment (see Chapter 22 for a discussion of ECT) has been used for severe depressive episodes in later life. An important benefit of this form of therapy is the prevention of suicide. Suicide rates are much higher in the older population (Neshkes and Jarvik, 1986). Because reversal of depressive symptoms is faster and safer with ECT than with drugs, ECT may be chosen for older people who are severely depressed (Blazer, 1982). One of its side effects, memory loss, is more common in the elderly than in younger people.

Pharmacological treatment of the elderly includes drugs similar to those used at other stages of life. But it is important to note that:
1. Drugs act differently in elderly clients than in younger people—unusual reactions to drugs

are more likely with the elderly (Age Page, 1987). Reasons for the differences include decreased ability to excrete drugs because of chronic renal failure and a diminished volume of body water that occurs as we age. This latter phenomenon makes the standard dose of a medication less diluted in the smaller volume of fluid and overdose therefore more common (Bennet, 1987; Blazer, 1982).

2. Elderly people are at greater risk for medication errors due to declining sensory acuity and memory as well as misunderstanding about directions that can occur with the preoccupation of depression.

3. Periodic review of all of an elderly person's medications is a must. One writer suggests the "paper bag" method for seeing all the drugs that are being taken. This is especially important when there is more than one specialist treating the person (as is usually the case). The client (or family member) simply puts all the medications being taken, including nonprescription drugs, into a paper bag and presents it to the physician for review (Bennet, 1987). Periodic testing of blood levels for some drugs is necessary, and periodic surveillance of blood electrolytes in elderly persons taking Lithium is especially important for those with cardiac or renal problems (Matteson, 1984).

4. Many drugs are used to treat the elderly for physical and psychological problems whose side effects can mimic or precipitate dementia. Combined with the fact that depression in the elderly can also mimic dementia, this presents a danger for tragic misdiagnosis in the elderly client.

Emergency intervention with the elderly client

Some guidelines for dealing with elderly clients in emergency situations include:

1. Poor nutrition and dehydration can exacerbate psychological symptoms—they should be assessed. The elderly are at risk for hypothermia. Attention to the physical subsystem cannot be neglected when intervening in the psychosocial subsystem.

2. Depression and dementia must be differentiated, since the symptoms of one can mimic the symptoms of the other.

3. Adverse medication reactions in the elderly are endemic. This is a crucial area in assessing the elderly client in crisis.

4. Members of the older age group, particularly elderly men, are at highest risk for suicide. Elders in crisis in emergency clinics or outpatient facilities need to be assessed for lethality of suicide risk or to determine if the crisis situation is a product of a suicide attempt.

5. With elderly people, an emergency crisis situation often reflects other underlying problems (Butler and Lewis, 1973).

6. The elderly person's recovery from any emergency crisis will generally take longer than will a younger client's.

Nursing Intervention
PRIMARY PREVENTION

A helpful way to look at primary prevention and the health problems of the elderly is to consider the heterogeneity of the population and to refer again to Rowe and Kahn's (1987) concept of "usual vs. successful aging." Primary prevention of problems associated with "usual aging" would imply a prevention of pathophysiological and psychopathological changes, while primary prevention of impediments to "successful aging" would imply prevention of some or all of the expected (so-called age-related) physiological changes and all or some of the blocks to continuing psychosocial/spiritual development in the elderly. Accidents, being accidental, are particularly hazardous to the elderly and can occur to an individual who is involved in a "successful" as well as a "usual" process of aging. Table 18-3 illustrates the areas of primary prevention for the elderly from this dual approach.

SECONDARY PREVENTION

As the population of elderly people increases, nurses who care for the aged are growing in num-

TABLE 18-3   Primary prevention with common physical, psychological, and spiritual coping patterns in the elderly

Usual aging		Successful aging	
Pattern	Primary prevention	Pattern	Primary prevention
Osteoporosis	Adequate diet; exercise program; life-style changes (decrease alcohol, caffeine; stop smoking)	Decreased bone density of "aging"	Sustained physical fitness program; maintenance of optimal diet; life-long health habits concerning smoking, drinking, and caffeine intake
Diabetes	Proper diet to correct carbohydrate intolerance; adequate exercise; periodic physical check-ups; obesity control	Carbohydrate intolerance	Sustained physical fitness program; maintenance of optimal diet; life-long health habits concerning weight control
Cardiovascular disease	Adequate diet; exercise; life-style changes (smoking, alcohol, caffeine); stress management, appropriate medications for other existing conditions (e.g., high blood pressure), periodic physical check-ups	High serum cholesterol, high blood pressure, increased body weight	Sustained physical fitness program; maintenance of optimal diet; life-long health habits concerning smoking, drinking, and weight control
Accidents	Monitoring and correction of physical health and sensory acuity; environmental modification (lighting, furniture placement, etc.); client learning and awareness, adequate social/family/peer networking	Accidents	Monitoring and correction of physical health and sensory acuity; environmental modification; client learning and awareness; adequate social/family/peer networking
Depression, substance abuse	Bereavement counseling; adequate networking; group living concept*; pet therapy; attention to cultural factors specific to client; periodic review of medication regimen	Inability to master life task of integrity vs. despair, decreased self-esteem	Logotherapeutic use of past, reminiscing, Life Review; enhancement of the client's cultural heritage; bereavement support
Anxiety and helplessness	Adequate social/family/peer networking; maintenance of sense of autonomy and control; attention to cultural factors specific to client; combat immobility due to physical or social reasons	Blocked creativity and inability to self-actualize	Creative arts program; learning experiences: e.g., Elderhostel† program and Eldercraftsmen, Inc.‡; careers and jobs; enhancement of the client's cultural heritage
Confusion	Periodic review of medication regimen; adequate social/family/peer networking; monitoring of physical condition and appropriate treatment; use of clocks and calendars	Benign memory loss	Mnemonic devices; memory training; lists and environmental manipulation; word skill games (e.g., crossword puzzles, Scrabble)

*Group living concept: "Shared housing" for the elderly—single, elderly people are able to pool finances, share the necessary chores and cooking, perhaps even hire a manager or director to relieve them of some of the work. Some group homes are private endeavors, others are supported and managed by social agencies. Loneliness and isolation are greatly relieved by group living units (Evans, 1988).

†Elderhosteling: A network of over 700 participating colleges and universities in all 50 states and some foreign countries. Older people take brief summer courses in subjects that interest them and explore new places. All of this is available for a reasonable fee that includes course, room and meals (MacLean, 1987).

‡Eldercraftsmen, Inc.: An organization that "educates, encourages and advises older people in the making of fine handicrafts, thereby improving the quality of their lives and adding to their dignity, their creative satisfaction and their incomes" (MacLean, 1987).

ber. One of the new ANA certification offerings to be introduced in 1989 is for clinical specialists in gerontological nursing (*American Nurse*, April, 1988, 3). Our country has never had so many elderly citizens, and according to Dr. Jane Chandler, a certified geriatric nurse, geriatric nursing is the "new frontier." Dr. Chandler (1987) describes some necessary attributes of anyone who would care for the aged: "It requires a working knowledge of the aging process, and understanding of the etiology and treatment of chronic conditions and an appreciation of the losses experienced by most aged persons." Gillin (1973) was talking specifically about group work with the elderly, but her prerequisite for working with older adults is applicable for all models of intervention: ". . . a firm belief that personality growth and behavioral change can take place at any time of life." The complexity of the aging process and the vast heterogeneity of experience and attributes that the elderly population presents make it imperative that we also maintain the view of aging as an asset that can be enhanced and not simply a degenerative process (Zarit and Zarit, 1984). While there are identifiable themes, aging is a unique experience for each individual. It may also be particularly difficult for younger people to empathize with. The powerful denial that surrounds death, dying, and the aging process contributes to this. Nursing theorist Margaret Newman, in her ongoing study of subjective time as experienced by the elderly, suggests that, as one grows older, one's inner experience changes. What younger people may view as evidence of slowing down or deterioration (for example, inactivity or increased reverie) is really an expanded sense of time. Because there is a natural difficulty in getting in touch with another person's inner experience and because, as younger people, we have not yet experienced it, we may tend to think that the elderly person's behavior is unhealthy. It is *not* our own reality—Newman suggests that it is *beyond* our reality (Newman, 1987).

Nursing process

The nursing process is the framework for nursing intervention with elderly clients. This section will focus on secondary prevention through intervention into clients' unhealthy patterns of coping with stress. This requires of the nurse an open attitude that is on guard against the many stereotypes imposed upon elderly people as well as an understanding of Maslow's concept of *self-actualization* (see Chapter 6) and of Erikson's life crisis of *integrity* vs. *despair* as the appropriate developmental task of old age. Eliopolous (1982) has outlined some basic principles of gerontological nursing. They include:

1. Aging is a *natural* process, common to all living organisms.
2. Heterogeneity of experiences and attributes influences the aging process and results in a unique experience for each individual.
3. The elderly peron's basic needs are similar to all other people's.
4. In fulfilling basic needs, each elderly person has unique self-care abilities and limitations.

ASSESSMENT

Irene Mortenson Burnside, a respected pioneer in the field of gerontological nursing, tells us that, in interviewing the aged client, three very important areas to assess are (1) physical and psychological distance, (2) hearing, and (3) comprehension.

1. The physical distance a person maintains is, in the elderly, affected by hearing and vision impairment and, particularly in the institutionalized elderly, by feelings of territoriality. The psychological distance in the elderly is affected by diminished attention span, physical exhaustion related to debilitating illness, the effects of medication, and a past history of poor interpersonal relations.
2. Assessment of hearing is naturally relevant in interviewing anyone, and, with the increased rate of impairment in the elderly, it becomes more important. Distance between interviewer and interviewee is necessarily shorter with the hearing impaired. Making lip reading more accessible and placing chairs beside the best hearing ear are helpful measures.
3. Assessment of comprehension—much of what Burnside writes for this area concerns the organically impaired elderly and does not really apply here. But some things that should be considered include *pacing oneself to the*

client, which usually means going more slowly and remembering that *reminiscing* and an *expanded time sense* may impose a slower pace. Burnside sees the real value of reminiscing as enhancing self-esteem, promoting healthy adaptation through social relations, maintaining a consistent self-concept, working through losses and changes, and reaffirming a sense of identity. As Burnside points out it can also provide many of the answers about the life style of the person being sought in the interview (Burnside, 1973).

The following section assists students in assessing elderly clients in institutions and in the community.

A *Life Review* done by the client can add to the scope of the nursing assessment as well as provide a valuable and therapeutic effect in itself. Included should be the client's assessment of his or her own strengths.

The nurse, in assessing elderly clients, should include the following areas:

1. Presenting symptoms or patterns of behavior; depression, confusion, substance abuse, inability to maintain adequate nutrition, susceptibility to accidents, degree of any self-care deficit.

2. Emotional state; feelings of loss and vulnerability, isolation, anxiety, helplessness, despair.

3. Stimulus situations; stressful life situations that are characterized by a threat to one's security and the frustration of one's attempts to satisfy needs (these stressful life situations may be engendered by maladaptive behavior or by the realities of life as an elderly person). What losses and changes have occurred and when?

4. Coping patterns; how effective are they? What coping behavior and strategies were used habitually in the younger years? They may be exaggerated in the present. Which coping patterns are newly developed in response to current stressful situations or problems?

5. Available support systems and resources. What services are available and which are appropriate? Possible services needed would include:

counseling
consumer education and cultural enrichment
employment, retirement
health care
housing
food (shopping, meal planning, meal provision)
financial and financial aid
legal
tax counseling and preparation
recreational
transportation
volunteer opportunity
chore assistance
home care
day care
respite care for families (adapted from Eliopolous, 1982)

6. *Holistic health status*—the physical, intellectual, emotional, sociocultural, and spiritual status of the client. These factors may either facilitate wellness (for example, a supportive and effective extended family system that can assist a moderately disabled elderly person to retain a degree of independence while living in the community), or these factors may impede wellness (for example, the poverty and isolation of some elderly clients prevents them from participating in programs that foster self-actualization through chosen and meaningful activities). Physical status assessment of the elderly is particularly important as it is the crucial basis for a person's other four subsystems. Physical losses, disabilities, chronic diseases, and medication regimen are all significant areas for the nurse to assess.

ANALYSIS OF DATA

Nurses, in assessing presenting symptoms, emotional status, stimulus situations, past and present coping patterns, and holistic health status of the client system can begin to understand the client's (and sometimes, the family's) perception of the presenting problem. The nurse's understanding is increased by participating with the client in any formalized life review or spontaneous reminiscing that may occur. Knowledge and understanding of the available community services for the elderly render the nursing assessment more valuable. The complexity of the aging process and the problems faced by the elderly can provide a challenge to nurses who are interested in providing comprehensive care to their clients. The following section will focus on some nursing diagnoses particularly relevant to the elderly client. With the understanding that one chapter in a book cannot do adequate justice to all nursing care problems in the elderly, it should be noted that the focus is primarily psychosocial. Other excellent texts and articles on geriatric nursing and medical-surgical nursing texts can provide insight and understanding about the physical disabilities and chronic illnesses of the elderly. Depression is a major problem with the elderly population—the reader is referred to Chapter 22 for nursing diagnoses associated with this maladaptive pattern of coping. Substance abuse is covered comprehensively in Chapter 20. The nursing diagnoses discussed here will be:

1. Altered family processes related to the situational crisis of nursing home placement.
2. Potential for injury related to sensory-perceptual alteration (vision, hearing, temperature-sensitivity); altered thought processes (memory deficit/problems); impaired home-maintenance management.
3. Sleep pattern disturbance related to sensory alterations; internal (illness, psychological stress), external (environmental changes, social cues).
4. Altered nutrition, less than body requirements, related to social isolation, inadequate finances, inadequate support system, cultural dissonance, altered taste sensation, misinformation and misconceptions.
5. Altered thought processes evidenced by memory deficit.
6. Powerlessness related to learned helplessness, sensory loss, role loss, situational loss of autonomy and control.
7. Spiritual distress related to inability to master the developmental task of integrity vs. despair.

An important goal in interviewing clients is to safeguard their autonomy in decision making whenever possible. This is particularly important with the elderly client who often experiences an erosion of decision making in many areas.

PLANNING AND IMPLEMENTATION

The nursing care plans on pp. 543-546 reflect a realistic approach to secondary preventive intervention. The nurse may initially establish goals; but as therapy progresses, the client may enter into goal-setting to ensure the client's commitment to accomplishing these goals.

▶ **Sample interaction**

The following sample interaction demonstrates logotherapeutic use of the past and the life review.

Client is a 75-year-old widow, no children. She is in the hospital for an extended stay because she broke her hip in a fall on an icy sidewalk. She also complains of "never feeling up to par—even before I broke my hip." Tests have disclosed no serious physical problems. She has been discussing her concerns with a psychiatric nurse doing liaison work from the psychiatric unit. They have set up a regular twice-weekly schedule of meetings, and they are in the beginning stages of a working relationship.

Client *I don't think I'm depressed; I just don't feel good—I don't know what it is.*

Nurse *Can you describe it to me?*

Client *It feels kind of—I don't know—blah! I have no energy for anything.*

Nurse *How long have you felt like this?*

Client *Well, when Joe died, I did feel terrible, I guess I was depressed then. But I couldn't go on that way forever—I mean I have to keep on with my life now. I cried a lot and people were good to me. My sister's daughter Suzy helped me a lot (pause: thinking about what she's said), but I feel like I'm in the way—over there so much! They ask me for every holiday and lots of times in between. I guess I feel like a fifth wheel with Suzy and Jim—they have their own family—four kids, and she's so busy!*

Nurse *Tell me about Suzy—were you both close in the past?*

Client *(smiling) Oh yes! We didn't have children of our own—we tried but we never could. Joe and I were crazy about Suzy!*

Nurse *What did you do, then?*

Client *We used to take her places—you know, the zoo and to movies! We even took her with us on vacation once or twice. She loved staying at our house—even when she was a teenager.*

Nurse *Really?*

Client *Yes, (quietly) she had some trouble with my sister* and her husband, Bill . . . he used to drink too much (pause) but that's all behind him now—he really worked on his problems. Suzy even lived with us for several months; we loved having her but we also felt very sorry for the whole family.

Nurse Sounds like you were pretty helpful to Suzy when she needed you.

Client Yes, you know I hadn't really thought about all of that for a long time. You know, I guess Suzy really does care about me. Joe always said we were important to her.

Nurse It sounds like you've got a lot of good memories about that—maybe some painful ones too—about your sister and her husband.

Client Yes, I guess I do. I'll have to think about that (silence).

Nurse Sometimes when we get caught up in the present we forget about the important things that happened in the past—I know that happens to me.

Client You know, you're right; I haven't been thinking about much lately except how to get through a boring day (looking at the clock). I guess time is up isn't it? Can we talk about this some more? I mean, next time you come by?

Nurse Yes, to both questions! I'll be back on Thursday. Why don't you write down some of your thoughts and memories—whatever comes to mind between now and Thursday. We can go over it together.

Client I'll do that! You know, I feel better talking about this stuff from the past.

Nurse I'm glad. See you Thursday!

EVALUATION

The evaluation of the problems in coping that elderly clients experience requires an ongoing assessment of the client's physical, emotional, mental, social, and spiritual status. The client, and when appropriate the client's family, should be included in evaluating the progress made toward attainment of short- and long-term goals:

1. Estimating the degree to which unhealthy coping patterns have decreased (e.g., depression, substance abuse, powerlessness, noncompliance with medication regimen).
2. Estimating the degree to which goals have been achieved and client has improved life patterns. This may be demonstrated by improved management of activities of daily living, decrease in maladaptive coping patterns, and/or incorporation of behaviors indicative of

effective coping (e.g., use of relaxation techniques and moderate exercise rather than reliance on sleeping pills). Increased decision making with decreased feelings of powerlessness are other indications.
3. Identifying goals that need to be modified or revised.
4. Referring the client to support systems other than nurse-client relationship:
   a. people in client's social network who are willing to serve as supports
   b. community agencies that help clients cope with patterns of aging. For example:
      1. financial counseling
      2. elder-education programs
      3. senior citizen centers/day care
      4. health care, including appropriate, periodic physical/medical assessment
      5. housing authority
      6. transportation services
      7. home care and chore services
      8. respite care for family caregivers

TERTIARY PREVENTION

Many of the elderly already suffer from the disabling effects of changes and losses in their lives. Many are in need of help with the everyday task of living. Such tasks as bathing, walking, dressing, and eating become formidable for some, and self-esteem is often eroded along with independence. A recent article by Joseph Califano, Jr. (Secretary of Health, Education and Welfare from 1977 to 1979) highlights this important area of concern in our health-care system. Dr. Califano advocates an expanded research effort to combat the threats to elderly independence. He also suggests major improvements in community programs to help the elderly person maintain as much self-care as possible—to be able to function safely at home. This could improve the quality of life and the self-esteem of many elderly people. It could also ease the burden of family members who are often stressed by the caregiver role. Califano estimates that it would also be cost effective; an economic advantage for our overburdened health care system. According to Califano, "Each reduction of one month in the average period of dependence means

Text continued on p. 547.

NURSING CARE PLAN
Elderly Clients

Long-term Outcomes	Short-term Outcomes	Nursing Strategies

Nursing diagnosis: Altered family processes related to the situational crisis of nursing home placement (NANDA 3.2.2)

Long-term Outcomes	Short-term Outcomes	Nursing Strategies
Achieve an optimal adjustment to nursing home setting Maintain a mutually supportive relationship with family members	Identify stressors in the immediate situational crisis Verbalize feelings associated with the stressful situation (when consistent with client's cultural orientation) Clarify information related to admission, adjustment, and relocation Collaborate with family in admission process and subsequent adjustment to relocation	Provide separate, private atmospheres where • client can discuss feelings and concerns about placement; • family members can discuss feelings and concerns about placement Provide an atmosphere where client-family can talk without outside interruption Help the client and family members identify stressors in the crisis situation Provide information about admission, adjustment, and relocation Facilitate discussion between client and family members about impending placement Allow client to make all possible decisions about relocation Support client in all possible decision making about relocation

Nursing diagnosis: Potential for injury related to sensory-perceptual alteration (vision, hearing, temperature-sensitivity); altered thought processes (memory deficit/problems); impaired home maintenance management (NANDA 1.6.1)

Long-term Outcomes	Short-term Outcomes	Nursing Strategies
Prevent injury through accidents Follow a safety-oriented life style	Identify potential hazards in: • physiological states of self • psychological/mental status of self • home environment • community environment • medication regimen Increase knowledge of safety mechanisms, environmental modifications, and accident prevention Begin to institute some appropriate safety mechanisms Explore alternative mechanisms for enlarging social support network Explore array of available community services	Provide atmosphere where client and nurse can talk Assess the client and the client's environmental potential for accidents* Assess the client's understanding of risk potential and use of safety mechanisms Discuss possible use of appropriate safety mechanisms and environmental modifications Discuss alternative means for enlarging social support network Describe available community services (e.g., financial, housing, counseling, transportation, homemaker services, visiting nurse, emergency response services, physical assessment/health care) Refer client to appropriate and available community services

*For an excellent home-safety tool, see Parsons and Levy (1987).

Continued.

NURSING CARE PLAN—cont'd

Elderly Clients

Long-term Outcomes	Short-term Outcomes	Nursing Strategies

Nursing diagnosis: Sleep pattern disturbance related to sensory alterations: internal (illness, psychological stress), external (environmental changes, social cues) (NANDA 6.2.1)

Long-term Outcomes	Short-term Outcomes	Nursing Strategies
Reach a level of sleep pattern equilibrium that is optimal for self	Identify any possible • physical stimuli • psychological stimuli • environmental stimuli to sleep pattern distrubance Follow through with any appropriate referrals for physical, psychological, medication regimen disturbances Increase knowledge of the various appropriate means to counteract particular problems of sleep pattern disturbance	Assess the client's • physical status • psychological status • environmental situation • medication regimen for possible stimuli to sleep pattern disturbance Assess the client's configuration of sleep patterns (e.g., early wakening? interrupted sleep? can't fall asleep? not fully rested? [Kim and Moritz, 1982]) Rule out depression and substance abuse as possible factors in sleep pattern disturbance Refer if necessary for specific treatment of depression, substance abuse, medication review, physical illness, and for review of medications Discuss possible measures for enhancing healthful sleep—(e.g., relaxation techniques; use of "white noise"; L-tryptophan–containing foods; avoidance of alcohol as a "nightcap"; avoidance of overly stimulating TV programs; use of a good mattress; placement of bed in relation to any light source; use of darkening shades for early a.m.; maintenance of fresh air source)

Nursing diagnosis: Altered nutrition, less than the body's requirements, related to social isolation, inadequate finances, inadequate support systems, cultural dissonance, altered taste sensation, misinformation, and misconceptions (NANDA 1.1.2.2)

Long-term Outcomes	Short-term Outcomes	Nursing Strategies
Maintain an optimal level and quality of nutrition	Identify specific problem areas related to state of altered nutrition Verbalize feelings associated with any specific problem area (e.g., cultural dissonance); this is done when it is consistent with the client's cultural orientation Increase knowledge about optimal diet for health and best ways of preparing food for health Increase knowledge of alternative means of achieving	Provide an atmosphere where client and nurse can talk without interruption Assess the client's nutritional status and differentiated altered status as it related to: • acute or chronic physical illness or disability • severe psychological disorder (e.g., depression, substance abuse) Refer client if necessary for appropriate treatment for acute or chronic illness or disability and/or severe psychological disorder Assess the client's nutritional status as it relates to social support system; financial status; cultural background; altered sense of taste, misinformation, and misconceptions

Long-term Outcomes	Short-term Outcomes	Nursing Strategies

Nursing diagnosis: Altered nutrition, less than the body's requirements, related to social isolation, inadequate finances, inadequate support systems, cultural dissonance, altered taste sensation, misinformation, and misconceptions (NANDA 1.1.2.2)—cont'd

| | optimal nutrition within the existing biopsychosocial boundaries
Explore array of community services available for possible assistance in achieving optimal nutrition | Provide nutrition information about constituents of optimal diet; best ways of preparing food for health
Discuss alternative ways and means for achieving optimal nutrition within the client's biopsychosocial boundaries (e.g., meals on wheels; home health aide; nutrition education programs; use of cooking herbs to enhance taste)
Refer client for resolution of any physical impediment to obtaining optimal nutrition (e.g., repair of teeth, dentures; vision examination and prescription) |

Nursing diagnosis: Altered thought processes evidenced by memory deficit/problems (NANDA 8.3)

| Maintain a problem-solving approach in coping with problems of *benign senescent memory loss*
Maintain self-esteem throughout process of benign senescent memory loss
Achieve an optimal adjustment to the process of benign senescent memory loss | Identify specific problems in living related to *benign senescent memory loss*
Verbalize feelings associated with the process of benign senescent memory loss (when consistent with client's cultural orientation)
Increase knowledge of mnemonic devices, environmental aids to memory, and use of word-skill games as aids for memory training
Begin to institute some appropriate mnemonic devices or memory aids and mind-skill games
Explore array of available home and community resources for exercising the mind | Provide an atmosphere where client and nurse can talk without interruption
Assess client's memory loss pattern to differentiate *benign senescent memory loss* from possible organic impairment or depression
Help client to identify concerns and specific problems in living related to benign senescent memory loss (be particularly cognizant of effects of memory loss on medication regimen)
Discuss various memory aids such as mnemonic devices; environmental aids (e.g., lists, calendar notes to self, placement of objects); word-skill games such as crossword puzzles and Scrabble that may be suited to client
Discuss available resources that might provide mind exercising: Elderhostel program; continuing education programs in local high schools
Encourage client to participate in appropriate, available home and community resources for memory training and mind exercising |

Continued.

Long-term Outcomes	Short-term Outcomes	Nursing Strategies

Nursing diagnosis: Powerlessness related to learned helplessness; sensory loss; role loss; situational loss of autonomy and control (NANDA 7.3.2)

Increase level of decision making in life Increase feelings of autonomy and control within appropriate and realistic biopsychosocial boundaries	Identify feelings of powerlessness Verbalize feelings of powerlessness (when consistent with client's cultural orientation) Connect feelings of powerlessness to factors (a) within the self (b) within the environment Identify factors connected with feelings of powerlessness that can be changed or modified Identify possible ways for modifying factors within the self that induce feelings of powerlessness Explore resources available for strengthening the ability to exercise autonomy and control Decide which ways and resources are appropriate and acceptable for particular situation	Provide atmosphere where client and nurse can talk without interruption Establish a working relationship between client and nurse Help client identify feelings of powerlessness Help client verbalize feelings of powerlessness and other feelings related to it (e.g., low self-esteem, helplessness, anger) Help client to explore relationship of feelings of powerlessness to factors within the self and environment Help client to identify powerlessness-inducing factors within self and environment that can be changed or modified and those that cannot Protect/respect client's autonomy and control within the nurse-client relationship and in relation to decision making Discuss available resources for strengthening client's ability to exercise autonomy and control (e.g., housing authority, legal aid, psychotherapy, family therapy, job training, career choices, consumer advocacy assistance)

Nursing diagnosis: Spiritual distress related to inability to master lifestage task of *integrity* vs. *despair* (NANDA 4.1.1)

Develop a positive sense of self Develop a realistic appraisal of past joys, losses, and failures Work through an acceptance of past losses and failures Integrate various aspects of past and present life Begin a process of acceptance of death	Verbalize concerns about self and past and present life (when consistent with client's cultural orientation) Participate in reminiscing and life review Increase self-esteem Develop an attitude of openness toward self and past life Verbalize feelings and beliefs about death	Provide an atmosphere where nurse and client can talk without interruption Establish a working nurse-client relationship Help client to identify concerns about present life Help client to review past life through reminiscing, a formal life review, logotherapeutic use of the past* Help client to connect past life events, accomplishments, losses, and failures to present-day concerns Encourage client to participate in an ongoing process of review of past life with connections to the present Provide therapeutic climate wherein client can verbalize thoughts and feelings about death

*See sample interaction on pp. 541-542.

a saving of up to $4 billion in health care and custodial costs" (Califano, 1988). While there certainly needs to be more effort in this direction, there are some helpful programs available in community and inpatient settings: day care, home care, and respite care.

Day care

Adult day care has been growing steadily in this country for the past 10 years (Ohnsorg, 1981). Day care helps to enhance the daily living of the elderly and to keep them involved in the community. Adult day care is coordinated with other services such as senior citizen centers, home care services, and inpatient care. According to Ohnsorg, day care programs all vary, but they do have a common goal: "To provide a noninstitutionalized support system for persons who would otherwise have difficulty in maintaining their independent living status in the community setting."

Day care centers can be found in several locations such as senior centers, hospitals, nursing homes, churches, and remodeled elementary schools. Most centers operate from 8 AM to 4:30 PM and from Monday to Friday. They will accept clients for the full period of time if they can secure their own transportation. Other clients can attend for specific hours or for specific days depending on their needs and their transportation resources. Day care programs can provide socialization, nutritional supplementation and education, coordination of health care services, a program of therapy, social services, and respite care for caregivers (Ohnsorg, 1981).

Day care treatment is a valuable alternative to inpatient or nursing home care, but it does require that the individual be able to manage at home with self-care or have someone available as a caregiver. It may also require that the individual have transportation available (Shanas and Maddox, 1985). The focal point for adult day care in the country has been the National Institute on Adult Day Care, which is a unit of the National Council on Aging. It promotes the concept of community-based day care for older Americans, and it provides assistance for establishing new programs. It also promotes research aimed at achieving practical solutions to many of the problems of providing care to elderly people (MacLean, 1987).

Home care

In today's cost-conscious society, home care for the elderly is being seen as a feasible alternative to nursing homes. The National Council on Aging estimates that home care costs an average $5,000 per year per recipient—the cost of a nursing home ranges from $20,000 to $50,000 per year. Recently there has been an improvement in the availability of state- and community-sponsored home care. Family members are still the most likely caregivers, but changing social norms (such as smaller families, greater mobility, and more women in the workforce) complicate the lives of families and their ability to provide care. Home care can include a range of services from occasional visits by visiting nurses to live-in health aides. A partial list of services that may be provided through Medicare, Medicaid, or private insurance companies follows:

1. Physical therapy (i.e., after a stroke or accident)
2. Speech therapy (i.e., after cancer surgery or a stroke)
3. Respiratory therapy (for a person with impaired lung function)
4. Occupational therapy (for a disabled person to learn new ways to accomplish activities of daily living)
5. A registered nurse to assess health status and to provide some part-time skilled nursing services
6. A home health aide to help with grooming, safety, and various kinds of personal care
7. A homemaker to shop, cook, and do light cleaning

Respite care

Family members (especially female family members) remain the biggest resource for the care of elderly people who are dependent in some way (Looney, 1987). Caregivers can become exhausted and severely stressed by their responsibilities. Respite care is a concept that began to gain acceptance in the mid 1970s. It is defined as "care provided on an intermittent basis to provide relief to the family or caregiver from the responsibility of caring for a chronically ill or disabled person" (Looney, 1987, 18).

Respite care can be provided right in the home or in an institution such as a nursing home, acute care hospital, or congregate care facility. Respite care may provide a combination of medical and social services based on the person's particular needs. It is *not* reimbursable by Medicare or by most private insurance companies, but it is a service that is being increasingly sought by caregivers. The "catastrophic" law referred to earlier in this chapter will provide a respite care benefit after January 1, 1990 (AARP Bulletin, September 1988). The help, the "time off," and the emotional support that respite care provides for the caregiver can combat the stress associated with continuous responsibility and involvement with a disabled or ill relative. It enables an elderly person to remain at home longer.

Before an elderly person is admitted for respite care for a week or a weekend, an assessment of his or her status is completed. This includes medications and over-the-counter drugs that are usually taken, treatments used (physician-ordered or family treatments), dietary preferences, self-care abilities, and limitations. This assessment can help the respite care program provide continuity of care during the respite period.

CHAPTER SUMMARY

Growing successfully into old age is a developmental task that Erikson has called *integrity* vs. *despair*. It can be another opportunity for continued self-actualization. Growing old can also be the source of much stress and conflict as people cope with age-related losses and changes and the negative stereotyping that is part of a youth-oriented culture. Such a determined preference for youth may give little credit to the growth in wisdom that aging can represent. Our population of elderly people is growing rapidly, as is the proportion of old people to young. Because of unique situations and characteristics, there is a vast heterogeneity of ag-

ing experiences among the elderly. "Successful vs. usual aging" is a concept that should be considered along with "pathological vs. normal"—particularly in the process of primary prevention with the elderly.

Myths about aging abound and can lead to the stereotyping and unfair discrimination of *ageism*. The self-esteem and autonomy of elderly people can reflect the negative view of aging that is often present in the culture. Legislation to protect the rights of the elderly in the workplace and in nursing homes continues to improve. Some elderly people are also active in fighting for their rights through groups such as the Gray Panthers, the A.A.R.P., and O.W.L. (Older Women's League). Others among the elderly feel lost and powerless in a complicated health care system and with their own declining financial security. Maladaptive patterns of coping include depression, substance abuse, poor nutrition, sleep disturbances, and susceptibility to accidents. Loss and change are major themes of aging, as most people must adapt to declining sensory acuity, declining health, and decreased mobility.

Retirement can represent the "golden years" for many aging people, or it can be a frightening loss of status, finances, and meaning in life. Social Security income and the health care provided by Medicare is available to some of our senior citizens, but not all.

The assessment of an elderly client's needs, resources, abilities, and limitations is essential to an adequate program of therapy. Treatment modalities such as individual, group, activity, family, and somatic therapies may need to be modified, but principles remain the same. The strain that family members and other caregivers can experience in caring for the frail elderly is a problem that needs to be addressed. Support through such programs as day care, home care, and respite care may help to ease the burden and can enable the elderly person who is partially independent to remain at home.

SELF-DIRECTED LEARNING

Sensitivity-Awareness Exercises

The purpose of these exercises is to:
- Develop awareness about the subjective experience of elderly clients who are experiencing some of the losses and changes associated with the aging process.
- Develop awareness about the subjective experience of the families and/or caregivers involved with the elderly.
- Develop awareness about your own feelings and attitudes when working with elderly clients.
- Develop awareness about your own feelings and attitudes toward aging.

1. Spend 2 or 3 hours of your day pursuing your usual routine, but make the following modifications:
   a. Wear dark sunglasses
   b. Place cotton in your outer ear canal
   c. Purposely move at approximately half your usual speed

   Keep a diary of your thoughts and feelings as you go through this exercise.
2. Spend an afternoon with a friend (family member, classmate). Have your friend wait on you for everything you need, including lunch or supper. As you remain seated in one place for this exercise, jot down your thoughts and feelings. Discuss your feelings and your friend's feelings about the experience after it is completed.
3. Develop a plan for supporting and counseling the family members of an elderly person who is about to move in with the family because of declining independence. The elderly person is reluctant to do so, and the family members are concerned about the effects of the change on their household. Compose a cast of characters with names and role descriptions for the plan.
4. As a group (clinical group, classmates in theory course), act out a counseling session using the cast of characters from the preceding exercise.
5. Write a short essay on how you imagine you will be living your life when you are 93. Describe any ailments you might have. What will your interests be? Where will you live? What activities of daily living will be difficult? Which ones will not be difficult? Before writing the essay, do some observing of and thinking about your family and any older

members to get some inspiration for your projection into the future.
6. Spend an entire day with an elderly friend or family member. Ask this person to talk to you about his or her younger days. Take some notes (with permission) when this process is occurring. After the reminiscing, make a mental note of how the person seemed to react. Ask the individual about thoughts and feelings in doing this for you.

Questions to Consider

1. *Ageism* is a term used to describe:
   a. *Learned helplessness* in the elderly and results in attempts to maintain autonomy through control of others.
   b. An overconcern with one's age that begins in mid-life and inhibits the elder's participation in the task of *generativity* vs. *stagnation*.
   c. A philosophy of ancient times and of some present-day primitive cultures that consistently favors the elderly over the younger members of a society.
   d. A form of stereotyping and discrimination practiced against elderly people.
2. *The Life Review* is:
   a. A professional journal that is specifically geared to gerontological health care professionals.
   b. A facilitating technique for clinical staff of geriatric institutions—it is used to plan comprehensive, appropriate care for the elderly clients at staff conferences.
   c. A universal process of remembering, appreciating, accepting, and integrating that is beneficial to the elderly person who carries one out.
   d. An individual form of therapy that should not be used in groups that are homogeneous for age. In this situation, the Life Review should be differentiated from *logotherapeutic use of the past*.
3. According to Erik Erikson, the life stage that is particularly related to the psychosocial development of the elderly is:
   a. Active mastery vs. Learned helplessness and passivity
   b. Integrity vs. Despair
   c. Egocentricity vs. Narcissism
   d. Generativity vs. Stagnation

Continued.

SELF-DIRECTED LEARNING—cont'd

Questions to Consider—cont'd

4. Medicaid, Title XIX of the Social Security Act, is the legislation that is:
   a. A federal program providing health care insurance for elderly people through transfer of payments.
   b. A voluntary health care insurance for the elderly—"Part B."
   c. A system of emergency services for homebound frail elderly people.
   d. A federal-state program that helps finance health care for the medically needy of all ages.
5. The theory of disengagement is:
   a. A universally accepted theory of natural and mutual societal/individual withdrawal.
   b. A theory that contends that as we age, intellectual functions decline slowly and social extroversion increases.
   c. A theory that is the basis for combatting the decline of physical and mental abilities in the aged through the encouragement of mind-skill games, memory devices, and cultural activities.
   d. A controversial theory of aging that includes a belief in a natural and desirable decrease in the social involvement of the elderly.

Match each of the following terms with the statement associated with it:

6. Respite care
7. Day care
8. Medicare
9. Elderhostel

a. Health care insurance for the elderly
b. Usually requires daily transportation resources
c. Temporary, scheduled inpatient hospitalization may be part of it
d. Continuing education system for older people

Answer key
1. d
2. c
3. b
4. d
5. d
6. c
7. b
8. a
9. d

REFERENCES

AARP News Bulletin: New focus on minority aging, AARP News Bull 29(1):6, 1988.

AARP News Bulletin: Answers to key questions about "catastrophic law," AARP News Bull 29(8):14-15, 1987.

AARP News Bulletin: When the mind falters, AARP News Bull 28(9):6-7, 1987.

AARP News Bulletin: AARP leads drive to put 'care' issue in '88 race, AARP News Bull 28(10):1 and 4, 1987.

AARP News Bulletin: AARP News Bull 28(11):2 and 4, 1987.

Achenbaum W: Societal perceptions of aging and the aged, In Binstock R and Shanas E, editors: Handbook of aging and the sociel sciences, ed 2, New York, 1985, Van Nostrand Reinhold Co.

Abrahams J and Crooks V, editors: Geriatric mental health, Orlando, Fla, 1984, Grune & Stratton, Inc.

Age Page: Minorities and how they grow old, Age Page, US Dept of Health and Human Services, April, 1987a.

Age Page: Finding good medical care for older Americans, Age Page, US Dept of Health and Human Services, April, 1987b.

Age Page: Heat, cold and being old, Age Page, US Dept of Health and Human Services, April, 1987c.

Aizenberg R and Treas J: The family in late life, In Birren J and Schaie K, editors: Handbook of the psychology of aging, ed 2, New York, 1985, Van Nostrand Reinhold Co.

Allen M: A holistic view of sexuality and the aged, Holistic Nurs Prac 1(4):76-83, 1985.

American Nurse, April, p. 3, 1988.

Antonucci T: Personal characteristics, social support and social behavior, In Binstock R and Shanas E, editors: Handbook of aging and the social sciences, ed 2, New York, 1985, Van Nostrand Reinhold Co.

Baltes P and Willis S: Toward psychological theories of aging and development, In Birren J and Schaie K, editors: Handbook of the psychology of aging, ed 2, New York, 1985, Van Nostrand Reinhold Co.

Barry P: Iatrogenic disorders in the elderly: preventive techniques, Geriatrics 4(9):42-47, 1986.

Bennet W: Monitoring drugs for the aged, The New York Times Magazine, December 13, 1987.

Beram G and Chauncey C: Money matters: the economics of aging for women, In Doress P and Siegal D, editors: Ourselves growing older: women aging with knowledge and power, New York, 1987, Simon and Schuster.

Binstock R and Shanas E, editors: Handbook of aging and the social sciences, ed 2, New York, 1985, Van Nostrand Reinhold Co.

Bird C: The shape of work to come, Modern Maturity Magazine, June/July, 1987.

Birren J: Relations of development and aging, Springfield, Ill, 1964, Charles C Thomas.

Birren J and Abrahams J: Contributions of the experimental psychology of aging to geriatric mental health, In Abrahams J and Crooks V, editors: Geriatric mental health, Orlando, Fl, 1984, Grune & Stratton, Inc.

Birren J and Renner V: Research on the psychology of aging: principles and experimentation, In Birren J and Schaie K, editors: Handbook of the psychology of aging, New York, 1977, Van Nostrand Reinhold Co.

Birren J and Schaie K, editors: Handbook of the psychology of aging, New York, 1977, Van Nostrand Reinhold Co.

Birren J and Schaie K, editors: Handbook of the psychology of aging, ed 2, New York, 1985, Van Nostrand Reinhold Co.

Blazer D: Depression in late life, St. Louis, 1982, The CV Mosby Co.

Blazer D and Maddox G: The use of epidemiological survey data in planning for geriatric mental health services, In Whanger A, editor: Mental health assessment and therapeutic intervention with older adults. Rockville, Md, 1984, Aspen Systems Corp.

Blenker M: Social work and family relationships in later life with some thoughts on filial maturity, In Shanas E and Streib G, editors: Social structure and the family: generational relations. Englewood Cliffs, NJ, 1965, Prentice-Hall.

Bower F and Patterson J: A theory-based nursing assessment of the aged, Topics Clini Nurs 8(1):22-32, 1986.

Brickfield C: Executive director's report, AARP News Bulletin, 28(8):3, 1987.

Brickfield C: Time to take stock as a milestone nears, Modern Maturity Magazine, October/November, p. 15, 1987.

Brody E: Aging parents and aging children, In Ragan P, editor: Aging parents, Los Angeles, 1979, University of Southern California Press.

Brody J: Alcohol and alcohol abuse, White House Conference on Aging background paper, Bethesda, Md, 1981, National Institute on Aging.

Burnside I: Interviewing the aged, In Burnside I, editor: Psychosocial nursing care of the aged, New York, 1973, McGraw-Hill, Inc.

Burrus-Bammel L and Bammel G: Leisure and recreation, In Birren J and Schaie K, editors: Handbook of the psychology of aging, ed 2, New York, 1985, Van Nostrand Reinhold Co.

Butler R: The life review: an interpretation of reminiscence in the aged, Psychiatry, 26:65-76, 1963.

Butler R: Why survive? being old in America, New York, 1975, Harper & Row.

Butler R and Lewis M: Aging and mental health: positive psychosocial approaches, St. Louis, 1973, The CV Mosby Co.

Califano J: The health-care chaos, The New York Times Magazine, Sunday, March 20, pp. 44-58, 1988.

Callahan D: The case for natural aging, The Hartford Courant, Sunday, October 4, pp. B1 and B4, 1987.

Carlson J: Executive director's report, AARP News Bull 29(1):3, 1988.

Cattell R: Theory of fluid and crystallized intelligence: a critical experiment, J Educ Psychol 54:1-22, 1963.

Chae M: Older Asians, J Gerontol Nurs 13 (11):11-17, 1987.

Chandler J: Editorial: long-term care challenges nursing's capacity to care, Am Nurse, November/December, pp. 4 and 22, 1987.

Chen Y: Economic status of the aging, In Binstock R and Shanas E, editors: Handbook of aging and the social sciences, ed 2, New York, 1985, Van Nostrand Reinhold Co.

Chown S: Morale, careers and personal potentials, In Birren J and Schaie K, editors: Handbook of the psychology of aging, New York, 1977, Van Nostrand Reinhold Co.

Clark R and Baumer D: Income maintenance policies, In Binstock R and Shanas E, editors: Handbook of aging and the social sciences, ed 2, New York, 1985, Van Nostrand Reinhold Co.

Coleman B: Congress enacts landmark bill, AARP News Bull 29(7):1 and 12-13, 1988.

Collins G: Graying of America: growth industry, New York Times, Saturday, December 5, p. 8, 1987a.

Collins G: Wanted: child-care workers, age 55 and up, New York Times, Tuesday, December 15, pp. I and A18, 1987b.

Comfort A: Sexuality and the elderly, In Abrahams J and Crooks V, editors: Geriatric mental health, Orlando, Fla, 1984, Grune & Stratton, Inc.

Crooks V: Impact of policy and planning issues on geriatric mental health care, In Abrahams J and Crooks V, editors: Geriatric mental health, Orlando, Fla, 1984, Grune & Stratton, Inc.

Cumming, E. Further thoughts on the theory of disengagement. Int Soc Sci J 15:377-393, 1963.

Cumming E and Henry W: Growing old, New York, 1961, Basic Books.

Davis K: Health care policies and the aged: observations from the United States, In Binstock R and Shanas E, editors: Handbook of aging and the social sciences, ed 2, New York, 1985, Van Nostrand Reinhold Co.

Deets H: Executive director's report, AARP News Bull 29(7):3, 1988.

Denning J: Older workers and their rights, Modern Maturity Magazine, October/November, p. 14, 1987.

Doress P and Siegal D: Ourselves, growing older: women aging with knowledge and power, New York, 1987, Simon & Schuster.

Eisdorfer C: Models of mental health care for the elderly, In Abrahams J and Crooks V, editors: Geriatric mental health, Orlando, Fla, 1984, Grune & Stratton, Inc.

Eglit H: Age and the law, In Binstock R and Shanas E, editors:

Handbook of aging and the social sciences, ed 2, New York, 1985, Van Nostrand Reinhold Co.

Eliopolous C: Assessment and action in gerontological nursing, In Spradley A, editor: Readings in community health nursing, Boston, 1982, Little, Brown & Co.

Encyclopedia of Social Work: Aging, Washington, DC, 1977, National Association of Social Workers.

Erikson E: Childhood and society, New York, 1950, W W Norton.

Evans O: Group living for the elderly, New York Times, Thursday, January 7, pp. CI and C12, 1988.

Ferris S et al: Recent developments in the assessment of senile dementia, In Abrahams J and Crooks V, editors: Geriatric mental health, Orlando, Fla, 1984, Grune & Stratton, Inc.

Fordham F: An introduction to Jung's psychology, Middlesex, England, 1966, Penguin Books.

Fozard J: Psychotherapy and the optimizing of adult development, In Horton A Jr., editor: Mental health interventions for the aging, New York, 1982, Praeger Publishers, Inc.

Frankl V: Psychotherapy and existentialism: selected papers on logotherapy, New York, 1968, Simon & Schuster.

Frazer J: Of time, passion, and knowledge, New York, 1975, George Braziller, Inc.

Gatz M et al: Psychological intervention with older adults, In Birren J and Schaie K, editors: Handbook of the psychology of aging, ed 2, New York, 1982, Van Nostrand Reinhold Co.

Gillin L: Factors affecting process and content in older adult groups, In Burnside I, editor: Psychosocial nursing care of the aged, New York, 1973, McGraw-Hill, Inc.

Goldenburg B: Depression in the elderly patient: recognition and treatment, Psychiatr Nurs Forum I(4), 1984.

Gollub J: Psychoactive drug misuse among the elderly: a review of prevention and treatment programs, In Kayne R, editor: Drugs and the elderly, EP Andrus Gerontology Center, University of Southern California, 1978.

Gutmann D: The cross-cultural perspective: notes toward a comparative psychology of aging, In Birren J and Schaie K, editors: Handbook of the psychology of aging, New York, 1977, Van Nostrand Reinhold Co.

Hall C and Nordly V: A primer of Jungian psychology, New York, 1973, New American Library, Inc.

Hatter J and Nelson D: Altruism and task participation in the elderly, Am J Occupational Ther, 41(6):379-381, 1987.

Havighurst R and Albrecht R: Older people, New York, 1953, Longmans Green & Co.

Henig R: How a woman ages, New York, 1985, Ballantine Books.

Henthorn B: An ecological view of gerontological mental health, In Lancaster J, editor: Community mental health nursing: an ecological perspective, St. Louis, 1980, The CV Mosby Co.

Herman S: Anxiety disorders, In Whanger A, editor: Mental health assessment and therapeutic invention with older adults, Rockland, Md, 1984, Aspens Systems Corp.

Herr J and Weakland J: Conducting family therapy with elderly clients, In Abrahams J and Crooks V, editors: Geriatric mental health, Orlando, Fla, 1984, Grune & Stratton, Inc.

Horton A: Introduction to the psychotherapy of aging, In Horton A, editor: Mental health interventions for the aged, New York, 1982, Praeger Publishers.

Horton A and Linden M: Geriatric group psychotherapy, In Mental health interventions for the aged, New York, 1982, Praeger Publishers.

Jennings J: Elderly parents as caregivers for their adult dependent children, Social Work 32(5):430-433, 1987.

Johnson D: Expressive group psychotherapy with the elderly: a drama therapy approach, Int J Group Psychother 35(1):109-126, 1985.

Johnson D: The developmental method in drama treatment with the elderly, Arts Psychother 13:17-33, 1986.

Kahn C: Companies help in care for aged, New York Times, Thursday, December 10, pp. CI and C10, 1987.

Kastenbaum R: New thoughts on old age, New York, 1971, Springer Company, Inc.

Kim M and Moritz D, editors: Classification of nursing diagnoses: proceedings of the third and fourth conferences, New York, 1982, McGraw-Hill.

Kline D and Schreiber F: Vision and aging, In Birren J and Schaie K, editors: Handbook of the psychology of aging, ed 2, New York, 1985, Van Nostrand Reinhold Co.

Kral V: Benign senescent forgetfulness, In Alzheimer's disease: senile dementia and related disorders, New York, 1978, Raven Press.

Labouvie-Vief G: Intelligence and cognition, In Birren J and Schaie K, editors: Handbook of the psychology of aging, ed 2, New York, 1985, Van Nostrand Reinhold Co.

Lancaster J: Community mental health nursing: an ecological perspective, St. Louis, 1980, The CV Mosby Co.

LaRue A: Aging and mental disorders, In Birren J and Schaie K, editors: Handbook of the psychology of aging, ed 2, New York, 1985, Van Nostrand Reinhold Co.

Lear M: The pain of loneliness, New York Times Magazine, Sunday, December 20, pp. 47-48, 1987.

LeBray P: Providing clinical geropsychology services in community settings, In Abrahams J and Crooks V, editors: Geriatric mental health, Orlando, Fl, 1984, Grune & Stratton, Inc.

Leszcz M et al: A men's group: psychotherapy of elderly men, Int J Group Psychother 35(2):177-196, 1985.

Longino C and Lipman A: Married and spouseless men and women in planned retirement communities: support network differentials, J Marriage Family 43:285-295, 1981.

Looney K: The respite care alternative, J Gerontol Nurs 13(5): 18-21, 1987.

LoPata H: Women as widows, New York, 1979, Elsevier.

Louden D et al: Common psychological illnesses in the elderly, West Indian Med J 34(3):148-153, 1985.

Lowenthal M: Toward a sociological theory of change in adulthood and old age, In Birren J and Schaie K, editors: Handbook of the psychology of aging, New York, 1977, Van Nostrand Reinhold Co.

McLane A, editor: Classification of nursing diagnoses: proceedings of the seventh congress, National Association of Nursing Diagnoses, St. Louis, 1987, The CV Mosby Co.

MacLean H: Caring for your parents: a sourcebook of options and solutions for both generations, Garden City, 1987, Doubleday & Company, Inc.

Martin E: Eldercare is good business for workers and employees, AARP News Bull 29(4), p. 11, 1988.

Masters W and Johnson V: Human sexual response, Boston, 1966, Little, Brown & Co.

Matteson M: Affective disorders, In Whanger A, editor: Mental health assessment with older adults, Rockland, Md, 1984, Aspen Systems Corp.

Mishara B and Kastenbaum R: Alcohol and old age, New York, 1980, Grune & Stratton, Inc.

Modern Maturity Magazine: Modern Maturity Magazine, October/November, 1987.

Myers A: Understanding the aging process, In Whanger A, editor: Mental health assessment with older adults, Rockland, Md, 1984, Aspen Systems Corp.

Natow A and Heslin J: Geriatric nutrition, Boston, 1980, C.B.I.

Neshkes R and Jarvik L: Depression in the elderly: current management concepts, Geriatrics 4(9):5-58, 1986.

Neugarten B: Age groups in American society and the rise of the young old, Ann Am Acad Polit Soc Sci 415:187-198, 1974.

Newman M: Aging as increasing complexity, J Gerontol Nurs 13(9):6-18, 1987.

New York Times: Study says nursing home costs impoverish many, New York Times, November 9, p. A20, 1987.

New York Times: Older men better off, study says, New York Times, November 26, p. B12, 1987.

New York Times: Retirees resettling in college towns, New York Times, November 29, pp. 1 and 12, 1987.

New York Times: For America's aged: a better break, New York Times, December 26, 1987, p. 22, 1987.

Ohnsorg: Burgeoning daycare movement prolongs independent living, Persp Aging 10(1):18-20, 1981.

Olsho L, Harkins S, and Lenhardt M: Aging and the auditory system, In Birren J and Schaie K, editors: Handbook of the psychology of aging, ed 2, New York, 1985, Van Nostrand Reinhold Co.

Omenn, G: Behavior genetics, In Birren J and Schaie K, editors: Handbook of the psychology of aging, New York, 1977, Van Nostrand Reinhold Co.

Parsons M and Levy J: Nursing process in injury prevention, J Gerontol Nurs 13(7):36-40, 1987.

Pascarelli E: Drug abuse and the elderly, In Laurenson J and Ruiz P, editors: Substance abuse, clinical problems and perspectives, Baltimore, 1981, Williams & Wilkins.

Pasquali E: The impact of acculturation on the eating habits of elderly immigrants: a Cuban example, J Nutrition Elderly 5(1):27-36, 1985.

Pear R: Rising costs of health care still outstrips medicare gains, New York Times, November 1, p. 7, 1987A.

Pear R: Protecting family assets: a new breed of Medicaid counselors steps in, New York Times, November 26, p. B12, 1987B.

Pear R: New law protects rights of patients in nursing homes, New York Times, pp. 1 and 18, 1988.

Poon L: Memory training for older adults, In Abrahams J and Crooks V, editors: Geriatric mental health, Orlando, Fla, 1984, Grune & Stratton, Inc.

Poon L: Differences in human memory with aging: nature, causes and clinical implications, In Birren J and Schaie K, editors: Handbook of the psychology of aging, New York, 1982, Van Nostrand Reinhold Co.

Quinn J: Eldercare emerging as an issue, Times Herald Record, Ulster County Edition, Monday, December 7, p. 34, 1987.

Rogers M: An introduction to the theoretical basis of nursing, Philadelphia, 1970, FA Davis Co.

Rosin A and Glatt M: Alcohol excess in the elderly, Q J Stud Alcoholism 32:53-59, 1971.

Roth H: Shifting landscape, Philadelphia, 1987, Jewish Publication Society.

Roth M and Mountjoy C: States of anxiety in late life: prevalence of anxiety and related emotional disorders in the elderly, In Burrows G and Davies B, editors: Handbook of studies on anxiety, New York, 1980, Elsevier.

Rowe J and Kahn R: Human aging: usual and successful, Science 237: 10-149, 1987.

Ryff C: Successful aging: a developmental approach, J Gerontol 22: 209-214, 1982.

Schulz J: The economics of aging, Belmont, Calif, 1980, Wadsworth.

Schwartz D et al: Medication errors made by elderly chronically ill patients, Am J Public Health 52:2018-2029, 1962.

Seligman M: Helplessness: on depression, development and death, San Francisco, 1975, W H Freeman Co.

Shanas E and Maddox G: Health, health resources and the utilization of care, In Binstock R and Shanas E, editors: Handbook of aging and the social sciences, ed 2, New York, 1985, Van Nostrand Reinhold Co.

Slimmer L et al: Perceptions of learned helplessness, J Gerontol Nurs 13(5):33-37, 1987.

Smith A: Age differences in encoding, storage and retrieval, In Poon L et al, editors: New directions in memory and aging: proceedings of the George A. Talland memorial conference, Hillsdale, NJ, 1980, Lawrence Erlbaum Associates.

Soldo B: American elderly in the 1980's, Population Bull 35(4): 3-4, 1980.

Solomon B: Minority elderly in mental health settings: clinical issues, In Abrahams J and Crooks V, editors: Geriatric mental health, Orlando, Fla, 1984, Grune & Stratton, Inc.

Sorenson M: Narcissism and loss in the elderly: strategies for an inpatient older adults group, Int J Group Psychother 36(4): 533-547, 1986.

Stern D and Kastenbaum R: Alcohol use and abuse in old age, In Abrahams J and Crooks V, editors: Geriatric mental health, Orlando, Fla, 1984, Grune & Stratton, Inc.

Sterns H et al: Accidents and the aging individual, In Birren J and Schaie K, editors: Handbook of the psychology of aging, ed 2, New York, 1985, Van Nostrand Reinhold Co.

Streib G: Social stratification and aging, In Binstock R and Shanas E, editors: Handbook of aging and the social sciences, ed 2, New York, 1985, Van Nostrand Reinhold Co.

Tavris C: Old age is not what it used to be, New York Times Magazine, Sunday, September 27 (The Good Health Magazine), pp. 24, 25, 91, 92, 1987.

Taylor S: TV grows up, Modern Maturity Magazine, October/November, pp. 36-39, 1987.

Verwoerdt A: Anxiety, dissociative and personality disorders in the elderly, In Busse E and Blazer D, editors: Handbook of geriatric psychiatry, New York, 1980, Van Nostrand Reinhold Co.

Walgren D: Nursing home patients need 24-hour R.N. staffing, Am Nurse November/December, p. 5, 1987.

Walker B: The crone: women of age, wisdom and power, San Francisco, 1985, Harper & Row.

Warner S: A comparative study of widows' and widowers' perceived social support during the first year of bereavement, Arch Psychiatr Nurs 1(4):241-258, 1987.

Wells C: Pseudodementia, Am J Psychiatr 139:895-900, 1979.

Whanger A: Substance abuse disorders, In Whanger A, editor: Mental health assessment with older adults, Rockland, Md, 1984, Aspen Systems Corp.

Winter A: Lucy's legacy, Modern Maturity Magazine, August/September, pp.42-43, 1987.

Wolinsky M: Marital therapy with older couples, Social Casework 67(8):475-483, 1986.

Wood J: Labors of love, Modern Maturity Magazine, August/September, pp. 27-34, 1987.

Woodruff D: Arousal, sleep and aging, In Birren J and Schaie K, editors: Handbook of the psychology of aging, ed 2, New York, 1985, Van Nostrand Reinhold Co.

World Health Organization: Preventing disability in the elderly: report of a WHO working group, Cologne, 1982, EVRO Reports and Studies.

Zarit J and Zarit S: Depression in later life: treatment, In Abrahams J and Crooks V, editors: Geriatric mental health, Orlando, Fla, 1984, Grune & Stratton, Inc.

ANNOTATED SUGGESTED READINGS

American Association of Retired Persons: A portrait of older minorities, AARP Minority Affairs Initiative in Cooperation with the Program Resources Department (AARP), 1986.

This valuable publication, available from the AARP, discusses demographics and specific problems of minority group elderly—poverty, discrimination, living arrangements, education, and employment. Ethnic groups surveyed include the elderly members of black, Hispanic, Asian/Pacific Islanders, and Native American populations.

Birren J and Schaie K, editors: Handbook of the psychology of aging, ed 2, New York, 1985, Van Nostrand Reinhold Co.

One of a set of three encyclopedic works. The other two are Handbook of the Biology of Aging, C. Finch and E. Schneider (eds.), and Handbook of Aging and the Social Sciences, R. Binstock and E. Shanas (eds.)—both second editions also. This comprehensive book covers a range of topics related to the psychology of aging including theory, research issues, biological influences on behavior, social influences on behavior, cultural aspects of aging, memory and cognition, therapy, and rehabilitation.

Consumer Reports: Who can afford a nursing home? Consumer Reports Magazine, May 1988.

A useful and complete guide to the economics, politics, and issues surrounding long-term institutional care for the elderly. Nursing home insurance plans are reviewed. Differences in Medicare, Medicaid, private health insurances, and Veteran's Administration policies are explained. The various types of long-term care facilities available are defined.

Doress P and Siegal D: Ourselves, growing older: women aging with knowledge and power, New York, 1987, Simon and Schuster (in cooperation with the Boston Women's Health Book Collective).

In the same format as Our Bodies, Ourselves, *first and second editions and the other books by the Boston group, this large and spirited book explains many aspects of aging as it is experienced by women in our society. Physical, psychological, health, sexual, economic, social, and ethical issues are all covered here. Even the illustrations and photographs are effective in setting the tone for the authors' message of women aging with power.*

MacLean H: Caring for your parents, Garden City, NY, 1987, Doubleday & Co.

This helpful book is clearly written, and it offers a complete guide for the caregiver involved with an elderly parent. The sections on home safety and health problems of the elderly are particularly helpful. Alternatives to institutionalization are outlined and discussed, and the book provides clarification of the "health care insurance maze" that faces elderly people and their families.

CHAPTER 19

Patterns of psychophysiological responses

CHAPTER FOCUS

This chapter focuses on psychophysiological responses to stress. It emphasizes the fact that such responses have many causes—including environment, genetic considerations, and interpersonal and intrapersonal factors—and that they all require equal weighting in the assessment process. Nurses as health care providers must begin to view the psychophysiological response as a two-way rather than a one-way process of interaction. Psychological factors such as anxiety, guilt, and shame affect the development of physiological responses. The reverse also occurs: a physiological response may then reinforce or intensify the feelings of anxiety, guilt, or shame. The two components act together to maintain a psychophysiological dysfunction.

The chapter includes a classification of dysfunctions. For each dysfunction, the underlying dynamics and the methods of expression of anxiety and communication of needs are described briefly. Specific etiological theories are presented in detail in a section devoted to that topic. Emphasis is placed on an *integrative* approach to the understanding of clients who express their needs through psychophysiological responses. The modalities of treatment described in this chapter reflect the fact that persons who exhibit psychophysiological responses to stress are seen more frequently in general hospitals than in psychiatrists' offices. This fact has implications for primary, secondary, and tertiary levels of prevention. Primary prevention deals with the identification of high-risk individuals or groups—for example, persons with type A personality (individuals who continually subject themselves to high levels of stress, such as high-powered business executives) and persons whose families used psychophysiological responses as appropriate methods of communicating needs. The chapter emphasizes the importance of parental counseling in relation to early interactional patterns within the family group and the significance of unmet needs and the eventual expression of those needs or feelings in later years. Secondary prevention directs attention to behavioral problems and appropriate nursing responses. Tertiary prevention involves the use of values clarification to help clients understand the origins of the stress they are experiencing. In addition, the use of adaptive methods to express needs should be encouraged by the nurse. The family and other significant social support systems are necessary components of tertiary care. Clients who communicate needs through psychophysiological responses should be assessed from a multifactorial frame of reference. Nurses must consider all relevant information to determine a nursing care plan that reflects the interaction of predisposing factors and precipitating events.

HISTORICAL PERSPECTIVES

Traditionally, the intricate interrelationship of physiology and psychology has been a question of interest and consternation. Cannon (1929) demonstrated that changes in organ secretion and muscle tension occur as a result of arousal of emotions. Selye (1956) suggested that stress causes the arousal of psychological and physiological responses and that the two responses combine to cause organ changes. Freud, in his study of conversion reactions, also noted the significance of the interrelationship of emotions and physiological responses.

We can no longer consider the dichotomy between mind and body appropriate when we assess an individual's health status. Nor can we predict that a stressor will lead to a certain set of responses. Each human being represents a complex interrelationship of internal and external factors. As we propose in the section on explanatory theories that appears later in this chapter, cognitive, genetic, communication, learning, and psychoanalytic theories all must be used to explain psychophysiological

responses, because experience, environment, personality type, and defense and coping strategies all combine to produce the responses. It is from such a perspective that nurses must work to determine an appropriate and comprehensive nursing care plan.

UNDERLYING DYNAMICS

Illness frequently is related to personality type and predetermined patterns of response to stress. Various physical symptoms may be related to the experience of stress in the environment. As we pointed out before, however, such a process does not operate in isolation from other significant factors. It is important to identify issues such as dependence, hostility, and self-esteem that arise as nursing problems in connection with the care of clients experiencing psychophysiological dysfunctions.

Dependence

Some clients are unable to express feelings of dependence and to feel comfortable being taken care of. Early patterns of interaction may have prohibited the expression of dependence needs. These needs then may have been translated into "words" that were expressed through the autonomic nervous system. Implicit messages from significant others and from society as a whole may prevent a person from acting out his or her dependence needs. For example, an active middle-aged man who experiences a heart attack may be unable to accept staying in bed. Denial of dependence needs is often a key issue in such a situation.

Hostility

Inability to express anger or resentment is another critical behavioral problem. Unacceptable hostile impulses and frustrations may be chronically repressed. This repression may be a response learned from early interactions with significant persons. Environmental factors may further accentuate the repression of these emotions. Expression of anger or resentment through psychophysiological responses may have been implicitly encouraged through the very same interactional patterns that prohibited the verbal expression of such emotions. Nurses need to remember that the development of a psychophysiological response is the result of a complex interaction among many factors.

Self-esteem

Self-esteem is a significant factor in a person's health status. When an individual is unable to communicate needs directly, there is a resulting loss of self-esteem. The degree of loss depends on the length of time such a pattern has existed, the repertoire of coping mechanisms and their efficiency, the availability of active support systems, and the number and type of stressors operating at any given time. Loss of self-esteem may result from a client's inability to accept a less independent state. Increasing the client's ability to directly express needs will increase the likelihood that the client will feel better about himself or herself.

• • •

Through the process of exploring issues of dependence and anger, the client can identify his or her role in the interaction with significant others. With the support of others, the client can be assisted to deal with the anger and hostility associated with dependence. He or she can be helped to see that anger or resentment can be discussed during interactions with others.

It is important to reemphasize the complex interrelationship of factors that results in a psychophysiological response. Intrapsychic issues, life stresses, personality organization, environmental supports, and biochemical factors act in conjunction to *increase the probability* that a psychophysiological response will occur.

CLASSIFICATION OF PSYCHOPHYSIOLOGICAL DYSFUNCTIONS
Gastrointestinal disorders
PEPTIC ULCER

Peptic ulcer disease in many cases represents what we consider to be the prototype of the "stress disorder" in American society. Oken (1985) notes the use of slang to describe the worry and frustra-

tion that ultimately cause ulcers. Such statements as "You're going to give me ulcers if you continue to behave like that" or "My boss is going to give me ulcers if he keeps piling on the work" are indicative of the perception of the correlation of stress and ulcers. Statistics compiled by Oken indicate that about 12% of males and 6% of females are afflicted with peptic ulcer disease. Differences are apparent in the incidence of duodenal and gastric ulcers: The incidence for gastric ulcers is approximately the same for men and women, while the incidence of duodenal ulcers is three times greater for men than for women. Thompson (1988) believes that the incidence in general of ulcers seems to be decreasing in American society. He notes further, however, that prisoners-of-war demonstrate an increased level of depression and a greater tendency toward the development of duodenal ulcers.

The client experiencing peptic ulcer disease does not necessarily demonstrate any one particular personaltiy type. Magni et al. (1986) conducted a study utilizing personality profiles and was able to categorize clients into three homogeneous subgroups: dependent and anxious clients, neurotic and anxious clients, and those with a balanced personality. They also noted that there were no significant differences among groups on the variables of age, sex, illness duration, fasting total serum pepsinogen levels, or number of cigarettes smoked per day. Thus it can be said that certain psychological factors may be significant for some types of peptic ulcer for some patients but not for others. Thompson indicates that duodenal ulcer disease may be more responsive to emotional stimuli. He reports that three psychological attributes—independence, achievement orientation, and expressiveness—have been positively correlated with gastrin levels and depression in ulcer disease. Further indications suggest that a recent loss or separation from a significant other may be correlated with the onset of peptic ulcer disease.

Alexander (1987) described the ulcer-prone client as one who unconsciously has a need to be cared for and loved, is quite dependent on others, and often feels frustrated and ungratified when excessive dependency needs are left unmet. When needs for love are thwarted, there is a continual sense of emotional "hunger," which is then converted into the wish to eat. Cheren and Knapp

(1985) suggest that the wish to be loved and cared for is equated with the ingestion of food. The unmet dependency needs may then be related to increased parasympathetic activity, which increases gastric acid secretion, gastric motility, and fragility of the mucosal lining—ultimately leading to ulcerative disease.

It must be noted that no single factor is responsible for ulcer formation. Genetic predisposition, strong oral-dependent traits, and increasingly high levels of stress in life experiences as well as a limited repertoire of effective coping strategies must be considered as variables leading to increased incidence of ulcer formation.

Thompson notes that Alexander's observations were made predominantly on men; women with ulcer disease do not necessarily fit these personality profiles. Prominant personality variables seem to include defensive emotional styles, relatively high levels of hostility, and an intense reaction formation against being taken care of. Thompson also cautions that lower socioeconomic groups may have different personality variables. This group tends to be less aggressive, less ambitious, and less goal-directed.

ULCERATIVE COLITIS

Studies indicate that clients who develop ulcerative colitis tend to have unmet dependency needs, have increased anal and obsessive-compulsive traits, and have poor ego integration. Thompson notes that ulcerative colitis clients are under continual psychological stress, fearing that a recurrence may lead to soiling and possibly even death in extreme circumstances. Alexander describes the ulcerative colitis client as one who experiences increased oral aggressive feelings when dependency needs are frustrated. Guilt is experienced, which then produces persistent parasympathetic overstimulation and leads to colitis.

Engels (1955) suggests that interpersonal relationships are more critical in the development of ulcerative colitis. He found that the mother-child relationship was characterized by a mother who continually demanded conformity and submissiveness from the child. In later life, that adult feels that he or she is a failure in attempting to satisfy mother or mother substitute. Feelings of hopeless-

ness ensue, accompanied by a "giving-up given-up" complex, which then leads to the onset of ulcerative colitis.

Thompson suggests that there may be several types of precipitating factors such as separation, loss, feeling slighted in relationships, and inability to meet expectations of self and others; however, there has been nothing to suggest specific factors. Stressful situations may cause disequilibrium in the immune system, which in turn generates the movement of the anticolon antibodies. As a result, the bowel becomes increasingly irritable and hyperactive, which may in turn lead to diarrhea. In the case of ulcerative colitis, a heightened immune response may be a significant factor.

Cardiovascular disorders
CORONARY ARTERY DISEASE

Coronary artery disease (CAD) has frequently been said to be stress related. Thompson notes that less than half the risk of CAD is secondary to cigarette smoking and elevated cholesterol levels. Friedman (1969) indicated that coronary-prone individuals or those with type A behavior were characterized as hardworking, competitive, aggressive, and constantly striving for success. They easily lost patience with others, were frustrated readily, and were hostile and angry. These individuals were said to be controlling; they did not express emotions readily, and dependency needs were often repressed. More recent studies by Reich (1985), Williams (1985), and Scherwitz (1983) suggest that personality factors related to coronary artery disease must be studied more closely. Reich notes in his findings that the nature of arrhythmias may not be solely related to sympathetic arousal. He found that some patients were experiencing relief from prolonged tension when they developed an arrhythmic episode. Further data suggest that it is not necessarily the magnitude of the stress but rather the particular susceptibility of the client. Clients who have had a greater number of stressful events that they perceived to be stressful appear to be at greater risk for CAD as well. Reich also indicates that ventricular tachycardia was most often precipitated by surges of anger and fear, while ventricular fibrillation was precipitated by prolonged periods of stress.

Williams found that the most severe cases of CAD were related to individuals who were rated high in hostility levels but who were also prone to repress hostility. The combination of increased hostility levels and the inability to release anger and hostility seems to be a major psychological precipitant of CAD. Scherwitz also noted increased levels of hostility accompanied by impatience as positive correlates of CAD.

Stressors in the environment—social, economic, cultural—may threaten an individual's sense of control, leading to increased incidence of cardiovascular dysfunction. However, it is important to note that stress may not be a relevant risk factor in all cases. In the psychosocial assessment, nurses can determine prior emotional reactivity as a basis for further psychosocial intervention such as stress management or supportive counseling.

Mr. James, a 42-year-old stock broker, was admitted to the coronary care unit of a major teaching hospital with a diagnosis of ventricular tachycardia. He described himself as having a "short fuse," spent 12 hours daily at the office, did not participate in leisure activities, was married, and had two children, ages 14 and 16. The vignette portrays the interaction between client and nurse two days post admission.

Nurse *Good morning, Mr. James, I'm Ms. D. and I'll be your primary nurse while you are in the unit.*

Mr. James *I just need to use a telephone—I have some business to take care of that can't wait.*

Nurse *I understand that your business is quite important to you; there is no phone in the unit, but I can make arrangements to convey information for you.*

Mr. James *I appreciate that, but I can't stay here for too long—I have things I must do.*

Nurse *I'd like to ask you a few questions that will help me to understand what brought you here and how we can best facilitate your recovery— would that be all right with you?*

Mr. James *I guess so—how long will it take?*

Nurse *Not long—I'd like to know if this is the first time you have had episodes of arrhythmias and if so, what did you do about them?*

Mr. James *Actually, the first time was several months ago—about the time of Black Monday—do you*

remember the day the bottom fell out of the market?

Nurse *Yes, I do—what physical symptoms did you experience at that time?*

Mr. James *I blacked out for about 30 seconds, my heart was beating so fast, and I was hyperventilating. My secretary found me at my desk, but I made her promise not to call the ambulance or tell anyone what had happened.*

Nurse *Have there been any episodes since then?*

Mr. James *Two that I can think of, but I seemed to pull out of them on my own—I've been trying to ignore them.*

Nurse *Were there any particular similarities in what was happening in your life at those times—any precipitating event?*

Mr. James *I was really being bugged by this one client—he makes me so angry—but I can't tell him that because I'd lose his business. Things have been somewhat shakey in my business since that crash.*

Nurse *Would you say that you generally don't express angry feelings—whether it has to do with business, family, or other facets of your life?*

Mr. James *I guess I don't—no one in my family ever did; my dad still never shows his feelings. That type of thing was just a given.*

Nurse *What do you do then when you feel angry—do you have any way of releasing that tension?*

Mr. James *I used to run, but I just don't have the time any longer—I really don't have any outlet.*

Nurse *Can you tell me what situations generally make you angry?*

Mr. James *Probably those times when I feel as though things are not going the way I want them to— whether it be in relation to business or my family.*

Nurse *It sounds as though it might be helpful to learn a more effective way of coping with some of those angry feelings you have. Often our emotions influence the way we feel physically. By learning a more effective way of releasing feelings, physical symptoms can be reduced.*

Mr. James *I don't know—I've never done that before.*

This vignette introduces the client to a more effective way of coping with angry feelings. It is important for the nurse to understand that long-standing methods of coping may be difficult to modify and may require continuing education and support on the part of the nurse.

ESSENTIAL HYPERTENSION

Hypertension can be defined as a persistent blood pressure elevation that remains above 140/90 mm Hg (Thompson, 1988, 501). Historically, it was thought that clients who developed hypertension were hostile, driven individuals who repressed their rage, which then led to vascular constriction and hypertension. However, hypertension cannot develop in the presence of repressed hostility alone—there must be a physiological susceptibility, which may be related to inherited autonomic hyperactivity, a potential illness antecedent. It seems that these individuals tend to be more chronically angry, and family styles reflect avoidance measures to cope with family conflict. Thompson notes that affective correlates are common: Depression and sadness tend to be related to higher blood pressure levels.

Stress as well as other environmental and physiological factors must be considered as epidemiological factors in the development of essential hypertension. Lower socioeconomic groups tend to have an increased incidence of hypertension, as do those individuals who have high-risk, high-responsibility jobs. Conditions that produce chronic stress such as unemployment, overcrowding, high crime rates, and pollution may in fact cause a chronic state of sympathetic arousal. Those individuals whose personalities are more susceptible may tend to be at greater risk for essential hypertension.

MIGRAINE HEADACHES

Walker, Brown, and Gallis (1987) describe factors that seem to be precipitants of migraine: fatigue, onset of menstruation, stress, lack of sleep, too much sleep, changes in the weather, alcohol, and bright sunshine. The authors note that this group of individuals share certain emotional and sociocultural characteristics. For example, perfectionism, compulsion to detail, repression of hostility, depression, anxiety, feelings of guilt, difficulty in relaxing, inability to delegate responsibility, and a lack of emotional maturity are frequently observed in clients presenting with migraine symptoms. Socially, clients have difficulty experiencing sexual satisfaction through intimate relationships. Relationships in general are limited, as migraine sufferers tend to be overly critical of others, which frequently causes distancing.

Physiologically, Walker notes that vascular stretching in the headache phase itself is responsible for the sensation of pain. However, it must be noted that both Walker and Alexander believe that the prodromal symptoms—zigzag flashing lights, scotomata, strange odors, paresthesias, vertigo, inhibited coordination, and hemiparesis—originate in the visual cortex as a vasoconstrictive mechanism. Vasodilation occurs as a compensatory mechanism that attempts to counteract the effects of the initial vasoconstriction. Migraines are also frequently associated with nausea and vomiting, which may be precipitated by monosodium glutamate and tyramine found in foods that sufferers consume. Nursing assessment reveals in many cases a family history of headaches (supportive of the belief that there is a genetic predisposition), ineffective coping behaviors reflected in temper tantrums and other childish behaviors, marital stress, and occupational, social, and environmental stress. Hypersensitive allergic responses have also been found to correlate with migraine headache sufferers. As in the case of psychophysiological illness in general, nurses must rule out the possibility of organicity in all assessments of clients presenting with migraine symptoms. The following sample interaction illustrates assessment of a client experiencing a migraine headache.

This client, a 28-year-old female, presented at the emergency room with complaints of dizziness, nausea, and profuse perspiration. She indicated that she had had a severe headache for the past two hours that would not go away.

Nurse *I'd like to spend some time with you to ask you a few questions; would that be all right?*

Client *No one ever believes that these headaches are as bad as they are—especially my mother.*

Nurse *I do believe you—you appear as though you are experiencing some real discomfort.*

Client *I've had these since I was 16 years old—they only seem to get worse.*

Nurse *Can you tell me what seems to start these headaches?*

Client *When I seem to get frustrated; I want things to go well, to be perfect all the time. Whether it's at work or with relationships. To be honest, I really don't have many relationships. People aren't interested in things I like, and I guess I have little tolerance for that.*

Nurse *When you get the headache, where does it start?*

Client *It starts like it did today—with some dizziness, nausea, and my head feels like it's going to split open.*

Nurse *How long does the pain last usually?*

Client *Anywhere from an hour to three or four—I generally have to lie down.*

Nurse *How often do these headaches occur?*

Client *I would say at least once every two weeks—maybe more depending on what's going on.*

Nurse *What do you mean "what's going on?"*

Client *Well, it seems as though they come when I'm working really hard—say I have a deadline to meet. It gets so frustrating because I have to get these things taken care of for work, and I can't.*

Nurse *What happens when you can't get things done?*

Client *I've had to get some help from others in the office, which I really don't like to do.*

Nurse *I'd like to ask a few more questions about the actual pain that you experience because understanding how you experience the pain is important. Then I'd like to continue with how you cope with the pain as well as how you cope with other matters in your life.*

In this vignette, the nurse first assesses the pain the client is experiencing, which validates its importance for the client. In subsequent interviews, the nurse would focus on perceptions of precipitating events, methods of successful and unsuccessful coping, significant others, moods, family relationships, and history.

Respiratory disorders
ASTHMA

The influence of emotions on the functioning of the respiratory system is evidenced in such statements as "The scenery was breathtaking" or "The experience took my breath away." As in the case of other psychophysiological disorders, multiple contributory factors must be considered. No definitive personality type has been described. Asthmatic clients have been portrayed as aggressive-compulsive; hypersensitive to others; shy and withdrawn; angry and hostile; and excessively compliant. Alexander suggests that there is a recurrent theme of maternal rejection, or attempts on the part of parents to make the child independent too quickly are often apparent. He believed that asthma attacks were precipitated by a fear that rejection would

occur, or, worse yet, rejection did occur in reality. Suppressed grief would then precipitate an asthma attack.

Thompson indicates that emotional factors are critical in the assessment of asthma precipitants; however, he notes that physiological susceptibility is critical as well. The presence of a respiratory tract infection or depressed immunological system may potentiate the effects of an otherwise insignificant emotional episode. For example, an asthma-prone adolescent is fatigued and has a sore throat on a Friday night when she has planned to go out with her friends. As she is getting ready to leave for the evening, her boyfriend calls to say he won't be able to join them because he has to work later than usual. She initially experiences a sense of hurt but continues her preparations for the evening. As she is driving to pick up her other friends, the adolescent begins to experience some palpitations and hyperventilation. In this case an asthmatic situation may occur that would otherwise not have occurred. Asthmatic clients may attempt to blunt their emotional responses to events to prevent the asthma attack—even to the point of not experiencing normal emotional responses such as happiness, joy, elation. In this sense, asthmatics restrict their pleasure in life, which may in turn precipitate increased stress and increased incidence of asthmatic attacks. In some cases, asthmatic attacks may occur as a conditioned response to a conditional stimulation (the stressful event).

Immune disorders
CANCER

The correlation between psychological stress and the onset of neoplastic disease has been suggested by several research studies. LeShan (1977) and Bahnson and Bahnson (1966) noted in their early research that loss of a significant, intensely dependent relationship often occurs within a 12-month period of onset of symptoms. The loss may reactivate unmet dependency needs that were generated in the early mother-child relationship. Hostility resulting from the loss cannot be expressed and leads to increased anxiety levels, which cannot be adequately resolved through individual coping strategies. Thompson indicates that depressed individuals may be more prone to develop cancer, yet there is a question as to whether there is a sense that something is wrong, i.e., the individual is experiencing physical changes that may be indicative of cancer. The individual then becomes depressed, yet the cancer may already be present. Persky, Rawson, and Shekelle (1987) found in their 20-year follow-up study of personality and risk of cancer that psychological depression as measured by the MMPI was positively correlated with mortality from cancer for the entire 20 years. The authors suggest that depression may, in fact, promote the development and spread of malignant growths. Their hypothesis that repression of feelings would be positively correlated with the risk of cancer was not supported. Stein (1985) suggests that individuals who have difficulty expressing their anger and hostility directly may be more prone to developing breast and lung cancer. Other studies indicate that selected subclinical cancers may be producing a metabolic substance that does in fact have an impact on affective status. There is also some evidence to suggest that there is a correlation between stressful life events and the incidence of cancer of the cervix and some forms of leukemia (Greene, 1966). The nature of the relationship between stress and the onset of cancer remains unanswered and acts as a challenge for further study.

Simonton (1980) discusses the impact of belief systems on the ability of cancer victims to cope with their illness and to increase their survival rate. He has found in his work with cancer victims that those individuals who have a more positive outlook, a feisty attitude, and were able to effect some measure of control in their own lives tended to have longer survival rates. Often these individuals were more assertive and aggressive in an effort to effect some influence over the environment and current life situation. These behaviors frequently earned them the label of "difficult" client by health professionals who cared for them. Simonton notes that these individuals did not ignore the facts of their situation but rather accepted the challenge of their illness and chose to participate actively in their lives until their death.

Behavioral characteristics of cancer-prone individuals have been described by LeShan (1977). These characteristics include a negative outlook on life, lack of validation as human beings, lack of assertiveness, need for conformity, and lack of

emotionally satisfying relationships with others. Life is often characterized by what "ought" to be rather than enjoying life for what it is. Socially distant relationships tend to reinforce feelings of loneliness and isolation, which in turn reinforce a sense of hopelessness and helplessness. Further studies must be conducted to determine the relationship, if any, among behavioral characteristics, stressful events, and the onset of symptoms.

Kiecolt-Glaser and Glaser (1986) indicate that stress may increase or decrease the effectiveness of the immune system. T-cells, which protect the body and assist in the control of abnormal cells, may be influenced by stress level. Thompson notes that T-cell levels were lower in monkeys who had experienced early maternal separation. It was also noted that stressful life situations, particularly loneliness, were correlated with significantly lower natural killer cell activity, which is an indicator of immune response. Stein found that stressful environmental conditions such as overcrowding and excessive noise levels also contributed to suppression of the immune system. Current immunological research would support a tentative relationship between stressful events such as loss or separation, decrease in T-cell levels, and the potential for the development of cancer.

The sample interaction below is an example of guided imagery used with cancer clients to enhance positive attitudes in relation to their disease process. The purpose of guided imagery is to create a scene that promotes peace and serenity as well as a sense of control over one's environment, in this case over one's disease process. This example is adapted from B. Weschler, "A new prescription: mind over malady," *Discover*, Feb. 1987.

To set the scene, the client must be in a quiet comfortable place where there are no interruptions. The nurse participates by assisting the client to create a visualization that enhances positive thinking.

Nurse: "Close your eyes and imagine that you are in a beautiful garden of flowers—smell the roses, feel the breezes blow gently. Hear the sounds of the birds singing." (Observe the client's position, breathing patterns. Reinforce client's participation in the exercise as the exercise continues.)

"As you lie sleeping in the garden you are protected by armed guards and a group of white attack dogs who patrol the area. Someone attempts to climb over the garden walls but is spotted by the guards and dogs. The guards fire at the intruder who tries to escape but cannot get away from the dogs. The dogs attack the intruder, ripping him apart. Once they have finished with him, they take his bones away from the garden."

"Now I would like you to awaken—you will feel healthy, in control of your disease. The dogs are your immune system which is keeping your cancer in remission. You can be in charge of your illness state."

The imagery exercise can be completed in 15 to 20 minutes. This type of exercise should be repeated at least two times daily for the visualization to become an effective measure of coping with stress. The imaging can then be called to mind to recreate the scene and initiate a relaxation and control response in a much shorter time frame.

ACQUIRED IMMUNE DEFICIENCY SYNDROME (AIDS)

Since the first cases of AIDS were diagnosed in 1981, the disease has assumed the position of a major health problem not only in the United States but in other countries of the world. Curtin (1987) indicates that in 1985 10,000 people had AIDS; at this time over half of those are dead. The incidence, as Larson (1988) suggests, will continue to increase, and a prevalence of over a quarter of a million cases will develop. Bennett (1987) notes that a substantive number of those cases will be children—infants who were born with AIDS, those who received contaminated blood, and abused children who were infected by their abuser. AIDS is known to be caused by a virus—human immunodeficiency virus or HIV—which attacks the body's natural immune system and infects the T-cells as well as certain brain cells. The invasion of the AIDS virus causes a weakening of the immune system, which results in the body's inability to fight off opportunistic infections such as pneumocystis carinii pneumonia (PCP) and Kaposi's sarcoma (KS). As in the case of cancer, researchers are attempting to define a link among emotions, the immune system, and

disease. Weschler (1987) states that PNI researchers Nick Hall and Candace Pert believe that AIDS is a psychoneuroimmunological disease. Hall indicates that AIDS victims who have been told of their diagnosis often become depressed, which in turn adversely affects their already depleted immune system. Further data gathered by Pert point toward a link between neuropeptides and AIDS.

Although AIDS has not been classified as a psychophysiological response, it is important to note the interaction of biopsychosocial factors that potentiate this deadly disease. It is a disease that evokes moral, ethical, religious, and value-oriented questions and issues. It is a disease that has stigmatized an already stigmatized population—gay and bisexual men. It has reached into the heterosexual population, mothers, and children. The psychosocial issues relative to AIDS assume an even greater proportion of import if we are to support the notion that emotions influence the course of illness. Feinblum (1987) and Flaskerud (1987) describe feelings of abandonment and isolation by others, particularly family members who are unable to accept the fact that these individuals are homosexual if that be the case. Overwhelming hopelessness, helplessness, discouragement, loss of control, dependence, and suicidal ideation are reported by AIDS victims and their families and friends. Some clients experience extreme fear and anxiety relative to their sense of impending death. Guilt and shame for their sexual preference and a belief that they are now being punished for their sexual behavior is also reported by some. Not only do these victims experience a range of emotions, but they are also often embroiled in social issues that impact on their sense of self as human beings. AIDS victims have been fired or have been unable to obtain employment. Flaskerud notes that in some cases clients have lost insurance coverage or have been denied insurance, thus being left with no long-term disability coverage after having contributed for the duration of their employment. Social relationships may be drastically curtailed. Sexual activity may be reduced, which in turn leaves both the victim and the partner feeling a lack of intimacy and sharing at a time when that supportive relationship is most necessary. Social support for AIDS victims may be limited for a variety of reasons: geographic distance from family and friends, incorrect belief on the part of the family and others that AIDS is caused solely by homosexual behavior, desire to avoid social stigma attached to the AIDS diagnosis. Thus, feelings of isolation, depression, abandonment, and rejection are reinforced, which then further depresses an already compromised immune system.

Farrell (1987) challenges nurses to examine their own belief systems through values clarification to address the needs of those affected by AIDS. She suggests that an effective nurse-client relationship can reduce the sense of alienation, isolation, and rejection and increase a positive sense of self for this population. However, nurses must first identify their own values and beliefs regarding sexuality, alternative sexual preferences, and their impact on care of clients who hold beliefs different from their own. Resolution of ethical dilemmas relative to the care of AIDS victims and their significant others will enhance the potential for positive outcomes for those individuals.

Although AIDS was originally described as a disease of gay men and thought to be isolated in the homosexual populations of large urban areas, research has demonstrated that AIDS is impacting on the heterosexual population at large. Parker (1987) emphasizes the need for health care professionals to recognize that AIDS has appeared in European cities as well as in central Africa and Haiti. His research with Brazilian AIDS victims further supports Parker's hypothesis that an understanding of AIDS in a cross-cultural perspective is imperative, as is the need for more extensive cultural analysis of the epidemiology of the AIDS virus.

The following is a sample interaction involving an AIDS client, his lover, and the psychiatric liaison nurse assigned to the medical unit.

The client is 32 years old and was diagnosed with AIDS six months ago. He was most recently admitted to the hospital with an exacerbation of PCP. His lover is spending much of the day with him and would like to be a participant in the client's care. The nursing staff have asked the liaison nurse to see the client because they felt that his mood was quite depressed and they feared he might be suicidal.

Nurse *Hello, Peter, I'm Ms. P.—I'd like to spend a little time with you today.*

Client *Well, you're really the only person who dares to come in here other than my friend Tom. Everyone else treats me like I have the plague—it feels like I do. (looking down at his hands, voice is trembling)*

Nurse *It sounds as though you're feeling very alone.*

Client *I've never felt this abandoned; I feel like a leper must have felt. It's not right—I did nothing to hurt anyone.*

Nurse *The feelings you're experiencing are shared by others who have AIDS—the anger, the isolation—what can I do to help you cope with some of those feelings?*

Client *Tom, my lover (points to Tom who is sitting quietly on the other side of the room) is ignored by the nursing staff every time he asks for something for me—it's as though neither one of us exist. It's depressing to see this happen*

Nurse *Tom, I'm glad you're here—it's important for Peter to have support from those he cares about.*

Tom *It's very hard to sit here and watch someone you love experience physical pain—but it's much worse to see him treated as a nonentity. We both have feelings; we're human just like those nurses out there at the desk.*

Nurse *I'd like to share some of the feelings you both are experiencing right now to help the nursing staff understand how to best meet your needs—both physical and emotional. I know they were concerned about your depression, Peter.*

Client *I don't mind you doing that, but please let them know that I need Tom and I'd like to have him participate in my care; it's important to me. I don't think I'd feel quite so depressed if I didn't feel as though he and I were being persecuted for who we are.*

Nurse *I will plan to do that with the staff. I'd also like to suggest a support group for AIDS clients and their lovers that is run by the psychiatric nursing liaison staff and a social worker. It often helps to share with others; one often learns more effective ways to cope with some of those feelings you've identified. You and Tom can think about that option and let me know. I will be back to see both of you tomorrow about the same time. I enjoyed our visit.*

After this interaction, the nurse met with the staff to discuss care issues as well as to identify dilemmas that staff were experiencing in relation to caring for a homosexual client and allowing his lover to participate in his nursing care.

Nursing staff need to be supported to facilitate their understanding of the impact of their feelings on their clients and clients' significant others. Educa-

NURSING CARE PLAN

Client with AIDS

Long-term Outcomes	Short-term Outcomes	Nursing Strategies

Nursing diagnosis: Social isolation related to a lack of family support following diagnosis of AIDS* (NANDA 3.1.2; DSM-III-R 316.0)

Long-term Outcomes	Short-term Outcomes	Nursing Strategies
Establish relationship with family that is satisfying to client and family Develop network of social support as an adjunct support to family	Identify and describe situations that precipitate feelings of isolation Describe previous methods of family coping Develop alternative methods of reducing social isolation in family-client relationship	Provide an environment where client and family can feel comfortable sharing emotions within culturally acceptable limits Assist client and family to discuss previous issues such as homosexual behavior of client that are influencing current family behaviors Encourage client to express need for support in a direct way Discuss fear of contagion and social stigma attached to AIDS victims and their families Educate family about transmission and course of AIDS virus Assist family and client to resolve conflicts generated by AIDS virus, i.e., drug use, homosexual behavior Involve community resources such as clergy, home health care, hospice as necessary Encourage client and family to participate in a support group Provide honest, concise information relative to health care Encourage family to participate in the daily care of the client as they are able Reinforce the value of satisfying relationships in reducing depression and alienation Educate client and family about the relationship between depression and the immune system Give positive feedback for new, more adaptive behaviors Provide an environment where client and family can prepare for a dignified death

*NANDA diagnosis stems relating to AIDS include: body image disturbance (7.1.1); situational low self-esteem (7.1.2.2); anxiety (9.3.1); chronic pain (9.1.1.1); knowledge deficit (8.1.1); ineffective individual coping (5.1.1.1); altered role performance (3.2.1); altered sexuality patterns (3.3); ineffective family coping: compromised (5.1.2.1.2); potential for injury (1.6.1.3); impaired gas exchange (1.5.1.1); potential for infection (1.2.1.1).

tion as to the transmission of AIDS and preventive measures is essential.

Endocrine disorders
PREMENSTRUAL SYNDROME (PMS)

Gise (1988) notes that PMS is not a discrete entity but rather is a heterogeneous group of symptoms. The National Institutes of Mental Health have attempted to delineate PMS more clearly by identifying two characteristic criteria: marked increase in the intensity of symptoms measured intermenstrually as compared to those measured premenstrually and documentation of these changes for a duration of at least two menstrual cycles (Gise). The DSM-III-R (1987) has included a category in the appendix of its current edition to represent the symptomatology of PMS which is to be referred to as "late luteal phase dysphoria (LLDD)." Although there may be as many as 150 different symptoms, the major symptomatology follows:

Psychological/behavioral	Physical
Anxiety, depression, poor impulse control, social isolation, irritability, labile mood, indecision, sensitive to rejection, crying, paranoid ideation, and decreased motivation	Headaches, bloating, decreased urination, joint and muscle pain, breast engorgement, craving for sweets and other appetite changes, increased perspiration

Gise does note that it is difficult to make a clear-cut diagnosis; she also suggests that there are no scientific data to make LLDD a mental disorder, since neither postpartum depression nor menopausal depression are classified as psychiatric disorders. Siegel (1987) supports Gise's position that the research on PMS does not clearly define PMS; further, there is little evidence as to the true incidence of PMS due to the lack of clarity of definition. Despite the controversy, PMS remains a significant issue for many women in this country.

As in the discussion of other psychophysiological disorders, there is a mutual interaction of multiple factors that are considered contributory in the development of PMS. Woods (1985) found in her

study of 100 subjects that stressful life events moderately potentiated negative affect, pain, and the ability to perform on a daily basis. The authors note, however, that psychological factors alone do not cause PMS; women who do lead more stressful lives did seem to be at higher risk to develop PMS symptoms.

Gise describes the etiology of PMS in terms of biochemical, social, and psychological determinants. A variety of biochemical suppositions has been put forth as etiologial factors, including vitamin deficiencies, hypoglycemia, alterations in central neurotransmitters, and alterations in hormonal balance. Sondheimer, Freeman, and Rickels (1988) suggest that the hormonal link, particularly the influence of progesterone, remains the most substantive. However, no empirical data exist to support this hypothesis.

Support for the influence of the psychological and social factors is presented by several researchers. Rose and Abplanalp (1983) and Siegel conclude that environment, through stressors and supports, impacts on the woman's experience of PMS symptoms. Siegel further hypothesizes that there is a moderate correlation between marital distress and premenstrual symptoms. Gise notes that predisposing factors may also exist such as family history of alcoholism, depression, and sexual abuse. Precipitating factors may include stopping birth control pills, tubal ligation, life-style, diet, and exercise. Last, cultural perspectives must be considered in the discussion of PMS. From one dimension, a lack of empirical data to support physiological etiology leads many to believe that PMS is merely a "woman's disease"—indicative of women's lesser abilities and intellectual functioning. Siegel notes the indignation of feminist groups regarding the inclusion of "late luteal phase dysphoric disorder" in DSM-III-R. They believe that this decision further emphasizes the negative perception of PMS in the medical community and tends to discredit women who have PMS. In conclusion, PMS must be viewed as resulting from a mutual interaction of multiple factors; it may not at this point be considered a specific emotional disease, as relatively few data exist to support that hypothesis. To provide comprehensive nursing care for these clients, nurses must seek to understand its multifactorial nature.* Intervention may then be directed toward providing treatment in the form of individual counseling as well as encouraging clients to become involved in support groups, to participate in regular exercise and stress-management programs, and to modify diet appropriately.

Miscellaneous psychophysiological disorders
ARTHRITIS

Rheumatoid arthritis has been considered related to increased levels of corticosteroids secondary to prolonged periods of stress. Thompson indicates that corticosteroids lower the immune response and increase physiological susceptibility to joint disease as well as other disorders. Chronic stress may also potentiate the effects of muscle tension at the site of joints, leading to the arthritic process, and may also cause changes in gammaglobulin levels.

Solomon (1981) found that particular individuals have a vulnerability to rheumatoid arthritis irrespective of emotional precipitants. In some cases, emotional factors do play a role in the progression of the disease when it seems related less to biological factors than to the emotional components of the individual's life situation. Engels (1985) reports that women with this disease tend to view their mothers in a more negative light than those without it and are less able to express their hostility directly. Another pattern of dynamics suggests that these individuals tend to hold their hostility in, portray an outward appearance of calm, and attempt to be all things to all people. Often in marriages where the wife has rheumatoid arthritis, there is an unusually high level of aggression. As has been noted by Solomon and Engels, research reflecting the above results was conducted after the individuals had been diagnosed; thus, it is difficult to deter-

mine whether the aggression, depression, and anxiety existed prior to the onset of the illness.

ACCIDENT-PRONE BEHAVIOR

Freud suggested that there was a relationship between self-mutilating behavior and severe neuroses. This view emerged as an extension of Freud's belief that mistakes have meaning—for example, that the proverbial "slip of the tongue" does in fact have roots in the unconscious. He further proposed that individuals who are accident prone have an underlying need to punish themselves that is basically operative at the conscious level. Physical circumstances within the environment tend to influence the impulse to hurt oneself. Freedman et al. (1980) note that individuals who are accident prone tend to place themselves in situations that reflect a high risk and that are likely to result in self-destructive behavior. These individuals have difficulty expressing aggressive drives directly and experience overwhelming feelings of guilt when confronted with their aggressive impulses. Freud supplies the basic rationale for the behavior: such an individual experiences self-punishment by virtue of the accident itself. In such a case, underlying dependence needs can be met in an acceptable manner because the person is in fact in the "sick role."

In conclusion, it must be noted that mind and body have a significant impact on one another. One cannot be separated from the other when assessing contributory factors. Thompson suggests that psychological and sociocultural factors may play several roles in the development of psychophysiological responses including predisposing, initiating, and sustaining those responses. Although this section has identified certain physiological disorders as having psychological correlates, it must be clarified that there are emotional/psychological facets to all disease processes. The question arises in this area as to the initiation of the physiological changes by psychological as well as sociocultural factors. Thompson states that in some cases the physical disorder would not exist if it had not been triggered by psychological factors. He identifies three components that must be present for an individual to develop a psychophysiological disorder: biologic predisposition, i.e., genetic correlates; personal

---

*NANDA diagnosis stems relating to PMS include: body image disturbance and situational low self-esteem (7.1.1, 7.1.2.1); anxiety (9.3.1); chronic pain (9.1.1.1); knowledge deficit (8.1.1); ineffective individual coping (5.1.1.1); altered role performance (3.2.1); urinary retention (1.3.2.2).

vulnerability to stressors; and sustained psychosocial stress in the vulnerable areas. The simultaneous presence of these factors increases the potential incidence of psychophysiological disorders. It must also be noted that the DSM-III-R does not identify the disorders as psychosomatic or psychophysiological; instead, this classification of disorders is termed "psychological factors affecting physical illness." Although Thompson and others believe that there may be disadvantages to this term, it would seem that the classification supports the notion of a delicate interrelationship among biopsychosocial factors.

EXPLANATORY THEORIES
Psychoanalytic

In the early 1900s, Freud introduced the concept of conversion hysteria whereby physical changes occurred as a result of prolonged psychic distress. Alexander (1987) notes that one of the most significant of Freud's findings was the fact that when emotion could not be expressed through healthy channels, it became a source of chronic psychic and physical disorders. The issue of "functional" versus "organic" began to come to the medical forefront. Psychiatry gained entry into the medical field through the treatment of functional disorders; however, it became recognized that organic disturbances might also result from prolonged psychological distress. Alexander describes the early principles of the psychosomatic approach as relative to three major categories: voluntary behavior, expressive innervations, and vegetative responses to emotional states. Voluntary behaviors such as seeking food or other maintenance functions are carried out under the guidance of psychological factors or motivations. Expressive innervations such as crying, laughing, and blushing are utilized as measures of tension relief as well as mechanisms to express emotions. Different from voluntary behaviors, expressive innervations do not have any utilitarian purpose other than to relieve tension. Last, vegetative responses to emotional disruption can be described as a disturbance in the mechanisms of the nervous system, which then lead to neurotic behaviors. (For further discussion, see Chapter 23.) Thus, the premise set forth by Alexander and oth-

ers was based on the belief that physiological responses, whether adaptive or maladaptive, were specifically related to the personality state of the individual.

Psychodynamic

Classic studies by Flanders Dunbar (1954) propose that individuals have "personality profiles" that can be statistically correlated with certain disease processes. For example, the client who is most likely to develop peptic ulcers is high-powered, goal-oriented, aggressive, and a long-term planner. Those who suffer from hyperthyroidism are often described as high-strung and excitable, while those who experience hypothyroidism are sluggish, more prone to depressive moods, and dull. Dunbar's studies of coronary-prone individuals reveal characteristic traits such as persistence in accomplishing tasks and reaching long-term goals, success orientation, and great control. She contrasts this personality type with the accident-prone individual who lacks discipline, is impulsive, lives for the moment with little concern for future ramifications, and has severe guilt feelings, which may then be manifested in self-recrimination and punishment. This personality profile is often found among hobo types or those who need to exist in situations that provide little external regulation or authority.

Dunbar's work has come under criticism due to the lack of firm statistical methodology. Most of Dunbar's research was based on anecdotal notes rather than empirical data. However, it is important to state that there does seem to be a correlation between personality type and disease process. Recognition of other factors, such as cultural mediation, must also be considered in the assessment of contributory factors.

Stress and change

As has been discussed in Chapter 8, stressors may have a profound impact on physical health. The fundamental concept of stress as described by Selye is that of a nonspecific response to a demand made on the body by environmental stressors, which lead to increased wear and tear on the body. A critical factor in the understanding of Selye's seminal work is that stress is a necessary component of everyday life. It prepares the body to react and function. It enhances learning, concentration, and attention to task. However, the nature, duration, and intensity of the stressor in conjunction with the individual's genetic predisposition, personality, previous coping style, family coping styles, and the individual's perception of the stressor itself must be considered within the framework of the stress-illness model. Each of these factors must be assessed as it relates to the individual and the particular situation. What may be considered stressful for one individual may be a normal course of events for another.

Change and loss are considered important antecedents to psychophysiological disorders. Change and loss occur throughout the life cycle; as the infant becomes more mobile, individuation and separation become the primary focus. Individuation continues through adolescence into young adulthood. Further change and adaptation are required as individuals enter careers, marriage, and parenting. Those measures of coping—both successful and unsuccessful—are carried into the marital relationship where unhealthy measures may be reinforced. Children may then be exposed to unhealthy coping styles, which may impact on their future coping styles. Thus the facilitation of healthy coping within the context of the family system is necessary to reduce the potential for psychophysiological disorders.

Conflict is a second issue that merits consideration in the discussion of psychophysiological disorders.

Conflict arises within the family system—among siblings, between the members of the parental dyad, and between parent and child. It also exists in the work environment; for example, staff members may be in conflict regarding the management of the time schedules, or nursing administration may be in conflict with nursing staff regarding the operationalization of the philosophy of the institution at the patient care level. Conflict can also exist on an intrapersonal level: Internal conflict generates feelings of helplessness, and a lack of an adequate solution is the overwhelming sense. When conflict continues, maladaptive methods of coping are employed, yet the conflict is never truly resolved.

Conflict may be a positive stimulus for change. As one might suspect, conflict occurs as a natural evolution from incompatible values, expectations, or beliefs. Viewed within the context of healthy collaboration, conflict resolution is seen as a productive end.

Conflict resolution that fosters growth and respects the rights and needs of both parties produces the most positive ends. Participants who choose to meet only their own hidden agendas and who behave in a hostile or passive-aggressive manner influence conflict resolution in a negative fashion. Conflict resolution can only occur when participants are willing to compromise and to reach a mutually determined end result.

Stress, change, and conflict are major concepts that need to be understood within the context of psychophysiological responses such as those that are addressed here. Intrapsychic conflict plays a major part in the development of these responses, as do genetic predisposition, personality traits, and familial influence.

Conditioned or learned response

Nurses need to consider how and if learning affects a response. Does the behavior result in dependence needs being met? Does it provide positive reinforcement from significant others in the environment? For example, does the onset of ulcer symptoms engender caring responses that the client cannot normally accept? Behavior may be learned from significant others such as family members. A child finds that one parent "uses" his or her ulcer pains to gain attention from others in the family. Others take care of the parent and perform the tasks that are part of that parent's responsibility. The child "learns" that such a technique is an effective way to be dependent while maintaining a facade of independence. This may be particularly true for men, since men generally are permitted neither to express emotions nor to be dependent—although this attitude does seem to be changing as society continues to emphasize the importance of sharing feelings openly. It is imperative that we recognize that the expression of tension through the autonomic nervous system may be a learned response that is well entrenched by the time a person reaches a point where he or she seeks treatment.

Biochemical

In his early work, Selye introduced the belief that stress may lead to differential changes in the functioning of the hypothalamic-pituitary-adrenal cortex. Increased adrenal cortical hormones, as a by-product of stress, may then mediate the function of the general adaptation syndrome. Selye suggests that when sufficient stress occurs, anxiety arises, causing the arousal of psychological and physiological responses. If coping strategies are unable to deal with the increased stress, a change in somatic functioning results. Selye further suggests that the organ of choice is dependent to a greater extent on physiology and genetic predisposition than psychological factors.

A new field of study is that of psychoneuroimmunology (PNI). In the recent past those who believed in the concept of "holistic therapy" felt that attitudes had a definitive effect on the course of an illness. However, these physicians and other health care providers were considered less than scientific. The Simontons, in the early 1970s, proposed that cancer patients must learn to be in charge of their illness, must be hopeful about its outcome, and must undergo counseling to learn how to cope with emotional and social issues in their daily lives. Since that time, the contingent of holistic health practitioners has been growing yet still lacks empirical data to support the link between the immune system and the body.

This link is currently being explored by those in the field of PNI. Wechsler (1987) reports that researches have found that the brain is capable of sending signals along neurons to enhance the body's defense system against infections and increase the ability to give off chemicals to fight against disease. Due to the nature of this mechanism, emotions can be said to alter the course of an illness. Studies conducted by PNI researchers indicate that the brain and immune system are in fact a closed system that functions in a mutual reciprocal manner. The brain regulates the immune response, while the immune system can function in similar fashion to a sensory organ. Signals from the immune system are capable of reaching both the rational and emotional centers of the brain, thus giving plausible explanation for why individuals become irritable when they are sick. Further research in the area of PNI supports the notion that the brain, through nerves and hormones, is communicating with the immune system about emotions, and the reverse is also possible. The immune system could be influenced by emotions and, in fact, alter the susceptibility to disease. Weschler notes that PNI researcher Candace Pert has done much in this area to identify the mechanism that facilitates the brain–immune system linkage. She discovered neuropeptides, small protein-like chemicals that include endorphins, which she believe are the biochemical units of emotion. Pert suggests that neuropeptides may contribute to the individual's mood and emotional state. She further notes that neuropeptides could attach themselves to macrophages and influence the speed and activity of the macrophage—different moods accounted for by different neuropeptides may then affect the manner in which the macrophage functions. A depressive mood may then reduce the macrophage's ability to control infection and result in a depleted immune system. This notion would support the Simontons' belief that the immune system could be strengthened by the client's positive attitude and sense of control over illness outcomes. Kiecolt-Glaser and Glaser also support the theory of psychosocial mediation of immune responses. Stressful life situations and isolation, depression, and feelings of powerlessness may significantly depress natural kill cell activity, which is indicative of cellular immune response. As has been noted in the discussion of cancer, several studies have demonstrated data that suggest a correlation between depression and the development and spread of malignancies.

Thompson notes that several factors have been identified as instrumental in determining the susceptibility of individuals to particular diseases. Interferon, in particular, has been found to be related to increased resistance to viral illness. In turn, psychosocial stressors have been noted to influence interferon production.

Last, autoimmune disorders must be considered in the discussion of immunologic theory of psychophysiologic disorders. The disruption of T-cell or

B-cell function may lead to autoimmune disorders such as rheumatoid arthritis, myasthenia gravis, psoriasis, and systemic lupus. Thompson also suggests that schizophrenia may have an autoimmune component. Lowered levels of immunoglobulin were found in schizophrenic patients; however, it is not clear whether this finding was due to the effect of major tranquilizers.

Family

The concept of family has become increasingly important over the last 20 years. The family transmits the mores and values of society to its members. The child is influenced by the manner in which parents communicate to one another and by the coping mechanisms they use to reduce stress and anxiety. The family structure provides an arena in which the offspring develop a sense of identity or a lack of identity. They learn to communicate with others, and they learn to relate in a healthy manner to others in their environment and in society as a whole. Satir (1972) points out not only that the family is charged with helping a child to accomplish these tasks but also that the child emerges as a mentally healthy adult as a result of their successful achievement. Satir therefore views the family as a complex, continuous interaction of individuals who assume various roles at various times, accomplish developmental tasks, cope with conflicts, and become active members in society. When discussing this concept of family, we often do not realize the full impact the family has on its individual members. As discussed earlier, adaptive behavior that clients use in response to stressors such as changes in body image, pain, immobilization, sensory overload or deprivation, and loss or change are greatly influenced by previous experiences with these stressors in the family setting. Parents act as role models for the handling of conflict situations. Communication patterns used by parents are adopted by children to be transmitted to future generations. As we know, this role modeling may be either positive or negative.

How is the concept of family related to the use of psychophysiological processes as modes of adaptation? How can it not be related? Minuchin (1978) believes that there is a "psychosomatogenic fami-

ly." Reviewing what has previously been discussed, we see that the child's adaptation mechanisms, as well as his or her roles, are learned through the family process. Within the psychosomatogenic family, the child learns that his or her psychophysiological dysfunction serves as a source of concern for family members. This allows the family to focus on something other than family conflict. Minuchin feels that there is a particular type of family organization that submerges or denies outright conflict; conflicts are never resolved in such a family. As the psychophysiological dysfunction continues to mask the conflicts within the family, the child receives positive reinforcement for his or her symptoms, which in turn serves to maintain the ritual of conflict avoidance. Minuchin also discusses the question of physiological vulnerability. The child may have a particular physiological weakness that determines the organ of choice, but the operation of the family and its impact on its members is a crucial aspect of the dysfunction.

Ackerman (1966) supports the concept that a psychophysiological dysfunction in a child serves to control conflict within the family. The dysfunction maintains patterns of communication and prevents the occurrence of psychosis.

Systems

Psychophysiologic disorders may be viewed within the context of systems theory as resulting from the simultaneous interaction of biologic, psychologic, and social processes. This group of disorders, in particular, represent the delicate, reciprocal interaction of biochemical factors such as depressed T-cell levels; biologic factors such as constitutional vulnerability, age, sex; psychological and social factors such as family conflict resolution style, ability to express emotions, coping skills, enculturation into particular ethnic groups, and unmet emotional needs. From the perspective of systems theory, there is no linear causative model of illness.

Precipitating stressful events such as loss, chronic unemployment, family conflict, or disturbances in hormonal balance may act to decrease effective coping methods, which then result in psychophysiologic disorders. Within the context of significant

TABLE 19-1   Theoretical orientations and nursing implications

Orientation	Implications for practice
Psychoanalytic	Nurses teach parents to facilitate healthy expression of emotions and to resolve conflict in an open, honest manner. Nurses educate clients to develop more effective methods of coping with loss and change.
Psychodynamic	Nurses can assist clients to understand the relationship of personality traits to the development of psychophysiologic disorders. Nurses can help clients to modify these traits in an effort to reduce unhealthy coping.
Stress and change	Nurses educate clients about stress theory and its impact on physical health. Nurses assist clients to develop more effective coping measures to deal with stress and change.
Learned response	Nurses educate parents about the effect of their behavior and coping styles on their children's coping styles. Nurses assist clients to understand the relationship between behaviors and responses elicited from others in the environment.
Biochemical	Nurses educate clients about the influence of emotions on the immune system. Nurses teach clients the use of guided imagery, relaxation, visualization.
Family	Nurses recognize that clients exist within the context of a family system and may maintain family equilibrium through their symptoms. Nurses can facilitate clients' and families' utilization of more effective coping measures.
Systems	Nurses recognize that psychophysiological disorders result from the simultaneous interaction of biopsychosocial factors. Strategies to assist clients in the development of more effective coping measures are based on the understanding of this complex interaction.

relationships, as in the case of the family system, the behavior of one individual impacts on all other members. This reciprocal function affects the total system, often generating a maladaptive equilibrium. Thus, utilizing a systems perspective, attempts to modify client behavior must be made within the context of that system.

A summary of the explanatory theories for psychophysiological responses to stress and their implications for nursing practice are presented in Table 19-1.

TREATMENT MODALITIES
Emergency intervention

Crisis-oriented intervention skills may be utilized to assist clients with psychophysiological disorders to develop more effective coping strategies. Initial intervention is directed toward assessing the physical sympytomatology and planning intervention to alleviate those symptoms. Since these clients are most frequently seen in the medical environment, the psychiatric liaison nurse may be the

initial point of contact for mental health services. Clients can be educated about the influence of emotional and psychological factors on physical health. Measures such as progressive relaxation, guided imagery, and visualization are useful tools to enable clients to monitor and reduce their own stress levels. Through the use of crisis-intervention skills, the client can gain an increased sense of control over environment and illness outcomes. The nurse can facilitate the client's understanding of the interaction among dysfunction, stress, life-style as well as other factors. Clients are then able to develop more effective methods of expressing feelings in an open, direct manner.

Pharmacology

A primary goal of the nurse is to assess the meaning that a dysfunction holds for the client. Why does he or she choose to adapt to stress in this manner? However, it is often necessary to deal with the high levels of anxiety and the symptoms of depression that precipitate and exacerbate psychophysiological dysfunctions. Tranquilizers, antidepressants, and sedatives are the drugs most frequently indicated. They should be administered judiciously and according to the needs of each individual client. Medications are not replacements for therapy but should be used in conjunction with appropriate modes of intervention. Other types of medication, directed toward specific disease processes, are often indicated as well.

Individual and group therapy

There are various psychological modalities for the treatment of psychophysiological dysfunctions. Treatment plans are based on the theory that is most relevant to the client's situation. Psychotherapy is directed toward the long-term goal of initiating new adaptive measures. Intensive psychotherapy is successful in the treatment of most psychophysiological dysfunctions. However, the decision to engage in this interpretive form of therapy depends on the fragility of the client's ego. This type of therapy is not recommended for clients with ulcerative colitis or peptic ulcers, since the exacerbation of symptoms may be potentially life threatening.

Supportive one-to-one therapy is essential until clients are able to accept themselves and their roles in their environments. They then will no longer "need" psychophysiological dysfunctions and will seek more realistic and self-satisfying modes of coping.

Anaclitic therapy may be used, but only in a well-controlled situation. This form of therapy involves the regression of the client to an earlier stage of development—a stage where he or she feels comfortable. The client then is gradually moved back through the developmental eras and helped to deal with feelings of dependence and/or guilt when appropriate.

Rest, diet, and other supportive measures, as well as medical intervention, are also used, as needed, in individual therapy.

Group therapy may be used as an adjunct to the supportive or psychotherapeutic one-to-one relationship. Initially, a client needs to feel comfortable with one helping person. He or she may then move into a group situation with greater self-confidence.

It is important to note that clients rarely seek psychiatric help for any of the dysfunctions discussed in this chapter. Frequently it is in the general hospital setting that nurses deal with clients who are experiencing stress-related dysfunctions. Society may, in fact, subtly condone the occurrence of such dysfunctions as ulcers or coronary artery disease as part of becoming successful—they are often seen as the mark of an aggressive, ambitious individual. Although therapy is important, it is more relevant for nurses to assist clients to gain an understanding of the interaction among dysfunction, stress, and life-style. In many instances, nurses can provide short-term supportive therapy that can enable a client to gain more control over his environment and to express needs in a more open, direct fashion.

Family therapy

Proponents of systems theory view the individual as a subsystem that is in continuous interaction with many other subsystems in the environment. The underlying premise is that one cannot successfully treat an individual client without considering him or her as an integral part of the total system. Family therapy involves all family members or significant others in the client's environment. As was previously discussed, the goal of family therapy is to enable the *family*, not just the individual client, to resolve the conflict and express needs directly, rather than force the client to use maladaptive behavior to maintain family patterns. (For further discussion see Chapter 14.)

Nursing Intervention
PRIMARY PREVENTION

Primary prevention is a key concept in the area of psychophysiological dysfunctions. As Chapter 8 pointed out, it involves the identification of potential stressors and the education of individuals and families to enable them to develop healthy patterns of adaptation.

Nurses need to be aware of the following principles when developing goals for primary prevention of psychophysiological responses.

1. Psychophysiological responses are a means of coping with unconscious conflicts in order to maintain functional ability.
2. Change, loss, and conflict are major stressors in the current societal situation.
3. Anxiety occurs as a result of encountering stressful situations.
4. Behavioral responses are directed toward maintaining psychological equilibrium and reducing anxiety.
5. Awareness of feelings is limited during periods of increased anxiety.
6. Vulnerability to rejection and criticism is heightened during periods of increased anxiety.

Goals for primary prevention of psychophysiological disorders include:

1. Minimizing the effects of factors that predispose people to psychophysiological disorders.
2. Identifying measures to prevent high-risk individuals from developing psychophysiological disorders

These goals can be implemented by identifying high-risk individuals and initiating family and marital counseling. (Refer to Chapter 8 for an in-depth discussion of change, loss, anxiety, and stress.)

It is important to identify high-risk groups, such as members of families in which one or both parents express needs primarily through psychophysiological behavior. This task may seem monumental, particularly since such clients do not usually seek psychiatric treatment. Nurses often see these clients in general hospital settings and physicians' offices. Assessment data should reflect the fact that the client is an integral part of his family and community system. Nursing intervention can be directed toward identifying the significance of early patterns of interaction within a family in which physical illness is directly affected by psychological factors. Since these issues are often quite emotionally charged, a client may deny that he or she has any difficulty expressing needs or feelings.

Through involvement with families on the community and school levels, the nurse is able to observe both children's and parents' responses to change. Indications as to the level of adaptability can be readily observed. Methods of maladaptive coping with stressful situations may be apparent in the parental dyad. Families in which parent-child relationships prohibit the expression of dependence needs, as well as the expression of anger, guilt, fear, and anxiety, are a target population. Relationships that are founded on unrealistic expectations that can never be fulfilled set the stage for maladaptive coping strategies, as exemplified by the cancer-prone individual.

A major aspect of primary prevention is parental and family counseling. As has been noted elsewhere, children learn within the context of their environments, particularly from their parents and/or significant others. It is at this level, then, that we must direct our attention. Nurses can act as facilitators by assisting parents in the open expression of feelings—anger, frustration, and anxiety. Learning adaptive methods to exist in a society that promotes and expects change is a must. Those children who learn to be flexible, to use many different ways to handle change, and who are not threatened by change are the ones who will be most successful in confronting and resolving the issues that arise in society. Families need to be active participants in stress reduction measures such as biofeedback, progressive relaxation, and assertiveness techniques. It is through these measures that open communication is fostered and feelings are authentically experienced.

Parental education on an informal level may stimulate parents to become more aware of the role they play in influencing their children's methods of coping with stress—particularly the use of psychological behavior. As was discussed in Chapter 8, the family is the target client system for nursing intervention. Nurses can enable clients to provide an atmosphere in which their children can feel safe and comfortable in sharing their needs to feel taken care of and to feel that they are whole, interdependent, unique beings. In such an atmosphere, expressions of anger, fear, and rage are dealt with in an open, honest manner. Providing open lines of communication may be difficult for a parent who has never experienced such a situation himself or herself. In spite of the significance of early parental interaction and direct lines of communication, it is important not to neglect the impact of genetic predisposition, personality factors, and precipitating factors that may interact to increase the use of psychophysiological responses as coping mechanisms.

Primary prevention is concerned with the identification of potential stressors and the education of the individual to deal with them. If a client has already developed a psychophysiological response as an adaptive measure, the focus of primary prevention shifts to the children of the client, with an increased emphasis on the influence of parental adaptive measures.

SECONDARY PREVENTION

Secondary prevention involves meeting the following objectives:

1. Early identification of cases of psychophysiological responses in the community
2. Obtaining cost-effective and prompt treatment that will assist clients in returning to their optimal levels of functioning
3. Assessment of available resources such as assertiveness training and stress management seminars
4. Participation with community groups and business organizations in developing expanded resources

Early identification of health deviations resulting from psychophysiological responses is particularly important. Many of these individuals do not actively seek help from health resources until symptoms are quite severe. At this point hospitalization for the physical symptoms is necessary. It is in this setting that nurses can become actively involved in assisting clients in identifying relevant stressors, assessing effective and ineffective coping strategies, and determining appropriate measures to resolve stressful issues. Nurses in occupational and community health are in key positions to identify and assess behavior patterns indicative of maladaptive coping measures. For example, the occupational health nurse may be the one individual that a young management trainee seeks out to discuss chronic intestinal problems that seem to be related to the beginning of the management program.

These initial assessments are tentative and need to be further validated with the client and with other health care resources before further intervention is implemented. The goal of early identification in secondary prevention is the referral of the client to further mental health resources. In the case of persons with psychophysiological disorders, individual therapy is not usually cost effective or actively sought by clients. A supportive nurse-client relationship may be the primary vehicle for assisting the client in developing more effective coping strategies. These individuals are often resistant to therapy because they do not believe that it could be helpful. Nurses should refer these clients to resources that provide stress management techniques and support their efforts to communicate their feelings and needs more directly and to assume active control over their lives with the responsibility that accompanies that control.

The focus of intervention in the secondary prevention phase is on resolution of internal conflict and identification and management of stressors. Through intervention, clients will be able to experience reductions in psychophysiological symptoms and to increase their levels of functional adaptation to both internal and external stressors. Nurses need to keep in mind the following principles, regardless of the symptom picture:

1. The focus must be on the client as a person rather than on symptoms.
2. Anxiety is an underlying concept whether it is observable or not.
3. The symptom is a mechanism of defense that is designed to control anxiety and preserve ego integrity.
4. Nursing intervention needs to recognize these behaviors as compensatory until clients are more able to develop effective adaptation measures.
5. Secondary gains may be powerful motivators relative to psychophysiological responses.
6. Clients are vulnerable to rejection and need to feel control over the environment.
7. Stress management techniques enable clients to manage their own stressors, including change and conflict. Knowledge of these principles will facilitate intervention.

Nursing process

The nursing process is the mechanism that provides the framework for therapeutic intervention.

ASSESSMENT

The assessment should reflect a comprehensive consideration of stressors, their impact, and the client's methods of coping. Although each disorder may impact on a different biological system, all clients share maladaptive coping strategies that prevent effective coping with their environments. The following areas should be assessed:

1. Presenting symptoms—systems involved (GI tract; respiratory tract; cardiovascular system)
2. Coping strategies—use of appropriate denial; general effectiveness; perception of precipitating event; past effectiveness of coping measures; level of communication of needs; origin of maladaptive coping strategies through past experiences
3. Emotional state—level of self-worth; degree of feelings of helplessness, hopelessness; feelings of frustration, anger, anxiety; degree of disruption incurred
4. Stimulus situations—stressful situations that create psychophysiological responses within the environment (social, work, school situations; within the context of familial relationships; client perception of stressors and methods of coping)
5. Support system—available support systems (family, significant others; individuals within the context of other relationships with client)
6. Holistic health status—biological, psychological, intellectual, sociocultural, and spiritual status of the client. These factors may impede or facilitate wellness. Expectations of unrealistic performance may, for example, generate angry feelings which are then repressed. These feelings are ultimately expressed through physical symptoms such as ulcerative colitis and asthma. In psychophysiological disorders, the primary mechanism of expressing feelings is through physical symptomatology.

ANALYSIS OF DATA

Nurses begin to understand their clients within the context of their relationships with family and significant others in their environment through a comprehensive health assessment. Following this assessment, nurses may formulate nursing diagnoses.

PLANNING AND IMPLEMENTATION

Diagnoses reflective of internal conflicts relating to psychophysiological responses include dependence and hostility. These diagnoses are presented in Chapter 22 with appropriate plans of care and implementation. Physical symptoms must be addressed and acute conditions must be treated; however, the physical symptoms are not the focus. It is important for readers to refer back to Chapter 8 for an in-depth discussion of stress management techniques, which are critical to effecting change in psychophysiological responses.

EVALUATION

Evaluation must reflect client participation in goal attainment and the impact of the client's family and significant others on the achievement of goals. The following areas must be considered:

1. The degree to which internal conflict has been resolved
2. The degree to which goals have been achieved and client functioning has improved—that is, decrease in physical symptomatology
3. Identification of goals that need to be modified or revised
4. Level of involvement in stress management techniques on an ongoing basis
5. Referral to support systems outside the nurse-client relationship
   a. Individuals within the client's network who will act as support systems
   b. Community agencies that provide services to assist clients in the management of their stressors (e.g., assertiveness training)
   c. Centers that specialize in treatment of specific psychophysiological disorders

NURSING CARE PLAN

Client with Ineffective Individual Coping*

Long-term Outcomes	Short-term Outcomes	Nursing Strategies

Nursing diagnosis: Ineffective individual coping related to sense of powerlessness to effect control over cancer outcomes (NANDA 5.1.1.1; DSM-III-R 316.0)

Long-term Outcomes	Short-term Outcomes	Nursing Strategies
Establish more effective coping measures to increase sense of power Develop positive sense of self	Identify and describe situations that precipitate powerlessness Identify uncontrollable situations related to cancer diagnosis Identify situations that can be controlled Implement more effective coping measures to increase sense of adequacy Implement measures to increase sense of control, i.e, guided imagery	Develop a trusting relationship where client can feel comfortable expressing feelings within culturally acceptable boundaries Accept feelings of anger and rage when client is able to share these Provide opportunities for client to participate in decision making re quality of life and treatment regimen Provide unbiased arena where choices are accepted regardless of one's own personal values. Support client in decision-making process Provide alternative measures such as guided imagery Provide client with honest information re course of life, treatment measures, etc. Identify any significant losses and/or depressive responses within recent past Assist client to develop more positive strategies of coping with stressors Encourage client to review own behaviors that may reinforce isolation and distancing Assist client to develop more effective skills in building relationships with others

Nursing diagnosis: Ineffective individual coping resulting in elevated blood pressure related to the inability to express angry feelings (NANDA 5.1.1.1; DSM-III-R 316.0)

Long-term Outcomes	Short-term Outcomes	Nursing Strategies
Develop more effective methods of coping with stress Renegotiate roles within the family system to facilitate expression of feelings	Identify and describe situations that precipitate elevated blood pressure Identify current methods of coping with family conflict Implement measures to reduce family conflict Implement relaxation program Participate in appropriate diet and exercise program	Establish a climate where the client can feel comfortable expressing feelings within appropriate cultural boundaries Encourage client to identify factors that may increase blood pressure Review family history to determine patterns of high blood pressure, methods of coping, history of depression Identify current successful methods of coping Reinforce the notion that physical health is directly related to psychological health Encourage client to try alternative measures of coping Reinforce positive attempts of client to modify behavior Encourage client to have a complete physical examination Include family in resolving conflictual issues that may be enhancing hypertension Encourage client to participate in support group for clients with essential hypertension

*Other applicable diagnoses such as those dealing with anxiety, hostility, and dependence may be found in Chapters 8, 9, and 22.

TERTIARY PREVENTION

Tertiary prevention is directed toward the avoidance of further impairment of a client's physical, psychosocial, and emotional status. The nurse-client interaction continues, with the focus of intervention being placed on efforts to understand the client's need for the particular mode of adaptation.

Nurses are also concerned with how a client's perception of himself and his roles is related to the mode of adaptation. As mentioned previously, certain psychophysiological responses are perceived as status symbols or marks of success, as in the case of ulcers. The issue that arises is the extent to which such an adaptation mechanism impairs the individual in his or her current life situation. The primary focus of tertiary prevention then becomes one of clarification of values and life goals. The nurse does not step in and immediately imply that the client must change value systems and reorder priorities. Instead, nurses can facilitate the understanding of the relationship between stress, personal life-style, and a psychophysiological dysfunction. The client must then decide whether to commit himself or herself to the long-term process of change. Active support of the use of alternative methods of expressing needs and coping with stress becomes the focus of the nurse during this phase of prevention.

CHAPTER SUMMARY

Physical symptoms cannot be viewed simply as reflections of physiological dysfunction. A delicate interweaving of physiological, psychological, and sociocultural factors can result in psychophysiological illness. This chapter has presented a discussion of the dysfunctions that have been traditionally identified as psychophysiological. Predominant behavioral problems have been identified, and nursing intervention has been presented in terms of the three levels of prevention—primary, secondary, and tertiary. Every day nurses in general hospital settings meet clients who exhibit physical illnesses that are related to psychological factors. These clients' cases are frustrating yet also most challenging! Such clients are not candidates for traditional therapeutic approaches. In fact, clients may be unwilling to acknowledge that they are experiencing any difficulty. Society compounds an already frustrating situation by subtly condoning a number of psychophysiological dysfunctions as being "job-related" or "success-related" hazards. The challenge for nurses, therefore, is to assess the physiological, psychological, and sociocultural components of dysfunctions. A nursing care plan must reflect a complete portrait of a client in the context of his own world. Nurses have the knowledge and skills to enhance a client's potential for change, through the use of short-term, flexible treatment measures. In the future, nurses will continue to be instrumental in assisting clients to assess their values, to identify and manage actual and potential stressors, and to develop alternative methods of coping.

SELF-DIRECTED LEARNING

Sensitivity-Awareness Exercises*

The purposes of the following exercises are to:
- Develop awareness about the vulnerability of client-families to psychophysiological disorders
- Develop awareness about the interrelationship of factors in the etiology of psychophysiological disorders
- Develop awareness about the subjective experience of clients who are suffering from psycho-

physiological disorders and of the experience of clients' families.
- Develop awareness about your own feelings and attitudes when working with clients who are suffering from psychophysiological disorders.

1. Try to imagine that you are suffering from one of the following disorders and explain why you selected that particular disorder. Then describe

*For other relevant exercises, refer to Chapter 9.

related to the uncertainty the illness situation presents. Health care providers can also encourage supportive sharing with others in a similar situation as the research demonstrated that this sharing affirmed client beliefs.

Moore I, Gilliss C, and Martinson I: Psychosomatic symptoms in parents 2 years following the death of a child with cancer, Nurs Res 37(2):104-106, 1988.

The article presents the findings of a longitudinal study of mothers and fathers following the death of a child with cancer. The purpose was to investigate psychosomatic symptoms experienced by parents after this type of loss. Data suggest that parents do demonstrate greater levels of somatization as well as increased anxiety, depression, hostility, and interpersonal sensitivity as compared to nonbereaved parents. The bereaved parents are less symptomatic than psychiatric patients, however. Nurses can reassure bereaved parents that psychosomatic symptomatology can be expected and is not related to mental illness. The authors also suggest that nurses be cognizant of the fact that the grieving process is not necessarily resolved in a neat 12-month package. They indicate that further data relative to psychosomatic distress 9 years postdeath are in the analysis phase currently and will provide useful information in the future.

Psersky V, Rawson J, and Shekelle R: Personality and risk of cancer: 20 year follow-up of the Western Electric study, Psychosom Med 49:435-449, 1987.

The authors present the results of a 20-year follow-up study of the relationship of depression and psychologic repression to the incidence of mortality from cancer. It was found that depression as measured by the MMPI was associated with incidence solely during the first 10 years of follow-up; however, depression was correlated with mortality for the entire 20 years. Adjustments were made for age, number of cigarettes smoked, alcohol, occupational status, family history of cancer, body mass, and serum cholesterol levels. There did not seem to be a relationship with any one particular type of cancer. The hypothesis that psychologic repression would be positively correlated with increased risk of cancer was not supported. The authors' findings are consistent with previous findings that depression may, in fact, promote the development and spread of various types of cancer. Implications for nurses lie in the realm of facilitating the development of a more positive sense of self; to enable clients to perceive themselves as active participants in decisions regarding their lives; and to mediate those factors which may increase depressive responses.

FURTHER READINGS

Blumenfield, M et al: Survey of attitudes of nurses working with AIDS patients, Gen Hosp Psychiatr 9:58-63, 1987.

Blumenthal J et al: Social support, type A behavior, and coronary artery disease, Psychosom Med July/August (4):331-340, 1987.

Brown M and Tanner C: Type A behavior and cardiovascular responsivity in preschoolers, Nurs Res 37(3):152-155, 1988.

Cousins N: The anatomy of an illness, New York, 1979, W.W. Norton.

Fava G and Wise T, editors: Research paradigms in psychosomatic medicine, New York, 1987, Basel-Karger.

Greenstadt L, Yang L, and Shapiro D: Caffeine, mental stress, and risk for hypertension: a cross-cultural replication, Psychosom Med 50:15-22, 1988.

Kubler-Ross E: AIDS: the ultimate challenge, New York, 1987, MacMillan Publishing Co.

Masters W, Johnson V, and Kolodny R: Crisis: heterosexual behavior in the age of AIDS, New York, 1988, Grove Press.

Nunes E, Frank K, and Kornfeld D: Psychologic treatment for the type A behavior pattern and for coronary heart disease: a meta-analysis of the literature, Psychosom Med March/April (2):159-173, 1987.

Pancher P et al: Life stress events and state-trait anxiety in psychiatric and psychosomatic patients, Issues Mental Health Nurs 7(1-4):367-395, 1985.

Shannon A: A nursing opportunity? psychological factors affect patients' physical recovery, Senior Nurse 7(3):42-44, 1987.

Siegel B: Love, medicine, and miracles, New York, 1986, Harper & Row.

Steiner H et al: Defense style and the perception of asthma, Psychosom Med 49(1):35-45, 1987.

U.S. Department of Health & Human Services: Understanding AIDS: a message from the Surgeon General, Washington DC, May 1988.

Van Riper S: Helping your patient to emotional recovery, Nurs 1988 18(4):32-34, 1988.

Walton J et al: Effects of support group on self-esteem of women with PMS, JOGNN 16(3):174-178, 1987.

Williams D et al: MMPI and headache: a special focus on differential diagnosis, prediction of treatment outcome, and patient-treatment matching, Pain 24(2):143-158, 1986.

Patterns of substance and practice abuse

CHAPTER FOCUS

Everyone lives within a social system, and every social system is based on a set of values and rules. These values and rules serve as standards to which members of society are expected to conform.

Some people try to cope with stress and tension through substance or practice abuse. These people behave in ways that deviate from society's standards. Such socially aberrant behavior often harms others and is condemned by society.

Various theories have been formulated to explain substance and practice abuse. These theories fall into four categories: biological, psychological, sociocultural, and systems. It is probable that a combination of interrelated factors leads to the development of substance and practice abuse. Some type of substance and practice abuse is known to all societies, but its form, meaning, and incidence are culturally influenced.

Persons who are substance or practice abusers are usually content with their behavior and may not seek treatment voluntarily. When treatment is instituted, a combination of therapies is usually indicated. The goals of therapy are to supplant the aberrant behavior with acceptable behavior and to facilitate an individual's reentry into society.

Although nurses may not directly participate in all treatment modalities, they do participate in all three levels of preventive intervention. A nurse's insight into his or her own attitudes, values, and behavior is essential in helping substance and practice abusers confront their aberrant behavior. By clarifying their own attitudes and values, nurses can accept people who abuse substances or practices without condoning their life-styles.

Everyone lives within a social system, and every social system is based on a set of values and rules. These values and rules serve as standards to which members of society are expected to conform. Social standards evolve to deal with problems that have arisen or to prevent the development of anticipated problems. Social standards also function to make more predictable and more controllable the behavior of members of society. When people try to cope with tensions by acting out against society through substance or practice abuse, they often harm others and are condemned and stigmatized by society.

In his classic work on stigma, Goffman (1963) describes two types of socially condemned or stigmatized individuals: the discredited and the discreditable. Discredited people are those who, because their deviance is visible or known, are devalued by society. For example, people who are arrested for driving while intoxicated and subsequently lose their licenses are vulnerable to social disapproval. Discreditable people are those who, if their behavior were generally known, would be devalued and condemned by society. For instance, "secret" alcoholics are discreditable people. However, once their "secret" is exposed as a result of drunken driving, being discovered drunk on the job, etc., discreditable people become discredited people. Obviously, the families and social networks of discreditable people are often instrumental in ensuring that their secrets are not made public. A wife who calls her husband's place of employment and says that he is too ill to go to work, when in reality he is too drunk or too "hung over" to go to work, is helping to keep her husband's alcoholism secret. Therefore, by preventing the visibility and exposure of his alcoholism, the wife is helping her husband to remain a discreditable, rather than to become a discredited, person.

People who abuse substances or practices are often content with their behavior and may not seek treatment voluntarily. When they are seen in mental health treatment centers, their behavior can be classified into one of the following DSM-III-R cat-

egories: psychoactive substance use disorders, pathological gambling, and sexual disorder.

UNDERLYING DYNAMICS

Many people who abuse substances or practices have failed to internalize the social values and standards of society at large; they may habitually operate outside the norms of society. Such individuals tend to be egocentric and oriented toward the immediate present. They strive for satisfaction of immediate needs and are unwilling to tolerate delayed gratification. They often perceive other people as objects through which personal strivings may be satisfied. Interpersonal relationships tend to be superficial. Such people attempt to cope with the world and the people in it through alienation, manipulation, rationalization, blame placing, hostility, and poor judgment.

Alienation

Alienation can best be defined as a failure in reciprocal connectedness between a person and significant others. Alienation is the estrangement of self from others.

Urban life is marked by decentralized and depersonalized living. Work is a major source of economic gratification, social interaction, and personal esteem. Operating within this context is egalitarian disparity. There is often a disjunction between aspiration and opportunity. This is especially true for members of minority groups who may be discriminated against and denied access to opportunities.

Coterminous with egalitarian disparity is a need to succeed. Success is measured in terms of the possession of "things"—money, material goods, services, education, and power.

Partially resulting from the aforementioned factors and certainly interrelated with them is a lack of caring. Both men and women compete in society. This competition often produces fatigue and irritability. There may be little time for meaningful interpersonal relationships.

Because alienated individuals feel powerless to alter the aspects of life from which they feel alienated, they tend to withdraw from personal relationships or to give them minimal attention and servicing. Alienated individuals have a sense of boredom, isolation, and futility. They may try to alter this alienated affect by abusing chemical substances or by striking out against people and/or social institutions with hostile, even criminal, behavior (e.g., prostitution, possession of a controlled substance) (Klinger, 1977).

Manipulation

Manipulation is the act of using the social environment for personal gain. The classic works of Horney (1937) and Fromm (1947) refer to people who habitually manipulate as exploitative. People who are alienated tend to repeatedly use others to gratify their own needs and desires. Other people are perceived merely as means to ends. Substance and practice abusers may manipulate others through force or guile. The can be domineering and ruthless, or they can be cunning and charming. Either approach is designed to allow them to use others. No one is exempt from being used. Family members, friends, and strangers are all fair game. Manipulative people feel little or no guilt about exploiting others and often behave as if they had a right to expect others to give them the good things in life.

Rationalization

Rationalization is a mechanism frequently used by socially deviant individuals. Rationalization is the process of constructing plausible reasons to explain and justify one's behavior. It allows a person to avoid looking at the actual reasons behind behavior. Underlying the rationalized explanation there is usually a shred of truth that is enlarged upon. For example, an alcoholic may tell himself that it is acceptable to drink three or four martinis at lunch: "Everyone has a drink at lunch. It relaxes a person." By accepting this explanation for his behavior, he denies the compulsive nature of his drinking; he denies the fact that he *must* have those martinis and that he becomes increasingly tense until he has had them.

Blame placing

Substance and practice abusers tend to use the mechanism of blame placing in their interpersonal relationships. Responsibility for their behavior, and especially their misbehavior, can be placed on others. Such persons usually experience alienation in conjunction with the blame placing. They feel alienated from the persons they blame.

By placing blame on other people, substance and practice abusers are able to avoid dealing with their roles in and responsibility for what happens to them. Blame is assigned to other people rather than to themselves. Blame placing is a way of manipulating the social environment. People tend to project blame when they feel powerless to control their social environments to the extent they consider necessary. Since being blamed is an extremely uncomfortable experience, even the threat of being an object of blame can often effectively control the behavior of many people.

Hostility

Hostility underlies all the interpersonal themes mentioned thus far. Hostility is a state of animosity. It is a response that endures; it builds up slowly and dissipates slowly. By reducing anxiety that is engendered by threats to one's security, hostility functions as a self-preservation mechanism. Hostility is expressed covertly in physical and verbal behavior that delivers some degree of injury or destruction to either animate or inanimate objects. In substance and practice abuse, hostility is directed both at oneself and at others. Because tensions are acted out in socially unacceptable ways, hostility is also directed at society.

Impaired judgment

People who are substance or practice abusers usually evidence poor judgment. Many do not show any insight into their behavior, nor do they indicate any concern about the consequences of that behavior. They may not learn from experience. They express little remorse or guilt for the damage they do to themselves or to others. They may convincingly promise to repent and mend their ways, but at the first opportunity they usually repeat the same behavior. The socially aberrant acts tend to be impulsive, and their perpetrators often take unnecessary risks of being caught.

• • •

The dynamics of alienation, manipulation, rationalization, blame placing, hostility, and poor judgment interrelate. A hypothetical clinical situation will demonstrate this interrelationship.

A student nurse had established a therapeutic relationship with an adolescent male drug addict. Student and client had been interacting twice a week over a 12-week period. During one of these interactions the client lit up a reefer and began to smoke. Possession of any drug was grounds for being asked to leave the drug treatment center. When the student nurse reminded the client of the center's rules, he responded: "I've really been trying hard to get off drugs. I've just been so tense and pot helps me relax. It's harmless enough. It's even going to be legalized. Everyone smokes it. You or your friends might even smoke it. It's less harmful than cigarettes. Anyway, I promise I won't do it again. If you report me, I'll get kicked out of here and I won't be able to complete the program. You know if I'm sent out into the streets now I'll get hooked on drugs again."

The student nurse was faced with a dilemma: should she ignore the client's infraction of the drug center's rules, or, knowing that he might be made to leave the center for breaking the rules, should she report him?

This clinical situation demonstrates many themes common to people who are substance or practice abusers. By smoking a reefer in front of the student nurse, the client was ignoring the center's rules and was taking an unnecessary risk at being caught (poor judgment). The client had not learned from past experience and was repeating the same type of unacceptable behavior. The client's explanation that he was tense and needed to relax, that everyone does it, that marijuana is less dangerous than tobacco, and that marijuana might soon be legalized were rationalizations. Promising not to repeat the offense and reminding the student nurse that if she reported him he would be expelled from

the treatment program were attempts at manipulation and blame placing. To the client's way of thinking, his expulsion from the treatment center would be a result of the student nurse's action and not a consequence of his misbehavior. The client would not accept responsibility for what might ensue. He placed the student nurse in a dilemma and showed neither concern nor remorse for the anxiety he caused her. Underlying his behavior were hostility and alienation. This clinical situation shows the interplay of themes that characterizes the behavior of substance and practice abusers.

TYPES OF SUBSTANCE AND PRACTICE ABUSE

People who are substance or practice abusers are responding to and trying to cope with tension and stress. However, the techniques they use for reducing tension and stress are usually socially unacceptable. We will examine two categories of aberrant behavior that represent major social problems: substance abuse and practice abuse.

Substance abuse

In an attempt to cope with the stresses of daily living and to achieve a feeling of well-being, a person may use chemical substances. These substances may be introduced into the body through inhalation, ingestion, or injection. People who use chemical substances beyond the point of voluntary control are referred to as *substance abusers*. If certain chemical substances are used often enough, *tolerance* is encountered. Larger and larger amounts of the substance are then required to produce the desired effect. *Psychological dependence*, also referred to as "habituation," is marked by a craving for drug-induced effects or mood changes (e.g., euphoria, relaxation) and by emotional withdrawal symptoms when the substance is abruptly terminated. *Physical dependence*, often referred to as addiction, is marked by a physiological need for the substance and by physical withdrawal symptoms when the substance is abruptly terminated.

Helman (1984) suggests that substance abuse must be viewed within a matrix of social values and expectations. For example, people may take tranquilizers, smoke, or drink alcoholic beverages to conform to social norms and expectations, to alter their moods, to improve their social relationships, or to cope with social demands and expectations. Table 20-1 looks at some of the social aspects of substance abuse.

Substance abusers are often members of a drug subculture. The degree of integration into such a subculture often is influential in a person's ability to give up substance abuse.

Troy, a 16-year-old high school student, has been smoking marijuana on a daily basis since he was 12 years old. Although he smokes in the morning before school, most of his smoking is in the company of friends who listen to music and get "high" together. Troy admits occasionally feeling lonely, anxious, and depressed and that marijuana makes him feel "good" again. However, he states that he smokes marijuana primarily to intensify his perceptions of music and sex. Since he has started smoking marijuana daily, Troy has stopped associating with peers who do not use marijuana because "They are nerds. They bore me. I can't relate to them."

As the above vignette indicates, Troy is involved in a peer subculture that accepts and encourages marijuana use. Giving up marijuana smoking would probably mean giving up those friends.

DRUG ABUSE

Family dynamics are a factor in drug abuse. The family may be the locus of the problem or it may contribute to the persistence of the problem. Drug abuse may be a symptom of a dysfunctional family system (see Chapter 14 for a discussion of family dysfunction). Textor (1987) describes communication within the families of drug abusers as (1) being vague and unclear in both message giving and information giving, (2) including little eye contact, (3) containing frequent interruptions, (4) routinely speaking for others, and (5) offering little praise, validation, or positive reinforcement. Emphasis is on impulse control rather than on expression of feelings. Expression of hostility is usually not permitted. Sometimes it is only through the experi-

encing of a drug "high" that a person can feel and express any intensity of emotion.

Chemical substances may also be used to defend against such feelings as loneliness, alienation, boredom, rage, depression, guilt, and anxiety. Parents and older siblings may serve as role models for the use of chemical substances. These family members may rationalize their use and abuse of medications and legal drugs. The parent-child relationship (especially the relationship with the opposite-sex parent) may be very intense and characterized by parental overprotection, control, and indulgence of the child. Sexual intimacy between parent and child may be present. Some studies (e.g., Stanton 1979; Wolper and Scheiner, 1981) have shown that as many as 50% of female addicts were sexually abused as children. Drug abuse maintains the balance in this intense parent-child relationship. By abusing drugs, the child stays dependent on the parent and does not have to assume adult responsibilities. At the same time, the parent sees the child's drug abuse as evidence of a need to nurture and protect the child. A cycle of overinvolvement and enmeshment persists that allies opposite-sex parent and substance abuser in a coalition against the same-sex parent. Resentment and retaliation of the same-sex parent against the child may develop, as well as conflict between the spouses (Textor, 1987). Drug abuse can be viewed, then, as a way of coping within a dysfunctional family system.

The following are some of the chemical substances on which people become dependent:

Narcotics. The term narcotics refers to opium and its derivatives. Users commonly call these drugs "hard stuff." Included in this group are heroin ("horse," "smack"), morphine ("white stuff," "morpho"), and codeine ("pop," "school boy").

Sedatives and depressants. These drugs have a quieting and sometimes sleep-producing effect. Bromides and barbiturates are frequently used. Alcohol, which is a central nervous system depressant, is so widely used and abused that it will be discussed separately. Street names are frequently used for barbiturates ("barbs," "downers," "yellow jackets"), Quaaludes ("ludes"), and sopor ("soapers").

Tranquilizers. These drugs reduce anxiety with-

TABLE 20-1 Social matrix and substance abuse

Social context promoting substance abuse	Social context inhibiting substance abuse
Emotions such as anger, loneliness, anxiety, and sadness should be denied or masked; they are negative human feelings; they are not socially acceptable feelings.	Emotions such as anger, loneliness, anxiety, and sadness should be acknowledged and expressed; emotions are not innately negative or positive; emotions accompany life experiences
Social relationships should be harmonious; disturbances in social relationships indicate failure to live up to cultural standards, emotional instability, or mental illness	Social relationships encompass periods of harmony and disharmony; it takes time and hard work to make relationships work
There is a socially acceptable drug culture (physician-prescribed or over-the-counter drugs) that treat specific medical conditions; if these socially acceptable drugs are overused, it is a bad habit; there is a socially unacceptable drug culture (illegal drugs); if these socially unacceptable drugs are used, it is drug abuse	There is no socially acceptable drug culture; regardless of its legality or source, any drug can be abused
Altered states of consciousness are undesirable; altered states of consciousness can only be attained through illicit drug use	Altered states of consciousness are not innately desirable or undesirable; altered states of consciousness can be attained without the use of drugs (e.g., through meditation)
Drug abuse results from defective personality structure and/or pharmacological properties of the drug	Drug abuse results from an interrelationship of the person, the sociocultural environment, the setting in which the drug is administered, and the pharmacological properties of the drug

Sources consulted include Lancaster (1980) and Helman (1984).

out producing sleep. Diazepam (Valium) and chlordiazepoxide (Librium) have become increasingly abused, and there is growing evidence of tolerance and habituation. Because of their long half-lives, withdrawal symptoms may not appear until a week or more after discontinuing the tranquilizer.

Stimulants. These drugs produce mood elevation and a feeling of boundless energy. Included in this group are cocaine ("crack," "coke") and amphetamines ("pep pills," "bennies," "cart wheels") and nicotine ("coffin nail").

Hallucinogens or *psychedelics.* The effect obtained from these drugs is frequently referred to as "tripping." A sense of unreality is experienced, and distortion in time, hearing, vision, and distance perception is produced. Actual hallucinations and delusions may occur. Other reactions include hypersensitivity to visual and auditory stimuli, vacillation between withdrawal and extreme agitation or violence, and schizophrenic-like psychosis. LSD flashbacks may happen days, weeks, or months after a dose. Included in this group are D-lysergic acid diethylamide ("LSD," "acid," "cubes," "royal blue"), mescaline ("mesc"), psilocybin ("God's flesh," "mushrooms"), marijuana ("Mary Jane," "tea," "grass"), and phencyclidine ("PCP," "angel dust").

Inhalants. These include such substances as glue, gasoline, paint thinner, and lighter fluid. Their fumes are inhaled. The immediate effects are similar to those of alcohol intoxication. Thirty to forty-five minutes later, drowsiness, stupor, and sometimes unconsciousness occur. The user retains no memory of the episode. The majority of solvent inhalers are children between the ages of 10 and 15.

Because drug abusers do not necessarily restrict themselves to one category of drug, cross addiction is common. The substances that are most commonly used in combination are as follows: opiates and barbiturates; opiates and cocaine; opiates and marijuana; barbiturates and amphetamines; barbiturates and alcohol; marijuana, amphetamines, and hallucinogens; and tranquilizers and alcohol. These combinations are dangerous. Because they are both central nervous system depressants, alcohol and barbiturates used together may be life-threatening.

Drug intoxication occurs when a person has ingested a toxic amount of a chemical substance. If a person combines substances, adulterates substances, or experiments with new substances, it may be difficult to assess and treat drug intoxication. A person experiencing drug intoxication may appear disoriented, depressed, giddy, excited, inattentive, sleepy, or irritable. Body functions may be altered. (Tables 20-2 and 20-3 summarize the effects of chemical substances.)

People who use chemical substances are often engaging in illegal as well as socially aberrant behavior. Most of these substances are "controlled" drugs. Under the Controlled Substances Act of 1970, unless these chemical substances are prescribed by a licensed physician, their possession is illegal. Table 20-4 gives the classifications, descriptions, and substances included under the Controlled Substances Act.

ALCOHOLISM

One very common type of substance abuse is alcoholism. People who are addicted to ethanol, or ethyl alcohol, come from all socioeconomic classes. Alcoholism may develop at any age. The popular stereotype of an alcoholic as an unkempt person living on skid row is true for fewer than 5% of all alcoholics. The majority of alcoholics are employed and living with their families. More men than women are diagnosed as alcoholic. The greater social acceptability of heavy drinking for men than for women probably contributes to "secret" women alcoholics who are protected by their families and concealed from society (Orford, 1985).

Alcohol is a central nervous system depressant. The exact action of alcohol on the brain is not completely understood, but it (1) lowers inhibitions, (2) even in moderate amounts, may cause memory lapses ("blackouts"), and (3) may produce headache, nausea, and fatigue ("hangover"). Because alcohol decreases inhibitions, it not only produces a transient feeling of well-being but also allows a person to act out impulses that ordinarily would be "held in check." It is because of this lack of impulse control that alcoholism is implicated in such violent acts as rape, battering, and homicide. However,

TABLE 20-2   Chemical substances: uses and effects

Chemical substances	Side effects	Hazardous effects	Withdrawal signs and symptoms
Narcotics	Euphoria, drowsiness, respiratory depression, constricted pupils, nausea	Slow, shallow breathing; clammy skin; convulsions; coma; brain and liver damage; possible death from overdose	Watery eyes, runny nose, yawning, decreased appetite, irritability, tremors, chills and sweats, cramps, nausea, panic
Sedatives and depressants	Slurred speech, disorientation, appears drunk but no odor of alcohol, drowsiness, impaired judgment and performance	Shallow respirations; clammy skin; dilated pupils; weak, rapid pulse; coma; possible death from car accidents, overdose, or interaction with alcohol	Anxiety, insomnia, tremors, delirium, convulsions, possible death
Tranquilizers	Drowsiness, fatigue, lethargy, ataxia	Somnolence, confusion, respiratory depression, coma	Seizure activity, symptoms similar to barbiturate withdrawal
Stimulants	Increased alertness, excitement, euphoria, increased pulse and blood pressure, poor appetite, insomnia, intense, short-term anxiety followed by depression	Agitation; increased body temperature; hallucinations; convulsions; cancer of lungs, throat, mouth, or esophagus (nicotine); nasal passage damage (cocaine); possible death from cardiac arrest, ventriular fibrillation, accidents, suicide, or cancer	Apathy, long periods of sleep, irritability, depression, disorientation
Hallucinogens	Illusions, hallucinations, poor perception of time and distance	Long, intense "trips;" psychosis; paranoia; possible death from accident or overdose	None reported
Inhalants	Poor motor coordination; impaired vision, memory, and thought; lightheadedness; drunk appearance; violence	Brain, liver, and bone marrow damage; anemia; possible death from suffocation or choking	

Sources consulted include Clayton (1984), "Drug Abuse" (1985), "Common Drugs and Symptoms of Abuse" (1986), Cohen (1987), Gawin and Ellinwood (1988).

these are only a few of the effects of alcohol. Alcohol affects the biological, psychosocial, and spiritual dimensions of a person. Table 20-5 summarizes some of these effects. In addition, many drugs interact with alcohol to potentiate many of the systemic effects listed in Table 20-5. Table 20-6 describes some of these alcohol-drug interactions.

Because alcohol affects every dimension of a person, it is important for nurses, especially nurses in general hospitals, to be alert for signs of alcoholism and to holistically assess clients.

Mr. Frink was admitted to his community hospital after he had suffered a stroke. Family members who accompanied Mr. Frink to the hospital were not asked about his drinking behavior. Mr. Frink was placed in an intensive care unit, and his condition was closely monitored. Forty-eight hours after admission to the hospi-

TABLE 20-3 Usual reactions to chemical substances

Signs and symptoms	Sedatives and depressants	Stimulants	Narcotics	Hallucin- ogens	Tranquil- izers	Inhalants
BEHAVIORAL						
Aggression	A*	A		A		
Depression	A	W				
Disorientation	A, W	A		A		
Euphoria		A	A	A		A
Drowsiness	A		A	A^1	A	W
Hallucinations	A, W	A		A		
Inattentiveness	A		A			
Irritability	A	A				
Suspicion	W	A		A		
Restlessness	W	A	W	A		
PHYSICAL						
Slurred speech	A		A			
Gastrointestinal			A		A	
Respiratory	A	A	A			
Nasal			W^2		A^3	A
Lacrimation			W	A		A
Pinpoint pupils			A			
Dilated pupils	A	A	W	A		
Tachycardia		A	W	A	A	
Hypotension	A, W		A		A	
Skin rash	A	A			A	
DANGERS						
Suicidal tendencies				A		
Convulsions	W					
Death^4	W					A
Organ damage			A	A		A

*A, acute phase; W, withdrawal phase.

^{1}Occasional.

^{2}Runny nose.

^{3}Nasal stuffiness.

^{4}Death from overdose can occur with most substances.

tal, Mr. Frink became increasingly restless, and muscle tremors began. Suddenly, he had a convulsion.

• • •

Mrs. Johnson had been in the hospital for three days. The morning of surgery, when the nurse brought Mrs. Johnson her preoperative medication, he noticed that she was restless, shaking, and speaking rapidly. The nursing history indicated that Mrs. Johnson drank "occasionally." No attempt had been made to clarify how often and how much "occasionally" meant. Because the nurse had not questioned Mrs. Johnson further, he did not know that she was an alcoholic. He attributed Mrs. Johnson's condition to preoperative anxiety.

In both situations, delirium tremens was neither anticipated nor recognized, but it was present. These vignettes illustrate the importance of thorough history taking and of being alert for signs and symptoms of alcoholism.

Once alcoholics start to drink, they tend to become progressively unable to control their con-

Text continued on p. 594.

TABLE 20-4 Classification of controlled substances according to the Controlled Substances Act of 1970

Classification	Description	Specific substances
Schedule I	Drugs that have high potential for abuse and no accepted medical use. Containers are marked C-1.	Heroin, LSD, peyote, marijuana, *NN*-dimethyltryptamine
Schedule II	Drugs that have high potential for abuse but have accepted medical use. Dependence may include strong physical and psychological dependence. Containers are marked C-II.	Amobarbital, amphetamine, codeine, dextroamphetamine, meperidine, methadone, hydromorphone, methaqualone, morphine, opium, pentobarbital, phenazocine, methylphenidate, secobarbital
Schedule III	Medically accepted drugs that may cause dependence but are less prone to abuse than drugs in Schedules I and II. Containers are marked C-III.	Codeine-containing medications, butabarbital, hexobarbital, paregoric, nalorphine
Schedule IV	Medically accepted drugs that may cause mild physical or psychological dependence. Containers are marked C-IV.	Chloral hydrate, chlordiazepoxide, diazepam, meprobamate, phenobarbital
Schedule V	Medically accepted drugs with very limited potential for causing mild physical or psychological dependence. Containers are marked C-V.	Drug mixtures containing small quantities of narcotics, such as over-the-counter cough syrups containing codeine

From Clark, Queener, and Karb (1986).

TABLE 20-5 Effects of alcohol: a holistic view

Personal dimension	Effect of alcohol	Description
Behavioral system	Decreased impulse control	Acting out, talkativeness, giddiness, risk-taking behavior, impaired judgment
	Mood change	Free-floating anxiety, shame, guilt, anger, jealousy, depression, worthlessness, self-pity
	Self-destructive behavior	Violent behavior to self (e.g., suicide) or others (e.g., homicide, assault, rape)
	Psychological disorders	Severe depression, alcohol psychoses (e.g., delirium tremens, Korsakoff's syndrome, Wernicke's syndrome)
Central nervous system	Impaired vision	Problems with tracking moving objects, coping with glare, and distinguishing colors
	Poor coordination	Problems with balance, staggering gait, slurred speech

Sources consulted include Clark, Queener, and Karb (1986), Leikin (1986), "What Everyone Should Know About Alcohol and Health" (1987). *Continued.*

TABLE 20-5 Effects of alcohol: a holistic view—cont'd

Personal dimension	Effect of alcohol	Description
	Memory lapse	Block of time may be forgotten ("blackout"), permanent memory loss (with prolonged and heavy use of alcohol)
	Loss of sensation	Weakness, numbness, stupor, coma, and death (with ingestion of large amounts of alcohol)
	Brain damage	Seizures, permanently impaired judgment and ability to learn
Digestive system	Oral cavity damage	Cancers of mouth, tongue, and throat
	Esophageal damage	Difficulty swallowing, esophageal varices, cancer
	Stomach damage	Nausea and vomiting. gastritis, ulcers
	Intestinal problems	Diarrhea, malnutrition (with prolonged and heavy use of alcohol)
	Pancreas damage	Pancreatitis
	Liver damage	"Fatty liver," alcoholic hepatitis, cirrhosis (chronic, irreversible disorder), clotting factor deficiency
Cardiovascular system	Heart damage	Cardiomyopathy, cardiac arythmias, increased risk of hypertension, angina, and heart attack
	Blood deficiencies	Anemia (due to red blood cells not being produced by bone marrow, blood loss, or lack of folic acid), decreased white blood cells and platelets
	Vasodilation	Permanent reddened nose and cheeks (with chronic heavy alcohol use)
Metabolic system	Inhibited glucose production	Hypoglycemia (with chronic, heavy alcohol use)
	Carbohydrate and fat metabolism problems	High lipid, lactic acid, uric acid, and ketone blood levels (with chronic alcohol use)
Reproductive system	Reproductive and sexual problems	Menstrual difficulties, miscarriages, Fetal Alcohol Syndrome (low-birth-weight babies, fetal anomalies, and fetal central nervous system damage), and infertility (with chronic, heavy alcohol use) in women, impotency and sterility (with chronic and heavy alcohol use) in men
Muscular-skeletal system	Muscle weakness	Muscle tenderness and cramping (with chronic, heavy alcohol use), muscle tremors (precipitated by abrupt abstinence from alcohol after chronic, heavy use)

TABLE 20-5   Effects of alcohol: a holistic view—cont'd

Personal dimension	Effect of alcohol	Description
	Joint inflammation	Gout (from excess uric acid, a waste product of alcohol metabolism)
	Bone fracture	Aggravation of osteoporosis (with chronic, heavy alcohol use, there is interference with calcium absorption)
Spiritual system	Ethical problems	Lying about drinking behavior to others, lying about need to drink to one's self, blaming others for one's problems
	Alienation	Loss of interest, caring, and/or love for others; self-centeredness; selfishness; boredom

Sources consulted include Clark, Queener, and Karb (1986), Leikin (1986), "What Everyone Should Know About Alcohol and Health" (1987).

TABLE 20-6   Drug interactions with alcohol

Effect	Interacting drugs	Comments
Increased CNS depression	Barbiturates Meprobamate Hypnotics Antihistamines Narcotic analgesics Monoamine oxidase inhibitors Tricyclic antidepressants Benzodiazepines Chlorpromazine and other sedating phenothiazines	Any drug causing sedation or drowsiness is potentiated by alcohol. Most of these drugs carry warnings not to drive or operate dangerous equipment and state that the situation worsens if alcohol is ingested. Alcohol can cause coma or death by respiratory depression when combined with CNS depressants even when the dose of either drug is not lethal by itself.
Increased liver metabolism	Barbiturates Phenytoin Tolbutamide Warfarin	When taken over a long period, alcohol induces the liver microsomal enzyme system for drug degradation. This speeds up the metabolism of drugs metabolized by these enzymes, so that the effective therapeutic dose must be increased. Alternatively, if an alcoholic person receiving one of these drugs becomes detoxified, the drug dose may have to be lowered.
Gastric and mucosal irritation	Aspirin Nicotine	Aspirin and alcohol act synergistically to irritate the stomach and cause bleeding. Alcoholic smokers have up to a 15-fold greater incidence of oral cancer.
Hypoglycemia	Insulin	Alcohol acts to lower blood glucose levels independently of insulin and may cause marked hypoglycemia when taken with insulin.
Disulfiram reaction	Disulfiram Sulfonylureas (oral hypoglycemic agents) Nitroglycerin	Disulfiram inhibits the degradation of acetaldehyde, which then accumulates and causes hypotension, gastrointestinal distress, and headache.
Vasodilation	Guanethidine Nitroglycerin	Alcohol acts centrally to produce vasodilation, which can potentiate the action of these drugs.

From Clark, Queener, and Karb (1986).

TABLE 20-7 Phases of alcoholism

Phase	Behavioral characteristics
Early phase	Gulps drinks, drinks before going to a social event, every event is an occasion for drinking, has habitual times each day for drinking (e.g., after work), justifies drinking behavior (e.g., everyone drinks, need to relax), may have blackouts but is able to hide them from others, makes promises to himself or herself to drink less
Middle phase	Early-phase behavior intensifies, breaks promises to self and others to stop drinking, ensures a ready supply of alcohol by hiding liquor and/or carrying it with him or her, drinks alone, becomes irritable when not drinking, frequency and duration of drunkenness and blackouts increase
Late phase	Unable to control drinking; risks drinking regardless of legal, work, or home-life consequences; sporadic sleep and eating patterns (may skip meals or go for days without eating); may steal to get money for alcohol; becomes nauseated and vomits when drinks but continues to drink; increasingly impaired reality testing and sense of time; blackouts may last for several days

Adapted from Mann (1981).

sumption of alcohol. However, not all alcoholics "lose control" and go on a drinking "spree" after only one drink. In addition, alcoholics do not all follow the same drinking pattern. Some alcoholics periodically go on drinking sprees and become noticeably intoxicated. Others drink consistently day in and day out. These alcoholics rarely show signs of intoxication but are continuously under the influence of alcohol. Authorities agree that the development of alcoholism usually occurs in three stages.

1. Social drinking. A person starts to drink socially to relax, to be less inhibited, and to be more convivial.
2. Escape drinking. Gradually, a person progresses from drinking to be sociable to drinking to escape stress and feelings of insecurity, inadequacy, and anxiety.
3. Addicted drinking. Ability to control the consumption of alcohol decreases, and the need to ingest alcohol increases. At this point, interpersonal relationships, work, and health are noticeably affected.

In addition to the aforementioned developmental stages of alcoholism, Mann (1981), the first female member of Alcoholics Anonymous, describes behavioral characteristics associated with the phases of alcoholism. Table 20-7 summarizes these phases.

Families may contribute to the alcoholism of family members by facilitating or "enabling" their drinking.

Whenever her husband had a hangover and could not go to work, Mrs. Thompson called his boss. She would say her husband had "the flu," a "stomach virus," or "a toothache." Mrs. Thompson would then try to keep the children quiet so that they would not disturb their father. She excused her husband's behavior, telling herself that his sales job put him under a lot of pressure and that he drank to "unwind." On one occasion, when Mr. Thompson was arrested for drunk driving, Mrs. Thompson bailed him out, because "how could I sleep knowing he was in jail. Anything can happen to a person in jail." Mrs. Thompson never confronted her husband about his drinking, nor did she share her feelings or problems with anyone.

• • •

Whenever Jessie's mother was too drunk to care for the children, Jessie would make breakfast, pack the school lunches, and get her school-age siblings off to school. Jessie would then stay home from school and take care of her mother and her toddler sister. Jessie was afraid that if she did not do this, the family would fall apart. She told herself that there were plenty of other teenagers worse off than she was—teenagers who were homeless or abused by their parents. Jessie never talked about her home life or her feelings with friends, family, or teachers. She would compulsively overeat when the tensions and pressures of home life escalated.

The above vignettes illustrate such enabling behaviors as covering up (making excuses), taking over (caring for siblings and mother), minimizing (there are others worse off), avoiding (compulsive overeating), rescuing (bailing out of jail), and enduring (keeping feelings inside). The vignettes also show that alcoholism is a disorder that affects the entire family. Families of alcoholics try to maintain equilibrium in the family system even when the alcoholic's behavior threatens to throw the family system into disequilibrium. Each member tries to carry out roles so that balance will be restored. Members of an alcoholic's family usually assume one of the following four survival roles to maintain equilibrium (even though it tends to be a precarious and unhealthy equilibrium) in the family system:

The family hero. Often this role is assumed by the oldest child in the family. By overachieving or becoming unusually responsible or successful, the hero makes the family proud.

The scapegoat. Often the second-born child assumes this role. By focusing the family's attention on his or her defiant or rebellious behavior, the scapegoat shifts the family's attention away from the alcoholic member. The concern that family members feel about the scapegoat's problems becomes a unifying element.

The lost child. This child characteristically appears withdrawn and assumes the role of a loner. The family views this child positively, as one member about whom there is no cause for concern.

The family mascot. Often the youngest child or the child that the family tends to overlook assumes this role. In an attempt to get attention, the mascot uses hyperactive, clowning, or obnoxious behavior.

In large families, several members may assume the same roles. Because family members tend to become entrapped in one role, so that role and role occupant become fused, all these survival roles are potentially destructive. Family "heroes" may become workaholics and encourage dependency in family members. It is not uncommon for the spouses and children of family heroes to be substance abusers. Family "scapegoats" may eventually engage in criminal behavior or abuse drugs or alcohol. "Lost children" frequently demonstrate low self-esteem, psychosexual difficulties (sexual identity problems or promiscuous behavior), and

suicidal behavior. Family "mascots" tend to experience difficulty coping with stress. Their maladaptive coping behavior may contribute to the development of ulcers or substance abuse. Many "mascots" marry "heroes" who will indulge their dependency needs. With treatment, the destructive aspects of survival roles can be prevented or reversed (Wegscheider, 1981).

Family members who try to cajole, beg, or intimidate alcoholics into sobriety soon become discouraged and frustrated. Alcoholics can only give up alcohol for themselves. Should an alcoholic decide to "swear off the bottle" for spouse or children, at the first argument he or she will return to drinking.

Even though alcohol reduces tension, awareness of deteriorating interpersonal relationships, knowledge of alcohol-associated physiological damage, and the realization that one may be drinking to cope with tension tend to increase an alcoholic's stress (Carruth and Pugh, 1982). Since use of alcohol is an alcoholic's primary way of coping, a vicious cycle is perpetuated.

If alcoholism is allowed to progress, an alcoholic may develop delirium tremens ("d.t.'s"), a form of acute psychosis sometimes precipitated by abrupt abstinence from alcohol. It is characterized by delirium, gross tremors, irritability, hyperactivity, and hallucinations. While the hallucinations may be of any type, they are most often visual, in color, and threatening. A "pink elephant" is a popular stereotype of an alcoholic hallucination. Alcohol-induced hallucinations differ from those experienced during a schizophrenic episode (see Chapter 25). Unlike most persons with schizophrenia, alcoholics are usually aware that they are hallucinating. Prolonged alcoholism can also lead to Korsakoff's syndrome—a type of chronic brain syndrome characterized by amnesia, disorientation, confabulation, and peripheral neuropathy—or to Wernicke's syndrome—a type of encephalopathy characterized by amnesia, ophthalmoplegia, confabulation, and ataxia. Wernicke's syndrome sometimes culminates in coma.

These three disorders are usually seen only in chronic alcoholism. These syndromes seem to be related to the toxic effects of prolonged use of alcohol and the nutritional deficiencies (especially of thiamine and niacin) associated with chronic alcoholism. Alcohol consumption is especially harmful during pregnancy. Physical and mental birth defects are found more frequently in the babies of drinking women than in the babies of nondrinking women. Also, neonates of alcoholic mothers have to be monitored for symptoms of alcohol withdrawal, neurological difficulties, respiratory distress, and fetal alcohol syndrome.

The controversy over whether alcoholism is a disease or learned behavior (nature vs. nurture) recently was debated by the United States Supreme Court. The American Medical Association, the World Health Organization, and the National Counsel on Alcoholism have stated that alcoholism is a disease brought about by conditions largely beyond the control of the alcoholic. Despite these statements, in April 1988, the Supreme Court ruled (in a 5-4 decision) that alcoholism may be viewed as "willful misconduct" and that the Veterans Administration may legally deny benefits (e.g., educational benefits) to alcoholic veterans (Cooke, 1988).

NICOTINE ADDICTION

Tobacco smoking tends to start at a very young age, and tobacco appears to be the drug of choice for adolescents. Approximately 90% of all tobacco smokers started smoking before they were 19 years old, 60% before age 14, and 49% before age 12. In comparison with other addictive behaviors, 20% of all adolescents smoke a minimum of one cigarette a day as compared to 15% who use marijuana every day and 5% who drink alcohol daily (Kids Target of . . ., 1987).

Until relatively recently, concern over tobacco smoking dealt with its medical effects rather than its addictive effects. Then in 1988, on the basis of two decades of research, United States Surgeon General C. Everett Koop declared that nicotine in tobacco is similar in its addictive nature to heroin, cocaine, or alcohol. People who suddenly stop smoking experience withdrawal symptoms.

After her sister, a smoker, died of lung cancer, Mrs. Simpson decided to stop smoking. She had smoked two packs of cigarettes a day for 30 years. After giving up cigarettes for three days, Mrs. Simpson complain- *ed, "I am fighting with everyone, pacing the floor, unable to concentrate at work, thinking about nothing but having a smoke, and even dreaming of cigarettes." Because Mrs. Simpson snacked on cookies and candy whenever she craved a cigarette, she had already gained two pounds.*

The preceding vignette illustrates the addictive quality of nicotine. The symptoms experienced by Mrs. Simpson are part of a nicotine withdrawal syndrome (see Table 20-8).

Many people repeatedly and unsuccessfully try to quit smoking. Relapse rates are approximately 50% within the first six months of giving up smoking and 70% within the first year. Factors contributing to the difficulty of breaking a smoking habit include the unpleasantness of nicotine withdrawal, the pleasant effects elicited from smoking, the longstanding nature of the smoking habit, and such environmental cues as people smoking and ready availability of nicotine products (DSM-III-R, 1987). The medical dangers and addictive nature of nicotine for smokers, as well as the damaging effects of "side smoke" for nonsmokers who inhale smoke-filled air (Why Smokers Should Quit . . ., 1987), have resulted in smoke-ending programs, antismoking campaigns, and antismoking laws. For example, many theaters, restaurants, and some forms of public transportation are beginning to segregate smokers from nonsmokers, and many establishments completely prohibit smoking. Despite the growing awareness of the addictive nature of nicotine and the health hazzards associated with smoking, a recent study by the Centers for Disease Control found that a majority of respondents (56%) reported that their physicians had not advised them to stop smoking, even when they had medical conditions that could be aggravated by smoking (Doctors Not . . ., 1987). In addition, a study of 1,000 nurses found that 22% of them smoked. Of those nurses who smoked, 50% did not view it as part of the nurse's role to encourage clients to quit smoking, and 25% believed that a smoking client has a right to smoke in a hospital room even if his or her roommate is a nonsmoker (Goldstein et al., 1987).

TABLE 20-8   Nicotine withdrawal syndrome

Diagnostic criterion	Withdrawal signs and symptoms
Daily use of a nicotine product for a minimum of several weeks Development of at least four withdrawal symptoms within 24 hours of having abruptly stopped using nicotine or decreasing the amount of nicotine used	Craving for nicotine Feeling of irritability, frustration, and/or anger Sense of anxiety Problems with concentration Restlessness Decreased heart rate Increase in appetite and/or weight

Adapted from DSM-III-R (1987).

Practice abuse

In an attempt to cope with day-by-day stress and to achieve a sense of well-being, people may compulsively rely on or overuse a practice. People who rely on a practice beyond the point of voluntary control and who experience habituation (emotional withdrawal symptoms when that practice is abruptly terminated) may be termed practice abusers. Compulsive gambling and compulsive working are examples of practice abuse. These practices usually start out as generative in regard to the physical and psychological well-being of the person. Initially, the person is able to exert control over the amount of time that the practice is indulged in, and the practice offers the person a short-term "escape" from stresses of daily living. Over time, however, the practice becomes habituating. The practice encompasses the individual's entire experiential self. The increased dependence on the practice limits the person's ability to grow and change. What began as a generative practice evolves into a destructive practice.

COMPULSIVE GAMBLING

Unlike people who occasionally gamble as a form of recreation and who usually frequent gambling spots with friends, compulsive gamblers bet excessively and uncontrollably and usually gamble in isolation. Bergler (1970), Martinez (1978) and Custer (1982) identify some characteristics of compulsive gamblers: predisposition to risk taking; involvement with gambling to the exclusion of other interests; unrealistic optimism that is not altered by consistent losses; frequent fantasizing that they are prestigious, wealthy, or able to outsmart rivals; ability to derive an emotional "high," or euphoria, from gambling; powerlessness to stop gambling when they are winning; and compulsion to bet beyond their means.

Although research into the effects of compulsive gambling on families is sparse, some effects are known. Wives of compulsive gamblers often experience the following feelings (1) low self-esteem and guilt about being unable to financially manage the household and/or control their husband's gambling, (2) anger about lies, unfulfilled promises, and debts, and (3) magical hope that a "big win" will end their financial problems. This emotional turmoil may contribute to a loss of sexual interest in their husbands, depression, and/or suicidal ideation. The effects of compulsive gambling on husbands (when the wife is the gambler) or on children have not been investigated. However, it is realistic to anticipate that compulsive gambling will generate emotional and behavioral problems in family members. Support groups such as Gam-Anon and Gam-A-Teen can provide peer support (Gaudia, 1987).

Compulsive gamblers usually do not want to stop gambling but do wish that the undesirable side effects of losing could be changed. While there are no physical withdrawal symptoms associated with the cessation of compulsive gambling, psychological withdrawal symptoms include anxiety, irritability, depression, and suicide (Orford, 1985; Lesieur and Blume, 1987).

TABLE 20-9 Profile of a work addict

Characteristic	Description
Technical skill oriented	Seeks situations where technical skills can be applied; applies technical skills in situations that do not warrant them; feels uncomfortable in situations calling for emotion, fantasy, or spontaneity
Analytically oriented	Approaches all situations by trying to define, measure, identify, categorize, or develop goals, procedures, and strategies for them; avoids situations that cannot be analytically approached; tries to force nonanalytical experiences into an analytical framework
Aggressively oriented	Tries to manipulate and control all situations; approaches concentration and self-discipline as self-directed manipulation and control; gains a sense of satisfaction and pride from the ability to manipulate and control self, others, and things
Future oriented	Focuses on future goals; unable to enjoy the present; experiences that are not "productive," such as leisure, are not valued
Efficacy oriented	Stresses the accomplishment of goals as quickly and efficiently as possible; becomes upset if time, material, or control is lost or wasted; because of the reluctance to delegate work (represents loss of control) and a tendency toward perfectionism, often expends more energy in accomplishing goals than is necessary

Adapted from Rohrlich (1980).

WORK ADDICTION

There are two types of compulsive workers: chronic work addicts and binge workers. *Chronic work addicts* make work the center of their lives. All other activities, including interpersonal relationships, take a back seat to work. The chronic work addict responds to all situations, regardless of their nature (e.g., success or failure, joy or stress), with work. The *binge worker* turns to work as a way of dealing with particular stressful situations. Periods of binge working are related to periods of situational stress and emotional responsibility. The binge worker is sporadically addicted to work (Rohrlich, 1980). Table 20-9 presents a profile of a work addict. Whether a person is a chronic work addict or a binge worker, if the opportunity to work is denied, withdrawal symptoms are experienced (see Table 20-10).

Many work addicts also abuse alcohol, nicotine, and other drugs. Often substance abuse is the only way they are able to relax and escape from their compulsion to work. Sometimes they may approach physical fitness programs with the same compulsiveness with which they approach work. Very often, however, exercise, nutrition, and sleep are sacrificed for work, and illness and/or accidents may occur (Rohrlich, 1980).

PROSTITUTION

Persons who engage in coital or extracoital sex in return for money are engaged in prostitution and are referred to as prostitutes. Although much of the general public considers prostitution strictly an adult female activity, prostitutes may be children or adults, men or women, heterosexuals, homosexuals, or bisexuals. Today many prostitutes are youngsters (16 years of age and younger) who have run away from home in an attempt to escape from intolerable home situations that often include alcoholism or drug addiction on the part of parents (Miller, 1986).

People engage in prostitution for many reasons Broken homes, parental promiscuity, and a social network that accepts prostitution can predispose people to prostitution. Economic incentives, opportunity for diverse types of sexual activity, and the expectation of a more leisurely and exciting life may attract people to prostitution. Economic difficulties, inducement by a pimp or by other prostitutes, or ready opportunity may precipitate entry into prostitution. By examining the reasons why people become prostitutes, the classic work of Benjamin and Masters (1964) divided prostitutes into two types: voluntary and compulsive. *Voluntary prostitutes* freely select prostitution as a way to

TABLE 20-10   Addiction to work: withdrawal symptoms

Symptom	Manifestations
Anxiety	Shortness of breath; tremors; anorexia; diaphoresis; cold, clammy hands (refer to Chapter 8 for further discussion of anxiety)
Depression	Hopelessness; despondency; guilt; insomnia; anorexia; disinterest in all activities, including sex (refer to Chapter 22 for further discussion of depression)
Psychophysiologic dysfunction	Migraine headaches; colitis; asthma, ulcers; etc. (refer to Chapter 19 for further discussion of psychophysiolgic dysfunctions)

Adapted from Rohrlich (1980).

support themselves, because of the advantages associated with it. *Compulsive prostitutes* enter prostitution because of a strong impulse to engage in sex for money. The classifications of voluntary and compulsive prostitutes are based on the *predominant* reasons people become prostitutes. These categories are not mutually exclusive, and most prostitutes have a combination of reasons. The attractive features of prostitution play an important role in the case of voluntary prostitutes. Predisposing elements play an important role in the case of compulsive prostitutes. A precipitating event or events usually increases the strength of attractive and predisposing factors. For example, when conflict or abuse in a dysfunctional family becomes unbearable, a child may run away from home and turn to prostitution as a means of financial support.

Clients, like prostitutes, can be divided into voluntary and compulsive categories. Voluntary clients engage in sex with prostitutes for such utilitarian reasons as sexual unavailability of a mate due to distance or illness, limited opportunity (or no opportunity) to find a mate, and desire to prove one's "maleness" to male friends.

Clients compulsively engage in sex with prostitutes for such psychophysiological reasons as inability to compete with others for a mate because of age or physical handicap, need for variety, sadomasochism or fetishism, and desire to avoid interpersonal relationships.

An important aspect of prostitution is the prostitute-pimp relationship. Mutual exploitation is a predominant theme. Prostitutes turn their earnings over to their pimps and often take their pimps as lovers. Pimps act as intermediaries between prostitutes and clients, drug dealers, police, and/or crime syndicate members. Pimps handle payoffs and protection money. From their relationship with pimps, prostitutes extract protection, the illusion of a caring figure, and a defense against loneliness. From their relationship with prostitutes, pimps extract money and the status symbols that money can buy. These status symbols plus the awareness of being a lover to a woman who has sexual relationships with many men increase the self-esteem of many pimps (Cohen, 1980; Miller, 1986).

In addition to the utilitarian nature of pimp-prostitute relationships, sadomasochism may be a common theme. Pimps may viciously beat "their" prostitutes. However, not all abuse is at the hands of pimps. Clients ("Johns" or "tricks") may also abuse, and even kill, prostitutes. The illegality of prostitution encourages such degradation and violence because the abusers know that few prostitutes will report abusive incidents to the police (Carmen and Moody, 1985).

Deviant street networks facilitate prostitution as an income-producing activity. These networks are composed of people engaged in prostitution (e.g., prostitutes and pimps). The networks tend to be flexible. Often members of a street network form a fictive family. For example, a pimp may be regarded by a prostitute as "my man," and prostitutes who are working for the same pimp may refer to each other as "wives-in-law" (Miller, 1986).

Drug dependency does not usually precipitate involvement in prostitution. However, prior to becoming a prostitute, many prostitutes may have used drugs or have been exposed to their use by members of their domestic networks. If prostitutes do become drug dependent, it is less likely that they will leave their street networks and prostitution than if they do not become drug dependent (Miller, 1986).

EPIDEMIOLOGY

The exact incidence of substance and practice abuse is unknown. Health professionals usually treat only a small portion of the people who display such behavior. Many such individuals do not receive any treatment but instead are sentenced to criminal justice institutions for their behavior.

Although many incidents of practice abuse are not reported (for example, work addiction) or are reported as crimes rather than as psychosocial disorders (for example, prostitution), the prevalence of different types of substance abuse has been estimated.

Drug abuse is found among all age groups. Drug use in general has increased in recent years. Moynihan (1984) estimates that 35% of the population has used illicit drugs. This represents a 31% increase in illicit drug use over the past 20 years. The incidence of drug abuse (including alcoholism) is reportedly two to three times higher among men than among women (Belle and Goldman, 1980; Klerman and Weissman, 1980). Greater societal acceptance of substance abuse in men than in women may partially account for this finding. Other reasons include (1) the reluctance of physicians to label women as having alcoholic cirrhosis; (2) the tendency for women to seek professional help for alcohol-related problems of depression, insomnia, and anxiety, rather than for alcoholism; (3) the tendency of some alcohol studies to use male prison populations, to focus on male-oriented questions and problems, or to focus on male alcohol consumption. Because of lower body weight and various hormonal fluctuations, women tend to become drunk even when they consume less alcohol than men (Efinger, 1983).

Alcohol is the most commonly abused drug in the United States. Alcoholism ranks with cancer and heart disease as a major health problem. There are approximately 18 million alcoholics in the United States. Each year, the direct and indirect effects of alcoholism cost industry an estimated $116.7 billion. The majority of vehicle accidents are caused by people who are driving while intoxicated. Many instances of homicide, assault, rape, suicide, and child abuse are associated with alcohol intoxication (Redeker, 1985-1986; Task Force on Substance Abuse Nursing Practice, 1987).

Alcoholic clients should be a major concern of health professionals. Not only are more than 20% of all hospitalized clients suffering from alcoholism, but 30 to 50% of all hospital admissions are to treat alcohol-related diseases. In addition, approximately 50,000 babies born each year suffer from Fetal Alcohol Syndrome (Redeker, 1985-1986; Brody, 1986).

A decrease in one type of substance abuse, nicotine, has been noted. There has been a 36% decline in smoking over the past 23 years. It is estimated that smoking will continue to decline until it reaches a plateau where between 10 and 15% of the adult population will smoke (Smoking at Lowest . . ., 1987).

Chemical dependency in nurses is the primary cause for disciplinary action taken against nurses. Nurses must be caught using or stealing drugs to be reported to their state boards of nursing. It has been estimated that 40,000 nurses may be suffering from alcoholism. Nurses also abuse other drugs. In addition to general risk factors, risk factors inherent in the practice of nursing, such as stress in the clinical setting, rotating shift work, and inadequate professional relationships, may increase the vulnerability of nurses to substance abuse. The effects of substance abuse on the professional careers of nurses includes impaired client care, job loss, and disciplinary action by a state board of nursing. This disciplinary action may result in the loss of one's nursing license (Sullivan, 1987).

SOCIOCULTURAL CONTEXT

Substance and practice abuse must be viewed from a sociocultural perspective. Special attention should be paid to the fact that cultures define aberrant behavior in various ways. For example, in 18th-century China, where opium smoking was customary, the custom in India of opium eating and opium drinking would have been considered aberrant (Orford, 1985).

The use of psychoactive substances is found in

TABLE 20-11 Sociocultural factors and drinking behavior

Factor	Criteria
Parental drinking pattern	Evidence of parental drinking, frequency of parental drinking, existence of a parental "drinking problem," parental approval of children drinking
Family structure	Style of decision making (e.g., who makes decisions regarding child rearing? Is decision making egalitarian or authoritarian?), extent of open affectual display and support among family members
Personality orientation	Orientation toward achievement, authority, and efficiency; degree of escape drinking (drinking to escape personal problems)
Spousal drinking pattern	Extent of spouse's drinking, frequency of spouse's drinking, existence of a spousal "drinking problem"
Drinking environment	Prevalence of drinking, availability of alcoholic beverages, types of occasions for which drinking is sanctioned (e.g., social gatherings such as holidays, ceremonials, or rituals), type of setting (e.g., drinking within a family milieu vs. drinking alone vs. drinking in bars)

Sources consulted include Bell (1970) and Greeley and McCready (1978).

most societies. Each society decides which substances will be approved and which will be condemned. Over time, a substance that originally was socially approved may become socially condemned. This is best exemplified by the Arab attitude toward the use of alcohol. Originally, the Revelations of the Prophet Muhammed differentiated between the beneficial and harmful uses of alcohol. Over time, successive revelations of the prophet (1) first cautioned against the use of strong drink, (2) next disallowed the drinking of alcohol before praying, and (3) finally completely prohibited the drinking, brewing, transporting, selling, purchasing, and serving of alcoholic beverages. Punishment for disobedience included scoldings and beatings with palm branches (Baasher, 1981).

A similar attitudinal change toward smoking is occurring in the United States today. After years of social acceptance of smoking and governmental subsidizing of the tobacco industry, antismoking campaigns and antismoking laws are being initiated. Thus, the way a society views a drug determines what constitutes drug abuse.

The concept of integrated drinking may explain why some societies have a lower incidence of alcoholism than do other societies. Integrated drinking refers to the incorporation of drinking alcoholic beverages into the life-style of a cultural group. Societies that have integrated drinking into their

way of life usually have a high rate of alcohol consumption but not necessarily a high rate of alcoholism.

Drinking patterns in the United States illustrate the concept of integrating drinking. Although Jewish Americans, Italian-Americans, and Chinese-Americans tend to drink alcoholic beverages more frequently than do people from other ethnic groups, these three groups have low incidences of alcoholism. The factor most readily discernible is the family-oriented drinking patterns of these three ethnic groups.

In Jewish culture, the primary alcoholic beverage is the sweet wine served at family gatherings and especially on religious holidays. In Italian culture, drinking is usually limited to the wine served during meals and at social activities. Similarly, in Chinese culture, drinking is done within the family milieu. In these cultures, alcohol tends to be viewed as a social beverage, and drinking patterns tend to be family oriented. Rarely do persons of Jewish, Italian, or Chinese heritage view alcohol as a way to escape from personal problems (Bell, 1970).

Therefore, specific sociocultural factors, such as those described in Table 20-11, seem to influence an individual's drinking behavior, including whether that behavior will be socially acceptable or abusive.

The incidence and types of practice abuse found in a society are also culturally influenced. For example, gambling is found in many societies, but the form it takes is culturally variable. Betting on cockfights is popular in Latin America and the Philippines; betting on jai alai is popular in Latin America and Southern Europe, and betting on poker games is popular throughout the United States. While most societies outlaw some types of gambling, other types of gambling may be approved. As an example, cockfights are illegal in the United States, but lotteries are permitted in a majority of the states.

Therefore, while some type of substance or practice abuse is known to all societies, the form it takes and the meaning it is given are related to other aspects of the social system. Also, the incidences of particular types of substance or practice abuse vary from society to society.

EXPLANATORY THEORIES

Explanatory theories fall into four major categories: psychological, biological, sociocultural, and systems. It is important to keep in mind that no definitive "cause" has been found for substance and practice abuse. It is probable that a combination of interrelated factors leads to the development of substance and practice abuse. We will look at some of these factors and at how they interrelate.

Psychological theories

Attempts to explain why individuals abuse substances or practices have focused on psychological vulnerability, interpersonal relationships, and learned responses. Some substance and practice abusers are thought to have antisocial personalities (see Chapter 21 for a discussion of antisocial personality). Various psychological theories try to explain why some people become substance or practice abusers and others do not.

PSYCHODYNAMIC THEORIES

Freud (1930, 1959) identified three agencies of the mind: id, ego, and superego (see Chapter 6). He believed that human infants are dominated solely by the id. Only through the process of social-ization do the ego and superego develop. The ego, through its appraisal of reality, and the superego, through its use of guilt, make people conform to social standards and thereby curb id behavior. Freudian theory holds that substance or practice abusers have defective egos and weak or immature superegos. Superego formation or "conscience" is acquired through identification with the values of significant others, especially parents. In individuals who abuse substances or practices, this identification has not occurred, or identification has been made with socially undesirable traits. In either case, a child is unable to internalize socially approved roles or socially acceptable values. Such a child grows into adulthood with an inadequately socialized superego. Social acceptance and disapproval then prove to be ineffective motivators or constraints. Such individuals operate for pleasure. They are impulsive; they are unable to arrive at successful compromise between society's standards and their own impulsive desires.

Adler (1927) looked at dependency. He suggested that the child situation is fraught with insecurity and inadequacy. Some children may focus on their own shortcomings and develop feelings of inferiority. Other children, especially first born children who are subsequently displaced by siblings, may also develop feelings of inadequacy. If parents are unable to reassure their children, then the feelings of inferiority persist, and a need to prove superiority may develop. As new problems arise and generate anxiety, instead of trying to problem solve, individuals may try to achieve a sense of superiority. Abuse of alcohol or other substances or practices succeeds in temporarily decreasing awareness of such feelings as insecurity, anxiety, and inferiority.

INTERPERSONAL THEORIES

Another psychoanalyst, Horney (1937), criticized Freud for not recognizing the role that anxiety and inner conflict play in the development of substance and practice abuse. Horney saw quests for power, prestige, and possessions as attempts to find reassurance against anxiety. She also realized that these quests are culturally specific and that they are not found in every society. She argued that in trying to obtain power, prestige, and possessions, some people become exploitative and manipulative.

Fromm (1947) defined character or personality as the way human energy is "canalized" or directed in the process of living and relating to the world. Once energy is directed into a specific character orientation, behavior becomes fairly consistent or "true to character."

Fromm's term *exploitative orientation* can be used to describe many individuals who are substance or practice abusers. Such people perceive the source of good and bad to be outside themselves. The only way to obtain the good things of life is to take them—through manipulation, guile, and/or force. This orientation pervades an individual's life-style. Everyone and everything is subject to exploitation. People and things are valued only for their usefulness.

No one psychological theory is adequate for explaining all types of substance and practice abuse or why some members of a family display such behavior and others do not. We cannot speak of a psychological "cause."

Biological theories

Biological theories purport that individuals abuse substances because they are biologically predisposed to such behavior. For instance, a person may have a physiological, biochemical, or genetic predisposition to alcoholism or heroin addiction. Such reasons are often given for substance abuse running in families.

BIOCHEMICAL THEORIES

Biochemical theories suggest that there may be metabolic differences in the way the bodies of alcoholics handle alcohol as compared to the way that the bodies of nonalcoholics handle it. It is not certain whether these metabolic differences are genetic or related to an alcoholic predisposition. For example, an early research study found that those individuals who have a low tolerance for alcohol are more accurate in their ability to discriminate blood alcohol level (BAL) than are those individuals who have a high tolerance for alcohol. The researchers concluded that "the development of tolerance may relate to the inability to discriminate BAL" (Lip-

scomb and Nathan, 1980). Other studies have focused on the blood level of the hormone cortisol. In nonalcoholic individuals, the blood level of cortisol has been shown to increase after drinking large amounts of alcohol and to remain high even as tolerance to alcohol develops. Recent research suggests that the level of cortisol in the bloodstream of sons of alcoholic fathers does not increase as dramatically as it does in sons of nonalcoholic fathers (Greenberg, 1987). Another study found that decreased epinephrine responsiveness may be associated with familial alcoholism (Swartz, Drews, and Cadoret, 1987).

PHYSIOLOGICAL THEORIES

The process by which physiological dependence on substances occurs is not completely understood. There is some indication that the central nervous system is involved in the development of dependency to specific drugs. For example, early studies on mice showed that there are at least two receptor sites for narcotic drugs in the brains of mice. One site intervenes in the pleasurable action associated with drug use, while the other site intervenes in the pain-controlling action (Pert and Synder, 1973). More recent studies on alcoholism indicate that chronic alcoholics may have a brain-wave deficiency (Benowitz, 1984). This apparent neurological involvement in substance abuse does not explain whether these factors generate a craving for a specific substance or whether they are related to emotional or behavioral disorders that contribute to substance abuse.

GENETIC THEORIES

Genetic predisposition may be involved in some types of substance abuse. For example, research suggests that a genetic factor may be implicated in alcoholism. Much of this research has focused on twins, half-siblings, and adoptees (children adopted at birth and raised by nonalcoholic parents apart from their alcoholic biologic relatives). Findings include: (1) There may be a genetic load in severe alcoholism. (2) There is a significant correlation between having an alcoholic biologic relative and alcoholism in adoptees. In one study, there was a fourfold increase in adoptee alcoholism when one biologic parent was alcoholic as compared with adoptees with nonalcoholic biologic parents. (3) There is a significant association between childhood conduct disorder in adoptees and alcoholism in adulthood. (4) Individuals with a family history of alcoholism (familial alcoholics) experience more severe alcoholic symptoms (both behavioral and physical), increased antisocial behavior, and poorer school and employment performance than do nonfamilial alcoholics. (5) Sons of alcoholics have lower blood cortisol levels after ingesting alcohol and are at greater risk for developing alcoholism than sons of nonalcoholics. (6) A low blood cortisol level after ingestion of alcohol may possibly act as a biological marker ("vulnerability marker") for intensity of response to ethyl alcohol (Goodwin, 1979, 1985; Cadoret, Cain, and Grove, 1980; Frances, Tim, and Bucky, 1980; Schuckit, 1985; Schuckit, Gold, and Rich, 1987).

Although rapid advances in biochemistry, neurophysiology, and genetics are providing increasing amounts of evidence for a relationship between biology and substance abuse, we cannot speak of a biological "cause" of such behavior. However, because people's perceptions of and responses to the environment must be filtered through their brains and implemented by their total bodies, we should not negate the role of biology in substance abuse. Although little research has focused on biological input into practice abuse, Custer's (1982) discussion of compulsive gambling acknowledges that biology probably is part of a confluence of factors responsible for the problem. The same may be true for other types of practice abuse.

Sociocultural theories

Sociocultural theories look to the broad social environment or to society-at-large for explanations for substance and practice abuse. While society stresses certain values, roles, and standards of behavior, the social structure often makes it difficult for a person to act in accordance with them. There may be a disjunction between socially approved goals and access to legitimized ways of achieving those goals, or the social situation may make the rules contradictory and meaningless. For example, while humanitarianism, honesty, and success are socially valued, many people find that they can succeed only through egocentric, aggressive, and cutthroat behavior.

SOCIAL STRAIN THEORY

Social strain theory views people as basically moral and desirous of following the rules of society. This theory maintains that since people want to internalize society's rule system, only major disjunctions in society can produce frustration, alienation, and socially aberrant behavior.

A sociocultural disjunction often cited as contributing to substance and practice abuse is rapid social change. Rapid social change tends to disrupt the values, standards, and social roles that govern socially acceptable behavior. Rapid social change may also affect the relationship of a person to self and others. Alienation may appear. In modern society, alienation tends to be pervasive. It may characterize the relationship of people to work, to things, and to other people. Feelings of boredom, hostility, isolation, and futility may develop. People may try to alter their alienated affect by abusing substances or practices. For example, some people may become addicted to drugs or to work. Others may experience an emotional "high" from compulsive gambling. Still others may show their hostility to and alienation from society through prostitution (Klinger, 1977; Rohrlich, 1980; Mann, 1984; Gaudia, 1987).

Social disintegration may be the result of a confluence of sociocultural disjunctures. Individuals often aspire to middle-class goals and life-style, but, because of such sociocultural disjunctures as dysfunctional families and inadequate opportunities for education or employment, they are unable to achieve them. People with low access to legitimate means of achieving goals or high access to illegitimate means of achieving goals may develop socially aberrant behavior. For example, underclass women may engage in prostitution as a means of obtaining economic and material gains otherwise unavailable to them (Miller, 1986).

Since it is not possible to directly measure social integration-disintegration, specific sociocultural indicators are useful. By employing a set of indices, social disintegration can be operationally defined. Using Leighton's (1959) classic criteria, as well as those of Ashcraft and Scheflen (1976), a community can be characterized as disintegrated if it contains many of the following sociocultural disjunctures:

1. A high incidence of "broken" homes (malfunctioning families). Little social control is exerted among family members.
2. Rapid social change. This leads to ambiguous standards of behavior.
3. A rapidly changing value system. This leaves people confused about the values around which to organize their lives.
4. Inadequate associations. There is little actual grouping of people around such common interests as religion, work, or recreation. Those groups that do exist are marked by low group cohesiveness.
5. Inadequate leadership. Leaders who live in the community are relatively ineffective in establishing meaningful, ordered social behavior.
6. Inadequate opportunities for recreation. Few opportunities exist for such group diversions as sports and hobbies. Recreation tends to take such individualistic forms as drinking and sexual promiscuity.
7. A high degree of hostility. There are many instances of physical and verbal abuse.
8. A high incidence of crime and delinquency. Criminal acts such as child abuse, robbery, physical aggression, and sexual assault are frequent.
9. Inadequate communication. Poor communication may be caused by such physically isolating factors as poor transportation systems or absence of telephones, or it may result from poor or nonexistent interpersonal relationships.

These disjunctions threaten the efficient functioning of a social system. Sociocultural disjunctions may result in inadequate socialization of children. Family patterns, kinship obligations, child-rearing practices, and economic activites may be disrupted. Value systems and role relationships may become confused, fragmented, or conflicting. Children may fail to learn socially sanctioned values, standards, and roles.

SOCIAL LEARNING THEORY

Social learning theory holds that substance and practice abuse are learned from role models and are reinforced by peer pressure and/or paternal and sibling influence. In environments where there is a high incidence of substance and practice abuse, novices learn deviant behavior by associating with social deviants. Individuals observe that they and/or their role models are rewarded with prestige and material gains for their socially deviant behavior. With every occasion of reward, the pattern of deviance is reinforced. A process of increasing attachment to the abuse of substances or practices develops. As the attachment increases, so does the risk of incurring costs. Costs refer to the personal and social hazards of abusing a particular substance or practice, and they are both personally and socially relative. Costs may either reinforce the deviant behavior or moderate the behavior. For example, an individual may respond to the costs involved in prostitution (e.g., police threats and competition from other prostitutes) by becoming a member of a deviant street network and thereby increase the attachment to prostitution. On the other hand, an individual may respond to the costs involved in heroin abuse (e.g., risks involved in obtaining the drug and contracting AIDS) by deciding to get help to break the heroin attachment. The balancing of increased attachment to a substance or practice with the incurring costs may generate ambivalence and an approach-avoidance conflict. At this point change, involving information processing, self-reconstruction, and the utilization of change-supporting therapies, may occur (Orford, 1985).

Because no single sociocultural theory is adequate for explaining all types of substance and practice abuse or why different people display different types of such behavior, we cannot say there is a definitive sociocultual "cause."

Systems theory

A systems approach to substance and practice abuse has a dual orientation. (1) It integrates biopsychosocial factors. (2) It emphasizes the family as a system. (Refer to Chapters 5 and 14 for discussions of the family as a system and dysfunctional families.)

Substance and practice abuse relates to all dimensions of self. A poorly developed physical potential interferes with a person's ability to enjoy life. This not only becomes a source of stress but also makes a person more vulnerable to other stressors. In addition, a person may fear expressing feelings. Inability to express emotion may result in manipulating others rather than relating in an open, compassionate manner. The intellect bridges the past (through memories) with the present and the future. Intellectual impairment may interfere with interpretation of the body's physical cues, channeling the expression of emotion, regulating interpersonal relationships, and giving the spiritual domain opportunity for expression. A person may turn to substance or practice abuse as a means of coping with the stress engendered by defective dimensions of self, as an anesthetic for emotions, as a way to end spiritual malaise, and as an attempt to boost faltering self-esteem.

If a family member is a substance or practice abuser, that family member's behavior may be a symptom of dysfunction in the family system. Behavior and interactions among all family members contribute to the development of problematic behavior. Therefore, understanding the problem and how it is being maintained, as well as intervention into the problem, must focus on the system rather than on the individual.

Family interdependence and interaction are constantly in a state of flux in an attempt to maintain system stability. When change occurs with one family member, it affects all members of the family. This informational flow, or feedback, may promote system stability (negative feedback) or promote system change (positive feedback). When a family system is functioning well, then positive feedback may be utilized for family growth. If there is a family problem, such as substance or practice abuse, then some types of positive feedback may further stress the family system.

Mr. Jackson, an insurance salesman, is a compulsive gambler. His gambling has put the family in debt. In addition, because of the time that Mr. Jackson spent away from his job gambling, Mr. Jackson's salary became inadequate to support the family's life-style. Initially, Mrs. Jackson tried to economize on groceries and clothes to make ends meet. Finally, she took a job as a bank clerk, and the two teenage children got part-time jobs. These actions (positive feedback) only en-

abled Mr. Jackson to continue gambling. Eventually, their indebtedness became so great that the family lost their home, and Mrs. Jackson divorced her husband.

However, not all positive feedback stresses a dysfunctional family system into further dysfunction. For example, if in the preceding vignette, Mrs. Jackson and the children had attended Gam-Anon and Gam-A-Teen, they would have received some support and guidance. They would have had opportunities to verbalize such feelings as anger and shame, prioritize their needs, and learn to plan for and meet some of those needs. The family might also have been able to find ways to assist Mr. Jackson in seeking help. Their behaviors would not have facilitated Mr. Jackson's gambling and would have increased the likelihood of his seeking professional help to stop gambling.

The more that substance or practice abuse threatens a family, the more anxious family members become. They tend to deal with their anxiety by blaming and scapegoating the abuser. Family stress level increases. The abuser tries to cope with increased family tension through greater reliance on chemical substances or compulsive practices. The abuser's increased dependency on the substance or practice escalates family tension. The situation continues to spiral.

The family of a substance or practice abuser directs most of its energy into covering up the problem, trying to force the abusing member to reform, and/or compensating for the abdicated role performance of the abusing family member. The family becomes a closed system. There is little family energy available for processing input from other systems (e.g., work, school, social network) that interact with the family or for growth (Estes, Smith-Dijulio, and Heinemann, 1980; Wegscheider, 1981; Textor, 1987).

Systems theory emphasizes the interrelationship among self, others, and the environment. Systems theory also shows how, in families with substance or practice abusing members, feedback can be used to promote system stability or to promote system change and growth.

TABLE 20-12   Theoretical orientations and nursing implications

Orientation	Implications for nursing practice
Psychodynamic	Nurses teach parents ways to facilitate healthy personality development in their children so they can develop the internal controls necessary to curb impulsive behavior. With clients who are abusing substances or practices, external controls should be used until internal controls can be developed.
Interpersonal	Nurses teach clients to communicate their needs for power, prestige, and possessions and to develop assertive rather than exploitative and manipulative behavior to fulfill their needs.
Biochemical	Nurses recognize that the bodies of alcoholics may metabolize alcohol differently than the bodies of nonalcoholics. Nurses utilize this knowledge in health teaching and counseling with alcoholic clients.
Physiological	Nurses recognize that central nervous system involvement in chemical dependency may mean that some substance abusers need external aids (e.g., antabuse and methadone) to control their behavior.
Genetic	Nurses recognize that genetic factors may predispose some individuals to substance abuse. Nurses counsel clients with family histories of alcoholism about their increased vulnerability to alcoholism.
Social strain	Nurses recognize that modification of the sociocultural environment may help prevent substance and practice abuse. Toward this end, nurses lobby elected officials for social programs that address such problems as poverty, homelessness, and unemployment.
Learning	Nurses recognize that when increased attachment to a substance or practice is weighed against its incurring costs and ambivalence develops, a client may be ready for behavioral change. Nurses provide a structured environment that rewards socially acceptable behavior but does not reward or reinforce manipulative, exploitative, or addictive behavior.
Systems	Nurses view substance and practice abuse as complex behaviors with multifactorial origins that signal dysfunction in the family system. Nurses assess the biopsychosocial aspects of a situation before making a nursing diagnosis. Nursing intervention focuses on the family system and not on the individual.

The various theoretical orientations toward substance and practice abuse impact on the practice of nursing. Table 20-12 gives examples of some of the implications of these theoretical orientations for nursing practice.

TREATMENT MODALITIES

Once a decision to begin treatment has been made, the question arises: *what type of treatment setting is appropriate?* Frequently, because of the medical problems associated with substance and practice abuse (for example, malnutrition, sexually transmitted disease, infection, or personal injury), a general hospital may be chosen. Abusers usually wish to have their medical problems treated and will cooperate with a medical regimen. Unfortunately, once the medical problems have been cor-

rected, referrals are only infrequently made for psychosocial therapy.

Individuals who are transferred to psychiatric treatment centers or who are remanded there by the courts are often poorly motivated to deal with their psychosocial problems. Since rationalization is a mechanism that is used frequently by such persons, they sometimes enter into treatment only halfheartedly. Ulterior motives may be operating. For instance, an addict may seek detoxification to reduce the severity of a habit rather than to kick it.

Individuals who are placed in psychiatric hospitals that also treat psychotic persons may resent it. In all probability, they not only will try to keep themselves apart from psychotic individuals but also may ridicule, attempt to provoke, and exploit them.

Specialized treatment centers may be the best setting in which to treat persons who abuse substances or practices. In such centers, rehabilitated former offenders may constitute part or most of the treatment team. A combination of professionals and former offenders is uniquely able to deal with the dynamics underlying substance and practice abuse.

Alternatives to hospitals and specialized treatment centers include such self-help groups as Alcoholics Anonymous, Gamblers Anonymous, and Narcotics Anonymous. The support and intervention offered by these groups have proven effective in helping many individuals. Of course, not everyone is a candidate for such a group. Those people whose behavior poses serious threats to society cannot safely be treated on a voluntary basis. Self-help groups usually provide a support system that functions 24 hours a day and 7 days a week to help sustain members through the periods of treatment, recovery, and rehabilitation. Any combination of the options mentioned may be used. For example,

---

Laura was a middle-aged housewife. Her children were grown and had set up households of their own. She complained of feeling "edgy and jumpy." She would begin with one drink each morning to help her get started with her housework. By the time her husband, Jim, came home for dinner, she was usually drunk. Jim recognized that Laura drank too much, but he did not want to "humiliate" her by placing her in an alcohol treatment center. Instead he consulted their family doctor, who had been Laura's physician for many years. The doctor told Jim that Laura was very tense and anxious, and he prescribed Valium to help her relax. Laura took the Valium but cut down on her drinking very little.

One day, Jim came home and found Laura hemorrhaging from the mouth. She was rushed to their community hospital, where she underwent detoxification and was treated for esophageal varices, gastritis, and malnutrition.

After her medical problems had been corrected, Laura was sent to a treatment center for alcoholics. There she was helped to recognize that she was cross-addicted to alcohol and Valium. While at the center, weekly Alcoholics Anonymous meetings were held. At discharge, Laura was referred to AA for rehabilitation.

This situation demonstrates that a combination of medical, psychological, and social therapy may be indicated. Once the decision to initiate treatment has been made, a number of settings may be used: general hospital, psychiatric hospital, specialized treatment center, and self-help groups. It is in these settings that the treatment modalities that facilitate recovery are instituted. We will now explore some of the most frequently used modalities.

Aversion therapy

Aversion therapy, or negative conditioning, makes use of learning theory to help a person to stop behaving in a socially unacceptable way. Some unpleasant consequence is attached to the undesirable behavior. Aversion therapy is applied in a systematic manner. First, the unwanted behavior is identified. Next, its baseline frequency is established. Then, any environmental factors supporting the behavior are discerned.

A common type of aversion therapy for alcoholism involves the use of the drug disulfiram (Antabuse). Disulfiram remains inert in the body unless alcohol is ingested. Once an alcoholic beverage (or any medicine or food with an ethyl alcohol base) is taken, a physiological reaction similar to a severe hangover occurs. The reaction includes throbbing headache, dizziness, nausea, vomiting, facial flushing, heart palpitations, difficult breathing, and blurred vision. These symptoms last for 1 to 2 hours. Disulfiram must be taken regularly to be an effective deterrent to alcoholism. If people wish to drink, they can simply discontinue the use of disulfiram and thereby avoid its effects.

John's employer had given him an ultimatum: either stop drinking or be fired. John decided to enter a veteran's hospital. He had heard about disulfiram and requested it. While he was in the hospital he took the drug regularly. After he was discharged, he continued to take disulfiram. John's job performance and interpersonal relationships improved. However, December came, and with it the office Christmas party. John decided to enter into the Christmas spirit—or should we say "spirits." He discontinued his use of disulfiram so that he would be able to "drink socially." He did not suffer any of the effects of disulfiram, but he did become intoxicated.

As the vignette shows, there clearly are drawbacks to treatment with disulfiram. The use of the drug can be discontinued at any time. Disulfiram therapy requires self-motivation to be successful.

Aversion therapy has been criticized because it inflicts noxious stimuli on clients without providing opportunities for pleasurable reinforcement of positive behavior. In addition, critics argue, only overt behavior is dealt with: aversion therapists are not concerned with the dynamics underlying behavior.

Proponents of aversion therapy emphasize that such therapy often works in cases in which other types of therapy have failed. They maintain that noxious stimuli are administered only in an attempt to change behavior that both the client and society have defined as unacceptable. Proponents argue that a short period of aversion therapy is preferable to a lifetime of socially unacceptable and inevitably self-destructive behavior.

The ultimate choice must be the client's. Nurses should ensure that candidates for aversion therapy have enough information to be able to weigh the advantages and disadvantages of negative conditioning and to compare it to other available treatments.

Drug therapy

Because of the addictive nature of substance abuse, the use of drugs as a treatment modality is extremely restricted. Many treatment programs are drug free: no drug, even aspirin, is permitted.

Some drugs have been found to have limited value in the treatment of specific types of behavior. In the discussion of aversion therapy, the use of disulfiram (Antabuse) for the treatment of alcoholism was mentioned. Two hundred fifty milligrams of disulfiram each day is an average maintenance dose. Disulfiram must be taken daily. Many alcoholics will intentionally discontinue use of the drug so that they can return to drinking. Therefore,

motivation for sobriety is very important. If disulfiram therapy is to be effective, concurrent psychotherapy is usually advisable.

People who take disulfiram need to avoid all substances containing ethyl alcohol, including not only alcoholic beverages but many medications, mouthwashes, and food preparations. Even inhaling alcohol fumes can cause a disulfiram reaction.

John had been discharged from an alcohol treatment program. He was taking disulfiram. One day he became violently ill; he had all the symptoms of a disulfiram reaction. He telephoned a counselor at the treatment center and made an appointment for the next day. John swore that he had not been drinking, and the counselor believed him. After discussion and data collection that bordered on detective work, the counselor discovered that John had bought a new mouthwash and had begun using it the day before he became ill. The mouthwash had a high alcohol content. No one had thought to discuss such a potential problem with John before his discharge.

This vignette illustrates the importance of education. It is not enough to dispense medication; a medication's action and side effects, as well as any contingencies affecting the action, should be made known to a client.

Opiate-blocking drugs have been found to be useful in preventing the pleasurable, tension-reducing effects of narcotics. Methadone (Dolophine) and cyclazocine (WIN) are two opiate-blocking agents. Dolophine, the best known of these drugs, is a synthetic opiate. Like an opiate, it is an addicting drug. Treatment based on the administration of dolophine involves the substitution of a legal addiction (to Dolophine) for an illegal addiction (to narcotics). Dolophine has two functions. It enables addicts to stop opiate usage without the usual painful withdrawal symptoms, and it helps addicts stay off opiates because they no longer get "high" from them. Dolophine is administered orally. It is long acting and has to be taken only once a day. An average maintenance dose is 140 mg daily. This dosage level effectively eliminates withdrawal symptoms, blocks the pleasurable effects of opiates, and lessens the desire for narcotics.

Dolophine maintenance has been instrumental in the successful treatment of many "hard core" addicts—those who have not responded to other therapies. Many such addicts have been able to resume their normal social roles and to remain gainfully employed. However, because their addictive personality patterns have not been altered, many of these addicts may take nonopiate drugs along with Dolophine. As opponents of treatment through Dolophine maintenance point out, people using Dolophine are still addicted, even though their addiction is legal. Thus it is important that psychotherapy accompany Dolophine maintenance. Otherwise, addictive personality traits and socially deviant patterns of coping and communicating may remain unchanged.

Group therapy*

One of the most commonly used treatment modalities for substance and practice abuse is group therapy. The utilization of a group approach recognizes the need of individuals for group identification.

Because substance and practice abusers demonstrate much hostile and aggressive behavior, they tend to threaten neurotic and psychotic persons. People who abuse substances or practices are better able to check one another's behavior than are outsiders. Therefore, such individuals may be treated more effectively in homogeneous groups than in heterogeneous groups. In a homogeneous group, limits are set by people who are experiencing or have experienced the same difficulties. Such a group setting permits individuals to reveal their true selves without fear of retaliation. Authority, restraint, and controls arise from within the group. Because they may be deriving gratification from the group experience, individuals may begin to submit to group pressure. Satisfying group experiences may ultimately lead to the capacity to become integrated into groups. Rules and norms may be internalized, and, eventually, other people and society may no longer be perceived as antagonistic.

---

*Refer to Chapter 13 for an in-depth discussion of group therapy.

Family therapy

Intervention with family members is essential to the treatment of substance and practice abuse. Families may mirror or facilitate and reinforce such behavior. It is thus necessary to intervene on the level of the family as well as on the level of the individual. Examples of nursing diagnoses that may be used for families of substance and practice abusers are:

1. Altered family processes related to inability to deal with substance abuse (specify type) of family member (NANDA 3.2.2)
2. Altered family processes related to inability to deal with practice abuse (specify type) of family member (NANDA 3.2.2)

Table 20-13 identifies some objectives of family therapy.

Substance and practice abuse can be very destructive to families. At the same time, family members can facilitate and reinforce a member's abusing behavior. For change to occur, the family should be part of the therapeutic process.

Educational therapy

Educational therapy has many purposes. It provides information. It facilitates group identification. It promotes self-esteem. Educational and vocational training programs offer opportunities for substance and practice abusers to learn skills and direct energy into socially acceptable channels. Educational therapy also provides information about substance and practice abuse and about activities of daily living that can facilitate personal and occupational adjustment. Educational therapy often also includes instruction in such personal matters as grooming, dress, and etiquette.

Lisa, an adolescent girl, had been admitted to a drug treatment center. She had been doing poorly in school and thought of herself as a "dummy." She planned to drop out of school as soon as it was legally permissible. The treatment team decided that Lisa was definitely a candidate for educational therapy. While at the drug center, Lisa not only attended daily classes but also received tutoring in subjects of special weakness. She was shown how to budget study time, how to take notes, and how to outline chapters. In addition, she

TABLE 20-13   Objectives of family therapy

Objective	Rationale
Initiate detoxification	The addict needs to accept responsibility for substance abuse and abstinence.
Promote a sense of family responsibility	Family members need to understand that the problem is a symptom of family dysfunction, that they have all contributed to its development and maintenance, and that change needs to occur with all family members and family relationships.
Promote open, clear communication	Family members need to be aware of the impact of verbal and nonverbal behavior. Family members need to acknowledge and correct ambiguous communication and doublebind messages. Family members need to learn to confront, argue, and express anger constructively. Family members need to increase their behavioral repertoire to include expression of humor, joy, sadness, etc.
Promote mutuality between spouses	Spouses need to learn to relate as partners. The alliance between the addict and the opposite-sex parent needs to be broken. The same-sex parent needs to become more involved with the addicted child. Time needs to be set aside for spouses to mutually participate in activities and discussions. Same-sex parent and addicted child need to discover common interests.
Promote effective parent-child interaction	Opposite-sex parent needs to stop overprotecting the addicted child. Same-sex parent needs to stop scapegoating the addicted child. Parents need to jointly engage in limit setting, to recognize and change unrealistic expectations of the addicted child, and to focus attention on and reward the positive qualities of the addicted child.
Resolve marital conflicts	Parents need to accept the spouse of a married addicted child. Parents and addicted child need to clarify the boundaries between the family of origin and the conjugal family. The addict and the addict's spouse need to identify role relationships and marital patterns transmitted from the families of origin to the conjugal family. The addict's spouse may need to join a support group (e.g., Alanon, Gam-Anon) that provides a social and/or fictive kin network.
Restructure the social network	The addict must give up friends who are addicted. Integration of the addict into a network of nonaddict peers provides the addict with support to individuate from parents and opportunities to discuss values and conflicts, problem solve, and make decisions. The addict may need to join a support group (e.g., Alcoholics Anonymous, Gamblers Anonymous) that provides a social and/or fictive kin network.
Strengthen relationships with other social systems	The addict may need to examine stressors associated with work or school. The addict may need to learn more effective ways of interacting with employers, teachers, and/or peers. Services may need to be coordinated among social agencies serving the addict and the addict's family.

Sources consulted include Textor (1987) and Gaudia (1987).

was placed in a personal development group that included other adolescent girls. With the assistance of a nurse, the group regularly discussed clothing styles and experimented with hairstyles and cosmetics. By the time Lisa was ready to leave the center, she felt able to return to junior high school and was confident that she could at least pass her courses. She also felt more comfortable with her appearance.

The preceding vignette shows how educational therapy can be designed to facilitate the social and academic reentry of substance or practice abusers into society. In an attempt to help individuals reconstruct lives that have been damaged by substance or practice abuse, educational therapy helps clients look at past failures and ascertain what contributed to those failures. In this way, those experiences can provide opportunities for learning and growth.

Emergency therapy

Clients who are in crisis because of substance intoxication need to be carefully assessed for

1. Chemical substance used: route, amount, type(s) (many substance abusers are polydrug users)
2. Pattern of use: habitual or crisis use
3. Nature of support system: availability of family and friends, community resources
4. Degree of motivation: history of previous treatment, amenability to discontinuing substance abuse

A physician should be summoned immediately. If the substance is known, nurses can make use of standing orders for antidotes. Because of the danger of polydrug abuse, all medications should be administered judiciously. Otherwise, nursing therapy involves the relief of symptoms or the administration of life-sustaining measures (for example, maintenance of an airway). In cases of alcohol or barbiturate abuse, abrupt withdrawal from the substance may precipitate convulsions. Table 20-14 outlines emergency intervention guidelines for clients with some types of substance intoxication or overdose.

Clients should be assured of the confidential nature of treatment. Rationale for treatment and the expected outcomes should be explained. In addition, before discharging any client, referral for ongoing treatment should be made (Seymour, Gorton, and Smith, 1982).

Sample interaction: talking down a client

Nurse (speaking slowly, softly and calmly). Tell me what is happening with you.

Client (speaking rapidly and appearing in a panic). Lions and tigers with grotesque red and green masks are coming towards me. They want to hurt me. They are attacking me! Dismembering me!

Nurse Red and green are Christmas colors.

Client (still speaking rapidly but with less panic). Christmas is my favorite holiday.

Nurse Tell me about your favorite Christmas.

The nurse spoke calmly, slowly, and softly in order not to inadvertently threaten the client and thereby increase his sense of panic. Because of the client's heightened state of suggestibility and distractibility, the nurse was able to refocus the client onto the topic of Christmas colors and Christmas. By focusing on a nonthreatening aspect of the client's hallucination, the nurse was also trying to lower the client's anxiety level. Since "talking down" may go on for several hours, the client's relatives, who had accompanied the client to the emergency room, periodically became involved in the talking down process.

Milieu therapy

A therapeutic community* is a form of milieu therapy. A therapeutic community for substance abusers attempts to correct behavior and to prepare residents for reentry into society. Every activity is designed to teach residents to live by society's standards and to function in a socially acceptable manner. A therapeutic community serves as a real-life reference group. As one resident of such a community explained.

We use a yardstick approach here. We figure that most of the people in society function at 24 inches. We try to bring ourselves up to 36 inches because we know when we leave here we'll slip back a little. But even with slipping back we'll be okay.

This "yardstick approach" explains why, in a therapeutic community, exacting behavior is expected and infraction of rules carries heavy penalties. Residents who do not clean their rooms may have to wear a sign that says "I'm a slob." Residents whose attitudes are manipulative or sullen may be verbally "blown away." Residents who run away from the therapeutic community and then want to return may receive a "haircut"—their heads may literally be shaved as a constant reminder of their immature behavior. These measures are taken to inculcate society's values and norms into people who have been operating outside society's rule system. Society may expect its members to function at "24 inches," but because many substance and practice abusers start out with little or no social conscience, they have to be brought up to "36 inches."

---

*See Chapter 12 for a general discussion of milieu therapy and the therapeutic community.

TABLE 20-14 Emergency intervention guidelines: substance intoxification

Chemical substance	Guidelines
Depressants (e.g., barbiturates)	Treat immediately any central nervous system, cardiovascular, and/or respiratory depression (e.g., gastric lavage; administration of IV fluids; forced diuresis; alkalinization of urine; maintenance of body temperature, blood pressure, and airway). Monitor vital signs. Keep client physically active (until barbiturate is metabolized). Use a firm, nonconfrontative, supportive approach. Refer for gradual detoxification (to avoid detoxification-related seizures).
Depressants (e.g., alcohol)	Assess for alcohol-drug interactions. Assess for methyl alcohol ingestion (methyl alcohol is often used as a cheap substitute for ethyl alcohol). Treat methyl alcohol intoxification with ethyl alcohol (prevents metabolism of methanol). Observe for metabolic acidosis, retinal damage, and central nervous system damage (e.g., hyperventilation, vision loss) caused by methanol. Monitor vital signs. Treat symptomatically effects of alcohol-drug intoxication. Manage assaultive or aggressive behavior (refer to Chapter 21).
Narcotics (e.g., opiates)	Administer naloxone (Narcan), a narcotic antagonist. Maintain a clear airway. Maintain body temperature. Treat any respiratory distress. Monitor vital signs. Monitor for opiate withdrawal symptoms (Narcan may precipitate opiate withdrawal). Use a firm, nonconfrontative, supportive approach.
Stimulants (e.g., amphetamine and cocaine)	Monitor the environment (e.g., low light and noise levels, minimal activity). Approach client with caution (may misinterpret any action as an attack). Speak slowly and calmly. Do not whisper (may increase client's paranoia). Explain all procedures and actions before initiating them. Decrease the level of stimulant in client's system (e.g., vomiting in conscious client, acidic gastric lavage in unconscious client, acidification of urine). Treat hypertensive crisis with an α-adrenergic blocking agent. Administer antipsychotic drugs (e.g., haloperidol). Treat anxiety with benzodiazepines (propranolol may increase the risk of cardiovascular toxicity). Monitor vital signs. Observe for depression associated with stimulant withdrawal.
Hallucinogens (e.g., LSD)	Manipulate the environment (e.g., allow friends to remain with client, low light and noise levels, minimal activity). Use a nonthreatening, nonauthoritative approach. "Talk down" the client (see Sample Interaction: Talking Down a Client).
Tranquilizers (e.g., diazepam and haloperidol)	Treat respiratory depression (e.g., maintenance of airway, methylphenidate or caffeine administration). *Do not* give barbiturates to treat tranquilizer-induced excitation. Treat hypotension (e.g., levarternol or metaraminol administration, IV fluids, vasopressors). Monitor vital signs. Use a firm, nonconfrontative, supportive approach.

Sources consulted include Yowell and Brose (1977), Seymour, Gorton, and Smith (1982), Clayton (1984), Gawin and Ellinwood (1988).

Frequently, the staff of a therapeutic community is composed entirely of former substance abusers. Professionals may be only tangentially involved. The rationale for such a staffing policy includes three elements:

1. Former offenders have experienced the problem and have overcome it. They therefore can serve as role models.
2. Since former offenders have used all the mechanisms common to substance or practice abuse, they can recognize and confront these mechanisms in newcomers.
3. Former offenders are considered peers by residents of a therapeutic community. Structure, challenge, confrontation, and discipline are more readily accepted when meted out by peers.

Many substance and practice abusers have become expert manipulators. Some are highly skilled at manipulating groups and have even been "gang" leaders. Most professionals do not have this kind of personal history. Professional education often focuses more on intervention with individuals than on intervention with groups. Many professionals have not learned confrontation techniques. Therefore, a former offender is often better able to deal with substance or practice abusers than is a health professional.

• • •

Substance and practice abuse may be treated in a variety of treatment settings and with a variety of treatment modalities. The goals of therapy are to supplant socially aberrant behavior with socially acceptable behavior and to facilitate reentry into society. Although nurses may not directly participate in all treatment modalities, they do participate in all levels of preventive intervention: primary, secondary, and tertiary.

Nursing Intervention

The behavior of substance and practice abusers is often challenging to a nurse's value system. Frequently such persons not only resist treatment but also attack the treatment process. They may try to "con" their therapists and "work" the system. In view of these difficulties, what qualities should nurses who work with these people possess? The Task Force on Substance Abuse Nursing Practice (1987) suggests that the knowledge and skills in Table 20-15 are fundamental for administering direct care (clinician role).

Addictions nursing encompasses diverse roles. In addition to the clinical role of the nurse, it includes the following roles: supervisor, administrator, consultant, researcher, and educator (see Appendix F for the ANA Standards of Addictions Nursing Practice).

PRIMARY PREVENTION

The alleviation of conditions that contribute to substance and practice abuse is vital for primary prevention. The ANA Task Force on Substance Abuse Nursing Practice regards the following interventions as essential to any program of primary prevention:

1. Education about addiction (e.g., addictive nature of specific substances, recreational substance abuse, signs and symptoms of addiction, factors contributing to substance and practice abuse)

TABLE 20-15   Addictions nursing: knowledge and skills

Knowledge/skill	Description
Theoretical and clinical	Knowledge consistent with a generalist level of nursing education.
Comprehensive nursing assessment	Interviewing, psychosocial assessment, taking a health history, conducting physical and mental status examinations.
Self-assessment	Foundation for understanding nurse-client relationships and addiction-related maladaptive interpersonal styles.
Patterns of addiction	Knowledge about physiological and behavioral responses associated with addiction.
Counseling skills	Formal and informal techniques; individual, group, marital, and family therapies; approaches specific to abuse and addiction; counseling goals. Establishment of goals should be a participatory process between nurse and client. Goals should be nonjudgmental. Goals should recognize the implications of addiction for health, identify maladaptive coping patterns, alter client's dysfunctional perceptions of self and the world, foster new and adaptive behaviors and coping styles, and modify the social environment so that the client receives positive reinforcement for new learning about abuse and addiction.
Health teaching	Done at the levels of primary, secondary, and tertiary prevention intervention.
Evaluation	Effectiveness of the treatment plan (periodic reassessment of client's status, modification of goals or priorities).

2. Identification of high-risk individuals (e.g., children of alcoholics, children raised in disorganized communities)
3. Recognition of early behavioral manifestations of addiction
4. Participation in social change (e.g., lobbying for and supporting laws directed at modifying conditions that contribute to substance and practice abuse)
5. Application of knowledge about addiction to client health teaching (e.g., effects of tobacco smoking on respiratory and cardiovascular systems, effects of compulsive gambling on family members)
6. Application of knowledge about the compulsive and dependent nature of addiction to health maintenance teaching (e.g., recognition that the course of recovery is often marked by periods of improvement and relapse, identification of stressors that precipitate relapse in order to prevent it)

Because the children of substance and practice abusers often experience guilt, shame, and confusion and may feel socially isolated, Schilit (1986) suggests that they be taught the interpersonal and assertiveness skills necessary to establish and maintain relationships. Since community health nurses and school nurse-teachers work with families and observe family interactions, they have opportunities to assess children's needs for such skills. Nurses can refer the children of substance and practice abusers to self-help organizations that provide supportive relationships and teach social skills.

Allison, a 16-year-old high school student, was receiving poor grades. She did not hand assignments in on time, and she frequently fell asleep in class. The school nurse-teacher recognized that Allison was a troubled youth and established a supportive relationship with her. Allison revealed that she had many family problems. Allison's father was a compulsive gambler, and her mother was an alcoholic. Allison had two younger brothers. The 15-year-old was "running around with a loose crowd and drinking." The 12-year-old seemed well-adjusted. Allison was trying to hold the family together, straighten out her 15-year-old brother, and protect the 12-year-old. She had as-

sumed the parenting role. Allison had not spoken about her situation with anyone except the school nurse-teacher. She felt ashamed and was afraid that if her classmates knew about her parents, they would not want to associate with her. As a consequence, Allison never invited classmates to her house and spent most of her time alone.

The school nurse-teacher referred Allison to Alateen, where she was helped to express her feelings of shame and anger. She also learned that her situation was not unique and that many adolescents were in similar predicaments. Allison learned that although she could not change her family's behavior, she could change the way she reacted. Toward this end, she learned assertiveness skills. Allison also made some friends in the group and generally found the Alateen group very supportive.

As the preceding vignette illustrates, when a family member is a substance or practice abuser, other family members may experience role confusion and role overburdening and may have difficulty establishing supportive interpersonal relationships. Referral to self-help organizations may provide networks of nonprofessional support.

Because substance and practice abuse develop out of a confluence of interrelated factors, only a multifaceted primary prevention program that encompasses a range of strategies will be effective.

SECONDARY PREVENTION

Secondary preventive intervention, aimed at assisting substance and practice abusers to achieve a higher level of wellness, should be begun when individuals are first identified as substance or practice abusers or when they are first seen in detoxification or treatment centers. Nurses should view clients as holistic human beings and should take a systems approach to nursing care.

A head nurse was orienting Gary to his nursing responsibilities on an alcohol detoxification unit. After giving Gary a tour of the unit and introducing him to the clients, the head nurse and Gary sat down and discussed the role of a nurse in a detoxification unit. Gary stated that he was aware that many of the clients would be malnourished and/or poorly hydrated and that at frequent intervals nourishing foods and fluids should be available to clients. The head nurse agreed and added, "Initially, bland foods are most easily tolerated. Because caffeine may increase tremors, only decaffeinated coffee and caffeine-free sodas should be offered."

Gary further recognized that client's vital signs would have to be monitored and that clients would have to be observed for confusion, tremors, seizures, hyperactivity, and hallucinations. Gary knew that a safe environment should be provided in order to prevent self-injury and that seizure precautions should be instituted. Clients should also be supported through their hallucinatory experiences (see Chapter 25).

Gary was aware that because of the physiological effects of chronic alcoholism, these clients were at high risk for many ailments, including gastritis, gastrointestinal bleeding, cirrhosis, pancreatitis, esophageal varices, impaired renal function, and neurological disorders. Gary knew that besides closely monitoring clients and administering medication to minimize the effects of withdrawal or the complications associated with alcoholism, he would have to alert a physician to any newly developed symptoms or changes in a client's condition.

The head nurse thought that Gary's view of the role of the nurse was limited. The head nurse pointed out that not only clients' physical problems, but also their psychological, social, and spiritual concerns needed to be considered. The head nurse reminded Gary that clients who are withdrawing from alcohol may be disoriented, anxious, hostile, beligerent, or depressed. Nurses on an alcohol detoxification unit may have to reorient clients to time, place, person, and situation. Nurses also have to assess the degree of client anxiety, hostility, aggression, and depression, and the lethality of any suicidal ideation and appropriately intervene. The emotional support of ex-alcoholics or pastoral counselors can be helpful. Nurses should be nonjudgmental of clients and should not try to reform or chastise them.

The head nurse also explained to Gary that clients who are experiencing severe withdrawal symptoms may have to be assisted with their personal hygiene. Other clients may have to be helped to develop routines of personal hygiene. In addition, the head nurse cautioned Gary that, because social network members often facilitate an alcoholic's drinking, during visiting hours nurses need to be alert to the possibility of visitors smuggling liquor to clients. The head nurse cited one instance in which a wife concealed whiskey in plastic bags in her satchel-type pocketbook. During visiting hours, the wife gave the whiskey to her hus-band. The head nurse pointed out that referral of social network members to such support groups as Al-anon and Alateen is important if nurses in detoxification units are to assist clients to reach their potentials for high-level wellness.

The preceding vignette illustrates that when nurses take a holistic, systems approach to client care, they can be instrumental in guiding clients as they learn about the process of wellness and in assisting and supporting clients as they try to achieve higher-level wellness.

However, when nurses work with substance and practice abusers, problems may arise that impede effective nursing care. For example, when clients use ingratiation and charm, nurses may not recognize that they are being manipulated.

Mrs. Graff, who had been admitted to a hospital with drug-related hepatitis, was very charming and witty, She confided to one of the nurses. "You are the only one in this hospital who treats me like a person. All the other nurses try to avoid me. They don't like me very much." The nurse was flattered by this comment. Even though he did not approve of Mrs. Graff's drug abuse, he felt that of all the staff, he alone was able to relate to Mrs. Graff as a person. In an attempt to compensate for the rejecting attitudes of the other nurses, he tried to be available to Mrs. Graff and to comply with her requests. One day over coffee, several nurses began discussing Mrs. Graff's feeling of rejection. They discovered that Mrs. Graff had told each of them that the other nurses were avoiding her and that he or she was the only nurse who cared. Each had felt flattered and had responded by going out of the way to give Mrs. Graff extra attention.

Thus, when nurses fail to recognize manipulation, they may unwittingly reinforce it. On the other hand, when nurses do recognize manipulative tendencies in clients, they may sometimes respond defensively. They may begin to see manipulation in the actions of all clients, or they may reject or show hostility toward manipulative clients. It is important for nurses to be aware of these possible responses to manipulative clients. Such responses may reinforce a client's low self-esteem and increase his or her need to engage in exploitative behavior.

Another area of potential difficulty concerns the communication theme of hostility. Because some nurses may fear the repercussions of dealing with a client's hostility, they may try to repress its expression or try to diffuse it.

Tony, a student nurse who was working with a drug addict began to realize that hostility was one of the client's predominant interpersonal themes. Although the student frequently assured the client that it was "all right to feel hostile" and encouraged him to talk about his hostile feelings, the client continued to deny any feelings of hostility. An instructor helped the student nurse look at his mode of intervention. Even though the student verbally encouraged the client to express hostility, his nonverbal communication (which included a very soft voice, hunched shoulders, and arms clenched around himself) amounted to "I'm afraid of your hostility." Once this situation was pointed out, the student nurse was able to talk about his fear of expressed hostility. He said that his family had always repressed and denied hostile feelings.

With this newly gained insight into his own behavior, the student nurse's nonverbal communication no longer belied his words. The client then began to express his hostile feelings. The instructor was able to support the student nurse through the experience, and the student nurse was able to tolerate and understand the client's expression of hostility—even when it was verbally directed at him.

In the preceding vignette, the student nurse was unaware of his feelings about hostility. When nurses are unaware of their own feelings about hostility or are afraid of hostile feelings, they may be unable to understand or intervene in a client's hostility. Client treatment and recovery may be impeded.

We will now discuss secondary preventive intervention as it pertains to the treatment and recovery of substance and practice abusers. Two aspects will be stressed: case finding and direct intervention.

Case finding

Nurses—especially community health nurses, school nurse-teachers, occupational health nurses, and staff nurses in general hospitals—have unparalleled opportunities for case finding. Awareness of the early signs and symptoms of addiction help nurses to identify individuals with problems of substance or practice abuse.

An occupational health nurse noticed that Mr. McCabe frequently called in sick on Mondays. His work performance during the rest of the week was sporadic. Mr. McCabe worked conscientiously in the morning, but in the afternoon he became lackadaisical about his work and irritable with his coworkers. During the past few months Mr. McCabe had experienced a number of minor industrial accidents. Each accident had occurred in the afternoon.

The occupational health nurse suspected that Mr. McCabe had a drinking problem. By observing his behavior and talking with him, the nurse confirmed this diagnosis. Mr. McCabe drank several beers with his lunch and took frequent afternoon work breaks for additional beers. He drank heavily on weekends "to relax and forget the rat race."

Mr. McCabe was told that if he did not seek treatment he would be fired. At the same time, he was assured that if he completed a treatment program his job would be waiting for him. The occupational health nurse helped Mr. McCabe find an appropriate treatment program.

The preceding vignette exemplifies how nurses may be able to identify incipient substance and practice abusers and refer them for treatment. Many times the substance or practice abuser, as well as family and friends, denies the problem. Denial needs to be worked through so that referrals for treatment will be acted upon.

Eliciting the cooperation and participation of client and family in a treatment program is often facilitated by nonjudgmentally confronting them with a realistic assessment of the problem. Presenting parallels between the client's behavior and patterns of abuse and/or addiction may be helpful. Explanations of types of programs and treatment modalities should be given. The use of self-help groups as treatment adjuncts should also be explained (Task Force on Substance Abuse . . ., 1987).

Nursing process

Nursing process provides the framework for nursing intervention. The focus of this aspect of secondary prevention is twofold: (1) intervention into maladaptive behavior patterns and (2) supplanting socially unacceptable behavior with socially acceptable behavior.

ASSESSMENT

When they work with a client who is a substance or practice abuser, nurses have to begin their assessment with the identification of the problem given by the client or members of the client's social network. The following areas should be assessed:

1. Presenting symptoms—substance abuses and/or practice abuses that are creating problems for the client (or for members of the client's family) even though the abuse behavior is serving as a defense against an emotional state that the client is experiencing
2. Emotional state—such feelings as anxiety, hostility and alienation that are responses to a stimulus situation
3. Stimulus situations—stressful life situations that constitute threats to the client's security. Quests for power, prestige, and possessions are attempts to find reassurance against the anxiety aroused by threats to one's security. In trying to obtain power, prestige, and possessions, some people use maladaptive coping behaviors
4. Maladaptive coping behaviors—substance abuse and practice abuse and coping patterns of manipulation, rationalization, and blame placing that are used in relating to others, in attempting to satisfy needs, and in protecting oneself from hurt
5. Origin of maladaptive coping behaviors—identification of childhood experiences (e.g., inadequate interpersonal relationships, inadequate opportunity for superego socialization, or the perception that society's norms are ambiguous, weak, or conflicting) that contributed to the development of or learning of maladaptive coping behaviors
6. Holistic health status—biological, intellectual, psychological, sociocultural, and spiritual status of the client. These factors may facilitate wellness—e.g., in cultures where alcohol is viewed as a social beverage and drinking patterns tend to be family oriented, rarely do people view alcohol as a way to escape from personal problems—or these factors may impede wellness—e.g., society may stress certain values and standards of behavior but the social situation may make it difficult to achieve these ideals in a legitimate way. In addition, many substance and practice abusers may have physiological disorders (e.g., compromised immune system with drug users, respiratory disorders with tobacco smokers, cardiovascular disease with workaholics)

The following guide may assist nurses in making assessments:

1. Behavioral observations
   a. State of consciousness
   b. State of orientation
   c. Thought and sensory functioning
   d. Motor activity
   e. Perception of time and space
2. Psychosocial observations
   a. Degree of alienation
   b. Ability to perform social roles
   c. Quality of interpersonal relationships
   d. Emotional state: depressed, hostile, anxious, etc.
   e. Coping behaviors: manipulation, rationalization, blame placing, etc.
   f. Threat to self-security* (intentional or inadvertent self-injury potential)
   g. Degree of self-awareness about the effects of substance or practice abuse on self and significant others
   h. Nature of social network: supportive, facilitative (of socially deviant behavior), uninvolved
   i. Purpose of substance or practice abuse: to escape problems; to achieve a sense of well-being; to avoid feeling emotional pain (e.g., anxiety, loneliness, worthlessness, depression); to improve self-esteem; to punish self/others

*Refer to Chapter 22 for discussion of assessment of suicidal potential.

3. Physical observations
   a. Vital signs
   b. Skin color and integrity
   c. Appearance of eyes
   d. Odor of breath
   e. Muscle tremors
   f. Elimination patterns
   g. Nutritional status
   h. Personal hygiene
   i. Speech patterns
   j. Sleep patterns
   k. Evidence of infection
   l. Known health problems
4. Contextual observations
   a. Substances or practices abused
   b. Alteration in life-style
   c. Changes in personality
   d. Changes in spirituality
   e. Deterioration in physical appearance
   f. Nature of stressors (e.g., sociocultural dysfunctions, family dysfunction, physical problems)
   g. Motivation for behavior change: eager to change behavior; ambivalent about changing behavior; resistant to changing behavior

ANALYSIS OF DATA

The analysis of presenting symptoms, emotional states, stimulus situations, maladaptive coping behaviors and their origins, and the holistic health status of the client leads to the formulation of nursing diagnoses. Through the interpretation and appraisal of the data, the nurse is able to better understand the interrelationship among predisposing and precipitating factors and the client's coping behaviors. Nurses may now be ready to formulate nursing diagnoses.

PLANNING AND IMPLEMENTATION

The following are nursing diagnoses that are frequently made for substance and practice abusers. Following each nursing diagnosis is a plan of care that reflects a realistic approach to secondary preventive intervention. The care plan also incorporates many of the process and outcome criteria suggested by the American Nurses' Association standards for addictions nursing (1988). The nurse may initially establish goals, but as therapy progresses the client should enter into goals setting to ensure commitment to their accomplishment.

NURSING CARE PLAN

Client with Impaired Social Interaction

Long-term Outcomes	Short-term Outcomes	Nursing Strategies

Nursing diagnoses:
- Impaired social interaction related to manipulation (NANDA 3.1.1; DSM-III-R 303.90-305.90, 312.31, 302.90)
- Impaired social interaction related to hostility (NANDA 3.1.1; DSM-III-R 303.90-395.90, 312.31, 302.90, 301.70)
- Impaired social interaction related to alienation (NANDA 3.1.1; DSM-III-R 312.31, 302.90, 301.70)

Develop a positive self-image (see Chapters 6 and 22)	Express feelings of anxiety, inadequacy, alienation, anger, and/or frustration (when consistent with client's cultural orientation)	Establish a relationship where client can feel free to verbally express feelings (see Sample Interaction with a Hostile Client)
Learn to relate to others openly and assertively	Identify interpersonal situations that arouse these feelings	Set limits about abuse of substances or practices while in treatment
Develop a	Develop awareness of manipulative, alienated and/or	Set limits on manipulative behavior (e.g., identify instances of attempted manipulation, state what behavior is expected, explain reasons for limits, state consequences of ignoring limits, enforce consequences [see Situation: Limit Setting])

Continued.

NURSING CARE PLAN—cont'd

Client with Impaired Social Interaction

Long-term Outcomes	Short-term Outcomes	Nursing Strategies
sense of "belonging"	hostile behavior Relate how behavior(s) affects relationships Decrease the use of manipulation, alienation, and/or hostility Follow rules and regulations in the treatment setting Develop impulse control Develop more effective coping behaviors and interpersonal skills Become actively involved in the treatment plan	Help client acknowledge the way he or she uses manipulative, hostile or alienated behavior (e.g., explore client's perception of how needs are gratified, discuss ways that other people gratify needs, point out instances of rationalization, blame placing, and/or anger) Encourage client to identify objects of manipulation, hostility and/or alienation Help client to evaluate effectiveness of current coping behaviors (e.g., point out instances of poor judgment, explore the damaging effects of manipulation, hostility and/or alienation on relationships) Support current effective coping behaviors Explore alternative coping behaviors Teach client assertive communication techniques Give immediate feedback or rewards for nonmanipulative, nonhostile, nonalienated coping responses Encourage client to evaluate the effectiveness of new behavior Remind client when he or she slips back into manipulative, hostile, and/or alienated patterns

Sample interaction with a hostile client

Client (frowning and sounding sarcastic) Well, I see you got here bright and early for our talk.

Nurse You are frowning and you sound angry. Do you feel angry?

Client What do you expect. I'm in this place. I can't drink. I can't go to work. How would you feel?

Nurse Let's talk more about how you feel.

Client I feel like having a drink! That's how I feel. Do you know what it's like to want a drink so bad and not be able to have one? Everyone's telling me what to do and when to do it. I get so angry I just want to drink and get away from it all.

Nurse Tell me about the last time you drank to "get away from it all."

Client I got mad at my boss. He wanted everything done yesterday. I went to lunch and had a few beers and didn't go back to work. I guess you'd say I got drunk. My boss fired me. I could have beaten him to a pulp. I was that angry.

Nurse It sounds like you drank to relieve your angry feelings. But your drinking got out of control and got you into a situation that only made you angrier.

The nurse was alert for indirect expressions (clues) of hostility and pointed them out to the client. The nurse also encouraged the client to validate the nurse's assessment of hostility. The nurse then helped the client look at the relationship between his hostile feelings and his drinking behavior.

Situation: limit setting

A unit for male adolescent substance abusers used a card system to reinforce socially acceptable behavior. The unit's environment was highly structured. Strict adherence to routine and rules was required. When an adolescent was admitted to the unit, he had no privileges. Through the card system, privileges could be

NURSING CARE PLAN

Client with Potential for Injury

Long-term Outcomes	Short-term Outcomes	Nursing Strategies

Nursing diagnoses:
- Potential for injury related to sensory-perceptual alteration (NANDA 1.6.1; DSM-III-R 303.90-305.90)
- Potential for injury related to poor impulse control (NANDA 1.6.1; DSM-III-R 303.90-305.90, 312.31, 302.90)
- Potential for injury related to low self-esteem (NANDA 1.6.1; DSM-III-R 303.90-305.90, 312.31, 302.90)
- Potential for injury related to withdrawal from addictive substances (NANDA 1.6.1; DSM-III-R 303.90-305.90)
- Potential for injury related to inducements of secondary gains as characterized by sympathy, lowered role expectations, prescriptions for drugs, etc. (NANDA 1.6.1; DSM-III-R 303.90-305.90, 312.31, 302.90)
- Potential for injury related to poor judgment (NANDA 1.6.1; DSM-III-R 303.90-305.90, 312.31, 302.90)

Long-term Outcomes	Short-term Outcomes	Nursing Strategies
Increase self-esteem (see Chapters 6 and 22) Develop impulse control Remain free of addiction	Remain injury free Safely withdraw from addictive substances or practices Develop insight about the consequences of one's behavior Demonstrate appropriate judgment Demonstrate orientation to time, place and person Learn new coping behaviors Avoid secondary gains associated with self-injury	Remain alert for types of self-inflicted injury (inadvertent injury during the acute phase or withdrawal phase of substance abuse, intentional injury for secondary gains, injury from suicidal attempts) Provide a secure environment (e.g., monitor vital signs, monitor restlessness and disorientation, institute such protective measures as side rails on bed and padded rooms) Keep addictive substances locked up (including cough medicine and alcohol-based mouthwash) Observe for mood alterations. Alternating euphoria ("high") and severe depression ("let-down") often accompany substance abuse. Suicidal attempts may be made when coming out of depression (refer to the discussion of suicide in Chapter 22) Orient client to time, place, and person Reassure client that staff will help the client control his or her behavior (client may fear losing control of own actions and hurting self) Help client to evaluate effectiveness of current coping behaviors (e.g., explore damaging effects of substance or practice abuse to self and others, point out instances of poor judgment or poor impulse control) Support current effective coping behaviors Explore alternative ways of coping Explore any secondary gains associated with client's behavior Establish a therapeutic environment free of secondary gains (e.g., expectations of client participation in activities of daily living and treatment modalities should be clearly stated, avoid giving client special privileges or dispensations because of potential for self-injury) Provide opportunities for gradually increased responsibility Give immediate feedback or rewards for behavior that shows good judgment or impulse control Encourage client to evaluate effectiveness of new behavior Remind client when he or she slips back and uses poor judgment or little impulse control

earned. Card 1 meant that an adolescent could use free periods (nontherapy periods) for activities of his choice. Card 2 carried grounds privileges: during free periods an adolescent could go outside unaccompanied by a staff member for walks, or lounge about. Card 3 carried weekend privileges: it allowed an adolescent to go home for weekends.

Just as cards could be earned for socially acceptable behavior, they could be lost for socially deviant behavior. If a card was taken away, a nurse would discuss the reasons for the penalty with the adoles-

cent. The possibility of reearning the card and the behavior required to accomplish this were discussed.

The preceding vignette shows how a client can be made aware of limits, the rewards for following routines and rules, and the consequences for ignoring established limits. At the same time, the nurse does not reject the client as a person.

NURSING CARE PLAN

Client with Altered Health Maintenance

Long-term Outcomes	Short-term Outcomes	Nursing Strategies

Nursing diagnosis: Altered health maintenance related to poor health habits (NANDA 6.4.2; DSM-III-R 303.90-305.90, 312.31, 302.90)

Long-term Outcomes	Short-term Outcomes	Nursing Strategies
Understand the relationship between good health habits and high-level wellness Develop health habits that promote high-level wellness Remain drug free	Establish an exercise program Establish a program of nutrition and hydration Establish routines that promote rest and sleep Establish routines of personal hygiene Stop using addictive substances Seek treatment for existent health problems	Provide an atmosphere that is conducive to health promotion (e.g., manipulate the environment so that it is quiet at bedtime, relaxed and without distractions at mealtime, affords privacy for hygiene). Promote adequate nutrition and hydration (e.g., offer small portions of food and fluid frequently, offer favorite foods and fluids that are consistent with client's cultural orientation). Promote a regular sleep pattern (e.g., establish a regular bedtime, provide relaxing and nonstimulating activities prior to bedtime, provide a light snack, avoid caffeine-containing beverages, offer herbal teas, teach relaxation techniques). Promote personal hygiene (e.g., establish routines of bathing, shampooing hair, brushing teeth, and laundering clothes). Promote regular exercise (e.g., establish a regular exercise time, include client's favorite exercise(s), exercise to music, exercise in groups, discuss the role of exercise in physical health and as a way of coping with stress). By exerting control over his or her body, the client can gain a sense of power that had previously been achieved primarily through manipulation. Assist client to seek treatment for existent health problems. Discuss health problems associated with the specific type of substance or practice abuse (see Situation: Education about Health).

Situation: education about health

*For more than a year, Joanna had been using halluci-nogenic drugs. In addition, after she had run away from home, much of her food supply had come from begging and scavenging. Joanna's physical examination revealed malnutrition and gonorrhea. A nurse talked with her about nutrition and sexually transmitted diseases. Joanna was unaware that untreated gonorrhea could cause permanent sterility. Moreover, in talking with the nurse, Joanna revealed much misinfor-*mation about AIDS. Joanna was also surprised to learn that long-term patterns of poor nutrition could limit her body's ability to fight infection, affect the health of any children she might bear, and eventually shorten her life.*

As the preceding vignette indicates, nurses can be instrumental in educating clients who abuse substances or practices about good health habits.

NURSING CARE PLAN

Client with Knowledge Deficit

Long-term Outcomes	Short-term Outcomes	Nursing Strategies

Nursing diagnoses:
- Knowledge deficit (learning needs) related to substance abuse (specify type) (NANDA 8.1.1; DSM-III-R 303.90-305.90, 312.31, 302.90)
- Knowledge deficit (learning needs) related to practice abuse (specify type) (NANDA 8.1.1; DSM-III-R 303.90 305.90, 312.31, 302.90)

Long-term Outcomes	Short-term Outcomes	Nursing Strategies
Understand addiction as a disease	Verbalize the addictive nature of substance or practice abuse	Provide an atmosphere that is conducive to learning (e.g., manipulate the environment so it is quiet, free of distractions, relaxed, and affords privacy)
Understand the effects of substance or practice abuse on an abuser	Verbalize the effects of substance or practice abuse on an abuser	Provide information to client and family about substance or practice abuse (e.g., characteristics of addiction, effects on abuser and on family, effects of substance abuse on fetal growth and development)
Understand the effects of substance abuse on a fetus	Verbalize the effects of alcohol and drugs on a fetus	Provide information to client and family about the process of recovery
Understand the effects of substance or practice abuse on a family	Verbalize the effects of substance or practice abuse on a family	Provide information to client and spouse about contraceptive measures and implications for contraceptive measures if abusing alcohol or drugs
	Identify an appropriate treatment program	Provide information to client and family about treatment programs and supportive self-help groups
	Verbalize plans to participate in an appropriate treatment program	Encourage client and family to participate in the learning process
	Participate in an appropriate treatment program	Help client and family to apply learning to their specific situation
	Use contraception until alcohol or drug abuse abates	Use behavioral objectives to measure client and family learning
		Encourage client and family to evaluate the learning experience

Nursing diagnoses pertaining to other problems associated with substance and practice abuse are addressed in the following chapters: potential for violence (Chapter 21), grieving (Chapter 9), anxiety (Chapter 8), altered family processes (Chapter 14 and Family Therapy section of this chapter), altered thought process (Chapter 25), sensory-perceptual alterations (Chapter 25), pain (Chapter 9).

EVALUATION

The client and, whenever feasible, the client's social network should be included in estimating the client's progress towards attainment of goals. Any evaluation should encompass the following areas:

1. Estimation of the degree to which anxiety and conflict have been decreased
2. Estimation of the degree to which goals have been achieved and client functioning has improved (demonstrated by a decrease in socially deviant coping behaviors and the learning of socially acceptable coping behaviors)
3. Identification of goals that need to be modified or revised
4. Referral of the client to support systems other than the nurse-client relationship
   a. People in the client's social network who are willing to serve as a support system and who will not act as facilitators of substance or practice abuse
   b. Community agencies that help clients learn to live with a vulnerability to substance or practice abuse that may never be completely eliminated (e.g., Alcoholics Anonymous, Gamblers Anonymous)
   c. Centers that specialize in the treatment of specific substance or practice abuses (e.g., drug or alcohol treatment centers, smokers' withdrawal clinics)

TERTIARY PREVENTION

Because social networks and communities change slowly, substance and practice abusers may be discharged from treatment and returned to the environments that contributed to the development of their unacceptable behavior. Following discharge from treatment programs, ongoing support in the form of *rehabilitative* or *after-care* services may be needed.

Although most people agree that tertiary prevention is a necessary part of treatment for socially aberrant behavior, after-care is not a major priority in the United States. Many communities may resist having treatment centers in their midst.

A drug treatment center puchased a large house in a suburban community. The plan was to establish a drug-free day treatment program for former addicts. Community members, however, were concerned and angry; they did not want former addicts passing through the streets on their way to the day treatment center. Parents, clergymen, and educators feared that the former addicts would serve as antiestablishment role models, try to peddle drugs, or in some other way adversely influence children and adolescents. After three fires of suspicious origin occurred, the treatment center sold the house and dismissed the idea of establishing a day treatment program.

Limited tertiary prevention programs are available in the following settings.

Transitional services

Transitional services involve the gradual severing of ties with a treatment center. Substance abusers spend ever-increasing amounts of time away from the center. They may start with an overnight pass, go on to weekend privileges, and finally work up to a week away from the center. Skills for community living and help in locating work and housing are provided. Once they are living in a community, many transitional programs encourage individuals to return to the treatment center for weekly, semi-monthly, or monthly "rap" sessions. At these sessions, problems of adjustment and daily living and ways of coping are discussed.

After-care centers

After-care centers are designed for substance abusers who have a place to live and an accepting, supportive family or social network but who are not yet ready to return to work. At a day center, some clients receive medication (such as methadone or Antabuse). All clients receive structure and organization. Social skills and activities of daily living are taught, and assistance is given in looking for a job and preparing for a job interview. Opportunities for socializing are provided. Many day care centers achieve a high degree of autonomy. A system of peer group control may develop, and members may actively set and reinforce rules. If a member experiences a crisis, other members may institute a 24-hour-a-day support system.

Self-help groups

Self-help groups support substance and practice abusers in their readjustment to community living and intervene in crisis situations. Such groups are composed of former substance and practice abusers who have successfully learned to live by society's standards. Alcoholics Anonymous, Narcotics Anonymous, and Gamblers Anonymous use a repressive-inspirational approach (see Chapter 13). Women for Sobriety attempts to teach women to live without alcohol. A self-help group known as Scapegoat helps prostitutes leave their pimps, learn marketable skills, and find employment.

CHAPTER SUMMARY

Substance and practice abusers use a large number of seemingly disparate and incongruous ways of relating to people. Individuals are characterized by such deeply ingrained maladaptive personality patterns and restricted emotional responses that they develop life-styles that often bring them into conflict with society.

Many theories have been formulated to explain substance and practice abuse. These theories fall into four major categories: psychological, biological, sociocultural, and systems. It is likely that a combination of interrelated factors leads to the development of substance and practice abuse. Some types of socially aberrant behavior are known to all societies, but its form, meaning, and incidence are culturally influenced and culturally relative.

Substance and practice abusers may be treated in a general hospital, a specialized treatment center, or a self-help group. Some of the most frequently used treatment modalities include aversion therapy, group therapy, and milieu therapy. A combination of therapies is often indicated.

Although nurses may not directly participate in all treatment modalities, they do participate in all three levels of preventive intervention.

Primary prevention focuses on identification of and intervention with high-risk individuals. Attempts are also made to rectify such environmental factors as community disorganization. Secondary prevention involves case finding and application of the nursing process to human responses associated with substance and practice abuse. Secondary prevention is most effective when it involves a collaborative and consistent team approach. Tertiary prevention requires that nurses, reformed substance and practice abusers, clients, and family members work toward a unified rehabilitative approach.

SELF-DIRECTED LEARNING

Sensitivity-Awareness Exercises

The purpose of the following exercises are to:

- Develop awareness about the vulnerability of people to substance and practice abuse
- Develop awareness about the interrelationship of factors in the development of substance and practice abuse
- Develop awareness about the subjective experience of clients who are substance or practice abusers and of the experience of clients' families
- Develop awareness about your own feelings and attitudes when working with clients who are substance or practice abusers
- Develop awareness about your own vulnerability to substance and practice abuse

1. Try to imagine that you use one of the following addictive disorders to cope with stress. Explain why you selected that particular addictive disorder. Then describe what you think it would be like to suffer from that disorder.
   a. Drug abuse
   b. Alcoholism
   c. Compulsive tobacco smoking
   d. Compulsive gambling
   e. Work addiction
   f. Compulsive prostitution
2. Describe what you think it would be like to have a family member who is a substance or practice abuser (specify which type). Which behavior do you think would be easiest to tolerate in a family member? Why? Which behavior would be hardest to tolerate? Why?
3. What might be some of your feelings and reactions as a nurse caring for a client who is a substance or practice abuser? Would your feelings and reactions vary with the type of abusive behavior used by clients? Explain why.
4. Imagine that you are a community health nurse engaged in health supervision with new parents. What high-risk factors (biological, psychological, and sociocultural) would you observe for that might predispose parents and their children to substance or practice abuse?
5. Develop a plan for counseling parents about child-rearing that incorporates principles and goals for primary prevention of substance and practice abuse.

6. The following substance abuse self-assessment guide* may help you assess whether you have a problem with substance abuse. Do you . . .
   a. Use substances (e.g., tobacco, drugs, or alcohol) to deal with personal problems (e.g., quarrels, disappointments, pressure situations)?
   b. Lose time from your job or school because of your use of a substance?
   c. Become very defensive or deny everything when criticized about your substance use?
   d. Use drugs or alcohol routinely every day?
   e. Have physical symptoms that may be related to your substance use (e.g., insomnia, confused thinking, lack of coordination, shortness of breath, "smoker's cough")?
   f. Cause family members embarrassment, hurt, or concern by your substance use?
   g. Need larger quantities of drugs or alcohol to obtain the same effect as when you first started using the substance?
   h. Feel uncomfortable at or avoid social functions where drugs or alcohol are not available? Where tobacco smoking is not permitted?
   i. Regret or feel guilty about the way you overindulged in a substance (e.g., got drunk)?
   j. Break promises made to yourself or others about decreasing or controlling your substance use?
   k. Avoid family and/or friends when you are high on drugs or alcohol or smoking too many cigarettes?
   "Yes" answers to one or more of these questions may indicate a problem with substance abuse and the need for prompt help.
7. The following practice abuse self-assessment guide† may help you assess whether you have a problem with practice abuse. Do you . . .
   a. Compulsively engage in a practice to deal with your personal problems (e.g., quarrels, disappointments, pressure situations)?
   b. Lose time from your job or school because of this practice?

*Sources consulted in preparation of this guide include Drug Abuse (1985), What Everyone Should Know . . . (1987), DSM-III-R (1987).
†Sources consulted in the preparation of this guide include Orford (1985), Rohrlich (1980), and Lesieur and Blume (1987).

c. Hear complaints from family members that your dependence on this practice is causing unhappiness at home?

d. Feel that dependence on this practice is ruining your reputation?

e. Feel regret or remorse because of this practice?

f. Experience a strong or irresistible urge to continue engaging in this practice?

g. Find yourself lying or sneaking in order to indulge this practice (e.g., understating the amount of money lost by gambling; making excuses for bringing work along on your vacation)?

h. Ever contemplate suicide because of the effect this practice has had on your life?

i. Find yourself so dependent on this practice that it takes priority over other aspects of your life (e.g., family responsibilities, job obligations, your reputation)?

j. Become very defensive or deny everything in the face of criticism about your dependence on this practice?

k. Experience depression, guilt, and/or anxiety when you try to give up this practice?

l. Break promises to yourself or others about decreasing or controlling this practice?

"Yes" answers to a majority of these questions may indicate practice abuse and the need for prompt help.

Questions to Consider

1. Jason Smith and Martin Jones are both alcoholics. Jason only drinks in the privacy of his home and has never missed work because of his drinking. Martin drinks on his lunch break and often goes back to the office too drunk to work. According to Goffman's categorization of stigmatized individuals, Martin is a(n)
a. Discreditable person
b. Discredited person
c. Incredible person
d. Secret alcoholic
e. Reformed alcoholic

2. Tracy Jackson was admitted to the emergency room with slurred speech, disorientation, drowsiness, shallow respirations, and dilated pupils. She appeared drunk, but there was no odor of alcohol on her breath. Tracy's friends said she had taken some pills. From Tracy's symptoms, the nurse would be correct in suspecting that Tracy had taken
a. Depressants

b. Stimulants
c. Narcotics
d. Hallucinogens
e. Tranquilizers

3. All through her pregnancy, Noreen Jameson drank wine and beer. Her alcohol intake was high. Her infant was born with low birth weight, several fetal anomalies, and some central nervous system damage. This syndrome is referred to as
a. Fetal Alcohol Syndrome
b. Alcohol Withdrawal Syndrome
c. Fetal Withdrawal Syndrome
d. Alcohol Toxicity Syndrome

4. Anthony Marston is a junior partner in a law firm. Anthony is a chronic work addict. Should Anthony be unable to work, all *but* which of the following withdrawal symptoms might appear?
a. Shortness of breath
b. Disinterest in sex
c. Watery eyes
d. Migraine headaches

5. In counseling children who have an alcoholic parent, it is important for nurses to realize that
a. Children of alcoholics have the same risk for developing alcoholism as children of nonalcoholics
b. Research has not implicated genetics in alcoholism
c. A family history of alcoholism does not play a role in alcoholic symptomatology
d. Children of alcoholics may be at four times greater risk for developing alcoholism than children of nonalcoholics

Match each of the following terms with the statement that is associated with it:

6. Aversion therapy — a. Larger and larger amounts of a substance are needed to produce the desired effect
7. Opiate blocker — b. Habituation
8. Tolerance — c. Methadone
9. Psychological dependence — d. Antabuse
10. Nicotine withdrawal — e. Anxiety, irritability, depression, suicide
11. Withdrawal from compulsive gambling — f. Craving, decreased heart rate, anxiety, concentration problems

Answer key

1. b   4. c   7. c   10. f
2. a   5. d   8. a   11. e
3. a   6. d   9. b

REFERENCES

Adler A: Understanding human nature, (Translated by WB Wolfe). New York; 1927, Greenberg Publisher, Inc.

Alcoholics' odd blood suggests genetic disease, Sci News 124(12):180, 1983.

American Nurses' Association: Standards of addictions: nursing practice with selected diagnoses and criteria, Kansas City, Mo, 1988, The Association.

Ashcraft N and Scheflen AE: People space: the making and breaking of human boundaries, Garden City, NY, 1976, Anchor Press/Doubleday.

Baasher T: The use of drugs in the Islamic world, Br J Addiction 76:233-243, 1981.

Belle D and Goldman N: Patterns of diagnoses received by men and women. In Guttentag M, Salasian S, and Belle D, editors: The mental health of women, New York, 1980, Academic Press.

Bell R: Escape from addiction, New York, 1970, McGraw-Hill Book Co.

Benjamin H and Masters REL: Prostitution and morality, London, 1964, Souvenir Press Ltd.

Benowitz SI: Studies help scientists hone in on genetics of alcoholism, Sci News 126(13):196, 1984.

Bergler E: The psychology of gambling, New York, 1970, International Universities Press, Inc.

Brody JE: Personal health, New York Times, January 15, 1986.

Cadoret RJ, Cain CA, and Grove WM: Development of alcoholism in adoptees raised apart from alcoholic biologic relatives, Arch Gen Psychiatr 37:561-563, 1980.

Carmen A and Woody H: Working women: the subterranean world of street prostitution, New York, 1985, Harper & Row.

Carruth GR and Pugh JB: Grieving the loss of alcohol: a crisis in recovery, J Psychiatr Nurs Mental Health Serv 20(3):18-21, 1982.

Clark JB, Queener SF, and Karb VB: Pharmacologic basis of nursing practice, ed 2, St. Louis, 1986, CV Mosby Co.

Clayton BD: Mosby's handbook of pharmacology in nursing, St. Louis, 1984, CV Mosby Co.

Cohen R: Deviant street networks, Lexington, Mass, 1980, D.C. Heath & Co.

Cohen S: The cocaine problems, Drug Abuse and Alcoholism Newsletter 27(8):1-3, 1987.

Common drugs and symptoms of abuse, Division of Substance Abuse Services, State of New York, Albany, NY, 1986.

Cooke R: A disease or not? Discover (Part III), Newsday, pp 1 and 3, May 3, 1988.

Custer R: An overview of compulsive gambling, In Kieffer S, editor: Addictive disorders update, New York, 1982, Human Sciences Press.

Diagnostic and statistical manual of mental disorders (DSM-III-R), Washington, DC, 1987, The American Psychiatric Association.

Doctors not urging quitting, ASH Smoking Health Rev 27(3):13, 1987.

Drug abuse, US Department of Justice and Drug Enforcement Administration, Washington, DC, 1985, Government Printing Office.

Efinger JM: Women and alcoholism, Topics Clin Nurs 4(4):10-19, 1983.

Estes NJ, Smith-Dijulio K, and Heinemann MC: Nursing diagnosis of the alcoholic person, St. Louis, 1980, CV Mosby Co.

Frances RJ, Tim S, and Bucky S: Studies of familial and nonfamilial alcoholism, Arch Gen Psychiatr 37:564-566, 1980.

Freud S: Civilization and its discontents, (Translated by J Riviere). London, 1930, The Hogarth Press Ltd.

Freud S: Collected papers of Sigmund Freud, (Edited by E Jones). New York, 1959, Basic Books, Inc., Publishers

Fromm E: Man for himself, New York, 1947, Holt, Rinehart & Winston, Inc.

Fromm E: The sane society, New York, 1955, Holt, Rinehart & Winston, Inc.

Gaudia R: Effects of compulsive gambling on the family, Social Work 32(3):254-256, 1987.

Gawin FH and Ellinwood EH: Cocaine and other stimulants, N Engl J Med 318(18):1173-1182, 1988.

Goffman E: Stigma: notes on the management of spoiled identity, Englewood Cliffs, NJ, 1963, Prentice-Hall.

Goldstein AO et al: Hospital nurse counseling of patients who smoke, Am J Public Health 77(10):1333-1334, 1987.

Goodwin DW: Alcoholism and heredity: a review and hypothesis, Arch Gen Psychiatr 36:57-61, 1979.

Goodwin DW: Alcoholism and genetics, Arch Gen Psychiatr 42:171-174, 1985.

Greeley AM and McCready WC: A preliminary reconnaissance into the persistence and explanation of ethnic subcultural drinking patterns, Med Anthropol 2:31-51, 1978.

Greenberg J, editor: Reactions to alcohol: cortisol clues, Sci News 132(21):324, 1987.

Helman C: Culture, health and illness: an introduction for health professionals, Bristol, England, 1984, John Wright & Sons Ltd.

Horney K: The neurotic personality of our time, New York, 1937, WW Norton Co.

Kids target of tobacco industry, ASH Smoking Health Rev 27(3):4, 1987.

Klerman GL and Weissman MM: Depressions among women: their nature and causes, In Guttentag M, Salasin S, and Belle D, editors: The mental health of women, New York, 1980, Academic Press.

Klinger E: Meaning and void: inner experience and the incentives in people's lives, Minneapolis, 1977, University of Minnesota Press.

Lancaster J: Community mental health nursing: an ecological perspective, St. Louis, 1980, CV Mosby Co.

Leighton AH: My name is legion, New York, 1959, Basic Books.

Leikin C: Identifying and treating the alcoholic client, Social Casework 67(1):67-73, 1986.

Lesieur HR and Blume SB: The South Oaks Gambling Screen (SOGS): a new instrument for identification of pathological gamblers, Am J Psychiatr 144(9):1184-1188, 1987.

Lipscomb TR and Nathan PE: Blood alcohol level discrimination, Arch Gen Psychiatr 37:571-576, 1980.

Mann CR: Female crime and delinquency, Montgomery, 1984, The University of Alabama Press.

Mann M: Marty Mann's new primer on alcoholism, New York, 1981, Holt, Rinehart, & Winston.

Martinez T: Cited in Hyde MO, Addictions: gambling, smoking, cocaine use and others, New York, 1978, McGraw-Hill Book Co.

Miller EM: Street woman, Philadelphia, 1986, Temple University Press.

Morton PG: Assessment and management of the self-destructive concept of alcoholism, J Psychiatr Nurs Mental Health Serv 17:8-13, 1979.

Moynihan DP: Drugs: where we've come from, where we're going, Newsday, Ideas section, p 5, June 24, 1984.

Orford J: Excessive appetites: a psychological view of addictions, New York, 1985, John Wiley & Sons.

Pert CB and Snyder SH: Opiate receptor: demonstration in nervous tissue, Science 179(4077):1011-1014, 1973.

Redeker MA: Alcoholism: a slow descent into darkness, The Magazine, Winter:3-18, 1985-1986.

Rohrlich JB: Work and love: the crucial balance, New York, 1980, Simon & Schuster.

Schilit R: Childhood social support deficits of alcoholic women, Social Work 67(10):579-586, 1986.

Schuckit MA: Genetics and the risk for alcoholism, JAMA 254:2614-2617, 1985.

Schuckit MA, Gold E, and Risch C: Plasma cortisol levels following ethanol in sons of alcoholics and controls, Arch Gen Psychiatr 44:942-945, 1987.

Seymour RB, Gorton JG, and Smith DE: The client with a substance abuse problem, In Gorton JG and Partridge R, editors: Practice and management of psychiatric emergency care, St. Louis, 1982, CV Mosby Co.

Slater P: Society's pressure causes drug dependency, In Debner CB, editor: Opposing viewpoints: chemical dependency, St. Paul, Minn, 1985, Greenhaven Press.

Smoking at lowest level ever, ASH Smoking Health Rev 27(5):16, 1987.

Stanton MD: Family treatment approaches to drug abuse problems: a review, Fam Process 18:251-280, 1979.

Sullivan EJ: A descriptive study of nurses recovering from chemical dependency, Arch Psychiatr Nurs 1(3):194-200, 1987.

Swartz CM, Drews V, and Cadoret R: Decreased epinephrine in familial alcoholism, Arch Gen Psychiatr 44:938-941, 1987.

Task Force on Substance Abuse Nursing Practice: The care of clients with addictions: dimensions of nursing practice, Kansas City, Mo, 1987, American Nurses' Association.

Textor MR: Family therapy with drug addicts: an integrated approach, Am J Orthopsychiatr 57(4):495-507, 1987.

Wegscheider S: Another chance: hope and health for the alcoholic family, Palo Alto, Calif, 1981, Science & Behavior Books, Inc.

What everyone should know about alcohol and health, Nassau County Department of Drug and Alcohol Addiction, South Deerfield, Mass, 1987, Channing L. Bete Co., Inc.

Why smokers should quit and nonsmokers should help, ASH Smoking and Health Review 27(4):12, 1987.

Wolper B and Scheiner L: Family therapy approaches and drug dependent women, In Beschner GM, Reed BG, and Mondanaro J, editors: Treatment services for drug dependent women, vol 1, Washington, DC, 1981, US Department of Health and Human Services.

Yowell S and Brose C: Working with drug abuse patients in the ER, In Backer BS, Dubbert PM, and Eisenman EJP, editors: Psychiatric/mental health nursing: contemporary readings, New York, 1977, D. Van Nostrand Company, Inc.

ANNOTATED SUGGESTED READINGS

Orford J: Excessive appetites: a psychological view of addictions, New York, 1985, John Wiley & Sons.

This book is divided into two sections. Part I discusses such "excesses" as alcoholism, gambling, drug abuse, overeating, and hypersexuality. Historical as well as current studies and cross-cultural examples are included. Part II develops a psychological model around the concepts of inclination, restraint, attachment, conflict, decision, and self-control.

Sullivan EJ: A descriptive study of nurses recovering from chemical dependency, Arch Psychiatr Nurs 1(3):194-200, 1987.

This descriptive study identifies characteristics of nurses who abuse substances and then looks at the progression of the disease and the process of recovery. Suggestions for further research include development of longitudinal studies that focus on risk factors, as well as recovery factors, in chemically dependent nurses.

Task Force on Substance Abuse Nursing Practice: The care of clients with addictions: dimensions of nursing practice, Kansas City, Mo, 1987, American Nurses' Association.

This booklet starts out by discussing the development of and need for addictions nursing. It proceeds to explain episodic phenomena and chronic phenomena associated with substance abuse. Strategies for primary, secondary, and tertiary preventive intervention are explored. In addition, role diversity in addictions nursing is described.

FURTHER READINGS

Adams FE: Drug dependency in hospital patients, Am J Nurs 88(4):477-481, 1988.

Arneson SW, Schultz M, and Triplett JL: Nurses' knowledge of the impact of parental alcoholism on children, Arch Psychiatr Nurs 1(4):251-257, 1987.

Becker PH, editor: Addictions, Holistic Nurs Prac 2(4):1-83, 1988.

Cannon BL and Brown JS: Nurses' attitudes toward impaired colleagues, Image 20(2):96-101, 1988.

Heggenhougen HK: Traditional medicine and the treatment of drug addicts: three examples from southeast Asia, Med Anthropol Q 16(1):3-6, 1984.

Hersch P: Coming of age on the streets, Psychol Today 22(1):28-37, 1988.

Peele S: The cultural context of psychological approaches to alcoholism: can we control the effects of alcohol? Am Psychol 39(1):1337-1351, 1984.

Sereny G: The invisible children: child prostitution in America, West Germany and Great Britain, New York, 1985, Alfred A. Knopf.

Sullivan EJ: Which nurse is likely to become chemically dependent? Am J Nurs 88(6):791-794, 1988.

Patterns of human abuse

CHAPTER FOCUS

Human abuse refers to physical abuse and neglect or emotional abuse. Abusive or violent behavior may be in the form of criminal violence, domestic violence, or sexual molestation. Although various theories have been formulated to explain human abuse, it is likely that a combination of biological, psychological, and sociocultural processes interrelate in the development of and response to abusive behavior. To understand the dynamics of human abuse, abuse must be viewed as a complex phenomenon involving both the abuser and the victim.

Treatment for abusers and victims often involves a combination of therapies. Treatment goals focus on reinforcing client strengths, decreasing sources of stress, and teaching more adaptive ways of dealing with stress. The most frequently employed modalities in the treatment of human abuse are emergency interventions, crisis intervention, family therapy, group therapy, and educational therapy.

Nurses engage in all three levels of preventive intervention. When working with abusers and victims of abuse, nurses may respond in various ways. Nurses may treat abusers with anger, avoidance, or punishment. Nurses may fail to question the source of an abused victim's injuries or ignore cues that domestic violence has occurred. Nurses may derogate the victim or make the victim feel guilty or responsible for having been abused. By clarifying their own attitudes and values, nurses can work more therapeutically with both abusers and victims of abuse.

Abusive or violent behavior may be perpetrated by strangers, friends and acquaintances, and family members. Violent behavior is behavior whose intent is to inflict harm on people or property. This harm may be in the form of physical abuse and neglect and/or emotional abuse. The damage inflicted by emotional abuse tends to be more subjective than the damage inflicted by physical abuse. Emotional abuse may also contribute to the expression of physical violence. The types of human abuse that will be discussed in this chapter are criminal violence, domestic violence, and sexual molestation.

UNDERLYING DYNAMICS

To understand the dynamics of human abuse, abuse must be viewed as a complex phenomenon involving both the abuser and the victim. Many abusive people and their victims experience feelings of low self-esteem, dependency and powerlessness, blame placing (or self-blame), frustration, and anger.

Low self-esteem

Assertive behavior is mature behavior. It is incompatible with assaultive or abusive behavior. Greenleaf (1978) points out that self-esteem, self-confidence, and assertiveness are interrelated. Without self-esteem and self-confidence a person is unable to behave assertively. Yet when one does not behave assertively, self-esteem and self-confidence are further eroded.

Many abusive individuals have themselves been victims of child abuse. Often the only attention a child may have received from a parent or a significant other was when that person was abusing the child. Such children grow up feeling unloved and devoid of adults on whom to depend. Growing up in an environment of family violence and personal abuse may generate a sense of inadequacy and failure and feelings of being unloved, unwanted, and rejected (Winters, 1985; Shupe, Stacey, and Hazlewood, 1987).

Victims of nonfamilial abuse also have had their self-systems attacked. Assault alters a victim's view of self and the world. Victims usually feel powerless

and vulnerable and experience a loss of self. Some victims may blame themselves for the abuse in an attempt to reinstate a sense of control, while other victims may try to minimize the assault to reestablish the world as a just and orderly place (Rieker and Carmen, 1986).

Dependency and powerlessness

Because of low self-esteem, abusive individuals are often emotionally dependent on others for affection and security. Since previous relationships, especially those in childhood, have not met their emotional needs, abusive individuals are often fearful of being hurt in their current emotional relationships. Their adult intimate relationships are usually characterized by ambivalence: wanting emotional closeness but being fearful of trusting those who might give it to them. Many abusive men and women are jealous and suspicious of their spouses or lovers. This lack of trust evidences itself in the abusive person's attempts to dominate or monitor the actions of significant others. Inability to communicate their feelings generates frustration that may not be expressed until it explodes in violent behavior. Violence becomes a means by which abusers reassure themselves that they are strong and in control (Shupe, Stacey, and Hazlewood, 1987).

A sense of powerlessness and dependency also may be operative in the victims of chronic abuse. Many victims of abuse exemplify Seligman's (1975) concept of learned helplessness. Past failed attempts to escape from an abusive situation as well as biopsychosocial forces that inhibit action combine to make victims feel hopeless about anyone or anything extricating them from the abusive relationship. Although he was referring to battered women, Hilberman's (1980) statement that "this expectation of powerlessness and inability to control one's destiny, whether real or perceived, prevents effective action" can apply to many victims of abuse.

Blame

Abusive individuals tend to use the mechanism of blame placing to avoid assuming responsibility for their behavior. They give many reasons for their violent behavior. They are always able to justify their actions. Circumstances or other people are always at fault. By rationalizing, minimizing, and placing blame on others, abusive individuals are able to avoid dealing with their roles in and responsibility for their violent actions (Shupe, Stacey, and Hazlewood, 1987).

At the same time, victims of abuse may engage in self-blame or self-scapegoating. For example, many adult victims of rape blame themselves for being in the situation where the rape occurred or for not being able to fight off the rapist. Significant others may reinforce this self-blame by blaming the victim for her poor judgement or by viewing the rape as a consensual sexual encounter. When the victim of abuse is a child, self-scapegoating also may occur. Because an abused child is often dependent on the abuser for nurturing, protection, and comforting, the child must distort the perception of the "bad" parent (or significant other) into the "good" parent. This enables the child to continue to look to that parent for assistance with day-to-day survival and for help with dealing with the feelings of fear and rage that are engendered by abusive events: "The bad has to be registered as good. This is a mind-splitting or mind-fragmenting operation" that facilitates self-blame (Shengold, 1979).

Frustration and anger

Witnessing family abuse and inability to protect one's self from being abused generate frustration and helpless rage. During early childhood experiences of emotional and physical abuse, a child is usually unable to respond to the hurt in any way other than through helpless rage. Frustration and anger become integral parts of the personality.

Victims of abuse, both children and adults, may repress their angry feelings because they (1) fear that expressing such feelings might alienate them from the persons on whom they are dependent (as in many instances of spouse abuse and elder abuse), (2) feel a sense of shame,* (3) fear that family and friends will be nonsupportive, and/or (4) perceive

*Refer to Chapter 16 for a discussion of shame as a dynamic in the moral system of Asian-Americans.

their anger and rage as potentially dangerous and uncontrollable. When victims of abuse do express feelings of anger, frustration, and rage, the feelings are usually displaced onto situations where the abuse has not occurred, and onlookers often perceive the display of angry, aggressive behavior as irrational. Partially because of sex-role socialization, male victims of abuse usually direct their anger in aggressive behavior toward others, while female victims of abuse usually direct their rage against themselves (Carmen, Rieker, and Mills, 1984; Mills, Rieker, and Carmen, 1984).

PATTERNS OF ABUSIVE BEHAVIOR

People who use violent or abusive behavior are responding to and trying to cope with tension and conflict. However, their repertoire of techniques for reducing tension and conflict usually include few, if any, nonviolent strategies. Table 21-1 outlines some factors that are associated with abusive behavior and that may serve as warning signs that an individual has potential for violence. However, the best indicator that a person may use violent behavior in the future is the knowledge that the person has used physically abusive behavior in the past. We will examine three categories of abusive behavior that represent major social problems: criminal violence, domestic violence, and sexual molestation.

Violence may be viewed as a response to stress. This response consists of five phases. Table 21-2 describes these phases. The following vignette exemplifies the phases of violence.

For the past two years, Tracy, now a junior in high school, had been extorting protection money from her classmates. One day while making a protection payment, a classmate referred to Tracy as a "butch." Tracy had long been in conflict about her sexual orientation. The word "butch" tapped into this conflict and triggered the violent episode. She became red in the face, began trembling, and started screaming obscenities (escalation phase). Tracy's behavior became increasingly uncontrollable as she began kicking and slashing out with a Swiss Army knife. The victim of Tracy's extortion was cut on the face and shoulder. Following this violent outburst (crisis phase),

TABLE 21-1 Predictor factors associated with abusive behavior

Factor	Characteristics
Childhood history	Bedwetting, arson, cruelty to animals, intimidating other children, impulsiveness, drug or alcohol abuse, school problems (e.g., truancy, discipline problems), temper tantrums, parental deprivation, parental abuse, social isolation from or interpersonal difficulties with peers
Situational	Dysfunctional family, unemployment, job dissatisfaction, personal history of violence, current family problem (e.g., family argument, separation from family members)
Behavioral	Depression, increased drug or alcohol use, increased visits to physician or emergency room, threats of violence

Sources consulted include Monahan (1981), Burckhardt (1981), Shupe, Stacey, and Hazlewood, 1987.

TABLE 21-2 Phases of violence

Phase	Description
Triggering	A stress-producing event precipitates the cycle. The abuser derogates or threatens the victim. The victim may try to placate the abuser by being compliant or getting out of the way.
Escalation	The abuser continues the derogation and/or threats. The abuse gradually escalates as the abuser becomes more enraged and exercises less and less self-control. Behavioral responses (e.g., increased muscle tension, raised pitch and volume of voice, emotional and physical agitation) lead to a violent outburst.
Crisis	Suddenly the abuser loses all control of anger and erupts in physically abusive behavior that may produce serious injury or death.
Recovery	Assaultive responses decrease as the abuser returns to a base-line level of behavior. In cases of domestic violence and rape, the victim may try to hide, mask the injuries, and/or deny the seriousness of the injuries to self and others.
Postcrisis	Abuser's emotional and physical responses become subnormal. The abuser may apologize and or use other forms of reconciliatory behavior. For example, a wife batterer may feel remorse and try to make amends to the victim. The batterer may promise not to be assaultive again and may beg forgiveness. At the time, the batterer may be sincere and believe that self-control of anger can be accomplished. The victim may agree to a reconciliation or to drop legal charges.

Sources consulted include Brown (1981b), Smith (1981), Steinmetz (1978, 1980), Collier (1987).

Tracy began to recover. Although she continued to curse her victim, Tracy's agitation gradually decreased. By this time school security guards were on the scene, and Tracy let herself be led away. She appeared very subdued and mumbled an apology to the guards for "losing my cool" (post crisis depression phase).

Associated with the concept of violence as a response to stress are behavioral cues that may indicate impending violent behavior. These behavioral cues occur during the escalation phase of the five-phase assault cycle and include such indices of

readiness for "fight or flight" as are described in Table 21-3.

Violence is not always a discrete behavior but is often a facet of the behavior pattern of people who engage in antisocial behavior. The DSM-III-R (1987) describes an antisocial personality disorder as a persistent behavior pattern that begins before the age of 15 and that continues into adulthood. In adolescence, it is characterized by lying, stealing, truancy, vandalism, promiscuity, initiating fights and physical assaults, running away from home (at least twice), substance abuse, and/or physical cruelty. In adulthood, this antisocial behavior pattern also may include failure to honor financial obliga-

TABLE 21-3 Behavioral cues associated with impending assault

Type of cue	Description
Verbal	Sarcasm, obscenities, derogation, threats, shouting, statements about previous violent outbursts
Kinesic	Angry faces, rigid posture, tremors, clenched fists, pacing, hyperactivity, throwing objects
Awareness	Impaired sense of orientation, heightened level of reality testing, impaired degree of situational insight, impaired ability to perceive, interpret and respond to environmental stimuli

Sources consulted include Clunn (1981) and Shupe, Tracey, and Hazlewood (1987).

tions, inability to function as a parent, violence against family members, intimidation of others, and involvement in illegal acts. Antisocial individuals usually feel little remorse about their behavior and often justify their abuse of others.

Criminal violence

For violent behavior to be considered criminal, it must conform to the definition delineated by the society in which it occurs. There are times when this delineation is relative. For example, in some societies, wife beating is not considered criminal behavior until it extends beyond the parameters established by that society. In the United States, police tend to be reluctant to become involved in instances of spousal violence, preferring to define such episodes as domestic disputes rather than as criminal violence. However, many locales are beginning to enact legislation that requires spouse abusers to be arrested for their violence. Furthermore, in the United States it is more socially acceptable for women to assault men than for men to assault women. It is also more acceptable for a small person to assault a big person than vice versa. Children in our society are admonished to "pick on someone your own size." These are all instances of ambiguous or unclear parameters delineating criminally violent behavior. On the other hand, there are times when the violation of social norms clearly constitutes criminally violent behavior. For example, in many societies premeditated murder is unequivocally defined as a violent crime (Smith, 1981).

Although a history of mental illness does not correlate with violent crime, a history of substance abuse, parental deprivation or abuse, intimidation of others, and/or an impulsive personality is associated with criminal violence. Discharged psychiatric clients who do engage in violent crime frequently have engaged in criminal violence prior to their treatment for psychiatric problems (Burckhardt, 1981).

Criminal violence cannot be readily predicted. A previous history of violent behavior is the most consistently shared factor among people who engage in criminal violence. However, a combination of situational and personal factors seems to be implicated in criminal violence. Table 21-4 summarizes these factors.

Delinquency and *criminal activity* are two common types of behavior that may involve criminal violence. Delinquents and criminals tend to be estranged from society and its predominant cultural themes. Juvenile delinquents and criminals often have grown up in environments in which socially approved role models and societal values, purposes, and goals are weak or absent. This is not to say that juvenile delinquents and criminals have no standards or values. Quite to the contrary, many belong to a countersociety—a society that runs counter to or against the established society in which it exists. This countersociety has its own role models, goals, and system of values and norms (Birenbaum and Sagarin, 1976; Halliday, 1976). In a sense, then, delinquent and criminal behavior can be viewed as adaptive. Birenbaum and Sagarin (1976) believe it helps a person obtain a positive self-concept and a sense of belonging and relatedness.

Domestic violence

Domestic violence is a symptom of family dysfunction. In the United States, domestic violence has increasingly come to the attention of nurses and

TABLE 21-4 Situational and personal factors associated with criminal violence

Factor	Description
Situational	Unemployment, job dissatisfaction, school-related problems
Personal	Impulsive personality; low self-esteem; coping behaviors of drug or alcohol abuse; childhood history of bedwetting, arson, cruelty to animals, and intimidating other children; family history of social deviance; dysfunctional family system

Sources consulted include Roth (1972), Rubin (1972), Shupe, Stacey, and Hazlewood (1987), Burckhardt (1981).

other health professionals. Contrary to popular belief, family violence is not restricted to any social class, religion, race, ethnic group, or educational level. Societal attitudes that the family is sacred, that family matters should be kept private, and that the family should not be interfered with have contributed to society's tolerance of domestic violence (Lichtenstein, 1981).

CONSORT ABUSE

After years of silence, the media is making *spouse abuse* a visible problem. Victims of spouse abuse describe living in intimate relationships characterized by fear, anger, and frustration. Spouse abuse may begin on the honeymoon, at the time of the first pregnancy, when there are financial problems, when a spouse has been drinking too much—at any time when domestic life becomes very stressful (Victims Information Bureau of Suffolk, Inc., 1986).

Although wife battering is the most commonly reported type of spouse abuse, husbands may also be victims of abuse. Wives are as likely to initiate assault to resolve marital conflicts as are husbands, and many spouses engage in reciprocal violence. However, because of differences in strength, wives often receive more serious injuries than do husbands. Possibly to compensate for a man's superior strength, women tend to use weapons more frequently than do men (McLeod, 1984; Strauss and Gelles, 1986).

Strauss and Gelles (1986) found that while the incidence of wife battering is decreasing, the incidence of husband battering is on the increase. They attribute the increased incidence of husband battering to a lack of public awareness of and concern about the problem of husband abuse and to nonexistent funding for programs to help husband bat-

terers reform. Because of the social stigma attached to a man being beaten by a woman, many husbands hesitate to tell anyone that they are being abused. The following statements of male clients speak to this reticence:

"My wife used to tie me up while I was sleeping and then beat the hell out of me. For years, I didn't tell anyone because I was afraid they would think I wasn't a real man."

• • •

"About 6 months after we were married, my wife started to beat me. It's been going on now for 2 years. I really love her, but I can't go on like this. I'm too ashamed to tell people about it. I would go to a support group where there are other men who are experiencing the same thing, only I don't know of any such groups."

Battered women, like battered men, experience considerable stress in their marital relationships. Situational crises such as economic problems and pregnancy may be contributing factors. Should a battered woman decide to dissolve her marriage, Turner and Shapiro (1986) have described the period of grief she will likely experience as she mourns the death of the abusive relationship. Table 21-5 describes this mourning period.

Abuse in an intimate interpersonal relationship may begin before marriage. Some couples are involved in a series of abusive dating relationships. As with spousal abuse, men and women may be either the initiators of or the victims of *dating violence* or *premarital abuse*. Many dating couples engage in reciprocal physical abuse. After an abu-

TABLE 21-5 Mourning the death of an abusive relationship

Phase	Characteristics
Denial	She denies that the abuse occurs or the seriousness of the abuse. She makes excuses to herself and others for the physical signs of abuse out of a feeling that she is responsible for her husband's violence, an association of abuse with love, and/or fear of losing an otherwise valued relationship. This stage may last for years, and denial may be more apparent at some times than at other times.
Anger	She feels angry toward her abusing husband, significant others who never offered help, and/or herself for not having resolved the situation sooner. If the anger is suppressed, the woman may turn it inward onto herself, and she may become accident prone or chronically ill. It is during this stage that a woman is most likely to seek professional assistance for help in leaving her husband.
Bargaining	She feels ambivalence about her decision to leave her battering husband. She vacillates between a desire to be cared for and a desire to be free of the threat of violence. She may also be swayed by the battering husband's promises to reform and his pleas for forgiveness. She may respond with a plan to return "if" her husband will comply with such demands as an end to the battering and marital counseling. If the husband complies with the demands, it is in this stage that a reconciliation may be effected.
Grief	She feels grief only when anger has been worked through and the losses associated with the relationship become apparent (e.g., loss of security, role loss, loss of an idealized relationship). Because of society's expectation that a battered wife should feel only anger and relief at the end of an abusive relationship, the grief is often suppressed. It is during this stage that she may attempt to avoid the feeling of grief by contemplating returning to the abusive relationship or by becoming involved in a new intimate relationship.
Acceptance	She decides to leave the abusive relationship and to establish a new way of life that includes new living arrangements and plans to be self-supporting. She feels secure in the decision she has made and is able to discuss the abusive relationship without feeling guilty or intensely angry. Periodic feelings of sadness over the losses will surface, but they will be experienced with ever-lessening intensity. It is during this stage that the professional helping relationship is usually terminated.

Adapted from Turner and Shapiro (1986).

sive episode, couples may experience feelings of sadness, remorse, confusion, and anger. Although they may discuss the relationship, unless serious injury was experienced, fewer than 50% of the couples dissolve the relationship. Jealousy is a predominant theme in the relationships of couples who engage in premarital abuse. A sense of insecurity within the dating relationship, changing sex norms and roles, and ambivalence about these changing sexual standards and expectations generate feelings of possessiveness and insecurity. Cohabitation, a family history of violence, and alcohol consumption are other contributing factors in dating violence (Lane and Gwartney-Gibbs, 1985; Makepeace, 1986; Carlson, 1987).

CHILD ABUSE AND NEGLECT

Child abuse refers to the deliberate injury of a child by a parent or caretaker. The abuse may be physical and/or emotional. *Child neglect* refers to lack of care in the provision of necessities such as food, clothing, and shelter. The legal definitions of child abuse and neglect vary from state to state.

Dr. C.H. Kempe coined the term *battered child syndrome*. He described the physical abuse experienced by infants and preschoolers who were defenseless and unable to communicate what was happening to them. Abused children have little sense of self—deriving what they can from parents who also have an underdeveloped sense of self. This poor sense of self is projected downward to the

TABLE 21-6   Types of elder abuse

Type of abuse	Description
Material	Theft or misuse of money or property (e.g., stealing Social Security checks, using retirement savings for the caregiver's needs rather than the elder's needs)
Physical	Deprivation of medical care, personal care, and/or food; misuse of medications (e.g., withholding medication or overmedicating); battering; misuse of physical restraints
Psychological	Verbal assaults, threats, and/or derogation; other-imposed emotional and/or social isolation

Sources consulted include Hickey and Douglass (1981) and Beck and Ferguson (1981).

child, and the cycle goes on. Abused children have few peer contacts, often remaining socially isolated because parents are not happy with any of their friends. They may tend to be very close to parents, yet withdrawn. There is a suspiciousness on the part of these children when they are in contact with other adults, particularly when questions are asked about their injuries. The parent-child relationship often confuses diagnosis because there seems to be a deep concern for one another. In contrast to neglected children who may be inappropriately dressed (for example, no socks and shoes in winter), malnourished, dirty, and have unattended health needs, abused children may be well fed and well dressed and have their injuries attended to appropriately. Parents will bring the abused child to various clinics—never using one consistently—thus making it more difficult for health professionals to fully assess the situation. Parents frequently reflect concern about their child's status as well as ambivalence about their role as parents. The child's body becomes a battleground for the simultaneous feelings of love and hate experienced by the abusing parent. Gladston (1979, 589) states that "child abuse is an act that reflects the human capacity to entertain two intense and mutually contradictory emotions simultaneously." He further suggests that child abuse lies on the spectrum of human violence somewhere between homicide and suicide.

Both physical and emotional child abuse and neglect are parental responses to frustration and anger. It is evidence of parental inability to fulfill parenting responsibilities whether from lack of energy, parental overburdening, or emotional stress. The effects of growing up in a violent family, in terms of physical and emotional neglect and abuse,

may take their toll in long-lasting physical and psychological problems.

ELDER ABUSE AND NEGLECT

For many frail elderly people who are living in the community, a relationship with a family care giver is an essential aspect of their lives. While many of the relationships with family caregivers are warm and caring, others are abusive and neglectful. Elder abuse and neglect refers to material, physical, and/or psychological deprivation or injury of an elderly person by a caregiver. Table 21-6 describes these types of abuse. Because elderly people are aware of their dependency on family caregivers, they may conform to the demands of abusive family members. Fear about moving into a new and strange living arrangement (e.g., a nursing home), fear of retaliation from abusive family members, and a desire to avoid the shame and humiliation that they may associate with being abused may keep aged family members from disclosing the neglect and abuse that they are experiencing. Stereotypes of the elderly as "forgetful" or "confused" may cause people to disbelieve accounts of abuse when they are disclosed.

An individual may abuse an elderly family member to control the elderly person's behavior or to express frustration and anger. Benign neglect is the most common form of abuse. Often adult caregivers are overburdened with household, child care, and occupational responsibilities, and the care of a dependent elderly family member aggravates the situation. In such situations, an elderly person may be left in his or her own feces, may be minimally fed, or may be left for hours in one position in bed. Decubiti, nutritional deficiencies, and contractures

TABLE 21-7 Types of rapists

Rapist type	Description
Anger rapist	Displaces anger toward a significant woman or women onto the rape victim; uses more physical force than is needed to subdue the victim; brutalizes the victim; may degrade the victim by forcing her to engage in oral sex, by masturbating on her, or by urinating on her; the victim is usually old or in some other way vulnerable
Power rapist	Most common type of rapist; uses only the amount of force necessary to subdue the victim; aim is to get the victim into his power and thereby "prove" himself as a man; intimidation rather than physical force is used to gain control over the victim; rapist may fantasize that his victim will be sexually attracted to him because of the sexual prowess that he will show during the rape; frequently asks the victim, while raping her, if she is enjoying the experience; at the conclusion of the rape, may ask the victim for a date
Sadistic rapist	Seeks sexual gratification and an outlet for aggression through rape; sexuality and aggression are blended together; rapist receives erotic excitement from the victim's death; instead of penetrating the victim with the penis, an instrument may be used; rapist may ejaculate at the moment of the victim's death; rapist may have intercourse with the victim's dead body; there may be a ritualistic aspect to the rape; least common type of rapist

Adapted from Burgess and Holstrom (1974).

may develop. Additional factors that contribute to elder abuse are

1. denial of the social needs of the elderly
2. role reversal among adult and elderly family members
3. inadequate understanding of the meaning of loss to the elderly

Because of the series of losses that people experience with aging (e.g., loss of spouse and friends, loss of physical health, role loss), such seemingly insignificant losses as the death of a pet or the surrendering of a driver's license may precipitate a grief reaction. Adult family members may become intolerant of the depression, despair, stubbornness, physical complaints, and criticism of elderly family members and may not recognize these signs as responses to multiple losses.

In addition, physical and psychological changes associated with aging may result in the withdrawal of some elderly people from social interaction and activity. Adult family members may think that their aged parents should be more socially involved. They may feel uncomfortable sitting, listening, and being with these elderly family members. They may assume parental roles and assign child roles to aged family members. Such role reversal tends to encourage dependency and helplessness and deny the sexuality, self-sufficiency, and dignity of the

elderly. Adult family members may be overburdened by this role reversal. At the same time, elderly family members may refuse to relinquish authority in the family. These factors tend to generate family conflict. Family conflict increases the potential for elder abuse (Johnson, 1979; Hickey and Douglass, 1981; Beck and Ferguson, 1981).

Sexual molestation
RAPE

Men who engage in forcible sexual intercourse with an unwilling partner are committing rape. Oftentimes, sodomy, (penis to mouth, penis to anus, or mouth to vulva) is part of the rape incident. Rape is *not* an act of passion; it is an act of violence. Rape serves the nonsexual purposes of venting anger and hostility and exercising control and power. These themes—anger, hostility, control, power— are present in every rape, but in any given rape one theme or combination of themes may predominate. In their classic study, Burgess and Holstrom (1974) used these themes to identify three types of rapist: the "anger rapist," the "power rapist," and the "sadistic rapist" (see Table 21-7).

Most rapists seem to follow an identifiable pattern. First, a rapist selects a woman who is perceived as vulnerable (e.g., old, living alone, or hitchhiking). Then he tests his potential victim. For example, a rapist may approach a woman, ask her for a match, make insinuating remarks, and then direct her to remove her clothes or tell her not to scream. In this way, he determines whether she can be intimidated. Next, he threatens her. He tells her what he wants her to do, that he will harm her if she does not submit, and that she will be spared if she cooperates. However, not all rapists are strangers. Women may be raped by spouses and acquaintances.

A woman who has been raped feels a sense of powerlessness, a sense of helplessness, and a sense of loss. She may feel unable to determine her life's course. She may also feel isolated from family, friends, and colleagues. She may be afraid to return to her home or to walk alone, whether it be day or night. The greatest assault, however, has been against the self. Her personal space has been violated by a violent act. Loss of her personhood, her self-esteem, results. The rape victim experiences a wide range of feelings, from anxiety and fear to profound depression. Rape victims should be allowed to grieve for the loss of self.

Burgess and Holstrom (1974, 1979) describe a two-phase response to rape—the rape trauma syndrome. The first, or acute, phase is characterized by disorganization. The second stage is characterized by reorganization. Table 21-8 describes these stages.

Burgess and Holstrom also describe the compounded reaction that can occur in women who have had previous psychological difficulties. This reaction is characterized by psychotic behavior, depression, acting-out behavior, and suicide. In addition, women who have been raped at a previous time, have denied their feelings about the rape, and have not revealed the rape to anyone may experience a *silent rape reaction*. Because the second rape reactivates the experience of the first rape, the victim's reactions to the first attack must be dealt with if the woman is to work through the present rape crisis.

Significant others may feel angry, helpless, and/or ashamed when they learn about the rape. They may respond to the rape by blaming the victim (believing the woman provoked the rape), by pressuring the victim not to report the rape, or by emo-

TABLE 21-8   Two-phase response to rape

Phase	Characteristics
Disorganization	Feelings of embarrassment, anger, humiliation, fear, and self-blame; may release angry, anxious feelings by talking, shouting, crying, or pacing (expressed style); or may maintain a calm, subdued affect, acting as though nothing out of the ordinary has occurred (controlled style)
Reorganization	Phase begins at a different time for each victim, depending on the availability of healthy coping methods, social support systems, and previous experiences with loss; phobic reactions (e.g., fear of entering house or apartment alone, fear of being followed, fear of sexual intercourse); increased motor activity (e.g., changing residence, job, or telephone number, taking trips); nightmares (occur in two stages—in stage one, the woman relives the rape but awakens before she can fight off the rapist; in stage two, the woman is able to successfully fight off the rapist)

tionally or physically (including sexually) distancing themselves from the rape victim. Such responses deprive the victim of the support that she desperately needs during the crisis. Long-term studies indicate that rape victims benefit from extended follow-up counseling, which can frequently continue as long as two years.

Because rape is a crime, a physical examination is required immediately after the assault. In addition to providing measures to prevent pregnancy and venereal disease, the physical examination documents physical trauma and the presence of semen. This documentation may be used as evidence in court to support the victim's case. Because the physical examination may cause additional stress for women already in crisis, supportive intervention by health care workers and rape crisis teams is essential.

SEXUAL ABUSE

Sexual abuse refers to sexual contact between a minor (or a developmentally immature person) and a developmentally mature person regardless of the kinship relationship. The sexual contact may include sexual intercourse, fondling, disrobing, sodomy, rape, showing pornographic pictures, and masturbation. In approximately 75% of sexual abuse, the child knows the abuser. *Incest* is a type of sexual abuse that refers to sexual contact between kin. Culture defines which relationships are considered incestuous. In our society, although there is variability in state laws, incest usually refers to sexual activity, not limited to intercourse, with a child by a member of the child's nuclear family. The most common form of incest occurs between father and daughter. Often more than one child in a family is victimized. The perpetrator may shift his or her sexual attention to a younger child when the older child matures or leaves home. The relationship between abuser and victim is one of dominance-submission. The abuser may use intimidation, manipulation, threats, endearments, and bribes to engage the child in sexual activity and to maintain the child's silence. The child may be told that no one will believe his or her accusations, that he or she will be punished, or that there will be retaliation against a significant other if the child reveals the "secret" (Winters, 1985).

The reactions of children who have been sexually abused are influenced by the support that they receive when they disclose the abuse as well as the degree of family disruption that occurs after the disclosure. Wolf and Mosk (1983, 707) suggest that "disturbances in the child's social and behavioral development may be more a function of family events and interaction patterns than isolated abusive episodes." The young age at which much sexual abuse occurs and the malfunctioning families in which it often occurs interfere with these children reestablishing a sense of self-esteem and integrity and may make them more vulnerable to subsequent sexual abuse (Hartman, Finn, and Leon, 1987).

EPIDEMIOLOGY

No one segment of society can be held accountable for abusive behavior. It is found in all social classes, age groups, and genders. For example, although reporting of domestic abuse tends to be more common among families in the lower socioeconomic bracket, this may reflect reluctance of people to report abuse in middle- and upper-income families (Gladston, 1979; Shupe, Stacey, and Hazlewood, 1987).

The exact incidence of abusive behavior is not known. Although instances of criminal violence are usually reported, many instances of domestic violence and sexual molestation go unreported. The Centers for Disease Control (CDC) report that the incidence of child abuse in the United States is on the increase. It is estimated that at least 1 million children in the United States are abused each year. Twenty percent of the cases involve children who have been abused before, and 22% involve multiple trauma. Child abuse is the second leading cause of death for children between the ages of infancy and 5 years (Winters, 1985). The incidence of spouse abuse also can only be estimated. Extrapolating from research findings, approximately 25 to 50% of all couples admit to the occurrence of physical abuse at some point in their marriages (Strauss and Gelles, 1980; Appleton, 1980; Goldberg and Tomlanovich, 1984).

Until recently, sexual abuse and incest have been considered taboo subjects. Dr. Ann Burgess has brought the issue of child molestation to the public's attention. In 1981 at the second annual Psychiatric Mental Health Symposium, she presented statistics showing that sexual abuse of children is on the rise. Frequently the abuser is an acquaintance of the family, and many times that person holds a respected position in the community. Dr. Burgess further noted that men who molest young boys are often involved with the boys in Boy Scouts, Little League, church groups, or other group activities. In 1987, several instances of child molestation were uncovered in day care centers.

SOCIOCULTURAL CONTEXT

Human abuse must be viewed in a sociocultural perspective. Special attention should be paid to the fact that sociocultural factors influence not only the definition of and response to violence but also the assessment and treatment of human abuse. Human abuse is a culture-bound issue.

A classic anthropological study has suggested that there is a correlation between increased homicide rates and periods of social stress. Nash (1967) found that in response to social change among the Teklum, in Mexico, charges of witchcraft increased with an associated rise in homicide. Among the Teklum, murder was a strictly male activity. Both perpetrators and victims were men. Men who were murdered had usually been suspected of witchcraft. Most of the Indian community felt that these homicides were justified. This situation also shows that while homicide might be perceived as a deviant form of behavior, members of a particular society might not always interpret it as criminal behavior.

Other anthropologists have related human abuse to family structure and family roles. Nuclear families, with their lack of alternative caretakers, often are characterized by parental overburdening and punitive, abusive parenting. On the other hand, societies with extended family households that have older children, relatives, or neighbors who serve as alternative caretakers or societies that have state-run child care facilities tend to be characterized by more nurturing and less punitive, abusive parenting (Korbin, 1978).

In the United States, violence and abuse are subject to cultural and subcultural variations. Historically, women have been viewed as property. First they were the property of their fathers. Then, in marriage, they were "given" by their fathers to their husbands. Although the view of women as the property of men began to change with the Industrial Revolution, the influence of this patriarchal tradition is still present in the Bible. Although most organized religions have always urged that people control their anger, some people use the patriarchal authority referred to in the Bible to rationalize domestic violence. A man may reason that it is his right to make all the decisions in the family. If his wife does not submit to his authority, then a beating is justified as a husband's biblical right to discipline his wife. A battered wife may rationalize that her abuse is a result of her own worthlessness and

failure to submit to her husband's demands instead of placing the responsibility for the abuse on her assaultive husband. She may look to God to help and protect her and not report the abuse and seek professional intervention. Parents may justify child abuse as their parental responsibility to "drive out the devil" from their children and thus excuse their violent behavior as necessary discipline (Jacobs, 1984; Long, 1986; Shupe, Stacey, and Hazlewood, 1987).

Subcultural variations related to ethnicity and population density also influence people's orientations to violence and abuse. Long (1986), a nurse who practiced in the rural northwestern United States, reports that among Native Americans child and spouse abuse are viewed as family matters in which nonfamily members should not become involved. In fact, it is customary for women and children to leave the house when a husband-father is angry or drunk, thereby placing the responsibility for avoiding abusive behavior on the potential victims. Among the Native Americans with whom Long has worked, abuse is determined more by the degree and permanency of damage that the violence inflicts and by the circumstances surrounding the incident than by the type of violent behavior used. In addition, confidentiality for informants is often difficult to maintain. For example, in instances where abuse is reported to a tribal court, loyalty to one's clan may result in a member of the tribal court revealing the name of the informant. Even when neighbors or relatives acknowledge that a person's behavior is violent, contacting the tribal court or the local white legal authorities may be viewed as interference in private matters (if the informant is outside the family) or as intolerable disloyalty to one's family or clan (if the informant is a family member). In either case, the informant may be derogated and ostracised. Long (1986, 133) states that "sanctions within a tribal clan or other subgroup are often more severe in relation to the informant than in relation to the abuser." Long's findings support those of others who have looked at human abuse within rural communities (Delaney and Woods, 1975; Soloman, Hiesberger, and Winier, 1981).

Health care professionals experience problems in defining, assessing, and intervening in human

TABLE 21-9 Sadistic and self-defeating personalities

Personality type	Characteristics
Sadistic	Uses physically violent, demanding, and aggressive behavior; lies to humiliate or cause suffering to others; dominates others and restricts their autonomy by using such tactics as intimidation and terror; has a fascination for violence, weapons, martial arts, injury, or torture
Self-defeating	Seeks out situations or relationships that cause disappointment, failure, or mistreatment; avoids opportunities for pleasurable relationships or situations; rejects offers of help; responds to positive personal events with depression or guilt; provokes anger or rejection from others and then feels hurt when they retaliate; fails to accomplish tasks necessary for personal goals despite ability to do so; avoids or rejects people who are consistently caring; engages in excessive and unsolicited self-sacrifice

Adapted from Diagnostic and Statistical Manual of Mental Disorders (DSM-III-R), 1987.

abuse. The DSM-III-R classifications of sadistic personality and self-defeating personality are criticized by some mental health professionals for cultural bias. DSM-III-R stipulates that a sadistic personality is a pervasive personality pattern that is not directed solely toward one person (as in spouse abuse or child abuse). DSM-III-R also states that a self-defeating personality pattern does not refer to a person who is responding to or anticipating physical, sexual, or emotional abuse. Despite these stipulations, there is concern among some health professionals that these constraints will not be observed. Critics of these personality classifications say that the diagnosis of sadistic personality will be given primarily to men and the diagnosis of self-defeating personality will be made almost exclusively with women (Boxer, 1987). The Council on Psychiatric and Mental Health Nursing (Pacesetter, 1987) criticizes the category of self-defeating personality disorder for discounting sociocultural factors that might generate such behaviors and for being potentially harmful to battered women who are seeking custody of their children. Rather than diagnosing the psychopathology of individuals, these diagnoses reflect sexism and pathology within American society. In addition, such diagnoses may suggest that perpetrators of human abuse are not responsible for their violent behavior while victims of abuse have sought it out. Table 21-9 summarizes the characteristics associated with sadistic and self-defeating personality types.

Further complicating the problem of assessment and intervention into human abuse is the tendency of some health care professionals to deny, ignore, or otherwise fail to report violent or abusive behavior in a colleague. The basic assumption of these health care workers is that abuse does not occur among the subculture of health care professionals (Long, 1986).

Sociocultural research and literature indicate that when violence occurs, the meaning it is given is related to aspects within the social system. Not only the definition of and response to human abuse but also its assessment and intervention are subject to cultural and subcultural variations.

EXPLANATORY THEORIES
Psychological theories

Psychological theories trace the origins of abusive and violent behavior patterns to psychological and maturational processes of early childhood. The reenactment of abusive and violent behavior in an adult, sometimes referred to as a generational transfer or a proclivity for violence, may be the legacy of adults who were traumatized by violence and abuse as children. However, not all children who are abused grow up to be abusers. Many factors decrease the risk of a legacy of violence being transmitted across generations. People who do not repeat the cycle of abuse with their own children tend to differ from those who do in the following ways:
1. Have more extensive social support systems
2. Are less ambivalent about pregnancy
3. Have physically healthier babies

4. More overtly express anger about their own abuse as children
5. Had only one abusing parent
6. Had one supportive and nurturing parent
7. Have an emotionally supportive spouse/mate
8. Have fewer life stressors
9. Consciously decide not to abuse their own children (Hunter and Kilstrom, 1979; Egeland and Jacobvitz, 1984)

PSYCHODYNAMIC THEORY

Many psychodynamically oriented therapists view violence as an innate and naturally dominant response to the frustration of a blocked goal. In psychologically mature individuals, this innate response to frustration is inhibited. Individuals who use violent behavior are viewed as having defective egos and immature superegos. The ego is unable to control and regulate behavior. Because social standards have not been internalized, the superego is unable to use feelings of guilt to make people conform to social standards and inhibit their impulsive id behavior. For example, from a feared parent figure, a child often internalizes the parent's socially undesirable violent behavior. Many abusive men and women have experienced their fathers as abusive, emotionally unresponsive, or indifferent. The only instances of paternal attention may have been instances of paternal abuse. Comforting, emotional warmth, protection, and feelings of self-esteem were only experienced from their mothers. Such family conditions produced hostile individuals with poor self-esteem who try to control their social environments by using violent behavior similar to the violence they initially encountered from their abusive, powerful fathers (Marmor, 1978; Shupe, Stacey, and Hazlewood, 1987).

INTERPERSONAL THEORIES

Children reared in an atmosphere of family violence witness the use of violence as a means to win arguments and to dominate others. Parents resort to violence rather than verbally express their feelings or negotiate as equals with others. The children in such families have little opportunity to learn how to verbally communicate their needs, opinions, and feelings. As a result, they become frustrated and enraged and turn to violence to settle disagreements and to get their own ways (Shupe, Stacey, and Hazlewood, 1987).

In Berne's (1961) transactional analysis model, the goal of interpersonal communication is to interact on the level of the "adult" ego state, a level that promotes open communication with the least risk of emotional pain. In this model, assertive behavior is mature behavior, and it is incompatible with assaultive or violent behavior. Therefore, assertive behavior should be the goal of interpersonal communication.

Biological theories

Biological theories purport that violent or abusive individuals are biologically predisposed to such behavior. Deschner (1984) believes that the rage that generates violence and abuse is primitive, unlearned, and instinctual. She holds that violent behavior patterns are "wired" into the brains of human beings as a survival response. Others (e.g., Montagu, 1975; Marmor, 1981) postulate that the human race has not yet evolved internal controls over violent behavior even though violence no longer is an effective survival mechanism.

BIOCHEMICAL THEORIES

Food colorings, diet, food allergies, and abuse of such substances as alcohol, barbiturates, hallucinogens, cocaine, amphetamines, and other sympathomimetics have all been associated with the development of violent behavior. Because substance abuse tends to produce emotional lability and irritability, decrease impulse control, and release inhibitions, assaultive behavior that is disproportionate to environmental stimuli may develop. For example, alcohol intoxication is implicated in 64% of all murders, 41% of all assaults, 34% of all rapes, 29% of other sex crimes, and 60% of all child abuse (Report of the National Council on Alcoholism, 1976). In addition, Deschner (1984) found that, in men with hypoglycemia, blood sugar and neurochemical imbalances seem to trigger depression and violence.

PHYSIOLOGICAL THEORIES

Mark and Ervin (1970) suggest that malfunctions in the brain may be responsible for violent behavior. Brain mechanisms both for expressing and controlling violent impulses are believed to be located in the limbic system, especially in the amygdala. Removal of the amygdala in violent individuals, with ensuing control of violent behavior, has reinforced this theory.

Such specific physical conditions as frontal or temporal lobe brain tumors, temporal-lobe epilepsy, cerebral vascular accidents, and head injuries are implicated in some cases of violent behavior. At the 1979 annual meeting of the American Academy of Neurology, Pincus (1979) suggested that neurological disorders may contribute to violent behavior in juvenile delinquents. Pincus found that 96% of the violent delinquents studied had some neurological impairment, as compared to 22% of the nonviolent delinquents.

Sociocultural theories

Sociocultural theories look to the broad social environment or to society-at-large for explanations for abuse and violence. Culturally defined sex-role stereotypes, which tend to be reinforced by mass media, often portray men as powerful and physically aggressive. Assaultive behavior and sexual misbehavior may be included in an exaggerated stereotype of the male role. In addition, power, decision making, and resources still tend to be disproportionately allocated to men, and this situation affords women relatively little control over their environments. To be "masculine" in Western society, less powerful and secure men have to "prove" themselves by taking what more powerful and secure men either already have or can readily obtain. Little in the media-reinforced cult of violence contradicts these impressions. Children reared in such an environment learn the appropriateness of using violence as a strategy for getting what they want. At the same time, social institutions that are characterized by unequal distributions of power and status influence patterns of victimization. In our society, women, children, and the elderly tend to be denied access to power and also tend to be vulnerable to domestic violence and all forms of sexual abuse

(Chesler, 1972; Lengermann and Wallace, 1985; Shupe, Stacey, and Hazlewood, 1987).

COMMUNITY DISINTEGRATION THEORY

Sociocultural factors often cited as contributing to violence include rapid social change and family disorganization. Rapid social change tends to disrupt the values, standards, and social roles that govern socially acceptable behavior, leaving people confused about the guidelines around which to organize their lives. For example, changes related to the women's movement, such as women attaining some of the opportunities and material goods and services that have previously been controlled by men, elevate the status of women from dependency to independency and provide women with roles other than wife and mother. At the same time, many men tenaciously try to hold onto their traditional positions of power in the family.* In the wake of such social change, the family may be used as a "battleground" (Prince, 1980).

In addition, societal norms have long held that the family is the guardian of children and that parents act in the best interests of their children. Such a social context gives parents a great deal of power over their children and provides a social context that tolerates abuse. When instances of abuse occur, it becomes difficult for children to violate social norms and disclose abuse or for children's reports of abuse to be believed. Children thus are "denied the right to protest" (Miller, 1984). Until recently, professionals (e.g., health care givers, teachers, clergy) and law enforcers have themselves been reluctant to disregard social norms concerning the inviolate nature of the family and intervene in domestic violence.

SOCIAL STRAIN THEORY

Rapid social change and family disorganization may contribute to inadequate socialization of children. Family patterns, kinship obligations, child-rearing practices, and economic activities may be disrupted, and social strain may increase. Social institutions may no longer support the family as it tries to fulfill its social and emotional functions.

---

*Refer to Chapter 3 for an in-depth discussion of power and gender bias.

TABLE 21-10 Support institutions

Institution	Conditions	Outcomes
School	Inadequate financial resources; achievement may be judged primarily by student performance on verbal and written examinations; large class size; decrease in teacher autonomy	Increased teacher-student ratio and educational pressures may generate low self-esteem, boredom, depersonalization, frustration, and anger in students and teachers; students and teachers may risk expulsion, disciplinary actions, or referral to health professionals if they openly display anger about the school situation; anger may later be displaced as aggressiveness or human abusiveness
Work	World economy limits upward mobility; mass production and piecework decrease sense of relatedness and sense of accomplishment	Occupational pressures, job shortages, and/or limited job opportunities may generate boredom, powerlessness, low self-esteem, frustration, and anger in workers; displaced anger may be expressed in abuse and violence
Health care facilities	Inadequate funding curtails delivery of comprehensive or personalized services	Sense of low self-esteem, frustration, powerlessness, and anger may be generated in recipients of health care; client expression of anger may be met with defensiveness or avoidance from health care providers and thus reinforce client anger; displaced anger may be expresssed as aggression and abuse against others

Sources consulted include Prince (1980) and Shupe, Stacey, and Hazlewood (1987).

Instead, these institutions may generate conditions that contribute to low self-esteem, powerlessness, frustration, and anger in family members (see Table 21-10). Family members may become estranged from socially approved purposes and goals and may deal with social strain through violence. For example, the unemployment rate among violent men is almost two times higher than the national average (Halleck, 1978; Prince, 1980; Shupe, Stacey, and Hazlewood, 1987).

SOCIAL LEARNING THEORY

Learning theorists believe that violence is learned from observing role models who use violent behavior as a means of achieving desired goals. For example, children often witness domestic violence and observe that the violent parent is able to control other family members and get his or her own way. Children may also observe that they and/or their role models are rewarded with prestige and

material gains for violent behavior. With every occasion of reward for violent behavior, the violent behavior pattern is reinforced. Both the observation of violence and its reinforcement by rewards in the environment are necessary for violent behavior to be learned (Brown, 1981a; Shupe, Stacey, and Hazlewood, 1987).

Systems theory

Systems theory hypothesizes that violent behavior is generated by biological, psychological, and social processes that are in constant simultaneous interaction with one another. This means that abusive behavior is a product of reciprocal interaction among such factors as personal resistance or vulnerability to a stressor, the nature and duration of the stressor, the presence and potency of a precipitating event, and the cultural expectations governing interpersonal relationships. The rage that precedes

646 *Client behavior and nursing practice*

TABLE 21-11 Characteristics of a family system

Characteristic	Examples
Social environment	Employment opportunities, marital tensions, crises such as unemployment and pregnancy
Personal traits of family members	Temperament, parental history of having been a victim of child abuse, ability to express anger and frustration nonviolently
Cultural heritage	Attitudes and values about violence and sex-roles, norms governing role expectations and role behaviors
Community context	Opportunities for recreation, type of community leadership, incidence of crime and delinquency

Sources consulted include Millor (1981) and Shupe, Stacey, and Hazlewood (1987).

an episode of violence may have been generated by abusive relationships in the past. The person may never have learned to nonviolently communicate feelings, opinions, and needs. Neurological impairment, biochemical factors, and/or substance abuse may interfere with the person's ability to tolerate need frustration in the present and to inhibit a violent response. Violence may be the only way the person has learned to communicate his or her intense needs and feelings.

Within a family system, each member's abusive behavior or response to abuse may be influenced by the characteristics of the family system. Table 21-11 summarizes some of the characteristics that simultaneously interact to either promote or deter domestic violence.

Usually abusive families have established an equilibrium that includes the abusive relationship. Disclosure of the abuse poses a threat to the homeostasis of the family system. For example, Solin (1986) describes the effect of incest disclosure on a family. The father's repentance, pleas for forgiveness, and promises to change tend to make family members feel sorry for him. The sexually abused children want the abuse to stop, but they may also feel a sense of loyalty to both parents. Moreover, they may be fearful of losing any nurturing that the father provided and may fear that the strain of being a single parent would decrease their mother's ability to meet their needs. The mother, who typically is characterized by low self-esteem, dependency, and depression, tends to compartmentalize and rationalize her husband's incestuous

behavior: Her husband is "sick," and the sickness is causing his incestuous behavior. The family consensus may be that rehabilitation of the father is more feasible than trying to survive as a single-parent family. Therefore, following the disclosure of incest, the family often tries to maintain equilibrium in the family system by using the defense mechanism of displacement. Anger toward the father is typically displaced onto helping professionals who are trying to intervene in the incestuous family relationship. Only when helping professionals demonstrate concern for all family members does the family begin to trust and work with the professionals. Should the helping professionals treat the father disparagingly, the use of displacement usually increases.

The various theoretical orientations toward violence and abuse impact on the practice of nursing. Table 21-12 summarizes some of the implications of these theoretical orientations for nursing practice.

TREATMENT MODALITIES

The therapeutic modalities used to treat abusers and victims of abuse include many of the measures employed in the treatment of other emotional disorders. Most of the modalities focus on reinforcing client strengths, decreasing sources of stress, and teaching more adaptive ways of dealing with stress. The most frequently employed modalities in the treatment of human abuse are emergency interventions, crisis intervention, family therapy, group therapy, and educational therapy.

TABLE 21-12 Theoretical orientations and nursing implications

Orientation	Implications for nursing practice
Psychodynamic	Nurses teach parents ways to facilitate healthy personality development in their children so they can develop the internal controls necessary to curb impulsive id behavior. With clients who are using violent behavior, external controls should be used until internal controls can be developed.
Interpersonal	Nurses teach clients to communicate their needs, opinions, and feelings and to develop assertive behavior. Nurses recognize that the risk of abusive behavior is greater with withdrawn or verbally aggressive clients than with communicative, assertive clients.
Biochemical	Nurses teach clients about the importance of good nutrition and avoidance of alcohol intoxication in the prevention of violence.
Physiological	Nurses recognize that clients with specific physical conditions may be unable to control their behavior without such external controls as medications and/or physical restraints.
Community disintegration	Nurses recognize that modification of the sociocultural environment may help prevent violent behavior. Toward this end, nurses work with disorganized families in family therapy and refer them to appropriate social service agencies. Nurses also become involved in planning and implementing programs addressing the effects of rapid social change.
Learning	Nurses provide a therapeutic milieu that rewards assertive behavior with attention, privileges, and/or tokens but does not reward violent behavior with increased attention or other interventions that may reinforce violent behavior.
Systems	Nurses view violence as complex behavior with multifactorial origins. Nurses assess biopsychosocial aspects of a situation before making a nursing diagnosis. Intervention in domestic violence involves the entire family unit.

Sources consulted include Weaver, Broome, and Kat (1978), Brown (1981a), and Shupe, Stacey, and Hazlewood (1987).

Emergency interventions

Crisis centers and hotlines provide short-term, emergency measures for dealing with frustrations that may lead to abuse or for dealing with the trauma of having been abused. Child-Help, a national child abuse hotline, offers counseling, referral to community services, and educational information for both the abused and the abuser.

Gerry, a single parent, felt overwhelmed and frustrated by the demands of parenting. One day, she found herself violently shaking her crying infant. She became frightened by what she was doing and the feeling that she was losing control. She called a crisis hotline that she had seen advertised on television. Gerry found a trained volunteer to whom she was able to vent her feelings. The volunteer listened empathetically, assisted Gerry to identify some nonviolent ways of coping with her problems, and then referred her to Parents Anonymous.

As the above vignette illustrates, hotlines provide short-term immediate measures aimed at reducing the incidence of violence.

Hot lines, such as Shelter Aid, a national domestic violence hotline, assist callers to explore options, obtain information, and find shelter. Shelters not only provide temporary safe housing for victims of domestic violence but may also provide individual counseling, group therapy, legal counseling, and employment counseling.

Crisis intervention*

Crisis intervention is a treatment of choice for victims of abuse. Crisis intervention should be initiated as soon after the abusive event as possible. Goals of crisis intervention include increasing physical safety, increasing self-esteem and trust, and decreasing fear, powerlessness, and alienation.

*Refer to Chapter 15 for further discussion of crisis intervention.

TABLE 21-13 Crisis behavior and intervention

Behavior	Description	Crisis intervention
Fear	Feels threatened; appears frightened, pale, tense, and hypervigilant; pupils may be dilated; may alternately open and close fists	*Tasks:* decrease client's fear; establish trust; increase client's sense of control *Approach:* walk slowly and diagonally in front of the client (position of indirect control); speak slowly and calmly about choices and alternatives; apprise client of all proposed staff actions
Frenzy	Feels frustrated; appears flushed and has constricted pupils; makes facial grimaces; hyperventilates; unable to problem solve	*Task:* establish control *Approach:* walk directly in front of the client (position of direct control) but out of range of client's arms and legs; other staff members fan out in a semicircle around client; provide medication, seclusion, or physical restraint as needed; reassure client that violent behavior will be controlled
Uproar	Feels in conflict (dependency needs vs. fear of merger with nurse); appears hyperactive, noisy, and demanding; behavior may quickly shift from object violence to person violence	*Tasks:* set limits on client's dependency; establish clear boundaries between nurse and client *Approach:* focus on process, not content, of client's verbalization; clearly state that client is responsible and accountable for own behavior; speak calmly and clearly; avoid dealing with the client in an angry, rejecting, or punitive manner

Adapted from Wommack (1982) and Morton (1987).

Within the framework of crisis intervention, a victim is helped to deal with the trauma of the present abusive experience. When physical safety is an issue, alternate living arrangements may be made (e.g., temporary shelters, foster care). The victim's coping style, decision-making ability, and support resources are assessed. Past events are dealt with only in terms of previously effective or ineffective coping skills. When indicated, the victim is helped to decide whether or not to take legal action against the abuser, and then the victim's decision is supported by the crisis counselor. The degree of personal disorganization and the strength and availability of support systems should be considered when determining the frequency and duration of therapy sessions. Generally, crisis intervention lasts for 6 to 8 weeks. If at the end of that time the victim is still experiencing profound disorganization and upset, referral should be made for longer-term psychotherapy. Referrals may also be made to such self-help support groups as rape crisis centers, women's centers, or crime victims' services.

Abusers may also profit from crisis intervention. Crisis intervention with physically abusive individuals focuses on management of assaultive behavior. Individuals who are in Stage III of the assault cycle (full-blown violent episode) are displaying crisis behavior. Three of the most frequently encountered forms of crisis behavior are fear, frenzy, and uproar. Table 21-13 presents these crisis behaviors and the appropriate crisis interventions. Prior to deciding that physical intervention is needed, attempts to deescalate the situation by "talking the client down" should have been made. Also, before initiating physical intervention, staff should be sure that they have removed all sharp or otherwise dangerous articles from their clothing (e.g., name pins, pens, jewelry).

Family therapy*

Many mental health professionals view domestic violence and neglect as symptoms of dysfunctional family systems. However, Bogard (1984) cautions that, because such an approach implies that the responsibility for abuse is shared within the family system, it may take the focus off the abuser and may not offer abused family members adequate support and affirmation outside the family system.

The goals of family therapy are to increase self-disclosure and assertive communication among family members and to help family members establish clear personal boundaries. To achieve these goals, family therapists point out dysfunctional coping behaviors that are evidenced in the family therapy session, emphasize the need to change these dysfunctional coping patterns, and assist family members to find more direct, assertive, and nonviolent ways of communicating and dealing with stress and anger. Family members are taught to view conflict within the family as both inevitable and beneficial. Within family therapy sessions, family members are helped to decide whether they want to continue dealing with conflict indirectly and violently or to learn to handle it directly and assertively. Children in the family system may be helped, through play therapy, to deal with the trauma of abuse and neglect, to express their needs and feelings, and to learn nonviolent ways of expressing anger and frustration.

Group therapy†

One of the most commonly used treatment modalities for abusers and victims of abuse is group therapy. The utilization of a group approach recognizes the needs of both the abuser and the abused for

1. identification with people who have shared similar experiences, thereby reducing the sense of intense isolation
2. opportunity to disclose a powerful and over-

---

*Refer to Chapter 14 for an in-depth discussion of Family Therapy.

†Refer to Chapter 13 for an in-depth discussion of group therapy.

whelming "secret" to an empathetic support group that has kept a similar secret

In addition, group therapy offers victims of abuse an opportunity for validating the reality of victimization and for sharing feelings that are often denied both by victims of abuse and their significant others.

Because of the traumatic nature and sequelae of human abuse for both perpetrators and victims, group treatment often elicits high anxiety. As one group member after another recounts the details surrounding the abusive situation, affect-laden memories may be aroused. Table 21-14 suggests areas in which potential group members should be assessed.

Group therapy techniques include *monitoring* (group members bring the group up to date on any important events that have transpired since the last group session), *feedback* (group members share their perceptions about how each member is responding to the session), *grounding* (therapist helps group members keep in touch with present-day reality so that they do not become overwhelmed by or "stuck" in past abusive experiences), and *reinterpretation* (therapist clarifies and ameliorates feelings that are overwhelmingly conflict-laden or distressful for group members).

Educational therapy

Educational therapy provides abusers with information about the biopsychosocial origins of abusive behavior and teaches skills for controlling stress and anger as well as problem-solving strategies. The goal of educational therapy is to increase self-esteem and teach ways of dealing with everyday stressors without resorting to violence.

A nurse working with a group of child abusers taught the parents about childhood growth and development. The nurse's rationale for teaching abusive parents factual knowledge about growth and development was to help parents develop realistic developmental expectations of their children. Parents who have unrealistically high expectations of their children may become frustrated and angry when the children do not meet those expectations. Because the nurse knew that many abusing parents have themselves been abused as

TABLE 21-14 Assessment criteria for potential group members

Criteria	Rationale
Coping behaviors (adaptive and maladaptive)	A client's repertoire of coping behaviors will be called upon when the group experience elicits high anxiety. The therapist needs to help the client strengthen or learn adaptive coping behaviors so that maladaptive coping styles (e.g., denial, blame placing, violence will decrease).
Crises (other than the abuse situation)	Additional situational or maturational crises will add to the client's stress level, tax coping behaviors, and decrease the client's ability to tolerate anxiety elicited by group sharing, thereby decreasing the client's ability to profit from the group experience.
Substance abuse (past or current)	A client may try to deal with anxiety elicited by the group experience through substance abuse. Current substance abuse should be treated before group therapy is initiated, and substance abuse treatment should then continue concurrently with group therapy.
Quality of social support network	The number and availability of significant others to lend support to the client can influence the client's ability to tolerate stress generated by the group experience.

Sources consulted include Cole and Barney (1987) and Bennett (1987).

children and have not experienced adequate parental nurturing, the nurse included role playing of appropriate parenting behaviors as part of the group experience. In addition, the nurse taught the parents such stress-reduction techniques as progressive relaxation and guided imagery and arranged for the parents to attend an assertiveness training workshop.

The preceding vignette shows how educational therapy can be designed to facilitate learning about one's self as well as learning skills for dealing with frustration and anger.

• • •

Abusers and victims of abuse may be treated in a variety of settings and with a variety of treatment modalities. The goals of therapy are to increase physical safety; increase self-esteem; decrease fear, powerlessness, and alienation; and facilitate self-expression in nonviolent ways.

Nursing Intervention

The behavior of abusers and the abused may challenge nurses' value systems. Assumptions based on these value and belief systems are often reflected in nursing care.

Nurses may treat abusers with anger, avoidance,

or punishment. Nurses may fail to question the source of an abused victim's injuries or ignore cues that domestic violence has occurred. Nurses may derogate the victim or make the victim feel guilty or responsible for having been abused. Reasons involved in such staff responses toward violence include lack of knowledge about abuse and violence, rigid stereotypes and prejudices about victims of violence, feelings of frustration and powerlessness about changing situations of long-standing domestic abuse, and covert fear about one's own potential for similar victimization. Also, previous personal experience with abuse may lead to resistance in recognizing abuse or to nontherapeutic responses of anger or avoidance. Kohan, Pothier, and Norbeck, (1987, 263) attribute such staff reactions to countertransference and state that "without assistance to examine and process these feelings, staff may be vulnerable to recapitulating interactional dynamics of the troubled family within the clinical setting."

In view of these difficulties, what efforts should be made to help nurses work with abusers and the abused? Consciousness raising and education about the dynamics of abuse and the factors contributing to its development may be effective in correcting staff knowledge deficits and sensitizing staff to the responses and treatment needs of abusers and their victims. Because long-standing attitudes, stereotypes, and prejudices are difficult to change, staff feelings about working with human abuse as well as personal fears and anxiety concerning their own experiences with or potential for victimization should also be explored.

PRIMARY PREVENTION

Primary prevention of human abuse should focus on enhancing self-esteem, facilitating nonviolent expression of feelings, increasing problem-solving ability, and promoting a social environment that allows people to grow and function to their maximum potentials.

Parental counseling

Early exposure to parental brutality has been associated with the development of violent behavior. Child abuse may develop when a parent has inadequate support in the parenting role. An abusing parent is usually isolated from a supportive social network and is not receiving support from the marital relationship. Such a parent may have unrealistically high developmental expectations for children and may become frustrated and angry when, at a young age, children cannot be toilet trained, for example, or feed themselves. Because many abusing parents have themselves been abused as children, they may not have personally experienced parental nurturing. Since child-abusing parents often have low self-esteem, nonsupportive relationships, and unrealistically high developmental expectations of their children, treatment should focus on these areas. For example, prenatal and child health clinic nurses might initiate programs that explore ways to improve parental self-esteem, to develop a relationship of support and assistance between spouses, to educate parents about childhood growth and development, and to explore with parents alternative methods for coping with their children's disruptive behavior.

Moreover, nurses might facilitate bonding between parents and their children by encouraging hospital policies that treat childbirth as a family-centered experience. Broome and Daniels (1987) note that during the postpartum period, failure to talk about a newborn in positive terms, failure to name an infant, and infant feeding problems should be viewed as cues to potential parenting problems. To prevent child abuse from occurring, referral should be made to community health nurses for family follow-up.

Family counseling

Family disorganization and overburdening may precipitate abusive behavior in a family member. Disorganized households are characterized by insufficient income, food, fuel, and clothing. There may be instability regarding place of residence, child-rearing practices, and interpersonal relationships. Role conflicts may develop and increase the potential for domestic violence. Nurses need to be aware of factors operating in situational crises that may make families violence prone.

The Schroeder family lived on a limited income. Because Mr. Schroeder worked as a landscaping assistant, not only was his income minimal but the work was also seasonal. The job did not provide such fringe benefits as paid vacations or health insurance. Mrs. Schroeder augmented the family's income by baby sitting two children of working mothers. The Schroeders had five children of their own.

When Mr. Schroeder's 79-year-old invalid mother came to live with the family, household tensions increased. Mrs. Schroeder became the primary care taker of her mother-in-law. She resented that this responsibility was added to those of homemaker and childrearer. She was constantly tired and irritable. Mr. Schroeder appreciated the care his wife was taking of his mother, but he felt unable to participate in the care. It was his busy season, and it was ''embarrassing for a man to do such things for a woman—especially his mother.'' The mother-in-law felt the tension in the household and resented that she was viewed as a burden by the family. She reacted by being critical and derogating.

Over time, Mrs. Schroeder became increasingly abusive in her ministerings to her mother-in-law. She would make her mother-in-law wait for the bed pan, would roughly turn her in bed, would pinch her when she complained, and would tell her that she was ''an old nuisance who had outlived her usefulness.''

As the above vignette points out, there is a need to help disorganized and overburdened families on several levels. If families are not already involved with social service agencies, referrals should be made. If disorganized families are involved with social service agencies, nurses should act as liaisons to assist those families to communicate with the social service agencies so that feelings of frustration, anger, and alienation are not evoked. Nurses also need to help disorganized and overburdened families with problem solving. For example, in the previous vignette, referral to a visiting nurse agency or respite program might help alleviate the problem, or the family might need support in selecting a "good" nursing home that will care for the elderly family member compassionately and with dignity.

Affordable child care facilities and homemaker services for families with working mothers could lessen family disorganization by decreasing role conflict and role overburdening. Nurses need to petition their elected representatives for legislation and funding that will provide adequate child care facilities in the community and at the workplace.

Modification of sociocultural environment

Society is partly responsible for human abuse. Earlier in this chapter we discussed the correlation among community disorganization, social strain, social change, and violence. Funding cuts for such federal and state programs as unemployment benefits and public assistance affect the environment in which people function and grow to their greatest potentials. All nurses can become involved in informing their elected officials about the potential for such funding cuts to increase the incidence of human abuse. Community health nurses can counsel unemployed workers to help them find employment and to cope with stressors associated with unemployment such as decreased self-esteem, frustration, and anger. School nurse-teachers, in their interactions with children and their parents, can screen unemployed parents for risk factors associated with domestic violence and refer them for preventive intervention. Industrial health nurses can be vigilant about reducing occupational health and safety hazards contributing to employee stress and thereby decrease the risk of domestic

violence. Industrial health nurses might also screen for violence-prone individuals and offer counseling and referral as part of on-the-job health services.

Through public education programs, nurses can increase public awareness about the incidence of violence in society, the sociocultural factors that contribute to the development of violence, and ways of making one's self less vulnerable to violence.

A female faculty member who taught a course on human sexuality approached the director of university health services with concerns that had arisen from class discussions of dating behavior. A large portion of the class had shared their experiences with abuse in dating relationships. After class, two female students had told the faculty member that they had been victims of date rape. The director of health services, who was a nurse, met with university officials and student leaders. Together they developed a formal policy about reporting interpersonal violence and regulating alcohol consumption on campus (because of the correlation between alcohol consumption and violence). In addition, the director of health services and her staff conducted workshops to educate students about violence in intimate relationships. These workshops presented factual information about interpersonal violence as well as experiential sessions for developing nonviolent interpersonal skills and skills in problem-solving.

Nurses can also lobby elected officials for enactment of strong gun control laws and laws mandating the arrest of spouse and child abusers. Sherman and Berk (1984) found that recidivist violence decreases when domestic abusers are jailed. Further, nurses can petition media executives to decrease the incidence of media violence and to stop glamorizing violence in the media.

A multifaceted approach, encompassing the range of strategies discussed in this section, is necessary for an effective program of primary prevention of human abuse.

SECONDARY PREVENTION

Changing patterns of health care and the expanding role of the professional nurse in community

TABLE 21-15 Behavioral evidence of effective bonding

Behavior	Description
Exploration and locomotion	Moves away from mother and interacts visually, verbally, or manually with other people and objects but returns periodically to mother
Head turning	Turns head toward door after mother leaves the room
Following	Crawls or walks to the door after mother leaves the room
Crying or distress	Whimpers or cries when mother leaves the room (if child had been crying before mother left the room, crying intensifies with mother's departure)
Positive greeting	When mother reenters room, child smiles, laughs, bounces, jiggles, leans toward mother, lifts arms, or stands up

Adapted from Ortman (1980).

health and mental health are placing increasing demands upon nurses to participate in secondary prevention of human abuse. Such prevention involves meeting the following objectives:

1. early identification of cases of abuse in the community
2. prompt and effective treatment for abusers and their victims so that they may be restored to optimum mental health
3. participation with community groups in expanding needed resources

Case finding

Early identification, or case finding, is important in instances of human abuse. Many individuals who have been victims of violence do not seek professional help until or unless the symptoms severely inhibit their ability to function or the situation becomes life-threatening. Educating relevant segments of the population about human abuse and its consequences is essential if case finding is to be effective. This would include educating not only health care professionals but also peer counselors, police and security personnel, and school and university staff.

An essential feature of such an educational program involves teaching personnel about signs suggesting impending violence or indicating that abuse has occurred. For example, a community health nurse or a pediatric nurse may be the first to recognize distorted bonding between parent and child. Ortman (1980) suggests that nurses look for specific behaviors in children aged 9 to 23 months

that evidence effective bonding when assessing for functional and dysfunctional mother-child relationships. While nonabused children exhibit approximately all or most of these behaviors, the behaviors are significantly absent with abused children. Table 21-15 summarizes the behaviors that suggest that effective bonding between mother and child has been established.

Nurses who suspect abuse or neglect need to thoroughly assess the situation. In most cases of child abuse and neglect, the degree and type of impairment do not correspond with parental explanations of how it developed. For example,

---

Miriam and Jack were the parents of three children, aged 5 years, 3 years, and 13 months. The 13-month-old baby was a boy, Jackie Jr. Jackie physically resembled his father. Following the birth of Jackie, Miriam had become very depressed and was experiencing difficulty fulfilling her roles as wife and mother.

Jack's employment pattern had been sporadic, and the family was living on unemployment benefits. Jack was preoccupied with looking for a job. He offered little emotional support or child-rearing assistance to Miriam.

One day while Miriam was bathing Jackie, a public health nurse unexpectedly visited. Although Miriam hurriedly dried and dressed Jackie, the nurse noticed what appeared to be burns on Jackie's back. Miriam explained the burns by saying that she often smoked while bathing the baby: "Ashes from my cigarette must have fallen on his back." The nurse also noticed that Jackie showed little exploration behavior in his play, that he did not turn his head or try to physically follow his mother when she left the room, nor did he display any positive greeting when she returned. This constellation of behaviors signaled to the nurse possible child abuse.

Accurate and well-documented records of abuse are important. The name of anyone who has witnessed the abuse should be noted in such records. Suspected instances of violence or abuse should be reported to appropriate legal or social service agencies, and efforts should be made to protect individuals from further abuse. This may mean moving a child to a foster home, an elderly person to a nursing home, or a wife to a shelter.

The objectives of early identification, or case finding, in secondary prevention are (1) safeguarding victims of abuse and (2) referring clients (both abusers and the abused) for treatment. Nurses should keep the following crisis intervention principles in mind when counseling victims of violence:

1. The primary concern should be to secure safety for the client.
2. The focus should be upon the client as a person who is suffering and not upon the violent event.
3. Whether or not it is observable, underlying anxiety and anger may be present and should be assessed.
4. The client needs acceptance and approval and is vulnerable to any form of rejection. An alliance with the client needs to be formed before intervention can begin (see Sample Interaction: Establishing an Alliance).
5. The client needs to confront the crisis and verbalize feelings about the abuse. Feelings may include anger, anxiety, guilt, and self-blame (see Sample Interaction with a Victim of Abuse).
6. The client needs to gain an understanding of the crisis. This includes helping the client examine his or her role in the attack. For instance, if the client hitchhiked, then the client needs to look at the way he or she placed one's self in a position of vulnerability. Other times, the attack may have been at random, and the client needs to come to grips with the

Sample interaction: establishing an alliance

Client *(Five-year-old girl sitting quietly, hugging a doll to her and avoiding eye contact. She has been raped by her mother's boyfriend).*

Nurse *My name is Jean. I am a nurse. I want to help you.*

Client *What are you going to do to me?*

Nurse *I am not going to do anything to you. I want to know what happened to you.*

Client *(Continues to be nonverbal).*

Nurse *It's important for me to know what happened so I can help you. You just take your time and tell me in your own words. If you want, you can use these dolls to show me what happened (places two anatomically correct rag dolls—a male and a female—in front of the child).*

Client *(After looking at the dolls for several minutes, she begins to touch the dolls' genitalia).*

Nurse *Tell me what happened to you.*

The nurse was honest with the child about the reason she was talking with her, thereby creating a foundation of trustworthiness with the child. At the same time, the nurse conveyed to the child that this interaction had a specific focus. By using open-ended questions, letting the child proceed at her own pace, and using age-related props, the nurse tried to decrease the child's anxiety and establish an atmosphere where they could work together.

Sample interaction with a victim of abuse

Client *(Dressed in a long-sleeve turtleneck sweater and crying) I feel so empty.*

Nurse *Tell me what it's like to feel empty.*

Client *I failed my husband. If I had been a better wife—maybe if I had been more patient with him—he wouldn't have beat up on me. Now I can't go back there. I don't want to be beat up on any more. Now I have nothing and no one—no husband, no marriage, no home to go to.*

Nurse *Tell me what it was like to live with your husband.*

Client *When he wasn't drinking, he could be so sweet and considerate. He would call me "honey" and kiss me. He would even help me carry heavy bundles, and we would talk about what we would do when we had money and could afford nice things. But* *whenever things went wrong at work, he'd stop at the bar before coming home. Then he'd come home drunk and get mad at me because the dinner was cold or his shirt wasn't ironed or something. Then he'd hit me. But this last time was the worst. I thought he was going to kill me. I can't go back there any more. I don't know what to do.*

Nurse *You don't have to face this problem alone. You can stay here at the shelter where your husband won't be able to hurt you. I will be here to help you, and so will the other staff. You can think things out and begin to get your life in order.*

The nurse helped the client express her feelings and start to evaluate the positives and the negatives of her relationship with her husband. This helped the client begin to move beyond denial and the idealization of her relationship with her husband. At the same time, the nurse began assessing the degree to which the client had begun mourning the death of her marital relationship and offered the client support, understanding, and availability for assistance in the future.

---

reality of not always being able to control all aspects of one's life.

7. The client needs to utilize effective coping behaviors to deal with the crisis. Nursing assistance should be directed at helping the client learn new coping strategies when necessary and to consider the ramifications of various coping behaviors. For example, a raped woman's impulsive desire to move to a new neighborhood might have the negative consequence of geographically distancing her from her support network. Nurses should offer anticipatory guidance to a client so that the client has support prior to acting on an idea.

8. Nurses and other staff members may have emotional responses to the violent event or to the client's behavior. For example,

---

A 15-year-old girl was brought into the emergency room by her high school guidance counselor. The adolescent had told her guidance counselor that she had been raped. She explained that she had run away from home and had no place to sleep. The friend of a friend had offered to let her sleep on the couch in his apartment. During the evening, he had made sexual advances to her. The girl said: "I tried to keep him away from me. I told him 'no.' I even hit him over the

head with a lamp. But it didn't matter. He was stronger than me, and he raped me." Following the rape, the girl had stayed in the apartment "because I had nowhere else to go, and I was afraid to be out on the streets in that neighborhood at night." In the morning, she had left the apartment, gone to school, and reported the rape to her guidance counselor.

The nurses in the emergency room treated the girl in a cold, detached manner. The nurses felt that she had not tried hard enough to fight off the attack and that she had "asked for it" by staying overnight with a man she did not know. They also felt that if she had "really been raped" she would not have spent the rest of the night in his apartment.

The nurses needed to separate out their own problems and conflicts from those of the client. The psychiatric clinical nurse specialist helped the nurses acknowledge their feelings and work them through in supervision. In this way, their personal growth could be enhanced, and, in the future, they would be able to handle similar situations more therapeutically.

Knowledge of these principles will facilitate intervention with clients who are victims of human abuse. The goal of nursing therapy is to help clients work through the impact of a violent act on their lives so that they can achieve an optimal level of functioning in the future.

When the client is an abuser, ensuring the safety and dignity of all involved is an essential goal of nursing therapy. Nurses should keep the following principles in mind:

1. The safety of the client and the staff should be ensured (refer to "Crisis Intervention" discussed in an earlier section of this chapter). Whenever possible, attempts to let the client verbally ventilate feelings and to "talk the client down" should be made prior to initiating physical intervention (see Sample Interaction with an Abusive Client).

2. The client's personal space needs to be respected. Intrusion into the personal zone may be interpreted by the client as a threat. Violent or potentially violent individuals may have a personal zone up to four times larger than that of nonviolent persons.

3. The client needs to be involved in and kept in therapy. Initially, motivation to get into and stay in therapy may be external (e.g.,

Sample interaction with an abusive client

Client (speaking loudly and angrily). Why isn't anyone in this emergency room taking care of my hand? I think it's broken, and all you people are doing is paper work. I smashed one guy today. Do I have to start smashing this place up to get any attention? (He shakes his fist at an orderly). My hand hurts now, and I want attention now. If I start throwing a few punches, I bet that high and mighty doctor will get in here pronto.

Nurse Stop, Mr. Jones! (Several staff members hear the interaction and calmly gather in the nurses' station, prepared to "fan out" around the client if talking does not de-escalate the situation). We cannot let you hurt anyone. (The nurse is standing in front of the client but out of reach of his arms and legs).

Client I don't want to hurt anyone.

Nurse Let's talk about what you are feeling (calmly sits down with Mr. Jones).

The nurse's calm and authoritative statement that physical assault was unacceptable set limits on the client's acting-out behavior. The nurse was careful not to intrude on the client's personal space and to keep out of range of potentially flailing arms and legs. At the same time, the staff calmly moved into readiness for physical intervention should it be necessary. The nurse did not become defensive about keeping the client waiting, since that would have tended to escalate the situation. The nurse offered the client an opportunity to ventilate his feelings so that he would be less apt to act them out physically.

remanded by a court or a condition of staying with one's mate). As therapy proceeds, internal motivation (e.g., acknowledgement of how therapy is helping) may develop.

4. The client needs to learn assertive and nonviolent ways of expressing anger.
5. The client needs to learn assertive and nonviolent ways of communicating with others.
6. The client needs to engage in cognitive restructuring. Nursing assistance should focus on client expectations that generate anger and ways of developing more realistic expectations.
7. The client needs to look at the role of substance abuse in his or her life. For example,

some clients may use alcohol to try to control feelings of anger only to find that they have less control when drinking. Other clients may use overindulgence in alcohol as an excuse for their violent behavior.

8. The client needs to learn assertive and nonviolent ways of dealing with fear, hurt, and anger.
9. Nurses should communicate acceptance of the client's feelings but the unacceptability of the client's violent behavior.
10. Nurses may have emotional responses to client behavior. For example, nurses may experience anxiety or anger when working with child abusers or rapists. Nurses should not try to ignore their feelings. Instead, they should acknowledge those feelings and work them through in supervision or counseling.

Knowledge of these principles ultimately prevents or minimizes the incidence of assaultive client behavior in care-giving settings and facilitates intervention with clients who use violent behavior.

Nursing process

The nursing process provides the framework for nursing intervention. The focus of this aspect of secondary prevention is twofold: (1) intervention into behavior patterns (both patterns of abuse and the sequelae of abuse) and (2) facilitation of an optimal level of functioning.

ASSESSMENT

When they work with clients who are abusive or who have been the victims of abuse, nurses begin their assessments with the identification of the problem given by the client or the client's significant others. The following areas should be assessed:

1. Presenting symptoms—violent behavior that is creating problems for self or others or sequelae of having been the victim of violence
2. Emotional state—such feelings as anxiety, anger, alienation, guilt, or depression that are responses to a stimulus situation
3. Stimulus situations—stressful life situations

that constitute threats to the client's security. Such situations include threats to self-esteem and control, and physical, sexual, or emotional abuse

4. Maladaptive coping behaviors—coping patterns of substance abuse, denial, blame (blame placing or self-blame), and rationalization that are used in relating to others, in attempting to satisfy needs, and in protecting oneself from hurt

5. Origin of maladaptive coping behaviors—identification of childhood experiences (e.g., physical, sexual, or emotional abuse; socialization patterns that did not permit expression of anger; social network members that repressed anger or expressed anger through violent behavior) that contributed to the development of or learning of maladaptive coping behaviors

6. Holistic health status—biological, intellectual, psychological, sociocultural, and spiritual status of the client. These factors may facilitate wellness (e.g., extended family members

to assist with child care so that parental overburdening does not occur), or these factors may impede wellness (e.g., unemployment and role conflict that generates tension in the family system).

Tables 21-16 and 21-17 may assist nurses in making these assessments.

ANALYSIS OF DATA

The analysis of presenting symptoms, emotional states, stimulus situations, maladaptive coping behaviors and their origins, and the holistic health status of the client leads to the formulation of nursing diagnoses. Through the interpretation and appraisal of the data, the nurse is able to better understand the interrelationship among predisposing and precipitating factors and the client's coping behaviors. At this point, the nurse may be ready to formulate nursing diagnoses.

PLANNING AND IMPLEMENTATION

The following are nursing diagnoses that are frequently made for abusers or the victims of abuse.

TABLE 21-16   Assessment of an abusive individual

Dimension	Behavioral indicators
Behavioral	"Loner" who has few if any close ties with friends, relatives, or neighbors; substance abuser; unable to logically or convincingly explain how family member (child, spouse, or elder) was injured; responds to inquiries about victim's injuries with anger and defensiveness or disinterest; lashes out at family member(s) when frustrated or enraged; blames, ignores, discounts, or derogates family member(s); maintains a chaotic home life; unable to discuss own feelings and behavior
Attitudinal	Overly concerned with fear of "spoiling" or "giving into" a child; believes in harsh, physical punishment as way of disciplining a child and asserting authority over a child or adult family member(s) (this is usually the way the abuser was reared); has unrealistic expectations of a family member (adult or child); complains about the family member being difficult to control or manage
Feeling	Erupts in rage; seems to love the family member (child or adult) or to be emotionally cold and unconcerned about the family member; feels own childhood was devoid of love and emotional support; feels remorse and guilt about abusive behavior
Self-esteem	Low self-esteem; sense of failure; sense of being unloved, unappreciated, and unwanted; fears rejection
Environmental	Significant financial pressures on family; family is a social isolate in the community, workplace, and school; family history includes substance abuse or domestic violence; adult family members are overburdened; situational stressor of pregnancy, premature or disabled child, or elderly and infirm parent in the household

Sources consulted include Winters (1985), Whiteman, Fanshel, and Grundy (1987), and Broome and Daniels (1987).

TABLE 21-17   Assessment of a victim of abuse or neglect

Situation	Behavioral Indicators
Physical abuse	Unexplained fractured bones, soft tissue swelling, hematomas, burns, welts, bruises, spontaneous abortion or fetal injury, trauma to genitals and breasts, head and facial injuries (e.g., black eyes, broken or loosened teeth, concussions, bald spots), psychophysiologic complaints (e.g., dermatitis, ulcers, headaches, eating disturbances, insomnia, fatigue), human bite marks, visual or hearing defects, fear of specific persons (e.g., parents, spouse, care taker), fear of going home, overly aggressive or withdrawn, school problems (in children)
Emotional abuse	Speech problems, failure to thrive (in children), habitual biting or rocking behavior (in children), anorexia, sexual acting out, sleep disturbances, learning difficulties, emotional lability, depression, helplessness and hopelessness, guilt, shame, anxiety, hostility, suicidal ideation or attempts, social isolation, self-doubt, low self-esteem, aggressive or destructive behavior
Sexual abuse	Discomfort when walking or sitting, painful or itching genitals or anus, bruised or bleeding genitals or anus, torn or bloodied undergarments, enuresis, frequent bladder infections, venereal disease, pregnancy (in female who is sexually inactive), sleep disturbances, depression or social withdrawal, poor peer relationships, precocious knowledge of or interest in sex, sudden onset of behavior problems
Neglect	Malnourished, constantly hungry, constantly disheveled and unclean, inappropriately dressed for the weather, slow growth rate (in child), unattended medical problems, lack of adult supervision (for child or dependent adult), begging or stealing food, constantly tired, truancy from school, substance abuse

Sources consulted include Kadushin and Martin (1981) and Winters (1985).

Following each nursing diagnosis is a plan of care that reflects a realistic approach to secondary preventive intervention. The nurse may initially establish goals, but as therapy progresses, the client should enter into goal setting to ensure commitment to their accomplishment.

Nursing diagnoses pertaining to other problems associated with human abuse are addressed in the following chapters: blame placing, manipulation, and rationalization (Chapter 20); low self-esteem and grief (Chapter 22); human sexuality (Chapter 7); anxiety (Chapter 8).

EVALUATION

Whenever possible, evaluation should occur within the context of the family system. This reflects client and family participation in the achievement of goals. Any evaluation should encompass the following areas:

1. The degree that anxiety and conflict have decreased

2. The degree that threats to the self-system have decreased
3. The degree that behavioral symptomatology has decreased
4. The degree that feelings (e.g., anger, frustration) can be expressed (when this is consistent with a client's cultural orientation)
5. The degree that origins and sources of feelings can be identified (when this is consistent with a client's cultural orientation)
6. The degree that functioning has increased (evidenced by utilization of more effective coping behaviors, impulse control, and assertive communication)
7. Identification of goals that need to be modified or revised
8. Appropriateness of referral to support systems other than the nurse-client relationship
   a. People in the client's social network who are willing to be supportive

Text continued on p. 663.

NURSING CARE PLAN

Clients Who are Abusers or Victims of Abuse

Long-term Outcomes	Short-term Outcomes	Nursing Strategies
Nursing diagnosis: Potential for violence directed at others related to role conflict or role overburdening (NANDA 9.2.2; DSM-III-R V61.80, 312.34)		
Develop adequate support systems Renegotiate family roles	Identify stressors in the family situation Verbalize feelings associated with role conflict or overburdening Identify strengths in the family system Decrease role stress Stop incidents of abuse	Provide an atmosphere where client-family can talk without outside interruption Recognize the needs of client-family based on goal priorities and the life stages of family members Help client-family identify stressors Help client-family identify current ways of coping with stressors Help client-family evaluate effectiveness of current coping behaviors Support effective current coping behaviors Help client-family identify family roles and strengths Discuss coping strategies that are congruent with the life stages of family members and the cultural orientation of the family (e.g., respite program, redefining family roles, nursing care, or homemaking assistance) Support client-family in their decision making
Nursing diagnosis: Ineffective individual coping related to repression of anger (NANDA 5.1.1.1; DSM-III-R 312.34, 296.20-296.66)		
Develop nonviolent ways of expressing anger Decrease anxiety associated with expression of anger	Recognize feelings of anger Identify situations that arouse feelings of anger Learn to assertively communicate angry feelings	Provide a trust relationship so anger can safely be verbalized (when consistent with client's cultural orientation) Point out indirect expressions of anger (e.g., sarcasm, fist clenching) Assist client to identify and label anger Set limits and provide safeguards in the event that the client tries to act out angry feelings against self or others Discuss anger as a normal human response Provide physical outlets for angry feelings (e.g., jogging, tennis, hammering) Help client identify and describe objects of anger Explore current ways of coping with anger Support effective current coping behaviors Explore socially acceptable alternative ways of coping with anger, including acceptable limits and client's responsibility for own behavior Teach client assertive ways of communicating angry feelings Support client in trying out new ways of coping with anger Assist client to evaluate effectiveness of new coping behaviors

Continued.

NURSING CARE PLAN—cont'd

Clients Who Are Abusers or Victims of Abuse

Long-term Outcomes	Short-term Outcomes	Nursing Strategies

Nursing diagnoses:
- Rape-trauma syndrome related to recent rape experience (NANDA 9.2.3.1; DSM-III-R 309.89)
- Rape-trauma syndrome: compound reaction related to previous history of emotional, physical, or social problems exacerbated by recent rape experience (NANDA 9.2.3.1.1; DSM-III-R 309.89)
- Rape-trauma syndrome: silent reaction related to unresolved previous rape exacerbated by recent rape experience (NANDA 9.2.3.1.2; DSM-III-R 309.89)

Long-term Outcomes	Short-term Outcomes	Nursing Strategies
Work through issues and feelings associated with the rape Resume pre-rape activities Resume pre-rape level of functioning	Verbalize feelings about being raped (when consistent with client's cultural orientation) Evidence decreased anxiety Utilize support systems Comply with medical care	Establish trust relationship that permits client to verbalize feelings Accept client's feelings (e.g., do not negate feelings of fear, guilt or anger) Allow client to proceed at own pace (e.g., do not push to express anger, fear, or guilt or to discuss the rape incident) Be alert for indirect clues of anger, guilt, or fear Assist client to gradually verbalize feelings about the rape Assist client to describe the impact of the rape on her life Explore current coping behaviors Support effective coping behaviors Explore alternative coping behaviors (e.g., relaxation techniques, rape crisis group) Assist client to evaluate effectiveness of new coping behaviors Assist client to identify ways of telling significant others about the rape (role playing may be useful) Support client as she informs significant others about the rape Inform client about support groups for significant others Assist client with medical care (e.g., stay with client during physical examination, review home care instructions, explain signs or symptoms that require follow-up care, review information about any prescribed antianxiety or sleep-inducing medication)

Long-term Outcomes	Short-term Outcomes	Nursing Strategies

Nursing diagnoses:
- Potential for violence directed at others related to need for control (NANDA 9.2.2; DSM-III-R 300.90, 301.70, 309.30)
- Potential for violence directed at others related to poor impulse control (NANDA 9.2.2; DSM-III-R 305.00, 305.60, 305.90, 310.10, 312.34)
- Potential for violence directed at others related to a sustained experience of abuse (NANDA 9.2.2; DSM-III-R 301.70, 309.30)

Long-term Outcomes	Short-term Outcomes	Nursing Strategies
Learn to cope with stress in a nonviolent manner Follow social norms and limitations concerning nonviolence	Identify and describe feelings of anxiety, anger, and frustration (when consistent with client's cultural orientation) Identify and describe precipitating stressful life situations Develop effective and nonviolent coping behaviors Avoid secondary gains associated with violent behavior Develop impulse control	Establish a relationship where client can feel free to verbally express feelings Set limits prohibiting physical acting out Reassure client that staff will help the client control his or her behavior (client may fear losing control of own actions if he or she begins to express anger) Encourage client to identify current ways of coping with stress and anger Help client to evaluate effectiveness of current coping behaviors Support current effective coping behaviors Explore alternative coping behaviors Teach client assertive communication techniques Give immediate feedback or rewards for nonviolent coping responses Provide a nonstressful environment (e.g., decrease sensory stimuli by lowering radio and television volume and dimming lights; decrease social stimuli by modulating your voice, providing client with a place to be alone, and not intruding on client's personal space) Provide opportunities for client to expend the energy associated with angry or anxious feelings (e.g., through manual labor, exercise, working clay) Explore with client any secondary gains associated with his or her violent behavior Establish a therapeutic environment free of secondary gains (e.g., expectations of client participation in activities of daily living and treatment modalities should be clearly stated; avoid giving client special privileges, dispensations, or attention because of his or her violent behavior) Be alert to behavioral cues of impending violence Inform client of consequences of violent behavior before it occurs Carry out the consequences in a nonpunitive, matter-of-fact manner immediately after a violent episode occurs Carry out any necessary physical or chemical restraining in a quick and nonpunitive manner After a violent episode is over, encourage the client to express his or her feelings about the occurrence

Continued.

NURSING CARE PLAN—cont'd

Clients Who are Abusers or Victims of Abuse

Long-term Outcomes	Short-term Outcomes	Nursing Strategies

Nursing diagnosis: Altered health maintenance (abuse or neglect) related to ineffective family coping (NANDA 6.4.2; DSM-III-R V61.20, 62.81, 61.80)

Long-term Outcomes	Short-term Outcomes	Nursing Strategies
Increase level of parenting or care-taking skills Increase level of family individuation Reach optimal developmental potential Continue as an intact family system (if feasible and in the best interest of the abused family member(s)) Follow social norms for treating people with care and dignity	Verbalize feelings in an open, direct manner (when consistent with client's cultural orientation) Identify situations that precipitate abusive or neglectful behaviors Develop more effective coping skills	Report abuse (sexual, physical, or emotional) or neglect to authorities Treat symptoms of abuse or neglect promptly Provide a safe environment for the abused/neglected child or adult Explore alternatives for reducing environmental and social stressors (e.g., respite services; day care, periodic use of babysitters or other helpers; financial aid) Mobilize social support systems Educate parents or other care takers about age-appropriate development and behaviors Educate parents or other care takers about the influence of chronic illness or disability on age-appropriate development and behaviors Help parents or care takers identify current coping behaviors Help parents or care takers evaluate effectiveness of current coping behaviors Support current effective coping behaviors Explore alternative coping behaviors Support parental or care taker efforts to use more effective coping behaviors Develop nursing strategies to increase victim's self-esteem (see Chapter 22) Refer parents or care takers to abuse-intervention groups or hot lines

Nursing diagnoses:
• Posttrauma response related to rape (NANDA 9.2.3; DSM-III-R 309.89)
• Posttrauma response related to assault (NANDA 9.2.3; DSM-III-R 309.89)
• Posttrauma response related to a sustained experience of abuse (NANDA 9.2.3; DSM-III-R 309.89)

Long-term Outcomes	Short-term Outcomes	Nursing Strategies
Work through issues and feelings associated with rape, assault, or abuse Resume pretrauma activities	Verbalize feelings about being raped, abused, or assaulted (when consistent with client's cultural orientation) Evidence decreased anxiety or guilt Utilize support systems Comply with medical care	Establish trust relationship that permits client to verbalize feelings Accept client's feelings (e.g., do not negate feelings of fear, guilt, or anger) Allow client to proceed at own pace (e.g., do not push to express anger, fear, or guilt or to discuss the incident) Be alert for indirect clues of anger, guilt, or fear Be alert for self-destructiveness (e.g., substance abuse, suicidal ideation) or other-directed destructiveness (e.g., homicidal ideation)

Long-term Outcomes	Short-term Outcomes	Nursing Strategies

Nursing diagnoses—cont'd
- Posttrauma response related to rape (NANDA 9.2.3; DSM-III-R 309.89)
- Posttrauma response related to assault (NANDA 9.2.3; DSM-III-R 309.89)
- Posttrauma response related to a sustained experience of abuse (NANDA 9.2.3; DSM-III-R 309.89)

Long-term Outcomes	Short-term Outcomes	Nursing Strategies
Resume pre-trauma level of function-ing (e.g., ability to re-member, to concentrate, to sleep)		Assist client to gradually verbalize feelings about the rape, abuse or assault Assist client to describe the impact of the rape, abuse, or assault on his or her life Assist client to think through the consequences of actions based on feelings that are out of control (e.g., homicidal ideation engendered by rage) Explore current coping behaviors Support effective coping behaviors Explore alternative coping behaviors (e.g., relaxation techniques, victim crisis groups) Assist client to evaluate effectiveness of new coping behaviors Assist client to call upon supportive significant others Assist client with medical care (e.g., review information about any prescribed antianxiety or sleep-inducing medication)

b. Community agencies* that help clients learn to live with the reality of having been abusive or having been abused (e.g., hotlines, self-help groups, shelters)

c. Community services that help clients reduce social stressors in their lives (e.g., financial aid agencies, employment agencies, vocational training centers, respite services)

TERTIARY PREVENTION

The goal of tertiary prevention is to attain or maintain system stability. Tertiary prevention measures include progressive goal setting, reeducation, and optimum utilization of health services. Although most people agree that tertiary prevention is a necessary part of treatment for both abusers and victims of abuse, after-care is not a major priority in the United States. Victims of violence often are for-

gotten by society. In addition, many people fear that they or their families will be victimized by the abusers that after-care centers are designed to treat. Although people may give lip service to the ideal of rehabilitation, few people want after-care facilities for rapists or other abusers located in their neighborhoods. For these reasons, after-care is limited, but some tertiary prevention programs that are available will now be discussed.

Educational training

Depending on the age, interests, and abilities of clients (both abusers and victims of abuse), continued education, including college and vocational training (retraining in old skills or teaching of new skills), may be indicated. Education increases self-esteem and prepares clients to be as financially self-reliant as possible.

Self-help groups

Self-help groups support individuals in their readjustment to community living and intervene in crisis situations. Such groups are composed of peo-

---

*A client's cultural orientation (e.g., Asian) may inhibit disclosure of problems outside the family. In such instances, it may be necessary to work with the family elder(s) and gain elder cooperation and support to contact community agencies.

ple who have had similar experiences and yet have learned to function in society. For example, the Fortune Society helps former criminals learn to operate within society's standards, assists them to support themselves legitimately, and helps them cope with the social stigma attached to imprisonment. Parents Anonymous provides support for parents who have abused their children. VOCAL (Victims of Child Abuse Laws) assists people who have been falsely accused of child abuse fight a legal-social system that they believe is predisposed against them. Battered spouse and rape-victim support groups help women get on with their lives and once again function in society.

Professional rehabilitation services

The purpose of professional rehabilitation services is similar to that of self-help groups. What differentiates these services from self-help groups is that they are staffed by professionals, many of whom have not been personally involved with human abuse. Abused women's shelters provide emergency aid in the form of housing and food. In addition, counseling and assistance in finding employment and housing may be offered. Crime victim compensation services, often a division of state accident boards or district attorney offices, give financial assistance to victims of violent crimes so that they may obtain such necessities as medical care, occupational rehabilitation, and counseling.

The role of the nurse in tertiary prevention is varied. Nurses may provide ongoing individual, group, and family therapy for clients who present chronic behavioral and/or physical dysfunction as a consequence of abusing or having been abused. In addition, nurses may identify families that exhibit chronically disturbed patterns of functioning and help them get treatment. Finally, nurses may act as resource persons who provide referrals for various treatment modalities and act as links between clients and resource facilities. Thus, nurses play a valuable role in preventing or reducing the residual effects of the syndrome of abuse (for both the abuser and the victim of abuse) as well as in maintaining optimal levels of client functioning.

CHAPTER SUMMARY

Human abuse may be in the form of physical abuse and neglect or emotional abuse. Abusive or violent behavior may be perpetrated by strangers, friends and acquaintances, and family members. It is likely that a combination of biological, psychological, and sociocultural processes interrelate in the development of and response to abusive behavior. To understand the dynamics of human abuse, abuse must be viewed as a complex phenomenon involving both the abuser and the victim.

Primary prevention of human abuse focuses on enhancing self-esteem, facilitating nonviolent expression of feelings, increasing problem-solving ability, and promoting a social environment that allows people to grow and function to their maximum potentials. Nurses engage in parental counseling, family counseling, and modification of the sociocultural environment. Secondary prevention involves nurses in early identification of cases of abuse in the community, obtaining prompt and effective treatment for abusers and their victims, and participating with community groups in expanding needed resources. Tertiary prevention focuses on attaining or maintaining system stability. Nurses may provide ongoing individual, group, and family therapy for clients who present chronic behavioral and/or physical dysfunction as a consequence of abusing or having been abused. In addition, nurses may act as resource persons who provide referrals for various treatment modalities and act as links between clients and resource facilities.

When working with abusers and victims of abuse, nurses may respond in various ways. Nurses may treat abusers with anger, avoidance, or punishment. Nurses may fail to question the source of an abused victim's injuries or ignore cues that domestic violence has occurred. Nurses may derogate the victim or make the victim feel guilty or responsible for having been abused. By clarifying their own attitudes and values, nurses can work more therapeutically with both abusers and victims of abuse.

SELF-DIRECTED LEARNING

Sensitivity-Awareness Exercises

The purposes of these exercises are to:
- Develop sensitivity to your own values and attitudes about human abuse
- Develop awareness about your own responses to abusers and victims of abuse
- Develop awareness of the way that human abuse is perceived by society and depicted by the media

1. Select a character who is an abuser or a victim of abuse from a novel, a movie, or a television program. How many different types of theories (e.g., interpersonal, biochemical, social strain) can you use to explain the character's behavior?
2. Read accounts in your local newspaper about the incidents of violence and abuse.
   a. What are the messages that the newspaper accounts convey about human abuse? about abusers? about victims of abuse?
   b. Do the messages conveyed differ according to the nature of the abuse? age or sex of the abuser? age or sex of the victim? ethnicity or social class of the abuser? ethnicity or social class of the victim?
3. Values clarification: This exercise sets two attitudes at opposite ends of a continuum. Place an X at the point which most closely corresponds with your attitude. Then consider why you have chosen that particular response.
   a. What do you feel about family members hitting, shoving or punching one another?
   It is acceptable under   It is wrong under
   certain conditions   any conditions
   b. How do you feel about family members derogating and/or threatening one another?
   It is acceptable under   It is wrong under
   certain conditions   any conditions
   c. What are your feelings about having a one-to-one therapeutic relationship with an abuser?
   I am totally against it   I think it can be a
                              meaningful learning
                              experience
   d. What are your feelings about having a one-to-

one therapeutic relationship with a victim of abuse?
   I am totally against it   I think it can be a
                              meaningful learning
                              experience
5. Briefly describe what you would say and how you would feel in the following situations. These exercises can be used in small group settings after some level of trust has developed among group members.
   a. A stranger uses threats and physical force to get you to engage in sex.
   I would feel . . .   I would say . . .
   b. Your date uses threats and physical force to get you to engage in sex.
   I would feel . . .   I would say . . .
   c. Your spouse/significant other uses threats and physical force to get you to engage in sex.
   I would feel . . .   I would say . . .
   d. Your parent uses threats and physical force to get you to engage in sex.
   I would feel . . .   I would say . . .

Questions to Consider

1. The Jaspers had been married for 29 years, and, during that time, Mr. Jaspers had physically abused his wife. After receiving counseling at the women's shelter where she had sought refuge, Mrs. Jaspers decided to divorce her husband. Recently, Mr. Jaspers has been very apologetic for his behavior and has been pressuring his wife to return to him. Mrs. Jaspers has begun to say "If John gets psychological help, I might consider a reconciliation" and "If John stops drinking, I might try to save our marriage." The Jaspers' behaviors are indicative of which stage of grieving a relationship?
   a. Denial
   b. Anger
   c. Bargaining
   d. Grief
   e. Acceptance
2. A nurse-leader of an assault intervention team is conducting in-service education for the team. It is

Continued.

SELF-DIRECTED LEARNING—cont'd

Questions to Consider—cont'd

essential for the nurse-leader to stress that when intervening with a frenzied client the team should
  a. Approach the client diagonally from the front, speak calmly, and give the client choices about how the situation will be managed
  b. Approach the client from the front, "fan" out in a semicircle around the client, take all decision making from the client, and provide medication or physical restraint
  c. Approach the client from the rear, be authoritative in all communications, take all decision making from the client, and calmly state that the client is responsible for his or her behavior
  d. Approach the client diagonally from the front, focus on verbalizations, speak calmly, and clearly state that the client is responsible for his or her behavior
3. Which of the following are nursing strategies aimed at secondary prevention of child abuse?
  a. Assessing the nature and degree of emotional and physical signs and symptoms of abuse
  b. Educating parents about child growth and development
  c. Facilitating parent-child bonding
  d. Assessing factors in situational crises that may make families violence prone
4. Nurses working with potentially violent clients

should be alert for which of the following verbal cues of impending violence?
  a. Self-deprecating statements
  b. Assertive statements
  c. Dependent statements
  d. Sarcastic statements

Match each of the following terms with the statement that is associated with it:

5. Triggering phase of assault
6. Uproar behavior
7. Emotional abuse
8. Rape trauma syndrome

  a. Verbal threats, other-imposed social isolation, derogation
  b. A stress-producing event
  c. Two-phase response of disorganization and reorganization
  d. Hyperactive, noisy, demanding behavior

Answer key

1. c
2. b
3. a
4. d
5. b
6. d
7. a
8. c

REFERENCES

Appleton W: The battered wife syndrome, Ann Emergency Med 9:84-91, 1980.
Beck CM and Ferguson D: Aged abuse, J Gerontolog Nurs 7(6):333-336, 1981.
Bennett G: Group therapy for men who batter women: some promising developments, Holistic Nurs Pract 1(2):33-42, 1987.
Berne E: Transactional analysis in psychotherapy, New York, 1961, Grove Press, Inc.
Birenbaum A and Sagarin E: Norms and human behavior, New York, 1976, Praeger Publishers.
Bogard M: Family systems approaches to wife battering: a feminist critique, Am J Orthopsychiatr 54(4):558-568, 1984.

Boxer S: The parable of the cheek-turners and the cheek-smiters, Discover 8(8):80-83, 1987.
Briere J: The effects of childhood sexual abuse on later psychological functioning: defining a "postsexual abuse syndrome," Paper presented at the Third National Conference on the Sexual Victimization of Children. Washington, DC, April 27, 1984.
Broome ME and Daniels D: Child abuse: a multidimensional phenomenon, Holistic Nurs Prac 1(2):13-24, 1987.
Brown L: Theoretical frameworks for understanding violent behavior, In Babich K, editor: Assessing patient violence in the health care setting, Boulder, 1981a, WICHE.
Brown L: A model for understanding the muddle between the legal and health care systems, In Babich K, editor: Assessing

patient violence in the health care setting, Boulder, 1981b, WICHE.

Burckhardt C: Research on violence: principles and findings. In Babich K, editor: Assessing patient violence in the health care setting, Boulder, 1981, WICHE.

Burgess A and Holmstrom L: Rape, victims of crisis, Bowie, Md, 1974, Robert J. Brady.

Burgess A and Holstrom L: Rape crisis and recovery, Bowie, Md, 1979, Robert J. Brady.

Carlson BE: Dating violence: a research review and comparison with spouse abuse, Social Casework 68(1):16-23, 1987.

Carmen E(H), Rieker PP, and Mills T: Victims of violence and psychiatric illness, Am J Psychiatr 141:378-383, 1984.

Chesler P: Women and madness, New York, 1972, Avon Books.

Clunn P: Nurses' assessments of violence potential. In Babich K, editor: Assessing patient violence in the health care setting, Boulder, 1981, WICHE.

Cole CH and Barney EE: Safeguards and the therapeutic window: a group treatment strategy for adult incest survivors, Am J Orthopsychiatr 57(4):601-609, 1987.

Collier JA: When you suspect your patient is a battered wife, RN (May):22-25, 1987.

Delaney P and Woods J: Patient-neighbor: a dilemma of the community mental health nurse, J Psychiatr Nurs Mental Health Serv 13(4):18-21, 1975.

Deschner JP: The hitting habit: anger control for battering couples, New York, 1984, The Free Press.

Diagnostic and Statistical Manual of Mental Disorders (Third Edition-Revised), Washington, DC, 1987, The American Psychiatric Association.

Egeland B and Jacobvitz D: Intergenerational continuity of parental abuse: causes and consequences, Paper presented at Conference on Biosocial Perspectives in Abuse and Neglect, York, Maine, 1984.

Friedrich WN and Reams RA: Course of psychological symptoms in sexually abused young children, Psychotherapy 24(2):160-170, 1987.

Gilbert C: Sexual abuse and group therapy, J Psychosoc Nurs Mental Health Serv 26(5):19-23, 1988.

Gladston R: Disorders of early parenthood, In Noshpitz J, editor: Basic handbook of child psychiatry, vol 2, New York, 1979, Basic Books.

Goldberg WG and Tomlanovich MC: Domestic violence victims in the emergency department, JAMA 251:3259-3264, 1984.

Greenleaf N: The politics of self-esteem, Nurs Digest 6(3):1, 1978.

Guyer M: Child abuse and neglect statutes: legal and clinical implications, Am J Orthopsychiatr 52(1):73-81, 1982.

Halleck SL: Psychodynamic aspects of violence, In Sadoff R, editor: Violence and responsibility: the individual, the family and society, New York, 1978, SP Medical and Scientific Books.

Halliday MAK: Anti-language, Am Anthropol 78:570-584, 1976.

Hartman M, Finn SE, and Leon GR: Sexual-abuse experiences in a clinical population: comparison of familial and nonfamilial abuse, Psychotherapy 24(2):154-159, 1987.

Hickey I and Douglass RL: The mistreatment of the elderly in the domestic setting: an exploratory study, Am J Public Health 71:500-507, 1981.

Hilberman E: Overview: the 'wife-beater's wife' reconsidered, Am J Psychiatr 137(11):1336, 1980.

Hunter R and Kilstrom N: Breaking the cycle in abusive families, Am J Psychiatr 136:1320-1322, 1979.

Jacobs J: The economy of love in religious commitment: the deconversion of women from non traditional religious movements, J Sci Study Religion 23:155-171, 1984.

Johnson DG: Abuse and neglect—not for children only! J Gerontol Nurs 5:11-13, 1979.

Kadushin A and Martin JA: Child abuse: an interactional event, New York, 1981, Columbia University Press.

Kohan MF, Pothier P, and Norbeck JS: Hospitalized children with history of sexual abuse: incidence and care issues, Am J Orthopsychiatr 57(2):258-264, 1987.

Korbin J: Changing family roles and structures: impact on child abuse and neglect: a cross-cultural perspective, In Lauderdal M et al, editors: Child abuse and neglect issues on innovation and implementation, vol 1, Washington, DC, 1978, U.S. Government Printing Office (U.S. Department of Health, Education, and Welfare Publication No. OHDS-78-30147).

Lane KE and Gwartney-Gibbs PA: Violence in the context of dating and sex, J Family Issues 6:45-59, 1985.

Lengermann PM and Wallace RA: Gender in America: social control and social change, Englewood Cliffs, NJ, 1985, Prentice-Hall, Inc.

Lichtenstein VR: The battered woman: guideline for effective nursing intervention, Issues Mental Health Nurs 3:237-250, 1981.

Long KA: Cultural considerations in the assessment and treatment of intrafamilial abuse, Am J Orthopsychiatr 56(1):131-136, 1986.

Makepeace JM: Gender differences in courtship violence victimization, Family Patterns 35:382-388, 1986.

Mark VH and Ervin FR: Violence and the brain, New York, 1970, Harper & Row.

Marmor J: Psychological roots of violence. In Sadoff R, editor: Violence and responsibility: the individual, the family and society, New York, 1978, SP Medical and Scientific Books.

McLeod M: Women against men: an examination of domestic violence based on an analysis of official data and national victimization data, Justice Q 1:171-193, 1984.

Miller A: Thou shalt not be aware: society's betrayal of the child, New York, 1984, Farrar, Straus & Giroux.

Millor GK: A theoretical framework for nursing research in child abuse and neglect, Nurs Res 30(2):78-83, 1981.

Mills T, Rieker PP, and Carmen E(H): Hospitalization experiences of victims of abuse, Victimology 9(3-4):436-449, 1984.

Monahan J: Predicting violent behavior, Beverly Hills, Cal, 1981, Sage Library of Social Research.

Montagu A: Is man innately aggressive? In Fields W and Sweet W, editors: Neural bases of violence and aggression, St. Louis, 1975, Warren H. Green.

Morton PG: Staff roles and responsibilities in incidents of patient violence, Arch Psychiatr Nurs 1(4):280-284, 1987.

Nash J: Death as a way of life: the increasing resort to homicide in a Maya Indian community, Am Anthropol 69:455-470, 1967.

Ortman E: Nursing intervention in child abuse, In Lancaster J, editor: Community mental health nursing: an ecological perspective, St. Louis, 1980, CV Mosby.

Pacesetter, DSM-III Criteria 14(1):1, 1987.

Parker H and Parker S: Father-daughter sexual abuse: an emerging perspective, Am J Orthopsychiatr 56(4):531-549, 1986.

Pincus JH: Neurologic abnormalities in violent delinquents, Neurology 29(4):586, 1979.

Prince JB: A systems approach to spouse abuse, In Lancaster J, editor: Community mental health nursing: an ecological perspective, St. Louis, 1980, CV Mosby Co.

Report of the National Council on Alcoholism: Long Island Council on Alcoholism Fact Sheet, Garden City, NY, 1976.

Rieker PP and Carmen E(H): The victim-to-patient process: the disconfirmation and transformation of abuse, Am J Orthopsychiatr 56(3):360-370, 1986.

Roth M: Human violence as viewed from the psychiatric clinic, Am J Psychiatr 128:1043-1056, 1972.

Rubin B: Prediction of dangerousness in mentally ill criminals, Arch Gen Psychiatr 17:397-407, 1972.

Seligmen ME: Helplessness: on depression, development and death, San Francisco, 1975, WH Freeman & Co.

Shengold LL: Child abuse and deprivation: soul murder, J Am Psychoanal Assoc 27:533-559, 1979.

Sherman L and Berk R: The specific deterrent effects of arrest for domestic assault, Am Sociolog Rev 49:261-272, 1984.

Shupe A, Stacey WA, and Hazlewood LR: Violent couples: the dynamics of domestic violence, Lexington, Mass, 1987, Lexington Books.

Smith P: Empirically based models for viewing the dynamics of violence, In Babich K, editor: Assessing patient violence in the health care setting, Boulder, 1981, WICHE.

Solin CA: Displacement of affect in families following incest disclosure, Am J Orthopsychiatr 56(4):570-576, 1986.

Soloman G, Hiesberger J, and Wimer T: Confidentiality issues in rural community mental health, J Rural Commun Psychol 2:17-31, 1981.

Steinmetz SK: The battered husband syndrome, Victimology 2:499-506, 1978.

Steinmetz SK: Women and violence: victims and perpetrators, Am J Psychother 34:339-347, 1980.

Strauss MA and Gelles RJ: Societal change and change in family violence from 1975-1985 as revealed by two national surveys, J Marriage Family 48:465-479, 1986.

Strauss MA and Gelles RJ: Behind closed doors: violence in the American family, New York, 1980, Doubleday.

Turner SF and Shapiro CH: Battered women: mourning the death of a relationship, Social Work: 31(5):372-376, 1986.

Victims Information Bureau of Suffolk, Inc: Pamphlet prepared by the Victims Information Bureau of Suffolk, Inc., Smithtown, NY, 1986.

Weaver SM, Broome AK, and Kat BJ: Some patterns of disturbed behavior in a closed ward environment, J Adv Nurs 3:251-263, 1978.

Whiteman M, Fanshel D, and Grundy JF: Cognitive-behavioral interventions aimed at anger of parents at risk of child abuse, Social Work 32(6):469-474, 1987.

Winters R: Child abuse digest, Tampa, Fla, 1985, Winters Communications, Inc.

Wolf DA and Mosk MD: Behavioral comparisons of children from abusive and distressed families, J Consulting Clin Psychol 51:702-708, 1983.

Wommack A: The client with assaultive behavior, In Groton JG and Partridge R, editors: Practice and management of psychiatric emergency care, St. Louis, 1982, CV Mosby.

ANNOTATED SUGGESTED READINGS

Lambert CE Jr. and Lambert VA, editors: Human abuse (entire volume). Holistic Nurs Pract 1(2):V1-88, 1987.
This journal issue addresses a broad spectrum of topics of abuse; attitudinal abuse toward pregnant women, child abuse, spouse abuse, elder abuse, least restrictive psychiatric treatment alternatives, care giver perceptions of abuse in health care settings, and the medicolegal role in detection and prevention of abuse. The focus of the journal issue is on developing nursing insight into a range of situations that are acts of human abuse.

Morton PG: Staff roles and responsibilities in incidents of patient violence, Arch Psychiatr Nurs 1(4):280-284, 1987.
The article explores client violence in hospital settings and nursing interventions that are needed for prevention and safe, humane management of assaultive crises. The roles and responsibilities of three groups of staff (team leader, team members, supportive staff) in situations of client violence are discussed.

Shype A, Stacey WA, and Hazlewood LR: Violent couples: the dynamics of domestic violence, Lexington, Mass, 1987, Lexington Books.
This book discusses epidemiological data, explanatory perspectives, and the dynamics of domestic violence. Attention is also focused on breaking the cycle of family violence. This book provides an excellent introduction to the topic of domestic violence.

Turner SF and Shapiro CH: Battered women: mourning the death of a relationship, Social Work 31(5):372-376, 1986.
The authors describe the process of grieving a relationship and discuss the implications of each stage of the mourning process for therapeutic intervention. Although the article is written for social workers, the approaches described can be effectively utilized by nurses.

FURTHER READINGS

Burgess EJ: Sexually abused children and their drawings, Arch Psychiatr Nurs 2(2):65-73, 1988.

Davis DL and Boster L: Multifaceted therapeutic interventions with the violent psychiatric inpatient, Hosp Commun Psychiatr 39(8):867-869, 1988.

Dawson J et al: **Response to patient assault: a peer support program for nurses, J Psychosoc Nurs 26(2):8-15, 1988.**

Henson TK: **Medicolegal role in detection** and prevention of human abuse, **Holistic Nurs Pract** 1(2):75-84, 1987.

Phillips **LR and Rempusheski** VF: A decision-making model for diagnosing **and intervening** in elder abuse and neglect, Nurs Res 34(3):134-139, 1984.

Sammons LN: Battered and pregnant, Matern Child Nurs 6:246-250, 1981.

Van Scoyk S, Gray J, and Jones DPH: A theoretical framework for evaluation and treatment of child sexual assault by a nonfamily member, Fam Process 27(1):105-113, 1988.

Wirtz PW and Harrell AV: Victim and crime characteristics, coping responses, and short-and-long-term recovery from victimization, J Consult Clin Psychol 55(6):866-871, 1987.

Patterns of depression

CHAPTER FOCUS

Depression is currently one of the most prevalent mental health problems in the United States. Discussion of depression as a disorder dates back to 1500 BC. The term is well known to many yet has several different connotations: mood disorder, change in affect, clinical syndrome, or cluster of behavioral symptoms.

Depression accompanies a significant proportion of physical illnesses, particularly those which are severe. Suicide is positively correlated with depression. Few individuals have not been touched by depression, at least in its mildest form, as a reaction to loss or change.

An understanding of depression begins with an understanding of the concepts of grief and loss. Depression may occur as a response to any form of loss—loss of function, body part, status or responsibility, or significant other. Depression, of course, is also experienced by persons who learn that they are going to lose their own lives. Phases of mourning will be discussed, and implications of healthy and maladaptive responses to loss will be identified.

The presentation of major theoretical constructs provides a framework for a thorough understanding of the complex underlying dynamics of depression. Predominant themes, coping mechanisms, and nursing interventions are discussed in relation to the major affective disorders and suicide.

UNDERLYING DYNAMICS

The dynamics of mood disorders reflect a complex interaction of factors. To provide effective nursing care, an understanding of those factors is critical. In the following discussion factors such as low self-esteem, powerlessness, hopelessness, helplessness, anger, dependency, ambivalence, and guilt will be presented.

Low self-esteem

Depressed individuals experience a negative sense of self-worth, which results from a poorly developed ego and punitive superego as well as a lack of success in significant relationships. Depressed clients feel they have few, if any, capabilities to achieve goals in life. There has been little praise or gratification from others to reinforce a positive sense of being. Feelings of worthlessness prevent depressed individuals from engaging in social relationships, e.g., "Why should I ask someone to go the movies; I'm sure they'll say no." This belief reinforces social isolation and feelings of low self-esteem. Depressed clients view the world from a negative perspective—"the glass is half empty" versus "the glass is half full." This perspective only serves to distance the individual from others and, again, reinforces the self-fulfilling prophecy of "I am really worth nothing in this world."

Negative feelings associated with self-worth may also result in feelings of guilt. In early life experiences where parental expectations were not met, feelings of guilt related to lack of achievement were generated. The depressed client then develops a mode of thinking and feeling that reflects self-condemnation and self-blaming. There is a repetition over and over of actual or imagined shortcomings, which invites others to consider the depressed individual as deserving punishment. This action in turn reinforces the individual's belief that he or she is an unworthy person.

Powerlessness, helplessness, and hopelessness

Miller (1983) defined powerlessness as the perception the individual holds regarding the effect his or her actions will have on events in his or her environment. It is a lack of control over current situations or potential happenings. A sense of powerlessness may be said to be directly correlated with a lack of self-esteem. Individuals who feel unworthy often express this in terms of actions within their environment. For example, a depressed client might make statements such as "I don't know why I'm going to college—I won't get a job anyway" or "I didn't get the promotion because I'm not as good as the rest of the people who work here." Other behaviors indicative of powerlessness include the inability to seek information regarding care, the inability to set future goals, fear of alienation from others, and apathy. The perception of powerlessness is pervasive and is not based on definable facts but rather on an internal set that is based on low self-esteem that is repeated and reinforced over and over in the client's life experiences.

Helplessness may be considered a correlate of powerlessness. Seligman (1975) described helplessness as the belief that one has no ability to effect change; that one's actions do not matter; and that no one will be of assistance in times of need. He proposed that in situations where individuals learned they had no control, they eventually developed a sense of helplessness. Helplessness then generates hopelessness.

Last, hopelessness as defined by Miller (1983) results from a prolonged sense of powerlessness and helplessness as well as from a lack of positive sense of self-esteem. Individuals experiencing a sense of hopelessness believe that neither they nor anyone else has control over what happens. Engel (1962) describes hopelessness as a "giving in–giving up" complex that results in feelings of having nothing left in life—"being at the end of one's rope." Depressed individuals experiencing hopelessness are unable to participate in decision-making activities and self-care measures or to set goals for the future. They feel an overwhelming sense of isolation; they tend to withdraw further from others, including care givers; there is a loss of faith in self and others. Engel notes that the ultimate result of prolonged hopelessness is a psychobiologic condition that contributes to the occurrence of disease. Wetzel (1976) indicates that hopelessness is a critical correlate in suicidal intent.

The concepts of powerlessness, helplessness,

and hopelessness may be considered critical to the development of depressive responses. Depressed individuals find themselves with no sense of control over their lives, believe that no one else can help them, and ultimately feel that there is no hope for achieving control in the future.

Anger, dependency, and ambivalence

Some theorists believe that depressed clients turn their anger inward as a self-derogatory measure. Clients are often unable to express anger to the appropriate source; when they do, they may feel a sense of guilt for doing so. The internalization of anger in early development may serve as a model for the denial of anger as an acceptable emotion in later life. Depressed individuals may unconsciously utilize the denial of anger as a means to continue the depression. Freudian theory supports the relationship between repressed anger toward the lost love object (parent) and the feelings of ambivalence that the client experiences in regard to the loss of the significant relationship. In later relationships, depressed individuals experience a similar sense of ambivalence. This ambivalence creates a feeling of bewilderment for those involved with the depressed client—others do not know how to respond to the depressed client, for there seems to be no direct connection between client feelings and the response of others. Depressed clients may give the impression that they desire an intimate relationship; however, when others indicate a willingness to develop a relationship, the depressed client may withdraw in an effort to protect himself or herself from the prospect of being hurt.

Individuals with a lowered sense of self-esteem are often dependent emotionally on others for love, advice, security, and support. Previous relationships have not resulted in the gratification of emotional needs. Often these relationships were based on contingencies—that the child meet parental expectations such as being first in the class, being best in an activity, or gratifying the parent in some other manner. The need to be cared for as an emotional being was thwarted, leaving unmet dependency needs that would then influence future relationships. In some cases, depressed clients set themselves in the position of help-rejecting complainers for whom all attempts by others to meet their dependency needs are rejected. There remains an underlying fear that others will hurt them; thus, the depressed client will reject them before he or she can be rejected. Depressed clients may also behave in a demanding and manipulative manner in an attempt to force others to meet their need for affectional ties. In some cases, the dependency needs of these clients are so overwhelming that they cannot all be met. The client is engaged in a "meet all my needs or none at all if you really care for me" hypothesis. This premise leads to the further dissolution of social relationships because no one can meet all the identified needs.

TYPES OF MOOD DISORDERS
Grief and loss

Grief is a universal process that is generally taken for granted. According to Engel (1962), grief involves a series of subjective responses to the loss of a significant love object. Individuals may describe feelings of helplessness, loneliness, hopelessness, anger, sadness, and guilt. The frequency and duration of these responses depend upon several factors:

1. Amount of support received from the lost object
2. Degree of ambivalence toward the lost object
3. Anticipatory preparation
4. Extent to which the loss alters life-style
5. Other supportive relationships available to the bereaved

Mourning encompasses the psychological processes or reactions a person uses to assist him or her in overcoming a loss. In the case of the loss of a family member or friend, mourning includes the funeral ritual, the wearing of somber, dark colors, or the draping of purple or black cloth over doorways and windows. As we will discuss later, such rituals permit the survivors to acknowledge the loss of the significant person and to share the loss with others.

Loss can be defined as the relinquishing of objects, status, persons, or functions that are identified as supportive. Loss is very much a part of the

TABLE 22-1 Bowlby's phases of grieving

Phases	Characteristics
Disequilibrium	Isolation of affect, limited intellectual reponses, lack of acceptance of loss, anger toward self and others, feelings of ambivalence and guilt towards lost object. Crying is major component and elicits support from others.
Disorganization	Disorganized behavior; loss of self-esteem; feelings of despair, helplessness, loneliness. May use denial to protect self from painful acknowledgement of loss. Lack of ability to complete goals. Permanence of loss sets in. Catharsis is necessary to review events related to loss. Experiences, thoughts, and feelings related to the deceased generate crying, sadness, and desire to have the person return. Activities of life are carried on with little or no spontaneity.
Reorganization	Grieving process varies for each individual dependent upon culture, personality of survivor, relationship with deceased, past experiences with loss, and available support systems. Reinvestment in others and the environment occurs. Introjects both positive and negative aspects of deceased. Sets future goals and develops effective problem-solving techniques.

life cycle. It is imperative that nurses direct their energies toward helping people respond in a positive manner to the crises caused by loss. Obstacles to mental health generally arise when a person attempts to avoid intense distress and the expression of related emotions.

What does a bereaved person feel or experience? Is there an empathic route a nurse might select that would facilitate a genuine involvement with such a client? John Bowlby (1973) believes that the grieving process is set in motion by a loss or separation that leads to a feeling of emancipation from the lost object. The individual experiences a varying array of feelings, ranging from numbness and anger to healing and resolution. Eric Lindemann (1944), in his extensive studies of grief, has described the grieving process in detail. The process is characterized by (1) somatic distress, including tightness in the throat, an empty feeling, a loss of appetite, and even a lack of muscular power; (2) a sense of unreality—that the loss has not actually occurred; (3) an accompanying sense of purposelessness, as well as an inability to maintain any patterns of organization; (4) feelings of guilt; and (5) feelings of hostility.

Bowlby divides the grieving process into three phases (see Table 22-1). Each phase is characterized by a predominant form of behavior.

As a result of healthy coping by means of the mourning process, individuals are able to remember both the pleasures and the disappointments of the lost relationship. The identity of the bereaved individual remains intact for them. They are able to reorganize thoughts and consider new patterns of problem solving. The behavior of the bereaved in this final phase is characterized by readiness to move forward, openness to new avenues, and reconciliation with the fact that the loss has occurred.

The three phases occur not only in response to the death of a loved one but also in response to any situation involving loss. As was discussed previously (see Chapter 9), research demonstrates that loss may be a critical precipitating factor in both physical and emotional illness. For example, LeShan (1966) concluded that "the most consistently reported, relevant psychological factor [in the development of neoplasms] has been the loss of a major emotional relationship prior to the first-noted symptoms." Greene (1966) and Bahnson and Bahnson (1966) reported similar findings. Loss of a relationship through divorce, loss through change in job status, loss of a body part or alteration in body function, and loss of a particular life-style as a result of marriage or the birth of a child are examples of changes that may precipitate the grieving process. The response to such a change, however, is often not recognized as grieving. A vague feeling of distress and sadness may occur, as well as somatic symptoms.

A young business executive had been experiencing feelings of lethargy, frustration, and helplessness in his work situation, and he described muscle spasms in his neck and back. A discussion with a nurse revealed that the young man's superior had recently been transferred. He had had a close relationship with the superior and had expanded his role within the company while working for this individual. By identifying the feelings he was experiencing as valid responses to the loss of a relationship and to the possible loss of some of his current responsibilities, the young man was able to accept the feelings as normal. Healthy coping with the loss was facilitated, and the experience could then be integrated into the self as a basis for future coping with loss.

What characterizes a maladaptive response to loss? Should a depressive response to loss be considered normal? A maladaptive response may frequently be characterized as depression, yet such a characterization is not always accurate. Denial may be operating at such an intense level that thoughts and feelings related to the lost object are repressed. Reality is often rejected as being too painful to cope with. Restlessness, withdrawal, and disorganized patterns of behavior are predominant themes. Disintegration of ego functioning results. Why are some individuals able to make healthy adaptations, while others develop depression or physical illnesses? There is no one answer to this question. Nurses must consider the individual as a system that is part of a larger system and that responds to that larger system. It must be remembered that diverse external and internal factors cause each individual to be unique and worthwhile.

Each individual responds to loss in a different manner. The life cycle of individuals is characterized by a series of losses, beginning with the loss of the breast or the bottle. Reactions to loss are based on many factors, including previous experiences with loss, our repertoire of effective coping measures, support relationships, and changes in daily living patterns necessitated by the loss.

The emotions experienced after a loss are quite likely to be the most intense of our lives. Nurses, however, do not always recognize that clients are frequently responding to loss situations. Nurses do not readily view illness as a loss situation, even though clients routinely lose the ability to function in their own environments, to wear their own clothing, and to determine their own schedules. Depression may occur as a result of such loss, but this behavioral response often goes unrecognized.

Major depressive disorders

Nurses come in contact with clients experiencing some form of mood disorder in acute psychiatric settings, in general hospitals, in ambulatory and home care settings, and in nursing homes and hospice centers. Minot (1986) states that approximately 16 million people suffer from depression, yet less than one-third seek treatment. The prevalence of depression is striking. Perhaps widespread publicity regarding celebrities, those in the entertainment field and the arts, who have experienced depressive or manic responses in their lives and managed these responses successfully has heightened the public consciousness. Kaplan and Sadock (1985) note that twice as many women as men experience major unipolar depression in their lives. The question arises as to whether the acculturation of men in our society denies them permission to express emotions or to be depressed. The authors further indicate that bipolar disorders are found equally in the two sexes; that blacks and whites suffer from bipolar and major depressions at equal rates; and that the risk for developing some form of depression in a lifetime is approximately 10 percent for men and 20 percent for women.

Although the prevalence of depression in some form or other is notable, a major concern for health professionals is the plethora of terms utilized to describe various categories of mood disorders. Terms such as *reactive, endogenous, exogenous, psychotic,* and *clinical* depression have been utilized to describe depression. To reduce the redundancy found in previous descriptions of depression, DSM-III-R (1987) has organized the discussion around the central concept of mood disorders. A key characteristic of these disorders is a disturbance of mood, which may be accompanied by some form of manic or depressive syndrome. Mood

TABLE 22-2   Classification of mood disorders

MOOD EPISODES

Manic	Characterized by
Hypomanic	lack of known or-
Major depressive episode	ganic factors and
Chronic	not a part of non-
Melancholia	mood psychosis
Seasonal pattern	

MOOD DISORDERS

Bipolar disorders	Determined by pat-
Cyclothymia	terns of mood epi-
Bipolar disorders NOS	sodes
Depressive disorders	
Major depression	
Dysthymia	
Depressive disorder NOS	

Adapted from DSM-III-R (1987).

as defined by DSM-III-R is a prolonged emotion, either depression or elation, that impacts on the psyche. Table 22-2 presents the DSM-III-R terminology related to mood disorders.

The DSM-III-R provides discrete differentiation as much as possible to clarify the concept of mood disorders. Nurses must understand, however, that depression may mean an altered mood, or it may involve a complex interaction of themes such as dependency, low self-esteem, anger, or hopelessness. Within the framework of nursing, depression may be viewed as mild—where affect is characterized by feelings of sadness, dejection, and disappointment; moderate—progressive physical and psychological deterioration; or severe, which is characterized by distorted thought processes and profound psychological deterioration. The vignette below depicts a client experiencing a mood disorder.

Judy, a 25-year-old woman, came into a 24-hour emergency walk-in clinic at a large, urban hospital. She described herself as being a generally happy person, but during the past two weeks she had become increasingly dejected. She awoke early in the morning and was unable to fall back to sleep. Everyday activi-

ties became monumental tasks. She felt as though her whole body had come to a halt. Relationships with other people in her environment were also being affected. She no longer wanted to participate in social gatherings. She often found herself sitting alone, pondering her fate in life. She was prompted to come to the clinic by a co-worker who was concerned by her change in personality.

After several sessions at the clinic, Judy acknowledged that she had lost her mother a year ago. She had been coping "well" until recently, when she lost her cat. When discussing the two loss experiences, she said, "I never really cried it all out when Mom died." But the loss of the cat triggered the revival of the past loss. Judy began to experience again the angry and helpless feelings she had experienced when her mother died. These feelings had been repressed, only to surface later. Loss is one of the cornerstones of the dynamics of depression. Judy, in this vignette, not only felt the loss of her mother but also saw herself as no longer being important to anyone. These two factors acted as the foundation for the development of her depressive response.

The manic-depressive reaction has become one of the most widely discussed depressive responses in Western society. It is characterized by mood swings; a manic-depressive person's moods range from profound depression to extreme euphoria, with periods of normalcy in between. It is important to point out that mania is considered the mirror image of depression. The manic episode of a young housewife is depicted in the vignette below.

Mary K., a 34-year-old mother of three children, was admitted to a small, private psychiatric hospital. On admission, she was in a state of such hyperactivity that it required four people to assist her to her room. She was extremely hostile and was lashing out at all around her. Her husband described her as having progressed from being quite vigorous in her approach to tasks to being so aggressive in her actions that he could not control her. She had decided to build an addition to their house and had contacted four contractors. She had then ordered building supplies amounting to a total cost of $4,000. Flitting to another *project, she had taken the children shopping to buy clothes for camp and in one afternoon had spent more than $5,000. It was at this point that her husband sought psychiatric help.*

An understanding of the dynamics of mood disorders is necessary to assess clients accurately and implement effective strategies of intervention. Table 22-3 compares the grief response, dysthymic behavior, and unipolar and bipolar disorders.

In summary, there are both similarities and differences between manic depression and other types of depression. The influences of childhood on later life are significant in the understanding of any depressive state. Manic clients are often "the life of the party" or those who have the energy to accomplish everything. But is this pattern of response being used to escape from reality? Is the pain of loss so great? As in depression, a diminished sense of worth, a loss of dependence, and a fear of not being loved can be noted. Yet these feelings are hidden beneath a mask of pseudohappiness. Relationships are characterized by superficiality; manic-depressive persons manipulate their environments to continually receive the gratification and support they need. When anxiety increases, however, the mask no longer serves as an effective coping response. Individuals then turn to either the elative or the depressive response to preserve ego integrity.

Suicide

Suicide is the ultimate response to hopelessness, helplessness, and low self-esteem. It is the final escape from reality. For individuals who consider suicide, life has become so intolerable that previous mechanisms of dealing with stress are inadequate.

It is difficult to consider the possibility of ending one's life. It is also difficult to understand the dynamics of self-destructive behavior. Nurses who work with clients who have attempted suicide must understand their own feelings about and responses to such an individual. A relationship with a suicidal client can have a profound impact on a nurse. Health professionals devote much time and energy to the preservation of life. How can a nurse relate to

TABLE 22-3 Comparison of grief, dysthymia, unipolar, and bipolar mood disorders

	Grief	Dysthymia	Unipolar	Bipolar (manic phase)*
Causation	Sudden, unexpected loss of loved one; loss of function or body part; loss or change in role	Chronic stress, anxiety, inadequate coping; poor sense of personal capabilities	Genetic, biochemical, cognitive, psychodynamic, familial, role strain—a complex interrelationship of factors	Same as unipolar
Physical signs	Increased fatigue; somatization—tightness in throat; "empty" feeling; decreased appetite; cries easily; possible sleep difficulties	Increased somatization; appetite varies; weight gain may occur	Unkempt appearance, increased weight loss when not dieting; no appetite; constipation; loss of libido; loss of energy; purposeless, stereotypic movements (agitated depression); early morning awakening with unpleasant thoughts	Pressured speech; need for sleep decreases (2 to 3 hours); inappropriate dress; poor eating habits; increase in motor activity; use of profanity; excessive involvement in pleasurable activities, which may have serious consequences (i.e., excessive spending, engag-

Emotional signs	Feelings of sadness, guilt, anxiety, ambivalence, which decrease with time; self-esteem remains intact	Anxiety ranges to panic levels; self-esteem vacillates from low to high; decreased interest in social interactions	Low self-esteem reinforced by delusional system; increased suicidal risk; increased anxiety; helplessness, hopelessness, ambivalence, social isolation, and excessive dependency; underlying anger may not be expressed; cannot perceive others' needs; severely limited communications with others	ing in sexual indiscretions) Manipulative, outgoing, sometimes euphoric; inflated self-esteem on the surface; grandiosity, elation and pseudohappiness; interferes with lives of others; relationships characterized by emotional shallowness
Cognitive signs	Memory is poor; ability to concentrate is decreased but is able to make decisions when necessary; no delusions or hallucinations; oriented to surroundings	Unreliable memory; is able to make some decisions but vacillates on major issues; judgment and orientation vary with anxiety level; no hallucinations; limited delusions	Lack of orientation to surroundings; unable to make decisions; poor judgment; lack of concentration; negative perceptions of self, environment, and future	Generally no delusions/hallucinations; flight of ideas; feels thoughts are racing; marked disturbance of concentration, attention span, and ability to make rational decisions; inability to screen irrelevant stimuli
Duration intensity	Mild to moderate; lasts 6–12 months; is culture-bound and is connected to other variables; may be chronic but not harmful	Mild to moderate; may become chronic as a way of life with periods of depression and normalcy	If untreated may be indefinite—assumes chronic level; severe intensity—could lead to exhaustion and death.	Chronic if untreated; may lead to physical exhaustion and death; intensity may range from hypomania to delirious mania[†]

*Bipolar refers to both manic and depressive episodes. Clients may experience alternating periods of manic and depressive behavior with a period of euthymia or normal mood responses that separates the manic and depressive moods.

[†]Hypomania is characterized by elevated expansive behavior accompanied by some symptoms of mania but is generally not severe enough to warrant hospitalization. Delirious mania is rarely seen. (Clients often hallucinate and exist within delusional systems. Thoughts are incoherent, and clients may be dangerous to themselves and others.)

a person who constantly deprecates himself or herself, finds no happiness in living, and simply wishes to die? Working with such a client can be a frustrating, anxiety-provoking, discouraging experience. The client's negative perceptions may lead to negative responses by the nurse. A pattern may emerge in the interaction that increases the client's feelings of worthlessness.

In the past decade the trend toward the study of suicide (suicidology) and the development of suicide prevention centers and hot lines has been growing. The National Institute for Mental Health's Center for Studies of Suicide Prevention directs its efforts toward increasing the scope and amount of research in the areas of assessment of clues to suicidal behavior and the contributory factors in suicide. Suicidal behavior has many sources—biological, psychological, and sociocultural. A nursing care plan should incorporate all these factors. An integrated concept of depression, and of suicide as a possible outcome of depression, is essential to the assessment process.

EXPLANATORY MODELS OF SUICIDE

▶ Psychological Models

Freud believed that the instinct for life (Eros) and the instinct for death (Thanatos) exist in every human being. Self-destructive behavior results in hatred toward an internalized lost object. There is marked ambivalence, however, in a suicidal person. If the hatred becomes overwhelming, individuals literally have no choice but to kill themselves. Freud correlated suicide with the death instinct: Thanatos turned inward may cause individuals to take their lives.

Menninger, in his book *Man Against Himself* (1938), describes three basic components of the suicidal personality: the wish to kill (aggression), the wish to be killed (submission), and the wish to die (self-punishment). These components can be seen in overt acts or in the guise of addiction, antisocial behavior, impotence, or a tendency to have serious accidents.

Schneidman and Farberow (1957) group individuals who attempt suicide into four general categories: those who commit suicide as a means of saving their reputations; those who regard suicide as a release—for example, the old and the chronically ill; those who commit suicide in response to hallucinations and/or delusions; and those who wish to hurt others in their environment.

Loss of self-worth and resulting helplessness and hopelessness are critical factors in the precipitation of suicidal behavior. Suicidal people perceive themselves as failures in every aspect of their lives. They place little or no value on their own existence. They seemingly have no hope for the future.

LaGreca (1988) notes that there is an assumption that individuals who attempt suicide are suffering from such disorders as psychoses, severe neuroses, personality disorders, and depression. The latter factor, depression, can be viewed as an overwhelming sense of hopelessness. Wetzel (1976) points out that this sense of hopelessness is positively correlated with suicidal intent. It must be noted that not all depression is characterized by hopelessness; however, when this factor is present, suicidal behavior must be taken seriously. LaGreca found that when persons do not seek help or when they have enough energy to complete a suicidal act, hopelessness assumes a critical factor in the initiation of suicidal behavior. These individuals believe they have little or no impact on the course of their lives, do not consider themselves of value, and have no hope for changes in the future.

Neimeyer (1984) suggests that suicidal individuals severely isolate themselves from others, are unable to integrate positive feedback from the environment, and reject the support of significant others. Neimeyer also puts forth the premise that these individuals construct their own theory of understanding events and ultimately base their behaviors on this theory. A negative perception of others and their relationship to the individual continues in a downward spiral, which leads to a constriction of options. Suicidal behavior then results when options are so severely constricted that there is no option other than the act of self-inflicted death. A "presuicidal syndrome" described by Ringel (1976) consists of a constricted perception of options, autoaggression, or turning anger inward, and compulsive suicidal fantasies. Ringel believes that the combination of these factors increases significantly the potential for suicidal behavior. Other studies by Adams (1986) propose a relationship between instability in early life resulting from loss of a parent through death, separation, or divorce and suicidal behavior.

A relationship between alcoholism and suicide has been noted by Dr. Aaron Beck (1986). He indicates that as many as 50% of all suicides may be alcohol related. A recent article in a Harvard Mental Health Letter (1986) supports Beck's position and states that alcoholics who commit suicide tend to be men over the age of 30. Further data suggest that these individuals have more often than not experienced a major life trauma such as being fired, being arrested, or separating from a significant other. In many cases these individuals commit suicide after binge drinking when inhibition levels are reduced. The concept of hopelessness may serve to enhance suicidal ideation and increase impulsive behavior, which may lead to suicidal actions. Beck also suggests that low-lethality methods of suicidal behavior may be potentiated by the effects of alcohol, which may, in turn, increase success of suicidal behavior.

▶ Biologic and Genetic Models

Support for a biological basis for suicidal behavior has been noted by Dr. Marie Asberg of Stockholm, Sweden. Dr. Asberg (1986) reports that there is a definitive link between below-normal levels of 5-HIAA, a breakdown product of serotonin, and suicide attempters. Dr. Allen Francis (1986) concurs with Dr. Asberg and states that reduced serotonin levels may be a biological marker for both suicidal and aggressive behaviors.

Dr. A. Roy (1986) suggests that there may be a genetic component to suicide. Results from his study indicate that there is an increased incidence among twins and first-generation relatives. He also notes that there may be a correlation between suicidal behaviors and the genetic transmission of schizophrenia and manic depression.

▶ Sociocultural Models

Durkheim's (1951) sociological theory has been one of the fundamental constructs of suicide theory. He presents three basic forms of annihilative behavior: egoistic, altruistic, and anomic. The first, egoistic suicide, is related to a lack of integration in society—having an absence of shared beliefs, a

sense of belonging, and a feeling of support. He found that those individuals who were married and had children were less likely to commit suicide than married individuals without children. Single individuals committed suicide at a higher rate than those who were married but had no children. Durkheim also believed that suicide decreased as political and economic turmoil increased; that individuals drew together and supported one another.

Altruistic suicide, or that suicide which is demanded by society, seems to be in opposition to the dynamics of egoistic suicide. The individual's value is of less importance than the greater good of society. Durkheim viewed altruistic suicide as either obligatory or optional, although others do not support his position. LaGreca (1988) presents the example of Kamikaze pilots during World War II as an obligatory suicide, while soldiers throwing themselves on grenades to protect their comrades displayed optional suicide behavior.

Durkheim described suicide resulting from a lack of a clear understanding of the normative structure of society as anomic, coming from the term *anomie*, or sense of normlessness. He noted that anomie was incurred by positive or negative economic change, which left individuals without rules or structure for the society in which they live. Widows and divorced individuals may be more prone to suicide based on the sense of lack of meaning and role change they experience following loss. Other studies, however, such as that by Marshall and Hodge (1981), repudiate Durkheim's belief that *any* economic change causes anomie. Instead, they suggest that only periods of economic decline are positively related to increases in suicidal behavior.

Studies done by Platt (1984) and Stack (1982) suggest that there is a relationship between employment and suicide. Platt found that as unemployment increased, the suicide rate increased as well. Negative working conditions also precipitated a rise in suicide rate. Stack noted that, as Durkheim predicted, a strike tended to cause workers to band together; however, a critical factor was the size of the strike. He found that the larger the number of workers striking, the lower the suicide rate was for males. Duration of strike had no effect on suicide behaviors. Marshall (1981) found that Durkheim's hypothesis regarding decrease in suicide during war was rejected. His study of suicide during World War II, Vietnam, and Korea indicates that suicide did not decrease solely because of involvement in a war.

▶ Imitative Behavior and Suicide

Researchers share a concern that imitation, particularly among adolescents and young adults, may lead to "copycat" behaviors. This phenomenon was apparent in the 1987 multiple suicides in Westchester County, New York, followed by similar clusters of suicide behaviors in New Jersey, Illinois, and Indiana. Bollen and Phillips (1982) concluded that there was a sharp rise in suicides following highly publicized news reports of suicidal acts. In fact, by using national networks to conduct the survey, they were able to determine the number of days and peak times of the suicidal cycle.

▶ Rational Suicide

Finnerty (1987) defines rational suicide as taking one's life in a voluntary and intentional manner. The concept of rational suicide is a difficult one fraught with emotions and conflicting values. Suicide is most frequently perceived as the act of an individual who is experiencing some form of emotional disorder and not acting in a rational manner. Finnerty posits that those who choose nontreatment in a rational frame of mind are, in fact, intending to end their own lives—thus the perspective of rational suicide. However, moral, ethical, and legal issues must be considered in the determination of the individual's right to choose whether he lives or dies. The issue of rational suicide has come to the fore in this country as a result of more sophisticated medical technology, which prolongs biological life. LaGreca cites the case of Elizabeth Bouvia who went to court to get a legal injunction against being force-fed. She is a cerebral palsy victim who is quadriplegic and feels that her quality of life has diminished considerably as a result of her deteriorating illness. At this time, her case has been heard in several courts and has received positive attention in regard to her starvation plea; however, the case remains under appeal. Society has indicated a need to reconsider its position on the rights of the terminally ill to determine a course of treatment, or non-

treatment, that would promote optimal quality of life. Suicide within the context of our moral, religious, and ethical framework cannot at this point be considered a rational choice, yet we must be cognizant of those individuals who choose to specify what treatment and duration of treatment as it applies to their terminal situation.

Dr. Cynthia Pfeffer (1986) indicates that preventive measures for suicidal behavior must be the focus of future interventive strategies. She states that making it more difficult to carry out popular methods of suicide should be initiated as a means of primary prevention. Dr. Pfeffer believes that education of the public is critical to the proper recognition of suicidal behavior and the effective use of treatment services.

Capodanno and Targum (1983) establish guidelines, similar to those of Hatton, Valente, and Rink (1977), that identify a set of potential predictor variables that may improve prediction of risk. They also note that the relatively low incidence of suicide makes it difficult to obtain presuicide data. The following are attributes of suicidal behavior that can be further developed by scale construction to improve prediction:

1. Perception of social environment as alien and hostile
   a. Significant others
   b. General environment
2. Hopelessness
3. Previous attempts
4. Family history
5. Biological markers
   a. Dexamethasone suppression test
   b. Reduced platelet MAO
   c. Elevated urinary cortisol levels

Papa's (1980) study on predictors of suicidal behavior contributes relevant information for nursing assessment. She considers the complex interaction of predictor variables such as hopelessness; locus of control; preference for inclusion, control, and affection; and stress from life events in relation to degree of suicidal intent. The focus is no longer on a single variable as a precipitating factor but on a relationship among or between variables. Two conclusions are noteworthy: that hopelessness and preference for affection are significantly related to suicidal intent and that there are significant correlations between locus of control and hopelessness and between preference for affection and hopelessness. Papa indicates that the series of life events or the "life process" is such that individuals ultimately reach a point where there is an end to hope and suicide is the mechanism of resolution. In fact there is no one precipitating factor but rather a series of life events, which may originate in childhood and continue throughout life. Nursing should consider the interrelationships of these variables to formulate more accurate assessment tools and to provide appropriate treatment for this population.

DEMOGRAPHIC DATA AND SUICIDAL BEHAVIOR

It is difficult to obtain accurate data relative to completed suicides as well as suicide attempts. In some cases, relatives fear religious repercussions or stigmatization from society; thus, reporting does not reflect a valid assessment of the cause of death. Statistics from the Harvard Mental Health Letter indicate that close to 100,000 individuals commit suicide yearly. This demonstrates a significant increase since 1970. LaGreca notes that the suicide rates for American males is not as high as some countries', i.e., Austria, Denmark, Sweden, and Switzerland. Female suicide in this country is appreciably higher than in Ireland, Greece, Spain, and Northern Ireland.

Demographic variables such as age, gender, marital status, and race must be considered to understand the dynamics of suicidal behavior. Table 22-4 addresses these variables.

Last, it has often been said that the incidence of suicide increases during holiday seasons. The reasons offered for this rise included reinforcement of loss of family ties, feelings of isolation, disappointment, and anticlimactic feelings related to the holiday period. Blakeslee (1987) reports that studies on suicides on holidays indicate that the risk is actually greater before holidays, in particular, Memorial Day, Thanksgiving, and Christmas; however, there are no empirical data to suggest a correlation between the holidays and suicide. It was also noted that holidays might provide some type of psychological and social protection that would nullify the need for suicidal behavior. In each case, individual

TABLE 22-4 Demographic variables and suicidal behavior

Age	Suicide rates increase with age; sharp peak in adolescence. Projected rise in the elderly population.
Gender	Males commit suicide two to three times more frequently than females; females attempt suicide three to five times more frequently than males. Trends show that the gap between males and females is lessening.
Race	Whites have a suicide rate two to three times higher than the black population. Suicide rates decrease in the black population as age increases. The reverse is true for whites. Age 60 and over whites kill themselves three times more frequently than blacks. This premise also is applicable to nonwhite Hispanics and to American Indians.
Marital status	Suicide rate is highest among white males who have never married. Divorced and widowed individuals have the next highest rate. Generally, married individuals have the lowest suicide rate.

Sources include Linden and Breed (1976), Wilson (1981), and Seiden (1981).

personalities must also be considered in relation to increased incidence of depression with resulting increase in the suicide rate.

FAMILIAL DETERMINANTS

Richman (1971) has identified several characteristics of families with suicidal problems: family fragility, family depression, intolerance for separation, symbiosis without empathy, closed family relationships, scapegoating, poor patterns of dealing with aggression, double-bind communicating, and inflexibility in responding to crisis. Since the family network has profound effects on a person's integrative functioning, it plays an important role in the development of any maladaptive response. But the role of the family is especially important in the case of a suicidal client. Oftentimes, it is a perceptive family that identifies clues to impending suicidal acts.

SOCIOCULTURAL AND SPIRITUAL CONTEXT

American society is composed of various ethnic groups and subcultures. Each person is a unique being whose behavior reflects the environment from which he or she comes as well as biological and psychological factors. In this section the attitudes toward suicide held by several ethnic or cultural groups are discussed.

▶ Navajo indians

Suicide is not acceptable to the Navajo tribe, not because it is thought to be inherently bad, but because of its effect on the members of the family.

Webb and Willard, in Farberow's *Suicide in Different Cultures (1975)*, point out the Navajo's belief that any death other than that resulting from old age is unnatural. A violent death is certain to bring misfortune to the family of the person who died. The usual precipitating event in suicide is bad feelings among kin; frequently, a person who commits suicide does so near his or her own residence and contaminates the family with a ghost. An intense fear of ghosts is an important element in the Navajo attitude toward suicide. Navajos believe that the dead person does not leave the situation but merely takes a new status—that of ghost. The Navajo's fear of the dead, coupled with their attitude toward violent death, clearly makes suicide unacceptable.

Suicidal behavior is found among the Navajo most frequently in men between the ages of 25 and 39. Use of alcohol is often noted as a variable.

Santora and Starkey (1982) note the impact of sociocultural, spiritual, and intrapsychic variables on suicidal behavior. Several tribes were studied, and data revealed that victims were most typically young, single men who were in conflict with values, work, or significant others. The authors also note that little is known about the motives of the victims.

It is important to understand sociocultural variables. There is increasing conflict between values of the traditional culture and the Anglo culture. There is a need on the one hand to integrate into the larger society while at the same time maintaining and preserving a distinct culture. This vacilla-

tion may serve as the basis for identity crisis, anomie, and social isolation—and, ultimately, suicide.

▶ Scandinavian-Americans

Scandinavian-Americans, proud of their Viking heritage, do not look favorably on suicide. To kill oneself is a sign of weakness and an inability to cope with life's stresses. Survival of the fittest was a predominant theme among the Vikings, as was the idealization of the physically strong.

Scandinavian-Americans also carry with them the belief that suicide is a sin that cloaks the entire family with shame. Early Christian doctrine forbade the Church to give a eulogy for a person who committed suicide or to sprinkle the traditional earth on the coffin.

Petterstol (in Faberow, 1975) sees a change of direction in Scandinavian-American attitudes toward suicide. There is still great concern for physical health, vigor, and life. However, there also is a more empathic attitude toward persons who have attempted suicide and toward the survivors of persons who commit suicide. The survivors themselves are ashamed and unsure of how they should respond to others. There are still strong taboos against taking one's own life.

▶ Italian-Americans

For Italian-Americans, suicide is regarded as a grave sin; this belief is rooted in Catholic dogma. The family of an individual who commits suicide is dishonored; the avenues to certain occupations are closed to his or her survivors, and the body cannot be buried in consecrated ground. This attitude is so strong that physicians and members of the clergy will falsify death certificates. For example, mental illness might be listed as the cause of death, for this is acceptable to the Church.

According to Farberow (1975), an understanding of the family is of utmost importance to an understanding of the dynamics of suicide among Italian-Americans. The family is the primary support system. Individuals are encouraged to depend on others in their family constellation; the family provides nurturing in the form of love, help, and protection. With such a constant support system it may be difficult for individuals to feel worthless. Italian-

Americans believe that each individual should be accountable for the welfare of others. Although the family is a support system, it often places great demands on its members. Since the family provides nuturance, it may also attach strings. Feelings of rage and helplessness may arise, leading to overt conflict and, in some instances, suicide.

Italian-Americans exemplify the characteristic ambivalence of persons who are considering suicide as a way of relieving overwhelming stress. Their ambivalence results from the strong doctrine of the Church and from an inability to escape the intricately woven net of family and Church. Members of third, fourth, and successive generations of Italian-Americans may no longer feel as constrained by Catholic dogma. Their concern for life, however, remains strong.

▶ Asian-Americans

The people of the Orient do not normally disapprove of suicide. Suttee, or the suicide of a widow after her husband's death, was quite common in India until the last century. It was taught that this death would be a passport to heaven, would atone for any sins of the husband, and would even give distinction to the remaining family members. It must be noted that some aspects of Hindu philosophy encourage suicide for religious reasons. In China suicide is regarded as acceptable as a means of revenge because it not only embarrasses the enemy but permits the dead man to haunt him from the spirit world. Voluntary death has also been given a place of honor in Buddhist countries.

Suicide has been held in positive regard amongst all classes in Japan. Hara-Kiri, a ceremonial form of suicide, was taught as a means to avoid capture as well as to avoid disgrace and punishment in order to preserve one's honor. The suicide pact of lovers who choose to end their lives in this world and to go on to another is also not unusual.

▶ Judeo-Christian Americans

Clinard (1974) states that the attitudes of Western European peoples toward suicide originated primarily in the philosophies of the Jewish and Christian religions. Talmudic law looks upon suicide unfavorably and condemns the individual yet believes that comfort should be provided to the

family. The Christian position against suicide has its roots in the beliefs that human life is sacred; individuals do not have the right to usurp God's authority and take their own lives; and death is an entrance into a new life in which behavior in the old is important. The concept of life after death had a strengthening effect on the Church's position against suicide.

Interestingly, early Christian teachings sanctioned suicide when it was connected either with martyrdom or protection of virginity. However, it was eventually disapproved for any reason and became a crime.

Throughout the Middle Ages, suicide was denounced. Augustine stated that suicide precluded repentance, and Thomas Aquinas maintained that it was unnatural and an offense against the community. Special treatment was provided for bodies of those who had committed suicide—often they were not permitted in traditional graveyards. In some instances, the bodies were hung from gallows, burned, or thrown into the sewer.

During the Age of Enlightment, the belief that individuals should not transcend God's authority and take their own lives was challenged. David Hume, Montesquieu, Voltaire, and Rousseau spoke of the importance of choice, even on the issue of life and death. If one does not have control over all aspects of life, then who should?

At present both Catholics and Protestants oppose suicide; however, increasing consideration is being shown for individuals within the context of their lives and their motivations to commit suicide, and condemnation is decreasing.

Suicide as an act generates many questions for the care giver as well as for the client. One must confront one's own personal beliefs about suicide as a choice as well as about individual and societal responsibility.

EPIDEMIOLOGY OF DEPRESSION

Are some people more prone to depression than others? If so, do these individuals have similar characteristics? Persons most likely to be depressed can be described as shy, perhaps oversensitive, self-conscious, and worriers. Reaching a level of perfection is their ultimate goal. The results of not achieving this end are self-deprecation and self-doubt—primary characteristics of depressed persons.

Statistics indicate that depression occurs more frequently in females than in males. However, this may not be an accurate assessment. The overt expression of depression by males is frequently frowned upon. Statistics also show that the incidence of depression increases with age in both men and women. Depression cuts across social classes.

To understand the prevalence of depression, nurses must consider socioeconomic factors, availability of mental health services, the attitude of each class toward mental health, and at what point treatment is sought.

Depression affects all age groups, from childhood through senescence. Individuals may be born with a predisposition to depression; however, susceptibility to depression also depends on the many factors noted previously—familial, genetic, biological, and chemical—and on early life experiences.

Age determinants
INFANCY AND CHILDHOOD

There is no apparent agreement regarding the incidence of depression in infancy and childhood. Subsequent studies did not replicate Spitz and Wolf's (1946) findings that depression as a syndrome occurred in infancy. Rutter and Garmezy (1983) conclude that depression in infancy and childhood is rare. However, Chess, Thomas, and Hassibi (1983) contend that depression in this period is more widespread than has previously been acknowledged. They state that attempting to model measurements for the evaluation of depression in childhood after the adult model of depression is inappropriate and results in distortions of diagnosis. Trad (1987) suggests that a developmental model be utilized to conceptualize depression in infancy and childhood. This model would consider critical developmental milestones as a baseline measurement from which to analyze data. Those factors to be evaluated include temperament, attachment behaviors, object permanence and constancy, empathy, self-concept, neuroendocrinology, and learned helplessness phenomena. The value of this model lies in the framing of both normal and abnormal maturation as the measure of evaluation rather than the assessment of infant and childhood depression based on adult depression criteria. (For further discussion, see Chapter 17.)

ADOLESCENCE

Rutter and Garmezy (1983) indicate that age-related changes do occur around the time an individual moves into adolescence. They also found that depressive disorders occur much more frequently in females than in males. Beck et al. (1979) support the notion that there is an increase in depressive disorders and a change in sex ratio during adolescence for these disorders. Factors that increase the risk of depressive responses in adolescence include frequent changes in care takers, changes in family roles, break-up of the home, financial and social strain, death of a parent and the impact on the surviving parent, and the blending of stepfamilies. These factors are critical to the understanding of adolescent depression; however, there is no clear evidence to suggest that these changes have any direct contribution to the development of depression in adolescence. (For further discussion, see Chapter 17.)

THE ELDERLY

Depression in the elderly is most often misdiagnosed or not diagnosed at all. The lack of accurate diagnosis may be related to complications incurred by medical illness, medications taken, neurological impairment, or the belief that "all older persons are normally depressed." Shamoian (1985) suggests that all elderly clients should be assessed for depression rather than assume it is a normal component of the aging process.

One significant finding that bears noting is Leviton's (1973) hypothesis that sexuality in the elderly is directly correlated with the desire for death. He proposed that once an individual feels he has lost the capacity or the ability to engage in intimate, loving relationships, there is a concurrent loss of desire to live. This factor reemphasizes the need for the elderly to maintain a viable sexual identity and to participate in intimate relationships whenever this is possible. Elderly people's responses to altered physical abilities, psychological loss, and changes in environment are influenced by the availability of support systems, previous coping styles, and current physical and physiological assets. Sudden changes in mood may indicate a decrease in the individual's ability to cope with current situations or may reflect physiological changes. Assessment of individuals who were content and well adjusted may reveal physiological factors as responsible for mood alteration. Nursing intervention is directed toward alleviating anxiety by providing accurate information and responding to and correcting, if possible, those physiological alterations.

As in other groups, an extended grief response needs to be addressed as a depressive response. Symptoms indicative of depression that are not attributable to advanced age include decrease in usual interaction with significant others and families, excessive fatigue, anorexia, and general apathy. A thorough understanding of these changes must include a recognition of the elderly person's response to the process of aging and to the prospect of dying and death. (For further discussion, see Chapter 18.)

EXPLANATORY THEORIES
Psychoanalytic theory

Proponents of the psychoanalytic theory of depression believe that a depressive response has at its roots a significant loss, either real or imagined. Anger resulting from the loss is turned inward, and self-hate results. The original loss is repressed; however, subsequent losses reactivate the feelings associated with it. Freud, in "Mourning and Melancholia" (1917), postulates that the characteristics of the normal grieving process are similar to those of the pathological state of depression. Unlike individuals experiencing normal grief, however, those experiencing depression seem to be grieving over an inner loss that they are unable to resolve. It is this unresolved grief that depressed individuals carry with them.

Freud states that the initial lost love object is the parent. Individuals simultaneously feel both love and hate for the parent, yet it is the hatred that is incorporated or symbolically introjected into the self. The psychic mechanism of introjection serves as a basis for the development of the superego. For

individuals who later suffer from pathological depression, the embryonic superego is punitive in that it never permits the acceptance of praise. Individuals never learn to value their own sense of self, a situation that is carried on throughout the life cycle.

The psychoanalytic literature suggests that such individuals' self-derogatory behavior is a sign that hostility toward the lost object has been internalized. They then become narcissistic. They believe that no one else cares enough about them to take care of their needs; therefore, they must care for themselves. By not becoming involved in any relationship, depressed individuals limit the social failures they might experience. Strong dependence needs become apparent. It is literally impossible to meet the needs of such persons; they never seem to be fulfilled. A cyclical pattern develops. Dependent individuals are disappointed in their attempts to gain recognition. They pull back from relationships to save face while at the same time chastising themselves for being so inadequate. The depressive response is adopted and promoted.

Melanie Klein (1934) suggests that the depressive response can be traced to the early mother-infant relationship. Feelings of rage and hostility characterize the infant's response to a lack of gratification of needs. A weakened ego state results; feelings of helplessness, sadness, and dejection arise as a result of tension between ego and superego. The introjective mechanism acts to internalize the persecutor. Klein points out that children need to feel fully assured that parental love is genuine. Without this assurance, sadness, dejection, lack of self-esteem, and a sense of loss result.

Rene Spitz and K.M. Wolf (1946) and John Bowlby (1973) believe that the origins of depression can be found in the infant's responses to experiences of separation and loss. This "object loss theory," as it is commonly referred to, suggests that trauma results when separation from significant others occurs. Spitz and Wolf, in their studies of mother-infant responses, point out a particular pattern of behavior that occurs following separation. (It is important to note that these authors argue that for the first 6 months of life a mother-infant relationship exists, but that during the second 6 months of life the relationship is gradually severed.) Spitz and

Wolf describe infants reacting to separation as being withdrawn, stuporous, and anorectic; showing psychomotor retardation; and experiencing overall slowing of the normal growth and development process. They call this cluster of symptoms "anaclitic depression." Bowlby identifies similar patterns of response in older children. He proposes three phases:

1. Protest—crying, looking for mother
2. Despair—withdrawal from environment, apathy
3. Detachment—total lack of investment in any mothering figure

Bibring (1953), although psychoanalytically oriented, differs from other psychoanalytic theorists in his perception of the dynamics of depression. He suggests that depression is characterized primarily by a loss of self-esteem. This loss can be stimulated by inadequate fulfillment of needs for affection as well as by frustration of significant hopes and desires. Bibring's primary thesis is based on the assumption that all depressive reactions have one aspect in common—a sense of loss. He attributes much of the basis of depression to trauma during the oral phase. Bibring also postulates that attacks of the ego that result in feelings of loss can occur in any developmental phase. We know, for example, that during the toddler phase, children direct their energies toward increasing their mobility. Bibring believes that the inability to accomplish this task is viewed by the toddler as a personal failure, a loss. Nurses thus need to be alert to potential loss situations in any developmental phase. Primary prevention then can begin to make strides forward.

Cognitive theory

Cognitive theorists suggest that analysis of the depressive response too often becomes tangled in the web of the psyche. They point out that Freud's concept of hatred directed toward the introjected lost love object is difficult, if not impossible, to validate and that it seems to involve no actual connection between theoretical constructs and observable behavior.

Beck (1967) ascribes causal significance to illogical thinking processes. He believes that illogical thought patterns operate solely in relation to the self. These patterns generate self-doubt and self-deprecation. In essence, a person's thought processes determine his or her emotional reactions. Beck identifies a "primary triad" in depression—three major cognitive patterns that force individuals to view themselves, their environment, and their future in a negativistic manner.

First, individuals perceive themselves as unworthy and inadequate; they believe they are failures. They attribute their failures to some nebulous flaw, whether physical, emotional, or moral. Rejection of self occurs as a result of these perceptions.

Second, they view their interactions with the social world as being poor at best. They are particularly sensitive to any barriers placed in the way of the attainment of goals. Difficulties of any degree are interpreted as indicating total inadequacy on their part. (Depressed persons are programmed to respond with a sense of failure. A mildly depressed nursing student, for example, did poorly on one out of ten quizzes. She looked on this one quiz grade as an indication of total failure and considered dropping out of the nursing curriculum.)

Another facet of the negative interpretation of interactions is that of deprivation. Depressed persons perceive seemingly trivial events as serious losses. Beck gives the example of a depressed client on his way to visit his psychiatrist. The client felt he was losing valuable time by having to wait 30 seconds for the elevator. He then regretted the absence of companionship as he rode alone in the elevator. Then he discovered that he was not the psychiatrist's first patient, and he regretted not having the first appointment.

Other loss situations related to interactions with other people center around money or the comparison of others' possessions to one's own.

A young woman had just moved to a lovely new home in a new neighborhood. She had been quite upset over this move initially. Her husband held a very good job, and she was finally able to purchase the kinds of things she desired for herself, her children, and her home. Yet when friends bought items for their homes, she felt as though she were being deprived.

This woman, and the man in Beck's example, automatically interpreted their experiences negatively, even though more plausible explanations were available.

The third, and final, component in Beck's triad is depressed individuals' negative expectations of the future. Just as they hold negative interpretations of self and social relationships, so also do they perceive the future as being constantly overcast with large dark clouds. There are no silver linings for depressed individuals. Even short-range predictions are negative. Each day is viewed with trepidation: There is not a chance in the world that events will turn out positively. Thus the power of thought is clearly an overwhelming factor in depression. This factor is of great importance in the assessment of depressed clients and in the determination of nursing goals.

It is of value to posit a relationship among affect, motivation, and the cognitive triad. If individuals think they are worthless and base their behavior on this premise, mood will be negative. In addition, they will experience a loss of motivation—a primary characteristic of depression. They will consistently expect to meet with failure and humiliation; therefore, they will attempt nothing. Hopelessness and self-doubt will pervade thought processes. Depressed individuals envision themselves as being overwhelmed by tasks they had previously been able to cope with. It has been demonstrated that by changing such clients' thought patterns to a more positive track, a nurse can enhance their ability to actively solve problems.

Psychodynamic theory

Arieti (1974) describes depressed clients as those who have experienced a nurturing relationship that was later withdrawn. In its stead came a provisional relationship—a relationship based on the stipulation that the child must meet the expectations of the parents. In this relationship, praise and gratification were given, for example, when good grades or other symbols of prestige were achieved. Feelings of self-worth were not enhanced, since rewards were in the far distant future.

The failure to receive positive feedback can be perceived as a loss, even though the significant oth-

er may have been physically present. Again, the early beginnings of the inability to form relationships can be discerned. The expectations of an early significant relationship are not met; therefore, individuals believe that all other relationships will fail. Little by little, they stop trying to interact with the environment.

It is important to see depression as a reaction or response. It is something individuals are doing rather than something that is happening to them. Depression is a behavioral interaction, a response to environmental stimuli.

Individuals who suffer from depression are often perfectionists whose few relationships are characterized by manipulation and control. They are unable to accept anything other than "black and white" solutions to problems. Underneath the veneer of a high-powered executive type may be the fear of total failure and powerlessness. The depressive response becomes apparent when individuals feel they have not met their own goals or those of significant others in the environment.

The predominant themes in manic depression are similar to those encountered in the depressive response. Clients in the manic phase are outgoing; they easily involve themselves in relationships with others. They can be quite manipulative and controlling if a situation is not satisfactory in terms of their own interests. To feel important, they often attack the worth of others. Manic-depressive persons are unsure of their own worth.

Biochemical theory

As they have in many emotional disorders, investigators have looked for an alteration in physiological functioning as a possible contributory factor. The study of electrolyte metabolism has indicated that in individuals suffering from depression there is a disturbance in the distribution of sodium and potassium from one side of a nerve cell to the other. Gibbons (1960), who worked with a group of 24 clients exhibiting depressive reactions, discovered that every client had an elevated sodium level within the nerve cells. During recovery from depression, the excess sodium was excreted.

These findings are consistent with what is known about the effect of the use of lithium compounds in the treatment of manic depression. Lithium interferes with sodium exchange at the cellular level. With the resolution of the mania, the tolerance of the body for lithium is lowered, and the lithium, along with the excess sodium, is excreted.

We need to be aware, however, that electrolyte changes may be a *result* of depression rather than a causative factor. Changes in diet and motor activity during depression could lead to electrolyte imbalance.

The biochemical theory described by Kicey (1974) is worth noting. Her research suggests that the supply of norepinephrine at receptor sites is lowered when a person is depressed. There is an inhibition of the transmission of impulses from one neural fiber to another. The purpose of the monoamine oxidase (MAO) inhibitors is to increase the availability of active norepinephrine.

The biological theory of depression has gained support through the introduction of a diagnostic tool, the dexamethasone suppression test. The neuroendocrine disturbance indicated by an abnormal dexamethasone suppression test demonstrates a dysfunction in the limbic system and hypothalamus. A plasma cortisol level of 5 mEq/100 ml or greater indicates that the client has melancholia. In test results of depressed clients versus nondepressed clients, investigators noted that the test was abnormal almost exclusively for depressed clients. Researchers also found that abnormal results were not related to age, sex, psychotropic drugs, or severity of symptoms ("Testing for Melancholia," 1981).

The dexamethasone suppression test (DST) is the first test of its kind with practical and clinical application on a large scale. Since the depressive response may be elusive, a method that can determine biological alterations relating to depression can be an asset in diagnosis and treatment. The method, however, is not biologically specific to depression. Conditions that can generate a false positive are pregnancy, high-dose estrogen therapy, Cushing's disease, marked weight loss, uncontrolled diabetes, major physical illness, trauma, fever, use of narcotics, and withdrawal from alcohol. False-negative results may occur in clients who have Addison's disease, hypopituitarism, or are on corticosteroids. Although the test has significance for diagnosis of depressed clients, it is important for nurses to consider the above-noted factors and to complete a comprehensive physical assessment and health history. All data must be considered to ensure accurate medical and nursing diagnoses and nursing intervention.

It has been determined through longitudinal studies conducted on Amish families that there is a genetic marker for the manic-depressive gene for approximately 60% to 70% of those who inherit it. Researchers from MIT, University of Miami School of Medicine, and Yale School of Medicine indicate that at least some instances of manic depression are a result of the effect of a dominant gene on the tip of the short arm of chromosome eleven (Kolata, 1987). There is also an indication that one of the genes in the area of C-11-tyrosine hydroxylase is related to the synthesis of dopamine, a substance considered a factor in manic depression.

Mental health research, up to this time, has pointed indirectly to a genetic predisposition to manic depression. Kolata reports that previous studies indicate that if one identical twin has manic depression, the chances are as high as 80% that the other twin will also experience manic-depressive symptoms. Further data on adoptive families demonstrates that only 2% of adoptive parents of manic-depressive individuals had manic depression, while 30% of the biological parents had a history of manic-depressive illness.

If this theory is supported by further research, it opens up new avenues for understanding manic depression. As Kolata points out, tyrosine hydroxylase may not be the causative agent; however, it still provides strong evidence as to where the gene might be located. Studies can also be initiated to determine why those 30 to 40% who have the gene do not develop manic-depressive symptoms. These studies can then assist researchers to identify potential preventive measures.

Sociocultural theory
LEARNING THEORY

Can a depressive response be learned? Is assuming a helpless position a viable adaptive mechanism for some individuals?

Seligman (1973) proposes that depression is

learned helplessness. In his study with dogs, he found that the experience of having no control over what was happening interfered with the dogs' adaptive responses. The dogs actually learned that they were helpless, that no matter what the situation was, their actions did not matter. They could not succeed. Seligman suggests that, in humans, the precursor to depression may be the belief that individuals have no control over their situation—that they are unable to effect any change in life experiences, to reduce suffering, or to gain praise. According to Seligman, if individuals have little success in mastering their environment, hopelessness, helplessness, and lack of assertiveness eventually become primary characteristics and the susceptibility to depression is heightened.

To compensate for weaknesses in his theory, Seligman and his associates incorporated a cognitive perspective into the theory (Abramson et al., 1978). Seligman proposed that depression resulted from prolonged negative perceptions of self related to experiences of helplessness. These depressed individuals tended to perceive themselves in terms of longstanding personal inadequacies rather than in terms of the inability to cope effectively with short-term situations. Negative cognitions would be repeatedly reinforced by situations where the depressed individual would experience failure. This pattern assumed a cyclical nature, feeding back into negative cognitions with a resulting sense of helplessness.

FEMINIST THEORIES

Published studies indicate that two to three times as many women experience depressive responses as men. There has been much investigation of the relationship between female hormones and the occurrence of depression.

According to Phyllis Chesler (1972), few women have been able to develop a true sense of identity outside that of wife and mother. This fact can be seen vividly when the prestige levels of men and women in the male-oriented professional and business worlds are compared. Chesler proposes that "women are in a constant state of mourning, grieving for that which they never had or had too briefly." The concept of learned helplessness can be correlated with society's preconceived notion of how a

woman is to respond. It is more acceptable for a woman to adopt a depressive response than for a male to do so.

However, Corob (1987) notes that while the sex factor may account for a percentage of a woman's depression, it cannot be said that this factor is capable in and of itself of accounting for the much larger number of women who experience depression than men.

Corob suggests that traditionally held theories of depression are not sufficient to explain women's vulnerability to affective disorders. She states that the psychoanalytic model does not consider sufficiently current life circumstances; behavioral theories do little to address the impact of feelings and past experiences or behaviors; and, last, none of the theories considers the sociocultural context of women.

Corob utilizes Brown and Harris's studies to support her presentation of depression in women as occurring within a sociocultural context. Brown and Harris (1978) identified "traumatic" events in the form of loss or disappointment concerning a person, role, idea, or object as well as "vulnerability" factors that increase the possibility of women becoming depressed. Those factors include three or more children under the age of 14 living at home; loss of one's own mother in childhood; lack of an intimate, supportive relationship; and lack of employment outside the home. These factors in and of themselves enhance the sense of low self-esteem and inability to exert influence over one's life or environment and in turn cause women to be more vulnerable to the effects of loss and stress.

Corob proposes that early life experiences can be critical in the development of inner resources—women may in fact suffer from less than satisfactory early relationships more than men. She indicates that even at birth, girls may be perceived as being "second best"—a perception that may be implicitly conveyed. This perception may in turn generate feelings of inferiority and lack of importance. Further external reinforcement for the assumption of the traditional female role provides limited options. Women then become caught up in the demand to achieve goals that have been determined for them by others, in many cases males. Bem (1975) in her research demonstrated that women who assume traditional female behaviors tend to have increased levels of anxiety, low self-esteem, and poor emotional adjustment. Those women who were outgoing, creative, and successful professionally were found to be more androgynous and less prone to depression.

Throughout the life cycle, women experience situations that reinforce their vulnerability and low self-esteem. Corob suggests that in adolescence, women view themselves as they believe others want them to be; in young adulthood women are conflicted with the pressure to "get married and have children" versus choosing to have a career. In middle age, women may be left as "empty-nesters."

Are women predisposed to depression? Dr. Pauline Bart (1971) studied depression in middle-aged women in relation to role loss. She suggests that women who have invested all their time and energy in their children and their homes are more likely to experience a depressive response than women who have not done so. These women are unable to find new roles for themselves. They have suffered the greatest loss—the loss of a purpose in life. Their self-doubt and low self-regard prevent them from seeing themselves as anything other than wives or mothers. The fear of attempting to adapt to new roles because they may fail becomes paramount. However, women who begin early to define roles outside those of wife and mother will find it less difficult to adjust to the eventual loss of the nurturing role.

The onset of menopause may activate depressive responses related to the lost chance to have a child as well as decreased feelings of femininity, loss of youthfulness and attractiveness, and other physical changes indicative of the aging process. Older women often outlive their partners and are forced to live restricted, isolated lives, which may then reinforce perceptions of low self-esteem and worthlessness.

Other factors and situations potentiate the occurrence of depressive behavior in women. Corob delineates those as follows:

1. Potential dependence of women on men for satisfaction of needs
2. Decreased prestige associated with role of housewife—"woman's work"
3. Role confusion/conflict re: birth of children (postpartum depression)
4. Inadequate feelings related to socially identified role of "mothering"
5. Inability to conceive children
6. "Deviancy" associated with the role of being a "single" woman
7. Lack of reward related to position in the job force
8. Stressful life events such as rape, sexual assault, abortion, miscarriage, mastectomy, hysterectomy, disablement
9. Feelings of oppression related to one's ethnic background, i.e., Hispanic, black, Asian

In conclusion, the feminist theory of depression considers the psychological, behavioral, cognitive, and biochemical components of depression. However, this viewpoint supports the need to view women as they exist within the social and cultural context that shapes their lives.

Family theory

Individuals exist within many systems, one of the most powerful of these being the family. As has been noted in the discussion of psychodynamic theory, origins of depression may be related to inconsistencies in parent-child relationships resulting in lowered self-esteem. Family theory suggests that individuals who are depressed should be viewed within the context of the family process.

Exceptionally high expectations of self may be derived from the family. If praise and gratification are received only when appropriate behaviors are demonstrated, home becomes equated with meeting parental expectations. Unrealistic expectations are brought from the family into current relationships, in which the individuals who are significant are expected to provide unquantifiable amounts of love. A cycle ensues: expectations are unrealistic; significant others cannot provide requisite amounts of love; and lowered self-esteem and depression result. Individuals continue to expect unrealistic praise and love, which are the bases for their tenuous self-worth. Often these individuals cannot develop their own reservoirs of inner resources and must continue their dependence on others.

It should be noted that depressed individuals

may maintain a particular function in the family system. Other members may derive their roles from their relationship with the depressed individual. A sense of worth and personal identity may result from acting as a caretaker or as the overfunctioning member. In essence, the overfunctioner cannot permit the underfunctioning member to change and assume a more independent role. Equilibrium is actually maintained through dysfunctional behavior. Energy resulting from other family conflicts or individual emotional distress may be directed toward the identified client or the overt symptom bearer—the depressed client. Whatever the issue, roles of family members are interrelated, with each member's behavior affecting others. An understanding of family relationships and dynamics is essential in nursing assessment and designing a plan of care (see Chapter 14).

Systems theory

It is important to point out that *no one* theory is sufficient to explain depression. Any client is a complex, unique human being who cannot be understood through an assessment of only one factor. It would indeed be simple to say that biochemical changes or poor early relationships within the family system account for a depressive response. It would then be easy to develop a nursing care plan to facilitate the remediation of these problems. In reality, however, life is not that simple. A nursing approach based on one theory would not facilitate an understanding of the client as a total human being.

A systems approach reflects the interaction of genetic, biochemical, cognitive, social learning, and object loss theories, as well as sex-role stereotyping. Akiskal and McKinney (1975) suggest that depression results from many variables, including biochemical responses, previous experiences, and learning and behavioral responses. According to these authors, a behavioral response such as social withdrawal is not an isolated factor but has direct impact on biochemical levels in the body. The reverse is also true: Chemical imbalances may contribute to a person's perceiving situations in a distorted manner, thus leading to social withdrawal.

Nursing strategies must be based on an understanding of the various theories and their interrelationship with precipitating factors to be reflective of individual clients—their personalities, their expressions of needs, and their methods of adaptation—inclusive of physical, spiritual, and emotional modes.

Understanding the explanatory theories of depression is critical to developing a comprehensive care plan for clients. Table 22-5 outlines major theoretical orientations and their implications for nursing practice.

TREATMENT MODALITIES
Emergency interventions

Emergency intervention, based on crisis theory, provides short-term measures that can assist clients to cope with depressive and/or suicidal feelings. Crisis services are most frequently offered through community mental health centers, hot lines, and emergency room (ER) settings. The latter has become a major provider of crisis intervention services—a very different focus from the emergency room of a decade ago. The ER has become a major avenue of access to mental healthy services. Jones and Pelikan (1985) note that depression is the most commonly seen psychiatric problem in the ER. The ER is no longer just a place for accident victims with physical trauma but a setting for those individuals experiencing emotional trauma as well. The following is a vignette depicting a depressed client seeking crisis services in an ER.

Sara, a 23-year-old female, came to the ER at 8 PM Saturday evening with generalized complaints of "feeling terrible all over." Her movements were sluggish; her voice was barely audible; her appearance unkempt. Sara's common-law husband brought her because he felt she wasn't acting herself. He described her as "staying in her room most of the time and not wanting to eat anything." Routine blood work and urinalysis were completed. The nurse obtained a psychosocial history from the client and her husband. The history revealed the following data: two-week history of sleep difficulty and early morning awakening; weight loss; lack of desire to do anything and inability to concentrate on tasks; feelings of isolation. The couple indicated that they had recently moved and had

TABLE 22-5 Theoretical orientation and implications for practice

Orientation	Nursing implications
Psychodynamic	Nurses educate parents to give children positive feedback consistently throughout development to foster positive sense of worth. Educate parents to be realistic and consistent in setting expectations that are not based on contingencies. Assist clients to value self; reinforce coping measures that enhance self-esteem.
Psychoanalytic	Nurses assist clients in reviewing past losses and resulting feelings of anger, rage, guilt, shame, which may impact on current behavior. Educate clients to develop more effective measures of coping with loss and to become more able to identify self as worthwhile.
Cognitive	Nurses educate clients about the impact of illogical, negative thought patterns on perception of self, environment, and failure. Assist clients to reframe negative thought processed to reduce self-doubt and deprecation.
Biochemical	Nurses educate clients about physical changes that may affect behavior such as increased sodium levels, decreased norepinephrine. Clients need to be educated regarding the use of psychopharmacologic agents to alter physiologic imbalances.
Social learning	Nurses recognize that clients may have learned a helpless response through repeated experiences that reinforce lack of control over one's life. Assist clients to develop measures that promote mastery over the environment.
Feminist	Nurses assist clients to select appropriate roles that provide satisfaction and increased sense of self-worth. Clients can be assisted to develop coping measures that decrease cognitive dissonance associated with female roles in society.
Family	Nurses recognize that clients exist within the context of a family and may maintain family equilibrium through their symptoms. Nurses can facilitate clients' and families' utilization of more adaptive coping measures while maintaining family equilibrium.
Systems	Nurses recognize that affective disorders result from the interaction of multiple factors. Strategies to assist client adaptation are based on the understanding of the complex interrelationship of these factors.

few social contacts. Sara did not work outside of the home. Her husband held two jobs and was home very little. When asked if she had experienced these feelings before, Sara indicated she had seen a nurse psychotherapist two years previous when she had lost her first baby. The client began to sob: "I should have died too; my husband hasn't loved me since that happened." Sara denied any suicidal thoughts at the time. She revealed no previous suicidal history. Sara requested something to "lift her spirits and help her feel better," indicating that she had had medication previously. The ER nurse explored with Sara the idea of talking with the psychiatrist on call. A referral was made, and Sara was seen that evening.

As the vignette indicates, the ER setting is utilized to provide crisis intervention measures. The presenting symptoms were evaluated quickly and accurately; the client was connected to the appropriate resource immediately. Nurses must reframe their perceptions of the ER setting as an environment for the provision of crisis intervention services. Rund and Hertzler (1983) note that over 23% of those entering ER for service are diagnosed as depressed.

Crisis centers and hot lines also provide services to those in acute emotional distress who are contemplating suicide. These centers utilize trained volunteers who are able to respond to acute situations as well as being capable of identifying potential suicidal behaviors. The following is an adaptation of Wass et al.'s (1988) steps in a hot line interview:

1. Create an atmosphere where the client can share distress.
2. Assess reason for the client's call.
3. Identify perception of the problem.
4. Determine lethality of suicide plan.

5. Discuss alternative solutions.
6. Assist client to seek additional resources as appropriate.
7. Send help if face-to-face contact is necessary.

These centers may also offer suicide prevention education programs to the community, schools, and other interested groups. Individuals can be assisted to develop more effective coping measures as well as increase their ability to identify potential suicidal behavior in others through this type of program.

Individual and group psychotherapy

Individual psychotherapy is initially more fruitful than group psychotherapy. Depressed clients have difficulty seeing themselves as worthwhile people. Becoming part of a group may precipitate stress and be an overwhelming experience. These clients' greatest need is to be accepted as human beings. By relating to other individuals on a one-to-one basis, depressed clients can explore various ways to reach that goal. As they become more sure of themselves and cease to view trust as an unattainable goal, they will venture into a group setting. Groups may be strictly supportive, or they may be analytical and insight-directed. An effective group leader facilitates growth through interaction within the group setting. Each person needs to become what he or she is capable of becoming. This can be accomplished only when a group leader is warm, sincere, and, most important of all, sensitive to the nature of the client's depressive behavior. Through the group process, depressed clients can learn alternative approaches to problems they are encountering. They may even find that the areas they considered problematic are no longer of primary concern. Whether the approach is individual or group, nurse-therapists must place top priority on the worth of human beings and the uniqueness of their responses.

The usefulness of the group approach with depressed women has been documented by Gordon (1982). She noted that depressed women who were exposed to a series of support groups on a regular basis were able to explore their feelings of inadequacy with regard to meeting society's demands, their feelings of anger in relation to dependency on their husbands, fears of being failures as wives and mothers, failure to be assertive, loneliness, the burden of responsibility for the care of elderly parents, and the need to express their feelings and get support. She also noted that many of these themes were reflective not only of depression but also of anxiety and anger.

Recommendations from this study suggest that further studies are necessary to determine the effect of structured group sessions with specific goals in this population. Replication is essential to substantiate the presence of relevant themes and evidence of cohesiveness.

Groups have also emerged to meet the need of the silent victims of suicide—the survivors. In the past the stigma attached to suicide caused relatives and friends of suicide victims to experience a legacy of guilt, shame, and anger. Self-help groups such as Ray of Hope, created by a woman whose husband had shot himself, and A Safe Place provide an atmosphere where suicide survivors can express their grief, anger, and despair; where they can attempt to make some sense of this seemingly senseless act. Bergson (1982) notes that practical issues are also addressed such as how to tell children who are involved; what to tell friends, employers, and relatives; and as well as how to handle possessions. Measures to cope with the devastating loss as well as the repercussions of the suicidal act are the primary focus of the group process.

The importance of this type of group assumes even more relevance as the number of suicides in this country increases dramatically. The American Association of Suicidology notes that the ravages imposed on families and friends must be addressed. In particular, family members often express guilt, anger, and shame. In many instances, suicidal behavior begets suicidal behavior. Children may learn suicide as a viable coping measure or may identify with the parent or relative who commits suicide, thus leading to a suicidal path for themselves. Group intervention facilitates the healthy expression of emotions in the presence of others who have suffered similar experiences.

Bergson indicates that questions have arisen in regard to the nature and composition of the group. For example, should the group be composed of just survivors of suicide victims, or should the individuals involved be a blend of suicide survivors and the bereaved in general? Should the bereaved all be at similar levels of bereavement? Health professionals involved in the counseling of the bereaved indicate that groups can be very effective; however, those individuals who are not comfortable in a group setting, yet need support, should be referred to the appropriate resource. Further research needs to be directed toward understanding the needs of suicide survivors and the modalities that are best suited to meet those needs. (For further discussion of group therapy, see Chapter 13.)

Family therapy

The family is the basic unit in society. Within the context of the family such functions as nurturance, promotion of healthy growth and development, support for adaptation and change, enhancement of self-esteem, and modeling of positive social relationships occur. These functions exist in a mutual, reciprocal manner. For example, in the family with a new infant, the function of the parental system is to provide for basic physiological needs as well as to provide an environment where the infant feels loved and wanted. The dynamics of the parental system impact significantly in either a positive or negative manner on the developing infant. In reciprocal fashion, the arrival of a new being creates changes in the way in which the couple has related to one another. It may place emotional and physical demands on one or both parents that they feel unable to meet.

A severely depressed or extremely agitated manic client is not generally a candidate for involvement in family therapy initially. However, as the client responds to psychopharmacologic agents, he or she may be more able to participate in family therapy sessions.

The underlying themes—low self-esteem, anger, guilt, ambivalence, and social isolation—become the foci of treatment within the context of the family system. Members are assisted to view the behavior of the identified client as symptomatic of dysfunctional family dynamics rather than as one individual's illness. Patterns of ineffective communicating, inadequate methods of coping, nega-

tive interpersonal relationships, and role conflict are evaluated, and strategies to restore equilibrium are developed. Whatever the issues are, roles of family members are interrelated—each member's behavior affects and is affected by all other members in the family system. Family therapy then facilitates a change of behavior for the identified client while at the same time supports other members' needs to develop more effective coping strategies. (For further discussion of family therapy, see Chapter 14.)

Psychopharmacology

Antidepressants can be effective in the treatment of depressive states. These drugs produce the energy that a client needs to invest in the environment rather than retreat into isolation. Two basic categories of drugs are utilized—MAO inhibitors and tricyclic compounds. The drugs in each of these groups treat symptoms rather than underlying dynamics. The administration of medication is therefore not the total solution. Drugs must be utilized concurrently with a supportive relationship. Clients must receive active support from the environment once the medication has enabled them to move out of isolation.

The tricyclics are more widely used than the MAO inhibitors and have a higher success rate. The greatest difficulty encountered with the tricyclics is the premature removal of the client from the medication. Physicians often feel that the depression has lifted when the symptoms have been alleviated. In many cases, however, after a period of a month or more the client is again experiencing symptoms of the depressive response. Maintenance of an adequate dosage is the key to successful control of depression.

Tricyclics seem to affect the brain amine levels, although the specific response is not actually known. Unlike MAO inhibitors, tricyclics have little potential for causing hypertensive crisis. Most side effects can be regulated by adjusting the dosage as necessary.

MAO inhibitors inhibit the production of the enzyme monoamine oxidase, which is present in several vital organs, including the brain. This enzyme reduces the levels of norepinephrine, epinephrine, and serotonin, all of which serve to activate the body. MAO inhibitors counteract this reduction, thus permitting the reactivation of normal levels of these vital hormones.

Side effects and idiosyncratic responses must be considered in a comprehensive assessment of clients. The drugs in this group of medications can be lethal if they are not administered properly.

Lithium carbonate is utilized primarily for the manic phase of manic depression. Marked reduction in manic behavior has been demonstrated after a period of 2 weeks. Lithium carbonate interferes with the elevated levels of norepinephrine and also affects the electrolyte balance within the brain, particularly sodium and potassium levels. Studies have shown that levels of intracellular sodium are low during the manic phase. Lithium increases the ion exchange factor, thus leading to higher levels of intracellular sodium and less impulsive behavior.

Prior to the administration of lithium, the client must have a complete physical, which will provide a data base. It is critical to determine whether the client has a history of cardiovascular or kidney disease; the administration of lithium is contraindicated in those instances. There is a lag period of approximately 1 week between the initial administration and the subsiding of symptoms. Tranquilizers may be used until the lithium takes effect. The nurse's primary role in the administration of lithium is the education of the client to the side effects and the results of misuse of lithium. It is imperative that the client continue to take lithium even though he or she is "feeling fine."

In their study of compliance with lithium regimens Kucera-Bozarth, Beck, and Lyss (1982) reported that 45% of the sample reported compliance but actually were noncompliant based on lithium-level criteria. The unreliability of self-reporting was further demonstrated by the fact that 9% reported noncompliance but were within compliance parameters based on serum lithium levels.

Noncompliant clients tended to be from lower socioeconomic backgrounds and were less likely to hold an internal health locus of control. Data of this nature are of particular importance, since documentation of noncompliance among clients on lithium demonstrates compromise of the management of the disorder. Some clients may even show evidence of gross decompensation after missing only a few doses (Kucera-Bozarth, Beck and Lyss 1982).

Kucera-Bozarth, Beck, and Lyss suggest that nurses consider this data in their assessment and intervention with these clients. Self-reporting cannot be relied upon for accurate prediction of compliance; thus the risks are increased for ineffective management of the disorder and exacerbation of inappropriate behaviors. (For further discussion of pharmacology and nursing implications, see Appendix B.)

Electroconvulsive therapy (ECT)

ECT, the use of electric current to produce seizures, was introduced by Ugo Cerletti and Lucio Bini in 1938. The mechanisms of its actions remain obscure. Following the advent of psychopharmacologic agents in the early 1950s, the use of ECT declined significantly. Negative impressions of its use and side effects were conveyed through mass media such as the film "One Flew over the Cuckoo's Nest." Controversy regarding its effectiveness has led to limited usage of ECT; it is no longer used in public institutions but rather is utilized more frequently in private facilities. Sands et al. (1987) indicate that several studies have been done regarding the use of ECT. For example, a methodological review of 60 research studies on ECT concluded that ECT is effective in its treatment of severe endogenous depression, and its rapid action is useful with actively suicidal clients. Other studies demonstrated no changes pre and post ECT in serum myelin levels, thus indicating its safety for older adults. Furthermore, there has been a lack of strong evidence to suggest long-term residual effects on cognitive function such as memory. Sands did indicate that some studies revealed cognitive changes; however, those changes may have been confounded by other variables, e.g., increased anticholinergic drug levels, premorbid factors such as lack of social support, residual adversity, and symptom severity. Sands concludes that further studies need to be conducted to verify the safety of ECT, to determine the underlying action of ECT, and to identify those factors which enhance the action of ECT.

The care of clients receiving ECT parallels that of clients undergoing surgery. Prior to therapy, the nurse should explain the procedure thoroughly and simply. A complete physical, including spinal x-ray film, is required. A consent form must be signed. On the morning of the treatment, clients should eat or drink nothing. They should remove dentures, put on loosely fitting clothes, and void prior to the administration of the treatment. Tranquilizers may be given if anxiety levels are rising. Atropine may or may not be given to reduce secretions.

The client is placed on a stretcher in the treatment room, and a short-acting barbiturate is given intravenously, followed by a muscle relaxant. A rubber mouthpiece is inserted to maintain a patent airway. The shock is administered, and a grand mal seizure results. Nurses in attendance allow the client's body to move with the tonic and clonic spasms, rather than holding him or her down. Restraining the body often causes fractures rather than preventing them.

Following the treatment, routine postoperative care is the primary nursing goal. Positioning the client on the side, with the head tilted, facilitates the maintenance of an open airway and reduces the possibility of aspiration.

Although clients may be alert and awake immediately following the treatment, assessment of vital signs every 15 minutes for the first hour is necessary. Since periods of confusion may occur after the treatment, clients need to be protected from injuring themselves. Nurses should orient clients to their surroundings to enable them to feel in control of themselves and their environment.

Once clients are able to, they return to their own rooms. Nourishment is provided as well as an opportunity to rest. Electroconvulsive treatments are given in a series, ranging anywhere from 12 to 60.

Electroconvulsive therapy alone is not the solution to depression. As in other treatments, a client must be supported by a relationship with a significant other. Once the client's defensive barrier has been lowered, nurses need to be there to provide an atmosphere in which exploration of issues and problem solving are priorities.

Nursing Intervention
PRIMARY PREVENTION

Programs of primary prevention of depression are just beginning to be organized. Clinical research is providing nurses with steadily increasing amounts of data regarding the delicate interweaving of the factors underlying loss and depression. Major goals of primary prevention are the promotion of positive feelings toward the self and the facilitation of a healthy adaptation to loss. The focus of this level of prevention is the promotion of open lines of communication and freedom of expression of feelings.

Nurses need to be aware of the following principles as they engage in activities of primary prevention of the major affective disorders:

1. Patterns of withdrawal and elation are a means of coping with unconscious conflicts in order to maintain functional ability.
2. Loss is a fundamental theme in the origins of affective disorders because of its effect on feelings of self-worth and personal control.
3. Individuals exist within the context of relationships that have a reciprocal effect on all members of the relationship.
4. Awareness of feelings and social relatedness are decreased further during crisis situations.
5. Multiple variables are interrelated in their effect on coping strategies.
6. Crisis situations increase personal vulnerability and limit perceptions of internal control and sense of worth to self and others.

Goals for primary prevention of major affective disorders include:

1. Minimizing effects of factors that predispose individuals to affective disorders
2. Identifying high-risk populations

Nurses can implement these goals by assisting individuals in their ability to cope with loss and change through parental and family counseling and by identifying high-risk populations.

Coping with loss

Since loss is a fundamental theme in the origins of depression, primary preventive efforts need to be directed toward helping people to adapt to the various loss situations that occur throughout the life cycle. The crises of loss begin with the loss of the warm, uterine environment and end with the ultimate loss—the loss of one's own life. Programs such as those outlined in parent effectiveness training courses, health education curricula, and workshop presentations can identify potential loss situations and probable reactions to them. Individuals can learn to be managers of their lives rather than victims of circumstance. Loss situations can be turned into learning situations. Disappointments can be handled appropriately. Children can then be better equipped to react to crises in a healthy fashion in later life. Through positive appraisals from significant others, a child's self-esteem can be enhanced at particularly crucial times of development. The child will learn to be adept at using problem-solving faculties, a discovery that in turn reaffirms positive feelings of self.

Primary preventive programs are still new, yet they serve as the basis for the healthy development of tomorrow's generation.

Grieving is a healthy response to loss, whether it be of a love object, self-worth, status, or function. The resolution of this process ultimately leads to the investment of energy in new relationships and to positive feelings regarding the self. When grief is prolonged, however, and the loss is not resolved, anxiety arises. The depressive response is activated to contain and/or diminish the anxiety (Hauser and Feinberg, 1976). Nursing intervention therefore needs to be directed toward facilitating healthy adaptation to loss. The following principles are important in such intervention:

1. The primary goal is to promote catharsis. Verbalization enables clients to work through feelings of anger, sadness, relief, and helplessness. Be particularly cognizant of nonverbal communication and the client's cultural orientation concerning verbalization of feelings.

2. Recognize that ambivalence is common. There may be sorrow that the loss has occurred. Yet in the case of a client who is experiencing the loss of a relative, there may be a sense of relief that the process of dying is finally over. For example, a family may feel a sense of relief after the death of a loved one who has been chronically ill. These ambivalent feelings are quite common; however, they are also quite upsetting. Let the client know that these feelings are quite normal. Provide a setting in which these feelings can be shared.

3. Assess clients to determine what phase of the mourning process they have entered.

4. Assist clients in maintaining contact with highly valued objects or people. This is not the time for grieving clients to sell all belongings or give them away.

5. Support already existing coping mechanisms, such as denial. Denial is quite commonly utilized to deal with pain experienced in a loss situation. If this mechanism is removed, the client will replace it with another, more pathological one. Do not reinforce denial, however; present reality as it can be tolerated.

6. Help clients to control their environments to prevent additional losses. Encourage them to participate as much as possible in the normal activities of daily living. They will then be able to feel as though their life-styles have not been irreversibly altered. They will see that they are still able to perceive events occurring in the environment accurately and that they can actively deal with them as necessary.

7. Be patient and tolerant of the wide range of behavior that can be exhibited by the grieving client. Anger toward the lost object that is released into constructive channels during this phase will not likely be turned inward upon the self at a later time.

8. Provide a private, quiet room for grieving clients in order that they may feel comfortable in their unique expressions of grief.

9. Assist the grieving person and family to review previous encounters with loss and methods of coping with them. Often individuals are unaware of their repertoire of coping mechanisms. The nurse can identify them with the client. The grieving person thus can be helped to develop a healthy approach to

loss rather than to view it as a negative situation each time it occurs.

10. Allow enough space and time for the individual to grieve. Each person is unique in his or her responses, particularly in the response to loss. Healthy resolution may take as long as 2 years, depending on the extent and type of relationship with the lost object. Anniversaries, birthdays, a special song, or a type of food may cause a normal reactivation of sadness. It is important to point out that such a reaction is acceptable behavior and to encourage the sharing of feelings regarding the precipitating factor.

11. Since loss is inevitable in the developmental cycle, nursing intervention must involve anticipatory work, as was previously pointed out. Recognize that an individual is having a difficult time resolving a situation. There may be a continued state of denial; the person may be unable to progress to the awareness phase. Further supportive therapy is then necessary. In addition, nurses may want to consult resource people in the event that a depressive response is prolonged.

Identification of high-risk individuals

Community health nurses, family and pediatric nurse practitioners, and school nurses work with children and their families in a variety of settings. Through observation of family interaction—whether a marital dyad expecting the birth of a first child or a family visit to a well-child clinic—nurses can note predominant patterns of relating, personal and group coping strategies, and roles of various members. As nurses become more familiar with family structure and patterns of relationships, children who come from families where social withdrawal, elation, or self-destruction are characteristic behaviors can be identified.

Assessment of the family system should include recognition of:

1. Unrealistically high expectations of child in the parent-child relationship
2. Unmet dependency needs in parenting figures

3. Contingency-based expression of love and gratification from parent to child
4. Lack of consistency of parental response in regard to giving gratification
5. Consistent lack of positive reinforcement for attempts and achievements
6. Consistent use of social withdrawal or elated behaviors as a means of coping
7. History of losses that have never been fully resolved
8. Overfunctioning or underfunctioning dyad in family system
9. History of suicidal behavior in present family system or family of origin
10. Consistent inability to express feelings of anger, apprehension, and dejection to others
11. Persistent perception of self, environment, and future in a negativistic manner
12. Persistent lack of role-appropriate definitions of self in various stages of the life cycle

These factors must also be considered in relation to biological, sociocultural, emotional, and spiritual factors that may predispose individuals to major affective disorders.

Parental and family counseling

Family members are often not cognizant of their impact on one another. As noted earlier, individuals exist within the context of relationships. Roles are maintained and behaviors learned through these relationships. Coping styles are often learned from parental role models. Facilitation of expression of feelings in an authentic and direct manner by nurses may enhance coping behavior in the developing family members and reduce the possibility of old conflicts and expectations being played out in new relationships.

Prenatal classes, well-baby clinics, and even physicians' offices are important target areas. The central goal at this level is to facilitate the mothering response, not just physically but emotionally as well. Mothers who are anxious and fearful are unable to meet their own needs, let alone attend to those of their infants. Parents who feel positive about themselves are more capable of allowing their children the room to explore their territory, to develop a sense of their own personal space—in other words, to be! Children need positive reinforcement on a continuous basis—not sporadically, when expectations are fulfilled. Mistrust begins to develop, as do feelings of low self-worth, when reinforcement is only sporadic. A child, as he or she grows up in such an anxious, uncomfortable environment, is not able to relate successfully to others in his or her social world. Relationships are characterized either by withdrawal or by aggressive, manipulative behavior. These responses tend to separate the individual from others even more.

Initial assessments are tentative and must be validated through consultation with other health care providers. Intervention should not be planned based on single observations. Health professionals such as community health nurses, family nurse clinicians, and occupational health nurses have the opportunity to observe and interact with clients and families on repeated occasions. Rapport develops between health care provider and client-family. Out of this relationship emerges a foundation of trust and accurate observation that can result in referral to a mental health resource—the goal of early identification in secondary prevention. It must be remembered that some clients find it difficult to enter into a relationship with a mental health resource person—whether the person be nurse-therapist, psychologist, social worker, or psychiatrist. These ambivalent feelings can be explored in a supportive relationship provided by the referring nurse. An empathic relationship can allay many fears as well as create an atmosphere that motivates the individual to enter further treatment. Nurses must also be careful not to move individuals too quickly into the mental health delivery system. Anxiety and inaccurate observations on the part of the referring nurse can be detrimental in themselves.

SECONDARY PREVENTION

Intervention in secondary prevention is based on the nursing process. In this section individual patterns of behavior will be addressed, with specific strategies of intervention being identified. However, it is important for nurses to consider these principles of action regardless of the presenting behavior or symptom:

1. The focus is client-centered rather than symptom-centered.
2. Behavior and/or symptoms are mechanisms of defense and attempts to maintain a sense of self-worth.
3. Clients need acceptance and approval as vulnerability is increased.
4. Repressed hostility may be overtly expressed when pressure is increased.
5. Anger should not be provoked, since clients fear the impact of their own hostility on self and others.
6. Nurses and other staff members will have emotional responses to client behavior. These responses must be considered within the context of the current relationship as well as in relation to past experiences. Nurses cannot negate these feelings; rather, they must learn how to use their feelings in a positive manner with the client.

These principles will guide nurses in their observations, data analysis, decision making, and determination of appropriate intervention strategies.

Nursing process

The nursing process acts as a guide for therapeutic intervention.

ASSESSMENT*

Client identification of the problem is a key factor in the assessment process. Nurses need to begin at that point which the client deems appropriate. A mental status examination as well as information relating to social and family history provides a comprehensive base (see Chapter 11). Specific areas of assessment include:

1. Presenting symptoms—slowed cognitions, retarded or agitated psychomotor activity, sleep disturbances, lack of energy, fatigue, verbal paucity
2. Emotional state—feelings of helplessness, hopelessness, lack of purpose and self-worth, anger, self-destructive feelings

---

*For assessment of suicidal potential, see box on pp. 706-707.

3. Stress-producing situations—are these generated or potentiated by maladaptive coping strategies? (What changes or losses have occurred in the past six months?)
4. Coping behaviors—how effective are they? (What coping strategies were used in the family and how effective were they?)
5. Available support systems and resources—friends, parents, others
6. Client strengths—what can and does the client do for self and/or others—i.e., regularly employed? Able to meet own personal hygiene needs? (What does client expect of self? Is this realistic?)
7. Holistic health status—biological, psychological, intellectual, sociocultural, and spiritual status of client. (These factors will influence client's wellness either positively or negatively, and in some instances, in both ways. For example, conflict between one's expectations

of self and societal expectations may occur, generating guilt and ambivalence.)

ANALYSIS OF DATA

Careful assessment of data enables the nurse to have a *beginning* understanding of clients, the contexts in which they exist (families and other relationships), and their perceptions of the identified problems. At this point nurses may be ready to identify nursing diagnoses. (It is important to note that throughout the nurse-client relationship, data are gathered and nursing diagnoses reformulated as appropriate.)

PLANNING AND IMPLEMENTATION

Following are nursing care plans that reflect a realistic approach to secondary preventive intervention. The nurse may initially establish goals; but as therapy progresses, the client should enter into goal setting to ensure commitment to accomplishing these goals.

Text continued on p. 707.

NURSING CARE PLAN

Clients with Patterns of Depression

Long-term Outcomes	Short-term Outcomes	Nursing Strategies
Nursing diagnosis: 296.20-36)	Impaired social interaction related to unmet dependency needs (NANDA 3.1.1; DSM-III-R	
Develop relationships that are based on acknowledgment of unmet dependency needs Decrease feelings of poor self-esteem	Recognize feelings generated by unmet dependency needs Identify situations that arouse feelings related to unmet needs Develop more adaptive methods of communicating needs	Provide an environment that encourages the expression of feelings within the cultural context of the client Confront behaviors that are attention-seeking Support efforts to care for self Do not do what the client can do for himself or herself Reinforce the client's ability to make decisions and problem solve Explore what realistic dependency needs are in a relationship Teach assertiveness skills when appropriate Include family in exploration of potential role changes and more adaptive methods of coping

Long-term Outcomes	Short-term Outcomes	Nursing Strategies

Nursing diagnosis: Powerlessness (NANDA 7.3.2) and hopelessness secondary to depressed mood (NANDA 7.3.1) (DSM-III-R 296.40-70; 296.20-40)

Work through conflict *generating* feelings of helplessness, hopelessness, and powerlessness and creating feelings of inadequacy Build relationships with others on assertive, decisive behaviors	Verbalize feelings of helplessness, hopelessness, and powerlessness within the cultural context Identify current situations that create the above feelings Relate past situations that may have aroused similar feelings Describe expectations of self in five dimensions—biological, intellectual, psychological, sociocultural, and spiritual, and determine their appropriateness to situations; develop a realistic perception of self Develop more appropriate coping strategies and interpersonal skills	Assist clients in manipulating their environments so that they can effect change Recognize that helplessness may be a learned response; provide situations in which clients can exert some control over their environments In response to behavior that indicates hoplessness, do not become "Suzy Sunshine" and try to talk clients out of their depression; instead, work with them to develop experiences in which they will receive positive feedback Do not condemn the negative feelings of clients, since they have a right to those feelings; on the other hand, do not perpetuate those feelings by condoning them

Nursing diagnosis: Inadequate nutritional intake (NANDA 1.1.2.2), altered patterns of urinary elimination (NANDA 1.3.2), and constipation (NANDA 1.3.1.1) related to major mood disorder (DSM-III-R 296.40-70, 296.20-40)

Reach optimal level of nutritional status and eliminatory regularity Develop an awareness of the relationship of good nutrition and elimination to increased feelings of self-worth	Maintain adequate daily nutritional status Plan meals and snacks that are nutritionally sound Select times that are most pleasurable and will maximize good eating habits	Monitor eating patterns and fluid intake; calorie counts and intake and output need to be recorded Supplemental feedings may be necessary, i.e., high-protein foods Determine food preferences and have them available Provide fingerfoods for the hyperactive client Observe and record all bowel movements; offer laxatives as necessary to prevent constipation Provide large amounts of fluid to prevent constipation

Continued.

Clients with Patterns of Depression

Long-term Outcomes	Short-term Outcomes	Nursing Strategies

Nursing diagnosis: Dysfunctional grieving related to the loss of a parent (NANDA 9.2.1.1; DSM-III-R 296.40-70, 296.20-40)

Work through conflict that generates feelings of guilt Relate to others in a manner that is not based on persistent expressions of inappropriate guilt	Verbalize feelings about interpersonal relationships and behaviors without imposing excessive self-blame for their appropriateness or inappropriateness Identify current situations that arouse feelings of guilt Relate past relationships that may arouse similar feelings Realistically appraise five dimensions of self—biological, psychological, intellectual, sociocultural, and spiritual Develop more appropriate coping strategies and interpersonal skills	Do not negate client's guilt feelings, even though they seem unreasonable Avoid closing off avenues of communication by refusing to listen to the constant degradation of self; such a refusal will only serve to reinforce the client's already existing low self-esteem and self-doubt Encourage the client to accept the forgiveness of others and to look to the future instead of the past Explore alternatives to client's self-inflicted punishment; can the client experience joy in any activities? If there is even the slightest kindling of interest in an activity, facilitate the client's participation in it

Nursing diagnosis: Chronic low self-esteem related to feelings of inadequacy and loss (NANDA 7.1.2; DSM-III-R 296.40-70, 296.20-36)

Work through conflict that generates worthlessness Develop relationships that promote feelings of confidence and self-worth	Verbalize feelings of low self-worth Identify current situations that arouse feelings of guilt Relate past situations that may arouse similar feelings Realistically appraise five dimensions of self—biological, psychological, intellectual, sociocultural, and spiritual strengths and weaknesses will be put into proper perspective Develop more appropriate coping strategies and interpersonal skills	Accept clients as unique human beings with needs specifically their own; one of the most devastating factors in the depressed client's life has been a lack of praise and gratification for *being* Define goals that are attainable so that clients can begin to achieve positive feedback in relation to their capabilities; do not make situations so easy that success is achieved with little effort; this will only serve to reinforce feelings of worthlessness and the inability to function; start with simple activities and move to complex Accept but do not condone the feelings of worthlessness exhibited; avoid a power struggle; a shouting match between client and nurse as to the worth of the client will certainly not further any type of relationship Recognize clients' needs for privacy—do not "crowd" them; you must maintain a delicate balance; let clients know that you are concerned yet do not overwhelm them with your presence Attend to physical hygiene and nutritional needs (these most basic needs must be met before you can move on to the development of a positive concept of self)

Long-term Outcomes	Short-term Outcomes	Nursing Strategies

Nursing diagnosis: Potential activity intolerance related to manic phase of bipolar disorder (NANDA 6.1.1.3; DSM-III-R 296.40-46)

Return to situation-appropriate levels of activity Reestablish relationships with others within appropriate social contexts	Maintain a balance between activity and sleep Utilize physical energy in an appropriate manner to release tension	Decrease environmental stimuli Note behavior indicative of increased restlessness and limit stimuli by removing the client to a quieter area Administer medications as necessary Discuss expectations of client behavior as soon as it is appropriate; provide some sort of structured environment with well-defined expectations Encourage verbalization of feelings and seek more effective methods of coping through active problem solving Provide time for physical outlet of energy through structured activities—do not engage in extremely competitive activities Include time for a short nap or rest period during the day while encouraging night time sleeping Observe sleep patterns and determine fatigue levels Provide a quiet atmosphere prior to bedtime, i.e., restful music, warm milk, reading Determine the client's level of responsibility for limiting his or her own activity levels

Nursing diagnosis: Impaired verbal communication related to feelings of inadequacy and lack of self-worth (NANDA 2.1.1.1; DSM-III-R 296.20-36)

Verbalize thoughts and feelings relative to one's own life experiences, whether they be positive and/or negative Take on the responsibility of resolving feelings by finding others to talk to, and develop a network of support	Identify situations in which feelings can be shared in an appropriate manner Expand more fully a discussion of routine daily events	Provide for opportunities in which verbalization can take place, i.e., a quiet atmosphere with little environmental stimuli Encourage expression of thoughts and feelings regarding events and/or people that are described by client Validate client's nonverbal messages so as to encourage expression of feelings Provide structured time that is just for client and nurse or client and significant others to talk Accept client's limited verbalizations while recognizing potential for increased expression of thoughts and feelings Assess family for overfunctioning members and subsequent disconfirmation of client's expression of feelings

Continued.

NURSING CARE PLAN—cont'd

Clients with Patterns of Depression

Long-term Outcomes	Short-term Outcomes	Nursing Strategies
Nursing diagnosis: Ineffective individual coping related to repression of anger (NANDA 5.1.1.1; DSM-III-R 296.20-70)		
Develop non-violent ways of express-ing anger Decrease anx-iety associ-ated with expression of anger	Recognize feelings of anger Identify situations that arouse feelings of anger Learn to assertively commu-nicate angry feelings	Provide a trust relationship so anger can safely be ver-balized within the cultural context of the client Point out indirect expressions of anger (e.g., sarcasm, fist clenching) Assist client to identify and label anger Set limits and provide safeguards in the event that the client tries to act out angry feelings against self or others Discuss anger as a normal human response Provide physical outlets for angry feeligs (e.g., jogging, tennis, hammering) Help client identify and describe objects of anger Explore current ways of coping with anger Support effective current coping behaviors Explore socially acceptable alternative ways of coping with anger, including acceptable limits and client's responsibility for own behavior Teach client assertive ways of communicating angry feelings Support client in trying out new ways of coping with an-ger Assist client to evaluate effectiveness of new coping behaviors
Nursing diagnosis: Bathing/hygiene self-care deficit related to lack of self-esteem and feelings of inadequacy (NANDA Self-care-6.5.1, Hygiene-6.5.2, Dressing-6.5.3; Toileting-6.5.4; DSM-III-R 296.20-40, 296.40-70)		
Carry out ac-tivities of daily living on a regular basis Develop an awareness of the impor-tance of participating in self-care in relation to positive feel-ings of self-worth	Establish and maintain ade-quate personal hygiene, i.e., bathing, dressing, and caring for clothing Participate in keeping own personal space neat and clean	Assist the client in bathing and dressing when he or she is unable to do so Encourage the client to take responsibility for personal hygiene as is appropriate, based on mood level Provide positive feedback for personal care as the cli-ent assumes increasing responsibility Structure times for getting up, bathing, and dressing so that client does not spend excessive time in bed

Long-term Outcomes	Short-term Outcomes	Nursing Strategies

Nursing diagnosis: Potential for self-directed violence related to feelings of low self-esteem and lack of impulse control (NANDA 9.2.2; DSM-III-R 296.50-56, 296.20-40)

Long-term Outcomes	Short-term Outcomes	Nursing Strategies
Work through internal conflict relating to feelings of poor self-worth and inadequacy Acknowledge and accept hostile feelings and unrealistic expectations towards self and others Decrease impulsive self-destructive behaviors Develop an insight into self-destructive behavior and its relationship to feelings of poor self-worth, hopelessness, and personal inadequacy Develop more appropriate methods of coping with suicidal feelings	Increase ability to discuss feelings as they occur in response to specific situations Identify stressors that initiate self-destructive behaviors Identify ways in which life situations can be made less stressful Identify unrealistic expectations of self and/or others Identify and explore more effective problem-solving methods	The initial phase of implementation involves providing a safe environment and assessing suicidal potential (see box on pp. 706-707). • Locating the client's room in an area central to the nurses' station • Removing sharp objects and other items that could be potentially dangerous • Remaining with clients if they are using items such as razors, lighters, etc. • Knowing where the client is at all times during the day—particularly at times when staff is busiest (e.g., change of shift and team meetings) or when there is a smaller staff (nights and weekends) • Checking periodically throughout the night at irregular times so that clients cannot identify a pattern in *your* behavior • Noting client behavior patterns and changes (e.g., decreased communication; sudden mood lift; increased frustration, dependency, or hopelessness; lack of interest in surroundings; subtle discussions of activities, such as with family, that no longer include the client) • Being alert to storing of medications • Observing relationships with other clients, i.e., those that may *reinforce* self-destructive behaviors or those individuals who may become confidants of the suicidal client • Maintaining lines of communication and interest—respecting privacy while at the same time not allowing the client to remain socially isolated • Identifying positive aspects of self and assisting the client in their integration into self • Reinforcing positive accomplishments • Assisting the client to deal with expression of angry feelings—promoting an atmosphere in which clients can test out more effective methods of coping with anger • Incorporating clergy (pastor, priest, rabbi) into the treatment plan at client's request • Examining client behavior within the context of current relationships and identifying stressors and strengths within those relationships (family, job, etc.) • Exploring alternative methods of coping with feelings should self-destructive feelings occur again • Identifying "lifeline" persons to contact when clients begin to feel they cannot control impulsive behavior

Assessment of suicidal potential

Demographic data	The following information should be obtained: name, age, sex, race, education religion, and living arrangements.
Hazard	What happened within the 2 to 3 weeks prior to entry into the health care system? Have there been any significant developmental or situational crises? Were there potential loss situations that might have precipitated the threat? The most crucial task is to identify the meaning the individual ascribes to such an event.
Crisis	What is the client experiencing internally? What are the psychological and somatic symptoms, and how severe are they? Be alert to the fact that as depression lifts, clients are more apt to attempt suicide, because they are able to view it as a way to resolve problems. Is the level of hopelessness elevated to such a degree that the suicide potential is great?
Coping mechanisms	It is important to determine how an individual usually approaches a problem. What makes the present situation different from others he or she has encountered? Is there a dependence on alcohol or drug abuse present that might alter the client's level of impulse control? Find out what the client perceives as helpful in reducing stress.
Significant others	Who constitutes the primary support system or systems in the client's environment? What does the client feel would be the reaction of significant others to his or her current behavior? Is this perception real or distorted? Contact may have to be made with these persons in order to obtain a complete data base.
Social and personal resources	What social resources, such as shelter, food, and clothing, are available? Personal resources include money, time, physical and mental abilities, and job. Clients are more able to cope with a crisis when such resources are available.
Past suicide attempts	Any past suicide attempts must be evaluated. Their seriousness, the methods used, and the resources available prior to those attempts should be determined. The current risk may be great if past attempts have been frequent and serious.
History of psychiatric problems	If the person has been hospitalized for emotional difficulties in the past, the risk of suicide should be considered great. Has the client made contact with any other psychiatric agencies? How did the client respond to them? Such information gives the nurse an idea of what alternatives have been explored and of what has been useful and what has not.
Current medical status	Is the client being treated by a health professional at the present time? If so, why is he or she now seeking out other people for support? Counseling is an emotionally charged process and may engender many feelings that a client feels he or she cannot share with the current therapist. The client may simply need another listening ear at this time. He or she then could be referred back to the original therapist. Does the client have any physical illnesses, acute or chronic, that may precipitate a stress response? If so, has this illness been going on for a long time? What were previous methods of coping, and were they effective? What has caused these coping mecha-

Adapted from Hatton, Valente and Rink (1977).

Assessment of suicidal potential—cont'd

	nisms to be ineffective? Has there been any significant change in health status within the past 6 months? Has the client consulted a physician during that time? Often, a person's attempts at making needs known fall upon deaf ears. We need to be acutely alert for the underlying theme "Please help me."
Life-style	Is the individual's life-style fairly stable? Or does he or she move from one job to another, from one location to another, and from one group of friends to another? Such a life pattern offers no consistency, no certainty as to where a person might be or what he or she might be doing. Clients who have not had stable patterns of interaction with other people will be less able to cope with any significant crisis situations.
Suicidal plan	Four basic criteria are involved in the measurement of suicidal intent: method, availability, specificity, and lethality. Has the client selected a particular method? How available is that method? Assume, for instance, that a woman tells you she has four full bottles of barbiturates on the nightstand next to her and that she rattles them into the phone. This action alerts you to the fact that suicide could be readily attempted. If the individual has formulated a specific plan of action, right down to the exact time and place, then there is a marked increase in suicidal risk. How lethal is the method? Lethality can be expressed in terms of the time span between the suicidal act and death. The most lethal method is shooting; hanging is second. Slashing one's wrists is last. Ingestion of pills poses considerable danger, yet there is time to get help to an individual. Gunshot wounds and hanging have a more immediate effect. Assessment of a suicidal plan cannot be a one-time activity; the criteria must continually be reviewed if a nurse is to act effectively to prevent suicidal acts.

Hatton et al. (1977) have developed a system for rating suicidal risk; this system appears in Table 22-6. The types of behavior listed are not mutually exclusive, nor are they arranged in a hierarchy. The types of behavior are evaluated in terms of a hypothetical scale from 1 to 9. A rating of 1 to 3 indicates low risk. A rating of 4 to 6 indicates moderate risk, and a rating of 7 to 9 indicates high risk. All criteria are not necessarily relevant to all clients.

Particular groups are at risk because the nature and quantity of stressors they experience. Hankoff and Einsedler (1979) have defined the following groups as being at risk:

1. *Alcoholics*—these individuals are characterized by poor impulse control, dependency, depression, and excessive use of denial. Often

they drink and take drugs concurrently, which increases the possibility of an adverse reaction and death. The suicidal intent should be considered perhaps in a passive sense; however, over time the ultimate result remains the same—death.

2. *Elderly*—as noted previously, suicide in the elderly population represents 25% of the total of suicides committed. Those individuals are confronted with multiple life changes, including physical as well as psychological assaults on the sense of self. Previous coping strategies and available support systems are significant factors in determining depression and suicide risk.

3. *Adolescents*—during this time of rapid physi-

TABLE 22-6 Assessing the degree of suicidal risk

Behavior or symptoms	Intensity of risk		
	Low	**Moderate**	**High**
Anxiety	Mild	Moderate	High, or panic state
Depression	Mild	Moderate	Severe
Isolation/withdrawal	Vague feelings of depression, no withdrawal	Some feelings of helplessness, hopelessness, and withdrawal	Hopeless, helpless, withdrawn, and self-deprecating
Daily functioning	Fairly good in most activities	Moderately good in some activities	Not good in any activities
Resources	Several	Some	Few or none
Coping strategies/devices being utilized	Generally constructive	Some that are constructive	Predominantly destructive
Significant others	Several who are available	Few or only one available	Only one, or none available
Psychiatric help in past	None, or positive attitude toward	Yes, and moderately satisfied with	Negative view of help received
Life-style	Stable	Moderately stable or unstable	Unstable
Alcohol/drug use	Infrequently to excess	Frequently to excess	Continual abuse
Previous suicide attempts	None, or of low lethality	None to one or more of moderate lethality	None to multiple attempts of high lethality
Disorientation/disorganization	None	Some	Marked
Hostility	Little or none	Some	Marked
Suicidal plan	Vague, fleeting thoughts but no plan	Frequent thoughts, occasional ideas about a plan	Frequent or constant thought with a specific plan

From Hatton, Valente, and Rink (1977).

cal growth and psychological adjustment, a person is particularly vulnerable. Suicide as a solution to conflicts is the second leading cause of death in this age group (for further discussion see Chapter 17).

4. *Police and physicians*—these individuals often deal with multiple serious problems on a regular basis. Society expects them to "take care of" and protect its members. This expectation can cause conflict and role confusion when the expectation is not met. Neither police officers nor physicians are expected, however, to experience stress or have difficulties of their own, lest they be labeled as "unfit." Stressors are allowed to build; isolation from significant others because of job responsibility and a sense of personal failure may lead to the suicidal act.

5. *Help-rejecting clients*—clients of this category are those who are unable to accept treatment or follow prescribed treatment plans. This type of client produces conflict for nurses as well as a sense of frustration, anger, and guilt. In a sense these clients are attempting to maintain a sense of control over their lives as well as prevent further loss of self-worth. Changes in life-style required by a treatment regimen may cause feelings of dependence and a lack of being a viable, active self. For example, a cardiac client with a lethal arrhythmia was advised to reduce his physical workload. The possibility of altering his productivity led to feelings of apprehension and uncertainty as to his own worth. He proceeded to return to work at his previous pace. Upon 3-month follow-up, his work schedule

was noted by the clinical specialist. She was able to negotiate some changes in his work schedule, thus reducing both the risk of further heart damage and the loss of self-worth.

Responding to treatment plans also implies that one will indeed reach a higher level of wellness. In some cases, getting well may be threatening, since this change in role impacts on current relationships. It becomes important to determine the benefits of remaining in a "sick role" that could lead to self-destruction. Nurses also need to identify the risk to personal worth that is required by adhering to a prescribed treatment plan. The value of choice of a "good life" is a consideration for both the client and the health professional—particularly when life is at risk. The degree of helplessness is said to vary with the assumptions one has about causes of the uncontrollable events. Individuals who blame themselves are more likely to exhibit greater helplessness than those who blame external events or persons. Murphy (1982) suggests that learned helplessness results in cognitive, motivational, and emotional deficits. Cognitively, individuals expect uncontrollability. Lack of motivation ensues because of individuals' perceptions that things will not change, no matter what they do. Self-esteem is lowered and depressed affect results when individuals feel that events are beyond their control.

Murphy (1982) notes that there is considerable evidence that major life changes perceived and labeled as negative lead to increased risk for physical or psychosomatic illness. Learned helplessness seems to result when individuals are exposed to uncontrollable events and believe that nothing can be changed.

However, there are limitations to the theory. Further questions will need to be asked: When is helplessness adaptive or maladaptive; under what depressive conditions does helplessness exist; and during what situations do individuals seek causal information? Murphy concludes that psychiatric–mental health nurses have a vital role in determining expectations of control in their clients and in testing attributional theories. Strategies of intervention may then be designed to assist individuals in coping with situational and transitional events that generate feelings of helplessness.

EVALUATION

Client, family, and/or significant others in collaboration with the nurse should review client progress toward goal attainment. The following areas need to be included in the evaluation process:

1. Degree of resolution of internal conflicts relative to affective disorders
2. Level and degree of goal attainment, i.e., improvement in client functioning demonstrated by use of more adaptive coping strategies
3. Identification of goals that need modification and revision
4. Designation of appropriate support systems other than the nurse-client relationship
   a. Available support systems within the context of current client relationships, e.g., friends, co-workers, clergy
   b. Community mental health centers which provide walk-in treatment, day/night hospitals
   c. Specialized services for treatment of affective disorders, e.g., mood clinics, suicide prevention centers and "hot-lines," and lithium clinics

TERTIARY PREVENTION

Continued research in the area of family dynamics and the interrelationship of variables is an important concern of tertiary prevention. Nurses need to direct efforts toward modifying the environment to reduce the intensity of some of the stress factors that ultimately lead to depression.

What happens to an individual who has experienced loss? Where is the follow-up care? When symptoms disappear, the underlying dynamics may remain. A discussion of what significance the loss holds as well as its correlation with past losses can facilitate an individual's understanding of coping measures. Nurses need to be acutely aware of the need to provide follow-up care for clients who have experienced depressive responses, even though symptoms may have subsided. It is quite easy and comfortable for these clients to revert to maladaptive methods of coping when stress again becomes overwhelming. It is therefore of utmost importance that such a client, who may possess little self-worth, feels that there is always a link with someone who cares. Contact with family members and others in the community can help the client to develop a social network of support that can facilitate reentry into the community.

CHAPTER SUMMARY

Loss occurs throughout the life cycle. The grieving process can be a healthy, adaptive response to loss. Individuals develop a pattern of response to loss that is based on early childhood experiences. It is important to understand the significance of these early experiences with loss to facilitate the open sharing of feelings. Grief is a normal response. Nurses can encourage people to participate actively in the grieving process, whether the grief be for the loss of a person, status, self-esteem, a body part, or a bodily function. Through such active involvement, a person can lay a foundation for coping with future losses.

Recurrently unhealthy or maladaptive responses to loss situations may lead to a delayed grief reaction, depression, or even suicide. Nurses need to recognize that many variables may be responsible for the development of a depressive response. Several major theories of depression, manic-depressive reactions, and suicide have been presented. A nursing assessment must reflect an integration of these theories, since no one theory can explain depressive behavior.

Individual and group therapy, the administration of psychopharmaceuticals, electroconvulsive therapy, emergency interventions, and family therapy have been discussed as treatment modalities.

Nursing intervention has been discussed in terms of the three levels of prevention. Primary prevention is directed toward facilitating an individual's coping with loss. Secondary prevention involves the use of specific techniques in response to each of the predominant themes of depression. The goals of tertiary prevention are to minimize the effects of loss, through discussion of an individual's adaptive (or maladaptive) mechanisms, and to facilitate the reentry of the client into the community.

SELF-DIRECTED LEARNING

Sensitivity-Awareness Exercises

The purposes of the following exercises are to:
- Develop an awareness of the vulnerability of client-families to major affective disorders (mania, depression, suicidal behavior)
- Develop an awareness of the interrelationship of factors in the etiology of major affective disorders
- Develop an awareness of the subjective experiences of clients who are suffering from affective disorders
- Develop an awareness of your own feelings and attitudes that are aroused when working with clients experiencing major affective disorders

1. Try to imagine that you are experiencing one of the following disorders. Explain why you selected that particular disorder, and describe how you think it might feel to experience that disorder/behavior.
   a. Manic disorder
   b. Depressive disorder
   c. Self-destructive behavior
2. Describe what it would be like to have a family member or a significant other suffer from one of the major affective disorders. Which disorder do you think would be easiest to tolerate in a family member or significant other? Why? Which would be the hardest to tolerate? Why?
3. What might be some of your feelings and reactions as a nurse to clients who are suffering from major affective disorders? Helplessness? Frustration? Anger?
4. Examine your feelings toward clients who have attempted to take their own lives. Would your reaction vary from situation to situation? Why?
5. Imagine that you are a community health nurse engaged in health promotion and maintenance activities with new parents. What high-risk factors (biological, psychological, sociocultural, intellectual, and spiritual) would you observe for that

---

SELF-DIRECTED LEARNING—cont'd

might predispose parents and/or their children to a major affective disorder?

6. Develop a plan for counseling parents about child rearing that incorporates principles and goals for primary prevention of major affective disorders.

Questions to Consider

1. During which phase of Bowlby's grieving process would the nurse expect the client to repeatedly review the events related to the loss
   a. Disequilibrium
   b. Cathartic
   c. Disorganization
   d. Reorganization
2. Intervention with a depressed client based on a cognitive model would include
   a. Educating the client about his or her method of communicating
   b. Assisting the client to reframe negative interpretations of the environment
   c. Facilitating the resolution of unconscious conflicts
   d. Identifying the client's role within the family system

3. Tertiary prevention strategies include which of the following
   a. Support groups for survivors of suicide victims
   b. Identification of high-risk groups
   c. Assessment of presenting symptoms
   d. Facilitation of social networking to re-enter the community

Match the characteristics that best describe the disorder.

4. Dysthymia	a. Pressured speech, excessive spending, increased motor activity
5. Grief	b. Early morning awakening, physiologic vegetative signs
6. Unipolar	c. Ability to make some decisions but vacillates on major issues
7. Bipolar	d. Feelings of sadness, self-esteem intact

Answer key

1. c	5. d
2. b	6. b
3. d	7. a
4. c	

REFERENCES

Abramson L, Seligman M, and Teasdale J: Learned helplessness in humans: critique reformulation, J Abnormal Psych 87(1):49-75, 1978.

Adams: Chemical factor found among causes of suicide, Sci Focus 1(1):1 and 7, 1986.

Akiskal H and McKinney W: Overview of recent research in depression, Arch Gen Psychiatry 32:285-290, 1975.

American Psychiatric Association: Diagnostic and statistical Manual III-R, Washington, DC, 1987.

Arieti S: Affective disorders: manic-depressive psychosis and psychotic depression, In Arieti S, editor: American handbook of psychiatry, 1974, New York, Basic Books, Inc.

Asberg M: Chemical factor found among causes of suicide, Sci Focus 1(1):1 and 7, 1986.

Atchley R: Aging and suicide: reflection of the quality of life, In Haynes S. and Feinleib M, editors: Epidemiology of aging— second conference, U.S. Department of Health and Human Services, 1980.

Baer C and Williams B: Clinical pharmacology and nursing, Springhouse, Pa, 1988, Springhouse Publishing Co.

Bahnson C and Bahnson M: Role of the ego defenses: denial and repression in the etiology of malignant neoplasm, Ann NY Acad Sci 125:827-845, 1966.

Bart P: Depression in middle-aged women, In Gornick V and Moran B, editors: Women in a sexist society, New York, 1971, Basic Books, Inc.

Beck A: Depression: causes and treatment, Philadelphia, 1967, University of Pennsylvania Press.

Beck A: Chemical factor found among causes of suicide, Sci Focus 1(1):1 and 7, 1986.

Beck A et al: Cognitive theory of depression, New York, 1979, The Guilford Press.

Bem S: Sex-role adaptability: one consequence of psychological androgyny, J Personality Soc Psychol 31:634-643, 1975.

Bergson L: Suicide's other victims, NY Times Magazine, November 14, 1982, pp 100-105.

Bibring E: The mechanism of depression, In Greenacre P, editor: Affective disorders, New York, 1953, International Universities Press.

Blakeslee S: Holiday suicide warnings are reported in study to be misplaced, NY Times, July 4, 1987.

Bollen KA and Phillips DP: Imitative suicides: a national study of the effects of television news stories, Am Sociolog Rev 47:802-809, 1982.

Bowlby J: Attachment and loss: separation, anxiety, and anger vol 2, New York, 1973, Basic Books, Inc.

Brown G and Harris T: Social origins of depression, London, 1978, Tavistock Publishers.

Brownmiller S: Against our will, New York, Simon & Schuster, Inc.

Capodanno A and Targum S: Assessment of suicide: some limitations in the prediction of infrequent events, J Psychosoc Nurs Mental Health Serv 21(5):11-14, 1983.

Chemical factor found among causes of suicide, Sci Focus 1(1):1 and 7, 1986.

Chesler P: Women and madness, New York, 1972, Doubleday & Co., Inc.

Chess S, Thomas A, and Hassibi M: Depression in childhood and adolescence: a prospective study of six cases, J Nervous Mental Dis 171:411-420, 1983.

Clinard M: Sociology of deviant behavior, New York, 1974, Holt, Rinehart & Winston.

Corob A: Working with depressed women, Aldershot, England, 1987, Gower Publishing Co. Ltd.

Durkheim E: Suicide, New York, 1951, The Free Press.

Engel G: Psychologic development in health and disease, Philadelphia, 1962, WB Saunders Co.

Farberow N, editor: Suicide in different cultures, Baltimore, 1975, University Park Press.

Finnerty J: Ethics in rational suicide, Critical Care Nurs Q 10(2):86-90, 1987.

Francis A: Chemical factor found among causes of suicide, Sci Focus 1(1):1 and 7, 1986.

Freud S: Mourning and melancholia, In The collected papers, vol 2, London, 1917, The Hogarth Press Ltd.

Gibbons J: Total body sodium and potassium in depressive illness, Clin Sci 19:133-138, 1960.

Gordon V: Themes and cohesiveness observed in a depressed women's support group, Issues Mental Health Nurs, 4:113-125, 1982.

Greene WA: The psychosocial setting of the development of leukemia and lymphoma, Ann NY Aca Sci 125:794-801, 1966.

Hankhoff L and Einsidler B: Suicide: theory and clinical aspects, Littleton, Mass, 1979, PSG Publishing.

Hatton C, Valente S, and Rink A: Suicide: assessment and intervention, New York, 1977, Appleton-Century-Crofts.

Hauser E and Feinberg F: Operational approach to delayed grief and mourning process, J Psychiatr Nurs 2:26-29, 1976.

Hradek E: Crisis intervention and suicide, J Psychosoc Nurs Mental Health Serv 26(5):24-28, 1988.

Jones S and Pelikan L: Nursing management of the depressed patient in the E.R., Psychiatr Nurs Forum 2:6-12, 1985.

Kaplan H and Sadock B: Modern synopsis of psychiatry, ed 4, Baltimore, 1985, Williams & Wilkins.

Kicey C: Catecholamines and depression: a physiological theory of depression, Am J Nurs 74:2018-2020, 1974.

Klein M: A contribution to the psychogenesis of manic-depressive states, In Contributions to psychoanalysis 1921-1945, London, 1934, The Hogarth Press Ltd.

Kolata G: Manic-depressive gene tied to chromosome 11, Science 235(4):1139-1140, March 1987.

Kucera-Bozarth K, Beck N, and Lyss L: Compliance with lithium regimens, J Psychosoc Nurs Mental Health Serv 20(7):11-15, 1982.

LaGreca A: Suicide: prevalence, theories and prevention, In Wass H, Berardo F, and Neimeyer R, editors: Dying: facing the facts, ed. 2, Washington, DC, 1988, Hemisphere Publishing Co.

LeShan L: An emotional life-history pattern associated with neoplastic disease, Ann NY Acad Sci 125:780-793, 1966.

Leviton D: Significance of sexuality as a deterrent to suicide among the aged, Omega 4:163-174, 1973.

Lindemann E: Symptomatology and management of acute grief, Am J Psychiatr 101:141-148, 1944.

Linden L and Breed W: Epidemiology of suicide, In Schneidman ES, editor: Suicidology: contemporary developments, New York, 1976, Grune & Stratton, Inc.

McLane A, editor: Classification of nursing diagnoses, St. Louis, 1987, The CV Mosby Co.

Marshall J and Hodge R: Durkheim and Pierce on suicide and economic change, Soc Sci Res 10:101-114, 1981.

Menninger K: Man against himself, New York, 1938, Harcourt, Brace & Co.

Miller JF: Coping with chronic illness: overcoming powerlessness, Philadelphia, 1983, FA Davis Co.

Minot S: Depression, Am J Nurs 3:285-288, 1986.

Murphy S: Learned helplessness: from concept to comprehension, Perspectives Psychiatr Care 20(1):27-32, 1982.

Neimeyer R: Toward a personal construct conceptualization of depression and suicide, In Epting FR and Neimeyer RA, editors: Personal meanings of death, Washington, DC, 1984, Hemisphere Publishing Co.

Papa L: Responses to life events as predictors of suicidal behavior, Nurs Res 29(6):362-369, 1980.

Pfeffer C: Chemical factor found among causes of suicide, Sci Focus 1(1) 1986.

Platt S: Unemployment and suicidal behavior: a review of the literature, Sociol Sci Med 19:93-115, 1984.

Richman J: Family determinants of suicidal potential, In Anderson D and McLean L, editors: Identifying suicidal potential, New York, 1971, Behavioral Publications, Inc.

Ringel E: The pre-suicidal syndrome, Suicide and Life-Threatening Behavior 6:131-149, 1976.

Roy A: Chemical factor found among causes of suicide, Sci Focus 1(1) 1986.

Rund D and Hertzler J: Emergency psychiatry, St. Louis, 1983, The CV Mosby Co.

Russell D: The politics of rape, New York, 1975, Stein & Day, Publishers.

Rutter MA and Garmezy N: Developmental psycholopathology, In Hetherington EM, editor: Handbook of child psychology, vol 4, New York, 1983, John Wiley.

Sands D et al: Understanding ECT, J Psychosoc Nurs 25(8):27-30, 1987.

Santora D and Starkey P: Research studies in American Indian suicides, J Psychosoc Nurs Mental Health Serv 20(8):25-29, 1982.

Schneidman E and Farberow N, editors: Clues to suicide, New York, 1957, McGraw-Hill Book Co.

Schultz J and Dark S: Manual of psychiatric nursing care plans, Boston, 1982, Little, Brown & Co.

Seiden R: Mellowing with age: factors influencing the nonwhite suicide rate, In J Aging Human Development 13:265-284, 1981.

Seligman M: For helplessness: can we immunize the weak? Psychol Today 73:90-95, 1973.

Selkin J: Rape, Psychol Today 75:71-76, 1975.

Shamoian C, editor: Treatment of affective disorders in the elderly, Washington, DC, 1985, The American Psychiatric Press, Inc.

Spitz R and Wolf K: Anaclitic depression, In The psychoanalytic study of the child, New York, 1946, International Universities Press.

Suicide: part I, Harvard Mental Health Letter 2:1-4, 1986.

Stack S: The effects of strikes on suicide: a cross-national analysis, Sociol Focus 15:135-146, 1982.

Talan J: Testing for melancholia, Emergency Med 5:118-119, 1981.

Talan J: Suicide: talking may not help teens, Newsday, March 24, 1987, p 5.

Trad P: Infant depression: paradigms and paradoxes, New York, 1986, Springer-Verlag.

Wass H, Bernardo F, and Neimeyer R, editors: Dying: facing the facts, ed 2, Washington, DC, 1988, Hemisphere Publishing Co.

Wetzel R: Hopelessness, depression and suicidal intent, Arch Gen Psychiatr 33:901-908, 1976.

Wilson M: Suicidal behavior: toward an explanation of differences in male and female rates, Suicide Life-Threatening Behav 13:147-154, 1981.

ANNOTATED SUGGESTED READINGS

Finnerty J: Ethics in rational suicide, Critical Care Nurs Q 109(2):86-90, 1987.

This article presents a discussion of suicide as a rational act. Moral, legal, and ethical issues are considered within the context of society's trend toward increasing medical technology. The author points out that the ethics of suicide requires much more discussing, more clarifying, and more agonizing over the question of termination of one's life as a rational choice. Connotations regarding the word "suicide" imply irrational, illogical actions; however, the author suggests that suicide may be utilized to define those actions taken by an individual who refuses treatment rather than be kept biologically alive when in a terminal state. The author proposes that the concept of suicide must be understood within the more central concepts of life and death rather than the means—suicide—to death.

Harkness S: The cultural mediation of postpartum depression, Med Anthropol I (2):194-209, June 1987.

The author presents a synopsis of the three psychological theories of postpartum depression as a basis for understanding women's affective functioning in the postpartal period. She then critiques the theories based on anthropological and psychological research in a rural Kipsigis community of Kenya. She reports the results of the evaluation of affective functioning in a sample of ten women during pregnancy and the postpartal period. Harkness found that at both the cultural and the individual levels, there seemed to be no evidence of postpartum depression. She hypothesizes that culture has a significant impact as a mediating factor between the physiological processes related to childbirth and their psychological outcomes.

Mullis M and Byers P: Social support in suicidal inpatients, J Psychosoc Nurs Mental Health Serv 25(4):16-19, 1987.

The authors present a clear, concise discussion of research conducted on social support variables relative to suicidal inpatients. They found that social support did not differ significantly between suicidal and nonsuicidal male psychiatric patients. Psychiatric inpatients had lower functional and social network social support scores and increased loss of support scores than adult male hospital employees. It was noted by the authors that nursing intervention with suicidal inpatients can be directed toward increasing social support systems of these clients.

Phillips D and Carstensen L: Effect of suicide stories on various demographic groups, Suicide and Life-Threatening Behav 18(1):100-114, 1988.

This article describes a demographic study of the effects of suicide stories. The authors found that for nearly all demographic groups, suicide stories do have an effect. However, it must be noted that for most segments of society, the suicide story exerts an effect that must be considered along with other etiological variables. One point of interest identified by the authors related to the effect of suicide stories on teenagers. Teenagers seemed to be more affected by these stories. Thus, the authors noted that it would be most appropriate to develop measures to reduce the harmful effects of suicide stories. Strategies for this purpose were also identified.

FURTHER READINGS

Coupar A et al: Hospital admission for depression, J Adv Nurs 11(6):697-704, 1986.

Dreyfus JK: The prevalence of depression in women in an ambulatory care setting, Nurse Pract 12(4):34, 36-37, 1987.

Glazebrook CK et al: Sex roles and depression, J Psychosoc Nurs Mental Health Serv 24(12):8-12, 1986.

Hensley M et al: Shedding light on 'SAD'ness...seasonal affective disorder, Arch Psychiatr Nurs 1(4):230-235, 1987.

Holinger PC et al: Spotting the potential suicide, Patient Care 21(14):62-68, 73, 77, 1987.

Kelly D and France R, editors: A practical handbook for the treatment of depression, Park Ridge, NJ, 1987, The Parthenon Publishing Group.

Lipsey H: Depression in women, Can J Psychiatr Nurs 28(3):10-11, 1987.

Ronsman K: Therapy for depression, J Gerontol Nurs 13(12):18-25, 1987.

Ryan L et al: Impact of circadian rhythm research on approaches to affective illness, Arch Psychiatr Nurs 1(4):236-240, 1987.

Simmons-Ailing S: New approaches to managing affective disorders, Arch Psychiatr Nurs 1(4):219-224, 1987.

Thobaben M: What you can do for the depressed caregiver, RN 51(1):73-75, 1988.

CHAPTER 23

Patterns of compulsivity, somatization, and altered identity

CHAPTER FOCUS

People who experience chronic anxiety and conflict and who try to cope through compulsivity, somatization, or altered identity are often diagnosed as having an anxiety disorder, somatoform disorder, dissociative disorder, or eating disorder. Neurotic anxiety and conflict may be manifested in rigidity of personality and the development of interpersonal patterns of dependence, domination, or detachment.

Treatment often involves a combination of therapies. Treatment goals focus on decreasing sources of stress, teaching more adaptive ways of dealing with stress, and alleviating symptoms associated with the neurotic process.

Nurses engage in all three levels of preventive intervention. The fundamental aspect of nursing intervention is a supportive nurse-client relationship. By clarifying their own attitudes, feelings, and values, nurses can work more therapeutically with clients who are suffering from neuroses.

Responsiveness to societal attitudes has contributed to periodic changes in the classification of neuroses. For instance, neuroses have been included under such diagnostic categories as "psychoses," "other diagnoses," and "psychophysiologic autonomic and viseral disorders." In 1980, The American Psychiatric Association's *Diagnostic and Statistical Manual of Mental Disorders* (DSM-III) eliminated neuroses as a diagnostic category and included them instead under anxiety disorders, somatoform disorders, and dissociative disorders. However, neuroses nomenclature continued to be acceptable. The 1987 revision of the Diagnostic and Statistical Manual of Mental Disorders (DSM-III-R) reiterated this position.

We have attempted to focus on behavioral patterns that are symptomatic of neurotic disorders and that are distressing to clients and their families. Theoretical discussions are aimed at showing how a multiplicity of interrelated factors contribute to the following disorders:

Anxiety disorders
    Generalized anxiety disorder
    Panic disorder
    Phobic disorders
    Obsessive compulsive disorder
Dissociative disorders
    Psychogenic amnesia
    Psychogenic fugue
    Multiple personality
Somatoform disorders
    Hypochondriasis
    Conversion disorder
Eating disorders
    Anorexia nervosa
    Bulimia nervosa
    Compulsive overeating

UNDERLYING DYNAMICS

To understand the dynamics of neuroses, neuroses must be viewed as complex phenomena. There is a neurotic personality core consisting of (1) feelings of inadequacy and anxiety and (2) defensive and avoidant behavior manifested by dependency, domination, or detachment. Because much energy is directed toward the maintenance of defensive and avoidant behavior, there is little energy available for personal growth and meaningful interpersonal relationships. Rigidity, self-defeating behavior, and an inability to move toward self-actualization become evident.

Inadequacy and anxiety

Neurotic individuals usually perceive the world as hostile and threatening, and they often feel incapable of coping with internal and external dangers.

These perceptions engender a feeling of vulnerability. Dysfunctional cognitive processes further contribute to a sense of inadequacy. For example, an individual may underestimate personal strengths and focus on and magnify personal weaknesses. In addition, minor failures may be catastrophized. While failure reinforces the sense of inadequacy, success carries the threat of having one's inadequacy exposed (Beck et al., 1985). Therefore, all situations are perceived as threatening or as potentially threatening. Anxiety is ever-present (see Chapter 8 for an in-depth discussion of anxiety).

Dependence on others

Because of feelings of inadequacy and anxiety, acceptance by other people may be perceived as essential for personal security. To achieve this security, individuals may relate to others in a submissive, dependent manner. They may have excessive need for attention, affection, and approval. They may view other people as superior and may adopt the attitudes and opinions of others as their own. Since they consider the approval of others essential to their own security, dependent people may function in accord with other people's beliefs and judgments. In essence, the dependent person is saying, "If I depend on you, you will not hurt me."

Illness and hospitalization usually increase dependency. Initially, an individual may assume the "good patient" role. However, because of an underlying fear of abandonment, demands for attention, clinging behavior, and an inability to tolerate criticism and frustration may soon become evident (Barry, 1984).

Such submissive, dependent behavior does not resolve the underlying sense of inadequacy. Furthermore, the dependent role itself may generate resentment, anger, or despondency in the dependent individual.

Detachment from others

The individual who is detached from others usually appears aloof and uninvolved. Detached people have strong needs to maintain independence and self-sufficiency. They keep emotional distance between themselves and others and avoid becoming emotionally involved. Intellectualization and a superior manner are used to accomplish this emotional detachment. Superficial relations with others may be amicable. However, any effort to place an emotionally detached individual in a dependent or submissive position arouses uneasiness, rebellion, and further emotional withdrawal.

Illness and hospitalization may generate anxiety and resentment. A detached individual may spend much time alone. Because of the superficiality of interpersonal relationships, the individual may have few visitors. Personal questions asked during history taking are likely to be perceived as an intrusion. However, because of an inability to express feelings, anger—as well as other emotions—probably will not be displayed (Barry, 1984). Health teaching is apt to be perceived as an attempt to dominate and to be met with resistance.

Domination of others

The individual who has a strong need to maintain control over other people may express this need in a variety of ways. Taking command in any situation may threaten others and thus maintain control. Overt expression of anger when orders are challenged or not carried out may also effectively maintain control and, in addition, can serve as an outlet for anxiety. At other times, particularly when direct methods of control would be ineffective, forms of subtle manipulation may be employed. Such manipulation may take the form of flattery, excessive concern about the plight of others, or efforts to obligate people.

There is often an inability to admit to one's self or others any feelings or fears. There may be a strong need to prove one's self as strong and right. Because interpersonal closeness tends to be regarded as threatening, efforts to establish anything other than superficial relationships usually fail.

Although such an individual may not be aware of dependency needs, these needs are still present. Because illness and hospitalization place a person in a dependent position, they may be very threatening. The individual may try to cope with the anxiety engendered with increased attempts at domination. Nurses may respond with frustration. For example,

Mr. H. was admitted to a hospital in the small community where he lived; the diagnosis was peptic ulcer. Married and a father of two children, Mr. H. was in his late thirties and held an important position in a bank. While in the hospital, he continued to carry on business on the phone and through visits from employees of the bank.

Mr. H., on several occasions, shouted at an employee and made disparaging remarks about his intelligence in front of hospital staff and the other client in the room. At other times, Mr. H. was heard to flatter an employee and then send him off on a personal errand. When the charge nurse attempted to set limits on such business activities, Mr. H. became very angry and threatened to report her. Efforts to explain to Mr. H. that his own recovery was not being helped by the business activity and that the other client in the room was very ill and needed a quieter atmosphere only served to increase Mr. H.'s anger.

When the nursing supervisor appeared to discuss the matter with Mr. H., he became very conciliatory and expressed concern about the other client. He flattered the supervisor about the way in which she ran the unit and expressed interest in her personal likes and dislikes. The next day he sent her tickets to a play they had discussed. The unit staff received a large box of candy.

Mr. H. continued to conduct business from the hospital room. When the subject was raised with him again, Mr. H. explained to the staff that his position was very important and that he was unable to rely upon the people under him. He attempted to convince the staff that he rested easier knowing that things were under control at the bank.

Since all of the nursing staff members were becoming frustrated in working with Mr. H., a group meeting was held to work out a plan of care. Underlying anxiety was identified as one of the major problems, and a plan of care that emphasized emotional support and health teaching through a one-to-one relationship was developed and implemented. However, Mr. H. initially thwarted any efforts to establish anything other than a superficial discussion. He said that he regarded talking about his experience as "sentimental hogwash." He resisted just as adamantly any health teaching, and responded to the nurse's efforts to open any avenue of communication with sexually seductive remarks.

In a supervisory session with a mental health nurse, a staff nurse mentioned the frustration and humiliation she was experiencing in working with Mr. H. After a review of the content of the interactions, the nurse was able to identify Mr. H.'s responses as "distancing *maneuvers.'' Once a nursing diagnosis of impaired social interaction (domination) related to dependence-independence conflict had been formulated, the staff nurse was able to utilize an approach that encouraged the client to take the lead in discussing areas of concern to him. This approach was less threatening to the client and more effective in meeting some of the nursing care objectives.*

PATTERNS OF NEUROTIC BEHAVIOR

In general, people who use neurotic coping patterns are functioning members of society. Neurotic individuals remain in contact with reality. Neurotic behavior differs from "normal" behavior only in the degree of anxiety experienced and in the extent that defense mechanisms are needed or available to help a person cope with anxiety. The intensity of neurotic behavior patterns varies with circumstances, with biological and physiological factors, and with the culture in which a person lives.

Neuroses are classified according to observable symptoms. The primary symptom in a neurosis gives the neurosis its name. Symptoms predominantly represent either direct manifestations of anxiety or defense mechanisms utilized to control anxiety. We will now examine four categories of neurotic behavior: anxiety disorders, dissociative disorders, somatoform disorders, and eating disorders.

Anxiety disorders

This group of disorders is also known as anxiety and phobic neuroses. The disorders are characterized by a high degree of anxiety and/or avoidance behavior. Anxiety disorders are common in the general population. Table 23-1 compares the various types of anxiety disorders.

GENERALIZED ANXIETY DISORDER

An experience of excessive and unrealistic anxiety and worry about two or more life situations (e.g., worry about passing courses when one's grades are good, worry about becoming homeless when one is financially secure) that lasts for 6 months or longer is a chronic state of anxiety known as *generalized anxiety disorder*. The symptoms of

TABLE 23-1 Anxiety disorders

Disorder	Behavioral symptoms	Physical symptoms
Generalized anxiety	Feelings of awe, apprehension, dread; fear of impending disaster; irritatibility; insomnia; poor concentration; exaggerated startle response	Muscle tension, fatigue, restlessness, somatic complaints, twitching or trembling, tachycardia, sweating, dry mouth, dizziness, nausea, diarrhea, frequent urination, difficulty swallowing
Panic	Severe anxiety: complications include abuse of alcohol and anxiolytics	Rapid respirations and pulse, palpitations, muscle tension, restlessness, trembling, profuse perspiration, faintness, dizziness, nausea, vomiting, diarrhea, dilated pupils, paresthesia, flushing or chills, shortness of breath, smothering or choking sensation
Phobic	Anxiety, desire to avoid object of phobia	Pounding heart, rapid pulse, dry mouth, dizziness, nausea, faintness
Obsessive-compulsive	Obsessive thoughts or impulses enacted in repetitive, ritualistic, purposeful, and intentional behavior; phobic avoidance of situations related to content of obsessions (e.g., germs); complications include depression and abuse of alcohol and anxiolytics	Sequelae of compulsion (e.g., excoriated hands from frequent handwashing)

Sources include Beck et al. (1985) and DSM-III-R (1987).

generalized anxiety disorder fall into the following patterns: motor tension, autonomic hyperactivity, and vigilance and scanning (see Table 23-1). It is common for individuals to experience mild depression along with symptoms of generalized anxiety disorder. The disorder can occur at any age, but onset occurs most frequently in the 20s to 30s. Generalized anxiety disorder is equally prevalent in men and women and usually only mildly interferes with social or occupational functioning (Beck et al., 1985; DSM-III-R, 1987). Since a sustained high level of anxiety affects not only the autonomic nervous system but also all body systems, psychophysiologic disorders may coincide with generalized anxiety disorder or be precipitated by it (see Chapter 19).

PANIC DISORDER

Panic disorder comes on suddenly and overwhelms an individual with terrifying anxiety. The sudden onset, without apparent cause, often occurs when people are alone or away from home. Although the individual is acutely aware of the anxiety and its effects (see Table 23-1), the individual tends to be unaware of the situation that precipitated the panic. An attack may last from several minutes to, rarely, several hours. Frequently, agoraphobia or a depressive disorder is also present. Childhood separation anxiety disorder or sudden loss of or disruption of significant interpersonal relationships may predispose a person to panic disorder.

Panic disorder can occur at any age, but onset occurs most frequently in the late 20s. Once an attack occurs, panic attacks often recur several or more times a week. It is not uncommon for an individual to feel ongoing apprehension or fear about having another panic attack. While panic disorder without agoraphobia is equally prevalent in men and women, panic disorder with agoraphobia is approximately twice as prevalent in women. When agoraphobia coexists with panic disorder, there may be moderate to severe impairment of social and occupational functioning. Otherwise, panic disorder tends to interfere only mildly with a person's life-style (Beck et al., 1985; DSM-III-R, 1987). The following vignette illustrates some features of a panic attack:

Mary J., a young college student who was enrolled in a social work program, was very shy and retiring in class. She rarely participated in classroom discussion, and when called upon to express an idea or opinion, she became very tense, restless, and obviously uncomfortable. She readily acceded to the opinions and decisions of other students in the class, even on controversial issues about which she privately expressed different opinions. When course assignments required that she speak before the group or participate in panel discussions, her level of anxiety made other students uncomfortable. Mary's achievement on written assignments and examinations indicated that she was intellectually mastering the material, and she was receiving fairly high grades.

During the course of the semester Mary became very dependent upon the teacher, constantly seeking approval and guidance outside the classroom. When the teacher was unable to spend as much time with her outside class as Mary demanded, or when the suggestion was made that she discuss in class some of the points she brought to the teacher, Mary reacted with an outburst of anger at the teacher. The outburst was followed shortly by submissive and conciliatory actions, including excessive praise and compliments.

Mary, who had an older brother and a younger sister, described her family as "very strict." High moral standards and demands for achievement had been stressed throughout her life. Failure in either area had been severely punished. Mary believed that her parents favored her brother because he was a boy and her sister because she was prettier and more like her mother. Her mother and younger sister often went on vacations together and shared many other activities—a practice that at times left Mary with the feeling of being alone and abandoned. Mary often expressed envy of her college classmates, whom she described as being more independent and having more fun than she did.

When Mary was placed in a social agency for field work practice, she continued to seek out the former teacher. On one occasion, Mary attempted to have her teacher intervene on her behalf with her agency supervisor, whom she described as being very difficult and impossible to please. Mary described her efforts to memorize all the procedures and techniques the agency used, and she expressed the wish that she could exchange places with the clients she was serving. The agency supervisor described Mary as disorganized and unable to plan or conduct even the simplest interview.

Mary experienced an acute anxiety attack in her car while driving to the agency one day. Following the attack, she became so fearful of leaving her immediate neighborhood that she had to temporarily withdraw from the program and seek professional help in coping with her anxiety.

PHOBIC DISORDERS

A phobia is a persistent pathological fear. The stimulus for a phobia can be almost anything in the environment. Exposure to the object or situation elicits an immediate anxiety response (see Table 23-1). Anticipation of encountering the phobic stimulus engenders anticipatory anxiety. A phobia represents a transfer of internal anxiety to some object in the environment. The major defense mechanisms operating are projection and displacement. Fear of a specific situation or object (e.g., dogs) is referred to as *simple phobia*. Fear of social situations (e.g., speaking in public, urinating in a public lavatory) that may cause embarrassment or humiliation is referred to as *social phobia*. Fear of being in a place or situation (e.g., away from home alone, being in a crowd, traveling) that may impede escape or the availability of help, should it be needed, is referred to as *agoraphobia* (Beck et al., 1985; DSM-III-R, 1987). Manifestations of agoraphobia can vary in degree from an inability to leave one's home to the less restrictive inability to travel any distance from one's neighborhood. A recent study indicates that in people who suffer from both panic disorder and agoraphobia, panic attacks often predate agoraphobia by up to one year (Breier, Charney, and Heninger, 1986). Implications for early intervention into panic disorder are obvious.

The age of onset for phobias is variable. For example, with simple phobia, fear of animals usually appears in childhood; fear of blood and injuries in adolescence to early adulthood; and fear of heights, enclosed spaces, driving, and traveling in airplanes in the fourth decade of life. Social phobia usually appears in late childhood or early adolescence. Agoraphobia most often appears between the ages of 20 and 40.

School phobia, because it has unique features and is specific to childhood, is classified by DSM-III-R as a diagnostic criterion of separation anxiety disorder. School phobia is one common phobia of children and adolescents. It centers around some school situation, generates high anxiety and fear, and results in trying to or actually avoiding going to school. School phobia may be either acute or chronic (Paccione-Dyszlewski and Contessa-Kislus, 1987). Table 23-2 compares acute school phobia and chronic school phobia.

For an individual who is suffering from a phobia, some or many needs may have to be met by other people, and many of the onerous chores of living may thus be avoided. These effects and the additional attention often given the phobic individual by family and friends provide secondary gains that may reinforce the phobia.

OBSESSIVE COMPULSIVE DISORDER

The most important symptoms of this disorder are obsessions and compulsions. Compulsions are the enactment of obsessions (persistent ideas, thoughts, images, or impulses). Obsessions most frequently involve violence, contamination, and doubt. Compulsions involve repetitious and stereotypic performance of ritualistic acts and may be very time-consuming. They serve to neutralize, control, or prevent psychological discomfit. Should an individual try to resist carrying out a compulsion, tension will increase, but it will be dispelled as soon as the compulsive behavior is performed. Obsessive-compulsive disorder may be accompanied by depression and anxiety. Often, a phobia that centers around the content of the obsession (e.g., germs) may coexist. Obsessive compulsive disorder frequently appears in adolescence or early adulthood, but onset may be in childhood. It is equally prevalent in men and women DSM-III-R, 1987). The following vignette illustrates a severe form of obsessive-compulsive disorder:

Jane M., a young woman of 24, was brought to a mental health clinic by her husband, who said that she had developed such elaborate rituals for getting dressed each morning that she was unable to get to work on time. The rituals included repeated hand washing and a pattern of dressing and undressing that took several hours to accomplish. These activities were interfering not only with Jane's life but also with her husband's,

TABLE 23-2   School phobia

Factor	Acute phobia	Chronic phobia
Onset	Acute	Incipient
Precipitating event	Trauma or loss (e.g., death, illness, parental divorce)	No definitive precipitating event
History of phobias	None	History of previous episodes of school phobia
History of punctuality or attendance problems	None	Significant history often beginning in elementary grades
School performance	Average or above-average grades	Poor grades; retention in grade placement
Behavioral	Depressed; sense of isolation from peers	Broad range of affect; severe personality problems
Situational	Phobia is called to the attention of a professional by a family member (e.g., parent or guardian)	Phobia is made known by a source outside the family (e.g., school, court, hospital); poor communication between parents and between parents and child; history of ongoing family crisis

Adapted from Paccione-Dyszlewski and Contessa-Kislus (1987).

since he was unable or unwilling to leave home until she was ready to leave also.

Jane's compulsive behavior began shortly after their marriage. It started with an inability to throw away dirt after she swept the kitchen floor. The hand washing started shortly after that incident, and the other rituals soon after that. At the time of the visit to the clinic, Jane was unable to do any of the housework because of her preoccupation with dirt. As a consequence, her husband had assumed these chores. Her health history revealed that Jane had refused to have sexual relations with her husband after the first month of marriage.

Jane had always done well in school and had graduated from college with honors. She was currently employed as an accountant. Her employer thought highly of her work and, despite the current difficulties, continued to employ her.

Jane was the only child in a middle-class family that she described as being very strict and upright. Her mother took great pride in maintaining her home in an immaculate condition and was completely unable to understand Jane's current inability to do the same. Although her parents had always placed demands upon Jane to excel in school and to conform to their precepts, they were also very proud of her and rewarded her for her achievements.

During the course of treatment at the clinic, Jane was very consistent in arriving on time. However, her hand-washing ritual increased to the point that, even though she arrived at the clinic on time, she would be late for appointments. She also developed an additional ritual that symbolically expressed her anxiety and ambivalence. This ritual consisted of repeatedly walking up to the front door of the clinic and then retreating back to the sidewalk.

Psychotherapy and the administration of anti-anxiety drugs were combined in the treatment. Although Jane made some progress, the therapy was not completely effective in eliminating the symptoms.

Dissociative disorders

Dissociative disorders may be acute or chronic and represent a form of psychological flight from the self in which a part or all of the personality is denied or dissociated. While there may be a dysfunction in any of the integrative functions of identity, consciousness, or memory, identity is primarily affected.

PSYCHOGENIC AMNESIA

Psychogenic amnesia is a response to an extremely anxiety-provoking situation that often involves loss of or rejection by a loved one. Both onset and termination tend to occur abruptly. In amnesia, a part or all of a person's past life is forgotten. Recall may be affected in one of the following ways:

1. Localized amnesia: inability to remember all events that happened during a limited time frame (most often the first few hours after a traumatic event).
2. Selective amnesia: inability to remember some, but not all, events that happened within a limited time frame.
3. Generalized amnesia: inability to remember any aspects of past life, including such vital information as name, place of residence, names of family and friends, and occupation.
4. Continuous amnesia: inability to remember events, including the present, that occurred following a particular time (DSM-III-R, 1987).

People with amnesia usually appear disoriented and confused. Typically, people with amnesia come to psychiatric attention when they are brought to an emergency room or psychiatric hospital by the police, who have found them wandering aimlessly.

PSYCHOGENIC FUGUE

Sudden purposeful travel away from home accompanied by an inability to remember any aspects of past life and the assumption of a new identity is referred to as *fugue*. This disorder is rare and can occur at any age. Usually a fugue state follows extreme psychosocial stress, and it is seen most often in wartime or following natural or personal disasters.

James Brandon was a physician. During a violent quarrel, James pushed his wife, causing her to hit her head on the fireplace mantle. James' wife fell to the floor, her head bleeding profusely. James disappeared and was found days later in a town 50 miles from his home. James had taken on the identity of John

Browden, a carpenter. He had found a job and had rented an apartment. James had no memory of the fight with his wife or of the family he had left behind.

The preceding vignette illustrates two factors that differentiate psychogenic fugue from amnesia: purposeful travel and assumption of a new identity. While psychogenic fugue usually lasts only hours or days, it can continue for months.

MULTIPLE PERSONALITY

Multiple personality is a disorder characterized by a primary personality that is usually shy and introverted and two or more alter or secondary personalities, each exhibiting values, behaviors, and sometimes ages and sexual orientations that differ from each other and from the primary personality. At any given time, the personality that is "out" (dominant) controls the person's behavior (Coons, 1980). Popularized reports of actual case histories of multiple personalities include *The Three Faces of Eve, Sybil,* and *When Rabbit Howls.*

Amnesia is always present initially in the primary personality and may be experienced as "blackouts," "fainting spells," or "blank spells." Secondary personalities may have varying degrees of awareness of or interest in one another. A personality that has total awareness and memory of *all* coexisting personalities is said to have "memory trace." A personality that is aware of the thoughts, feelings, and behavior of at least one other personality is said to have "co-consciousness." The personality that has memory trace is often very helpful in psychotherapy. In addition to these characteristics, people with multiple personality disorder may experience headaches, conversion disorders, brief psychotic episodes, and difficulties with interpersonal relationships. (Coons, 1980; Greenberg, 1982; DSM-III-R, 1987).

During their childhood, people with multiple personality disorder have usually suffered severe physical and/or sexual abuse. The victimized child is coerced by threats of severe punishment into not divulging the abuse to others.

Dissociation may begin with the creation of imaginary playmates (a normal and not uncommon occurrence in childhood) who later evolve into alter personalities. As imaginary playmates (conscious level of functioning) or alter personalities (unconscious level of functioning) the purposes served are fundamentally the same—to help the primary personality cope with the loneliness, trauma, and hostility of life and to act out impulses (often of a hostile or sexual nature) that are not sanctioned by the primary personality (Coons, 1980; Greenberg, 1982; DSM-III-R, 1987).

Recent studies using electroencephalography indicate that there is as drastic a variation in the brain waves of the primary and secondary personalities inhabiting a multiple personality's body as there is from one "normal" person to another. This finding indicates that each personality of a multiple personality has a functionally different brain and a separate reality from the other personalities (Hale, 1983).

Complications of multiple personality include suicidal attempts, self-mutilation, human abusiveness (e.g., child abuse, rape), and substance abuse.

The goals of psychotherapy are for each of the personalities to become aware of and to communicate with the other personalities about the traumas that contributed to the disorder and, ultimately, for all of the discrepant personalities to become fused or integrated (Greenberg, 1982; DSM-III-R, 1987).

Somatoform disorders

The primary feature of somatoform disorders is the existence of physical symptoms without demonstrable pathophysiological processes. The physical symptoms are not intentionally produced or grossly exaggerated, as they are in malingering, and the symptoms are most readily explained by psychological means.

HYPOCHONDRIASIS

Hypochondriasis is a morbid preoccupation with the state of one's health. Such concern can range from preoccupation with bodily functions to exaggerated concern about minor physical abnormalities (e.g., a slight skin discoloration, an infrequent cough). Hypochondriasis may be demonstrated by a series of minor complaints or by a conviction that

one has a serious disease that persists despite medical reassurance to the contrary. Hypochondriasis appears most frequently between the ages of 20 and 30, and it is equally prevalent in men and women. A history of organic disease and psychosocial stress may predispose an individual to hypochondriasis (DSM-III-R, 1987).

Hypochondriacs are frequently seen in acute health care settings repeatedly complaining about the same, or similar, health symptoms. They also frequently "doctor shop." Such behavior often arouses anger or indifference on the part of health professionals. Physical illness should always be ruled out before labeling the complaints hypochondriacal.

Shelby Marston had a history of hypochonriasis that focused on kidney disease. Shelby frequently went to her family physician with complaints of low back pain. After numerous work-ups with negative findings, the physician had gotten into the habit of reassuring Shelby and prescribing "something for your nerves." After an episode of frequent visits to the doctor with complaints of severe low back pain, a neighbor, who was a nurse, suggested that Shelby get a second opinion. Shelby followed through on the advice. She was found to have kidney disease.

CONVERSION DISORDER

Conversion disorder is usually manifested as impairment of one of the senses or as paralysis of a limb or other body part. The symptom symbolically expresses some underlying conflict or need. Conversion disorder may appear at any period of life, but it is most common in adolescence or early adulthood. Predisposing factors include (1) severe psychosocial stress, (2) exposure to a physical disorder in self or others (may serve as a prototype for the conversion symptom), (3) histrionic or dependent personality disorder.

Conversion disorders produce self-limiting symptoms. The symptoms serve as emergency responses to situations that generate overwhelming anxiety.

A young woman on the maternity unit of a general hospital (she had given birth to twins) suddenly became blind. Physical examination and diagnostic testing revealed no pathology that could account for her blindness. The examining physicians were struck by her complete absence of concern or other emotional response to what could be presumed to be a terrifying experience. Following a psychiatric consultation, a diagnosis of conversion disorder was made, and the woman was treated by a psychiatrist. After a few days of supportive treatment, she recovered her sight and was discharged to an outpatient clinic. Her parents and in-laws arranged to take turns helping her care for the twins.

The woman had become blind a few hours before she was scheduled to be discharged from the maternity unit. She had previously said several times, "I don't see how I'm going to manage caring for twins."

The preceding vignette illustrates several points about conversion disorder. (1) It serves a primary gain (keeps conflict out of awareness and temporarily decreases anxiety). (2) It serves a secondary gain (avoids a noxious situation, elicits concern and support from others). (3) There is often a lack of observable concern about the severe nature of the symptom. Termed *la belle indifference*, this feature often serves as a clue that the problem is a psychological rather than a physical one. (4) The symptomatology is symbolic of the underlying conflict.

Eating disorders

Eating disorders are characterized by severe problems in eating behavior. Many of the dynamics involved in eating disorders have their origins in early childhood. These children develop a sense of inadequacy, ineffectiveness, and poor identity that may persist throughout adolescence and adulthood. Mastery over body weight, whether it is accomplished by losing weight or gaining weight, may be an attempt at asserting independence and mastery over their lives (Brone and Fisher, 1988).

Eating disorders are usually not included among the neurotic disorders. We have included them in this chapter because of the features eating disorders have in common with neuroses: (1) They are obsessive compulsive in nature. (2) There is little interference with intellectual functioning. (3) There is little impairment of reality testing. In this section, anorexia nervosa, bulimia nervosa, and compulsive overeating will be discussed.

ANOREXIA NERVOSA

Anorexia nervosa is characterized by refusal to maintain even minimal body weight, extreme fear of becoming obese, disturbed body image, and amenorrhea. Excessive exercising, purging, and dieting may be carried out to the point of severe malnutrition and emaciation. Even in the emaciated state, individuals tend to perceive themselves as overweight. In some instances, the disorder results in death (DSM-III-R, 1987; Oehler and Burns, 1987).

Anorexia nervosa usually has its onset in adolescence, and it may have been preceded by a slightly overweight condition. Although it can occur in men, the majority of people with this disorder are young women. Such women are often highly intelligent and well-educated.

BULIMIA NERVOSA

Bulimia nervosa is characterized by recurrent episodes of binge eating and purging. The foods that are rapidly consumed in large amounts (and often in secret) tend to be high-calorie foods. During binging, there is a sense of loss of control over eating behavior. Purging is usually accomplished through self-induced vomiting, excessive exercising, and the use of laxatives. There is also a preoccupation with body shape and size.

Bulimia nervosa usually has its onset in adolescence or early adulthood. It is more prevalent in women than in men. Bulimia tends to be a chronic and intermittent condition that extends over many years. In between episodes of binging, eating behavior may be normal, or normal eating may alternate with fasting. People suffering from bulimia nervosa, unlike those suffering from anorexia nervosa, are aware that their eating behavior is abnormal (DSM-III-R, 1987; Oehler and Burns, 1987).

COMPULSIVE OVEREATING

Compulsive overeating is characterized by an inability to stabilize body weight, obesity, and preoccupation with food (thoughts of food and eating—not eating). Because of poor interoceptive awareness, compulsive overeaters may interpret any discomfit (e.g., anger, anxiety) as hunger and as a need to eat. In an attempt to control their weight, compulsive overeaters may engage in cycles of dieting and fasting. Although DSM-III-R (1987) does not classify compulsive overeating as an eating disorder, compulsive overeaters who have psychological factors contributing to their obesity may be classified under the DSM-III-R category psychological factors affecting physical condition (Schneider, 1987; Brone and Fisher, 1988). Table 23-3 compares anorexia nervosa, bulimia nervosa, and compulsive overeating.

EPIDEMIOLOGY

Although there are few definitive demographic studies available, it is believed that neuroses are among the more prevalent functional disorders in society. Reliable data on incidence are difficult to obtain for a variety of reasons. The primary reason is that many people function effectively and successfully despite neurotic problems until or unless they are confronted with overwhelming situational stress.

It is estimated that 15% to 20% of the population of the United States suffers from some neurotic disorder (Colby and McGuire, 1981). Some neuroses (e.g., panic disorder with agoraphobia, agoraphobia without history of panic disorder, multiple personality disorder, anorexia nervosa, bulimia nervosa) tend to be more prevalant in women than in men (DSM-III-R, 1987). For example, it is estimated that 2% of school-age girls suffer from anorexia nervosa, 50% of female college students suffer from bulimia nervosa, and 60% of women (aged 15-45) suffer from compulsive overeating (Eichenbaum and Orbach, 1983). Besides affecting the quality of life of individuals, neuroses can be costly to the economy. For instance, triskaidekaphobia (fear of the number 13) costs industry approximately $1 billion a year in absenteeism, cancellations, and decreased business (Up Front, 1987).

SOCIOCULTURAL CONTEXT

Neuroses must be viewed in a sociocultural perspective. Problems engendered by often contradictory demands of society may be metaphorically expressed through such symptoms as somatization, phobias, and eating disorders. Viewed in this framework, neurotic symptoms become a communication form that synthesises nature, society, and culture (Scheper-Hughes and Lock, 1987). In Japan, for example, there is a culturally specific neurosis, *Taijin Kyofu*, which is a phobic fear *(kyofu)* of meeting people *(taijin)*. Japanese who suffer from this phobia experience feelings of inadequacy and a fear that their presence, specifically their gaze, can harm or cause discomfit to others. Therefore, they avoid looking at people. In addition, victims of this phobia stutter, emit foul-smelling body odors, look ugly, or otherwise do things that will produce discomfit in people with whom they are interacting.

If *Taijin Kyofu* is to be understood, it must be considered within the context of Japanese culture. Japanese mothers tend to be nurturing and soothing to their children. Infancy and childhood are characterized by ready gratification of needs and little need frustration. Furthermore, Japanese mothers use much eye-to-eye communication, unaccompanied by speech, as a primary mode of mother-child interaction. Such eye-to-eye communication may convey pleasure, displeasure, sadness, frustration, etc. This factor may partially explain why the eyes are the locus of this disorder. In addition, Japanese children are reared to be group-oriented and to conform to the many rigid social rules and formalities of Japanese society. Individuals who violate these rules and formalities are met with social ostracism and humiliation. "Saving face," the avoidance of shame and humiliation, is a primary guideline for social interaction. When victims of *Taijin Kyofu* avoid being among people, they also avoid the possibility of experiencing shame and humiliation (Nakakuki, n.d.).

TABLE 23-3 Comparison of major eating disorders

	Anorexia nervosa	Bulimia nervosa	Compulsive overeating
Onset	Any age but most frequently at puberty; small, consistent weight loss progressing to severe weight loss of 25-50% of body weight	Any age, but most frequently at puberty; often maintains "ideal" body weight through episodes of purging	Any age; unable to maintain reduction in body weight over time
Eating pattern	Reduction of food intake progressing to fasting and/or vomiting; abuse of diuretics, exercise, enemas; denies hunger pains	Consumption of large amounts of food, especially sweets and high-calorie foods, in 1-2 hours followed by purging through laxatives, vomiting, diuretics, amphetamines, enemas, exercise, fasting; experience hunger pains, but binge eating usually unrelated to hunger	Consumption of large amounts of food in short periods of time and often several times a day; often characterized by night eating, secret eating, lying about eating; diet-fasting cycles to control weight; occasional abuse of amphetamines, patent medicines for weight control, laxatives, enemas, diuretics; experiences hunger pains, but overeating usually unrelated to hunger
Thought pattern	Preoccupation with thoughts of food and eating—not eating; little interference with reality testing	Preoccupation with thoughts of food and eating—not eating; unimpaired reality testing	Preoccupation with thoughts of food and eating not eating; unimpaired reality testing
Body image	Distorted body image	Distorted body image	Distorted body image
Sexuality	Often avoids sexual relationships; often develops amenorrhea	Often sexually active, but sexual relationships tend to be short-term and superficial; menses may be regular, irregular, or absent	May be sexually inactive; oftentimes sexual relations are consciously desired but unconsciously avoided; menses may be regular, irregular, or absent
Affect	Frequent mood swings; fear of womanhood/adulthood; anxiety conflict concerning dependency and nurturence; fear of gaining weight	Frequent mood swings; may develop depression with suicidal ideation and attempts; fear of being fat	Frequent mood swings; covert anger; often a sense of interpersonal isolation
Behavior	Perfectionism; usually not a practice or substance abuser; avoids decision making; hyperactive	Often acts out through kleptomania, gambling, substance abuse, self-mutilation	Poor impulse control; often acts out through substance abuse, gambling, compulsive spending; desires to be liked and accepted
Physical signs	Frequent headaches; soft body hair on face, arms and stomach; grayish skin; sunken eyes and dark circles under eyes; brittle hair; leg cramps; interrupted sleep; premature osteoporosis	Split lips; mouth sores; sore throat; hoarse voice; loss of tooth enamel; receding gums; gastrointestinal problems	Progressive weight gain interrupted by periods of weight loss; obesity-related disorders (e.g., hypertension, shortness of breath)
Death	From sequelae of starvation	From electrolyte imbalance or hemorrhage	From sequelae of obesity (e.g., heart disease, stroke, diabetes.)

Sources include Oehler and Burns (1987), Schneider (1987), Maklen (1987), Levondron (1987), Brone and Fisher (1988), DSM-III-R (1987), Rigotti (1988).

In the United States today the technocratic nature of our society and the permeation of technology into our daily lives seem to be contributing to the development of a new phobia: compuphobia. Compuphobia, the fear of working with computers, in experienced by many people. This phobia has three aspects: (1) the general fear of using computers, which may stem from quantitative or linguistic anxiety, (2) the fear of failing when working with computers, which may arise from anxiety about loss of control, and (3) the fear of being replaced by technology, which may be related to a sense of inadequacy, helplessness, and loss of control (Suinn, 1983).

Cultures may also differ considerably in the traits they seek to encourage in their people. For example, in contemporary Western society, female attractiveness is equated with slimness. Anorexia nervosa may be a pathological response to the value put on female slimness as well as a pathological expression of dissatisfaction with body image. In contrast, in some traditional West African societies, plumpness was a culturally sought-after appearance. The daughters of wealthy men went to "fatting-houses," where they gorged on high-calorie foods and were allowed minimal exercise. Plumpness was equated with feminine attractiveness, wealth, and fertility (Polhemus, 1978; Garner and Garfinkel, 1980; Helman, 1984).

In many cultures, possession behavior is a socially acceptable way of expressing personal and interpersonal conflict without evoking retribution from members of the family or the community. Krippner (1987), who studied multiple personality disorder in Brazil, states that many Brazilian spiritists attribute multiple personality disorder to "involuntary possession." Involuntary possession involves long-term inhabiting and control of a person's body by malevolent or immature spirits. The spirits may be remnant personalities from a past life or personalities that have died and do not want to leave their earthly abode. This attitude toward multiple personalities reflects a traditional culture where people are defined within a context of social and kinship relationships. The idea of a singular, isolated self in the Western sense of "I" as an individual is not part of this world view.

Thus, there is much evidence that sociocultural factors not only contribute to people's vulnerability to neuroses but also contribute to the pattern behavior takes and the meaning that it is given.

EXPLANATORY THEORIES
Psychological theories

Psychological theories trace the origins of neuroses to psychological and maturational processes of childhood. Such factors as psychic trauma, pathological parent-child relationships, dysfunctional interpersonal relationships, and cognitive errors are viewed as especially relevant.

PSYCHODYNAMIC THEORY

Many psychodynamically oriented therapists believe neuroses originate during the period of psychosexual development (see Chapter 6). Such a Freudian (1936, 1960, 1969) orientation relates neuroses to innate drives or instincts, particularly libidinal (sexual) and aggressive drives, and to the struggle to express these drives in a socially acceptable manner. Thoughts or fantasies, termed *drive derivatives*, are considered primitive, since they have their roots in early developmental years. The overt expression of such primitive fantasies and wishes represents a danger to the person. The danger may come from external reality, or it may result from a conflict with the individual's moral standards and values. For example, acting out aggressive or sexual wishes impulsively against another person may result in punishment or pain. Such action may also result in feelings of shame and guilt.

In neuroses, there is imbalance between unconscious fantasies and wishes and ego defense mechanisms. The person with a neurosis has less variety of defenses and fewer options for gratification of unconscious strivings than does the "normal" person. Also, defenses are used more frequently and more rigidly than in the nonneurotic personality. Anxiety is aroused when unconscious wishes threaten to become conscious. Additional defenses are then needed to control anxiety.

INTERPERSONAL THEORY

According to Horney (1937, 1939, 1945), conflicts in neuroses center around meeting basic interpersonal needs for affection, attention, approval, recognition from others, and expression of aggression and sexuality. In meeting these needs, people are pulled or driven by a compelling striving to become dependent upon others (to move toward others). This striving may be blocked, however, by an equally compelling striving to move against others (to dominate them) or to move away from others (toward detachment). Trapped between such powerful and opposing forces in meeting fundamental needs, the individual is immobilized and unable to function unless some unconscious adaptive compromise can be achieved. Table 23-4 describes these compromise solutions.

Another compromise solution involves the creation of an *idealized image*. People who feel insecure and inadequate and who compulsively crave perfection and admiration may come to view their actual selves as unreal and may unconsciously create an idealized image. The qualities that are incorporated into an idealized image depend upon the ideals, beliefs, and needs of an individual. For example, some people may regard themselves as intellectually or morally superior to others. Efforts to point out discrepancies between the way people see themselves and the way others see them are strongly resisted.

Compromise solutions represent defensive maneuvers that serve to control anxiety and to enable an individual to function despite underlying conflict. Once a particular compromise solution has been adopted, it becomes part of the individual's personality structure and is used compulsively and indiscriminately in every interpersonal situation, whether it is appropriate or not.

COGNITIVE THEORY

In the cognitive model, activation of specific maladaptive cognitive patterns is viewed as a basis for neurotic symptoms. For example, individuals with anorexia nervosa who have episodes of bulimia have been found to be more cognitively impulsive than anorexic individuals who consistently restrict food intake (Toner, Garfinkel, and Garner, 1987). With anxiety disorders, Beck, Emery, and Greenberg (1985) believe there is cognitive malfunctioning in the activation and termination of a defensive

TABLE 23-4 Compromise solutions

Compromise solution	Description
Move toward others	Become compliant, submissive, and dependent
Move against others	Gain power and domination over people
Move away from others	Become detached and limit interpersonal interaction

response to threat. The cognitive set of "threat" is manifested by preoccupation with fears, loss of control, and inability to cope. The cognitive system may become preoccupied with the "threat," leaving little cognitive capacity available for other demands on the cognitive system. Some neurotic symptoms represent hyperfunctioning of the cognitive system (e.g., hypervigilence), while other neurotic symptoms represent inhibited cognitive functioning (e.g., memory loss).

People with neuroses usually apply the wrong rules to complex, ambiguous, or problematic situations. For example, a person with generalized anxiety disorder may act upon the following assumptions or rules (Beck, Emery, and Greenberg, 1985):

1. I should regard any unfamiliar situation as unsafe.
2. I should regard any situation or person as dangerous until shown to be safe.
3. I should always assume the worst.
4. I must anticipate and be prepared for danger at all times. My well-being depends on it.
5. I cannot rely on anyone else to keep me safe. I must secure my own safety.
6. I must be cautious and quiet in unfamiliar situations.
7. I must always stay capable and strong if I am to survive.
8. I know that strangers hate weakness.
9. I know that strangers will attack me if they notice any sign of weakness in me.
10. I know that an attack will mean that I seemed weak and socially ineffective.

The following verbatim illustrates how a person operating on the preceding assumptions might respond to the prospect of having elective surgery:

Assumption: *I should always assume the worst.*
Situation: *After my fall a few weeks ago, I had terrible headaches (actually had a mild headache for one day). There must be something seriously wrong with my brain. If I have the surgery, I will probably have a bad response to the spinal anesthesia. I might be left paralyzed. When I had oral surgery, I developed complications. I must be prone to complications. It is always safer to overestimate the danger than to underestimate it.*
Conclusion: *I had better not have the surgery.*
Self-instruction: *Keep vigilant. I cannot entrust my safety to strangers. I have to look out for myself.*

The preceding verbatim illustrates some of the thinking errors that neurotic individuals may make: (1) exaggeration (a one-day mild headache becomes "terrible" headaches), (2) catastrophizing (a headache means there is serious brain damage; spinal anesthesia will result in paralysis), (3) overgeneralizing (complications following oral surgery signify complication-proneness), and (4) ignoring the positive (personal strengths such as level of overall wellness, past positive experiences with surgery, or social support systems are overlooked).

Biological theories

Biological theories purport that people suffering from neuroses are biologically predisposed to such behavior. Familial patterns in panic disorders, for example, may be related to biological factors (Crowe et al., 1987), and administration of antidepressants, especially imipramine, has proven effective in the treatment of panic disorder (Gorman et al., 1983). Findings such as these suggest a biological dimension in the development of neuroses.

BIOCHEMICAL THEORIES

The lactate hypothesis suggests that alkalosis, hypocalcemia, and increases in both blood lactate and epinephrine stimulate the anxiety that is present in neurosis. Balon, Yeragani, and Pohl (1988) have been able to precipitate panic attacks with sodium lactate infusions. Other studies implicate abnormal brain chemistry in obsessive-compulsive disorder. The brains (especially the dominant-hemisphere orbital gyrus and caudate nucleus) of people with obsessive-compulsive disorder metabolize glucose at excessively fast rates. In addition, these two brain areas contain large quantities of serotonin. Serotonin-squelching agents are effective in decreasing obsessive compulsive behavior, while serotonin-stimulating drugs increase this behavior (Baxter et al., 1987).

Biochemistry is also implicated in eating disorders. For example, the body regulates the "set point" (stabilized ideal biological body weight) in people. Even when food intake varies substantially, the body regulates its expenditure of energy so that the set point is maintained as closely as possible. It may be that obese individuals have a higher set point than nonobese individuals (Keesey and Pawley, 1986; Krieshok and Karpowitz, 1988).

PHYSIOLOGICAL THEORIES

Physiological malfunctioning may be involved in the development of some types of neuroses. Kahn, Drusin, and Klein (1987) suggest that autonomic mechanisms may explain the association between idiopathic cardiomyopathy and panic disorder. The following autonomic mechanisms may be involved: (1) increase in centrally mediated cardiac sympathetic tone, (2) mitral valve prolapse, and (3) increase in peripheral catecholamines. The relationship among catecholamines, idiopathic cardiomyopathy, and panic is twofold: (1) panic, by increasing the level of catecholamines, may contribute to the development of cardiomyopathy and (2) congestive heart failure (found in end-stage idiopathic cardiomyopathy), by increasing the level of catecholamines, may exacerbate a panic disorder.

The autonomic nervous system may also be involved in obesity. Significant correlation has been found between decreased sympathetic and parasympathetic activity and obesity (Peterson et al., 1988). Another study has identified adrenergic receptors on the surfaces of fat cells. While β receptors stimulate the breakdown of fat, α_2 receptors stimulate the accumulation of fat. The ratio of glycerol to free fatty acids (products of fat cell metabolism) in peripheral tissues may be responsible for controlling appetite (Hirsch and Leibel, 1985).

GENETIC THEORY

Although there is not a clear genetic basis for all neuroses, genetics does seem to be implicated in some types. For example, monozygotic and dyzygotic twin studies have shown the influence of genetic factors for panic disorder and agoraphobia with panic disorder (Torgenson, 1983). Genetic factors are also implicated in degree of body fat as well as distribution of body fat. A correlation between the degree of fatness of adoptees and their biological mothers has been found that is independent of degree of fatness of adoptive parents (Price et al., 1987). Genetic factors have also been found to account for abdominal obesity and extremity-trunk fat ratio (Bouchard et al., 1985; Forbes, Prochaska, and Weitkamp, 1988).

The explanation for neuroses appears to be complex. Although biochemical, physiological, and genetic factors are being investigated, an organic explanation has not been definitely demonstrated. Future research may more clearly indicate what role biological factors play in the development of neuroses.

Sociocultural theories

Sociocultural theories look to the broad social environment for explanations of neuroses. There are several ways that society and culture can increase vulnerability to neuroses. These include (1) childrearing practices that promote feelings of shame or guilt, (2) role stress, and (3) socially unrealistic expectations. In addition, such social stressors as unemployment, acculturative pressures, and marital discord may significantly weaken people's social support systems and function either as predisposing or precipitating factors in the development of neuroses. Williams' (1988) statement that "cultural transmission (of risk factors) can be even

stronger than genetic transmission" can be applied to neuroses. While genetically dominant traits will affect only 50% of all offspring, culturally transmitted traits, such as eating patterns and ways of coping with anxiety, may be transmitted to nearly all offspring.

FEMINIST THEORY

Eichenbaum and Orbach (1983) look at the way that postindustrial American sex-role stereotypes influence gender identity. Culture effectively molds "needs, desires, and psychic life," which serve as a basis for concepts of femininity and masculinity. Personality is an outgrowth of gender identity. Within a cultural context, parenting, especially the mother-daughter relationship, teaches many daughters to be nurturers of others even at the expense of their own needs and autonomy. Neurotic symptoms may serve as pathological expressions of this upbringing. For example, through phobia, a woman may express her needs for dependency and connectedness. Through agoraphobia and claustrophobia, physical boundaries may substitute as psychological boundaries that protect a woman against loss of self. Through obsessive compulsivity, a woman may express thwarted dependency needs. She must take care of herself, but she feels incapable of doing so.

Eating behavior among women may express conflict about or rebellion against culturally defined sex-role stereotypes. To fulfill the female sex-role stereotype, women are socialized to be appealing to men. Emphasis is placed on dependence, nurturing, sensualness, coquettishness, and physical attractiveness. This idealized image of femininity is imposed by significant others, the media, and the fashion industry. Much of a woman's self-image reflects her dual social role of sex object and nurturer. Women may find these two roles unrealistic and conflicting. For many women, it is impossible to be both a thin, demure, dependent sex object/lover and a reliable, well-organized, giving wife/mother. For these women, fat may symbolize the sustenance necessary to fulfill the role of wife and mother. Compulsive overeating, for example, serves a dual purpose: While expressing a basic need for comforting, it also acknowledges an inability to be appropriately responsive to one's own

TABLE 23-5 Infant feeding patterns and maladaptive eating behavior

Hypothesis	Rationale
External caloric regulation	Association of environmental cues and hunger are learned early in life. When parents indiscriminately offer an infant food (food is offered whether the infant is hungry or not), presence of food becomes a stimulus to eat. Compulsive overeating may be triggered by such external cues rather than by internal hunger cues. When infant hunger cues are ignored (feeding is according to a fixed schedule), interoceptive hunger recognition and a sense of personal control may not be learned. Anorexia is often found in young women who, as infants, had fixed feeding schedules and whose mothers "anticipated" their hunger.
Internal caloric regulation	The ability to use internal cues of satiation is learned. Early introduction of solid food (before 3 months of age) may lead to overfeeding (e.g., amount of milk is not decreased when food is introduced; salt in baby food increases infant's thirst, so the infant drinks more milk). The infant does not learn to associate internal cues with satiation, and compulsive overeating may develop.

Sources consulted include Rodin (1980), Garner et al. (1984), Krinsky (1987).

emotional needs. Thinness may be equated with vulnerability; fatness, with protection. To give up fatness means emotional starvation. Robbed of the protective shield of fat, a woman's needs will be exposed and unmet. Bulimic women have similar ideas attached to food and eating. Binging is associated with emotional neediness; purging, with denial of need gratification. Anorectic women, on the other hand, try to gain control over the "self" by creating a new person—one who has no appetite and no needs. The rejection of food is associated with rejection of emotional neediness. Extreme dieting and excessive exercise create a barrier between the anorectic woman and her needs.

SOCIAL LEARNING THEORY

Social learning theorists view neuroses as conditioned or learned responses to painful stimuli. Urbanization, social insecurity, and overcrowding are examples of aspects of the environment that frequently serve as stimuli for anxiety. Because a stimulus produces anxiety and this anxiety, in turn, engenders more anxiety (neurotic anxiety), when the stimulus is again encountered, a reflex arc is established. Conditioned responses become self-perpetuating and circle back upon themselves. For example, the labeling of hunger is a behavior learned early in life. Maladaptive eating behaviors have been explained using social learning theory (see Table 23-5).

Systems theory

The explanation for neuroses appears to be complex and multifactorial. A systems approach to neuroses integrates the biopsychosociocultural dimensions of self and looks at how these dimensions are continuously interacting to contribute to neurotic behavior. For example, conflict between one's social behavior and one's cultural values and/or spiritual standards may generate neurotic anxiety, shame, or guilt. In addition, biological and psychological factors may predispose an individual for a particular neurosis. Moreover, physiological and emotional symptoms are found in all neuroses. The form that these symptoms take varies from society to society. Neuroses seem to develop when a confluence of interacting factors becomes so disrupted that a person cannot adaptively cope. Then maladaptive or neurotic coping behaviors emerge. This means that neurotic behavior is a product of reciprocal interaction among such factors as (1) personal resistance or vulnerability to a stressor, (2) the presence and potency of a precipitating event, and (3) the cultural expectations governing interpersonal relationships.

Anxiety disorder will be used to exemplify the constant simultaneous interaction of biological, psychological, and social processes that generate neurotic symptoms. Biochemical factors and/or genetic factors may interfere with a person's ability to tolerate stress. An imbalance in the regulatory functions of the individual's cognitive system may result in the inappropriate perception of an environmental stimulus as a threat. A sense of vulnerability develops, and anxiety is engendered. The anxiety further interferes with the individual's functioning in the following ways: (1) The affective symptoms of anxiety are distracting. (2) The anxiety is interpreted as a manifestation of dysfunction and loss of control. (3) The somatic symptoms of anxiety become frightening. (4) Others observe the manifestations of anxiety. The individual interprets these other-observations as evidence that he or she is viewed as weak, powerless, ineffective, etc. (5) The individual begins to question his or her ability to cope with the situation. A cognitive-affective-behavioral feedback loop is in effect. This feedback loop transports information concerning the individual's affect (e.g., anxiety), behavior (e.g., activated patterns and inhibitions), physiological responses (e.g., autonomic factors that facilitate somatic mobilization) and cognitive processing (Beck et al., 1985).

TREATMENT MODALITIES

The most frequently employed modalities in the treatment of neuroses are psychoanalytic psychotherapy, cognitive therapy, family therapy, group psychotherapy, behavior therapy, emergency interventions, and administration of psychopharmaceuticals. Goals of treatment include (1) exploration of feelings, thoughts, and assumptions; (2) teaching new ways of perceiving the environment; (3) teaching new and more effective ways of coping; and (4) intervening in life-style patterns that are reinforcing neurotic behavior.

Psychoanalytic psychotherapy

Psychoanalysis, a long-term and intensive form of therapy that is oriented toward restructuring the personality, emphasizes ego growth and resolution of unconscious conflicts. Psychoanalysis may last over a period of 2 or more years, with sessions held as often as three times a week. Psychoanalytically oriented psychotherapy, a modified form of psychoanalysis, strives for symptom reduction or change in areas of the personality that are troubling to a

client. Psychoanalytically oriented psychotherapy may extend over a period of a year or more.

Cognitive therapy

Cognitive therapy is a short-term therapy (from five to twenty sessions) that utilizes the Socratic method and is based on an educational model. With cognitive therapy, a structured, directive approach is taken to client problems, and therapy is task related. For example, focus may be directed to such specific target behaviors as teaching a client to recognize distorted automatic thoughts, correcting thinking errors (such as exaggeration, catastrophizing, over-generalizing, and ignoring the positive), and responding with logic and reason to distorted thoughts. Imagery-related interventions that help clients modify distorted fantasies, improve reality testing, and distance themselves from anxiety are frequently used. Clients are assigned homework that reinforces the educational process (Beck et al., 1985).

Family therapy

Family systems theory views the neurotic disorder of a family member as evidence of dysfunction within the family system. The family system becomes unbalanced. Anxiety is generated in a family member, and the family member develops a neurotic disorder. For example, Madanes (1981) suggests that a neurotic symptom in a spouse may be an attempt to alter the hierarchical nature of the couple's relationship and achieve a balance of power. The couple's method of interacting about the symptom is analogous to the way they interact about other situations in their marriage. The approach taken to neurotic symptomatology in the family system varies according to the therapist's theoretical orientation (see Table 23-6).

Group psychotherapy

Psychoanalytically oriented group psychotherapy is perhaps the most common type of group therapy used in the treatment of neuroses. Emphasis is on developing awareness of impulses, feelings, and needs. The long-range goal is to work through basic

TABLE 23-6 Family therapy approaches*

Family therapy approach	View of neurotic behavior	Therapeutic focus
Multigenerational	Evidence of a low level of self-differentiation from family members	Resolution of unresolved emotional attachments with one's parents, differentiation of self from one's family of origin, and identification and modification of one's role in the family triangle
Structural	Evidence of anxiety engendered by dysfunctional family transactional patterns	Establishment of new transactional patterns or scripts
Interactional	Evidence of anxiety and confusion produced by vague and ambiguous rules regulating family interaction	Clarification of rules regulating family interaction

*Refer to Chapter 14 for an in-depth discussion of family dysfunction and family therapy.

conflicts that provoke anxiety and that interfere with clients' ability to function. For example, Oehler and Burns (1987) found that, in a group composed of anorectic and bulimic clients, issues surrounding familial and social functioning, gender identity, and heterosexual concerns were addressed. The group provides a safe environment to explore these issues as well as fantasies, feelings, and behavior patterns. Group therapy with people who are experiencing neurotic disorders tends to be conducted in outpatient rather than inpatient settings. (Refer to Chapter 13 for an in-depth discussion of group therapy.)

Behavior therapy

One form of behavior therapy is desensitization therapy. There are two types of desensitization therapy: in vivo and fantasy. In vivo desensitization requires that a client be exposed to the real-life situation or object that produces anxiety. Exposure to the anxiety-producing event can be done in steps (a client is gradually exposed to anxiety-producing situations of increasing intensity) or all at once (a client is suddenly put in the anxiety-producing situation). The latter method is referred to as implosion or flooding. Fantasy desensitization, on the other hand, requires that a client actively imagine being exposed to the situation or object that generates anxiety. Muscle-relaxation techniques may be used as aids in both in vivo and fantasy desensitization.

Desensitization therapy is most frequently used to treat clients with phobias and anxiety disorders.

Behavior modification of a different type, where behavior changes are reinforced through rewards, is sometimes used in treating people with eating disorders. Although immediate change in eating behavior may be produced, long-term change seems poor (Brone and Fisher, 1988).

Emergency interventions

Crisis centers and hot lines provide short-term emergency measures for dealing with specific neurotic behaviors. For example, Binge Eaters Hot Line and ANAD (National Association of Anorexia Nervosa and Associated Disorders) are national hotlines that offer counseling and information for people with eating disorders.

Merker (1986) stresses that an individual who seems to be experiencing a psychiatric emergency needs to have a thorough medical work-up (health history, physical examination, laboratory testing) to be certain that pathophysiology is not responsible for the symptoms. For example, such medical conditions as arrhythmias, mitral valve prolapse, hypoglycemia, and pulmonary embolus may present symptomatology similar to some anxiety disorders. Clients should be assessed for (1) level of anxiety-panic, (2) evidence of underlying depression, (3) thought disorders (e.g., obsessions), (4) degree of care needed, and (5) urgency of need for care. For instance, if a client is helpless (e.g., suffering from severe psychogenic amnesia) or dangerously ill (e.g., manifesting severe physical sequelae of anorexia nervosa), or if a diagnosis is in question (e.g., reason for paralysis or blindness is undetermined), hospitalization may be indicated. If a client is able to participate with the nurse during crisis intervention in developing a plan of action and has an effective social support system, then outpatient care may be indicated. Emergency interventions for the anxiety underlying psychoneurotic emergencies are discussed in Chapters 8 and 15.

Psychopharmaceuticals

Nonamphetamine anorexigenic agents, minor tranquilizers (e.g., benzodiazepines and glycerol derivatives), barbiturates (e.g., phenobarbital, butabarbital), tricyclics (e.g., imipramine pamoate), and antihistamines (e.g., hydroxyzine) are often used in the treatment of disorders discussed in this chapter. For example, trazodone hydrochloride, a triazolopyridine derivative with antidepressant properties, and alprazolam, a benzodiazepine derivative, have been found effective in the treatment of panic disorder and panic disorder with agoraphobia (Mavissakalian et al., 1987; Ballenger et al., 1988; Noyes et al., 1988). (Refer to Appendix B for detailed information about these drugs.)

All the minor tranquilizers are central nervous system depressants. The degree to which central nervous system depression occurs depends upon dosage and varies according to the particular drug group. The barbiturates and the antihistamines have a greater sedative effect than the benzodiazepines and the glycerol derivatives. The benzodiazepines are among the safest and most effective in the treatment of anxiety. They also have anticonvulsant and muscle relaxant properties and produce little effect on autonomic functions such as blood pressure. All these drugs can produce physiological addiction, but the benzodiazepines are less addictive than the others and have fewer side effects. The side effects of the minor tranquilizers, which are often dosage related, are daytime drowsiness and sedation, decreased mental acuity, and decreased coordination. Overdoses produce muscle weakness, lack of coordination, sleep, and coma.

Because the tricyclic drugs have a sedative as well as an antidepressant action, imipramine has often proved more effective than tranquilizers in treating some phobias, such as the social phobias and agoraphobia (Clayton, 1987). The actions and side effects of imipramine are further discussed in Chapter 22.

Since the minor tranquilizers are central nervous system depressants, they should not be used in combination with other central nervous system depressants such as the phenothiazines and alcohol. They are also contraindicated in pregnancy, particularly in the first trimester, and, because of the potentially addicting effect, in people known to be addicted to alcohol or other drugs.

Clients should be alerted to the possible side effects of antianxiety medications, and they should be cautioned against the use of other sedatives such as sleeping pills and alcohol. They should also be alerted to the possible dangers involved in driving a car or operating tools or machinery that require alertness and attention—especially in the early weeks of administration, when side effects are most apt to appear. Withdrawal symptoms, which can occur if the administration of a drug is suddenly ended, can be avoided through a gradual decrease in dosage over approximately a week's time. Nurses are responsible for the administration of medication and the assessment of client responses, including side effects. Nurses are also responsible for health teaching in relation to dosage and side effects (see Appendix B).

Nursing Intervention
PRIMARY PREVENTION

Primary prevention of neuroses should focus on enhancing self-esteem and a sense of adequacy; promoting open, nondefensive communication; and increasing problem-solving ability. The goals for primary prevention of neuroses include (1) identifying high-risk individuals and (2) minimizing the effects of factors that predispose people to neurotic disorders. Nurses should keep the following principles in mind when they engage in activities of primary prevention of neuroses:

1. Interpersonal patterns of dependence, domination, and detachment are a means of coping.
2. Anxiety is present whether or not there are overt symptoms.
3. A behavioral response in any situation is aimed primarily at maintaining psychological security and keeping anxiety under control.
4. During periods of crisis, anxiety increases and symptoms may increase.
5. Awareness of feelings and interpersonal behavior is low during periods of crisis.
6. Crisis periods are characterized by excessive vulnerability to criticism, rejection, or abandonment.

Identification of high-risk individuals

Community health nurses and school-nurse teachers work with families and observe family interactions. This provides opportunity to identify children who are asymptomatic but who come from families where people habitually relate to others through dependency, domination, or detachment. Table 23-7 summarizes the characteristics of such high-risk individuals. In addition, nurses should be aware of such holistic health factors as family history of neuroses, family dynamics, childrearing prac-

tices that promote feelings of shame and guilt, role stress, and socially unrealistic expectations that may predispose people to neurotic disorders.

Parental and family counseling

An important activity of primary prevention of neuroses is helping families learn more adaptive coping behaviors. Families should be taught stress-reduction techniques (e.g., meditation, progressive relaxation, and physical exercise) as well as ways of expressing feelings of anxiety, fear, and apprehension directly and authentically.

A child born into a family in which one or both parents use neurotic coping patterns is in a vulnerable state.

A community health nurse was teaching Mr. and Mrs. Jefferson, who were new parents, to care for their prematurely born twins. Mrs. Jefferson had not gained adequate weight during her pregnancy, and her antepartum care had been sporadic. The Jeffersons had not expected twins. In addition, Mr. Jefferson had only recently begun working as an automobile mechanic. Although the family had accumulated many bills during Mr. Jefferson's period of unemployment and his new job paid poorly, they were glad that the new job's fringe benefits included a comprehensive health plan.

TABLE 23-7 Characteristics of high-risk individuals

Characteristic	Description
Interpersonal dependency	Consistently relates to others in a helpless or vulnerable manner; persistently and indirectly expresses dependency needs; repeatedly needs attention and approval from others; habitually evidences hypersensitivity to anything that may be perceived as rejection, criticism, or neglect; excessively complies with the wishes of others
Interpersonal domination	Always takes command of a situation; always projects an image of confidence; views the world as a hostile, threatening place; has difficulty trusting others; is unable to admit to self or to others feelings of apprehension, fear, and anxiety; repeatedly responds to anxiety-producing situations with angry outbursts or with sarcasm; habitually perceives any questions of a personal nature (including a health history) as prying and is resentful; habitually resists advice and suggestions
Interpersonal detachment	Habitually relates to others with indifference, disinterest, or an air of superiority; repeatedly uses intellectualization to cope with anxiety; has an excessive need for privacy (much value is attached to privacy and to being alone); habitually perceives questions of a personal nature (including a health history) as an intrusion of privacy and responds with evasion, withdrawal, or anger

The community health nurse observed that Mr. Jefferson frequently complained of his "heart skipping beats," shortness of breath, and a "strange feeling" in his chest. Mr. Jefferson was very concerned that he had heart disease.

The community health nurse suggested that these symptoms be medically evaluated. The medical examination was negative. Mrs. Jefferson revealed to the community health nurse that early in their marriage her husband had also been afraid that he had heart disease. Mrs. Jefferson told the nurse, "My husband always seems worried about his health, but it gets worse whenever changes come into his life. I hate to tell him if someone we know becomes seriously sick, because he immediately starts checking himself for the symptoms." Mr. Jefferson had a history of noticing some small irregularity in his health, interpreting it as a symptom, becoming increasingly concerned about what it might mean, and having it checked out by a doctor. The medical examinations had always shown no pathology.

The community health nurse referred the Jeffersons for family therapy. Referrals were also made to a Twins Club that had a loan closet and to social services for food stamps and the WIC program (supplemental food program for women, infants, and children at nutritional risk). These referrals helped modify the family's socioeconomic stressors.

As the above vignette illustrates, when a parental pattern of neurotic coping behavior (e.g., hypochondriasis) is observed, there is need to help the family on several levels.

Inadequate parental coping responses, poverty, or other environmental stressors that contribute to a chronic crisis situation may interfere with a child's ability to accomplish the tasks of normal development. Identification of and preventive intervention for such families are particularly pertinent in the prenatal and perinatal periods, during developmental crises in the child, in family developmental crises, and in situational crises. For example, a parent who has excessive dependency needs may be unable, without ongoing support, to meet the dependency needs of an infant. A parent who copes through interpersonal domination may be unable to allow a toddler the freedom necessary to develop autonomy, or an adolescent the degree of independence essential to the development of identity. Identification of such parents (or prospective par-

ents) and follow-up care during their children's early developmental years are essential aspects of primary prevention of neuroses.

SECONDARY PREVENTION

Although professional nurses have traditionally been involved in the treatment of the more severe psychiatric disorders, such as the psychoses, changing patterns of health care and the expanding role of the nurse in community health and mental health are placing increasing demands upon the profession to participate in secondary prevention of neuroses. Such prevention involves meeting the following objectives:

1. Early identification of cases of neurosis in the community
2. Obtaining prompt and effective treatment to restore the individual to optimum mental health
3. Assessment of available community resources for referral
4. Participation with community groups in expanding needed resources

Case finding

Early identification, or case finding, is important in neuroses since many individuals suffering from them do not seek professional help until the symptoms severely inhibit their ability to function. The professional involvement of nurses in many aspects of community life brings them into contact with families and individuals. Nurses thus have opportunities for case finding that may not be available to other health professionals. A community health nurse, for example, providing services to a family in the home, may be the first health professional to learn of a phobia in a mother that is undermining the mental health of the entire family. A school nurse may be the first to recognize an anxiety disorder in a parent that is interfering with a child's learning or to recognize school phobia in a child. An industrial nurse may be the first to recognize symptoms of an underlying neurosis that is contributing to alcohol abuse in an employee.

The objective of early identification in secondary prevention is the referral of the client to a mental health resource for treatment. Many neurotic clients, however, are highly resistant to any form of psychiatric intervention. In such a case, the person's right to refuse treatment must be respected. For persons who are reluctant to accept treatment or who are ambivalent about becoming involved, a supportive nurse-client relationship, with the time-limited goal of providing emotional support while the client is in crisis, may be effective in motivating the individual to accept further treatment.

The focus of this aspect of secondary prevention is on intervention into behavioral patterns associated with the neurotic process and restoration of functional patterns of client behavior. Nurses should keep the following principles in mind regardless of the symptom picture:

1. The focus should be upon the client as a person who is suffering, and not upon the symptom.
2. Whether or not it is observable, underlying anxiety is present and should be assessed.*
3. The symptom is a mechanism designed to contain anxiety.
4. Nursing interventions and activities should permit the client to carry out demands of the disorder, such as an obsessive-compulsive ritual.
5. The client needs acceptance and approval, and he or she is vulnerable to any form of rejection.
6. If the disorder is characterized by indecisiveness, any pressure to have the client make decisions should be avoided.
7. Although the client is in contact with reality and able to think logically, the client may be out of touch with his or her own feelings.
8. Repressed hostility may be overtly expressed when the client feels pressured or frustrated.
9. Since the client fears his or her own hostility and anger, and anxiety increases when these feelings become overt, actions that may arouse anger should be avoided.
10. Any attempt to rationally explain symptoms or underlying dynamics should be avoided. Such attempts would be met with resistance and increased anxiety.

Knowledge of these principles will facilitate intervention with clients who are experiencing neurotic disorders.

Nursing process

The nursing process provides the framework for therapeutic intervention. The focus of this aspect of secondary prevention is twofold: (1) intervention into neurotic behavior patterns and (2) facilitation of an optimal level of functioning.

ASSESSMENT

When they work with clients who cope with anxiety and conflict through compulsivity, somatization or altered identity, nurses need to begin their assessment where the client identifies the problem. The following areas should be assessed:

1. Presenting symptoms—phobias, compulsions, hypochondriacal behavior, etc. that are creating problems for the client even though they are serving as defenses against an emotional state the client is experiencing
2. Emotional state—such feelings as helplessness, anxiety,* or anger that are responses to a stimulus situation
3. Stimulus situations—stressful life situations that are characterized by a threat to one's security (These stressful life situations are engendered by maladaptive [neurotic] coping behaviors.)
4. Maladaptive coping behaviors—neurotic symptoms and coping patterns of dependency, domination, and detachment that are used in relating to others in protecting oneself from hurt
5. Origin of maladaptive coping behaviors— identification of childhood experiences that contributed to the development of or learning of maladaptive coping behaviors
6. Holistic health status—physical, intellectual, emotional, sociocultural, and spiritual status of the client (These factors may either facilitate wellness [e.g., a culturally approved belief in spirit possession may permit expression of personal and interpersonal conflict through

---

*Refer to Chapter 8 for a discussion of anxiety and its assessment.

*Refer to Chapter 8 for a discussion of assessment of anxiety

TABLE 23-8   Client assessment guide

Dimension	Behavioral indicator
Physiological	Cardiovascular (e.g., palpitations, tachycardia, hypertension, lightheadedness, syncope), respiratory (e.g., hyperventilation, shortness of breath, choking sensation), neuromuscular (e.g., tremors, twitching, increased reflexes, unsteady gait, generalized weakness), gastro-intestinal (e.g., constipation, diarrhea, heartburn, nausea, vomiting), genitourinary (e.g., polyuria, amenorrhea), skin (e.g., facial flushing or pallor, perspiration, dark circles under eyes, split lips), sensory-perceptual (e.g., psychogenic blindness, dazed appearance), nutritional-metabolic (e.g., disrupted fluid volume integrity, impaired nutritional status), endocrine-biochemical (e.g., imbalanced hormonal status, hypocalcemia, increased blood lactate level)
Behavioral	Restlessness, altered thought patterns (e.g., obsessions, preoccupation with thoughts of food and eating—not eating, preoccupation with health or body functions), disturbance in identity (e.g., distorted body image, amnesia, multiple personality states, idealized image), fear (e.g., of specific social situation, of specific object), impaired social interaction (e.g., excessive need to control others, excessive need to be independent and self-sufficient, excessive need for attention, affection, and approval), altered impulse control (e.g., compulsive or ritualistic behavior, rigidity, substance abuse)
Feeling	Anxious, frightened, uneasy, impatient, depressed, angry, ashamed, guilty, alexithymia (inability to "read" one's feelings—emotions are experienced as undifferentiated or as absent), mood swings
Self-esteem	Sense of inadequacy, underestimation of personal strengths, exaggeration of personal weaknesses
Environmental	Childbearing practices that promote shame or guilt, social stressors that generate anxiety, sex-role stereotypes that thwart or create conflict about expression of dependency needs, parental use of neurotic coping patterns, family and ethnic eating habits

Sources consulted include Beck et al. (1985), Bryant and Kopeski (1986), Mazlen (1987), DSM-III-R (1987), Brone and Fisher (1988).

"possession behavior"], or these factors may impede wellness [e.g., a conflict between one's social behavior and one's cultural values and/or spiritual standards may generate neurotic anxiety, shame, or guilt]. In addition, many neurotic disorders involve physical as well as emotional manifestations [e.g., clients who compulsively wash their hands may have excoriated hands; anorexic clients may have amenorrhea, malnutrition, etc.].)

Tables 23-1, 23-2, 23-3, and 23-7, presented earlier in this chapter, and Table 23-8 may assist nurses in making these assessments.

ANALYSIS OF DATA

As nurses assess the presenting symptoms, emotional states, stimulus situations, maladaptive coping behaviors and their origins, and the holistic health status of clients, nurses begin to understand the client's (and often the family's) perceptions of the presenting problem. The aforementioned assessments also aid nurses in understanding the interrelationship between family dynamics, predisposing and precipitating factors, and clients' maladaptive coping behaviors. At this point, nurses may be ready to formulate nursing diagnoses.

PLANNING AND IMPLEMENTATION

The following are nursing diagnoses that are frequently made when caring for clients with patterns of compulsivity, somatization, or altered identity. Following each nursing diagnosis is a plan of care that reflects a realistic approach to secondary preventive intervention. The nurse may initially establish goals, but as therapy progresses the client should enter into goal setting to ensure commitment to goal accomplishment.

Text continued on p. 747.

NURSING CARE PLAN

Clients with Impaired Social Interaction

Long-term Outcomes	Short-term Outcomes	Nursing Strategies

Nursing diagnosis:
- Impaired social interaction (dependency) related to dependence-independence conflict and a sense of inadequacy (NANDA 3.1.1, DSM-III-R 300.01-300.14, 300.21-300.30, 300.70, 307.10, 307.50, 307.51, 316)
- Impaired social interaction (detachment) related to dependence-independence conflict and a sense of inadequacy (NANDA 3.1.1; DSM-III-R 300-300.14, 300.21-300.30, 300.70, 307.10, 307.50, 307.51, 316)
- Impaired social interaction (domination) related to dependence-independence conflict and a sense of inadequacy (NANDA 3.1.1; DSM-III-R 300-300.14, 300.21-300.30, 300.70, 307.10, 307.50, 307.51, 316)

Long-term Outcomes	Short-term Outcomes	Nursing Strategies
Work through dependence-independence conflict Develop a sense of personal adequacy Relate to others in an assertive manner	Express feelings of dependency, anxiety, and inadequacy (when consistent with client's cultural orientation) Identify interpersonal situations that generate feelings of dependency, anxiety, and inadequacy Relate current stressful interpersonal situations to situations in the past that aroused similar feelings Develop more effective coping behaviors and interpersonal skills Realistically perceive strengths and weaknesses Build self-esteem (see Chapter 22)	Establish a relationship where client can feel free to express feelings Meet client's dependency needs *initially* (trying to force client to be independent or interdependent may increase the sense of anxiety and inadequacy) Identify the degree of client dependency and potential for interdependent functioning (e.g., use your own observations as feedback; obtain client's perceptions of how he or she functions with peers and authority figures and in structured and unstructured, competitive, and noncompetitive situations) Help client evaluate effectiveness of current coping behaviors and interpersonal skills (e.g., air of superiority, intellectualization, manipulation, approval-seeking, submissiveness) Support effective current coping behaviors and interpersonal skills Teach client necessary skills for independence (e.g., making lists and schedules, developing strategy plans, etc., that aid in organizing and carrying out tasks) Teach client assertive communication techniques (teach the difference between assertive behavior and domineering and detached behavior) Teach client stress-reduction techniques (e.g., progressive relaxation, meditation, guided imagery) Help client correct negative self-appraisals by (1) identifying personal strengths and weaknesses and (2) restructuring thinking errors (see Sample interaction: cognitive restructuring) Include client in a plan to (1) gradually progress from having things done for him or her to (2) accepting assistance with tasks to (3) taking independent action to accomplish tasks to (4) feeling comfortable with interdependent relationships Support client during the transition period from dependence to independence or interdependence Encourage client to evaluate the effectiveness of new independent or interdependent behavior Remind client when he or she slips back into patterns of dependency, detachment or domination

Continued.

Sample interaction: cognitive restructuring

Client I'll never be able to register for college by myself. If I did go by myself, I wouldn't know what to do. I would register for all the wrong classes. It would be a total disaster.

Nurse What are your reasons for thinking this?

Client I just know it. I've never been able to do anything on my own and have it turn out right.

Nurse You came here by yourself today and nothing went wrong. Are your thoughts always *right*?

Client I guess not always.

Nurse What benefit do you get from thinking negatively like this?

Client Well, I guess I don't have to do things on my own.

Nurse What disadvantages are there to thinking negatively?

Client I have to wait for people to help me, and sometimes I miss out on things because of waiting. I also sometimes feel like a baby or get mad when people won't help me.

Nurse Is this negative thinking helping you get what you want out of life?

Client I guess not.

Nurse What can you do to change your negative way of thinking?

Client I guess I can try to think more positively.

Nurse Let's start by looking at the way that your thinking exaggerates and catastrophizes.

The nurse helped the client begin to recognize thinking errors of (a) exaggeration (never able to do anything unassisted and have it turn out right) and (b) catastrophizing (registering unassisted would be a disaster) by pointing out that the client had gone to the therapy session without anything going wrong. The nurse then helped the client begin to question whether her thoughts were always logical and correct. Next, the nurse helped the client begin to look at the effectiveness of this negative way of thinking, so that the client could begin to change it.

NURSING CARE PLAN

Clients with Phobias

Long-term Outcomes	Short-term Outcomes	Nursing Strategies

Nursing diagnoses:
- Fear related to a specific object (e.g., an animal, germs) (NANDA 9.3.2; DSM-III-R 300.29)
- Fear related to a specific situation (e.g., gaining weight, speaking in public, having a serious disease) (NANDA 9.3.2; DSM-III-R 300.21-300.23, 300.70, 307.10, 307.51)
- Fear related to a specific place (e.g., a bridge, being outside alone) (NANDA 9.3.2; DSM-III-R 300.21, 300.22)

Long-term Outcomes	Short-term Outcomes	Nursing Strategies
Work through problems concerning sexuality, control, self-esteem, etc., that generate	Express feelings of fear, anxiety inadequacy, need for control, sexuality, etc. (when consistent with client's cultural orientation)	Establish a relationship where client can express feelings
	Identify situations and/or objects that generate fear and anxiety	Focus on the client as a person who is suffering and not on phobic behavior
		Support client efforts to avoid the feared situation or object *initially*
		Encourage client to examine the impact of phobic behavior on his or her life

Long-term Outcomes	Short-term Outcomes	Nursing Strategies
fear and anxiety Decrease phobic behavior (phobic behavior may never becompletely eradicated) Develop more effective social and/or occupational functioning	Relate current stressful situations and/or objects to situations and/or objects in the past that aroused similar feelings of fear and anxiety Recognize a relationship between stressful situations and/or objects and phobic behavior Learn more effective coping behaviors Become desensitized to the feared situation or object Avoid secondary gains associated with phobic behavior	Help client evaluate effectiveness of current coping behaviors Support current effective coping behaviors Explore any secondary gains associated with client's phobic behavior Plan with client and family for nonreinforcement of secondary gains related to phobic behavior Implement the plan for nonreinforcement of secondary gains (see Situation: nonreinforcement of secondary gains) Teach client stress reduction techniques Refer client to a phobia program for desensitization Support client during the period of desensitization Give immediate feedback or rewards for improved social and/or occupational functioning Refer to Chapter 8 for additional nursing strategies to intervene in stress and anxiety and to teach more effective coping behavior Encourage client to evaluate effectiveness of new behavior

Situation: nonreinforcement of secondary gains

A community health nurse had met several times with Mrs. M, the mother of three children, in her home. Because of a phobia, Mrs. M was unable to leave her home even when accompanied by her husband and children. She eventually had reached the point where she was motivated to contact a nearby mental health clinic. During each of the past two visits by the community health nurse, a plan to leave the home in the company of her husband and the nurse had been agreed upon by the client. But it had to be canceled each time because the client had an anxiety attack and could not follow through. During a supervisory meeting with a mental health nurse, the community health nurse expressed her frustration with Mrs. M and mentioned that she believed the client was enjoying her disability. After examining this idea for evidences of secondary gain in the situation, both agreed that the perception was valid. Together they developed a plan for intervention into secondary gains. In a subsequent meeting between the community health nurse and the client, the client agreed to the plan and with the nurse began to examine aspects of her lifestyle that might be subtly reinforcing her phobia. Several factors were identified. The husband regularly brought Mrs. M a variety of magazines and books, in addition to doing all of the shopping for the family, which the client admitted had always bored her. The husband also was very good about buying the foods and delicacies she preferred and about keeping her informed about affairs of the community. Many small comforts were provided by a friend who visited regularly and shared Mrs. M's interest in fashion and design. In the next session, in which both the husband and the friend participated, everyone agreed upon a plan that would eliminate all but necessities from Mr. M's shopping list. The friend's visits would be suspended for a time. The nurse would continue to hold regular sessions and would be available by phone for crises that might ensue from the plan. Several small crises did arise, but the husband and the friend, with the support of the nurse, held firmly to the agreed-upon plan. The client was eventually able to keep an appointment at the mental health clinic.

NURSING CARE PLAN

Clients with Anxiety or Somatoform Disorders

Long-term Outcomes	Short-term Outcomes	Nursing Strategies

Nursing diagnosis: Panic level of anxiety related to conflict (e.g., social role conflict, sexual conflict) (NANDA 9.3.1; DSM-III-R 300.01, 300.21)

Work through conflicts that are generating anxiety	Identify and describe feelings of anxiety (when consistent with client's cultural orientation)	Stay with client until anxiety subsides to moderate-mild level
Learn to cope with stressful life situations more effectively	Identify and describe the precipitating stressful life situation and the associated feelings	Maintain a calm, accepting manner
	Relate the precipitating stressful life situation to situations in the past that aroused similar feelings	Communicate in a brief, clear, concrete, and slow manner
	Reevaluate the stress potency of the precipitating life situation	Establish a relationship where client can feel free to discuss feelings that are being experienced
		Avoid asking probing questions
		Avoid making demands on client
		Provide comfort measures (e.g., loosen tight clothing, give caffeine-free fluids, provide calm, quiet surroundings)
		Administer antianxiety medications
		Encourage client to describe the situation that precipitated the panic attack and the associated feelings *(after anxiety has subsided to moderate-mild level)*
		Use open-ended questions to move from non-threatening issues to more threatening issues
		Provide opportunity for physical exercise
		Refer to Chapters 8 and 15 for other nursing strategies to intervene in anxiety/crisis and to teach more effective coping behavior
		Encourage client to evaluate effectiveness of new behavior

Nursing diagnoses:
- Impaired physical mobility (specify type—e.g., hysterical paralysis of right arm) related to psychological conflict (NANDA 6.1.1.1; DSM-III-R 300.11)
- Sensory/perceptual alterations (specify type—e.g., conversion blindness) related to psychological conflict (NANDA 7.2; DSM-III-R 300.11)

Work through conflict that is contributing to motor or sensory dysfunction	Express feelings of anxiety, shame, guilt, hostility, etc. (when consistent with client's cultural orientation)	Establish a relationship where client can feel free to express feelings
Develop coping behaviors other than motor or sensory	Identify the underlying conflict	Protect client's right to the symptom (premature attempts to convince client that medical evidence does not support the existence of the symptom or interpretation of the meaning of the symptom to the client will increase anxiety)
	Recognize a relationship between the conflict and the motor or sensory dysfunction	Accept client's need for the symptom but do not reinforce it (neither deny nor confirm symptom's existence)
	Learn more effective coping	Focus on client feelings and not on the symptom
		Encourage client to participate in occupational and rec-

Long-term Outcomes	Short-term Outcomes	Nursing Strategies
dysfunction to deal with conflict	behaviors to deal with anxiety, shame, guilt, hostility, etc. Avoid secondary gains associated with motor or sensory dysfunction	reational therapies that help focus client attention away from the symptom Encourage client to discuss stressful life situations; if the stressful life situation involves the family, family therapy is indicated (Refer to Chapter 8 for additional nursing strategies to intervene in stress and anxiety and to teach new coping behavior) Explore any secondary gains associated with client behavior Establish a therapeutic environment free of secondary gains (e.g., expectations of client participation in activities of daily living and treatment modalities should be clearly stated, avoid giving client special privileges or dispensations because of conversion symptom) Help client evaluate effectiveness of new behavior

Nursing diagnosis: Altered thought processes (obsessions) related to psychological stress (NANDA 8.3; DSM-III-R 300.30)

Long-term Outcomes	Short-term Outcomes	Nursing Strategies
Work through conflicts that are generating psychological stress Decrease obsessional thoughts and accompanying compulsive behavior (they may never be totally eliminated) Develop more effective social and/or occupational functioning Improve self-esteem (refer to Chapter 22)	Express feelings of anxiety, guilt, shame, etc. (when consistent with client's cultural orientation) Identify stressful life situations and the associated feelings Recognize a relationship between stressful life situations and obsessions and compulsions Learn noncompulsive coping behavior to deal with psychological stress Eliminate self-mutilating behavior	Establish a relationship where client can feel free to express feelings Maintain a calm, quiet approach Allow client to set the pace of interactions Focus on the client as a person and not on the symptomatology Recognize that symptomatology is a way of coping with stress Allow client to perform harmless compulsive behavior *initially* Recognize that client has a low tolerance for frustration and a strong need for control Include client in any decision to limit compulsive behavior Limit harmful compulsive behavior by substituting safe behavior for harmful rituals (e.g., allow client to pick the nap off a piece of woolly or fluffy material instead of picking at own skin) Promote client's physical well-being (e.g., treat dermatitis of hands related to compulsive hand washing; treat malnutrition related to rituals concerning food) Allot extra time for rituals *initially* Decrease the amount of time allotted for symptomatic behavior *gradually* (see Situation: limit setting) Refer to Chapter 8 for additional nursing strategies to intervene with stress and anxiety and to teach more effective coping behavior Give immediate feedback or rewards for noncompulsive behavior Encourage client to evaluate the effectiveness of new behavior

Situation: limit setting

Jessica, a 23-year-old woman, was obsessed with her postman, Tony. Jessica talked about Tony continuously. Jessica had never dated Tony and had only interacted with him in relation to mail delivery.

Initially, the staff at the mental health clinic permitted Jessica to compulsively talk about Tony. Gradually, and with Jessica's consent, they decreased the amount of time that she was permitted to talk about Tony. First, Jessica was allowed to talk about her obsession with Tony for 10-15 minutes of every hour. For the rest of the hour, Jessica was expected to engage in psychotherapeutic, occupational, and recreational treatment modalities. If she slipped, the staff would remind Jessica that it was not the time to talk about Tony. At the end of each hour, when she followed the limits, Jessica was praised by the staff. Jessica was also instructed in progressive relaxation and encouraged to do it whenever she felt the compulsion to talk about Tony. The time alloted to Jessica's obsession was gradually decreased, until it became completely unacceptable for her to talk about Tony.

The preceding vignette shows how a client with obsessive-compulsive disorder can be made aware of limits and included in limit setting. It also shows how staff can gradually decrease the amount of time allotted for symptomatic behavior as the client learns more effective ways of handling stress.

NURSING CARE PLAN

Clients with Dissociative or Eating Disorders

Long-term Outcomes	Short-term Outcomes	Nursing Strategies

Nursing diagnosis: Altered growth and development related to anxiety and severe childhood physical and/or sexual abuse and manifested by the development of primary and secondary personalities (NANDA 6.6; DSM-III-R 300.14)

Develop communication and cooperation among all the personalities Develop fusion or integration of all the personalities into one whole person	Recognize the existence of secondary personalities Learn about the traumas and repressed painful feelings that contributed to the development of secondary personalities Develop more effective coping behaviors to deal with anxiety and feelings of hositlity, loneliness, etc.	Establish a relationship where client can feel free to express feelings, conflicts, traumas, and needs Help client understand that he or she has a multiple personality Encourage client to work toward the goal of personality integration Work with each secondary personality on a cognitive level. This is a *gradual* process that necessitates (1) the trust of each secondary personality in the nurse, (2) some degree of trust of each secondary personality in the primary personality Encourage each secondary personality to tell the primary personality what it knows about past experiences and feelings of which the primary personality is unaware Help client verbalize painful feelings (as client becomes aware of past traumatic experiences) Refer to Chapter 8 for nursing strategies to intervene in stress and to teach more effective coping behaviors Support client as personality fusion and reintegration occur Assist client to mobilize support from friends, relatives, clergy, etc. Encourage client to evaluate the effectiveness of personality integration

Long-term Outcomes	Short-term Outcomes	Nursing Strategies

Nursing diagnosis:
- Personal identity disturbance in personal identity, related to severe psychosocial stress and manifested by psychogenic amnesia (NANDA 7.1.3; DSM-III-R 300.12)
- Personal identity, disturbance in personal identity, related to severe psychosocial stress and manifested by psychogenic fugue (NANDA 7.1.3; DSM-III-R 300.13)

Work through problems that are generating severe psychosocial stress Learn to deal more effectively with stress	Express feelings of anxiety, especially those surrounding the precipitating event (when consistent with client's cultural orientation) Identify life situations, both current and past, that arouse anxiety Recognize a relationship between stressful life situations, memory loss, and altered identity Develop new coping behaviors Avoid secondary gains associated with memory loss and altered identity	Establish a relationship where client can feel free to express feelings Carry out crisis intervention strategies (refer to Chapter 15) Employ physical stimuli (e.g., smelling salts) or cultural/spiritual stimuli (e.g., native healers) to at least partially arouse client from dissociative state Reinforce renewed level of awareness through activity (e.g., walking, talking) Recognize that alteration of identity and memory loss are means of coping with stress Refrain from telling client about his or her past life (provision of such information will increase anxiety and may precipitate psychosis) Focus on client feelings, especially those surrounding the precipitating event, and on stressful life situations Explore family dynamics, family roles, and feelings about family members Refer to Chapter 8 for additional nursing strategies to intervene in stress and anxiety and to teach more effective coping behaviors Help client identify secondary gains associated with memory loss and altered identity Establish a therapeutic environment free of secondary gains (e.g., assist family members to decrease behavior that fosters secondary gains, expectations of client participation in activities of daily living should be clearly stated, avoid giving client special privileges or dispensations because of memory loss) Support client as disassociative state lessens

Nursing diagnoses:
- Altered nutrition: more than body requirements related to distorted body image and conflict (NANDA 1.1.2.1; DSM-III-R 316, 307.51)
- Altered nutrition: less than body requirements related to distorted body image and conflict (NANDA 1.1.2.2; DSM-III-R 307.10, 307.50)

Work through conflicts Develop a positive self-image (refer to Chapters	Express feelings of anxiety, inadequacy, need for control, etc. (when consistent with client's cultural orientation) Identify life situations that	Establish a relationship where client can feel free to express feelings Supervise eating behaviors closely. Anorectic client may try to avoid food intake or to purge food from body. Bulimic client may try to binge and purge food. Compulsive overeating client may try to sneak food

Continued.

NURSING CARE PLAN—cont'd

Clients with Dissociative or Eating Disorders

Long-term Outcomes	Short-term Outcomes	Nursing Strategies

Nursing diagnoses:—cont'd
- Altered nutrition: more than body requirements related to distorted body image and conflict (NANDA 1.1.2.1; DSM-III-R 316, 307.51)
- Altered nutrition: less than body requirements related to distorted body image and conflict (NANDA 1.1.2.2; DSM-III-R 307.10, 307.50)

Long-term Outcomes	Short-term Outcomes	Nursing Strategies
6 and 22) Learn to cope with stressful life situations more effectively	generate feelings of anxiety, inadequacy, and need for control Recognize a relationship between stressful life situations and food-related coping behaviors Develop nonfood-related coping behaviors Decrease manipulative behavior (control tactics) Increase interpersonal skills Realistically perceive personal strengths and weaknesses Establish healthful habits of nutrition and elimination	Weigh anorectic client in clothes that do not permit the concealing of weights in the clothing or on the body Promote healthful patterns of nutrition and elimination (e.g., bulimic or anorectic client may have to be accompanied to the bathroom to prevent purging of food; compulsive overeating client may need information about physiological factors associated with obesity; anorectic client who refuses to eat may need nasogastric [NG] tube feeding or intravenous feeding, done in a nonpunitive manner, but remove NG tube immediately after feeding to prevent siphoning) Set limits on manipulative behavior (e.g., explain what behavior is expected, explain reasons for limits, state consequences of ignoring limits, enforce consequences). An eating disorder client often fears loss of control over his or her behavior and needs limits to be set Provide opportunities for client to have some degree of control (1) communicate that client has control over and responsibility for weight gain/weight loss (e.g., with an anorectic client, privileges may be increased for weight gain and decreased for weight loss), (2) offer choices whenever possible (e.g., between several foods of equal nutritious and caloric value) Explore client's feelings as weight is lost or gained Verbally recognize and reinforce authentic communication of feelings Explore client's feelings about family dynamics, family roles, and family alliances Explore client's perception of and feelings about self-image. Point out misperceptions in client's self-image Assist client to develop non-food-related coping behaviors to deal with stressful life situations (refer to Chapter 8) Explore secondary gains associated with client's eating behavior Establish a therapeutic environment free of secondary gains (e.g., expectations of client participation in activities of daily living and treatment modalities should be clearly stated, avoid giving client special privileges or dispensations because of anorectic, bulimic, or compulsive overeating behavior) Encourage client to evaluate effectiveness of new behavior

Nursing diagnoses pertaining to other problems associated with compulsivity, somatization, and altered identity are addressed in the following chapters: stress and anxiety (Chapters 8 and 15), mild depression (Chapter 22), low self-esteem and inadequacy (Chapter 22).

EVALUATION

The client and, whenever feasible, the client's family or significant others (e.g., housemate, very close friend) should be included in estimating the client's progress towards attainment of goals. Any evaluation should encompass the following areas:

1. Estimation of the degree to which neurotic conflicts have been worked through
2. Estimation of the degree to which goals have been achieved and client functioning has improved (demonstrated by a decrease in neurotic coping behaviors and the learning of more effective coping behaviors)
3. Identification of goals that need to be modified or revised
4. Referral of the client to support systems other than the nurse-client relationship
   a. People in the client's social network who are willing to serve as a support system
   b. Centers that specialize in the treatment of specific neurotic disorders (e.g., eating disorder programs, phobia clinics, centers for the treatment of multiple personalities)

TERTIARY PREVENTION

Relatively little attention has been given to the long-range effects of neuroses upon a person's ability to function. The level of maladaptive functioning that occurs in neuroses does not produce the severe psychological crippling that is seen in schizophrenia, for example, and the other psychoses. Except for individuals with hypochondriasis, which is sometimes a stage preliminary to schizophrenia, persons who have neuroses often function satisfactorily in society, although they may require some psychiatric intervention in times of crisis.

However, everyone approaches old age with the personality characteristics and coping patterns that have developed over a lifetime. The sociocultural

and physiological problems that beset people in the older age group may be made more severe by any neurotic coping patterns that, under less stressful circumstances, have been used to maintain the ability to function. When confronted with the loss of family and friends, who earlier provided needed support, and with decreasing economic status, a neurotic individual is often less able to cope with the problems of aging than the average person. Many such individuals can be found, somewhat isolated, in single-room dwellings and health-related facilities, where they are often viewed as problem clients by staff members and other residents.

Tertiary prevention includes identification of individuals in the community who have chronically displayed neurotic symptoms, and provision of support groups for them. Recovery, Inc. is one such support group. Recovery, Inc. uses a form of self-monitored behavior modification to help clients control anxiety and neurotic symptomatology.

CHAPTER SUMMARY

Neurotic disorders involve little or moderate distortion of reality or impairment of intellectual functioning. There is, however, an exaggerated use of various defense mechanisms and compromise solutions to control anxiety and maintain functioning. The utilization of interpersonal patterns of dependence, domination, or detachment is characteristic. When a neurotic person experiences stress, such pathological symptoms as compulsivity, somatization, or altered identity may develop.

Many theories have been formulated to explain neurotic disorders. These theories fall into four major categories: psychological, biological, sociocultural, and systems. It is likely that a combination of interrelated factors leads to the development of neurotic disorders. Although neurotic disorders can be found in many societies, the form, meaning, and incidence are culturally influenced and culturally relative.

Treatment for neuroses includes psychoanalytic therapy, cognitive therapy, family therapy, behavior therapy, and psychopharmaceutical therapy. Primary prevention focuses on identification of and intervention with high-risk individuals. For instance, intervention may deal with inadequate parental coping, poverty, and other environmental stressors. Adapting nursing intervention to meet the needs of at-risk clients during health-related crises is another aspect of primary prevention.

The role of the nurse in secondary prevention depends, to some extent, upon the type of neurosis and the setting in which the nurse intervenes. Central to nursing intervention, however, is case find-

ing and application of the nursing process to human responses associated with neurotic disorders. Secondary prevention is most effective when it involves a collaborative and consistent team approach. Tertiary prevention requires nurses, clients and family members, and community groups to work toward a unified rehabilitative approach.

SELF-DIRECTED LEARNING

Sensitivity-Awareness Exercises

The purposes of the following exercises are to:
- Develop awareness about the vulnerability of client-families to neuroses
- Develop awareness about the interrelationship of factors in the etiology of neurotic disorders
- Develop awareness about the subjective experience of clients who are suffering from neurotic disorders and of the experience of clients' families
- Develop awareness about your own feelings and attitudes when working with clients who are suffering from neuroses

1. Try to imagine that you are suffering from one of the following disorders and explain why you selected that particular disorder. Then describe what you think it would be like to suffer from that disorder.
   a. Anxiety disorder
   b. Obsessive-compulsive disorder
   c. Multiple personality
   d. Psychogenic amnesia or fugue
   e. Eating disorder (select one)
   f. Conversion disorder (select one symptom)
   g. Phobic disorder (select one phobia)
   h. Hypochondriasis
2. Describe what you think it would be like to have a family member suffering from one of the neuroses listed in Exercise 1. Which disorder do you think would be easiest to tolerate in a family member? Why? Which disorder do you think would be hardest to tolerate? Why?
3. What might be some of your feelings and reactions as a nurse caring for clients who are suffering from neuroses? Would your feelings and reactions vary

with the neurotic disorders experienced by clients? Explain why.
4. Imagine that you are a community health nurse engaged in health supervision activities with new parents. What high risk factors (physical, emotional, intellectual, sociocultural, and spiritual) would you watch for that might predispose parents and/or their children to a neurotic disorder?
5. Develop a plan for counseling parents about childrearing that incorporates principles and goals for the primary prevention of neuroses.

Questions to Consider

1. Doreen Johnson relates to people in an aloof, detached manner. Classmates often characterize her as "thinking she is better than everyone else." Doreen has difficulty expressing her feelings, and she frequently intellectualizes. According to Horney, Doreen's interpersonal behavior is an example of
   a. Moving toward others
   b. Moving away from others
   c. Moving against others

A community health nurse has been visiting the Greary family to help them care for Mr. Greary's bedridden mother. The community health nurse has noticed that Mr. Greary is a very controlling person who has difficulty getting in touch with and expressing his feelings. During this period of situational stress, Mr. Greary has become very fearful about his own state of health. Despite an extensive physical examination that revealed no pathophysiology, Mr. Greary is convinced that he has cancer. The following 2 questions refer to this situation.

SELF-DIRECTED LEARNING—cont'd

2. Mr. Greary's profile indicates that he may be suffering from which of the following neurotic disorders?
   a. Hypochondriasis
   b. Conversion disorder
   c. Generalized anxiety disorder
   d. Obsessive-compulsive disorder
3. When intervening with Mr. Greary's behavior, the community health nurse should be guided by which of the following goals of secondary preventive intervention?
   a. Early identification of neurotic behavior patterns
   b. Referral to available community resources for rehabilitative treatment of neurotic disorders
   c. Prompt intervention into patterns of vulnerability to neurosis
   d. Reduction of factors that predispose people to neurotic disorders
4. Clients with eating disorders have many characteristics in common. They tend to be preoccupied with thoughts of eating–not eating. They tend to have distorted body images. They tend to have problems and conflicts about sexuality. Psychodynamically, the client who tends to be a perfectionist and to avoid decision making is the client with
   a. Bulimia nervosa
   b. Compulsive overeating
   c. Anorexia nervosa
   d. Obesity
5. A psychiatric clinical nurse specialist was working with a client who had generalized anxiety disorder. The client exhibited anxiety-producing thought patterns of exaggeration, catastrophiz-

ing, overgeneralizing, and ignoring the positive. The nurse was helping the client to restructure these thought patterns. The nurse gave the client homework assignments that utilized imagery. The nurse was primarily using which of the following treatment modalities?
   a. Psychoanalytic therapy
   b. Behavior therapy
   c. Desensitization therapy
   d. Cognitive therapy

Match each of the following terms with the statement that is associated with it:

6. Phobic disorder	a. Unrealistic self-concept based on one's needs, beliefs, and values
7. Compulsive behavior	b. Alter personality that differs from a primary personality
8. Desensitization therapy	c. Repetitious, stereotypic, ritualistic behavior
9. Secondary personality	d. Persistent pathological fear of an object or situation
10. Idealized image	e. A form of behavior therapy

Answer key

1. b	6. d
2. a	7. c
3. a	8. e
4. c	9. b
5. d	10. a

REFERENCES

Ballenger JC et al: Alprazolam in panic disorder and agoraphobia: results from a multicenter trial: 1. efficacy in short-term treatment, Arch Gen Psychiatr 45(5):413-422, 1988.

Balon R, Yeragani VK, and Pohl R: Relative hypophosphatemia in patients with panic disorder, Arch Gen Psychiatr 45(3):294-295, 1988.

Barry PD: Psychosocial nursing assessment and intervention, Philadelphia, 1984, JB Lippincott Co.

Baxter LR Jr et al: Local cerebral glucose metabolic rates in obsessive-compulsive disorder, Arch Gen Psychiatr 44(3):211-218, 1987.

Beck AT, and Emery G with Greenberg RL: Anxiety disorders and phobias: a cognitive perspective, New York, 1985, Basic Books.

Bouchard C et al: Body composition in adopted and biological siblings, Hum Biol 57:61-75, 1985.

Breier A, Charney DS, and Heninger GR: Agoraphobia with

panic attacks: development, diagnostic stability, and course of illness, Arch Gen Psychiatr 43(11):1029-1036, 1986.

Brone RJ and Fisher CB: Determinants of adolescent obesity: a comparison with anorexia nervosa, Adolescence 23(89):155-169, 1988.

Bryant SO and Kopeski LM: Psychiatric nursing assessment of the eating disorder client, Topics Clin Nurs 8(1):57-66, 1986.

Clayton BD: Mosby's handbook of pharmacology in nursing, ed 4, St. Louis, 1987, CV Mosby Co.

Colby KM and McGuire MT: Signs and symptoms: zeroing in on a better classification of neuroses, The Sciences (November), pp 21-24, 1981.

Coons PM: Multiple personality: diagnostic considerations, J Clin Psychiatr 41(10):330-336, 1980.

Crowe RR et al: A linkage study of panic disorder, Arch Gen Psychiatr 44(11):933-937, 1987.

Diagnostic and statistical manual of mental disorders, ed 3, revised, Washington, DC, 1987, The American Psychiatric Association.

Eichenbaum L and Orbach S: Understanding women: a feminist psychoanalytic approach, New York, 1983, Basic Books, Inc.

Forbes GB, Prochaska E, and Weitkamp LR: Genetic factors in abdominal obesity: a risk factor for stroke, N Engl J Med 318(16):1070, 1988.

Freud S: The problem of anxiety, New York, 1936, WW Norton & Co.

Freud S: Group psychology and the analysis of the ego, New York, 1960, Bantam Books, Inc.

Freud S: A general introduction to psychoanalysis, New York, 1969, Pocket Books.

Garner DM and Garfinkel PE: Socio-cultural factors in the development of anorexia nervosa, Psycholog Med 10:647-656, 1980.

Garner DM et al: Comparison between weight-preoccupied women and anorexia nervosa, Psychosom Med 46(3):255-266, 1984.

Gorman JM et al: Effect of acute β-adrenergic blockade on lactate-induced panic, Arch Gen Psychiatr 40(10):1079-1082, 1983.

Greenberg WC: The multiple personality, Persp Psychiatr Care 20(3):100-104, 1982.

Hale E: Inside the divided mind, New York Times, p 100, VI, April 17, 1983.

Helman C: Culture, health and illness: an introduction for health professionals, Bristol, England, 1984, John Wright & Sons Ltd.

Hirsch J and Leibel R: Reported in Kolata G, editor: Why do people get fat? Science 227:1327-1328, 1985.

Horney K: The neurotic personality of our time, New York, 1937, WW Norton & Co.

Horney K: New ways in psychoanalysis, New York, 1939, WW Norton & Co.

Horney K: Our inner conflicts, New York, 1945, WW Norton & Co.

Kahn JP, Drusin RE, and Klein DF: Idiopathic cardiomyopathy and panic disorder: clinical association in cardiac transplant candidates, Am J Psychiatr 144(10):1327-1330, 1987.

Keesey RE and Pawley TL: The regulation of body weight, Ann Rev Psychol 37:109-133, 1986.

Krieshok SI and Karpowitz DH: A review of selected literature on obesity and guidelines for treatment, J Couns Dev 66(7):326-330, 1988.

Krinsky K: Childhood eating patterns and their relationship to later-life eating disorders, presented at The Psychological, Emotional, and Medical Aspects of Eating Disorders: Anorexia, Bulimia, and Compulsive Overeating, South Oaks Hospital, March 17, 1987.

Krippner S: Cross-cultural approaches to multiple personality disorder: practices in Brazilian spiritism, Ethos 15(3):273-295, 1987.

Levendron S: Anorexia and bulimia—the tip of the obsessional iceberg, presented at The Psychological, Emotional, and Medical Aspects of Eating Disorders: Anorexia, Bulimia, and Compulsive Overeating, South Oaks Hospital, March 17, 1987.

Madanes C: Strategic family therapy, San Francisco, 1981, Jossey-Bass Publishers.

Mavissakalian M et al: Trazodone in the treatment of panic disorder and agoraphobia with panic attacks, Am J Psychiatr 144(6):785-787, 1987.

Mazlen R: Medical aspects of eating disorders—metabolic and nutritional complications, presented at The Psychological, Emotional, and Medical Aspects of Eating Disorders: Anorexia, Bulimia, and Compulsive Overeating, South Oaks Hospital. March 17, 1987.

McGrory A: Women and mental illness: A Sexist Trap? J Psychiatr Nurs Ment Health Serv 18(10):17-22, 1980.

Merker MS: Psychiatric emergency evaluation, Nurs Clin N Am 21(3):387-396, 1986.

Nakakuki M: Japan's homegrown neurosis. In Psychiatric perspectives: Roche reports, frontiers of psychiatry.

Noyes R Jr et al: Alprazolam in panic disorder and agoraphobia: results from a multicenter trial: (2) patient acceptance, side effects, and safety, Arch Gen Psychiatr 45(5):423-428, 1988.

Oehler JM and Burns MJ: Anorexia, bulimia, and sexuality: case study of an adolescent inpatient group, Arch Psychiatr Nurs 1(3):163-171, 1987.

Paccione-Dyszlewski MR and Contessa-Kislus MA: School phobia: identification of subtypes as a prerequisite to treatment intervention, Adolescence 22(86):377-384, 1987.

Peterson HR et al: Body fat and the activity of the autonomic nervous system, N Engl J Med 318(17):1077-1083, 1988.

Polhemus T: Introduction, In Polhemus T, editor: Social aspects of the human body, Harmondsworth, 1978, Penguin Books.

Price RA et al: Genetic contributions to human fatness: an adoption study, Am J Psychiatr 144(8):1003-1008, 1987.

Rigotti NA: Reported in Biomedicine: anorexic bone: lost but not found, Sci News 133(20):312, 1988.

Rodin J: The externality theory in obesity. In Stunkard AJ, editor: Obesity, Philadelphia, 1980, WB Saunders Co.

Scheper-Hughes N and Lock MM: The mindful body: a prolegomenon to future work in medical anthropology, Med Anthropol Q 1(1):6-35, 1987.

Schneider G: Compulsive overeating—the silent killer, presented at The Psychological, Emotional, and Medical Aspects of Eating Disorders: Anorexia, Bulimia, and Compulsive Overeating, South Oaks Hospital, March 17, 1987.

Suinn RM: The fear of using computers is common, Part 11, Newsday, col 1, p 5, July 9, 1983.

Toner BB, Garfinkel PE, and Garner DM: Cognitive style of patients with bulimic and diet-restricting anorexia nervosa, Am J Psychiatr 144(4):510-511, 1987.

Torgenson S: Genetic factors in anxiety disorders, Arch Gen Psychiatr 40:1085-1089, 1983.

Up Front: Discover 8(11):16, 1987.

Williams RR: Nature, nurture, and family predisposition, N Engl J Med 318(12):769-771, 1988.

ANNOTATED SUGGESTED READINGS

Bryant SO and Kopeski LM: Psychiatric nursing assessment of the eating disorder client, Topics Clin Nurs 8(1):57-66, 1986.

The authors use a holistic framework, based on Gordon's functional health patterns, for assessing health care problems of clients with anorexia nervosa and bulimia. Among the patterns discussed are health-perception/health-management, nutritional-metabolic, elimination, activity-exercise, cognitive-perceptual, self-perception–self-concept, role relationship, sexuality-reproductive, and coping-stress tolerance.

Merker MS: Psychiatric emergency evaluation, Nurs Clin N Am 21(3):387-396, 1986.

Although this article does not deal exclusively with psychiatric emergencies experienced by individuals suffering from neurotic disorders, it frequently applies emergency guidelines to such persons. Clinical examples are used to illustrate guidelines.

Oehler JM and Burns MJ: Anorexia, bulimia, and sexuality: case study of an adolescent inpatient group, Arch Psychiatr Nurs 1(3):163-171, 1987.

This article looks at the issue of developing sexuality in anorexia nervosa and bulimia. The characteristics of these eating disorders and their etiology are briefly reviewed. The rationale for group therapy is given, and the treatment group, including its composition and issues covered in group sessions, is described.

FURTHER READINGS

Anderson G: Understanding multiple personality disorder, J Psychosoc Nurs 26(7):26-30, 1988.

Bulow BV and DeChillo N: Treatment alternatives for bulimia patients, Social Casework 68(8):477-484, 1987.

Dager SR: Mitral valve prolapse and the anxiety disorders, Hosp Commun Psychiatry 39(5):517-527, 1988.

Dattilo FM: The use of paradoxical intention in the treatment of panic attacks, J Couns Dev 66(2):102-103, 1987.

Ishiyama FI: Use of morita therapy in shyness counseling in the west: promoting clients' self-acceptance and action taking, J Couns Dev 65(10):547-551, 1987.

Marston AR et al: Characteristics of adolescents at risk for compulsive overeating on a brief screening test, Adolescence 23(89):59-65, 1987.

Minichiello WE, Baer L, and Jenlke MA: Behavior therapy for the treatment of obsessive-compulsive disorder: theory and practice, Compr Psychiatry 29(2):123-137, 1988.

Pearson JE: A support group for women with relationship dependency, J Couns Dev 66(8):394-396, 1988.

Perugi G et al: Relationships between panic disorder and separation anxiety with school phobia, Compr Psychiatry 29(2):98-107, 1988.

Reich J and Yates W: Family history of psychiatric disorders in social phobia, Compr Psychiatry 29(1):72-75, 1988.

Svec H: Anorexia nervosa: a misdiagnosis of the adolescent male, Adolescence 22(87):617-623, 1987.

Trueman D: The behavioral treatment of school phobia: a critical review, Psychol Schools 21:215-223, 1984.

CHAPTER 24

Patterns of emotional turbulence and primitive defenses

CHAPTER FOCUS

Borderline personality disorder is a relatively new diagnosis of mental illness that is receiving a great deal of attention today. Characterized by themes of anger, erratic and self-destructive behavior, and severely disordered interpersonal relationships, the syndrome is believed to be increasing in our society. In fact, it has even been suggested that this disorder is "a metaphor for our unstable society" (Sass, 1982, 12).

In terms of etiology, borderline personality disorder (also referred to as *borderline syndrome, borderline pathology,* and *borderline personality organization*) is viewed as a developmental arrest in the separation-individuation phase of the first year of life.

Until recently, most of the theoretical work on etiology and the treatment methods based on clinical experience have been presented by psychoanalysts who have treated borderline clients. For this reason, the focus of this chapter is necessarily influenced by a psychoanalytical viewpoint. While nurses in various psychiatric settings increasingly are interacting and intervening with borderline clients, to date very little material on the disorder has appeared in the nursing literature.

As with other forms of mental illness, nursing intervention with clients diagnosed as having borderline pathology is focused on therapeutic response to behavior. Material on nursing intervention that is quite relevant to manifestations of borderline pathology but that is also covered in detail in other chapters (for example, substance abuse and other addictive behaviors in Chapter 20; suicidal behavior and self-derogation in Chapter 22; brief psychotic episodes in Chapter 25) will not be repeated here. Seven major problems that the borderline client experiences will be reviewed in conjunction with the nursing process. These include five primitive defenses that Kernberg views as core underlying dynamics (splitting, primitive idealization, projective identification, rapidly shifting ego states, omnipotence of self with devaluation of others) and two recurring themes in the lives of borderline clients (the inability to tolerate aloneness, chronic boredom). This work is based on theoretical and clinical concepts from the literature and the author's [H.M.A.] clinical practice in intervening with borderline clients in inpatient and outpatient settings.

It is generally agreed that long-term treatment is necessary for meaningful changes in the personality organization and life-style of the borderline client. Most often this will be carried out by clinical nurse specialists and clinicians from other disciplines who are treating clients on an ongoing, outpatient basis. Long-term goals build on short-term goals, however, and the frequent hospitalizations and many crises that these clients experience make an understanding of the condition and its treatment important for all professional nurses working in psychiatric settings.

HISTORICAL ASPECTS AND DEFINITIONS OF BORDERLINE PERSONALITY DISORDERS

Borderline personality disorder, borderline personality syndrome, and *borderline personality organization* are various terms used to denote a condition that is capturing the attention of many writers and workers in the mental health fields. Thus, borderline personality is becoming increasingly familiar to nurses working in a variety of psychiatric settings. The category is controversial—some writers suggest that it is a "catch-all" or "wastebasket" term to cover a very large group of individuals who don't quite fit into the more conventional diagnostic categories (Klein, 1977; Freed, 1980; Lynch and

Lynch, 1977; Pine, 1986). Many others insist that it is a definite, recognizable syndrome (Arieti and Chrzanowski, 1975; Adler, 1975; Capponi, 1979; Freed, 1980; Gunderson and Singer, 1975; Rinsley, 1977). Currently the latter group seems to be in the majority, and the designation is not only an accepted one (for example, it is now included in DSM-III and DSM-III-R), but it also seems to be one of the most frequently discussed disorders in mental health journals today. There is a proliferation of books, workshops, panels, conferences, and "popular press" articles on the subject. Certainly, borderline disorder is more precisely defined than it has been, even in the fairly recent past. Wolberg, writing in 1973, pointed out that most of the material on the borderline client had been written in the past five or six years (Wolberg, 1973). While it may be receiving a good deal of attention and interest and while much of the clarification, description, terminology, and analysis are just evolving, the syndrome itself is probably not a new one, nor is it simply a contemporary development of new psychiatric thinking. It is quite probable that terms such as Freud's *narcissistic neuroses* (which he considered unanalyzable), Wilhelm Reich's *impulsive character disorder,* Helene Deutsch's *as-if personality,* and the later designations of *psychotic character, pseudoneurotic schizophrenia, ambulatory schizophrenia, latent schizophrenia,* and *nonpsychotic schizophrenia* all included a good number of people who would now be diagnosed as suffering from borderline personality disorder (Capponi, 1979; Mack, 1975). The earlier descriptions of pathology seem to parallel many of our current delineations of borderline personality. It can be seen from these early terms that at first the concept was used to characterize something that lay between schizophrenia or psychosis and neurosis. For example, Laplanche and Pontalis' definition (1973, 54) of *borderline case* states: "Term most often used to designate psychopathological troubles lying on the frontier between neurosis and psychosis, particularly latent schizophrenias presenting an apparently neurotic set of symptoms." Many modern writers affirm that there is such a thing as borderline or latent schizophrenia but that it is discrete from borderline personality disorder. Later contributions from a variety of theorists tend to place borderline personality disorder on a continuum, not simply between neurosis and psychosis but one that requires differentiating the diagnosis from several other pathologies (see Fig. 24-1). In 1975, Chrzanowski noted that while borderline pathology may still be considered something of a hybrid concept and that the state is often classified as early, ambulatory, transient, or latent forms of schizophrenia, this tendency is changing. He states: "In recent years, greater emphasis has been placed on the relatively specific pathology of borderline states compared to conceptualizations of either a continuum ranging from neurosis to psychosis and vice versa or to a halfway station between moderate and severe mental illness" (Chrzanowski, 1975, 147).

Perhaps, as many writers have suggested, a more appropriate word would be *borderland*. For example, Green states: "So the contradiction emerges. Our clinical experience tells us that the border of insanity is not a line; it is rather a vast territory with no sharp division: *a no-man's land* between sanity and insanity" (Green, 1977, 16).

The borderland has been explored by many, and the condition is differentiated from other forms of mental illness mostly in terms of *degree or severity of illness*. Papers have been written distinguishing borderline disorders from schizophrenia (Chrzanowski, 1975; Gunderson and Kolb, 1978); depression and other affective disorders (Gunderson and Kolb, 1978; Kibel, 1978); character disorders (Chrzanowski, 1975; Boyer and Giovacchini, 1967; Kibel, 1978); narcissistic personality (Adler, 1981; Goldstein, 1987; Grotstein, 1979; Kohut, 1971; Zander, 1984); neurosis (Kibel, 1978); and psychosis (Giovacchini, 1979; Kernberg, 1977; Kibel, 1978; Masterson, 1973, 1974; Pine, 1974).

Thus, borderline personality disorder can be viewed as "bordering" on several other psychopathological conditions (see Fig. 24-1), and the reason for so much confusion about the term becomes apparent.

Some definitions of the disorder that may help to clarify the concept include:

The borderline condition represents a degree of psychopathology that differs, on the one hand, from neurotic and character disorders, and, on the other hand, from the psychoses. Thus, borderline patients have ego im-

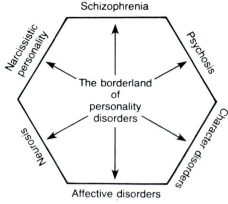

Fig. 24-1

pairment of a severity that lies midway between these and other conditions (Kibel, 1978, 342).

. . . patients with stable character structures who demonstrate the immature defenses stressed by Otto F. Kernberg*—splitting, primitive idealization, projection and projective identification—and the core conflicts related to primitive hostility and fear of abandonment (Adler, 1975).

Borderline people typically are harrowed by a sense of aloneness, and in their relations with others are tortured by alternating horrors of abandonment and engulfment. In order to relieve their exhausting inner despair, these patients exhibit a strong tendency to act impulsively and to defend with denial, projection and splitting (Maltsberger and Buie, 1975, 126).

. . . nonpsychotic character disorders who suffer from severe developmental failure, and who possess the potential for slipping in and out of psychosis . . . the ego of the borderline can be said to be preoccupied primarily with problems of a preoedipal nature centering around symbiosis and object relatedness (Leboit and Capponi, 1979, 5).

Chrznowski (1975, 147) described the borderline client as having a common denominator in these three aspects:

---

*Kernberg is considered one of the leading authorities on borderline pathology. See later parts of this chapter for discussion of some of his concepts and of those "immature defenses" mentioned here.

1. An inhibition to display overt anger and aggression
2. A tendency to maintain a certain amount of social distance
3. A tendency toward intense transference phenomena

The definitions all make serious attempts at the difficult task of illuminating the controversial concept of borderline personality disorder, but one is still left with a rather vague, and sometimes conflicting, understanding of the syndrome.

Gunderson and Singer (1975) presented an excellent overview of the literature on borderline personality disorder in which they were able to abstract six descriptive features of the disorder. They are

1. *Intense affect,* depression or, more often, anger
2. A history of *impulsive behavior* (self-mutilation, drug abuse, alcoholism, gambling)
3. A certain amount of *superficial social adaptiveness* (more of a mimicry)
4. *Brief, psychotic episodes* characterized by intact reality testing in the face of a poor sense of or relationship to reality
5. *Primitive personality organization* as revealed by psychological tests and loose thinking
6. Severely *disordered interpersonal relationships* vacillating between transient, superficial states and intense, dependent relationships. Relationships are marred by devaluation of others, manipulation, and a tendency to be demanding.

Kernberg would add another characteristic: *a negative and indistinct sense of self*, and Singer has noted that these individuals suffer from *rapidly shifting ego states* (Singer, 1979). Finally, many writers have pointed to another prevalent and important characteristic of the borderline personality: the greatly *diminished ability to use sublimation* as a defense mechanism. This difficulty in sublimating is an important factor in two recurring themes—*the inability to tolerate aloneness* and *chronic boredom.*

A similar listing of characteristics is found in DSM-III, which provides a detailed description of the disorder as a basis for making the diagnosis:

. . . the following are characteristic of the individual's current and long-term functioning, are not limited to episodes of illness, and cause either significant impairment in social or occupational functioning or subjective distress.

A. At least five of the following are required:
   1) impulsivity or unpredictability in at least two areas that are potentially self-damaging, e.g., spending, sex, gambling, shoplifting, overeating, physically self-damaging acts
   2) a pattern of unstable and intense interpersonal relationships, e.g., marked shifts of attitude, idealization, devaluation, manipulation (consistently using others for one's own ends)
   3) inappropriate, intense anger or lack of control of anger, e.g., frequent displays of temper, constant anger
   4) identity disturbance manifested by uncertainty about several issues relating to identity, such as self-image, gender identity, long-term goals or career choice, friendship patterns, values, and loyalties, e.g., "Who am I?," "I feel like I am my sister when I am good"
   5) affective instability: marked shifts from normal mood to depression, irritability, or anxiety, usually lasting a few hours and only rarely more than a few days, with return to normal mood
   6) intolerance of being alone, e.g., frantic efforts to avoid being alone, (being) depressed when alone
   7) physically self-damaging acts, e.g., suicidal gestures, self-mutilation, recurrent accidents or physical fights
   8) chronic feelings of emptiness or boredom
B. If under 18, does not meet the criterion for Identity Disorder (Diagnostic and Statistical Manual [DSM-III], 322).

UNDERLYING DYNAMICS

Otto Kernberg prefers the term *borderline personality organization* to describe these clients. He views the organization as a pathological one and has described some of the primitive and pathological defense mechanisms* that are frequently used. These include (1) splitting, (2) primitive idealization, (3) projective identification, (4) denial of ego

---

*The reader is referred to Chapter 6 for a review of defense mechanisms in general.

states, and (5) omnipotence of self with devaluation of others (Kernberg, 1977).

Splitting

Splitting is the failure to synthesize the positive and negative experiences and ideas one has of oneself and other people (or things). It is a normal developmental style when the infant is attempting to differentiate *self* from the rest of the world. Mother is seen as a separate, distinct person (object) who is powerful and *good* (brings food, comforts) but also as *bad* (doesn't come when she's needed). One way of conceptualizing this is to note the infant's self-protecting (keep the "bad" away from the "good") perception of mother as the "good mother" and the "bad mother," or "the good breast" and the "bad breast." Things become, in this *either-or* and *primitive* point of view, "good-bad" or "black and white"—there is no "gray" or ambiguous area tolerated. Since in reality, life is a mixture of good and bad, positives and negatives, this primitive defense, if overused in later life, can lead to rather severe problems in ego development and a decrease in the ability to function in a healthy manner. One's sense of identity and one's sense of others and other things tend to shift rapidly. There is a lack of integration, and the contradictory images of the world cause one to relate to *part objects* rather than *whole* (and therefore a mixture of "good" and "bad") persons, situations, or institutions. In healthier development, one's sense of identity and one's sense of the *other* are based on a synthesis of different characteristics of any personality. Being able to tolerate a certain sense of ambivalence in relating to the other (an imperfect human being or situation) is one of the important hallmarks of mental health.

Gerry is a 24-year-old young woman who has a long history of serious mental and emotional difficulties. She has been hospitalized several times, usually for brief periods only, and she has had two superficial suicide attempts and one serious attempt. After three years of intensive psychotherapy with a clinical nurse specialist (Anna), Gerry is just beginning to notice and to understand how "I do a number on people in my own head." In one recent session, her therapist point-

ed out that she seemed to be strongly degrading and expressing rage toward her mother, whom she "hated" and who was "no good for anything," and that last week she was experiencing very strong loving feelings toward her mother, praising her highly and wanting to be "close with her." Also in this particular session in which she was vehemently degrading her mother, Gerry told Anna that she loved Anna, wanted to be just like her, that she was sure that Anna was the "best therapist in the world," and that everything would be OK in her own life if Anna were only her mother. Gerry said that she has "a lot of trouble remembering any of the good" about people whenever she feels angry with them. She also remembered, with Anna's help, how she hates herself and feels like a bad person—"a piece of garbage" whenever she gets depressed. Gerry has a great deal of difficulty remembering or acknowledging any of her own good points when she is experiencing one of her frequent bouts with depression.

Primitive idealization

Primitive idealization is a derivative of *splitting* and in the clinical example described above, it is quite evident that Gerry uses primitive idealization in her reaction to her therapist ("things would be perfect if you were my mother—you do everything just right").

Primitive idealization is a defensive maneuver in which the person tends to see the external object (often the therapist, perhaps a new lover or friend) as *all good* and powerful and necessary for protection against all-bad objects. The idealized external object is also seen as all good to protect it from one's very bad and dangerous self-image. This mechanism is not like the higher-level defense mechanism of *reaction-formation*, where the other person is protected out of concern or regard for the individual's welfare. With primitive idealization, it is mostly derived out of a more basic need-fulfilling motivation ("I need the other to survive"). The object (friend, lover, therapist) can protect or serve by (1) protecting against bad objects in the world and (2) serving as a recipient for omnipotent identification; the person using this mechanism can "share" in the chosen one's greatness as a direct gratification of narcissistic needs.

Projective identification

Projective identification is a lower, or more primitive, level of the defense mechanism known as projection, and it is characterized by:

1. A tendency to experience impulses that are, at almost the same time as they are experienced, projected onto another person
2. A fear that this other person who serves as the recipient of the projection will act under the influence of that projected impulse and do harm
3. The felt need to control this person who is under the influence of this dangerous projection

This mechanism serves to externalize all-bad self and object images, but it leads to the perception of dangerous, retaliatory persons as populating one's world—persons whom one had better control (through manipulation, devaluation).

Gerry, in the course of her therapy, began to experience angry feelings toward her therapist and to experience therapy as "difficult," "no fun anymore," "not helping me at all." Partly she wanted to run away from this situation, where she felt very dependent on her therapist, yet she also felt unimportant—not counting for much with the therapist. Using the mechanism of projective identification, she began to suspect and verbalize that Anna wanted "to kick me out of therapy," that Anna was "tired of working with me." Gerry began to increase the number of phone calls to Anna, much past the pattern of contact they had both agreed on and with which they had been working for some time. Calls began to come at unusual times; demands for attention outside of the parameters of their working relationship increased. Gerry took comments or statements of Anna's out of context, interpreting and using them in such a manner as to "prove" negative feelings toward herself on Anna's part. Indeed, Anna began to experience a sharp increase in her feelings of frustration in working with Gerry (see discussion of countertransference, Chapter 11). In working with her supervisor, Anna was able to identify these negative countertransference feelings and the signs of projective identification in Gerry. This helped Anna to regain her perspective and begin to work more constructively with Gerry.

Denial of ego states

This is typically a "mutual denial" of two different and emotionally independent ego states or "areas of consciousness." This denial reinforces splitting. The person may be aware that two ego states are experienced with completely opposite perceptions, thoughts, and feelings. However, this awareness has no emotional impact. This awareness is not helpful in influencing present feelings toward an object at all. For example, a person may calmly convey a cognitive awareness of the situation while denying its emotional implications. As Kernberg states: "The patient is aware of the fact that at this time his perceptions, thoughts, and feelings about himself or other people are completely opposite to those he has had at other times; but this memory has no emotional relevance, it cannot influence the way he feels now" (Kernberg, 1977, 31). Again, there is a lack of integration in the person suffering from borderline pathology.

Omnipotence of self with devaluation of others

This is also linked to splitting. A highly inflated, grandiose, and omnipotent self relates to a depreciated, devalued representation of others. Underneath the feelings of insecurity and harsh self-criticism, the borderline person often experiences grandiose and omnipotent trends. There may be an unconscious belief that one has the right to expect to be treated as a special and privileged person. If another person no longer provides the narcissistic gratification or protection that is sought, that person is usually dropped. Devaluation of the other person is also used defensively and intrapsychically to control and protect oneself from this potentially dangerous person. Kernberg notes that the devaluation of significant people in the person's past (for example, the parents) can have very serious detrimental effects on superego development and integration. This is because devaluation of one's internalized object relations interferes with healthy identifications.

For a schematic representation of underlying dynamics, see box on p. 758.

A schematic representation of the dynamics of borderline personality disorder

Underlying dynamics	Effects on the psyche	Behavioral results

A. Abundance of intolerable rage (perhaps an inborn, higher level of aggressive feelings)
B. "Mothering failure"* in early life
  1. Failure to synthesize the "good" and the "bad"
  2. Failure to separate-individuate
  3. Failure to develop adequate sublimation—unable to derive pleasure from anything that is not a direct sensual pleasure (no pleasure, for example, in work performance)
	Negative, indistinct self-image; rapidly shifting ego states with use of denial; use of splitting, projective identification; primitive idealization, omnipotence of self with devaluation of others	Severely disordered interpersonal relations; brief, psychosis-like episodes; impulsive, self-destructive behavior; dependency on excessive use of drugs and alcohol and on promiscuity; poor work history

*For further discussion of these dynamics, see the section on explanatory theories in this chapter. Briefly, (1) is related to Winnicott's concept of the *good enough mother* (the mother who is not perfect but who is predominantly able to meet her infant's needs); (2) is related to Mahler's idea of the maternal failure to facilitate the toddler's developmental task of separation-individuation; and (3) can be related to Winnicott's views on the transitional object as a precursor to development of *sublimation*—the ability to substitute something for the original object.

CLASSIFICATION OF BORDERLINE PERSONALITY DISORDERS

Based on a thorough and systematic inquiry into the borderline syndrome, Grinker et al. (1968) have defined four subgroups of the disorder. These are descriptive of clustering symptomatology:

1. *Group I:* "the psychotic border"—characterized by inappropriate and negativistic behavior. Members of this group tend to be angry, withdrawn, depressed, and hostile.
2. *Group II:* "the core borderline syndrome"—negativistic, chaotic feelings and behavior are evident. Individuals seem unstable, labile, and vacillating emotionally. There is a high potential for acting out.
3. *Group III:* "the adaptive, affectless, defended 'as if' person." This person is schizoid, obsessional, detached, and withdrawn and has a bland and superficial adaptiveness with an "as if" quality to interpersonal interactions.
4. *Group IV:* "the border neurosis"—characterized by childlike, clinging behavior, anxiety, and depression.

Donald Klein (1977) has noted the similarity of the classification of Grinker et al. (1968) to some groupings he has made and, based on his own research, he believes that in some cases, specific medications are effective within each group. (See discussion of pharmacological treatment below.)

EPIDEMIOLOGY AND SOCIOCULTURAL CONTEXT

Millman et al. (1982) state (with no apparent validation) that the disorder is more common in women than in men. And it has been noted by a

Harvard Medical School professor that "some psychiatrists believe the disorder affects as much as 7 to 10 percent of the population of the United States and 25 percent of those who receive any kind of psychiatric or psychological treatment" (Sass, 1982, 12).

However, these unsupported statements and the general lack of epidemiological references in the literature point to the fact that an epidemiological approach to the problem of the borderline syndrome has not been taken at this time. Kaplan and Sadock (1981, 488) note that "no systematic studies of borderline pathology have been carried out."

In spite of this, the study by Grinker and his associates (1968) and another by Lazar (1973), concerning clients applying for therapy at the Columbia University Psychoanalytic Clinic, raise some important questions about the syndrome and its interaction with our present culture. These questions are:

1. Is the syndrome becoming more prevalent because of our particular culture's characteristics, such as the chaos of urban living, the increase in existential anxiety, and some profound changes in social structure and family life?

2. Do shifts in diagnostic categories (that is, the increase in diagnoses of "borderline") reflect real population changes or are they more apt to be due to increased attention by professionals to certain phenomena or diagnoses (Mack, 1975, 17)?

Freed (1980) suggests that our society is an etiological factor. To support her belief she cites a discussion of "the new narcissism" by Reiner (1979) and Christopher Lasch's book *The Culture of Narcissism* (1978). She points to such deep and pervasive disorders as "a sense of irrelevance in society, alienation, narcissistic 'deification of the isolated self,' 'lifeboat ethics,' social pressures and stresses, massive traumas (. . . the Holocaust, terrorism, the Viet Nam war, nuclear war, violence in families), inhuman environments in which people live, and widespread discrepancies between values and beliefs" (Freed, 1980, 552-553). Chessick, writing in 1977, agrees with this view and lists ten features of Western culture that may be contributing to problems in interpersonal relating and to the development of borderline pathology.

EXPLANATORY THEORIES
Psychoanalytic theories

An inborn, overabundance of aggressiveness that may have a biological basis is postulated by several theorists as an important factor in the borderline personality. Most of the investigation and theorizing, however, has been focused on early childhood development. The disorder is considered a *preoedipal* or *pregenital* disorder (see Chapter 6 for a review of the psychosexual stages of development according to Freud), and a *mothering failure* during this period is related to development of the syndrome. Five theorists who have added the most clear and cogent ideas to our present understanding of the condition include Melanie Klein, Margaret Mahler, D.W. Winnicott, Otto Kernberg, and James Masterson. Some relevant points that they make will be reviewed here, and Mahler's theory of the preoedipal stages of development will be treated with some depth. All five theorists focus on object relations and human development. *Object relations* is the term used to designate the way an individual (subject) relates to his world (object). Of course, the first object relationship is with the mothering one.

Melanie Klein's extensive contribution to the theory of object relations will not be reviewed here*, but it includes a view of the infant, very early in life, as defensively needing to deny the terror associated with a potential loss of the good object (mother). The child needs to deny the complexity (good and bad qualities together in one object) of the object, and this is done by splitting it into *either* all-good *or* all-bad. Depending on chronology, this can be seen as a normal developmental stage in object relations (Rinsley, 1977).

Otto Kernberg believes that the defects in ego

---

*The reader is referred to *Introduction to the Work of Melanie Klein*, second edition, by Hannah Segal, for a more detailed explanation of some of Melanie Klein's theories of infant development.

functioning, and most specifically in interpersonal relating, grow out of the interaction of the mother-child dyad. He sees them originating in the period toward the end of the first year of life. Kernberg cites early relationship problems with the mothering one as leading to an inability to internalize good interpersonal relating. This in turn affects the child's self-concept—the superego and ego-ideal are negatively influenced, and borderline pathology may be the result. Specifically, a synthesis of "good" and "bad" introjects* does not take place—there remains a split. The world is then something of an "either-or" situation. The person has defects in the ability to relate to *whole* (and therefore mixtures of "good" and "bad" qualities in) other persons. Trusting, meaningful, *reciprocal* interpersonal relationships are inhibited, and feelings of loneliness, emptiness, and depression result. The split is also in the image of the "self," as well as the "other." The image of a good, acceptable self is protected from the image of a bad, aggressive (and therefore dangerous) self, just as the image of a good other (mother) is protected from the dangerous other (mother). This is a normal developmental stage, but when inadequate mothering occurs and continues into the first year or two of life, the child fails to separate from the mother in a healthy way, and an integrated self concept does not evolve. The roots of the primitive defense mechanisms that Kernberg describes can be seen. Extreme, idealized images and an extremely sadistic superego to punish the "bad self" and a continued excessive use of splitting in later life are some of the results. Extreme dependency and desires to merge with powerful others are never worked through adequately and in fact are reinforced to become pathological factors in adult life. The development of healthy sublimation and other coping mechanisms is retarded because of energy being expended to control the good-bad conflict, anxiety, and frustration. The individual is in an intolerably painful position: the use of splitting and the feelings of rage

---

*An introject is a mental image of someone or something that becomes incorporated into one's ego system. The process of *introjection* is opposite to that of *projection*. An introject becomes emotionally invested for the individual and is involved in the process of *identification* and superego development.

tend to isolate the person, wreck interpersonal relationships, and cause feelings of aloneness and abandonment. The individual feels what Masterson has termed *abandonment depression* (see below for further discussion of this concept). Dependency and lack of development of sublimation (for substitute pleasures, interests, distractions) offer no solution to the powerful loneliness and emptiness and can lead to escape through alcohol and drugs. A failure to separate-individuate leads to a continuing need-fear dilemma as far as merging with the significant other is concerned, and this too may be defended against by seeking oblivion through drug and alcohol abuse.

D.W. Winnicott proposes a specific maternal task—the provision of a "holding environment"—to provide the matrix that can facilitate normal development in the infant. Winnicott has been called "the analyst of the borderline" (Green, 1977, 24). Winnicott, originally a pediatrician and later a renowned psychoanalyst, had long been interested in the maturation processes of childhood development. He believed that a necessary component of healthy development is a *maternal preoccupation* of the mother with her newborn infant. This preoccupation is necessary for the baby to form a healthy symbiotic attachment to its mother. Failure to enter into a symbiosis with her would lead to serious withdrawal—autism, childhood schizophrenia, or later schizophrenia depending on the degree and timing of the withdrawal. The mother, and to some extent the father who protects the symbiotic dyad, *is the facilitating environment* for healthy development. The *True Self* of the human organism, according to Winnicott, begins to have life through the mother's preoccupation. His term *the good enough mother* is relevant to the development of schizophrenia *and* borderline pathology.

Winnicott describes this good enough mothering: "The 'good enough mother' meets the omnipotence of the infant and to some extent makes sense of it. She does this repeatedly. A *True Self* begins to have life through the strength given to the infant's weak ego by the mother's implementation of the infant's omnipotent expressions" (Winnicott, 1965, 145).

Good enough mothering implies imperfect mothering, which is all any human mother can expect to provide. This fact of imperfection is not only realistic, it is necessary to provide an optimal level of frustration so that the infant can encounter the reality principle of life. But the encounter should be a gradual one; the frustration should not be more than the baby can tolerate. It should be, in the words of Winnicott (1965, 57): "here and there, now and then, but not everywhere all at once." If needs could be met without any frustration, it would be impossible for the child to gradually learn self-reliance. The *transitional object* helps to bridge the gap between extreme dependency and self-reliance. The transitional object is an important part of childhood development. The teddy bear or the favorite blanket substitutes for the absent and needed mother. The baby is beginning, in a sense, to sublimate through a primitive substitution of one object for another. It soothes and makes separation (frustration) tolerable.

Thus the small failures of mothering that must naturally occur facilitate growth and lead to a strengthening of the baby's ego. It is only when there are profound failures in mothering that borderline pathology develops. Specifically, these failures are seen as occurring in the separation-individuation stage of preoedipal development. Some discussion of this and Margaret Mahler's theory will follow.

Margaret Mahler's theory of human development has gained considerable attention in recent years as a basis for understanding the development of borderline personality syndrome. Much of the present treatment approach to the disorder has also evolved from Mahler's work. Basing her theory on her many years of therapeutic work with children and direct observation of mother-child dyads, Mahler has delineated the phases and subphases of preoedipal development. Mahler's theory incorporates an ego psychology* and an object-relations focus.

Ego psychology is a direct outgrowth of Freudian psychology and includes in its ranks such theorists as Heinz Hartmann, Ernst Kris, Rudolph Lowenstein, and Anna Freud; *object relations* is a school of psychoanalytic thought that is strongly influenced by people such as Melanie Klein, Donald Winnicott, W. Ronald Fairbairn, and Harry Guntrip. The reader is referred to their various works (see reference list) to gain a deeper understanding of their ideas.

The infant does not develop in a vacuum—it needs human contact and relationship to grow in complexity. The child grows normally, in a matrix of the *average expectable environment* (Hartmann, 1958). That is to say that the environment does not have to be a perfect one but that the frustrations should not be overwhelming. Severe failures in mothering may prevent the child from adequately negotiating with its environment and from successfully navigating through the preoedipal developmental stages. These stages are the autistic stage (birth to 1 month), the symbiotic stage 1 month to 5 months), the separation-individuation stage (5 months to 2½ years). The separation-individuation stage has been defined further by Mahler into four subphases, and these phases are important to our understanding borderline pathology. Depending on the particular preoedipal stage where developmental arrests occur, serious pathology may result. Just as failure to resolve the oedipal crisis is seen as resulting in psychoneurotic problems (see Chapter 23), a failure along the continuum of development from birth to the oedipal period results in an arrest in differentiation of both "self" and "object" (other). Ego functioning related to these important differentiations will also be arrested (Masterson, 1977, 476-477). For example, a failure to form a symbiotic bond with the mother is postulated as the defect leading to pathological *early autism*, whereas failure to work through the symbiotic phase and begin to separate-individuate leaves the individual stuck in symbiosis manifested by the various forms of schizophrenia (see Chapter 25 for further discussion). A brief description of Mahler's phases and subphases follows.

1. *The autistic phase.* The infant lacks cognitive awareness of any mothering agent. This is termed *normal autism*, and it gradually changes as the child becomes aware of needs that cannot be satisfied by oneself. To be stuck in this phase would imply pathological autism. At approximately 1 month of age (and it must be remembered that all Mahler's age estimates are approximate), the infant begins to be aware of the mothering one and enters into the next stage, the symbiotic phase of development.

2. *The symbiotic phase.* From 1 month to ap-

proximately 5 months of age, the child participates in what Mahler describes as the *symbiotic orbit*. This is a "magic circle" of the mother-infant world in which all parts of mother, including her voice, gestures, clothing, and even the space in which she comes and goes, are joined with the infant.

3. *The separation-individuation phase.* The third phase begins when the infant starts to psychologically "hatch" from the symbiotic orbit, to see and experience itself as separate from the mother. Mahler views the infant's *psychological birth* as occurring here. This happens over a period of time (5 months to 2½ years) and evolves through four distinct subphases. The subphases of the separation-individuation phase are:

a. Differentiation (5 months to 9 months). Maturation of partial locomotor functioning brings the first tentative moves away from mother, and interest in her as a separate being begins. Differentiation of a primitive but distinct body image seems to occur at this time.

b. Practicing (from 9 months to about 14 months of age). During the second subphase, the child is able to move away from mother and return to her (crawling at first, later through upright locomotion). Investigation of the environment and practicing locomotor skills become very important to the child, and *elation* is a common theme.

c. Rapprochement (from approximately 14 months to approximately 2 years of age or more). This is a stage that is characterized by a rediscovery of mother, now as a separate individual. The narcissistic inflation of the subphase of practicing, when the child is in love with the world, is replaced by the realization of separation and vulnerability. The *rapprochement crisis* occurs now, and this is seen as a very important developmental event. *Ambivalence* is the significant theme here. The child wants to be united with and, at the same time, separate from mother. This phase and its inherent crisis are seen as extremely significant in the development of bor-

derline pathology. Mahler believes that the collapse of the child's belief in its own omnipotence combined with the mother's emotional unavailability leads to a hostile dependency on the mother (Akhtar and Byrne, 1983, 1014).

d. Consolidation of individuality and emotional object constancy. The fourth subphase of separation-individuation begins toward the end of the second year and it is seen as open ended. A degree of object constancy* is accomplished, and separation of self and object representation is established. "Mother is clearly perceived as a separate person in the outside world, and at the same time has an existence in the internal representational world of the child" (Mahler et al., 1975, 289).

Of course, the battles of one's separation-individuation task continue throughout one's lifetime; it is an ongoing process. But within healthy psychological development, a firm beginning is established with this fourth and final subphase. Failure to attain object constancy in the process of separation-individuation is the *core problem of the borderline* states. Object constancy and clear ego boundaries are necessary for a strong sense of self-identity to develop.

James Masterson (1977) designates the rapproachement subphase as *the* most critical one in the development of borderline personality disorder. Rapprochement occurs after the child has practiced separating and has begun to assert the self and to individuate. The child now needs to return to the mother, to sort of "check in" with her.

---

*Object constancy occurs when the child is able to maintain a mental and emotional representation of mother. This definition has important implications for treatment goals for many borderline clients who enter a treatment situation at the level of need gratification. The therapeutic task becomes one of raising object relations to the level wherein the image of the object (for example, the therapist) is retained regardless of need state. This is a significant indication that the individual has synthesized the "good" and "bad" object representations, incorporated a healthy ambivalence, and can relate to a whole object (person). It also means the individual has become less dependent on the environment and is moving toward greater autonomy (Blanck and Blanck, 1979, 35).

Some children get confusing messages from a mother who may not have resolved her own separation-individuation. The mother is threatened by the child's efforts to separate and may react by rejecting the child at this period. According to Masterson, two messages may be given: *regression is rewarded* and *separation-individuation is punished by withdrawal* of the mother. This reinforces a maintenance of "split-object relations" in the child. Masterson terms these split-object relations:

1. The rewarding part unit. Feelings associated with the rewarding part unit are those of receiving unconditional love, feeling gratified, and being taken care of.
   a. The child maintains an image of the mother (part-object representation) that provides approval, support, and other rewards for regressive clinging.
   b. The child maintains a self-image (part-self representation) as being good and passive and compliant.
2. The withdrawing part unit. Feelings associated with this withdrawing part unit are rage, helplessness, and depression. The child feels that attention and concern from the parent must be paid for by conforming. The rapprochement stage is not adequately resolved, and object constancy is not achieved.
   a. The child maintains an image of a maternal part-object that is hostile and attacking and that withdraws supplies in the face of any efforts on the child's part to separate-individuate.
   b. The child maintains a part-self object that is bad, guilty, inadequate, and helpless.

Masterson points to an *abandonment depression* in the individual as what is being defended against by the primitive and pathological defenses of the borderline client. Abandonment depression is a major personality feature of the disorder (Lynch and Lynch, 1977, 74). The dilemma is one of striving for autonomy versus fear of abandonment, and the depression implies a helpless "giving up."

Masterson (1976), in his own work with borderline clients, found that many of the mothers and fathers of these clients suffered from borderline personality disorder themselves.

Systems theory

If a family member has a borderline personality disorder, that family member's behavior may be a symptom of dysfunction in the family system. Gordon (1987) notes that such family systems may be fragile and there may be much concern about family dissolution. There may also be a high degree of enmeshment among family members and personal growth, and individuation among family members may be prevented. Pseudomutuality may be evidenced. The family often presents itself as "normal," except for the borderline client who is the family scapegoat. Should only the client improve, then scapegoating may be transferred to another family member.

Zinner and Shapiro (1975, 105) believe that the primitive regressive defenses such as splitting occur as a family norm in the families of clients exhibiting borderline pathology. They point to a relationship between severity of the disorder in an individual and the following three variables within a family.

1. The parents' capacity to experience themselves as separate from a particular child
2. The parents' own dependence on such primitive defenses as projective identification, which leads to a necessary collusion on the part of the child (in the case of projective identification, for example, the child must serve as a container for the projection)
3. The level of maturity of the parent's own object relations (that is, self-object differentiation).

Zinner and Shapiro have also pointed out the four choices posed by the family group to the borderline adolescent:

1. To preserve good ties to family by repudiating one's own maturation
2. To choose autonomy with a persisting "bad" self-object relation with one's family
3. To oscillate between the two choices, while remaining in a state of conflict, anxiety, and uncertainty
4. To choose developmental progression—growth toward autonomy

Zinner and Shapiro see this fourth option as open to the borderline adolescent within a conjoint family therapy situation that provides a growth-enhancing "holding environment" that allows for separation of individuals.

TREATMENT

While some work has begun on pharmacological, family, and group therapy approaches, most of what has been written to date has focused on psychoanalytically oriented therapy for borderline clients. The following section will review some of the concepts relevant to the treatment of these individuals. The long-term goals for *any* treatment modality involving borderline clients have been well defined by Freed (1980, 554):

1. To heal the "split": to bring about integration of "good" and "bad" images; to work toward eliminating the need for excessive use of splitting mechanisms and patterns
2. To accept primary (healthy) ambivalence rather than fight it
3. To develop normal repression by bringing primitive idealization and projective identification within reality contexts
4. To develop a mature level of dependence through the experience of the therapeutic relationship
5. To develop increased mastery of the environment, impulse control, frustration control, and frustration tolerance
6. To develop an ability to use realistic planning and healthy coping behavior through the problem-solving process
7. To increase self-esteem and improve self-image through a reduction in self-defeating behavior and through a realistic recognition of achievements
8. To accept one's separateness and wholeness
9. To improve ability to relate to others; to permit closeness without fusion, separation without abandonment, and individuality within a social or family context
10. To use the therapeutic experience as part of relationship and trust building

Psychopharmacological treatment

Donald F. Klein (1975, 1977), one of the foremost experts in psychopharmacology in this country, believes that a psychiatric diagnosis that considers observable affects (e.g., mood) rather than the more abstract structural defects or drives is a more useful method of defining the appropriate drug treatment for clients who have been termed *borderline*. He has had a long-term interest in the diagnostic use of drugs in psychiatry. Comparing the four subtypes of Grinker et al. (1968) (see p. 758) to some groupings of his own, he has suggested specific medications as being helpful.

In studies carried out by Klein (1977) and his associates, they found that Group I individuals (who are characterized as angry, withdrawn, depressed, and hostile) were best treated with monoamine oxidase inhibitors.

Group II individuals, who are described as labile, vacillating, and emotionally unstable, seem to be improved by lithium carbonate for mood swings and phenothiazines for both anxiety with impulsivity and for depression with withdrawal. (See Chapter 22 for a discussion of monoamine oxidase inhibitors and lithium carbonate and their actions; see Chapter 25 for a discussion of phenothiazines.)

Group III individuals, characterized by schizoid, detached withdrawal, do not display clearly understood responses to medications. An exception to this was in a case where depression in a relatively well-integrated person was found. For this individual, antidepressant medications were found useful.

Group IV of Grinker's classification, which Klein closely compared to neurotic depressives and which are described by Grinker and his associates as characterized by clinging anxiety and depression, responded well to imipramine. (See Appendix B.)

Psychotherapy

Although one writer (Mendelsohn, 1982) has outlined an "active, short-term" approach to treatment for the borderline client, psychotherapy for these individuals is almost always seen as a long-term situation. Therapy is a combination of supportive approaches and psychoanalytically oriented psychotherapy. Boyer (1982), who uses these methods, has outlined six principles for effective treatment of the borderline client:

1. Initially, the client's negative reactions to the therapist should be discussed in a here-and-

now focus without attempts to relate them to the past.

2. The therapist should point out defensive maneuvers when they occur.

3. Limit-setting to control acting out of transferential feelings is important. (For a discussion of the phenomenon of transference, see Chapter 11.)

4. While positive responses toward the therapist are encouraged, any tendency to see the therapist as *all good* or *all bad* should be pointed out.

5. Distortions about the therapist's interventions or about real life events need to be clarified.

6. Any bizarre or psychotic-like fantasies about the therapist need to be worked through to facilitate the client's reexperience of actual childhood events.

Waldinger (1987), in his review and distillation of the literature on intensive treatment of the borderline client lists eight basic tenets of *safe* and effective treatment:

1. A stable framework of treatment—clearly stated expectations by the therapist about time limitations, missed appointments, reimbursement procedures, etc.

2. Increased activity by the therapist to anchor the client in reality and minimize distortions by the client.

3. Tolerance of the client's verbal hostility—examine and understand it within the therapeutic relationship.

4. Connection of the client's behavior to feelings in the *present*—the client needs to see that he or she uses action to communicate and that this is a defensive maneuver.

5. Consistently drawing the client's attention to adverse consequences of self-destructive behavior (drug abuse, promiscuity, inappropriate rages, manipulation in interpersonal relations). Motives are not focused on—the results of such actions are.

6. Acting out transference feelings is blocked—the therapist sets limits on behavior that threatens the client, the therapist, or the treatment.

7. Clarifications and interpretations are focused on the here-and-now. Reconstructions such as those done in psychoanalysis are counterproductive—they divert attention from possibly dangerous and pathological behavior patterns in the present.

8. A careful, persistent monitoring of countertransference feelings by the therapist is necessary.

Most of those who have written on the topic of psychotherapy for borderline syndrome agree that a *modified form of psychoanalysis* or *psychoanalytically oriented* psychotherapy is the treatment of choice. This involves parameters and techniques beyond a more conventionally structured psychoanalytic situation. Two important concepts related to this are Winnicott's "the holding environment" (1965) and "the transitional object" (see pp. 760–761). The *holding environment* implies that the therapeutic relationship, in a sense, provides a climate of "good enough mothering" while encompassing an "empathic awareness and response to adult strengths and self-esteem issue," rather than the therapist's omnipotent wish to save the client (Adler, 1977).

The *transitional object* is particularly relevant in matters of technique and in the necessary management of potentially self-destructive anxiety in the client. For an individual who has not adequately achieved object constancy and who has difficulty maintaining contact with an effective memory of the therapist during inevitable absences (for example, the therapist's vacation or unexpected illness), such times can become desperate ones and contribute to escalating anxiety. There is an increased risk of acting-out behavior as a coping mechanism. Some transitional objects that have been used by therapists or by clients on their own include the therapist's business card, a picture of the therapist, a copy of the monthly bill, and the client's own efforts to keep a journal of thoughts and feelings during the therapist's absence. Adler and Buis (1979) postulate that intense, painful aloneness is a theme in the lives of borderline clients. They see this aloneness as an intrinsic aspect of the disorder related to the inability to remember positive images of the significant, sustaining people in their lives *or* being overwhelmed by negative images and memories of these significant others. The developmental defect or arrest is in the rapprochement subphase and implications for treatment include the therapist's use of transitional objects (from those of an abstract, symbolic quality to actual ones, depending on the client's situation) during absences.

Relaxation therapy

Relaxation therapy that is adapted to work with borderline clients is seen by Glantz (1982) as a useful adjunct to psychoanalytic treatment. Deep and rhythmic breathing exercises are taught to the client. This therapy helps the client (1) to discover previously unrecognized anxiety that could be worked with in therapy and (2) to reduce anxiety to a level where difficult material can be discussed.

Relaxation therapy is begun only after a trusting relationship with the therapist has been well established; the timing for introducing it is a crucial factor. Relaxation therapy is used after the therapist has observed dissociated ego states (for example, immersion in angry, hostile feelings or pervasive feelings of affection) and repetitive alternation between two ego states with a concomitant denial of one while in the other. During these times the client's memory is affected and when angry, for example, there is no memory of pleasant feelings or events for the object of this anger. It is not used when the client is immersed in a particular ego state; it is used while the client is in the "zone of fear that lies between the two states" (Glantz, 1982, 345).

Family therapy

Family therapy for borderline clients involves moving the family structure from lower-level defensive patterning to a higher level of patterning (Mandelbaum, 1977, 437).

The same issues and problems arise in family therapy as they do in individual therapy. Use of primitive defenses such as splitting and issues of separation-individuation are all present and must be dealt with. While problems are similar, there may be (particularly in the case of the borderline adolescent) more opportunities for change. There may be another chance within the family of origin to resolve failures, thus reconciling good and bad

images, and to reach a point where ambivalence can be tolerated. Feelings of closeness and love need to be experienced without the threat of loss of identity, without risking merger and fusion. Separation and growth toward autonomy can be worked on through the individual and supported through working with all the family members.

Group therapy

Borderline clients who present severe weaknesses in ego functioning and object-relations development may benefit from group therapy. As an adjunct to individual therapy, group therapy is recommended by numerous therapists as providing the kind of mutual support and mutual control that severe borderline clients need (Freed, 1980, 357). A study by Kretsch et al. found that ego functions (as rated on Bellack's Ego Function Scale) of borderline clients were significantly and *markedly* improved after one year of group therapy. The authors suggest that there are factors in group therapy that can evoke processes conducive to change in borderline clients.

Freed (1980) notes that there are several advantages to group therapy that are specific to borderline pathology:

1. Group therapy helps the client learn to listen to others, to explore and begin to understand the communication of others.
2. There is much opportunity for reality testing within the group.
3. There is the possibility of a corrective emotional experience without the forced (and threatening) closeness of a one-to-one relationship.
4. Reactions can be somewhat diluted within the group. For instance, clients may not feel narcissistically devastated by any criticism when others in the group are hearing similar comments.
5. Defensive mechanisms like splitting and projective identification are ideally handled in the group situation.
6. There are opportunities for dealing with maladaptive behavior with the goal of learning new ways of coping within the protective atmosphere of a group.

7. A supportive, working group can enhance the formation of trust and the kind of closeness that can help foster individuation in each group member.

In conducting group therapy sessions with borderline clients, the basic principles of group therapy apply (see Chapter 13). Some principles adapted from Kibel (1978) that are specific to the disorder include:

1. Clarification of here-and-now relationships within the group is important to foster increased understanding of distortions and of the tendency to distort through projective identification, splitting, and primitive idealization. The client needs to distinguish what is "inside" (defensive distortions) from what is "outside" (the reality situation).

2. Improved reality testing in all areas needs to be fostered and supported.

3. Mutual support and mutual control of the group is facilitated by the leader's directing major interventions toward the group as a whole. The threat of closeness with, or harm from, the leader is also diluted through this process.

4. Aggressive drives are channeled through verbalization and problem solving.

5. Degree of confrontation of individuals needs to be modified from that for a group of neurotic clients, since there is the danger that harsh confrontation may serve as a narcissistic blow.

Hospitalization

According to most writers, hospitalization, when it is necessary for the borderline client, should be brief. This is to prevent a negative therapeutic reaction activated by a tendency to regress in situations of dependency. At least one group (Tucker et al., 1987) is studying the effects of long-term hospitalization on borderline clients. Preliminary results show that clients do show improvement for the first postdischarge year, but the data from the second postdischarge year indicated little difference between those hospitalized for shorter or longer stays. The authors view this as a beginning attempt to study the important question of hospital treatment for borderline clients.

Hospitalization most often occurs at times of crisis in the client's life and often around issues of dependency on significant others (for example, the breakup of a relationship). Hospitalization may be precipitated by threats of suicide. Regressed, suicidal individuals need a setting that provides Winnicott's ideal of a "holding environment." This implies an empathetic, nurturing yet appropriately limit-setting situation.

Borderline clients tend to repeat with the staff the interaction patterns they have employed in the past. This is the basis for a major problem—the development of negative countertransference by staff members. (See Chapter 11 for a discussion of countertransference.) Manipulation of others is a common life-style theme of borderline clients. Most often this manipulation serves unconscious needs, but the staff may interpret it as conscious, willful behavior and may respond with decreased empathy, increased anger, and withdrawal. Adler (1977) points out that hospitalization is a special problem because the chaotic behavior of borderline pathology can activate in the staff members themselves repressed, primitive defenses, such as splitting and projective identification. He emphasizes the importance of this potential and advocates continuing vigilance for the danger signals of countertransference.

Wishnie (1975, 43) lists three factors necessary for brief hospitalization to be effective as a therapeutic modality for borderline clients:

1. *Rapid identification* of the client as suffering from borderline pathology

2. *Clear limit setting*—goals, limits and what can be expected from the hospitalization all need to be defined

3. Administrative support of *consistency* from the staff members through education, supervision, and communication

Emergency interventions

The following points (adapted from Goldfinger, 1982) are important to consider in crisis intervention with the borderline client:

1. How significant is the danger of self-destructive acting out? Some borderline clients are chronically impulsive—suicidal gestures and attempts are possible dangers.
2. Can the client function outside a structured setting at this time? If admission to a structured setting is indicated, should it be a hospital or a less structured setting, such as a halfway house or a supervised group home?
3. Overnight hospitalization may be useful in certain situations. A number of borderline clients demonstrate a marked reduction in suicidal and homicidal ideation, anxiety, and depression after 12 to 24 hours. A transfer to another setting (halfway house, etc.) may then be considered.
4. The borderline client has the potential for rapid shifts in level of functioning—emergency intervention is aimed at assisting the client's rapid reintegration, and long-term care solutions should be postponed, if possible, until this has occurred.
5. Borderline pathology is characterological in nature—structural changes are carried out in long-term treatment not in brief, crisis intervention. The appropriate goals for emergency treatment are (a) reduction or elimination of immediate stress and (b) protection of clients from acts that can harm themselves or others.
6. The degree of anxiety, rage, or psychotic ideation may make verbal interaction with the client impossible. Such behavior has responded rapidly to low-dose neuroleptic medication.
7. The borderline client's tendency to use *splitting* as a defense can lead to a distorted view of the emergency care clinician as either "powerful" or "impotent," "all-loving" or "rejecting." This may be a problem when treatment plans are presented to the client—goals and purposes of the treatment may also be distorted. Self-awareness in the clinician and an understanding of the phenomenon of splitting may curtail countertransference responses that might escalate the problem.

Nursing Intervention
PRIMARY PREVENTION

Since the genetic roots of a borderline syndrome are believed to be in a disturbed, preoedipal period of development (roughly, before 3½ years of age) (Pine, 1986), primary prevention of the disorder naturally encompasses some sort of therapeutic intervention with the mother-infant dyad and the family. One example of this would be the group therapy program carried out with the borderline mothers of toddlers (Holman, 1985). A time-limited program that focused group content and process on the psychological issue of separation was effective in helping the mothers to increase their tolerance of the normal separation-individuation of their toddlers.

Bowen (1976) (see Chapter 14) has pointed out that mental illness results from a multigenerational transmission of disorder so that treatment of the parent becomes a means of primary prevention for the child. Grinker and his associates (see below) point out that maternal depression is an outstanding feature in the families of borderline individuals. Family therapy can be viewed as primary prevention. Minuchin (1976) points to the enmeshment patterns of a pathological family system. This includes overresponsiveness and overinvolvement as well as distancing maneuvers. Such a pattern can activate abandonment depression and seriously disturb issues of separation-individuation.

In addition to *treatment* of the parents as a primary prevention method, *education* of parents about their roles in fostering healthy object relations with the child is a means of primary prevention. Some work has been done on the need for and methods used to facilitate healthy parent-infant interactions (Brazelton and Als, 1979; Field, 1982). *Interaction coaching* is a term used to describe this. An intuitive and natural sensitivity of a mother to her child's needs is not present in everyone. Interaction coaching is an attempt to modify disturbed mother-infant interactions with the goal of improving the "fit" between them.

If primary prevention is to be possible, it is necessary that high-risk families be identified. Grinker and his associates (1968), in their research study of borderline pathology, have delineated ten recurring qualities that they found in the nuclear families of borderline individuals:

1. A highly discordant marital relationship
2. Relationships within the family that reflect chronic, overt conflict or competition
3. Parenthood rejected outright or conflict over parenthood
4. A lack of provision of nurturing care for the children
5. The mother's affect is predominantly negative
6. The marital couple is unable to achieve mutuality of purpose and their conflicting demands remain unresolved
7. Family goals do not include support of its members
8. Father's affect is predominantly negative
9. The couple engage in mutual devaluation and criticism
10. The husband and wife are unable to achieve reciprocal role relationships

To summarize, some important points under "primary prevention" would include

1. Identification of parent-child dyads and families at high risk for producing borderline offspring
2. Therapeutic intervention with, and support of, high-risk parents and family units
3. Education and interaction coaching aimed at facilitating healthy relationships within the nuclear family
4. Education of parents about the needs of the toddler for healthy separation-individuation

SECONDARY PREVENTION

Most writers agree that the borderline syndrome is a rather long continuum that includes varying degrees of pathology. The range is from severely impaired ego functioning, with severely disordered interpersonal relationships, to minimal impairment with relatively high functioning. It is important to remember that, because of the chaotic nature of the individual's inner and outer life, the course of treatment may also be chaotic.

Nursing process

This section focuses on secondary prevention through nursing intervention into clients' patterns of impaired ego functioning and object-relations development, alleviation of symptoms associated with borderline personality syndrome, and restoration of functional patterns of client behavior. It is important to assess an individual's level of functioning and coping in general.

Nurses, in establishing therapeutic nurse-client relationships with borderline clients, may be helped by the following guidelines (adapted from Masterson's four-stage guide for treating the borderline client [1974]):

1. In the initial phase of treatment, the client is defending against abandonment depression and needs assurance that this relationship will not intensify the terror of abandonment. The client's defenses may include acting-out behavior and other forms of "testing." When the client becomes more comfortable with the relationship, the second phase of the therapeutic relationship is begun.
2. In this "working through" phase, the abandonment depression is dealt with. The client's depression may deepen somewhat during this second phase, but the relationship provides a structure that makes it easier to cope with. Through the use of therapeutic communication techniques, the principles of psychiatric nursing, and the use of self as a therapeutic tool, the nurse helps the client to get in touch with the anger that is underlying the depression. There is the possibility of working through some of the feelings of hopelessness, rage, and loneliness that are the core of the developmental arrest.
3. The client begins to develop some ability to integrate "good" and "bad" images of people through a consistent, nonexploitative relationship with the nurse. The client's development of an internalized sense of identity and object representations is facilitated, while healthy separation-individuation is encouraged by the nurse. Examples of this would be allowing for and discussing "differences" be-

tween nurse and client and supporting the client's decision-making processes.

4. In the termination phase of the relationship, the client may experience regressive feelings and may need to be reminded of the differences between separation and abandonment. The goal is for the client to realize his or her potential for a separate but related life with others.

An understanding of potential problem areas and of the possibilities for healing within the context of the nurse-client relationship is important in working with borderline clients. The nursing process serves as a conceptual framework for this work.

ASSESSMENT

Based on some of the theoretical constructs of ego psychology and object relations development discussed earlier in this chapter, the following areas can be assessed when working with the borderline client:

1. Presenting symptoms. Brief, psychotic-like episodes; impulsive self-destructive behaviors; disordered, chaotic interpersonal relationships; drug and alcohol abuse; promiscuity; poor work history. These are the behavioral manifestations of the core problem—abandonment depression that is based on developmental defects (failure to synthesize "good" and "bad"; failure to separate-individuate; failure to develop *sublimation* adequately).

2. Emotional state. Feelings of rage, depression, helplessness, anxiety, and boredom in response to stimulus situations. An understanding of the tendency for the individual to rapidly "shift" emotional states is also important here.

3. Stimulus situations. Stressful life situations are often part of a vicious cycle wherein the person's self-defeating behavior perpetuates a life of poor functioning, disordered interpersonal relationships, and many painful crises.

4. Maladaptive coping behaviors. Coping patterns based on primitive defensive organization—splitting, projective identification, primitive idealization, omnipotence-devaluation in relating to others. These primitive

defenses are attempts to satisfy and protect oneself, but they are unsuccessful in that they perpetuate a painful, unsatisfactory life-style of disordered interpersonal relations and inadequate functioning in the world.

5. Origin of maladaptive coping behaviors. Identification of childhood experiences that contributed to the development or learning of maladaptive coping behaviors, to the continued reliance on primitive defenses, and to severe difficulties in separation-individuation.

6. Holistic health status. Physical, intellectual, emotional, sociocultural, and spiritual status of the client. These factors may either facilitate wellness (for example, an intact, nuclear family that is motivated to change through their desire to help the "identified client," may facilitate the client's growth through participation in family therapy), or these factors may impede wellness (for example, a seriously physically disabled borderline client who must necessarily be very dependent on others may find it extremely difficult to work through and resolve issues of separation-individuation).

ANALYSIS OF DATA

With some understanding of presenting symptoms, emotional state, stimulus situations, maladaptive coping behavior and their origins, and the holistic health status of these clients, the nurse will get a clearer and more empathetic understanding of the predicament these clients and their families face. This empathetic understanding is a prerequisite to formulating nursing diagnoses.

PLANNING AND IMPLEMENTATION

The following section will focus on nursing care plans which may be made for borderline clients. A discussion of short-term outcomes, long-term outcomes, and implementation of planning will be included with each nursing diagnosis. *Helplessness, dependency* and *feelings of worthlessness* as themes have been covered in Chapter 22; *manipulation, aggressive behavior* and *acting out through substance abuse* were discussed in Chapter 20; approaches to *psychotic behavior* are found in

Chapter 25. Since these are all important themes of the borderline personality, it will assist the nurse to review the principles discussed in these chapters. Nursing diagnoses based on themes of splitting, primitive idealization, projective identification, rapidly changing ego states, omnipotence of self with devaluation of others, boredom, and inability to tolerate aloneness will be discussed.

Since the borderline client is coping with the effects of an early developmental arrest with hopes of growing toward greater autonomy, the treatment of this disorder tends to be a long-term undertaking. Therefore, the long-term outcomes (as outlined in the nursing care plans that follow) will most often be undertaken or accomplished by clients working with a clinical nurse specialist (or other therapists) in an outpatient setting. The short-term outcomes support these long-term outcomes, however, and they are consistent with the work of the professional nurse working in a psychiatric setting. *Text continued on p. 778.*

NURSING CARE PLAN

Clients with Borderline Personality Disorder

Long-term Outcomes	Short-term Outcomes	Nursing Strategies

Nursing diagnosis: Sensory/perceptual alteration: defects in perception (splitting*) (NANDA 7.2; DSM-III-R 301.83)

Long-term Outcomes	Short-term Outcomes	Nursing Strategies
Develop more effective coping behaviors and interpersonal skills Accept ambivalence of self and ambivalence in the world Develop and strengthen an observing ego† Synthesize and integrate contradictory images of self and others to accept self and others as wholes	Develop awareness of *splitting* mechanisms and patterns when they are used Identify interpersonal and environmental situations that trigger the use of *splitting* mechanisms and patterns Identify difficulties in interpersonal relationships and in the ability to function that are related to the reliance on *splitting* mechanisms and patterns	Establish a working nurse-client relationship Point out the client's tendency to see only one aspect of self, others, and situations as it occurs within the course of the nurse-client relationship (for example, "You seem to have a great deal of difficulty remembering anything good about yourself when you get depressed"; "Today, it sounds like you are not able to accept anything positive about your mother—that's different from yesterday, when you said you felt very close to her") Relate specific occurrences of the client's *splitting* to any particular stimulus situations Support the development of active self-observation by the client when he or she is experiencing strongly positive or negative feelings (an "observing ego")

*Splitting can be defined as a defense mechanism that helps the individual cope with anxiety by keeping two opposite affective states separate—"bad" and "good" images cannot be integrated because of an early developmental arrest. At a very early age, it is a normal protective mechanism for keeping the "bad" mother image from contaminating the "good" mother image. However, in normal development, this becomes unnecessary and the representations merge.
†Strengthening an observing ego implies that there is (1) an increasing awareness of one's own behavior and its effects on self and the environment and (2) a decreasing tendency toward harsh, judgmental (punitive superego) reactions to oneself that only serve to escalate defensive, self-defeating behaviors. Instead, one is able to work toward realistic behavioral changes that will enhance separation-individuation. *Continued.*

NURSING CARE PLAN—cont'd

Clients with Borderline Personality Disorder

Long-term Outcomes	Short-term Outcomes	Nursing Strategies

Nursing diagnosis: Sensory/perceptual alteration: defects in perception (splitting*) (NANDA 7.2; DSM-III-R 301.83)—cont'd

		Respond verbally to the client's *splitting* in a manner that helps to integrate contradictory reactions (for example, "It sounds like you're saying that you like some of the things your mother does when she's being helpful, but sometimes you get angry with her when she tries to take over too much; I guess you have a mixture of feelings toward her, which is very natural") Remember, as a nurse, the importance of self-awareness to avoid identifying with the client's negative or positive split. The goal is for the client to accept self, others, and the world as a necessary mixture of good, bad, and indifferent

Nursing diagnosis: Sensory/perceptual alteration: distortions in perception with disturbed interpersonal relationships related to protection of self from dangerously perceived introjects (projective identification*) (NANDA 7.2; DSM-III-R 301.83)

Long-term Outcomes	Short-term Outcomes	Nursing Strategies
Develop more effective coping behavior and interpersonal skills Accept ambivalence in the self and ambivalence in the world Develop and strengthen an observing ego Relinquish dependency on projective identification as	Develop awareness of any distortions of others and their motives in interpersonal situations Identify interpersonal and environmental situations that trigger the use of projective identification as a defense Identify difficulties in interper-	Establish a working nurse-client relationship Observe the client for tendencies to overreact in interpersonal situations or to distort perceptions of others Explore the client's perception in situations of possible overreaction or distortion Clarify situations whenever possible†— provide additional input, examples of

*Projective identification is a lower-level or more primitive defense mechanism than projection. Projective identification serves to externalize (get rid of) all-bad, potentially dangerous images of the self, and all-good, potentially nurturing images of the self. However, its use leads to a view of the world as full of dangerous, powerful, and retaliatory persons whom one must control. In projective identification, attributes, tendencies, strengths, and weaknesses may be projected onto the person (1) to externalize and thus "control" the dangerous introject or (2) to achieve symbiosis with a powerful and good externalized introject. The result is a severe distortion of reality that can disorder interpersonal relationships and impair one's ability to function in life.

†A consistent clarification to reduce distortions as they appear in the nurse-client relationship is an appropriate and therapeutic nursing response. Self-awareness and nondefensive, objective stance on the part of the nurse is crucial because part of projective identification includes the client's unconsciously motivated efforts to manipulate the person to react in harmony with the projection.

Long-term Outcomes	Short-term Outcomes	Nursing Strategies
a defense and develop normal repression Synthesize and integrate negative and positive images of self and others to relate to self and others as whole persons	sonal relating and in ability to function related to reliance on projective identification as a defense	modifying circumstances, other viewpoints; use the communication technique of "reasonable doubt"; be a bridge to reality in this situation Support the development of active self-observation by clients when you suspect any hint of overreacting or distorting in interpersonal situations (an "observing ego") Remember the importance of self-awareness to minimize any manipulation by the client aimed at inducing you to react in harmony with the projection

Nursing diagnosis: Impaired social interaction related to primitive idealization* (NANDA 3.1.1; DSM-III-R 301.83)

Develop more effective coping and interpersonal skills Develop and strengthen an observing ego Realistically perceive the five subsystems of the self (biological, psychological, intellectual, sociocultural, and spiritual strengths and weaknesses will be put in perspective) Realistically perceive strengths and weaknesses of others Work through exaggerated and debilitating fears of living in the world Tolerate a probabilistic world and the possibility of ambivalent, negative, or indifferent feelings from or toward others Begin to relate to others on a more realistic level that incorporates healthy ambivalence	Verbalize feelings of loss, inadequacy, and fear Identify interpersonal situations that arouse fears of possible attack from the environment or from a harshly critical superego (review the concept of superego in Chapter 6) Relate current stress to stressful situations in the past that aroused similar feelings Build self-esteem (refer to Chapter 22 for a discussion of self-esteem)	Establish a working relationship with the client Allow the client to verbalize and explore the nature of fears about self and the world Clarify any distortions about you, the nurse, in an objective and dispassionate manner Use the communication techniques of "reasonable doubt" in response to the client's exaggerated claims about your attributes. (This is not to be confused with a "becoming modesty"—the goal is not to confess the ordinary nature of yourself so much as it is to help the client to see and tolerate an imperfect, human you. This should be done in combination with the acknowledgment of any realistic appraisal of your good qualities. Again, it is apparent that self-awareness on the part of the nurse is crucial) Explore with the client incidents, situations, and interpersonal relationships outside the nurse-client relationship where a tendency to use primitive idealization is evident

*Expressions of idealistic admiration for the nurse that are exaggerations or unrelated to any real situation are indications that a client is using primitive idealization as a defense.   *Continued.*

NURSING CARE PLAN—cont'd

Clients with Borderline Personality Disorder

Long-term Outcomes	Short-term Outcomes	Nursing Strategies

Nursing diagnosis: Impaired social interaction related to primitive idealization* (NANDA 3.1.1; DSM-III-R 301.83)—cont'd

Develop a mature level of dependence on others rather than immature dependence Develop a mature level of interdependence with others		Explore with the client a more realistically based appraisal of self

Nursing diagnosis: Impaired social interaction: grandiosity and devaluation of others* related to protection of self from self-derogating introjects and projections (NANDA 3.1.1; DSM-III-R 301.83)

Develop more effective coping skills Develop and strengthen an observing ego Realistically perceive the five subsystems of the self (biological, psychological, intellectual, sociocultural, and spiritual strengths and weaknesses will be put in perspective) Realistically perceive strengths and weaknesses of others Work through exaggerated and debilitating fears of living in the world Tolerate a probabilistic world Develop a realistic sense of self and others Accept oneself and others as separate, whole people Develop a mature level of dependence on another person	Verbalize thoughts of grandiosity and inadequacy Identify interpersonal situations that arouse defensive feelings of grandiosity of self or devaluation of others Relate current stressful situation to situations in the past that aroused similar feelings Identify current difficulties in interpersonal relations and in ability to function related to viewing the self as omnipotent and others as devalued Build self-esteem in a reality-based context	Establish a working nurse-client relationship Encourage the client's verbalization of thoughts of grandiosity and inadequacy Explore situations that arouse feelings of grandiosity of self and devaluation of others Assist client in relating current stressful situation to situations in the recent past that aroused similar feelings Assist client in relating current interpersonal difficulties and inability to function to the pattern of viewing self as omnipotent and others as devalued Maintain the limits of the relationship in an objective manner when grandiosity leads to testing behavior, manipulation, and acting out behavior Explore any examples of testing behavior and its consequences with the client Relate any devaluation of others back to the client (e.g., "Do you ever have any of these same complaints about yourself?")

*Feelings of insecurity and a harsh, punitive superego underlie the more obvious statements and actions of grandiosity. Devaluation of others is part of the same matrix of low self-esteem, but it is more likely to appear on a more subtle level.

Long-term Outcomes	Short-term Outcomes	Nursing Strategies
Develop a mature level of interdependence with others		Support the client's growth steps toward increasing independence and interdependence Expect a course of treatment that includes growth steps *and* periods of regression in between. Explore the regressions and encourage the growth steps

Nursing diagnosis: Ineffective individual coping related to rapid alterations in perceptions and feelings about self, others, or situations (rapidly shifting ego states with mutual denial*) (NANDA 5.1.1.1; DSM-III-R 301.83)

Synthesize and integrate contradictory inner images to relate to self and others as whole persons Accept a probabilistic world and healthy ambivalence in self and others Develop and strengthen an observing ego Develop a consistent sense of self-identity	Develop awareness of phenomenon of rapidly shifting ego states in self Verbalize the subjective experience of rapidly shifting ego states in self Develop awareness of the use of denial in relation to rapidly shifting ego states Identify stressful situations that seem to trigger rapid shifts in ego states Identify difficulties in interpersonal relating and in ability to function that are related to this phenomenon	Establish a working nurse-client relationship Be aware that the client may or may not be aware (on an intellectual level) that perceptions, feelings, and thoughts about self and others are quite opposite to those held previously. Even when intellectual awareness *is* present, emotional relevance is denied in the current situation Confront the client with any examples of rapidly shifting ego states as you observe their occurrence within the relationship. This should be done while the experience is still fresh but at a point when the client is able to be fairly calm Explore the client's subjective experience of the phenomenon of rapidly shifting ego states (what were your feelings and thoughts when this was happening?) Do some tracking of behaviors and experiences just prior to immersion in the ego state (e.g., what happened that might have triggered the shift from one state to the other; was there a threat to self-esteem, and, if so, what was it? Is this reaction to this particular stressor an identifiable pattern in the client's life?)

*The phenomenon of rapidly shifting ego states with mutual denial is engendered by the underlying defect in synthesizing contradictory internal images of the self and others. There may be intellectual awareness of two opposing ego states, but there is denial of the emotional relevance of one while immersed in the other.

Continued.

NURSING CARE PLAN—cont'd

Clients with Borderline Personality Disorder

Long-term Outcomes	Short-term Outcomes	Nursing Strategies

Nursing diagnosis: Fear of abandonment related to impairment in separation-individuation process and inadequately developed ability to sublimate (NANDA 9.3.2; DSM-III-R 301.83)

Long-term Outcomes	Short-term Outcomes	Nursing Strategies
Develop alternative ways of sublimating through substitute activities, interests, etc. Increase tolerance for times of "being alone" Work through issues of separation-individuation with growth toward object constancy Accept separateness and wholeness; tolerate closeness in interpersonal relationships without the need for fusion	Explore any underlying feelings of anger Explore fears of separation and aloneness Identify difficulties in relating interpersonally and in ability to function that are related to fears of abandonment and inability to tolerate aloneness Explore difficulties in sublimating the need for contact with others through substitute activities, interests, etc. Explore alternative ways of sublimating through activities, interests, etc.	Establish a working relationship with the client. Help client develop a tolerance for aloneness. The inability to tolerate aloneness is a long-term treatment issue and would arise with the clinical specialist who is involved in ongoing therapy with a borderline client. Short-term outcomes are relevant to the professional nurse working in a psychiatric setting. Consistency and trust in the nurse-client relationship are important to help the client deal with fears of abandonment and the underlying rage that is being defended against. The nurse will need "skill, empathy and the capacity to tolerate rage, confusion and disappointment" (Adler and Buie, 1979, 441) in helping the client to grow and develop a tolerance for inevitable periods of aloneness. The client's feelings of panic over aloneness can be manifested through a profound sense of emptiness, painful restlessness, and boredom and feelings of anger that may be displaced onto the nurse. When feelings of panic over isolation and aloneness escalate, this is generally the time of greatest danger for suicide attempts in the borderline client. Nurses in inpatient units and in outpatient settings must be aware and vigilant at this time to protect the client. Acknowledge the client's efforts toward successful mastery of these difficult periods. This can serve as a positive reinforcement and stimulate further growth in this area. Explore and, at times, offer concrete assistance in developing new interests, hobbies, and vocations that can encourage healthy sublimation and increased ability to cope with aloneness.

Long-term Outcomes	Short-term Outcomes	Nursing Strategies
		Failure to accomplish object constancy is a core problem underlying the difficulties borderline clients have with aloneness. Transitional objects may prove useful at times of separation from the therapist such as vacations or illnesses. Examples include structured telephone contacts and the client's keeping a journal of thoughts and feelings to evoke memories of the therapist.

Nursing diagnosis: Ineffective individual coping: boredom related to denial of feelings and inadequately developed ability to sublimate (NANDA 5.1.1.1; DSM-III-R 301.83)

Long-term Outcomes	Short-term Outcomes	Nursing Strategies
Increase awareness of underlying feelings and be able to cope with them in a healthy manner Develop meaningful interests, hobbies, or vocation—increase ability to sublimate	Explore feelings of boredom Explore underlying feelings (anger, emptiness, fear, hopelessness) when consistent with client's cultural orientation Identify times when there is a greater tendency to feel bored Relate any tendencies to "act out" with self-destructive behavior to attempts to cope with boredom Identify activities that help to decrease feelings of boredom	Establish a working nurse-client relationship. Assist the client in exploration of feelings associated with boredom (e.g., anger, emptiness, fear, hopelessness).* Help client identify the times when there is a greater tendency to be bored. Boredom implies a sort of hopelessness in the person who suffers from it. Therefore, patience on the part of the nurse is crucial. Clients who are experiencing chronic feelings of boredom tend to take a help-rejecting stance in response to any assistance toward constructive coping with it. Help the client develop a reality-based, problem-solving approach to the problem of boredom. This is more helpful than supplying pat suggestions for dealing with it. However, concrete direction in the form of client teaching or referral to outside sources can be beneficial and is often necessary in helping the client develop new interests in life.

*The client's awareness and verbalization of underlying (denied) feelings may be the most important aspect of dealing with chronic boredom. It is possible that the release of energy associated with even a partial resolution of conflict can provide the stimulus to the client's own successful efforts to counteract boredom.

EVALUATION

The client and, whenever feasible, the client's family or significant others should be included in estimating the client's progress toward attainment of goals. Evaluation should encompass the following areas:

1. Estimation of the degree to which conflicts around separation-individuation and defects in achieving object constancy have been dealt with (this would include *awareness* of conflicts and problem areas and beginning efforts toward working them through)
2. Estimation of the degree to which goals have been achieved and client functioning has improved (demonstrated by decreased disorder in interpersonal relationships; increased ability to function in society; decreased reliance on addictive behavior and increased inner harmony)
3. Identification of goals that need to be modified or revised
4. Referral of the client to support systems other than the nurse-client relationship
   a. People in the client's social network who are willing to serve as a support system
   b. Clinics or individuals for ongoing individual psychotherapy
   c. Community agencies or self-help groups that help clients learn to live with disorders that may never be completely eliminated (for example, Recovery, Inc.)
   d. Centers or organizations that specialize in the treatment of specific problem areas for some borderline clients (for example, Alcoholics Anonymous, Gamblers Anonymous)

TERTIARY PREVENTION

Borderline personality syndrome is a disorder that usually requires long-term treatment. Because of the chaotic life-style with poor impulse control, low frustration tolerance, and a tendency to act out internal conflicts, many borderline clients will need much in the way of supportive, rehabilitative services. Hospitalization, when it is necessary, is generally brief to prevent the tendency to regress that is a common feature of borderline pathology. Fol-

low-up care *after* hospitalization is important. Rosenbluth (1987), in his review of the implications of aftercare for borderline clients, suggests that the stabilization of the client, the outpatient therapy, and the aftercare system are important goals of hospital care. A more severely disturbed individual may benefit from a structured day hospital or partial hospitalization setting and from retraining through vocational rehabilitation programs. In those cases where acting out has taken the form of substance abuse or other addictive behaviors, referrals to such self-help groups as Alcoholics Anonymous, Narcotics Anonymous, Gamblers Anonymous, or Overeaters Anonymous should be explored. For the borderline client who suffers from debilitating, chronic anxiety, a group such as Recovery, Inc., which uses a form of self-monitored behavioral modification, can be very helpful. The client whose dysfunctional interpersonal relations have gravely affected marital and family harmony should be referred for marital or family therapy. During any brief psychotic-like episodes, it may be necessary for the client to be placed on a temporary regimen of major tranquilizers to prevent the deterioration of self-esteem to which one is vulnerable at these times.

CHAPTER SUMMARY

Borderline personality disorder is a DSM-III-R diagnostic category used to describe an ever-increasing number of clients. *Borderline syndrome* or *borderline personality organization* are terms also used to describe the condition. Much of the work on etiology and treatment methods has been carried out by psychoanalysts, but, more often, intervention with this group is carried out by social workers and nurses working in inpatient units and outpatient settings. It is a condition that can be viewed as being on a dynamic continuum of pathological functioning. Severely disordered interpersonal relationships, difficulties in functioning as evidenced by poor school and vocational histories, lack of impulse control demonstrated by addictive behaviors, and a general tendency to act out inner conflicts are some of the common features of the syndrome.

Behavioral symptoms of borderline pathology include a reliance on primitive-level defense mechanisms such as splitting, projective identification, and primitive denial; the dysfunctional interpersonal modes of primitive idealization and omnipotence of self with devaluation of others; and the subjective experience of rapidly shifting ego states with mutual denial, chronic boredom, and an inability to tolerate aloneness.

Borderline syndrome is believed to be rooted in the rapprochement subphase of the developmental phase of separation-individuation. Because of problems in the interaction of the mother-child dyad, a developmental arrest is believed to occur that interferes with the person's ability to synthesize the "good" and "bad" qualities (or contradictory images) of self and others. The important developmental task of object constancy is not adequately mastered. Excessive reliance on splitting has its genesis here, and most of the behavior and the other defenses are derivatives of this reliance on splitting.

Some theorists have pointed to profound sociocultural changes (such as the changes in values, family life) as being closely related to the increase in borderline pathology.

Primary prevention of the syndrome focuses on therapeutic intervention with parents *before* the rapprochement crisis and interaction coaching of mother-child dyads to improve the "fit."

Secondary prevention includes individual therapy as the treatment of choice, with adjunct services from family and group therapy for some clients. Treatment tends to be long-term. Tertiary prevention may encompass vocational rehabilitation, self-help groups, and structured treatment settings such as day care. Since the chaotic lifestyle and disordered interpersonal relationships of the borderline client may damage family and marital relationships, therapy in these areas needs to be considered, too.

SELF-DIRECTED LEARNING

Sensitivity-Awareness Exercises

The purposes of the following exercises are to:

- Develop awareness about the subjective experiences of clients who are suffering from borderline personality disorder and the experience of clients' families in relating to them
- Develop awareness about the interrelationship of factors from the past and in the present in perpetuating the syndrome
- Develop awareness about your own feelings and abilities when working with clients who are suffering from borderline disorder

1. Try to imagine what it would be like to experience one of the following (explain why you selected that particular problem area and what you think it would be like to experience it):
   a. Rapidly shifting states of thinking, feeling, perceiving; rapid and complete swings from one emotional state to the other (for example, angry and rageful to loving and affectionate)
   b. A need to see someone you are close to as *only* good, caring, comforting, brilliant
   c. A need to see someone you are interacting with as only bad, disgusting, frightening
   d. Recurring periods of *extreme* anxiety, bordering on panic, in response to the absence of someone with whom you are close (Try to imagine that this person has left temporarily and you are alone and that you have a great deal of difficulty remembering that person's qualities, voice, and even picturing his or her face in fantasy.)
   e. Chronic feelings of boredom with little or no desire or ability to engage in creative or even distracting activities
2. Describe what you think it would be like to relate to a close friend or family member who experiences several of the problem areas listed above.
3. What might be some of your feelings and reactions as a nurse caring for clients who are suffering from borderline personality disorder? Would some of the problems areas outlined above be more difficult to deal with than others? Might some (for example, the client's need to see you as all-good,

Continued.

SELF-DIRECTED LEARNING—cont'd

Sensitivity-Awareness Exercises—cont'd

caring and loving, and very bright) be fairly "easy to take"? (Explain your answers.)

4. What do you think might be some of the difficulties in establishing and maintaining a consistent, trusting relationship with a borderline client?

5. As a community health nurse engaged in health supervision with new parents, develop a plan of counseling parents about child rearing that incorporates principles and goals for primary prevention of borderline personality disorder.

Questions to Consider

1. A young mother of a 20-month-old toddler asks you for some advice. Her child has been "very clingy" lately, and she thinks she may be "babying" him too much. She tells you that he often cries when she leaves the room if they are away from home, in another house. She sometimes tells him to "act like a big boy," but he seems to be getting more and more upset when she does this. Your best action would be to:
   a. Support her in her efforts to foster his independence by not babying him in these situations.
   b. Suggest that she refrain from visiting other homes for awhile.
   c. Explain to her that this is a developmental stage and that she should allow him to fluctuate between acting independent and being "clingy."
   d. Refer her to a child psychiatrist.

Match the term with the appropriate phrase:

2. Splitting
3. Projective identification
4. Primitive idealization
5. Omnipotence of self and devaluation of others

   a. An unconscious belief in the right to special attention from others
   b. "My new friend is wonderful and perfect"
   c. An "either-or" point of view
   d. The need to control an intrapsychically feared person

6. A transitional object is:
   a. an unimportant part of a childhood phase
   b. a teddy bear
   c. the result of culture shock
   d. something to prevent sublimation

7. *Borderline personality disorder* is considered by most theorists to be:
   a. A preoedipal disorder
   b. An oedipal disorder
   c. A symbiotic disorder
   d. An autistic disorder

8. "Good enough mothering" is a concept that:
   a. Implies imperfect mothering
   b. Describes a state conducive to the development of borderline pathology
   c. Implies meeting all the needs of an infant without stimulating any frustrations
   d. Describes a state that is impossible to achieve in a realistic world

9. According to Mahler, the subphase (of the separation-individuation phase) that is related to elation and being "in love" with the world is:
   a. Differentiation
   b. Practicing
   c. Rapprochement
   d. Object constancy

Answer key
1. c
2. c
3. d
4. b
5. a
6. b
7. a
8. a
9. b

REFERENCES

Adler G: The usefulness of the 'borderline' concept in psychotherapy, In Mack J, editor: Borderline states in psychiatry, New York, 1975, Grune & Stratton.

Adler G: Hospital management of borderline patients and its relation to psychotherapy, In Harticollis P, editor: Borderline personality disorders: the concept, the syndrome, the patient, New York, 1977, International Universities Press, Inc.

Adler G: The borderline-narcissistic personality disorder continuum, Am J Psychiatr 138:46-50, 1981.

Adler G and Buie D: The psychotherapeutic approach to aloneness in the borderline patient, In LeBoit J and Capponi A, editors: Advances in psychotherapy of the borderline patient, New York, 1979, Jason Aronson, Inc.

Akhtar S and Byrne J: The concept of splitting and its clinical relevance, Am J Psychiatr 140(8):1013-1016, 1983.

Arieti S and Chrzanowski G, editors: New dimensions in psychiatry: a world view, New York, 1975, John Wiley & Sons.

Blanck G and Blanck R: Ego psychology, vol 2, New York, 1979, Columbia University Press.

Bowen M: Theory in the practice of psychotherapy, In Guerin PJ, editor: Family therapy, New York, 1976, Gardner Press, Inc.

Boyer L: Borderline personality disorder: psychoanalysis, In Millman H, Huber J, and Diggins D, editors: Therapies for adults, San Francisco, 1982, Jossey-Bass Publishers.

Boyer L and Giovacchini P: Psychoanalytic treatment of characterological and schizophrenic disorders, New York, 1967, Science House.

Brazelton T and Als H: Four early states in the development of mother-infant interaction, In the Psychoanalytic study of the child, vol 34, New York, 1979, International Universities Press.

Capponi A: Origins and evolution of the borderline patient, In LeBoit J and Capponi A, editors: Advances in psychotherapy of the borderline patient, New York, 1979, Jason Aronson, Inc.

Chessick R: Intensive psychotherapy of the borderline patient, New York, 1977, Jason Aronson, Inc.

Chrzanowski G: Recent advances in concepts and treatment of borderline cases, In Arieti S and Chrzanowski G, editors: New dimensions on psychiatry: a world view, New York, 1975, John Wiley & Sons.

Diagnostic and Statistical Manual of Mental Disorders, The American Psychiatric Association, 1980.

Fairbairn W: Psychoanalytic studies of the personality, London, 1952, Tavistock; reprinted as An object-relations theory of the personality, New York, 1954, Basic Books.

Field T: Interaction coaching for high-risk infants and their parents, Prev Hum Serv 1(4): 1982.

Freed A: The borderline personality, Social Casework 61(9):548-558, 1980.

Freud A: The ego and its mechanisms of defense, London, 1936, Hogarth Press.

Glantz K: Borderline personality disorder: relaxation technique as an adjunct to psychodynamic treatment, In Millman H, Huber J, and Diggins D, editors: Therapies for adults, San Francisco, 1982, Jossey-Bass Publishers.

Goldfinger S: The client with a borderline condition, In Gorton J and Partridge R, editors: Practice and management of psychiatric emergency care, St. Louis, 1982, CV Mosby Co.

Goldstein W: Current dynamic thinking regarding the diagnosis of the borderline patient, Am J Psychother 41(1):4-21, 1987.

Gordon S: The borderline patient: systemic versus psychoanalytic approach (Part III: commentary), Arch Psychiatr Nurs 1(3):176-179, 1987.

Green A: The borderline concept, In Harticollis P, editor: Borderline personality disorders: the concept, the syndrome, the patient, New York, 1977, International Universities Press, Inc.

Grinker R Sr, Werble B, and Drye R: The borderline syndrome, New York, 1968, Basic Books.

Grotstein J: The psychoanalytic concept of the borderline organization, In LeBoit J and Capponi A, editors: Advances in psychotherapy of the borderline patient, New York, 1979, Jason Aronson, Inc.

Gunderson J and Kolb J: Discriminating features of borderline patients, Am J Psychiatr 135:792-796, 1978.

Gunderson J and Singer M: Defining borderline states, Am J Psychiatr 132:1-10, 1975.

Guntrip H: Personality structure and human interaction: the development synthesis of psychodynamic theory, New York, 1961, International Universities Press.

Hartmann H: Ego psychology and the problem of adaptation, New York, 1958, International Universities Press.

Hartmann H, Kris E, and Lowenstein R: Comments on the formation of psychic structure, In The Psychoanalytic Study of the Child, 2, New York, 1946, International Universities Press.

Holman S: A group program for borderline mothers and their toddlers, Int J Group Psychother 35(1):79-93, 1985.

Kaplan H and Sadock B: Modern synopsis of comprehensive textbook of psychiatry, ed 3, Baltimore, 1981, The Williams & Wilkins Co.

Kernberg O: Borderline conditions and pathological narcissism, New York, 1975, Jason Aronson, Inc.

Kernberg O: The structural diagnosis of borderline personality organization, In Harticollis P, editor: Borderline personality disorders: the concept, the syndrome, the patient, New York, 1977, International Universities Press.

Kibel H: The rationale for the use of group psychotherapy for borderline patients on a short-term unit, Int J Group Psychother 28(3):339-364, 1978.

Klein D: Psychopharmacology and the borderline patient, In Mack J, editor: Borderline states in psychiatry, New York, 1975, Grune & Stratton.

Klein D: Psychopharmacological treatment and delineation of borderline disorders, In Harticollis P, editor: Borderline personality disorders: the concept, the syndrome, the patient, New York, 1977, International Universities Press, Inc.

Kohut H: The analysis of the self, New York, 1971, International Universities Press.

Kretsch R: Change patterns of borderline patients in individual and group therapy, Int J Group Psychother 37(1):95-111, 1987.

Laplanche J and Pontalis JB: The language of psychoanalysis (translated by D. Nicholson-Smith), New York, 1973, WW Norton & Co., Inc.

Lasch C: The culture of narcissism, New York, 1978, WW Norton & Co., Inc.

Lazar N: Nature and significance of changes in a psychoanalytic clinic, Psychoanaly Q 42:579-600, 1973.

LeBoit J and Capponi A: Advances in psychotherapy of the borderline patient, New York, 1979, Jason Aronson, Inc.

Lynch V and Lynch M: Borderline personality, Persp Psychiatr Care 15(2):72-87, 1977.

Mack J: Borderline states in psychiatry, New York, 1975, Grune & Stratton.

Mahler M, Pine F, and Bergman A: The psychological birth of the human infant, New York, 1975, Basic Books, Inc.

Maltsberger J and Buie D: The psychiatric resident, his borderline patient and supervisory encounter, In Mack J, editor: Borderline states in psychiatry, New York, 1975, Grune & Stratton.

Mandelbaum A: The family treatment of the borderline patient, In Harticollis P, editor: Borderline personality disorders: the concept, the syndrome, the patient, New York, 1977, International Universities Press, Inc.

Masterson J: The borderline adolescent, In Feinstein S and Giovacchini P, editors: Adolescent psychiatry, vol 2, New York, 1973, Basic Books.

Masterson J: Intensive psychotherapy of the adolescent with a borderline syndrome, In Arieti S, editor: American handbook of psychiatry, New York, 1974, Basic Books.

Masterson J: The splitting defense mechanism of the borderline adolescent: developmental and clinical aspects, In Mack J, editor: Borderline states in psychiatry, New York, 1975, Grune & Stratton.

Masterson J: Psychotherapy of the borderline adult, New York, 1976, Brunner/Mazel, Inc.

Masterson J: Primary anorexia nervosa in the borderline adolescent—an object-relations view, In Harticollis P, editor: Borderline personality disorders: the concept, the syndrome, the patient, New York, 1977, International Universities Press.

Masterson J: New perspectives on psychotherapy of the borderline adult, New York, 1978, Brunner/Mazel, Inc.

Masterson J and Rinsley D: The borderline syndrome: the role of mother in the genesis and psychic structure of the borderline personality, In Lax R, Bach S, and Burland J, editors: Rapprochement: the critical subphase of separation-individuation, New York, 1980, Jason Aronson, Inc.

Mendelsohn R: Borderline personality disorder: Short-term psychoanalytic therapy, In Millman H, Huber J, and Diggins D, editors: Therapies for adults, San Francisco, 1982, Jossey-Bass, Inc.

Millman H, Huber J, and Diggins D: Therapies for adults, San Francisco, 1982, Jossey-Bass, Inc.

Minuchin S: A conceptual model of illness in children, Arch Gen Psychiatr 32:1031-1038, 1976.

Pine F: On the concept 'borderline' in children: a clinical essay, Psychoanal Study Child 29:341-368, 1974.

Pine F: On the development of the borderline–child-to-be, Am J Orthopsychiatr 56(3):450-457, 1986.

Reiner B: A feeling of irrelevance: the effects of a nonsupportive society, Soc Casework 60(1):3-10, 1979.

Rinsley D: An object-relations view of borderline personality, In Harticollis P, editor: Borderline personality disorders: the concept, the syndrome, the patient, New York, 1977, International Universities Press, Inc.

Rosenbluth M: The inpatient treatment of the borderline personality disorder: a critical review and discussion of aftercare implications, Can J Psychiatr 32(3):228-233, 1987.

Sass L: The borderline personality, NY Times Magazine, pp 12-67, August 22, 1982.

Segal H: Introduction to the work of Melanie Klein, ed 2, New York, 1964, Basic Books, Inc.

Singer M: Some metapsychological and clinical distinctions between borderline and neurotic conditions with special consideration to the self experience, Int J Psychiatr 60:489-499, 1979.

Tucker L et al: Long-term hospital treatment of borderline patients: a descriptive outcome study, Am J Psychiatr 144(11):1443-1448, 1987.

Waldinger R: Intensive psychodynamic therapy with borderline patients: an overview, Am J Psychiatr 144(3):267-274, 1987.

Winnicott D: The maturational processes and the facilitating environment, New York, 1965, International Universities Press, Inc.

Wishnie H: Inpatient therapy with borderline patients, In Mack J, editor: Borderline states in psychiatry, New York, 1975, Grune & Stratton, Inc.

Wolberg A: The borderline patient, New York, 1973, Intercontinental Medical Book Corp.

Zander K: The fragile princess: midway on the borderline-narcissistic personality continuum, Persp Psychiatr Care 22(2):77-84, 1984.

Zinner J and Shapiro E: Splitting in families of borderline adolescents, In Mack J, editor: Borderline states in psychiatry, New York, 1975, Grune & Stratton, Inc.

ANNOTATED SUGGESTED READINGS

Adler G and Buie D: The psychotherapeutic approach to aloneness in borderline patients, In LeBoit J and Capponi A, editors: Advances in psychotherapy of the borderline patient, New York, 1979, Jason Aronson, Inc.
This is an exploration of the borderline client's difficulties in coping with aloneness. It includes a discussion of some of the developmental and psychodynamic aspects involved in an individual's reactions to aloneness. Issues in the clinical treatment of borderline clients, including the use of transitional objects (such as tape recordings of sessions, a postcard from a vacationing therapist), are reviewed. The importance of such themes as rage and regression are also dealt with.

Akhtar S and Byrne J: The concept of splitting and its clinical relevance, Am J Psychiatr 140(8):1013-1016, 1983.
Splitting is a central defense seen in borderline clients. The

literature on the concept of splitting is reviewed here, and several clinical manifestations of this primitive defense are described. These manifestations include (1) the inability to experience ambivalence, (2) impaired decision making, (3) oscillation of self-esteem, (4) egosyntonic impulsivity, and (5) intensification of effects. Differential diagnoses of personality disorders and treatment issues are explored.

Brobyn L, Goren S, and Lego S: The borderline patient: systemic versus psychoanalytic approach, Arch Psychiatr Nurs 1(3):172-182, 1987.

A three-part essay that uses the case-study format (Brobyn) with two possible approaches to treatment considered: the family systems approach (Goren) and the psychoanalytic approach (Lego). Underlying dynamics and strategies are included in this interesting article.

Horner T: Rapprochement in the psychic development of the toddler: a transactional perspective, Am J Orthopsychiatr 58(1):4-15, 1988.

This is a reinterpretation of the concept of rapprochement from a transactional perspective. The author suggests that rapprochement is a continuing process in life rather than a phase-specific process of early development. He contends that the concept is a useful metaphor for our understanding of the characterological dynamics of older children and adults. Rapprochement is seen as a process of restoring positive equilibrium in relationships after conflicts.

Kibel H: The rationale for the use of group psychotherapy for borderline patients on a short-term unit, Int J Group Psychother 28(3):339-358, 1979.

This article focuses on three topics: the borderline client, milieu therapy for the borderline client, and group therapy within that milieu. The author focuses on descriptions and treatment recommendations for the more severely disturbed borderline client. Theoretical concepts (for example, the work of Kernberg) are reviewed, and specific goals and methods for treating the client in group therapy are discussed. The topics of brief hospitalization and the problems it presents are addressed as they relate to these clients.

Sass L: The borderline personality, The NY Times Magazine, pp 12-15 and 66-67, August 22, 1982.

A well-written, comprehensive, yet concise overview of the borderline syndrome, including intrapsychic, familial, and sociocultural aspects. The author is a clinical psychologist. Differing theoretical viewpoints on etiology, differential diagnosis, and effective treatment are reviewed. There is some clinical case material presented.

Waldinger R: Intensive psychodynamic therapy with borderline patients: an overview, Am J Psychiatr 144(3):267-274, 1987.

Major controversies surrounding the techniques of intensive psychodynamic treatment for borderline clients are reviewed. Included are debates about the importance of content vs. process in the early stages of therapy, the origins of transference, the primacy of a positive transference in the therapy, the value of early interpretation of negative transference, and the role of the therapist in providing "corrective" experiences for the client.

FURTHER READINGS

Paris J, Nowlis D, and Brown R: Developmental factors in the outcome of borderline personality disorder, Compr Psychiatry 29(2):147-150, 1988.

Zanarini M, Frankenburg F, and Gunderson S: Pharmacotherapy of borderline outpatients, Compr Psychiatry 29(4):372-378, 1988.

Patterns of withdrawal and distorted perceptions

CHAPTER FOCUS

Schizophrenia is the most perplexing of all the psychopathologies. More has been written about its etiology, course, and treatment than about any other emotional disorder.

Schizophrenia is more properly called a syndrome than a disease (Shapiro, 1981). It can involve any of several combinations of symptoms, disturbances, and reactions. Some writers and investigators have suggested that it would be more accurate to refer to the schizophrenias rather than to a single entity. The condition has probably always been with mankind, at least since man became a social animal.

Because of the complexity of schizophrenia, many explanatory theories have been proposed, and many treatment modalities have evolved and are still evolving. This chapter will summarize several of these theories, including the psychodynamic, sociological, and biological views. Current and past treatment methods will be reviewed as well as the many dimensions of primary, secondary, and tertiary prevention.

Nursing intervention for schizophrenic individuals is based not on a reaction to a diagnostic category but on a therapeutic response to specific types of behavior. These forms of behavior, while maladaptive, are not unexplainable and awesome derivatives of madness, as they have been thought of in the past. They represent an individual's attempts to deal with a threatening environment and a disintegrating sense of self.

Schizophrenia is most often a chronic disabling disorder, and young people have the highest prevalence rates (Aiken, 1987). For these reasons, family intervention aimed at support and education is important.

HISTORICAL ASPECTS

There are ancient tomb writings that graphically describe what was most likely schizophrenia. Undoubtedly, many of the witches who were burned at the stake in medieval times for being possessed by the devil were suffering from schizophrenia.

The syndrome was termed *dementia praecox* by Morel, a contemporary of Sigmund Freud. Dementia praecox, as Morel used it, meant youthful (precocious) insanity. It was thus distinguished from the dementias of later life, such as senility. Kraepelin, who has been called the *Great Classifier* of mental disturbances, used the term when he set about developing his taxonomy. Another contemporary of Freud, Eugen Bleuler, reacted to the primary symptom of dementia praecox—a splitting off of the emotions ordinarily connected to thoughts—by inventing the term *schizophrenia*. The word comes from the Greek *schizo* (to split) and *phren* (mind). *Schizophrenia* is the term now in popular use.

SOCIOCULTURAL ASPECTS OF LABELING

The label *schizophrenia* has caused some difficulties. A minor difficulty is the confusion many people experience over the meaning of the word. Many have understood the word to mean "having more than one personality." This is really a description of another psychological disturbance—a severe psychoneurotic condition of the dissociative type called *multiple personality* (see Chapter 23). *The Three Faces of Eve* and *Sybil* are both accounts of persons with the disorder of multiple personality. *Dr. Jekyll and Mr. Hyde* is a fictional account of a person with multiple personality.

The difficulty in the average person's understanding of the term schizophrenia is inconsequential when compared to the problems it has caused for most of the people who suffer from the disorder.

These problems are inherent in the process of labeling. The fear and utter hopelessness associated with schizophrenia, which have grown throughout the history of the disease, remain with us even after more effective treatments for controlling the symptoms have evolved. Schizophrenia is still the most dreaded of all psychiatric disorders (Grinker, 1969; Hoffer, 1987). Being told that one is schizophrenic is akin to receiving a diagnosis of cancer (Holden, 1987). Yet, if one were to compare the prognosis for successful adaptation to life, a diagnosis of schizophrenia is more hopeful than one of *sociopathy*.

Another problem with the label of schizophrenia is that, as defined by Bleuler, it suggests "OK, here it is—live up to it!" In other words, expectation of pathological behavior tends to elicit pathological behavior. Through the expectations and interpretations of other people, symptoms that had been dormant or even nonexistent may be manifested. Any of a therapist's biases or distortions may be projected onto a client during a therapeutic relationship (Ivker and Sze, 1987); the effects of such projection should never be underestimated. It is particularly important to remember this point, in view of the studies (such as Sarbin, 1972) that have shown that many persons who have been labeled schizophrenic do not demonstrate one or more of the cardinal symptoms of schizophrenia. It has also long been known that anyone—schizophrenic, neurotic, or normal—who is under sufficient stress may demonstrate any of these symptoms (Ivker and Sze, 1987).

Another problem arising in connection with the use of diagnostic categories has to do with cultural differences between the labeler and the person who gets labeled (Ivker and Sze, 1987). For example, previously it was well known that in Great Britain, where the average citizen is more reserved than the average American, the label most frequently given at the time of admission to psychiatric facilities was manic-depressive psychosis. In the United States, where dynamic, gregarious characters are more common and withdrawal is less acceptable, the most frequent diagnosis upon admission to state hospitals was schizophrenia (see Andreason, 1987; Kendel et al., 1971). Now, scientific differences between cultures add another dimension to diagnostic variation. The narrow scope of description for schizophrenia found in DSM-III and DSM-III-R is reversing British-American differences, and fewer Americans are diagnosed as schizophrenic compared to British (Andreason, 1987).

The economic factor is also important in the diagnosis of schizophrenia. Psychiatrists are reluctant to give their private clients that label on admission. Upper- and middle-class clients admitted to psychiatric units in general hospitals are less apt to be called schizophrenic than the lower-class patients of the state hospital systems.

Much of the discontent with the diagnostic term schizophrenia is reflected in one prominent psychiatrist's statement.

The term schizophrenia should be abandoned. It has no priority, it misleadingly implies an understanding of a supposed basic disorder, and its two main subdivisions (process and reactive) are defined by responses to therapy, which is absurd! (Altschule, 1970)

At an 1986 international conference on schizophrenia, geneticist K. Kendler summarized his views on the important research findings on schizophrenia:

If you put everything that is known about schizophrenia into a pot and boiled it down, you would come up with these things—it seems to run in families, neuroleptics (antipsychotic drugs) make it better, and there may be something structurally abnormal in the brains of schizophrenics. (Cited in Barnes, 1987)

The validity of labeling people with psychiatric terms has been questioned by many. For example, Laing (Boyers and Orrill, 1971) and Szasz (1961) have both pointed out that such labeling has served a purpose for society—it has allowed society to explain away as "sick" any behavior that deviates from accepted norms.

A nurse working with psychiatric clients usually has an aversion to putting people into pigeonholes. Nurses are aware that such a practice can be destructive. However, there is another side to this question, and other factors need to be examined. Some would argue that it is not the label itself but the stigma attached to it that causes the damage. They see the label as a potentially *helpful* device (Hoffer, 1987). For example, proponents of the medical model of the etiology of schizophrenia suggest that we say to a client: "You have a biochemical disorder called schizophrenia. We have medications and other treatments to help you control your symptoms. We will work together." Proponents of the medical model thus believe that confronting the client with the disorder, in the same way in which a diabetic person must be confronted with the metabolic disorder, is more helpful than shrouding the term "schizophrenia" in mystery. They accuse the "radical therapists"* of not providing any real help to a person trying to cope with schizophrenia when they deny that it is a disease, as Szasz does, or define it as "the only way to be sane in an insane world," as Laing views it. Whichever side of the debate you agree with, an understanding of terms and diagnostic categories is necessary if you are going to be able to read the enormous amount of literature about the schizophrenic experience. With this point in mind, we will review several classification systems, along with the underlying dynamics and common symptoms of the schizophrenic syndrome.

UNDERLYING DYNAMICS
The schizoid personality†

The development of schizophrenia often follows a predictable course. The first stage of this course is the assumption of the schizoid personality. The schizoid personality is characterized by a tendency toward isolation and withdrawal, a bland affect, vagueness in communicating, and an overuse of the defense mechanism of projection. There seems to be an emptiness or poverty of personality, and the individual may appear rather eccentric to other people (see Diagnostic and Statistical Manual of Mental Disorders, Third Edition, Revised). While most schizophrenic processes may be shown to have developed in persons who have schizoid personalities, it does not follow that everyone who

---

*R.D. Laing is considered one of the "radical therapists" because of his beliefs, for example, that schizophrenia is a liberating experience. Thomas Szasz is also counted among the radical therapists because of such views as his denial of schizophrenia as a disease.

†DSM-III-R coding: Axis II, 301.20, schizoid personality.

demonstrates a schizoid personality will necessarily develop schizophrenia.

The preschizophrenic state

The next stage of the process is generally the pre-schizophrenic or prodomal phase (DSM-III-R, 190). This stage, which may last 1 or 2 years, is characterized by social withdrawal, role-function impairment, eccentric behavior, blunted affect, unusual perceptual experience, and a lack of initiative and energy. Friends and relatives often note a dramatic change in personality at this stage (Arieti, 1979; DSM-III-R; Shapiro, 1981).

THE NEED-FEAR DILEMMA

The individual has low self-esteem and a basic feeling of rejection combined with a fear of relating to others. This fear is a factor in the conflict that has been termed the *need-fear dilemma* (Burnham et al., 1969). The preschizophrenic person seems to suffer from an inordinate *need* for interpersonal closeness and an inordinate *fear* of that closeness. Since we all suffer from the need-fear dilemma, it is the adjective *inordinate* that sets the preschizophrenic person's experience apart from that of everyone else. Leopold Bellak (1958) has illustrated this dilemma by citing the philosopher Schopenhauer's parable of the porcupines:

On a cold winter day the porcupines move close to each other in order to take advantage of the warmth from their body heat. As they move closer and closer, they hurt each other with their quills. The porcupines had to move back and forth to find the best distance between each other in order to get the maximum body warmth while minimizing the hurts from their quills.

We only have to think of the instances when the need-fear dilemma has operated in our own lives. For example, we fall in love and experience fear because the loved one now has the power to hurt by leaving. An expectant mother experiences the need-fear dilemma: her desire for the new baby is combined with a fear of the baby's power to hurt her by becoming sick or dying.

THE "AS-IF" PHENOMENON

Feeling rejected by others leads to increased and painful isolation from others, which leads in a cir-

cular fashion to increased feelings of rejection. Gradually the person's whole existence takes on an "as if" quality (Laing, 1965a). One may go through the necessary actions related to job, family, and friends in a mechanical way—acting *as if* one was an interested worker, a loving husband and father. But there is little emotional involvement in the action.

INAPPROPRIATE AFFECT

The person's affect may be inappropriate. A few preschizophrenic persons may be depressed or euphoric, but most seem to have a bland affect. The bland, shallow affect that accompanies the preschizophrenic and schizophrenic states may be an indication of a withdrawal into the individual's inner world.

There is not always a clear line of demarcation between the preschizophrenic state and the schizophrenic state. Often an insidious development from one stage to the next occurs. With some individuals, however, there *is* a dramatic shift. Usually, when there is a florid and sudden psychotic "break with reality," the prognosis is better than it is when the break is gradual (DSM-III-R, 191).

The schizophrenic state

The symptoms of many emotional problems can be viewed as unconscious attempts to make the best of a bad situation; so can the symptoms of schizophrenia. They are unconsciously mediated attempts to halt the destructive process of the disease. It is useful to divide the symptoms of schizophrenia into primary and secondary groups. (The difference between primary and secondary symptoms becomes clear if we consider some examples from pathophysiology. In the physical disorder of rheumatic heart disease, the primary symptom is the stenosed mitral valve of the heart. Secondary or accessory symptoms include orthopnea, decreased renal function, and fatigue. In cirrhosis, a fibrotic, nodular, and therefore inefficient liver is the primary symptom. Secondary symptoms include jaundice, bone demineralization, cholesterol lesions of the skin due to high serum levels, and a tendency toward bleeding. In both rheumatic heart disease and cirrhosis, the secondary symptoms result from the primary symptom and are ways the organism compensates for the primary symptom.)

PRIMARY SYMPTOMS

The primary symptoms of schizophrenia were delineated by Bleuler and are usually remembered as *Bleuler's four A's*. They are autism, an associative looseness, ambivalence, and affective indifference or inappropriateness.

▶ Autism

The term *autism* refers to thought processes that are not used by the normal person in conscious thinking. They are similar to the thought processes of very young children or to those found in dreams. The ego judgments of time and place, of possible and impossible, are not used, and there is a strong element of unreality. In a case of autism that is so extreme that it leads to a break with reality, an individual might construct a private inner world, complete with characters. A person may then live in this dream world, which could become a nightmare (Shapiro, 1981, 20). Cameron (1963) has termed this phenomenon the *pseudocommunity*.

Autism is a compensating maneuver of the ego. It may be an attempt to deal with the pain of failing to relate to other people (Mendel, 1976). Autism is closely tied to the ability to think abstractly. When this function is impaired, as is often the case in schizophrenia, autism results. Words, objects, events, and even people may take on private, symbolic meaning for a schizophrenic person, and communication may therefore become difficult. Autism may be manifested in personally symbolic communication, concrete thinking (inability to think abstractly), or associative looseness, another of Bleuler's A's.

▶ Associative looseness

Associative looseness is characterized by verbalizations that are very difficult and sometimes impossible to understand. Associative looseness may seem similar to the *flight of ideas* that is seen in the manic phase of manic-depressive psychosis (see Chapter 22). Flight of ideas, however, is different in that even though it involves rapid jumping from one topic to another, there is some connection between one phrase or idea and the next. In asso-

ciative looseness, the connection between one phrase and another is apparent to the speaker but not the listener. Associative looseness may be diagramed as follows:

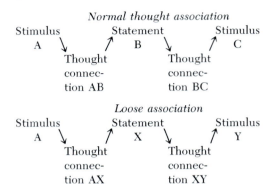

The logical sequence of A to B to C makes the normal thought processes easy to understand and follow. The esoteric or autistic connections of thought that characterize associative looseness make conversation difficult or impossible. Consider the following sample conversations:

Both persons normal
Person 1: "I'm late because the phone was ringing." (A)
Person 2: "Did you answer it in time?" (AB)
Person 1: "Yes." (B)
Person 2: "Who was it?" (BC)
Person 1: "My mother." (C)

One person schizophrenic
Person 1: "I'm late because the phone was ringing." (A)
Person 1: "Are you engaged?" ("ringing" is associated with getting a ring and being engaged.) (AX)
Person 1: "Excuse me?" (X)
Person 2: "I cannot teach you." (The association is that one is dismissed or "excused" in class by a teacher.) (XY)
Person 1: "I don't understand you." (Y)

Loose association is not limited to individuals who are suffering from schizophrenia. Anyone may at times demonstrate this dysfunctional communication—especially under conditions of stress. You may have witnessed this symptom if you have taken part in a lengthy telephone conversation in which the other person's way of communicating was unclear to you. Perhaps that person was upset about something, and you slipped into agreeing with some points along the way because of your reluctance to admit that you did not quite understand all of what was being said. At the end of the conversation you may have been disturbed to find yourself agreeing with a point when you were not at all sure that you actually did agree. At that point you may have been embarrassed to admit that you had not been "tuned in." It is quite possible that one reason you found yourself in this uncomfortable position was that the person you were listening to was demonstrating loose association.

▶ Ambivalence

We all experience ambivalent feelings at times. The difference between this "normal" ambivalence and that experienced by a schizophrenic individual lies not so much in the frequency or even the intensity of the ambivalence. It lies in the effect the ambivalence has on behavior (Mendel, 1976; Strahl, 1980).

A schizophrenic person may experience a powerful combination of conflicting emotions of love and hate toward his significant others. These strong and opposing emotions neutralize each other, leading to psychic immobilization and difficulty in expressing *any* emotion. The result is often inactivity and *apathy*, an extreme, defensive "blunting" of the emotions. Apathy is always a defense against possible pain—it has been described as the defense mechanism of the concentration camps (Frankl, 1959). Apathy is evident when a person is indifferent to what might be expected to cause emotional arousal. Affective indifference is part of another of Bleuler's four A's.

▶ Affective indifference or inappropriateness

A schizophrenic person may display indifference or apathy or express feelings that do not fit a situation, such as laughing loudly after being notified that one's mother has just died.

The term *inappropriate* may be misleading. Mendel (1976) maintains that if we were to understand the purely personal logic and thought processes of a schizophrenic individual, the behavior

would not seem inappropriate. He suggests that a better term would be *socially inappropriate*.

SECONDARY SYMPTOMS

The secondary symptoms of schizophrenia can be viewed as disturbances in thought, speech, mood, behavior, sensation, and perception.

▶ Anxiety

Anxiety, of course, is more than a secondary symptom. It is the basis for all emotional disturbances, and in that sense it might be considered the most primary, or fundamental, of all symptoms. However, it is a secondary symptom in schizophrenia because much anxiety is generated by the trauma and the social consequences of being schizophrenic. In addition, anxiety can occur in response to other secondary symptoms. For example, the experience of hallucinating can be very anxiety producing. Anxiety often occurs at various points in the natural history of schizophrenia, such as hospital admission and discharge, initial diagnosis, and exacerbation of symptoms.

▶ Depression

Because depression is in itself a psychiatric entity or category, nurses sometimes lose sight of the fact that schizophrenic clients can be and usually are depressed. Like anxiety, depression can occur in response to the schizophrenic experience. To feel that one is a failure in interpersonal relationships can be extremely depressing. In addition, schizophrenia is usually a chronic condition, and depression often accompanies chronicity.

▶ Social withdrawal

Shyness, isolation, fear of others, and withdrawal can be expressed in degrees. The extreme situation would be characterized by *mutism* and *stupor*.

▶ Loosening of external ego boundaries

Inappropriate identification, depersonalization experiences, and gender identity confusion can occur as a result of a loosening of external ego boundaries. External ego boundaries are those mental processes that help us differentiate between our inner subjective thoughts and stimuli that are coming from the outer environment.

Inappropriate identification. A client, involved in a therapeutic relationship with a nurse, might begin to dress like the nurse, verbalize a decision to become a nurse, use identical phrases, and so on. This behavior can vary in severity; an extreme example would be clients who are unable to distinguish their wants and needs from those of other people or to make their own decisions.

Depersonalization. Depersonalization results from feelings of change in self or environment. These feelings may be relatively mild—expressed by such phrases as "I don't look like I usually do" or "Somehow the room has changed—it seems completely different." The feelings and experiences may, however, be more extreme; believing that one has been "transformed" or that one has entered another dimension of the universe would be examples. The delusion* that one is someone else would be an even more extreme situation. Delusions of this kind and others often follow current cultural trends and facts. For example, it is not likely that a person would have the delusion of being Napoleon, as is often portrayed in comic situations. Today, clients are more apt to believe that they are the president, the godfather, Martin Luther King, Marilyn Monroe, or Elvis Presley reincarnated. The most common delusions of this kind are for a male to believe he is Jesus Christ and for a woman to believe she is the Virgin Mary. Many factors are operating within such delusions; feelings of evil versus good and of power versus impotence are among them.

Gender identity confusion. Sexual identification might become weak or confused. Instead of a comfortable acceptance of one's sexual orientation (heterosexual, homosexual, or bisexual), a labile, primitive, guilt-ridden stance in relation to sexuality might develop. In some instances this situation may be characterized by a wish to become a member of the opposite sex or by a fear that such a transformation might occur spontaneously and magically. In extreme cases there may be delusional and symbol-laden beliefs that one is actually half male and half female.

---

*A delusion is a belief that is contrary to fact.

► Loosening of inner ego boundaries

Inner ego boundaries are the borders between the repressed unconscious of an individual and conscious mental life. They help us to differentiate "real" from "unreal." Defective inner ego boundaries can lead to the *attribution of supernatural powers to self and others.* Symptoms of this phenomenon include ideas or delusions of reference, ideas or delusions of control, and religiosity.

Ideas or delusions of reference. Ideas or delusions of reference occur when individuals believe that others are referring to or communicating with them through newspapers, television broadcasts, or books (even books published many years ago) or in passing conversations. A mild form of this condition would be to believe that the people across the hall are talking about you (something that perhaps most of us have experienced). An extreme form is the belief that the headline of this morning's paper is actually a coded message about oneself.

Ideas or delusions of control and influence. Ideas and delusions of control or influence are demonstrated when there is a belief in the ability to control and influence other people through supernatural means. The belief that others can influence one's own mind or control one's behavior is another example. The following letter illustrates such a delusion.

Dear Sir:
My name is _____. I am writing to you in hope of some answers. My wife, three sons, and myself are being bugged by some kind of electronics, which I believe is in your field. I went to electronics experts for consultation, and they told me it would cost about $3,000 for them to help me. I don't have that kind of money, so I'm writing to you and pray that you can help me and my family. Here are some of the things that are taking place: (1) Using some kind of transmission to our heads, they can jam our memory so we can't think straight. (2) The equipment they're using can induce personality changes, such as increased friendliness or aggression. (3) They can keep us awake or make us sleep. (4) They can put words in our mouth, and make us say things we don't want to say. (5) At times I hear a high ringing noise in my ears that causes great pain. (6) It affects us mainly on our heads. (7) It appears that I can hear voices from the liquid in my stomach. (8) The fre-

quency they use affects our equilibrium and causes pain to our spinal column.

I would appreciate any help you can give me.

Thank you,

_____

(name and address)

Religiosity. Religiosity is a difficult symptom to assess in another person (Peterson and Nelson, 1987), since religious belief and degree of commitment are exceedingly personal and variable. It has been pointed out that it is extremely difficult for people to agree on the line of demarcation between normal and pathological religious investment (Field and Wilkerson, 1973).

An individual in a preschizophrenic state that is becoming steadily more severe may seek out religion to compensate for the cruelty of an increasingly alien world and to provide structure and guidelines for behavior (Arieti, 1979; Strahl, 1980). Religion and God thus become good parents, substituting for the real, "bad" parents (Arieti, 1955).

Field and Wilkerson (1973) view the schizophrenic's use of religiosity as a restitutive attempt to deal with two major pathological processes that are operating in the disorder—tendency toward withdrawal and lability of affect. They suggest that religious preoccupation helps support and rationalize this withdrawal and that it also helps to stabilize or control emotions.

▶ Autistic thinking and acting

Symbolic distortions and neologisms. Schizophrenic individuals may exhibit any of several forms of symbolic distortions: Overuse of generalization and universal pronouns (for example, "They" said . . .), vagueness, and inaccuracy are all relatively common patterns of communication. Neologisms are words that are invented to describe people, things, and events. They have completely personal meanings, and they may be egocentrically symbolic in nature. In extreme disorders of communication it may be necessary to "decode" the verbalizations of a client. This requires the establishment of a trusting relationship and may take a fairly protracted period of time.

Concrete thinking. Symbolic distortion often has its roots in another autistic form of thinking—concrete thinking. Concrete thinking involves the fairly consistent use of literal interpretation of others' communication; it is a regression to an earlier form of thinking. A person who thinks such a way has great difficulty in thinking abstractly. The belief that this symptom is frequently associated with schizophrenic thought disorders has led to the use of a "proverb test" in the diagnosis of schizophrenia. The individual is asked to give the meanings of some common proverbs, such as "A new broom sweeps clean" or "A rolling stone gathers no moss." Inability to give the abstract meanings of the proverbs is viewed as evidence of concrete thinking and becomes one of the factors in a diagnosis of schizophrenia.

Primary process thinking. Primary process thinking, a Freudian term, is an early, prelogical form of thinking that incorporates such elements as concrete thinking, the post-hoc fallacy,* and paralogical or paleological thinking. Dreams are examples of a type of primary process thinking that is considered normal experience. During a psychotic experience, a person may seem to be dreaming while in a waking state.

Paralogical or paleological thinking. Paralogical thinking is a term that has been adopted by clinicians (Von Domarus, 1944) to denote a type of logic that accepts identity based upon identical predicates—in contrast to normal logic, which only accepts identity based upon identical subjects. Arieti prefers to designate this type of thinking, which is a frequent correlate of schizophrenia, as "paleologic," from the Greek word for ancient, "palaios." This form of thinking is illogical according to normal logic, but it is really a logic of its own (Arieti, 1955, 1967). The following is an example of normal, or Aristotelian, logic:

All men are mortal.
Socrates is a man.
Therefore, Socrates is mortal.

Compare this with the following example of paralogical or paleological thinking:

*"After this; therefore because of it." The post-hoc fallacy is also an element in Sullivan's concept of *parataxic distortion* (Arieti, 1967).

The Blessed Mother Mary is a virgin.
I am a virgin.
Therefore, I am the Virgin Mary.

(For a more detailed examination of this complex and interesting phenomenon, see *Language and Thought in Schizophrenia*, edited by J.S. Kasanin, *Interpretation of Schizophrenia*, by Sylvano Arieti, or *The Intrapsychic Self*, also by Sylvano Arieti.)

Stereotypical actions, echopraxia, echolalia. Stereotypical actions involve the persistent repetition of a motor activity. A "normal" example of this is thumb twiddling or finger tapping. Such actions are often much more bizarre when used by a psychotic client; they may include posturing, intricate hand gestures, or facial grimacing. A stereotypical action is used to control anxiety, but it may also have symbolic, personal meaning. Echopraxia, which is also characterized by persistent movement, is the imitation of someone or something a person is observing; it thus involves the element of loose ego boundaries. Echolalia is the pathological repetition of the words or phrases of another person.

Lack of social awareness. A withdrawn, self-preoccupied person may exhibit some degree of social insensitivity and crudeness. An example would be engaging in such activities as nose picking and masturbation in public places, with little or no awareness of the impact on other people. The activities of daily living (ADL), such as body cleanliness, grooming, and proper attire, may be completely neglected. In a very extreme situation, there may be bizarre, repulsive behavior, such as coprophagia, the desire to eat feces. In fact, the habitual ingestion of various objects (for example, knives and spoons) is a symptom of the extreme or regressed stage of schizophrenia, which is not often seen today. This behavior is sometimes symbolic for the schizophrenic person. Before the advent of psychotropic drugs, it was not as rare an occurrence as it is now.

Somatic preoccupations. A person who is either preschizophrenic or schizophrenic may exhibit an excessive amount of concern about body functions and health. This behavior may be demonstrated in varying degrees—from vague fears about one's health, to hypochondria, to the extreme situation wherein the person suffers from bizarre somatic

delusions. The following are some somatic delusions that have been expressed by schizophrenic clients:

1. Complete body infestation by worms
2. Body infestation by snakes
3. Electrical wiring throughout the body
4. Electrical wiring of the brain
5. Depletion of energy and life force by others and through the eyes
6. Exposure of one's inner thoughts, to be read as if in a book, through the eyes
7. One side of the body being female, the other male
8. One side of the body being clean and healthy, the other filthy and diseased

It is evident that these delusions, like most other secondary symptoms of schizophrenia, may serve more than one purpose for a person with a threatened and crumbling ego. Symbolic statements, expressions of guilt, projection of blame onto others and outside forces, and rationalization of weaknesses and fear of others are a few explanations that are possible.

CLASSIFICATIONS OF SCHIZOPHRENIA
Classic

Several systems for categorizing schizophrenia have been devised. The oldest one—the classic one—was first described by Kraepelin. It included several types, four of which are still in use today: *catatonic, paranoid, hebephrenic,* and *simple*. Before Kraepelin devised this classification system, all the types of schizophrenia were considered to be one disease and were seen as that particular kind of madness that strikes at a young age—dementia praecox. Three of these four types (catatonic, paranoid, and hebephrenic) can be shown to involve specific patterns of defensive reactions to the threat of the ego-disintegrating schizophrenic process.

CATATONIC SCHIZOPHRENIA

Catatonic schizophrenia (DSM-III-R: schizophrenia, catanoic; see Appendix A for other DSM-III-R codings) is associated with motor disturbances. There are two stages in this type of schizophrenia: *catatonic excitement* and *catatonic stupor*.

Someone who is in the excited stage may exhibit a frenzied overactivity that is in many ways similar to the extreme state of mania that is part of manic-depressive psychosis (see Chapter 22). There is, however, more personality disorganization evident in this schizophrenic condition than in mania. Before the antipsychotic drugs were available, a person in the excited stage of catatonic schizophrenia was in danger of dying from exhaustion.

In catatonic stupor, the motor disturbance is underactivity, which can occur in varying degrees. In severe cases, a person may exhibit the symptom of cerea flexibilitas, or "waxy flexibility." The phrase describes a situation wherein the person's arms, legs, or any other body part can be moved about by another person and will remain in any position in which they are placed. The childhood game of "statues" is a little like this situation—it is as if the person has relinquished voluntary movement. Catatonic stupor was a fairly common occurrence in psychiatric wards before the availability of the major tranquilizers; there was an ever-present danger of such conditions as leg ulcers because of the impaired circulation that results from remaining in any one position too long. Hypostatic pneumonia was also a danger, as were accidental burns from radiators that were leaned against during the stuporous phase.

Hallucinations and delusions may be present in catatonic schizophrenia; the delusional system may be persecutory or mystical and magical. Catatonia, of all of the four Kraepelinian types, is most often the one to come on and clear up suddenly—it is thought to have the best prognosis of the four. Denial is the defense mechanism that is pathologically overused—the individual denies reality and the environment through complete withdrawal or through frenzied overactivity that shuts out the world and everyone in it.

PARANOID SCHIZOPHRENIA

The defense mechanism being used in a pathological manner by a paranoid schizophrenic person is projection. Fear, insecurity, or a hostile and threatening inner world are projected or blamed on the outside environment and on other people. Delusions are often persecutory or grandiose, and suspicion is a predominant theme. The paranoid schizophrenic (DSM-III-R: schizophrenia, paranoid; see Appendix A for other DSM-III-R codings) often appears more organized and better able to function within a psychosis than the catatonic schizophrenic, but the prognosis is considered less favorable.

HEBEPHRENIC SCHIZOPHRENIA

Hebephrenic schizophrenia was thought to represent massive regression to a primitive, childlike state. The word comes from the name for the Greek goddess of youth—Hebe. It was seen as a more extreme condition than the previously mentioned types of schizophrenia, with rapid disintegration of the personality. Hebephrenic schizophrenia was considered to have the poorest prognosis of the four types. Hallucinations and delusions are common, and it is described as childishness, silly giggling, and bizarre facial grimacing. Speech may be garbled—a person may exhibit "word salad," an unintelligible jumbling of words and phrases. Sometimes complete disorganization and dissociation from the self take place, and the person believes he or she is someone else. (Hebephrenia is not a term used in DSM-III-R. Schizophrenia, disorganized type, is used to describe the classification.)

SIMPLE SCHIZOPHRENIA

There is no predominant pattern of defensive reaction in simple schizophrenia—only the primary symptoms of schizophrenia appear. Loose association and poor attention span are usually present. Persons with simple schizophrenia are seen less often in psychiatric units and hospitals than in jails, skid rows, and isolating jobs. Such persons sometimes become "neighborhood eccentrics." Some heroin addicts may actually be simple schizophrenics, since heroin can have an encapsulating effect on a person's life. Simple schizophrenia is often described as a "poverty of personality." (Simple schizophrenia is not coded in DSM-III-R.)

The later classifications

Kraepelin's classification system has been enlarged and refined throughout the years. Several additional types of schizophrenia have been delineated.

SCHIZOAFFECTIVE SCHIZOPHRENIA*

Schizoaffective schizophrenia includes a pronounced affective element—there is much similarity to manic-depressive psychosis. The underlying thought disorder that characterizes schizophrenia is present, along with a marked lability of mood.

PSEUDONEUROTIC SCHIZOPHRENIA

Pseudoneurotic, borderline,† latent, residual, ambulatory, nonpsychotic—these are all terms that have been used by various writers and clinicians to describe approximately the same state. An affected person seems to have moderately severe neurotic problems, but there is actually an underlying schizophrenic process. Sometimes treatment that is traditionally used for neurotic symptoms (for example, psychoanalysis) will uncover the schizophrenic process.

CHILDHOOD SCHIZOPHRENIA‡

There is some debate in clinical circles as to whether early infantile autism and childhood schizophrenia are the same thing. However, most writers do distinguish between the two disorders. While the underlying basis of early *infantile autism* is not known, several theorists believe that it has a definite organic basis.

Childhood schizophrenia, which has also been termed *pathological symbiosis*, is thought to involve a pathological fusion of mother and child. Each is dependent upon the other, and independence in one is a threat to the other.

CHRONIC, UNDIFFERENTIATED SCHIZOPHRENIA

Reflecting the fact that no one ever fits into neatly delineated categories, the term *chronic, undifferentiated schizophrenia* has come into common use in recent decades. A sort of wastebasket term, it is probably the most common diagnosis for schizophrenia in large psychiatric facilities. *Burned-out schizophrenia* is another term used to

---

*Termed "schizoaffective disorder" in DSM-III-R.
†See Chapter 24 for contemporary beliefs about the differentiation of borderline schizophrenia and borderline personality disorder
‡For further discussion of childhood schizophrenia, see Chapter 17.

describe chronicity in schizophrenia. While it means that the condition has become chronic, it also implies that the rather dramatic, florid aspects of the process are not especially evident. There may be an element of docility in an affected person's approach to life. For this reason, many clinicians feel that such a person is more amenable to rehabilitation than someone who is actively psychotic.

Process schizophrenia and reactive schizophrenia

Another way of categorizing schizophrenia is to describe it as either "process" or "reactive." This broad system looks at schizophrenia in terms of the parameters of premorbid adjustment, timing and quality of onset of symptoms, progress, and prognosis. With the advent of DSM-III and DSM-III-R, there is a much narrower delineation of schizophrenia as a diagnostic category (Andreason, 1987; Harrow and Westermeyer, 1987; Herron, 1987). This has led some theorists and researchers to note that most currently diagnosed schizophrenics would be in the *process* category.

PROCESS SCHIZOPHRENIA

A person with process schizophrenia has had a relatively poor premorbid adjustment. In terms of ability to form and maintain interpersonal and sexual relationships, to function at school or in an occupation, or to master the environment, there has been very little success. The onset of symptoms is early (most commonly at or just after puberty), and the onset of the schizophrenic condition tends to be slow and insidious rather than sudden and dramatic. The precipitating events in the environment are not particularly obvious. This disorder is characterized by a steady, progressive worsening rather than an abrupt, florid exacerbation followed by remission. The prognosis for a person with process schizophrenia is considered to be poorer than for a person with reactive schizophrenia.

REACTIVE SCHIZOPHRENIA

A person with reactive schizophrenia probably has made a fairly adequate—in some cases, a rather good—premorbid adjustment. There is usually evidence of accomplishment in the areas of social, sexual, educational, and occupational adjustment. Perhaps the person has graduated from high school or college, for instance. The events that lead to diagnosis or hospitalization are fairly obvious, and the onset tends to be abrupt and dramatic. Often, remissions will follow acute exacerbations—there is a periodic quality to the course of the disorder. There is often evidence that one has developed insight into the effects of one's behavior on the quality of life. The prognosis for an improved adjustment to life is much more promising in reactive schizophrenia than in process schizophrenia.

Orthomolecular psychiatry

In the 1970s a group of psychiatrists adopted a system for categorizing schizophrenia based on the principles of orthomolecular medicine, a term that was coined by the biochemist and double Nobel laureate Linus Pauling. Orthomolecular medicine involves the provision of "the proper quantities of nutrients for the individual" (Pfeiffer, 1975). Orthomolecular psychiatrists believe that in schizophrenic persons, the blood (and therefore the brain) contain abnormal levels of histamine: *histapenic schizophrenics* have abnormally low levels, and *histadelic schizophrenics* have abnormally high levels. Histapenic schizophrenics comprise 50% of all schizophrenics, and histadelics comprise 20%. The remaining 30% are *mauve factor schizophrenics*, so called because of an abnormal factor that is excreted in the urine in greater frequency than is the case with normal persons (Pfeiffer, 1975). Orthomolecular psychiatrists have characterized persons who have schizophrenia-like clinical pictures as *facsimile schizophrenics*. Facsimile schizophrenia can result from such conditions as brain syphilis (dementia paralytica), pellagra, thyroid hormone deficiency, amphetamine psychosis, vitamin B_{12} deficiency, or wheat gluten sensitivity.

Persons with histapenic schizophrenia are apt to be excessively affected by inner stimuli and thus to have misperceptions of place, time, self, and other people, which result in confusion and distortion. They often hallucinate and suffer from delusions. There is hyperactivity and a high pain threshold. Histadelic schizophrenia is characterized by sui-

cidal depression, obsessive rumination, and loss of contact with reality. Hallucinations and delusions are much less frequent, but there is difficulty in thinking and an inability to concentrate. Frequent headaches may be a symptom.

In mauve factor schizophrenia, the classical symptoms of schizophrenia are often present, but insight and affect are better than in the other two types. This condition is now called *pyroluria* because pyrroles are found in the urine (Hoffer, 1987). Other symptoms may include white spots on the fingernails, stretch marks on the skin, memory problems, sweet breath odor, constipation, photosensitivity, impotence, and intolerance for barbiturates (Pfeiffer, 1975; Hoffer, 1987). The illness is viewed as stress-induced (Pfeiffer, 1975) or stress-related (Hoffer, 1987).

EPIDEMIOLOGY AND SOCIOCULTURAL ASPECTS OF THE SCHIZOPHRENIC SYNDROME

While schizophrenia can strike at almost any age, the usual range for onset is 15 to 45, and especially 25 to 35. For some unknown reason, significantly more schizophrenic persons are born in the first quarter of the year than in any other quarter (Barnes, 1987; Kety, 1978). Schizophrenia is a major health problem. Estimates of incidence range from .5% to 1.2% of the population (Barnes, 1987). Under the wider definition used in DSM-II, it was estimated that as many as 4,000,000 people in this country suffered from schizophrenia (Trotter, 1977). With the narrower DSM-III and DSM-III-R definitions, the range is from 100,000 to 200,000 people (Aiken, 1987; Ivker and Sze, 1987). The difference may reflect a greater number of *reactive* schizophrenics with the older system and a more homogeneous grouping of *process* schizophrenics in the current DSM-III and DSM-III-R diagnosed group of schizophrenics (Harrow and Westermeyer, 1987; Herron, 1987).

Schizophrenia is found in all cultures throughout the world and in all socioeconomic groups. However, the distribution is not equal: there is a definite correlation between poverty and the incidence of schizophrenia. The possible reasons for this are complex and debatable. Various workers cite economic, sociological, and genetic factors. For one thing, schizophrenia depletes financial resources, as any debilitating and chronic disorder does. Recent research suggests that people who are chronically mentally ill are 20 times as likely to be homeless as the general population (Aiken, 1987). Roman and Trice (1967) found, in their synthesis of several studies of the etiology and epidemiology of schizophrenia, that one generalization was possible—the positive correlation among life in the lower socioeconomic strata, excessive psychological stress, and schizophrenia. Certainly, the effects of poverty are felt in many areas of living. Poor people generally do not receive proper nutrition and health care, and they lack adequate living space. They also have little opportunity for socialization and self-actualization. These conditions may increase the chances that a person will develop a schizophrenic psychosis. Finally, there is an element of subjectivity inherent in the act of diagnosing: many clinicians are reluctant to condemn their middle-class clients with the label of schizophrenia, even when they believe the condition is present.

Sociocultural factors must be considered integral parts of the schizophrenic process. For example, which explanatory theory is accepted depends on culture. The Awilik Eskimos may attribute a case of catatonia to the machinations of a vengeful ancestral spirit (Carpenter, 1953), while a Washington psychiatrist may proclaim it to be the result of an escalation of multigenerational psychopathology.

Treatment also is related to sociocultural forces. In Israel, where a premium is placed on being a productive citizen, even the most passive, chronic psychotic is considered capable of some personal and social regeneration and is treated accordingly. Communal philosophy in China fosters the development of self-help groups for people, and reintegration into family and community groups is an important goal of treatment (Howells, 1975).

The content of delusions and hallucinations is shaped by sociocultural trends and current events. Presidential assassinations, moon landings, or the popularity of a movie star are all possible influences.

The severity of and prognosis for a case of schizophrenia depend in large part upon a socioeconomic or cultural group's reactions to the disorder. Since medieval times, ambulatory schizophrenics in the village of Gheel, Belgium, have easily made the transition from hospital to community because of the villagers' acceptance of them.

Anthropologists have pointed out that the incidence of mental illness seems to increase during the social unrest that accompanies periods of change and acculturation (Carpenter, 1953). Sometimes, according to medical anthropologist Edward F. Foulks (1975), schizophrenia may even be helpful to an individual or to society during times of social upheaval. The hallucinations and delusions of an individual can help to explain catastrophic events to the people or provide guidelines for change when social change is required. Foulks describes a New York Seneca Indian, called Handsome Lake, whose stress-induced hallucinations in the mid-eighteenth century told him of a new and useful code for his people to adopt. His society was in a period of rapid change and therefore of social disorganization with its potential for destructive trends. Thus, through his hallucinatory experience, Handsome Lake was able to assume the role of prophet or shaman.

The syndrome of schizophrenia has a long history in the development of mankind and a wide incidence throughout the world. Symptoms of the syndrome can be viewed as restitutional; they are extreme exaggerations of the defense mechanisms we all use. Useful definitions of schizophrenia acknowledge the complexity of the syndrome and of the correlated factors surrounding it. While several systems of classification have been devised and are used by clinicians and writers, it remains crucial to recognize and remember the concept of individuality in the treatment of schizophrenic clients. Mendel and Green (1967) have pointed this out succinctly:

Obviously, the patient does not have a diagnosis; we, the physicians, have the diagnosis. When the diagnosis and the patient do not fit we must feel free to abandon the diagnosis and return to the patient.

EXPLANATORY THEORIES OF SCHIZOPHRENIA

The exact basis of schizophrenia is unknown. There are, however, many theories about the origin of the disorder, and several of them will be reviewed here.

Genetic theories

Many studies concerned with the genetic basis of schizophrenia have been carried out, with various results. Some early studies reported a concordance as high as 76% (Slater, 1953) or 86% (Kallman, 1938) for monozygotic twins as compared to 14% to 15% for dizygotic twins. Other studies have reported lower degrees of concordance. Possible explanations for this variability in findings in studies of twins include the use of differing statistical methods, research designs, and diagnostic criteria.

In the 70s, adequately controlled studies of schizophrenic persons were carried out in Denmark. These studies, which involved schizophrenics who had been raised by adoptive families, showed a significant incidence of schizophrenia in the biological parents (Kety, 1978). This incidence was close to that described in earlier studies, which had shown an expectation of 16.4% that children of one schizophrenic parent would become schizophrenic (versus 0.85% for the general population) and an expectation that ranges from 38% to 68% when both parents are schizophrenic (Jackson, 1960). An 1983 update of the National Academy of Sciences–National Research Council Twin Registry continued to support the importance of genetic factors in schizophrenia (Kendler and Rolinette, 1983). A study in Finland by Tienari et al. (1985) of the adopted offspring of schizophrenic women (247 subjects: 112 index and 135 control adoptive families) explored the genetic and environmental factors in the development of schizophrenia. The data strongly support the role of genetic factors in the disorder (Goldstein, 1987).

Both early and recent studies show that nonschizophrenic relatives of schizophrenic persons have significantly more of the conditions, such as eye-tracking disorders, that are associated with schizophrenia than the general population (Holzman et al., 1974; Holzman, 1985).

Most theorists, whether they are concerned with organic, psychodynamic, or sociocultural bases for schizophrenia, do agree that a genetic factor is operating. There is no conclusive evidence as to the mode of genetic transmission—schizophrenia, like many other disorders, seems to be polygenetic.

Chapman and Chapman note that the evidence suggests that not all schizophrenic disorders have a strong genetic component and that even the more narrowly defined DSM-III schizophrenia "appears heterogeneous with respect to genetic contribution to etiology" (Chapman and Chapman, 1987).

At least one aspect of the genetic controversy that needs to be refined is the differentiation of genetic factors from perinatal and prenatal influences.

Biochemical and physical theories
PRENATAL AND PERINATAL INFLUENCE THEORY

Prenatal and perinatal influences have been cited as explanatory factors for schizophrenia. Explanations include a possible alteration of the fetal oxygen supply, passage of endocrine and toxic substances across the placental barrier, and the effects of maternal emotions on fetal endocrine balance and nervous system.

Birth trauma of one sort or another has been suggested as an explanation for schizophrenia. Significantly more prenatal and perinatal complications have been found in the histories of schizophrenics than in those of nonschizophrenics (Taft and Goldfarb, 1964), and stillbirth rate, rate of premature births, and incidence of serious congenital malformations in offspring have been found to be higher in schizophrenic mothers (Campion and Tucker, 1973). Some investigators suggest that some sort of trauma present at or before birth is the agent that interacts with a genetic predisposition to result in schizophrenia.

A group of researchers in California has suggested that subtle brain abnormalities occurring in the first trimester of pregnancy help to trigger chronic forms of schizophrenia (Greenberg, 1983). They found a high incidence of minor physical anomalies (which are known to develop during the first trimester) and evidence of neurological impairment among the schizophrenic males they studied. They propose an interaction model incorporating *functional* and *organic* defects as contributory factors in some forms of schizophrenia.

The Copenhagen High-Risk Project (from 1962 to 1986) demonstrated that perinatal trauma was one of the factors associated with an increased risk for the development of schizophrenia. This group theorized that neurological deviance may be produced by disruption occurring in the second trimester of fetal development (Mednick et al., 1987). Ventricular enlargement may be correlated with low birth weight and obstetrical complications (Andreason, 1988).

ANATOMICAL OR PHYSIOLOGICAL DEFECT THEORIES

One physiological defect that has been identified as a possible factor is an abnormally responsive autonomic nervous system. One group of researchers, who verified this finding in a large-scale study, found an overresponsive autonomic nervous system to be especially evident in schizophrenics who had suffered complications at birth. The researchers hypothesized that this overreactivity combines with a genetic predisposition for schizophrenia and results in expression of the disorder (Trotter, 1977).

In the past, anatomical and physiological defects have been hypothesized as the basis of schizophrenia. Until recently there has been no evidence to support these hypotheses. Now, however, investigators have announced findings that they view as a breakthrough in our understanding of the physical basis of schizophrenia. *Amphetamine psychosis* is a condition that closely mimics the schizophrenic process and symptomatology (Snyder, 1974). In this disorder, amphetamine stimulates the release of dopamine (a neurotransmitter catecholamine), and a possible flooding of the brain with dopamine may occur. Also consistent with the anatomical or physiological defect theory are aspects of another disorder—Parkinson's disease. In this disease the problem is that the individual's brain lacks many of the dopamine-producing cells, resulting in a scarcity of the substance. Treatment with L-dopa alleviates symptoms of parkinsonism. Another fact linking schizophrenia to a physiological defect is that antischizophrenic drugs, which are believed to act on the neurotransmitters in some way, possibly reducing the level of dopamine or blocking its transmission, also produce side effects that mimic the symptoms of Parkinson's disease.

Another model (Stein and Wise, 1971) suggests a possible deficiency in the level of the enzyme that converts dopamine to norepinephrine, and yet another model (Potkin et al., 1978) postulates decreased activity of the enzyme monoamine oxidase, which is involved in the degradation of chemicals such as dopamine. In addition, it was discovered through autopsy that the brains of schizophrenics contain about twice the normal number of receptor sites for dopamine. They theorized that schizophrenics are overstimulated with their own brain signals and thus are flooded with strange thoughts, hallucinations, and misperceptions (*Science News*, Vol. 112, p. 342, 1977). New data, reported by Wong et al. (1986), appear to resolve a long-standing dispute about whether dopamine receptors are increased in schizophrenics because of drug therapy or because of the disorder itself. Positron emission tomography (PET) scans of the brains of living, diagnosed schizophrenics show significantly increased levels of binding to D2 dopamine receptors in both treated and untreated subjects. They conclude that the increase seems intrinsic to the disease, not resulting from drug treatment.

The *dopamine hypothesis* was the second hypothesis to be derived from attempts to understand the physical bases of schizophrenia. The first was the *transmethylation hypothesis*, which was derived from the study of psychotomimetic drugs such as mescaline (Snyder, 1974). Mescaline, which is a methylated catechol, produces symptoms that mimic schizophrenia. It was theorized that a transfer of a methyl group to neurotransmitters or their precursors changes them into psychotomimetic substances. Methylated catecholamines and methylated indoles were looked for, but so far there has been no definitive evidence of elevated levels in schizophrenic persons. The difficulty of separating the effects of diet, drugs, stress, and environmental conditions has complicated the picture. It seems likely that excess dopamine is a fundamental factor in schizophrenia. Currently, the dopamine hypothesis is the most widely accepted neurochemical theory (Andreason, 1988).

In 1972, Murphy and Wyatt of the National Institute of Mental Health reported their findings that people with schizophrenic disorders have a low activity of the enzyme monoamine oxidase (MAO) in their blood platelets. Further investigations revealed a wide range of MAO activities in the disorder (Maugh, 1981). In 1981, Schildkraut (as cited by Maugh) reported that different ranges of MAO activity appear to be characteristic of certain subgroups of schizophrenia. Specifically, schizophrenics who do *not* hallucinate have normal range levels of MAO activity, whereas there is a below-normal level in schizophrenics who do hallucinate. Many in this latter grouping exhibit paranoid symptoms. An above-average level of MAO activity was observed in those schizophrenics who were characterized as asocial, depressed, markedly introverted, and exhibiting bizarre behavior.

Edelstein and his associates (1981) have estimated that 24–40% of schizophrenic-like, psychotic individuals may have a "lithium-responsive" type of illness. This conclusion was based on earlier work with individuals diagnosed as schizophrenic and who have an above-average *lithium ratio*. These people responded very well to lithium therapy. This lithium ratio has been described as a defect in the transport of sodium and lithium ions across the membrane of red blood cells. This can be quantitatively measured—the ratio of the concentration of lithium in the red blood cells to that in the plasma is determined. The defect leads to a higher than normal ratio and this condition responds to lithium therapy (Maugh, 1981).

A possible anatomical defect that is receiving a good deal of attention is cerebral atrophy that is demonstrated by enlarged ventricles in the brain (Andreason, 1988). Citing 10 years of studies conducted on the brains of living subjects and their own recent investigations of CT (computerized tomographic) scans of 71 chronic schizophrenics and 30 control subjects, Shelton et al. (1988) note that the schizophrenics showed larger ventricle-brain ratios and larger third-ventricle widths. Cerebral atrophy (especially lateral ventricle enlargement) correlated with the severity of illness, using such clinical measurements as cognitive impairment, poor premorbid adjustment, poor outcome, and persistent unemployment. The authors also note that brain changes have been found at the onset of overt symptoms, before any exposure to antipsychotic drugs, and they conclude that the studies "lend strong credence to the concept of brain

pathology in schizophrenia." Age, age of onset, duration of illness, and hospitalization were not demonstrated to correlate with brain changes in their own study, suggesting that the brain abnormalities they observed were independent of these variables.

Another study by Yates, Jacoby, and Andreason (1987) was carried out, using CAT (computerized axial tomography) scans of 108 people diagnosed as schizophrenic (DSM-III criteria) and 50 people with affective disorder (DSM-III) and 74 age- and sex-matched control subjects. The team was looking for global cerebellar atrophy and found no differences between control subjects and the two groups of diagnosed subjects. Schizophrenic subjects did show evidence of mild cerebellar atrophy, but it was not significantly different (for global atrophy of the brain) from the control group. While cautioning that different methods of examining brains, different guidelines for interpreting "global," and different sampling procedures require that their study be interpreted conservatively, the authors point out that their sample was a large and representative one and that it may indicate that young, nonchronically ill schizophrenics do not suffer from cerebellar atrophy.

Bogert et al. (1983) systematically examined the brains of 13 schizophrenics and 8 normals that had been collected before the discovery of antipsychotic drugs. They found that while the weight of the brains in both groups was approximately the same, tissue mass of the schizophrenic brains was reduced in five specific areas.

In the past decade neuropsychiatric studies that use modern brain-imaging techniques have rapidly changed the way we view schizophrenia (Taylor, 1987). Taylor notes that researchers at the National Institute of Mental Health (NIMH) classify schizophrenia as a "group of brain diseases." While the basis of the brain abnormalities is still largely a mystery, theories include genetic makeup, viral infection, damage due to chemicals or to hormonal dysfunction. Much of the research is focused on the temporal lobe of the brain and the limbic system (which includes the hypothalamus, the amygdala, and the septal and hippocampol regions). The frontal lobe and the limbic system are responsible for receiving, organizing, and integrating internal and external perceptions. The newer tools for observing the human brain are the CAT scan (computerized axial tomography), MRI (magnetic resonance imaging), rCBF (regional cerebral blood flow), the PET scan (positron emission tomography), BEAM (brain electrical activity mapping).

The following descriptions are adapted from Taylor (1987):

- *The CAT scan* produces a two-dimensional black and white x-ray of the surface and inner tissue of the brain.
- *MRI* produces cross-sectional, two-dimensional pictures of the brain. It has higher resolution images, and it can focus on more restricted areas of the brain than a CAT scan. MRI is replacing CAT scans in brain investigation because it is less interfered with by bony structures, allowing a more detailed study of hidden, preventricular structures. Also, MRI does not expose the individual to radiation so that studies can be updated more often.
- *rCBF* records the rate and volume at which blood moves through major areas of the brain. The radiation exposure is about equal to that of a routine dental checkup. The person breathes an inert isotope of xenon (a gas), and the amount of isotope passing each sensor (lightly touching the top and sides of the head) is recorded on a computer that converts the information mathematically.
- *The PET scan* produces high-resolution, sliced images of subcortical sections and colored indications of brain activity. This enables brain researchers to consider brain structure *and* the interactional dynamics of the working mind. Glucose is the primary energy source of the brain, and glucose responds as demands are placed on the organism. The time required, the complexity of the procedure, and its possible discomforts make it a difficult one for use with schizophrenic subjects, and it has not been used as frequently as other procedures. With refinement, it holds hope for future research because it records, pictorially, the brain's metabolism.
- *BEAM* has been used to corroborate rCBF studies. It turns EEG (electroencephalographic) signals into colored maps of brain activity.

In addition to all the imaging tools that are being used to study brains, other biochemical measure-ments are being taken in the research into schizophrenia. For example, the amount of dopamine sulphate in cerebrospinal fluid is being studied, and Kaufman et al. (1984) found a decreased level in chronic schizophrenics who respond poorly to treatment (cited in Taylor, 1987). Autopsy studies of schizophrenic individuals demonstrated a decreased number of neurons, diffuse cellular changes, and a difference in the size of the corpus callosum (Torrey, 1983). The levels of dopamine and dopamine receptors in the brain continue to be examined, and, as mentioned earlier, evidence points to an increase in dopamine receptors that is intrinsic to the disorder itself (Wong, 1986). Many researchers now believe that while abnormalities of dopamine neurotransmission may not cause schizophrenia, it is somehow important in the disease process (Barnes, 1987). There is strong evidence that the antipsychotic drugs act by blocking dopamine receptors (Holzman, 1987).

TOXIC SUBSTANCE THEORIES

A theory suggested by Heath et al. (1958) concerned a toxic or abnormal protein, called *taraxein*, in the blood of schizophrenics. When injected into nonschizophrenics, it produced behavior and symptoms similar to those of schizophrenia. This substance has been isolated by three different researchers, but it is not generally considered to be the fundamental factor in schizophrenia. The dopamine hypothesis seems more widely accepted as the biochemical basis for schizophrenia.

It has been hypothesized that food might contain a toxic substance—specifically, the protein gluten that is found in wheat. A research team found that when wheat was removed from the diet of schizophrenics, their symptoms improved dramatically. While the research team cautioned that this is not a simple cause-and-effect situation, it concluded that wheat gluten is a pathogenic factor in schizophrenia (Singh and Kay, 1976).

It has been suggested that a slow viral infection process may be responsible for the subsequent development of schizophrenia. This theory has received support because of the discovery that the organic brain syndrome known as Jakob-Creutzfeldt disease may be of viral origin and because of the fact that individuals suffering from herpes encephalitis have a clinical picture that is very similar to an acute schizophrenic episode (Wynne et al., 1978).

ORTHOMOLECULAR THEORY

Mescaline psychosis has been used as a model by the proponents of the orthomolecular theory of schizophrenia. Osmond and Hoffer studied mescaline psychosis and saw similarities to the delirium associated with the vitamin-deficiency disease pellagra (Pfeiffer, 1975). They noted that earlier findings had shown that vitamin B_3 (in the form of niacin or nicotinic acid) not only cured the physical symptoms of pellagra but also provided complete relief from the mental symptoms. They hypothesized that perhaps schizophrenia, with symptoms that are also similar to mescaline psychosis, represents an abnormally high requirement for vitamin B_3. They began treating people with megadoses of the vitamin—usually 3 g combined with 3 g of vitamin C and trace mineral supplements.

The orthomolecular psychiatrists prefer to designate the disorder in the plural—the schizophrenias. They have categorized them as histadelic schizophrenia, histapenic schizophrenia, and pyroluriacs. The histapenic schizophrenics are the ones who are treated with vitamin B_3. Pyroluriacs are treated with B_6 (Hoffer, 1987). Vitamin therapy is not the sole treatment; a combination of vitamins, psychotropic drugs, and psychotherapy is used. Young schizophrenic persons, whose symptomatology is still labile, are viewed as the most likely candidates for the treatment.

The theory is not widely accepted in established medical circles, and conflicting claims are made by proponents and skeptics.

Perceptual and cognitive disturbance theories

SENSORY INPUT DYSFUNCTION

Several theories have been postulated and explored concerning a possible defect in the schizophrenic's ability to perceive and organize experience effectively (Anscombe, 1987). The defect in controlling incoming stimuli from the environment results in overload. According to those theories, a schizophrenic person has an ineffective barrier be-

tween inner self and the parade of events he or she is exposed to in the environment. One theorist (Cameron, 1963) has termed this situation *overinclusiveness* and has described it as a failure to weed out irrelevant material, with a resultant flooding of the ego. The person is unable to organize perceptions appropriately. Loud voices, multiple conversations, a crowded room, a busy street, life changes, or simply too many activities are all examples of things that may be too difficult for the schizophrenic person to process. High stress and anxiety are the result, and psychotic symptoms may be precipitated (Pepper and Ryglewicz, 1986). Such theories are consistent with several studies of the effects of sensory deprivation, which indicate that chronic schizophrenics tolerate sensory deprivation much better than nonschizophrenics.

Another way of looking at sensory input dysfunctions and schizophrenia is to view the schizophrenic as being deficient in the ability to modulate sensory input. Two manifestations of this defect are possible—the overresponsiveness of the acute stage of schizophrenia and the underresponsiveness of the chronic schizophrenic (Epstein and Coleman, 1971).

LEARNING THEORY

One hypothesis concerning schizophrenia holds that the disorder is learned. According to this theory, an overresponsive autonomic nervous system, a genetic predisposition for schizophrenia, and a harsh environment all combine to encourage a person to learn to avoid stress by displaying schizophrenic symptoms—hallucinations, delusions, withdrawal, isolation from others, and so on (Trotter, 1977). If a sensitive caretaker (parent) shields the overresponsive nervous system from the harsh environment, the defect is compensated for and symptoms may not be expressed (Shapiro, 1981).

Psychodynamic theories

Harry Stack Sullivan did a good deal of his work with schizophrenic persons. His "interpersonal" theory of psychiatry pointed to an unhealthy relationship between the schizophrenic and his parents. His view of schizophrenia was more hopeful than Freud's; he believed that a later, more satisfying relationship could do much to erase the harm of the early, unhealthy ones.

Heinz Hartmann, a follower of Freud and the father of ego psychology, believed that schizophrenia is a defect in the capacity to neutralize the instinctual drives (Hartmann, 1964). He saw this as resulting in an interference with object relations* and the development of healthy defenses. He postulated a vicious circle of increasing frustration, mobilization of more aggression, and the incapacity to neutralize *instinctual drives*, leading eventually to schizophrenic symptom formation (Pao, 1979).

Fairbairn, an object-relations theorist, pointed to a crystallization of the conflict "to love or not to love," which he viewed as derivative of the infant's conflict of "to suck or not to suck." He saw the schizophrenic as stuck in the *schizoid position* or early oral stage of psychosexual development (Pao, 1979).

Margaret Mahler et al. (1975)† in outlining the preoedipal period of childhood point to the *symbiotic phase* as the crucial one in the subsequent development of the various forms of schizophrenia. The child with a pathological symbiotic orientation has not been able to grow adequately beyond that stage. The mother is viewed not as a separate being but as "fused with the self." The child is unable to integrate the mother's image as a whole object and, therefore, a split good object–bad object is perceived. There is a disabling alternation between the desire to incorporate the good and the desire to expel the bad.

Generally, the psychodynamic theorists argue that the roots of schizophrenia are in the oral stage of psychosocial development—the stage in which a child develops an ability to trust other people. These theorists believe that schizophrenia originates in problems in the mother-child relationship that develop during this period. There is a faulty development of the ego. In particular, the defense mechanism of repression is ineffective, a situation that constitutes the underlying psychodynamic problem. Clinicians have long noted that the schizophrenic's unconscious seems very close to

the surface. Since the defense mechanism of repression is weak and ineffective, unconscious material threatens to flood the ego and thus stimulates the psychotic symptoms as defense mechanisms. Freud viewed schizophrenia as a regression to a state of infantile narcissism with a withdrawal of the libido from the external world to the internal self. Freud did not work with many schizophrenics—most of his patients were neurotics. In fact, he was rather pessimistic about the value of psychotherapy for schizophrenics.

Carl Jung viewed schizophrenics as centripetal (inner-directed) in their relationships with the world rather than centrifugal (outer-directed).

Sylvano Arieti, an authority on schizophrenia, saw schizophrenia basically as a defensive reaction to severe anxiety that originates in childhood and recurs in later life. It is a restitutive attempt to make the best of a bad situation.

Eric Berne's transactional analysis system defines schizophrenia as a situation in which the "child ego state," rather than the "adult ego state," is in command of the ego functions. The child is frightened and "not OK." In the schizophrenic person the "parent ego state" participates sporadically, mostly in a harsh and oppressive manner. Berne believed that the only way to proceed with psychotherapy for a schizophrenic is to engage the child ego state and obtain its cooperation.

More recently, Kohut considers schizophrenia an example of a noncohesive self that is secondary to an inherent biological tendency. Kernberg believes it to be an example of the lack of differentiation of self and object representations. He views this lack of differentiation as leading to a failure of ego boundaries and reality testing (Munich, 1987).

Family systems theories

Family systems theorists have identified communication patterns and family relationship patterns (see Chapter 14) that may be contributory factors in schizophrenia. Murray Bowen (1976, 1977), a leading family systems theorist who did his original work with schizophrenic clients, argued that a *multigenerational transmission* may be oper-

---

*See Chapter 24 for more discussion of object relations.
†See Chapter 24 for an outline discussion of Mahler's theory of preoedipal development.

ating in the disorder. He postulated that in some families, a process that is based on the defense mechanism of projection is passed down from one generation to the next. If two people who are neurotic marry and have a child, their neuroses may "mesh" in such a way as to produce a more severe neurosis in the child. If this child eventually marries a neurotic person, once again neuroses will mesh to produce an even more severely impaired offspring. Bowen views schizophrenia as a severe emotional disorder. Whereas others see neurosis and schizophrenia as discrete entities, he considers schizophrenia to be on a continuum with neurosis and other emotional disorders. According to Bowen's theoretical system, schizophrenia is a product of several generations of escalating impairment, with increasing use of a *family projection process* and decreasing levels of differentiation between family members. As a treatment goal, Bowen stresses increased differentiation of each family member from the family system, as opposed to unhealthy "fusion" among family members. He sees a tendency to fuse or merge with others operating in all families. This is the "undifferentiated family ego mass." If this tendency is strong enough and pervasive enough, it can be pathological for individual family members, who lose their sense of self.

Thus, some family systems are viewed as being pathological to the point of being *schizophrenogenic*. That is, the family system itself fosters schizophrenia. The person who is identified as the client is simply the carrier of the family's illness.

Certain *family configurations* have been singled out by Lidz (1973) as being schizophrenogenic. According to Lidz, the *skewed family pattern* is most often seen in the development of male schizophrenics. While the mother is most apt to be termed schizophrenogenic, the father, through his ineffective role modeling and inability to counteract the actions of his wife, plays an equally important role. The mother is described as domineering and egocentric. She is unable to differentiate her own feelings and anxieties from those of the other members of the family—particularly those of her son. In the beginning she has great difficulty relating to her infant son. This situation leads to overprotection and then to symbiosis. Eventually, she

begins to use her son to make up for her own failures and disappointments in life.

In the *schismatic family pattern* there is usually overt conflict between the spouses—the father is dominant and perhaps overtly paranoid. He tends to downgrade his wife and her role as mother and wife. Both spouses undercut each other, and the child is competed for and used as a pawn in the conflict between the parents. Lidz believes that this pattern is more apt to produce schizophrenia in a girl than in a boy. There is overprotection, great concern about morality, and intrusiveness into the child's sexual behavior during adolescence.

There are some similarities between these two patterns—overprotection, a poor relationship with the parent of the same sex, and parental failure to establish proper and healthy boundaries between self and child. The child is unconsciously used by the parent of the opposite sex to fulfill needs and make up deficiencies.

Other patterns that family theorists see as particularly important in the development of schizophrenia include emotional divorce, coalition across generation boundaries, vagueness in communicating, tangentiality, double-bind communication, family myths, and mystification (see Chapter 14).

Existential theories

The existential psychologist Binswanger believed that the great philosopher Kierkegaard referred to schizophrenia when he described sickness of the mind as "the sickness unto death" (May, 1958). Existentialists point to altered perceptions of time, space, and causality as essential ingredients in the creation of the schizophrenic's world. Themes that existential psychologists and psychotherapists mention when they discuss schizophrenia include emptiness, nothingness, and painful internal vacuum. The schizophrenic's defect resembles a hole that requires constant filling; there is constant fear of annihilation. This need for constant filling and the fear of nonexistence are cited as reasons for obesity in some schizophrenics and latent schizophrenics. It has been suggested by clinicians, existential and otherwise, that a certain percentage of obese individuals should not attempt to reduce, since doing so may precipitate a schizophrenic break with reality.

The internal emptiness or lack of identity of the schizophrenic leads to strained interpersonal relations; the whole existence takes on the "as if" quality described earlier in this chapter. R.D. Laing, considered to be an existential psychiatrist, believes that schizophrenia is not an illness but a way of being in the world. He views it as a potentially growth-promoting state, a change to correct a developmental problem. He sees the submerging into a psychotic state as beneficial, with a higher and more insightful level of development being the eventual compensation. His Kingsley Hall experiment allowed individuals to enter psychotic states in a tolerant and drug-free atmosphere. This philosophy of treatment is not shared by more conventional therapists, who see the potential for residual damage to the personality inherent in each psychotic break.

Sociocultural theories

R.D. Laing also suggests that schizophrenia may be the only way to be sane in an insane world. Thus he implicates society in the development of schizophrenia.

Other theorists, notably Thomas Szasz, have proposed that schizophrenia is not a disease or a psychological disorder at all but rather a construct that has been invented by society to serve some of its needs—for example, to explain behavior that is deviant from the mainstream and to segregate persons who, in their deviance, make us uncomfortable. Proponents of this view remind us of the historical beginnings of care for the mentally ill, when the so-called mentally ill included what was considered the dregs of society—beggars, paupers, the physically disabled, and the diseased. They were an embarrassment to the more privileged classes, so they were warehoused in large institutions—at first mixed in with criminals. Szasz and theorists who agree with him maintain that the "treatment"—the warehousing of people—existed first and that it then became necessary to have the "patients" to fit the treatment. The furtherance of the modern mental health industry, which does indeed provide financial support and security for many workers, is pointed to as one of the pur-

poses the mentally ill serve for society.

One facet of society that has been implicated in the incidence of schizophrenia is poverty: poverty and schizophrenia are strongly correlated. Several explanations for this are possible. One that has been postulated is that poverty is an etiological agent through the medium of increased stress. Crowded living conditions, poor nutrition, inadequate or nonexistent prenatal care, and lack of meaningful recreation are only some of the concomitants of poverty that increase stress in everyday living. In their review of the massive literature on schizophrenia and social class, Roman and Trice (1967) hypothesized that a combination of child socialization patterns and patterns of environmental stress and social disorganization is related to the high incidence of schizophrenia in the lower social strata. One well-controlled study comparing schizophrenics with normal persons found that schizophrenics experience significantly greater stress in dealing with life events than do nonschizophrenics (Serban, 1975). An animal study that incorporated increasingly stressful conditions resulted in the delineation of three groups of animals—those that remain relatively disease-free, those that suffer from various psychosomatic disorders, and those that exhibit behavior that could well be described as psychotic (Stroebel, 1969).

Systems theory

A systems approach to schizophrenia integrates all the dimensions of self. Schizophrenia is considered to be the final outcome of complex, interrelated factors. Biopsychosocial processes are in simultaneous interaction with one another. For example, Ernest Hartmann cites the wealth of evidence that supports a theory of increased brain dopamine activity as a correlate of schizophrenia. The evidence is based on the ability of amphetamine and similar drugs* to induce schizophrenia-like processes, whereas the antipsychotic major tranquilizers all appear to be dopamine receptor blockers. His view is that the dopamine plays a role in the biology of

---

*Another example is PCP or "angel dust," which has been used as an animal model in the study of schizophrenia (Herbert, 1983a).

psychosis, that it may be related to unneutralized psychic energy (or, the unneutralized aggressive energy that Heinz Hartmann [1964] earlier postulated as the genesis of schizophrenia). Ernest Hartmann (1982) also states that the excess dopamine is responsible for the psychotic symptoms rather than schizophrenia as a whole, and he goes on to say that "clearly, the dopamine-blocking drugs reduce psychotic manifestations in schizophrenia, but do not cure an underlying schizophrenic defect." What Hartmann is saying implies a holistic approach to understanding the etiology and treatment of schizophrenia.

In addition, environmental stress, genetic predisposition, metabolic disorders, psychodynamic weaknesses, and family dysfunction mutually and simultaneously interact to produce the final outcome of schizophrenia. Contemporary researchers who investigate psychosocial variables in schizophrenia do so within the context of a vulnerability-stress model (Goldstein, 1987). The stress-diathesis model described by Eisenberg (1973) illustrates the mutual interaction of multiple factors in the development of schizophrenia:

Psychobiological stress acts on an individual with a genetic predisposition to psychosis and eventually leads to abnormal metabolic processes that cause disorders of mood and thought. Predisposition probably varies on a continuum.

Within this model, psychobiological stress and genetic predisposition both vary on a dynamic continuum. An individual with a strong genetic predisposition might succumb to moderate or even minimal stress—for example, the stress of adolescence (the process schizophrenic described earlier). A person with relatively little genetic predisposition might react to severe stress with a psychotic break (the reactive schizophrenic). This model for stress and genetic predisposition is compatible with Murray Bowen's view that schizophrenia exists on a dynamic continuum with neurosis and other psychological disorders (Bowen, 1976). While some theorists disagree and consider schizophrenia and neurosis as discrete and unrelated phenomena, Karl Menninger (1963) and others (see Ivker and Sze, 1987) also view neurosis and schizophrenia on a dynamic continuum of mental health and mental illness.

Carrying the dynamic continuum model a step further, Bahnson and Bahnson view all the human individual's disorders, psychological and physiological, as being on a continuum of psychophysiological complementarity. This particular construct seeks to identify alternate forms for the discharge of energy associated with stress experienced by the human organism. As the degree of stress increases, an individual becomes more vulnerable to physical or psychological disorders. Which type of disorder is chosen depends on habitual patterns of response. The extreme manifestation of disorder in a person who tends to somatize is cancer, while in an individual with a tendency toward emotional lability it is schizophrenia. The Bahnsons point to various studies that demonstrate an inverse relationship between cancer and schizophrenia (Bahnson and Bahnson, 1964). This approach represents an attempt to develop a monistic theory rather than a false splitting of "mind" and "body" (Bahnson, 1969, 1974). Such an approach is consistent with systems theory and emphasizes the interrelationship among self, others, and the environment.

The exact basis of schizophrenia is not known (Barnes 1987; Carpenter, 1987). The many theories that have been postulated focus on such areas as genetic endowment, biochemical abnormalities, anatomical differences, psychodynamic defects, family dysfunction, and social disorganization. The schizophrenic syndrome is a complex disorder, and while the findings of the 1980s continue to point to a biochemical-neurological defect (Barnes, 1987; Taylor, 1987), the most generally accepted view is that of a multifactorial disorder incorporating many or all of the holistic health elements that have been discussed in this section. A definition that addresses the complexity of explanatory theories and the insights of the 1980s is one proposed by Falloon and Liberman (1983). Schizophrenia is defined as "a biologically mediated, stress-related disorder of unknown etiology" (Falloon and Liberman, 1983, 134). A summary of the explanatory theories of schizophrenia from ancient times to the present is presented in Table 25-1.

TREATMENT
History

The treatment of schizophrenia has a history as long as the history of the disease itself. In ancient

TABLE 25-1 The evolution of explanatory theories of schizophrenia

Ancient	Mediaeval	1900	1930s, 40s and 50s	1960s	1970s	1980s
Possession by evil spirits	*Witchcraft*	*Organic* Kraepelin: Dementia Praecox; metabolic basis	*Psychoanalytic, psychodynamic and interpersonal* Freud: pathological narcissism; Sullivan: parent-child relations; Jung: "inner-directed"; Hartmann: unneutralized drives; Arieti: overuse of defense mechanisms and paleological thinking	*Family systems and communication* "Schizophrenogenic mother and family" Lidz: distorted family structure; Laing: "mystification process" Bowen: multigenerational transmission Wynne: pseudomutuality	*Developmental* Mahler: a preoedipal disorder—the symbiotic phase	*Early parent/child* "Poor fit" dyad *High EE families* Birley, Brown and Wing; Anderson
Natural causes and the mind/body link Hippocrates	*The will of God*		*Existential* Binswanger, Laing, May: Inner emptiness, divided self, fear of annihilation	*Society as causal factor* Laing, Szasz *Sensory input dysfunction* Stimulus barrier defect Cameron: overinclusiveness	*Brain chemical and structure* → Excess of dopamine; increased dopamine receptors; enlarged ventricles	*Brain imaging techniques* → CAT, PET scans; MRI, Beam, etc.—ventricle structure, brain atrophy, brain physiology and metabolism in the brain; increased dopamine receptors intrinsic to the disorder
			Genetic Early twin studies —————→		*Learning theory* Harsh environmental predisposition *Stress-diathesis model* High risk and vulnerability research	*Vulnerability/stress* Scandinavian and American studies ————→

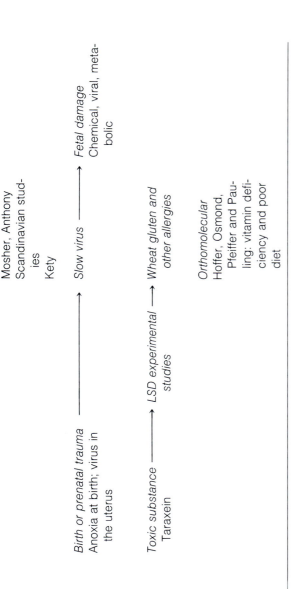

times, treatment was quite enlightened; it involved music, poetry, and dance therapy; rest; and "talking therapy." In ancient Greece temples were set aside for such treatments. In medieval times, when madness was thought to indicate possession by evil spirits or to be evidence of the practice of witchcraft, treatment took the form of exorcism and burning at the stake. After this period, but before any scientific approach to mental illness had evolved, treatment consisted of segregation from society in places like Bedlam in England or the prototype of the modern mental hospital, the Hôpital Général in France. In these large institutions people were kept in crowded, filthy conditions, and they were watched over by keepers who were at best apathetic and often cruel. Even at the beginning of the twentieth century, families of schizophrenics were told to forget about their hospitalized relatives. There was little hope for improvement.

When psychiatrists began to treat schizophrenia, their approach was mainly somatic. *Prefrontal lobotomy* is a brain operation that was used on many schizophrenics before the discovery of the phenothiazine drugs. In this procedure the tracts between cortex, subcortex, and basal ganglia are severed. It often resulted in a mitigation of aggressive, violent behavior, but it also left the patient* in a fairly deteriorated condition—docile, unmotivated, and demonstrating regressive, crude behavior. Thousands of lobotomies were performed on schizophrenics during the 1940s and early 1950s.

Hydrotherapy was a much less destructive modality. The purposes of hydrotherapy included sedation of the overactive patient (continuous tub baths and wet sheet packs) and production of tonic effects (needle spray and alternate jet showers). The wet sheet packs did seem to have a highly sedating action, and before effective psychotropic drugs were available, some patients would ask to be put into the packs when they realized that tension and anxiety were building up.

Isolation from others in seclusion rooms was a common treatment. There is a legitimate rationale for reducing environmental stimuli and allowing

---

*In this section the term *patient* is used because of the historical content.

the hyperactive patient to calm down. Unfortunately, the seclusion rooms were sometimes used as punishment in the manner of solitary confinement in prisons. Seclusion also became the easiest way to treat excited patients; some were kept in the same small, bare seclusion rooms for long periods—sometimes for years.

Insulin coma therapy, or *insulin shock,* was used, for the most part, in the 1940s and early 1950s. The patient was given insulin to induce coma; he became somnolent and pacified in the hypoglycemic state. There appeared to be some successes with the treatment, particularly in cases of young schizophrenics who had just experienced their first psychotic breaks. There were also some very real dangers attached to insulin coma therapy, and some fatalities resulted—one reason why it is no longer used as a treatment for schizophrenia. The apparent remissions that sometimes occurred were later attributed to the intensive and intimate nursing care required during the coma period—care that was described as a healthier and more loving reparenting (Schwing, 1954). Perhaps some of the remissions were ones that would have occurred in any group of young schizophrenics undergoing their first psychotic breaks.

Electroconvulsive therapy

Electroconvulsive therapy is sometimes called *electric shock therapy* or *electrostimulative therapy,* which is the currently preferred term. The rationale for using this treatment in cases of schizophrenia was originally based on a misconception. It was thought that schizophrenia and epilepsy do not occur together and that convulsions perhaps prevent schizophrenia (Rowe, 1975). This view was later shown to be untrue, since schizophrenia and epilepsy can occur in the same person. While the reason for the treatment was inaccurate, the treatment was helpful in some cases. Today electroconvulsive therapy is considered useful for schizophrenics who are in severe, life-threatening catatonic stupors (Hoffer, 1987; Shapiro, 1981) or for severely depressed and suicidal schizophrenics (Goldfarb and Goldfarb, 1977; Mendel, 1976; Rowe, 1975; Strahl, 1980). It also seems to be helpful for extremely confused and agitated postpartum psychosis clients. A

woman who is suffering from postpartum psychosis is actually experiencing an acute schizophrenic reaction.

Psychotropic drugs

The somatic treatment most widely used for schizophrenia today is the administration of psychopharmaceuticals. The major tranquilizers, which came into widespread use in the early 1950s, are called *antipsychotic drugs,* or *antischizophrenic drugs* by some. In some ways, "tranquilizer" is a misnomer, since the action of such a drug is to decrease the severity of psychotic behavior more than it is to sedate. In fact, the tranquilizers will stimulate or energize persons who are withdrawn and apathetic and calm those who are hyperactive—in other words, these drugs tend to normalize levels of activity. Chlorpromazine was the first of the phenothiazine drugs to be used. Other drugs were developed from the prototype. Some common phenothiazines that are used today include chlorpromazine (Thorazine), promazine (Sparine), butaperazine (Repoise), triflupromazine (Vesprin), trifluoperazine (Stelazine), perphenazine (Trilafon), prochlorperazine (Compazine), fluphenazine (Prolixin), and thioridazine (Mellaril). Haloperidol (Haldol), chlorprothixene (Taractan), and thiothixene (Navane) are not phenothiazines but are examples of some other major tranquilizers or antipsychotic drugs. Haldol is a butyrophenone, and Taractan and Navane are thioxanthenes.

A psychotropic drug that was used in India for several centuries, *Rauwolfia serpentina,* is used today to make the calming agent reserpine (Serpasil). However, the use of reserpine as a psychotropic drug is infrequent—it is more often used to lower blood pressure.

While it must be remembered that any drug can demonstrate a paradoxical reaction in any one person, some of the major tranquilizers (antipsychotics) tend to be sedating and some tend to be activating (see Table 25-2).

Characteristics specific to some of these drugs are as follows:

Haldol is believed to be especially helpful in decreasing the severity of hallucinations and delusions. It is also the drug of choice in *Gilles de la*

TABLE 25-2 Antipsychotic drugs

Generic name	Trade name	Average daily maintenance doses (by mouth)
I. PHENOTHIAZINES		
A. Aliphatic		
1. Chlorpromaxine	Thorazine	150-600 mg
2. Triflupromazine	Vesprin	150-400 mg
B. Piperidine		
1. Thioridazine	Mellaril	150-450 mg
2. Mesoridazine	Serentil	100-400 mg
C. Piperazine		
1. Trifluoperazine	Stelazine	6-30 mg
2. Fluphenazine	Prolixin	(1-10 mg. P.O: 25-30 mg IM every 2 to 4 weeks)
3. Perphenazine	Trilafon	6-32 mg
II. THIOXANTHENES		
A. Chlorprothizene	Taractan	45-400 mg
B. Thiothixene	Navane	20-60 mg
III. BUTYROPHENE		
A. Haloperidol	Haldol	3-20 mg
IV. DIBENZOXAZEPINE		
A. Loxapine	Loxitane	60-100 mg
V. DIHYDROINDOLONE		
A. Molindone	Moban	20-225 mg

Sources include Bassuk et al. (1983), Govoni and Hayes (1982), Grimm (1986), Matorin and Dechillo (1984).

Tourette's syndrome, a physiologically based disorder that is characterized by bizarre choreiform movements and the compulsive and uncontrollable utterance of obscene words—coprolalia. The syndrome is believed to be related to excess dopamine in the brain, and antipsychotic drugs are thought to somehow block the transport of dopamine.

Prolixin, in the form of Prolixin Decanoate, is a long-lasting phenothiazine. Intramuscular injections can be given in dosages that will last for 1 to 3 weeks, with an average of 2 weeks' duration. For this reason, Prolixin is believed to be an especially appropriate drug for persons who, for various reasons, resist taking their medication or are unreliable self-medicators. Among schizophrenics, failure to take drugs is one of the main reasons for readmission to hospitals.

Dosages of *Mellaril* should not exceed 800 mg per day. In high doses, Mellaril can cause pigmentary retinopathy and eventual blindness. Any complaints of decreasing visual acuity from clients who are taking phenothiazines should be investigated immediately, and this is particularly important for those who are taking Mellaril.

The major tranquilizers or antipsychotic drugs are relatively safe drugs for long-term use, and they are not addicting. Minor or moderate side effects occur fairly frequently; serious and life-threatening side effects except for tardive dyskinesia are rare. A summary of the side effects of drugs used to treat schizophrenia can be found in Tables 25-3 and 25-4.

Studies noted in *Science News* (1984, 126 [47]: 297; 1987b; 1988) reported on research that low dosages of antipsychotic drugs (as little as 1/10 of conventional dosages) have been used to decrease the risk of tardive dyskinesia in schizophrenics, but there is also an increased risk of exacerbating a

TABLE 25-3 Side effects of the antipsychotic drugs

Side effects	Nursing intervention
MINOR	
Menstrual irregularities	Inform client of possibility
Changes in libido	Inform client of possibility
Increased weight, increased appetite	Nutritional counseling
Constipation	Increased ingestion of bulk-producing foods; exercise; laxatives as needed
Dry mouth	Rinse with water; give sugarless gum (however, not advisable for elderly clients because of increased danger of choking—the phenothiazines can affect the swallowing reflex)
Postural hypotension	As a preventative, client should learn to sit up gradually from a lying position; to combat, have client lie down with feet elevated
Photosensitivity	Use sun hats and sunscreening lotions during the summer months
Allergic rash	May require an order to change to another drug
Contact dermatitis in staff members dispensing the drug in liquid form	Use of rubber gloves when the drug is being dispensed
MODERATE	
Extrapyramidal symptoms: drugs act on limbic area of brain to promote muscular dysfunctions (see Table 25-4)	Extrapyramidal symptoms, if they persist, require drugs to counteract them; such drugs as benzotropine (Cogentin), procyclidine (Kemadrin), trihexyphenidyl (Artane), and biperiden (Akineton) may be used; these drugs, however, are not without side effects of their own (e.g., constipation); the automatic prescribing of one of these is not an advisable practice, since extrapyramidal symptoms are sometimes transistory and thus may disappear after a few days
SERIOUS	
Agranulocytosis (often is manifested as a sore throat or high fever)	Stop giving the drug immediately; notify a physician when a client complains of a sore throat or has a fever; total and differential white cell counts are done, and in some cases reverse isolation may be used
Drug-induced jaundice (begins like influenza)	Periodic liver function tests should be carried out when clients are receiving phenothiazines
Tardive dyskinesia. Although one of the extrapyramidal symptoms, it is included here because unlike the other extrapyramidal symptoms it can become irreversible. It is a disfiguring and disabling syndrome characterized by involuntary twitching of the face, tongue, arms, and legs. Abnormally low levels of acetylcholine are believed to be responsible. Signs of such emotional disturbances as euphoria, unstable moods, and manic interactions with people have been associated with the worst cases of tardive dyskinesia, and several groups of researchers have suggested that this syndrome may be related to extensive use of the drugs. The terms used to describe the syndrome—*iatrogenic schizophrenia* and *tardive dysmentia*—point to the need for a close monitoring of major tranquilizers and to the strict avoidance of any inappropriate use (Herbert, 1983b).	A common early sign of tardive dyskinesia is wormlike movements detected in the tongue (Bassuk et al., 1983). Nurses should regularly inspect the tongues of clients who are taking antipsychotic drugs.

TABLE 25-4   Extrapyramidal symptoms

Akinesia	Akathisia	Dyskinesia	Pseudo-parkinsonism
Usually has slow onset	Usually has slow onset (most often occurs in middle-aged people)	May have sudden onset (most often occurs in younger people)	Slow onset (most often occurs in older people)
Reduced physical activity	Restlessness, pacing	Torticollis	Shuffling gait
Listlessness	Jittery movements	Carpal spasms	Masklike facies
Apathy (often not recognized)	Fine hand tremor	Opisthotonos	Increased salivation
Development of painful muscles and joints	Facial tics	Oculogyric crisis	Stooping posture
	Insomnia		"Pill rolling" tremor Cogwheel rigidity

return of severe psychotic symptoms on these lower dosages. The researchers concluded that there is no simple formula for selecting the best dosage for individuals. Driscoll (1985) concurs and in her search of the literature found no solid indicators of good prognosis or drug response from maintenance regimens of antipsychotic medication. She points out that there is value in protecting some chronically ill clients from relapse into such acute symptoms as hallucinations, delusions, and agitation with maintenance and medication. The schizophrenic symptoms that do not seem to respond to the regimen are the "defect state" symptoms of blunted affect, social withdrawal, volitional impairment, and other forms of underactivity. She notes that some theorists speculate that such symptoms serve an adaptive role by reducing stimuli input for schizophrenics. Because there are risks involved in long-term administration of antipsychotics, she advocates a risk/benefit assessment for deciding to use any maintenance regimen with chronic schizophrenics. Her assessment includes:

1. *Who:* An accurate diagnosis of schizophrenia—a history of repeated relapses with positive response to antipsychotic drugs is the only good prognostic indicator for long-term use of these drugs.
2. *When and for how long?:* The client's first year back in the community after an acute episode is a crucial adjustment period. The

regimen should be considered for anyone who has had more than two acute episodes. She suggests a maintenance regimen for at least 4 to 5 years.

3. *What are the benefits?:* Symptoms of acute psychosis respond, "defect state" ones do not, but medication can act as a buffer against stress.
4. *Dosages:* The usual range is 300–500 mg of Thorazine—for Prolixin decanoate, it is 25 to 62.5 mg at 2–4 week intervals. She notes that the data about very low dosage (1/10 of standard doses) and megadoses (4–5 times standard doses) are inconsistent.
5. *Risks:* The extrapyramidal symptoms of tardive dyskinesia and akinetic depression are possible side effects. Extrapyramidal symptoms other than tardive dyskinesia can be controlled with dosage reduction or anticholinergic medications. Tardive dyskinesia, if it is to occur, will most often show up after two years of drug theapy—earliest signs are reversible. Any client on long-term antipsychotic medication should be continuously assessed for these early signs (e.g., a wormlike movement of the tongue).
6. *Oral vs. depot* (injection of long-lasting doses): Depot neuroleptics (e.g., Prolixin Decanoate) are preferred for clients with a history of noncompliance or for those with dif-

ficulty in absorbing oral medications. Otherwise, flexibility of dosage and a possible decreased risk for side-effects favor oral administration (adapted from Driscoll, 1985).

Clozapine, a drug first synthesized in the 1960s but unavailable for prescription use in the United States of America, has been studied recently and found to be effective in treating severely ill schizophrenics who do not respond to other antipsychotic drugs. The drug has an increased risk for agranulocytosis so that weekly white blood cell counts are necessary (*The New York Times*, 1987; *Science News*, 1987a).

Carbamazepine (Tegretol) is an anticonvulsant used in the treatment of epilepsy and trigeminal neuralgia. Recently it has been reported as effective in reducing the symptoms of schizophrenia (Grimm, 1986; Rankel, 1988).

Nursing implications of selected drugs used to treat schizophrenia are found in Appendix B.

Psychotherapy

Forms of psychotherapy representing all the schools of psychology have been used in the treatment of schizophrenic clients. Many clinicians believe, as Freud did, that psychoanalysis is not the treatment of choice for schizophrenics because of its goal of freeing unconscious conflicts. They argue that the psychodynamic defect in schizophrenia is an impaired ability to repress and that the unconscious is all too close to the surface. It is the threat that unconscious material will flood the ego that stimulates the psychotic symptoms as defenses. Currently, many clinicians cite the increasing evidence of a biological defect in the disorder and the research that validates a more structured, supportive, and educational approach to the treatment of schizophrenia (Gunderson et al., 1984; Taylor, 1987).

Some notable clinicians, however, have worked with schizophrenics in a psychoanalytic manner: Harry Stack Sullivan (1953), Gertrud Schwing (1954), John Rosen (1953), Marguerite Sechehaye (1956), Harold Searles (1965), and Frieda Fromm-Reichmann (1950) are examples. All have written about their work. A well-known psychiatric nurse who works within the psychosis of a client is June

Mellow. She calls her in-depth approach *nursing therapy*. Mellow helps the client to relive the original mother-child symbiotic attachment, but the new emotional experience is a corrective one (Mellow, 1968).

Therapists who do work in this manner with schizophrenic clients point out that the clinician must be a healthy, well-integrated person in touch with thoughts, feelings, and reactions. The ethical practice of psychoanalysis mandates that the therapist be analyzed as part of the training process. Psychoanalysis is not an economical form of treatment, since one therapist can treat only a limited number of clients and there are many schizophrenics in need of help. Psychoanalysis is a specialized and expensive form of therapy. In comparison to the number of schizophrenics in need of treatment, there are *very* few psychoanalysts willing and able to treat them in this manner. Aside from this fact, as was mentioned before, many clinicians and writers believe that psychoanalysis, with its goal of uncovering unconscious conflicts, is not a useful or even safe treatment for schizophrenics, whose faulty use of repression may be the basic defect of the disorder. Evidence to date has not established the therapeutic effectiveness of insight-oriented psychotherapy in schizophrenia (Carpenter, 1986).

Several mental health workers point to supportive therapy as the most appropriate form of psychotherapy for schizophrenics (Carpenter, 1987; Gunderson, et al., 1984; *Science News*, 1984). Such therapy can be long term, and it can be crisis oriented at intervals when necessary. It can be modified over time to match the needs and the growth of the client. Rather than attempting to uncover the unconscious, the goal of supportive therapy is to gain insight into the effects of one's behavior on one's life and to encourage the development of ego strengths through the realization of successful changes in behavior. Mendel and Green (1967) describe this type of treatment and suggest that while the beginning stages of a relationship may require frequent meetings with the client, the number of meetings may gradually decrease.

Mendel and Green take the "as if" phenomenon, described earlier, and turn it around to use it therapeutically. For example, they suggest encouraging a person who feels unable to get up and face the world and a daily job as other people do, to act "as if" that was possible. After acting this way for a period of time, the client gains some ego strength from the realization of being able to accomplish this task every morning.

In supportive therapy, the nurse lends ego strength to the client to provide support while they both work toward the goal of developing the client's own ego strength. The nurse-client relationship in psychiatric nursing is ideally suited to relationship therapy.

Family therapy

Therapy that involves the families of schizophrenics is focused on clarifying mystifying forms of communication (Laing, 1965b), such as double-bind communicating and tangentiality, which were discussed in Chapter 14. Family therapy is also concerned with strengthening appropriate boundaries between family members. For instance, one approach to decreasing the debilitating hold of a mother and a son's symbiotic relationship might be to improve the relationship between the two spouses and the relationship between the son and his father. Insight into communication and relationship patterns within the family is encouraged, and alternate patterns are explored.

The initial and primary goal of the family therapist, according to Murray Bowen (1977), is to decrease the level of anxiety within the family system, since it is this anxiety that fosters development of the various types of pathological behavior. Bowen's definition of a mental health professional is "someone who helps decrease anxiety."

Pittman and Flomenhaft (1970) have described a marital configuration that is characterized by an unequal relationship between the spouses. One spouse's incompetence is required and encouraged by the other spouse, to verify his or her own competence. This "doll's house marriage"—the name comes from the situation portrayed in Ibsen's play *The Doll's House*—may involve a childlike wife and a masterful husband, although the roles can be reversed. Each spouse needs this system of relating to maintain inner equilibrium and the equilibrium of the marriage. Pittman and Flomenhaft view this type of unequal relationship as common in a poten-

tially schizophrenic population; they suggest that one or both spouses may be latent schizophrenics maintaining stability through the marriage. With the development of crises such as severe financial difficulties or the addition of children to the family, such individuals may come into a treatment situation. It is then that the tendency of a therapist to push for too much and too rapid change can precipitate a psychotic break. The great importance that the therapist places on individual growth may foster an attempt to promote more change than is necessary, thus destroying the family and precipitating illness in one or more family members. Pittman and Flomenhaft suggest that the therapist work with caution and develop an ability to tolerate a certain degree of inequality within a marriage, which may be the wiser choice for some couples.

Support groups for the spouses and parents of schizophrenic clients are an especially helpful form of family intervention. The goals of such groups (adapted from Iodice and Wodarski, 1987) include:

1. to identify separation-individuation issues for the relative and the schizophrenic client
2. to foster independence in the schizophrenic client
3. to explore spousal or parental guilt about the client's illness and the detrimental effects of such guilt on the management of the schizophrenic illness
4. to deal with feelings of loss over the expectations that relatives may have had for the client
5. to teach management skills for use while the schizophrenic individual is at home
6. to give parents and/or spouse the permission to meet their own needs and to ventilate any negative feelings

Anderson et al. (1980) have formulated a model for a long-term psychoeducational series for the families of schizophrenic clients. The model is based on the belief in a relationship between high EE levels and patient relapse. EE stands for the concept of "expressed emotion," and it is a term used to describe the emotional climate within the homes (Mintz et al., 1987) of families with a schizophrenic member. At present, it is not adequately defined (Goldstein, 1987; Hatfield et al., 1987) but

Table 25-5   Psychoeducation of the families of schizophrenic clients

Phase	Outcomes	Strategies
Phase 1 (connecting)	Family connects with therapy team Cooperation with treatment program is established Guilt, emotionality, negative reactions to client's treatment decrease Family's stress is reduced	Join with family Establish a treatment contract Discuss the crisis history Discuss feelings about client and illness Make specific and practical suggestions that mobilize family's concerns into effective coping mechanisms
Phase 2 (conducting survival skills workshops)	Family's understanding of illness and the client's needs are increased Family stress is reduced Social network of family is enhanced	Conduct multiple-family groups for education and discussion Present concrete information on schizophrenia Present specific management suggestions Foster basic communication skills
Phase 3 (facilitating reentry and application)	Client is maintained in the community The marital/parental coalition is strengthened Family tolerance for low-level dysfunctional behavior is increased Responsibilities are gradually resumed by the client	Generational and interpersonal boundaries are reinforced Specific tasks are assigned Low-key problem solving is encouraged
Phase 4 (maintaining the client community)	Client is reintegrated into community roles (e.g., work and/or school) General family processes will be increasingly effective	Infrequent maintenance sessions with family Traditional or exploratory family therapy

Adapted from Anderson et al. (1980).

described through scores on the *Camberwell Family Interview* (Hatfield et al., 1987). The concept of EE is, at present, controversial, since some believe that it might lead to the negative labelling of families of schizophrenics (Hatfield et al., 1987; Strachan, 1986) as in the past, when the concept of the "schizophrenogenic family" was paramount. Others cite a lack of real understanding of the EE concept as leading to its poor acceptance in some quarters (Strachan, 1986). One definition supplied by Snyder and Liberman (1981) explains the concept of EE as follows: "The number of criticisms together with the quality of emotional over-involvement expressed by relatives designates them as high or low EE."

Proponents of the usefulness of the concept (Anderson et al., 1981; Falloon et al., 1981; Imber et al., 1987; Iodice and Wardarski, 1987; Strachan, 1986) suggest that the schizophrenic's deficit in processing stimuli is particularly manifested in an overly stimulating family environment. Research

does seem to support the validity of a relationship between high EE scores and the tendency to relapse into acute schizophrenic symptoms (Mintz, et al., 1987; Strachan, 1986). Anderson's model for psychoeducation of families as part of the treatment for schizophrenia is summarized in Table 25-5.

Phase 1 begins at the hospital admission of the client and involves the family but not the client in at least two sessions per week throughout the hospital stay. Client and family meet for one session at discharge. Phase 2, which occurs early in treatment, is a day-long workshop conducted with multiple families. Phase 3 includes the client and starts as soon as the acute stage of illness has been controlled. This allows the client to participate fully. The sessions are bi-weekly for six months. Phase 4 begins once the family and professional goals for effective functioning are accomplished to the best degree possible. At this point, the family and client may choose to continue in more intensive family therapy aimed at dealing with unresolved issues and conflicts: developmental issues, sibling issues, marital discord, and increased differentiation of family roles (Iodice and Wodarski, 1987).

Group therapy

As in individual psychotherapy, few clinicians advocate psychoanalytically oriented group therapy for schizophrenics (Kanas, 1986). Group therapy should be focused *not* on probing the unconscious but rather on the development of insight into behavior and on helping clients to improve their social interaction skills. A more comfortable adjustment to life is a legitimate goal of group therapy for schizophrenic clients. Group therapy can promote socialization—or resocialization for a regressed schizophrenic—and can provide opportunities for a client to become more outer directed. Concern for other people can be positively reinforced, a development that can lead to increased self-esteem. Sharing of experiences and problems can provide the reassurance that comes from knowing that others have lived through similar situations. Support from a peer group during periods of crisis and attempted change can help to make experiments with new behavior less frightening.

The leader in group therapy for schizophrenics—particularly withdrawn schizophrenics—needs to take a more active role than the leader of another type of group might take, especially in the beginning stages of the group. But the same principles of group dynamics apply (see Chapter 13). Besides psychotherapy groups, various activity therapy groups, such as dance, music, and poetry groups, are helpful. *Remotivation groups* are often used to bring severely regressed schizophrenics back to a here-and-now orientation; such groups constitute a particularly useful tool for psychiatric nurses.

Certain self-help community groups are available for discharged schizophrenics; giving a client information about them would be an appropriate and helpful referral. Recovery Inc. is one such group—its method is a type of self-mediated behavior modification combined with peer group support. Schizophrenics Anonymous is another self-help group that is available in many communities.

Milieu therapy

Since disorganization in living is a major aspect of the schizophrenic experience, milieu therapy can provide schizophrenic clients opportunities to learn or relearn interpersonal skills and to become competent in the activities of daily living. Milieu therapy can also provide opportunities for satisfying recreation. An ideal milieu for schizophrenics is an active one and one that provides the structure that is so badly needed in a disorganized life.

Shapiro (1981) offers an important cautionary note. She states that clients may adapt very well to an active, supportive milieu only to face a rude shock when they leave the hospital. The highly structured environment does not prepare them for the social isolation and unstructured living of such placements as welfare hotels. Transitional services (such as support groups, supervision, and planned activities) aimed at bridging the gap are essential.

Brief hospitalization versus institutionalization

Many clinicians believe that much of the apparent deterioration in chronic schizophrenics is due not to the disease process but to the effects of long-term institutionalization. Some of the dangers of institutionalization have been pointed out by Mendel and Green (1967) in their excellent book on the treatment of chronic schizophrenics:

1. The client loses a "place" in the family and community. It is not so unusual for people who are discharged after many years of hospitalization to go back to their "roots" and find, for example, that a parking lot or a highrise has been built where the old neighborhood stood.
2. The fact that the person has failed in a developmental task is reified. Secondary guilt is an accompaniment of this realization.
3. The role of the person as a passive receiver of treatment is reinforced instead of the role of active participant in the individual's own treatment plan.
4. The person's energy and resources (for example, financial) go toward adaptation to the hospital rather than toward adaptation to living in society.

Mendel and Green argue that short-term hospitalization should be viewed as a coping mechanism or safety valve to be used when a person's anxiety approaches unbearable heights. They suggest that the person's knowing the hospital is there when needed may help to reduce anxiety.

Emergency interventions

In emergency intervention with the schizophrenic client, the following points are considered:

1. The client may be withdrawn or severely confused. Simple words, talking slowly, short sentences, and clear questions are helpful— repetition may be necessary with a very confused person.
2. For the relatively rare schizophrenic person who becomes combative in the emergency setting, a pre-existing procedure and staff teamwork are essential. Guidelines for obtaining and administering parenteral antipsychotic medication should be in place. It is important to avoid the use of long-acting parenteral medications at normal dosages until the client's sensitivity to small doses has been ascertained.
3. Interviewing of collateral persons—relatives or friends, if present—may be able to verify or supplement the client's account. The assessment of probable support for the client's return to the current living situation is also important.
4. The reasons for hospitalizing a client are as follows:
   a. The client's degree of confusion mandates supervision for the protection of the client and others.
   b. The client appears to need higher doses of medication than should be tried without careful and frequent supervision. Until stabilization has occurred, hospitalization is necessary.
   c. The family needs relief from bizarre or otherwise difficult behavior. Relief may prevent the family's withdrawal from or hostility toward the client.
   d. The client needs a structural program and

group involvement to prevent increasing social isolation and deepening psychosis.
   e. The client's behavior is so bizarre that acceptance in the community is jeopardized unless treatment gains are made and behavior modified.
   f. The family situation may be toxic for some clients—hospitalization is used to evaluate the possibility. With more data, the choice for family treatment or placement outside of the family can be made (adapted from Crockett, 1982).

Many forms of treatment are used to help schizophrenic clients live more comfortably in the world. While a few specially trained clinicians provide psychoanalytical therapy for schizophrenics, psychoanalysis is a comparatively rare form of treatment in schizophrenia, and the value and safety of it for schizophrenics are questioned by many clinicians. Supportive individual and group therapy, in combination with psychotropic drugs and supportive family therapy, seems to be the treatment of choice for schizophrenic clients.

Nursing Intervention
PRIMARY PREVENTION

Primary prevention of schizophrenia includes modification of the environment and strengthening of coping abilities. Only in recent years has much been attempted or even written as far as prevention of schizophrenia is concerned. This is probably because there has never been complete agreement on the basis of the disorder. Since the consensus is that it is of multifactorial nature, a multifactorial prevention program must be developed. Some work has begun. Clinicians have identified high-risk groups—this process is termed *vulnerability research*. Basically, it is the selection and study of children who are at risk for developing schizophrenia. This determination is based on the presence of the following factors:

1. Genetic predisposition
2. History of deprivation of some kind in the prenatal or neonatal period
3. Evidence of excessive disorganization in the family

4. A disordered sociocultural environment such as that found in poverty-stricken inner-city ares or that occurring after a massive natural or man-made disaster (Garmezy, 1971).

Through study of the vulnerable children, a group of children classified as "invulnerables" has been delineated. These are people who, through every indication, should have developed schizophrenia but did not—in fact, many excelled in various life tasks. The goal of researchers is to try to determine what factors helped to prevent these children from becoming schizophrenic and then to use this information to help prevent other children from developing the disorder.

Several areas have in the past been defined as providing possible approaches to the prevention of schizophrenia. *Premarital counseling* has been employed to help ensure a strong base for the future family or, in some instances, to prevent marriages from taking place. Most marriages are the result of "falling in love," which is an interweaving of the unconscious and often neurotic needs of two people. Later, it is the projection of these needs by one spouse onto the other that contributes to many marital problems. Some insight into the potential hazards may help to minimize marital discord or at least set a pattern for individual self-awareness and open communication between the spouses. Perhaps people need lessons in how to be married—it is not something that we know instinctively.

Marital counseling has been used for marriages that are showing signs of strain because of discord or dysfunctional family members. Alleviation of anxiety between married persons may prevent the conflict from being projected onto a child, a situation that can, according to family theorists, result in a schizophrenic reaction.

Family therapy that is instituted in the preschizophrenic stage of a child or adolescent's disorder may prevent a full-blown schizophrenic break. Alleviating anxiety within the family system, fostering insight into disordered patterns of communicating and relating, and encouraging the learning of new patterns are all parts of the family therapist's goal.

Prenatal care and *neonatal care* should be optimal to prevent the possible damage to fetus and infant that is significantly correlated with the incidence of schizophrenia.

Genetic counseling may be appropriate for families that are at extremely high risk of having schizophrenic offspring because numerous family members have the disorder. However, the exact mode of genetic transmission is unknown.

Child-rearing counseling can help alleviate such problems as "poor fit" between mother and child as far as stimulus barriers are concerned. A mother who enjoys giving and receiving stimuli might have a child with a low tolerance for stimuli, or vice versa. Developmental stages and the mother's need for rest, recreation, and time away from her children are also important aspects of this type of counseling. Just as people may need lessons in how to be married, preparation in parenting might prevent potentially harmful family discord.

There is rather extensive documentation in the literature that the children of schizophrenic women are at 10 to 15 times greater risk for developing the disorder than is the general population (Siefer and Sameroff, 1982, 87). The symbiotic phase of preoedipal development (which occurs approximately from 1 month to 5 months of age) is believed to be the crucial one in the subsequent development of schizophrenia. Mahler (1975) found that the most deeply disturbed schizophrenic children were never able to establish a healthy symbiosis with their mothers. Searles (1965) pointed out that, if they were able to establish it, they were never able to resolve it in a healthy way.

The infant's psyche takes shape in harmony and counterpoint to the mother's own particular ego and lifestyle. Spitz (1965) has called the mother *the auxiliary ego of the infant*. The important factor is whether the mother provides a healthy or pathological object for this adaptation of the infant. Strong ego boundaries can only be established by the mother at the phase-appropriate time. During the symbiotic phase, it is healthy for the mother to be preoccupied with her infant (Winnicott, 1965) to protect the child from inappropriate stimuli. Thus, the mother serves as a replacement for the earlier, inborn stimulus barrier and protects the child from undue stress and strain (Mahler, 1975). Mahler suggests that an infant who later becomes schizophrenic is unable to invest in its mother or to use her to establish affective-tension homeostasis and, instead, must resort to maintenance mechanisms that are pathological (schizophrenic) and lead to isolation and withdrawal (Pao, 1979). These are maladaptive mechanisms, but they help the baby to cope in the absence of "mutual cuing."* The lack of mutual cuing in the mother-child dyad is perhaps where efforts at primary prevention may best be focused. Field (1982) agrees and suggests that early intervention to facilitate healthy interactions between mother and child may be helpful. "Interaction coaching" is the term used to describe attempts to modify disturbed mother-infant interaction. Efforts are directed toward improving the "fit" or mutual cuing between the two. Field's set of interventions that are aimed at modulating arousal and improving the level of information processing in high-risk infants include:

1. Appropriate games for the age level
2. Coaching mothers through an earpiece microphone
3. Replaying videotapes for her viewing

Using "infant gaze" as the dependent variable in 14- to 18-week-old infants, the data suggested that mothers of high-risk infants can be taught other ways of interacting. The goal is a more harmonious relationship for mother and child. Field states:

The problem relates to finding the optimal level of stimulation since low levels do not seem to arouse or elicit responses from infants while high levels eventuate in gaze aversion or fussiness.

Field also points out that infant gaze avoidance and irritability and parental overactivity and overcontrol were revealed in a retrospective analysis of the harmonics of infants later diagnosed as schizophrenic.

To summarize, primary prevention of schizophrenia through intervention at or before the symbolic phase (Arnold, 1983) would include:

1. Identification of parent-child dyads and triads at high risk for producing schizophrenic offspring

2. Therapeutic intervention with, and support of, the high-risk mother and family unit, both pre- and postpartum
3. Education and interaction coaching aimed at facilitating a healthy symbiosis in high-risk mothers
4. Support of the sensitivity-facilitating preoccupation of the low-risk mother

The preceding material on possible avenues for preventive intervention makes it obvious that there is an important role for nurses in the prevention of schizophrenia, whether they work in the community, in maternal and child-focused agencies, in psychiatric settings, or in traditional hospital settings.

Traditionally the allocation of funds for research into the underlying factors and treatment of schizophrenia has been sparse—this area is sometimes called the stepchild of research in this country. Perhaps one of the reasons for this situation is that chronically ill schizophrenics have very little political power; they have neither the personal nor the financial resources to mount much of a protest movement. As concerned and informed citizens and as advocates of their clients, nurses can make their voices and their votes count. Social changes that lead to improved living conditions and to the availability of optimum health care for all people may be viewed as primary preventive measures for all mental illnesses, including schizophrenia. The reason for the strong correlation between poverty and schizophrenia is unclear, but that there is a strong correlation is undisputed.

SECONDARY PREVENTION

What constitutes nursing care for the schizophrenic client? Just as no person fits exactly into any of the diagnostic categories, there is no exact set of rules or techniques that nurses use to intervene in cases of schizophrenia. It is best to deal with the behavior manifested rather than with the client as a psychiatric category. According to Freud, all behavior has meaning, and the psychotic behavior of the schizophrenic is a form of communication.

The two areas that nurses can be particularly helpful in are interpersonal relationships and com-

---

Mutual cuing is defined by Mahler (1975, 290) as "a circular process of interaction established very early between mother and infant, by which they 'empathically' read each other's signs and signals and react to each other."

munication—these are usually the two areas that the schizophrenic has the most problems with in life. A well-known psychiatric nurse, Marguerite Holmes, believes that in the nurse-client relationship, the nurse should concentrate on learning about and understanding the way the client is experiencing the world. The client will then have been *heard* and *understood*, and because this communication will have taken place, may be able to move toward changing behavior.

The skills required of the nurse then, are that she be able to (a) help the patient accept and appreciate his own inner experiences, which means that she has to be able to tolerate sharing in some of these experiences, and (b) meet the patient in real encounter (Holmes, 1971).

Many things can happen to the nurse and the client through their attempts to relate to each other in a meaningful way. An important development is that the client may be able to increase trust in other people. One relationship is rarely, if ever, the remedy for many years of social withdrawal, but one relationship can lead to another.

Bleuler's "four A's"—his delineation of the primary symptoms of schizophrenia—were reviewed earlier in this chapter. While they may be helpful as a mnemonic device, they are basically a negative concept, since they focus on pathology. There is a danger in this. Expectation of pathological responses is a powerful stimulus for the production of pathological responses in people. A more helpful way of viewing the interaction between the nurse and the schizophrenic would be to focus on *four A's of therapeutic intervention* (Arnold, 1976). Unlike Bleuler's four A's, which are concepts that are often projected onto the client, the therapeutic four A's apply to both partners in the relationship. The therapeutic four A's are as follows:

1. Acceptance. Crucial to the relationship is the nurse's acceptance of self, of the client as he or she is in the present stage of development, and of the world as *he* or *she* sees it.
2. Awareness. Before nurse and client can begin to communicate effectively, the nurse must be aware of his or her own thoughts, feelings, and actions. This self-understanding, combined with an awareness of the client's verbal, nonverbal, and symbolic communication, is

an essential part of the therapeutic relationship.
3. Acknowledgment. The existence of a person whose communication is not acknowledged is disconfirmed. People need to know that they have been heard, and they need to know whether they have been understood.
4. Authenticity. Most important of all of the elements of a therapeutic relationship, whether they begin with "A" or not, is authenticity. The tool of a psychiatric nurse is *self*. The self can only be a useful tool if it is real. Because of the nature of their disorder, it is not unusual for schizophrenic clients to have a history of many hurtful relationships. For this reason they tend to be very sensitive interpersonally and can quickly detect any signs of dissembling or deceit.

Nursing process

Many approaches to the understanding and treatment of schizophrenia have been discussed. Psychiatric nursing is based on an eclectic theoretical approach and on appropriate responses to behavioral problems. This section will deal with secondary prevention through nursing intervention with clients' patterns of underactivity and withdrawal, overactivity and anxiety, autistic behavior, feelings and thoughts of unreality, low self-esteem, depression, and suicide. The nursing process will provide guidelines for our interventions.

ASSESSMENT

In using the nursing process to intervene with the schizophrenic client, the nurse should assess the following areas:

1. Presenting symptoms, or patterns of behavior—underactivity and withdrawal, overactivity and anxiety, verbal hostility and physical aggression, suspicion and fear of interpersonal relationships, autistic behavior (symbolic communication, inappropriate behavior, ritualistic behavior), feelings and thoughts of unreality (depersonalization, loose ego boundaries, delusions, hallucinations), low self-esteem, and suicide.
2. Emotional state—feelings of anger, fear, anx-

iety, helplessness, apathy. An understanding of the tendency toward a crippling ambivalence and the subjective experience of the "need-fear dilemma" is important here.

3. Stimulus situations—stressful life situations that threaten the self-system and engender an increased tendency to withdraw inwardly.
4. Maladaptive coping behaviors—coping patterns based on withdrawal from interpersonal relations and control of the environment and one's inner life through magical level thinking. Coping behaviors may also be influenced by thought and perceptual disorders. The behaviors are an attempt to maintain a cohesive sense of self in the face of overwhelming anxiety, but they are maladaptive in that they lead to further problems in relating and functioning in the world.
5. Origin of maladaptive coping behaviors—identification of childhood experiences that contributed to the development of or learning of maladaptive coping behavior.
6. Holistic health status—physical, intellectual, emotional, sociocultural, and spiritual status of the client. These factors may either facilitate wellness (e.g., a benevolent, protective marital relationship may shield the client from some of the stresses of life) or these factors may impede wellness (e.g., difficulties in concentrating can be exacerbated by poor nutrition and amplify any tendency toward a thought disorder).

ANALYSIS OF DATA

A clear and comprehensive assessment of presenting symptoms, emotional state, stimulus situations, maladaptive coping behavior and its origin, and the holistic health status of the schizophrenic client can assist the nurse who is formulating a nursing diagnosis.

PLANNING AND IMPLEMENTATION

The following section focuses on anxiety, depression, and on behavioral problems and nursing responses to these problems. Following each nursing diagnosis will be an appropriate care plan and its implementation.

▶ Anxiety

Anxiety is often a part of the schizophrenic experience. The times when a client is particularly vulnerable to acute anxiety attacks are as follows:

1. On admission to a psychiatric facility (and particularly on first admission—depression is more apt to accompany subsequent readmissions)
2. When the client begins to participate in any new activity, such as group therapy
3. When the staff member or therapist the client is accustomed to working with goes on vacation, is transferred, or resigns
4. Just before discharge from the hospital (Many hospitalized schizophrenics express feelings of ambivalence and anxiety about being discharged. The hospital may seem less threatening and more accepting than the outside world; the client may feel overwhelmed by the thought of increased responsibility.)

In working with an anxious client, a nurse must remember that anxiety can interfere with the client's hearing and comprehension; a nurse may have to repeat much of what he or she says. Complete but concise directions are best. The nurse's support of the client through his or her presence as the client begins to participate in new activities or try out new behaviors may help ease discomfort. Adequate preparation, with opportunities for the expression of concerns, will help a client during the anxiety-provoking predischarge period or when a trusted staff member is leaving.

▶ Depression

Schizophrenia is often accompanied by *anhedonia*, the inability to experience pleasure. The schizophrenic is quite apt to be depressed. The symptoms of the disorder, its incapacitating effects, the inhibition of personal growth, and the drain on financial resources are some of the reasons for depression. As in any chronic illness, depression is part of the process of the individual's acceptance of the disorder. In addition, low self-esteem is the common denominator of *all* emotional illnesses.

The therapeutic response to depression in the schizophrenic is the same as that for any depressed client (see Chapter 22). Realistic emotional support, activity, and gradually increasing interpersonal involvement are all helpful. Since depression can produce symptoms of psychomotor retardation, nurses must allow clients enough time to react to questions or statements and to verbalize. Like any depressed person, a depressed schizophrenic may attempt suicide. But factors other than depression may also lead to suicide attempts. Suicide attempts by schizophrenic persons are sometimes bizarre and are often quite unpredictable. A suicide attempt may occur in response to a hallucinated voice, or it may be a response to a delusional system. Since a break with reality affects an individual's judgment, the impossible—for example, "flying" out of a window of a tall building—may seem possible. A suicide attempt might be precipitated by loose ego boundaries. For example, a young, very psychotic man reacted to the successful and just-completed suicide of his roommate by jumping out of a window after him. He was badly injured, but he lived. His explanation of why he jumped was that the crumpled body lying on the ground was really *him* and that he was jumping to put himself back together again.

Since the suicides of schizophrenic persons are so unpredictable, with few if any "clues" being given, it is particularly important for nurses to be vigilant. A vague, subjective uneasiness about the possibility of the client committing suicide may be an important clue and should not be dismissed lightly.

▶ Socially inappropriate behavior

Some types of socially inappropriate behavior—ritualistic or stereotypical behavior—and nursing responses to them are shown in the following case studies.

One form of socially inappropriate behavior was demonstrated by a young schizophrenic girl who felt compelled to touch other females or stroke their hair. The behavior may have had its roots in an exceptionally strong symbiotic relationship with her mother. She would make such statements as "My mother is my only reason for living." The touching and stroking aroused anger among other clients—particularly those who felt threatened by physical closeness. She was sometimes assaulted. At best, her behavior alienated her from many of the ward residents. The nursing staff

members used a firm but gentle approach. They conveyed their expectations that she could indeed control her behavior. After a student nurse taught her how to crochet as a possible substitute activity for her hands, she was able to decrease the touching significantly, resorting to it only when anxiety was extremely high.

• • •

An elderly and chronically ill woman greeted every morning with her ritual of placing a cloth packet of salt she had made on her head and facing the east for 15 minutes. Her need for this strange but harmless ritualistic behavior was accepted by the nursing staff. After this ritual she would go about her business of the day.

• • •

One burly, middle-aged man controlled his anxiety by twirling about the room like a ballet dancer. Staff members responded by accepting his need for this behavior, but they also focused on developing his ability to control it at times. Eventually, the frequency of the behavior decreased to a point where the success of his placement in the community was ensured. His substitute behavior was an unspoken slogan that he would recall during times of increased anxiety.

▶ Delusions

More extreme feelings of unreality based in loose ego boundaries include delusions and hallucinations. In responding to these experiences of the client, the nurse can act as a bridge to reality.

Delusions are ideas that are contrary to culturally accepted facts. Delusions can be persecutory, grandiose, of control or of influence, somatic, or religious. There is a kernel of truth somewhere in a delusion, although, if it is a long-standing delusion that has been embellished through the years into a complex delusional system, it may be difficult to find. A delusion may be difficult to dispel. If a delusion is just beginning to form and is still rather fluid, it may be possible to intervene to prevent its adoption by the client. In the case of a rigid delusional system, however, some researchers suggest that the best way to work with it is to help the client see the importance of not verbalizing the delusional beliefs so that he or she can function acceptably in society.

The difference between these two approaches to the treatment of delusional beliefs can be illustrated by a comparison of the cases of clients with whom a student nurse worked.

One client was an elderly woman who had had numerous admissions to the hospital. She usually remained in the hospital for 3 to 4 months and then was able to function quite adequately in the community for several months. Her delusion was complex and quite fixed. Among other things, she believed that pigeons carried secret messages about her to the Nazis and that they, in collaboration with a Puerto Rican political group, carried out experiments on human beings in the apartment beneath her—no matter where she lived. When she was less anxious and ready for discharge, she was able to keep quiet about these beliefs. But they never really left her, and she would start to talk about them more as her anxiety began to increase.

In contrast to this woman, the other client the student was involved with had experienced her first psychotic break and was exhibiting obsessive-compulsive behavior and indications of low self-esteem. She washed her hands constantly after touching anyone or anything in her unit, and she dusted off any chair she intended to sit on. One day she greeted the student in an excited, worried state: "Don't touch me! I have all of these worms growing inside of me and you might catch them!"

By spending time with her and asking for details and clarification, the student learned the basis for this belief. The client had been eating almost constantly (probably because of a combination of anxiety and the appetite-increasing effects of thorazine), and an aide in the unit had jokingly said, "You must have a tapeworm, you eat so much!" Interpreting this remark concretely and in the light of her low self-esteem, she began to believe that she had worms growing inside of her. The student was able to explain what the aide really meant, and the client was able to accept the explanation.

In responding to a delusion that is already formed, a logical, rational confrontation is usually not helpful. In fact, in the cases of some clients it may stimulate a defensive argument. Usually it is best to respond to what is at the "core" of the delusion and to the feelings associated with it (Donner, 1969). For instance, at the core of a delusion of grandeur one might expect to find feelings of low self-esteem and powerlessness. Most likely at the core of a persecutory delusion are projected feelings of hostility toward other people.

Text continued on p. 836.

NURSING CARE PLAN

Clients with Schizophrenia

Long-term Outcomes	Short-term Outcomes*	Nursing Strategies

Nursing diagnosis: Activity intolerance: *underactivity* related to biochemical imbalance and/or anxiety (NANDA 6.1.1.2; DSM-III-R 295.1x through 295.9x, 298.80, 295.40, 295.70, 298.90)

Long-term Outcomes	Short-term Outcomes*	Nursing Strategies
Work through some of the fears of relating to other people Increase confidence in ability to function in the world Realistically perceive the five subsystems of self (biological, psychological, intellectual, sociocultural, and spiritual strengths and weaknesses) in perspective	Verbalize feelings of anxiety, inadequacy, helplessness (when consistent with client's cultural orientation)† Identify situations that arouse feelings of anxiety, inadequacy, and helplessness Relate current stressful interpersonal or mastery situations to situations in the past that aroused similar feelings Identify any effective coping behavior used during these past situations Develop more effective coping behavior and interpersonal skills Build self-esteem in a realistic manner Meet needs for adequate rest, exercise, food, personal hygiene, and leisure activity	Work toward establishing a trusting nurse-client relationship Encourage client's verbalization of feelings Explore with client situations that arouse feelings of anxiety, inadequacy, and helplessness Help client identify any effective coping behavior used in past Explore alternative coping behavior for the present and near future Encourage client in efforts to test out alternative coping behavior Encourage client to participate in available activities (e.g., remotivation group, dance, art, music therapy groups) Support client's participation in activities and groups (e.g., accompanying client to group, participate with client, etc.) Observe state of health and hygiene; client's subjective reports of physical condition may not be reliable when preoccupied and withdrawn Assist client, as needed, in meeting needs for personal hygiene Assume "mothering" role when necessary; avoid fostering excessive dependence Encourage client's own efforts in meeting needs for personal hygiene Consider the possibility that the underactivity may be evidence of an extrapyramidal reaction to antipsychotic medication and discuss with mental health team members (This is done concurrently with the preceding strategies.)

*Because the degree of underactivity and withdrawal varies, short-term goals may need to be modified. (For example, in the case of a mute client, short-term goals as stated here would be intermediate or long-term.)

†This should be encouraged at a rate and to a degree that are not overwhelming to the client or threatening to the self-concept. In other words, it should be facilitated but not "pushed." *Continued.*

NURSING CARE PLAN—cont'd

Clients with Schizophrenia

Long-term Outcomes	Short-term Outcomes*	Nursing Strategies

Nursing diagnosis: Impaired verbal communication: *mutism* related to biochemical imbalance and psychological barriers (psychosis) (NANDA 2.1.1.1; DSM-III-R 295.1x through 295.9x, 298.80, 295.40, 295.70, 297.30, 298.90)

Long-term Outcomes	Short-term Outcomes*	Nursing Strategies
Work through fears of relating to others Increase confidence in ability to function in the world	Begin to verbalize Verbalize feelings of anxiety, inadequacy, helplessness (when consistent with client's cultural orientation) Build self-esteem in a realistic manner	Work toward establishing a trusting nurse-client relationship Maintain an attitude of patience and quiet optimism with client Communicate in simple, precise terms that are so phrased as to require an answer from the client Avoid excessive details and limit the introduction of new topics Orient client to the proposed length of time for the interaction and schedule of future interactions (repeat for each following interaction) Ask for *description* of actions and events rather than thoughts or feelings Avoid making the client's mute behavior a power struggle in any way

Nursing diagnosis: Alteration in activity level: *over-activity* related to biochemical imbalance and/or anxiety (NANDA 6.1 (proposed); DSM-III-R 295.1x through 295.9x, 298.80, 295.40, 295.70, 298.90)

Long-term Outcomes	Short-term Outcomes*	Nursing Strategies
Work through some of the fears of relating to other people Increase confidence in ability to function in the world Realistically perceive the five subsystems of self (biological, psychological, intellectual, sociocultural, and spiritual strengths	Decrease level of activity Meet needs for adequate rest, exercise, food, personal hygiene, and leisure activity Verbalize feelings of anxiety, inadequacy, and helplessness (when consistent with client's cultural orientation) Identify interpersonal situations that arouse feelings of anxiety, inadequacy, and helplessness Relate current stressful interpersonal or mastery situations to situations in the past that aroused similar feelings Identify any effective coping behavior used during these past situations	Work toward establishing a trusting nurse-client relationship Assist client in reducing activity level (e.g., use of reduced-stimuli atmosphere; appropriate p.r.n. medications) Observe state of health and hygiene; client's subjective reports of physical condition may not be reliable when immersed in frenzied activity Assist client in meeting needs for adequate rest, exercise, personal hygiene and leisure activity (exercises and games that do not involve a great deal of concentration may help dissipate the tension and energy associated with a high state of anxiety for some clients) Plan to rotate staff members caring for client to prevent any one staff member from being overwhelmed by frenzied behavior and rapid speech that may be part of the client's symptoms Use complete but concise phrases when communicating with client; repetition may be necessary for a highly anxious client

*As in the case of underactivity, short-term goals may need to be viewed as intermediate or long-term, depending upon the degree of overactivity in the client.

Long-term Outcomes	Short-term Outcomes	Nursing Strategies

Nursing diagnosis: Alteration in activity level: *over-activity* related to biochemical imbalance and/or anxiety (NANDA 6.1 (proposed); DSM-III-R 295.1x through 295.9x, 298.80, 295.40, 295.70, 298.90)—cont'd

and weaknesses) in perspective	Develop more effective coping behavior and interpersonal skills Build self-esteem in a realistic manner	When client is able to, explore situations that arouse feelings of anxiety, inadequacy, and helplessness Help client identify any effective coping behavior used in the past Explore alternative coping behavior for the present and near future Encourage client in efforts to test out alternative coping behavior Encourage client, when ready, to participate in available activities (e.g., start with one-to-one situations, gradually progress to group) Consider the possibility that the overactivity may be evidence of an extrapyramidal reaction to antipsychotic medication and discuss with mental health team members (This is done concurrently with preceding strategies.)

Nursing diagnosis: Impaired social interaction related to biochemical imbalance and/or anxiety characterized by *verbal hostility* (NANDA 3.1.1; DSM-III-R 295.1x through 295.9x, and 297.10, 298.80, 295.40, 295.70, 298.90)

Work through any feelings of anxiety, anger, frustration, disappointment, and fear Learn to relate to others in a manner that is not	Verbalize feelings of anxiety, anger*, frustration, disappointment, and fear (when consistent with client's cultural orientation) Identify interpersonal situations that arouse these feelings Relate current stressful interpersonal situations to situations in the past that aroused similar feelings	Work toward establishing a trusting nurse-client relationship Assist client in verbalizing feelings Help client explore interpersonal situations that arouse feelings of anxiety, anger, frustration, disappointment, and fear Help client relate any current stressful interpersonal situation to past situations that aroused similar feelings Help client to identify any effective coping behavior that was used in past situations Explore alternative coping behavior and ways of relat-

*The expression of anger serves a purpose. It substitutes a more comfortable feeling for feelings of anxiety, and it provides relief from the tension that comes from being frustrated or disappointed or from a threat to self-esteem (Hays, 1963). Verbally expressed anger is a more mature form of behavior than the physically expressed anger that previously may have resulted in many unpleasant situations for the client. Jurgen Ruesch (1957) views communication as a continuum. Acting out one's feelings—a primitive form of communicating—is situated on one end of the continuum. Verbalizing one's feelings—a more developed form of communicating—is on the other end. Interestingly, Ruesch (1957) views psychosomatic illness as being in the middle, between acted-out feelings and verbalized feelings:

Acted-out	**Psychosomatic**	**Verbalized**
feelings	**illness**	**feelings**

The client who is able to express feelings of anger and hostility is demonstrating a healthier, more mature form of communicating.

Continued.

NURSING CARE PLAN—cont'd

Clients with Schizophrenia

Long-term Outcomes	Short-term Outcomes	Nursing Strategies

Nursing diagnosis: Impaired social interaction related to biochemical imbalance and/or anxiety characterized by *verbal hostility* (NANDA 3.1.1; DSM-III-R 295.1x through 295.9x, and 297.10, 298.80, 295.40, 295.70, 298.90)—cont'd

hostile and that allows for appropriate expression of anger Develop more effective coping behavior and interpersonal skills Realistically perceive the five subsystems of self (biological, psychological, intellectual, sociocultural, and spiritual strengths and weaknesses) in perspective	Identify any effective coping behavior used in the past under similar circumstances Try out more effective coping behaviors and interpersonal skills in present and near future Build self-esteem in a realistic manner	ing with client Support client in any efforts to try out alternative coping behavior and ways of relating to others Allow verbal expression of hostility toward you as the nurse when it occurs; adopt a *nondefensive stance* to avoid escalation of client's defensive reaction of verbal hostility; instead, use the situation to explore client's anger as described above Intervention on the part of the nurse may be necessary, at times, to protect the self-esteem of other clients when they are the recipients of the angry feelings and verbal hostility

Nursing diagnosis: Potential for violence: directed at others related to biochemical imbalance and/or paranoid ideation (NANDA 9.2.2; DSM-III-R 295.1x through 295.9x, 297.10, 298.80, 295.40, 295.70, 298.90)

Work through any feelings of anxiety, anger, frustration, disappointment, or threats to the self-system Learn to ex-	Identify feelings of anxiety, anger, frustration, disappointment, or threats to the self-system Verbalize these feelings over a period of time (and in a manner consistent with cultural orientation) Relate current stressful interpersonal situations in the past that aroused similar	Protect client, self, and others from harm* *Prevent* physical aggression from happening whenever possible (e.g., observe levels of tension and anxiety early; judicious use of p.r.n. medication—chemical restraints; the use of "quiet" rooms to cut down on threatening environmental stimuli; work with client in a way that encourages communication of a need for sedation *before* tension becomes unbearable) When a situation has reached the point where a client is clearly exhibiting signs of assaultiveness, some points are helpful to remember:

*Implies that the locus of decision making is no longer with the client (e.g., the client is exhibiting assaultive behavior).

Long-term Outcomes	Short-term Outcomes	Nursing Strategies

Nursing diagnosis: Potential for violence: directed at others related to biochemical imbalance and/or paranoid ideation (NANDA 9.2.2; DSM-III-R 295.1x through 295.9x, 297.10, 298.80, 295.40, 295.70, 298.90)—cont'd

press feelings verbally rather than resorting to a physical "acting out" Develop more effective coping behavior and interpersonal skills Realistically perceive the five subsystems of self (biological, psychological, intellectual, sociocultural, and spiritual strengths and weaknesses) in perspective	feelings Relate difficulties in interpersonal relationships and the inability to gain satisfaction from the environment to the reliance on physical aggression as a mode of expressing feelings Identify any effective coping behavior used in the past under similar circumstances Try out other, more effective coping behaviors and interpersonal skills in present and near future Build self-esteem in a realistic manner	• A unit should have a preplanned way of dealing with such incidents; all staff members should know what it is • The self-esteem of the client should be protected through the nurse's attitude and communication • Since anxiety is contagious, a calm attitude on the nurse's part may also help to soothe the client • Staff members should avoid smiling at the client. A suspicious, paranoid person may feel he or she is being laughed at • A sufficient number of staff members should be available to deal with the problem physically. Even the frailest of psychotic clients can exhibit tremendous strength under conditions of panic. But a nurse should not automatically use all staff members present at the scene to surround the client at close quarters. Sometimes the very sight of a number of staff members in the background will quiet an assaultive client, while a feeling of being surrounded can be a threat that increases panic Work toward establishing a trusting nurse-client relationship* Help client identify feelings of anxiety, anger, frustration, and disappointment or threats to the self-system Assist client in verbalizing these feelings over a period of time Help client to relate current stressful interpersonal situations to situations in the past that aroused similar feelings Assist client to relate difficulties in interpersonal relationships and inability to gain satisfaction from the environment to the reliance on physical aggression as a way of expressing feelings Help client identify any effective coping behavior used in the past under similar circumstances Explore alternative coping behavior and ways of relating to others with client Support client in any efforts to try out alternative coping behavior and ways of relating to others

*This and the following strategies are appropriate after the threatening situation has been resolved.

Continued.

NURSING CARE PLAN—cont'd

Clients with Schizophrenia

Long-term Outcomes	Short-term Outcomes	Nursing Strategies

Nursing diagnosis: Impaired social interaction related to biochemical imbalance, altered thought processes. Characterized by *fear and suspicion of others* (NANDA 3.1.1; DSM-III-R 295.1x through 295.9x, 297.10, 298.80, 295.40, 295.70, 298.90)

Long-term Outcomes	Short-term Outcomes	Nursing Strategies
Work through some of the fears of relating to other people Develop an increased ability to trust other people Realistically perceive the five subsystems of self (biological, psychological, intellectual, sociocultural, and spiritual strengths and weaknesses) in perspective	Verbalize feelings of anxiety, inadequacy, helplessness (when consistent with client's cultural orientation) Verbalize suspicions and fears of other people Learn to clarify any doubts, suspicions, or possible misinterpretations of other people's communications or actions Identify situations that arouse feelings of suspicion Relate current stressful situations to situations in the past that aroused similar feelings of fear and suspicion Identify any effective coping behavior used during these past situations Increase self-esteem in a realistic manner	Work toward establishing a trusting nurse-client relationship Help client to verbalize feelings Help client identify situations that arouse feelings of suspicion Help client relate current stressful situations to situations in the past that aroused similar feelings of fear and suspicion Identify any effective coping behavior used during these past situations A client who is habitually suspicious of other people requires a thoughtful and consistent nursing approach. The following are some helpful points: • A matter-of-fact attitude is better than one that is overly warm. While a nurse's warmth may be an asset with other clients, in this situation it can arouse even more of the client's feelings of suspicion ("Why is she pretending to be my friend?" "What does she really want?") • In situations in which an apology may be appropriate (for example, a nurse is delayed because of another client and is late for a scheduled appointment) offer the apology in a matter-of-fact way and avoid overdoing it; profuse apologies may elicit increased suspicion • Physical contact should be avoided—it can be interpreted by a paranoid client as a sexual advance or threat • Too much eye contact can be threatening, while too little can arouse suspicion • Nonverbal behavior is important—smiling may be misinterpreted by a suspicious client • Speak clearly and concisely and with sufficient loudness; there should be no chance for a client to misinterpret what is being said; the use of the communication technique of consensual validation may be helpful • Never hide medications in the food of any client but particularly that of a client who has difficulty trusting others; in situations in which the nurse is taking notes while talking with the client, the nurse should be prepared to let the client read them at any time he or she seems concerned

Long-term Outcomes	Short-term Outcomes	Nursing Strategies

Nursing diagnosis: Impaired social interaction related to biochemical imbalance and/or anxiety, characterized by *inappropriate, dysfunctional* and/or *stereotypical behavior* (NANDA 3.1.1; DSM-III-R 295.1x through 295.9x, 298.80, 295.40, 295.70, 298.90)—cont'd

		• The need to control and the fear of being controlled often characterize a suspicious client; avoid power struggles or situations wherein nurse or client is required to be dominant or submissive; the client should be allowed as many opportunities for decision making as possible; but avoid a situation wherein efforts to provide such opportunities result in being manipulated or feeling controlled by the client
		• Be aware of, and allow for, the need-fear dilemma of the client; the client should be allowed to set the pace for the closeness of the relationship and to backtrack whenever the degree of closeness becomes threatening
		• Nurses should be honest about their own feelings when asked about them by clients; a suspicious person is usually very sensitive in interpersonal situations and may "test" in this way to see if the nurse really can be trusted

Nursing diagnosis: Impaired verbal communication: inappropriate, *symbolic verbalization* related to biochemical imbalance and/or anxiety (NANDA 2.1.1.1; DSM-III-R 295.1x through 295.9x, 297.10, 298.80, 295.40, 295.70, 298.90)

Long-term Outcomes	Short-term Outcomes	Nursing Strategies
Work through some of the fears of relating to other people Increase ability to communicate effectively and directly	Identify difficulties in communicating with others • Increase awareness of the tendency to use symbolic forms of communication • Increase awareness of the difficulties others have in understanding one's symbolic communication Identify interpersonal situa-	Work toward establishing a trusting relationship with the client Assist client in identifying difficulties in communicating with others* • Confront client when symbolic forms of communication are used • Let client know of the difficulty you experience in trying to understand when symbolic communication is used† Use the communication techniques of *consensual vali-*

*The verbalizations of schizophrenics are often quite difficult to follow. Loose association of thoughts, the use of neologisms, a tendency to use pronouns in unusual ways, and pathological thinking all are elements in a way of communicating that is disguised, confusing, and ineffective in facilitating interpersonal relationships. Decoding this communication pattern and helping the client to learn clearer ways of communicating with others are important nursing problems. Some particularly helpful communication techniques include consensual validation, asking for clarification, exploring content, and asking for amplification (Hays and Larson, 1963).

†It is essential that you let the client know when you do not understand—don't let things slip by because of the fear of alienating the client by asking for clarification frequently. The client may be testing to see if you are interested enough to ask for this clarification. Also, not asking for clarification may reinforce a client's ineffective way of communicating with others.

It is important to avoid fostering the notion that either the nurse or the client can read the other's mind. Such notions are not at all uncommon among schizophrenics. Responding to hints, inferring meanings that are not obvious or intended, offering interpretive statements, and finishing the other person's sentences are all examples of communication techniques that are not therapeutic. *Continued.*

NURSING CARE PLAN—cont'd

Clients with Schizophrenia

Long-term Outcomes	Short-term Outcomes	Nursing Strategies

Nursing diagnosis: Impaired verbal communication: inappropriate, *symbolic verbalization* related to biochemical imbalance and/or anxiety (NANDA 2.1.1.1; DSM-III-R 295.1x through 295.9x, 297.10, 298.80, 295.40, 295.70, 298.90)—cont'd

with other people Realistically perceive the five subsystems of self (biological, psychological, intellectual, sociocultural, and spiritual strengths and weaknesses) in perspective	tions that elicit increased reliance on symbolic communication Relate current stressful interpersonal situations in the past that tended to elicit increased reliance on symbolic communication Relate difficulties in interpersonal relating, in the ability to function, and in the ability to gain satisfaction from the environment to the reliance on symbolic forms of communication Develop more effective communication and interpersonal skills (e.g., seeking clarification, asking for validation)	*dation, asking for clarification, exploring content* and *asking for amplification* (Hays and Larson, 1963) Help the client identify interpersonal situations that elicit increased reliance on symbolic communication Help client relate difficulties in relating and functioning to the reliance on symbolic communication Assist client in developing more effective communication and interpersonal skills

Nursing diagnosis: Impaired social interaction related to biochemical imbalance and/or anxiety, characterized by *inappropriate, dysfunctional* and/or *stereotypical behavior* (NANDA 3.1.1; DSM-III-R 295.1x through 295.9x, 298.80, 295.40, 295.70, 298.90)

Work through some of the fears of relating to people Increase level of social awareness Increase interpersonal skills Realistically perceive the five subsystems of self	Verbalize any feelings of anxiety and any fears of interpersonal relating (when consistent with client's cultural orientation) Increase awareness of effects of behavior in interpersonal situations Identify interpersonal situations that tend to elicit dysfunctional social behavior Develop more effective coping behavior and interpersonal skills Increase self-esteem in a re-	Establish a trusting nurse-client relationship For regressed schizophrenic clients who are hospitalized, masturbation in public is one possible form of dysfunctional social behavior; ritualistic or stereotypical behavior is another. The implementation of a helpful, cooperative nurse-client plan should include the following: • Nonjudgmental acceptance of the client • Awareness of the purpose the behavior serves on the part of both client and staff (usually the behavior is used to help decrease anxiety or to communicate something) • Expectations on the part of the staff that the client can control behavior • Protection of other people from the client's behavior,

Long-term Outcomes	Short-term Outcomes	Nursing Strategies

Nursing diagnosis: Impaired social interaction related to biochemical imbalance and/or anxiety, characterized by *inappropriate, dysfunctional* and/or *stereotypical behavior* (NANDA 3.1.1; DSM-III-R 295.1x through 295.9x, 298.80, 295.40, 295.70, 298.90)—cont'd

(biological, psychological, intellectual, sociocultural, and spiritual strengths and weaknesses) in perspective	ality-based context	when necessary • Substitution of activities for the behavior (helpful in some cases) Help client to verbalize any feelings of anxiety and any fears of interpersonal relating Assist client in identifying situations that tend to elicit dysfunctional behavior Some types of behavior of regressed schizophrenics, while serving very real purposes, may get them into trouble in social situations; for example, a client who is very anxious may masturbate openly in a crowded day room; masturbation, besides providing relief from tension for a psychotic client, may be a substitute for interpersonal relatedness and a way of maintaining reality contact (Gibney, 1972); this statement suggests several possible elements of nursing intervention: • The rest of the client population may need to be protected from a scene that could be anxiety provoking; the needs of the entire group are important to consider • The client's need to masturbate and for increased social awareness can best be served by suggesting, in a nonjudgmental way, that a more private place be found • A nurse can respond to the message that the client may need or wish greater interpersonal contact by increasing his or her efforts to relate to the client and by encouraging the client to relate to others in the unit • Masturbation that has become compulsive may indicate severe regression

Nursing diagnosis: Personal identity disturbance: *depersonalization* and/or *loose ego boundaries* related to biochemical imbalance and/or anxiety (NANDA 7.1.3; DSM-III-R 295.1x through 295.9x, 298.80, 295.40, 295.70, 298.90)

Work through some of the conflicts that are generating the underlying anxiety Develop a	Recognize the relationship between escalating anxiety and the subjective experience of depersonalization and other manifestations of loose ego boundaries Verbalize and explore feelings about current inner	Work toward establishing a trusting nurse-client relationship. Assist client in recognizing the relationship between escalating anxiety and feelings of depersonalization and other manifestations of loose ego boundaries: feelings of strangeness and estrangement or thinking that one's body or objects in the environment have changed are all highly anxiety provoking. They are

Continued.

NURSING CARE PLAN—cont'd

Clients with Schizophrenia

Long-term Outcomes	Short-term Outcomes	Nursing Strategies

Nursing diagnosis: Personal identity disturbance: *depersonalization* and/or *loose ego boundaries* related to biochemical imbalance and/or anxiety (NANDA 7.1.3; DSM-III-R 295.1x through 295.9x, 298.80, 295.40, 295.70, 298.90)—cont'd

Long-term Outcomes	Short-term Outcomes	Nursing Strategies
clearer, more consistent sense of self Increase the ability to cope with stress without the use of psychotic defenses or severe distortions of reality Realistically perceive the five subsystems of self (biological, psychological, intellectual, sociocultural, and spiritual strengths and weaknesses) in perspective	conflicts, current stressful situations in life (when consistent with client's cultural orientation) Recognize and differentiate inner (intrapsychic) stimuli and outer (environmental) stimuli Increase self-esteem in a reality-based context	also anxiety based. Such situations are examples of anxiety feeding upon itself. A nurse can combat this escalation by explaining that depersonalization is a by-product of increased anxiety, the nurse can remove the unknown, frightening quality and interrupt a vicious circle. Things that are unknown or unexplained are always frightening to the person experiencing them. Depersonalization increases with increasing anxiety, and it is a part of the phenomenon of loose ego boundaries. Assist client in differentiating inner from outer stimuli: • No clear concept of self, getting one's needs and desires "mixed up" with other people's, difficulty in forming opinions on any subject, and problems in differentiating internal stimuli from environmental stimuli are all manifestations of loose ego boundaries. The phenomenon can be thought of as a dynamic continuum on which manifestations range from indecisiveness and lack of clarity about one's own feelings to having a delusion that one has been transformed into someone else. • Sometimes loose ego boundaries will result in mild or intense identification with another person. For example, expressing a desire to be a nurse, stating that one really is a nurse, wearing the same sort of clothes, copying a hairstyle, and so forth may all be indications that a client is identifying with the nurse. Saying things like "You'd like to go down to the music room" when wanting to go there oneself is also an indication. It is important that a nurse use correcting, clarifying statements such as "Did you mean that you would like to go to the music room?" Differences between the nurse and the client should be pointed out whenever appropriate.

Long-term Outcomes	Short-term Outcomes*	Nursing Strategies

Nursing diagnosis: Altered thought processes: nonreality-based thinking related to biochemical imbalance and/or anxiety; characterized by *delusional thinking*† (NANDA 8.3; DSM-III-R 295.1x through 295.9x, 297.10, 298.80, 295.40, 295.70, 298.90)

Long-term Outcomes	Short-term Outcomes*	Nursing Strategies
Work though some of the conflicts that are generating the underlying anxiety Work through some of the fears of relating to other people Increase the ability to cope with stress without the tendency to severely distort, misperceive, misinterpret and exaggerate Realistically perceive the five subsystems of self	Recognize the relationship between escalating anxiety and the increased tendency to severely distort, misperceive, misinterpret, and exaggerate Identify any difficulties in interpersonal relating and in functioning in the world that are related to the tendency to severely distort, misperceive misinterpret, and exaggerate Verbalize and explore feelings about current stressful situations in life Increase self-esteem in a realistic manner	Work toward establishing a trusting nurse-client relationship. Assist client in recognizing the relationship between escalating anxiety and an increased tendency to distort, misperceive, misinterpret, and exaggerate. Assist client in recognizing any difficulties in interpersonal relating and functioning in the world that may be related to the tendency to distort, misperceive, misinterpret, and exaggerate. Encourage verbalization of feelings. The following are some points to consider in responding to the client who is experiencing delusions: • Collect data before formulating a response; in the beginning, noncommittal responses may be necessary. In some situations you may only suspect that a client is making a delusional statement. It is easy to make a judgment when the client says she is the Virgin Mary and that she is being controlled from the planet Mars, but a client who tells you she has 16 children may be telling you about an actual situation. Then again, she may not be, since this is a fairly common sort of delusion. Give the client the benefit of the doubt until you know whether he or she is suffering from a delusion, but remain fairly noncommittal in your responses. • In responding to the client's delusion, convey your acceptance of a need for the belief while letting the client know you do not agree with the delusion.

*For a client who has been delusional for many years, these long-term goals may never be achieved. See pp. 821-822 for different approaches to delusional clients based on this point.

†Because of the inevitable denigrating connotations that the term delusional can elicit, it is not a helpful term to use with a client in planning care (an exception might be a client, recovering emotional health, who has accepted that he or she has been delusional and refers to the experience in direct terms). Less threatening terminology for most clients would be distortions, misperceptions, misinterpretations, exaggerations.

Continued.

NURSING CARE PLAN—cont'd

Clients with Schizophrenia

Long-term Outcomes*	Short-term Outcomes†	Nursing Strategies

Nursing diagnosis: Altered thought processes: nonreality-based thinking related to biochemical imbalance and/or anxiety; characterized by *delusional thinking* (NANDA 8.3; DSM-III-R 295.1x through 295.9x, 297.10, 298.80, 295.40, 295.70, 298.90)—cont'd

Long-term Outcomes*	Short-term Outcomes†	Nursing Strategies
(biological, psychological, intellectual, sociocultural, and spiritual strengths and weaknesses) in perspective		• Do not argue with the client about the belief—incorporating reasonable doubt as a communication technique is more effective. • If possible, connect the belief to the client's feelings (for example, "It's possible to misinterpret things when anxiety is very high" or "Things can seem like they're out of control when you're frightened"). • Respond to the core of the delusion. If low self-esteem is at the core, try to help the client build self-esteem in a realistic way. An individual who thinks that there is a complex and well-controlled plot against him or her may need to express anger appropriately in everyday situations.

Nursing diagnosis: Sensory/perceptual alterations: *hallucinations‡* related to biochemical imbalance, anxiety, fears of interpersonal relating (NANDA 7.2; DSM-III-R 295.1x through 295.9x, 297.10, 298.80, 295.40, 295.70, 298.90)

Long-term Outcomes*	Short-term Outcomes†	Nursing Strategies
Work through some of the conflicts that are generating the underlying anxiety Increase the ability to cope with stress without the reliance on hallucinations Realistically perceive the five subsystems of self	Verbalize the content of any hallucinations (important especially in the case of command hallucinations) Identify the times and situations when the tendency to hallucinate increases Recognize the relationship between escalating anxiety and an increased tendency to hallucinate Identify any difficulties in interpersonal relating and in functioning in the world that are related to the reliance on hallucinating as a defense Verbalize and explore feel-	Work toward establishing a trusting nurse-client relationship. Approaches to hallucinations depend upon the need they are serving and upon the length of time the client has been experiencing them. If a client has been hearing voices for a short time, it is important to know what the voices say, since they could be command hallucinations (commands to commit suicide or homicide, for example). It is helpful to know if the hallucinations are frightening, degrading, or kind and helpful to the client. The therapeutic response in each situation would be different. In the case of a person who has hallucinated over a long period of time, a nurse might not be as concerned with content as with when the client tends to hallucinate. This information is useful if the nurse intends to distract the client back to reality or to attempt to decrease anxiety and thus the need for hal-

*For a client who has relied on (comforting) hallucinations for years, these long-term goals may never be achieved.
†Depending upon the degree of regression in the client, short-term goals may be intermediate or even long-term goals.
‡Hallucinations are false sensory perceptions. They can be auditory, visual, tactile, olfactory, gustatory, or kinesthetic. The majority of schizophrenic hallucinations are auditory. In fact, the occurrence of auditory hallucinations is correlated so strongly with schizophrenia that some suggest that it be considered a fifth "A" to be tacked on the Bleuler's original "four A's" (Hofling et al., 1967).

Hallucinations are seen in conditions other than schizophrenia such as those associated with very high fevers and toxic conditions. The nursing intervention is the same.

Long-term Outcomes	Short-term Outcomes	Nursing Strategies

Nursing diagnosis: Sensory/perceptual: *hallucinations*‡ related to biochemical imbalance, anxiety, fears of interpersonal relating (NANDA 7.2; DSM-III-R 295.1x through 295.9x, 297.10, 298.80, 295.40, 295.70, 298.90)—cont'd

Long-term Outcomes	Short-term Outcomes	Nursing Strategies
(biological, psychological, intellectual, sociocultural, and spiritual strengths and weaknesses) in perspective	ings about current stressful situations in life Increase self-esteem in a reality-based context	lucinations. Also, continually focusing on content that is already well known might reinforce the hallucinations. In general, the following points are helpful in the treatment of the hallucinating client: • An accepting approach will encourage the client to share the content and the times of hallucination. It is important to accept the client and the need for the hallucinations and to accept the fact that while you do not share these perceptions, the client does indeed experience them. • Determine the content of the hallucinations to prevent possible injury to client or to others from command hallucinations. • When discussing hallucinations, phrase your comments in such a way as to avoid reinforcing the hallucinations. For example, "What do the voices *seem* to be saying when you get anxious?" rather than "What are the voices telling you to do?" • Respond to and reinforce the aspects of reality that the client reacts to. Connect the hallucinations to anxiety as an explanation that might prevent the escalating sequence of increased anxiety, increased hallucination, increased anxiety. • Be alert for times of hallucinating. Arieti (1975) has identified a "listening pose" that a schizophrenic who is hallucinating may assume. Other workers identified mumbling or "subvocalizing" as indicators of hallucination (*Discover*, April, 1987). • Distract the client at times of hallucinating. Bring the client back to reality through interpersonal involvement and activities. • In cases of clients who have hallucinated chronically, instructions to "talk back" to voices, telling them to "shut up," have sometimes helped, since they can give the client a feeling of control over these symptoms and thus decrease anxiety. This technique must be used with a clear message that the voices are not awesome realities but symptoms of anxiety.

EVALUATION

The client, and, whenever feasible, the client's family or significant others should be included in estimating the client's progress toward attainment of goals. Evaluation should encompass the following areas:

1. Estimation of the degree to which there has been effective coping with any disorders of thought, mood, feeling, sensation, perception, and behavior. This would include *awareness* of tendency to use withdrawal from interpersonal relationships and from reality and beginning efforts toward modifying this.

2. Estimation of the degree to which goals have been achieved and client functioning has improved (demonstrated by decreased disorder in interpersonal relationships; increased ability to function in society; decreased reliance on withdrawal mechanisms, and increased self-esteem and increased interpersonal and social involvement)

3. Identification of goals that need to be modified or revised

4. Referral of the client to support systems other than the nurse-client relationship
   a. People in the client's social network who are willing to serve as a support system
   b. Clinics or individuals for ongoing individual, supportive psychotherapy
   c. Community agencies that help clients and their families learn to live with disorders that may never be completely eliminated (e.g., Recovery, Inc.; Schizophrenics Anonymous)
   d. Centers or organizations that focus on rehabilitation for the schizophrenic client and on specialized treatment of specific problem areas (e.g., vocational counseling, family therapy, family support groups, day hospitals, medication administration and supervision)

TERTIARY PREVENTION

While an individual may experience one schizophrenic break, recover, and perhaps never have another, schizophrenia is most often a chronic disorder.

According to Mendel and Green (1967), two elements that are most needed in the lives of chronic schizophrenics and that can be fostered through supportive relationship therapy are *organization* and *structure*. A chronic schizophrenic's whole life is unstructured and disorganized; the ordinary activities of daily living seem overwhelming. The goals of supportive therapy are to foster remission, to prevent complications, and to support the functioning of the schizophrenic client. Mendel and Green transform the "as if" phenomenon, a symptom that appears in the preschizophrenic state, into a concept that can be used as a therapeutic aid for the chronic schizophrenic. They suggest that a therapist say to a client, "OK, so you *don't* feel like you have the ability to get up, get dressed, and go to work every morning—act *as if* you can." After the client has done so for a number of mornings, ego strength will be gained from having accomplished something that seemed overwhelming.

Mendel and Green also advocate long-term involvement between a helping professional and the chronic schizophrenic. In some cases the amount of this involvement may be decreased, during times of low anxiety and adequate functioning, to a monthly or even yearly "check in" with the therapist. Of course, at times of developmental or situational crises, involvement would be increased again.

The schizophrenic, the community, and tertiary prevention

What was probably one of the most ideal communities for discharged schizophrenics ever to be devised existed at one time in the village of Gheel, Belgium. This town is situated near a shrine to St. Dymphna, the patron saint of the mentally ill, and a psychiatric hospital dedicated to her. During the Middle Ages and later, people from all over the world came to the shrine and hospital, hoping for saintly intervention in their illness. After treatment at the hospital they were often discharged into the town. Some lived in the village while they awaited admission to the hospital. The villagers were quite accepting of them; eccentric behavior was tolerated, and individuals were allowed to participate in the community to the degree that they were able.

Unfortunately, in the United States today there are few such friendly and accepting communities. An exception is *Fountain House* (Rehab Brief, 1982), a "club for former mental patients." Fountain House was started in the early 1940s by a small group of former "patients" from a New York State psychiatric hospital. Their goal was to achieve successful deinstitutionalization* through cooperative efforts. The club has grown tremendously, and the Fountain House concept has provided a model for other, similar efforts. For example, Plymouth House (on the grounds of Pilgrim State Hospital in Brentwood, New York) used the Fountain House model and offers its services not only to discharged clients but to those still hospitalized who choose to take advantage of them.

There are four primary beliefs in the Fountain House concept:

1. People with emotional disabilities, even severe ones, have productive potential.
2. Work is important for all people.
3. Everyone needs social relationships.
4. All people need adequate housing.

The staff of Fountain House continually conveys four basic messages to the members:

1. Fountain House is a club and its participants are members, not clients.
2. Members are made to feel that their participation is expected and that staff anticipate their arrival with pleasure.
3. Members are wanted as contributors to the club.
4. Members are needed by the club, staff, and other members.

Various community and professional and volunteer services are also provided. While more research needs to be done into the effectiveness of the Fountain House model, it does hold out some hope for successful adjustment to the community and for improvement in living for some schizophrenic clients.

However, a discharged schizophrenic too often faces a harsh, intolerant, and unwelcoming community situation. Aftercare for mental illness has not been a major priority in our country; it can only be described as inadequate. We have the knowledge

*For in-depth discussion of deinstitutionalization, see Chapter 16.

of what is required to provide optimum aftercare services for chronic schizophrenics, but most often only lip service is paid to the ideals. Partial hospitalization, a part of aftercare, has been found to be effective in treating severely disturbed clients, and it has been found to be cost-effective in many comparative studies with full hospitalization (Neal, 1986). It was estimated that approximately 40% of the cost was saved. Services that are available to a limited degree in some communities, include the following:

1. *Transitional services*—a concept that includes a gradual lessening of the client's dependent ties with the hospital. Clients are given lessons and help in tasks of everyday living. Particularly in the case of a client who has been institutionalized for a long time, many skills may not have been learned or they may have been long since forgotten. Helping a client to arrange for suitable living accommodations is another transitional service.
2. *Day care centers*—for the client who has a supportive, accepting home environment but who cannot yet function in a job. This service provides structure to the day, opportunities for socialization, and a chance to learn some skills. In addition, medication may be supervised in such a center.
3. *Night hospitals*—for the client who can function in a job but has no suitable living arrangements. Perhaps, as is so often the case with the chronic schizophrenic, there are no family ties. The client may also benefit from supportive therapy within the night hospital. For instance, group therapy sessions may be held in the evening as part of the hospital's program.
4. *Halfway houses and foster homes*—for the client who does not have a family or whose family can no longer support him or her. Such a client needs some supervision in such areas as diet, medication, recreation, and activities of daily living. Some foster homes in a community may be excellent; others may be deplorable. A system of inspection before placement is therefore crucial to the protection of the client's welfare.

5. *Rehabilitation, vocational training, and sheltered workshops*—retraining in old skills and training in new skills to help the client function to the maximum of potential and strengthen self-esteem.

6. *Token economy programs*—for severely regressed schizophrenics. These programs, which have been used in some psychiatric inpatient and outpatient facilities, involve a form of behavior modification. Tokens that can be exchanged for goods (snack foods or clothing) or privileges are given in return for participation in certain activities. For example, a token may be given for making one's bed in the morning or for attending group therapy sessions. Such a program can be useful if it is carried out in a way that protects the dignity of the client. Unhappily, this is not always the case.

Working with family and client

An important aspect of the tertiary care of schizophrenics is the supervision of medications. Failure to take prescribed drugs is one of the most common reasons for readmission to hospitals. A drug like prolixin, which can be given in two-week intervals, is very often useful. But the most important aspect of tertiary care is the continuing and regular involvement of the community mental health nurse with the client's family. Some hospitals provide "crisis teams" of hospital personnel—people the client has known while in the hospital.

Three important guidelines for a community mental health team to provide and monitor services such as medication supervision and psychosocial intervention are:

1. Services should extend over decade-length periods, since schizophrenia is so often a lifelong disturbance.
2. Since the clinical course of schizophrenia tends to be episodic, services should include a crisis-oriented component.
3. Services may be provided over decades, yet they need to be provided *precisely* enough to fit a widely fluctuating severity in the condition. This implies that the client must be enabled to take a role in regulating the medication (self-regulation through education) (Hansell, 1978).

Education of families is often as important as education of clients. A study at the University of Southern California School of Medicine reported that when families are taught to talk out their problems and to use the problem-solving method, identified clients are more likely to remain free of schizophrenic symptoms (*Newsday*, 1982).

Home visits at times of increased anxiety for the client may prevent rehospitalization. It is essential that a nurse engage the family of the chronic schizophrenic, along with the client, as part of the treatment team. It is especially important to avoid arousing any feelings of guilt in family members, since such feelings can lead to withdrawal from involvement with helping professionals and perhaps to a withdrawal from the client. Family members can be helpful in alerting professionals to increasing anxiety in the client, and they can assist in the supervision of medications. In addition, they can help modify environmental stress in the client's life and facilitate the client's necessary acceptance of his or her illness.

CHAPTER SUMMARY

Schizophrenia is a disorder of thought, mood, feeling, sensation, perception, and behavior. It is characterized by a disturbed ego, no clear concept of self, and inadequate ways of communicating with and relating to other people. Schizophrenia is a major health problem. It affects 0.5% to 1.2% of the population of the United States, and there is some evidence that the incidence is increasing (Aiken, 1987; Torrey 1983)

Schizophrenia was originally called *dementia praecox* (dementia of the young); its incidence seems to be highest among young adults, but it can occur at any age. *Schizophrenia*, the term invented by Bleuler, means "split mind"; it refers to a splitting apart of some of the functions of the mind. For instance, thoughts and feelings that normally go together may be split apart.

The disorder occurs in all cultures and all socioeconomic groups, but for complex reasons it is strongly correlated with poverty.

Several systems for classifying schizophrenia are

in existence. Some writers believe that schizophrenia is actually several disorders and therefore refer to "the schizophrenias."

The exact underlying basis of schizophrenia is unknown, but several theories have been postulated. These include genetic, biochemical, intrapsychic, interpersonal, family, communication systems, sociological, and adaptation theories. An eclectic or multifactorial approach that acknowledges a biological mediation of stress-related disorder is most widely accepted.

Treatment for schizophrenia includes somatic approaches (particularly the use of drugs), psychotherapy, group and family therapy, and occupational and recreational therapy. Primary prevention at this time is limited mainly to the identification of high-risk groups. Secondary prevention currently focuses on the belief that much of the deterioration

in the condition of a schizophrenic may result from institutionalization rather than from the disorder itself. A more active treatment approach has provided a much better prognosis for recovery. However, schizophrenia is often a chronic disorder. Tertiary prevention of schizophrenia involves a cooperative, rehabilitative effort from health workers, client, and family. Adding support, structure and organization to the client's life and providing support and education for the family are important aspects of treatment.

In working with a schizophrenic client, a nurse helps most by assisting in the improvement of *communication skills* and *interpersonal skills*. *Therapeutic use of self* in an authentic relationship with the client is the most important component of nursing intervention.

SELF-DIRECTED LEARNING

Sensitivity-Awareness Exercises

The purposes of the following exercises are to:
- Develop awareness about the subjective experience of clients who are suffering from schizophrenic disorders
- Develop awareness about the subjective experience of the families of clients who are suffering from schizophrenic disorders
- Develop awareness about your own feelings and attitudes when working with clients who are suffering from schizophrenic disorders
- Develop awareness about the interrelationship of underlying factors in the development of schizophrenia

1. Try to imagine what it is like to experience one of the following symptoms:
   Auditory hallucinations
   Delusional thinking
   Depersonalization
   Loose ego boundaries
   Tardive dyskinesia
   Mutism
   Explain why you selected that particular symptom. Then describe what it would be like to experience it.

2. Describe what you think it would be like to have a family member who is suffering from chronic schizophrenia. How do you think you might cope with this? Which schizophrenic symptom do you think it would be most difficult for you to accept in a family member?

3. Imagine that you are a community mental health nurse engaged in health supervision activities with new parents. What high risk factors would you observe for that might predispose children to developing a schizophrenic disorder?

4. Develop a plan for teaching and counselling parents about parent-child interaction that incorporates principles and goals for the primary prevention of schizophrenia.

Questions to Consider

1. The genetic research studies concerning the subsequent development of schizophrenia have demonstrated:
   a. a higher prevalence of the syndrome in the Scandinavian countries
   b. a higher degree of concordance for dizygotic twins
   c. that an unknown genetic factor is operating
   d. a significant decrease in eye-tracking disor-

Continued.

SELF-DIRECTED LEARNING—cont'd

Questions to Consider—cont'd

ders for the relatives of schizophrenic clients

2. Delusions are:
   a. false sensory perceptions related to paleological thinking
   b. evidenced in the individual by subvocalizations and the assumption of the "listening pose"
   c. usually built on a partly true premise
   d. the perceptual misinterpretation of an actual object or event

3. A classification of schizophrenia that is characterized by suspicion and overuse of the defense mechanism of projection is termed:
   a. paranoid schizophrenia
   b. simple schizophrenia
   c. catatonic schizophrenia
   d. hebephrenic schizophrenia

4. The prevalence of schizophrenia in the population is generally estimated to be:
   a. 1–1.5% of the population
   b. 10–15% of the population
   c. rapidly decreasing with the use of antipsychotic drugs
   d. approximately 10 times as common in children born in the autumn

Match the terms and descriptions:

5. Ideas of reference
6. Auditory hallucinations
7. Concrete thinking

   a. Difficulty with innuendo, sarcasm, abstract thinking
   b. "The devil made me do it"
   c. *Life Magazine* is a chronicle of my existence

8. Ideas of influence
   d. "They are saying I've given up my rights as the Virgin Mary and must become a prostitute."

9. The current, most widely accepted theory to explain schizophrenia is that it is:
   a. a definite physiological disorder
   b. a psychodynamic, functional disorder
   c. caused by the *schizophrenia mother*
   d. a biologically mediated, stress-related disorder

10. In responding therapeutically to the delusional client, the nurse should remember to *first:*
    a. give a logical, rational explanation for events that the client perceives as threatening
    b. respond to the client's feelings—the "core of the delusion"
    c. administer a prn antipsychotic medication
    d. refer the client to the most experienced team member

11. Tertiary prevention of schizophrenia includes:
    a. halfway houses, transitional services, and family support
    b. interactional mother-child coaching
    c. high-risk vulnerability studies
    d. brief hospitalization for initial episodes and antipsychotic medication

Answer key

1. c	7. a
2. c	8. b
3. a	9. d
4. a	10. b
5. c	11. a
6. d	

REFERENCES

Aiken L: Unmet needs of the chronically mentally ill: will nursing respond? Image: J Nurs Scholarship 19(3):121-125, 1987.

Altschule M: In Cancro R, editor: The schizophrenic reactions: a critique of the concept, hospital treatment and current research, New York, 1970, Brunner/Mazel, Inc.

Anderson C et al: Family treatment of adult schizophrenic patients: a psycho-educational approach, Schizophrenia Bull 6(3):490-497, 1980.

Andreason N: the diagnosis of schizophrenia, Schizophrenia Bull 13(1):490-497, 1987.

Andreason N: Brain imaging: applications in psychiatry, Science 239(4846):1381-1388, 1988.

Anscombe R: The disorder of consciousness in schizophrenia, Schizophrenia Bull 13(2):241-260, 1987.

Arieti S: Interpretation of schizophrenia, ed. 1, New York, 1955, Basic Books.

Arieti S: The intrapsychic self. New York, 1967, Basic Books.

Arieti S: Interpretation of schizophrenia, ed 2, New York, 1975, Basic Books.

Arieti S: Understanding and helping the schizophrenic: a guide for family and friends, New York, 1979, Simon & Schuster, Inc.

Arnold H: Working with schizophrenic patients, four A's: a guide to one-to-one relationships, Am J Nurs 6:941-943, 1976.

Arnold H: Is schizophrenia preventable? a psychoanalytic view, A paper presented at the Annual Nurse Scholar Series, First Endowed Hildegard E. Peplau Lecture, Rutgers College Alumni Association, April 15, 1983.

Bahnson CB: Psychophysiological complementarity in malignancies: past work and future vistas, Ann NY Acad Sci 125(3):827-845, 1969.

Bahnson CB: Epistemological perspectives of physical disease from the psychodynamic point of view, Am J Public Health 64(11):1036, 1974.

Bahnson CB and Bahnson MB: Cancer as an alternative to psychosis: a theoretical model of somatic and psychological regression. In Kissen DM and LeShan LL, editors: Psychosomatic aspects of neoplastic disease. Philadelphia, 1964, JB Lippincott Co.

Barnes D: Biological issues in schizophrenia, Science 235(4787):430-433, 1987.

Bassuk E et al., editors: The practitioner's guide to psychoactive drugs, ed 2, New York, 1983, Plenum Medical Book Co.

Bellak L: The schizophrenic syndrome: a further explanation of the unified theory of schizophrenia, In Bellak L, editor: Schizophrenia: a review of the syndrome, New York, 1958, Logos Press.

Bogerts B et al: A morphometric study of the dopamine containing cell groups in the mesoencephalon of normals, Parkinson patients and schizophrenics, Biol Psychiatr 18(9):951-969, 1983.

Bowen M: Theory in the practice of psychotherapy, In Guerin PJ, editor: Family therapy, New York, 1976, Gardner Press, Inc.

Bowen M: Workshop in family therapy, Mercy Hospital, Rockville Center, NY, 1977.

Boyers R and Orrill R, editors: R.D. Laing and anti-psychiatry, New York, 1971, Harper & Row, Publishers.

Burnham DL, Gladstone AI, and Gibson RW: Schizophrenia and the need-fear dilemma, New York, 1969, International Universities Press.

Cameron N: Personality development and psychopathology: a dynamic approach, Boston, 1963, Houghton Mifflin Co.

Campion E and Tucker G: A note on twin studies, schizophrenia and neurological impairment. In Cancro R, editor: Annual review of the schizophrenic syndrome, New York, 1973, Brunner/Mazel, Inc.

Carpenter E: Witch-fear among the Aivilik Eskimos, Am J Psychiatr 110(3):194-199, 1953.

Carpenter W: Thoughts on the treatment of schizophrenia, Schizophrenia Bull 12(4):527-539, 1986.

Carpenter W: Approaches to knowledge and understanding of schizophrenia, Schizophrenia Bull 13(1):1-8, 1987.

Chapman L and Chapman J: The search for symptoms predictive of schizophrenia, Schizophrenia Bull 13(3):497-503, 1987.

Crockett M: The client with a schizophrenic disorder, In Groton J and Partridge R, editors: Practice and management of psychiatric emergency care, St. Louis, 1982, The CV Mosby Co.

Diagnostic and Statistical Manual of Mental Disorders, ed 3, revised, American Psychiatric Association, Washington, DC, 1987.

Discover Magazine: Hushing the voices schizophrenics hear, Discover Magazine 8(4):4-5, 1987.

Donner, G: Treatment of a delusional patient, Am J Nurs 12:2642-2644, 1969.

Driscoll P: Maintenance mediation for chronic schizophrenics: risk/benefit assessment, Persp Psychiatr Care 23(3):104-110, 1985.

Edelstein P et al: Physostigmine and lithium response in the schizophrenias, Am J Psychiat 138:1078, 1981.

Eisenberg L: Psychiatric intervention, Sci Am 229(3):117-127, 1973.

Epstein S and Coleman M: Drive theories in schizophrenia, In Cancro R editor: The schizophrenic syndrome: an annual review, New York, 1971, Brunner/Mazel, Inc.

Falloon I et al: Family therapy of schizophrenics with high risk of relapse, Family Process 20(6):211-221, 1981.

Falloon I and Talbot R: Achieving the goals of day treatment, J Nervous Mental Dis 170:279-285, 1982.

Falloon I and Liberman R: Behavioral family intervention in the management of chronic schizophrenia, In McFarlane W, editor: Family therapy in schizophrenia, New York, 1983, Guilford Press.

Ferris P and Marshall C: A model project for families of the chronically mentally ill, Soc Work 32(2):110-114, 1987.

Field T: Interaction coaching for high-risk infants and their parents, In Prevention in human services, I(4), New York, 1982, The Haworth Press.

Field WE and Wilkerson S: Religiosity as a psychiatric symptom, Persp Psychiatr Care 11(3):99-105, 1973.

Foulks EF: Schizophrenia held useful for evolution, NY Times, December 9, 1975.

Frankl V: Man's search for meaning: an introduction to logotherapy, New York, 1959, Washington Square Press.

Fromm-Reichman F: Principles of intensive psychotherapy, Chicago, 1950, University of Chicago Press.

Garmezy N: Vulnerability research and the issue of primary prevention, Am J Orthopsychiatr 41:101-116, 1971.

Gibney H: Masturbation: an invitation for an interpersonal relationship, Persp Psychiat Care 10(3):128-134, 1972.

Goldfarb C and Goldfarb S: Multiple monitored electroconvulsive treatment, In Masserman JH editor: Current psychiatric therapies, vol 17, New York, 1977, Grune & Stratton, Inc.

Goldstein M: Psychosocial issues, Schizophrenia Bull 13(1):157-172, 1987.

Govoni L and Hayes J: Drugs and nursing implications, ed 4, Norwalk, Ct, 1982, Appleton-Century-Crofts.

Greenberg J: Fetal brain damage linked to schizophrenia, Sci News 124(11):164, 1983.

Grimm P: Psychotropic medications: nursing implications, Nurs Clin North Am 21(3):397-411, 1986.

Grinker R Sr: An essay on schizophrenia and science, Archi Gen Psychiatr 20:1-24, 1969.

Gunderson J et al: The Boston psychotherapy study II comparative outcome of two forms of treatment, Schizophrenia Bull 10(2):564-598, 1984.

Hansell N: Services for schizophrenics: a lifelong approach to treatment, Hosp Comm Psychiat 29(2):105-109, 1978.

Harrow M and Westermeyer J: Process-reactive dimension and outcome for narrow concepts of schizophrenia, Schizophrenia Bull 13(3):361-367, 1987.

Hartmann E: Toward a biology of the mind, In The psychoanalytic study of the child, 37. New York, 1982, International Universities Press.

Hartmann H: Contributions to the metapsychology of schizophrenia, In Essays on ego psychology by Heinz Hartmann, New York, 1984, International Universities Press.

Hatfield A et al: Expressed emotion: a family perspective, Schizophrenia Bull 13(2):221-226, 1987.

Hays DR: Anger: a clinical problem, In Burd S and Marshall M, editors: Some clinical approaches to psychiatric nursing, New York, 1963, Macmillan, Inc.

Hays JS and Larson KH: Interacting with patients, New York, 1963, Macmillan, Inc.

Heath R et al: Behavioral changes in nonpsychotic volunteers following the administration of tarexein, the substance obtained from the serum of schizophrenic patients, Am J Psychiat 114:917-920, 1958.

Herbert W: Schizophrenia clues in angel dust, Sci News 123(26):407, 1983a.

Herbert W: Mental illness from psychiatric drugs? Sci News 124(14):214, 1983b.

Herron W: Evaluating the process-reactive dimension, Schizophrenia Bull 13(3):357-359, 1987.

Hoffer A: Common questions on schizophrenia and their answers, New Canaan, Ct, 1987, Keats Publishing, Inc.

Hofling CK, Leininger MM, and Bregg E: Basic psychiatric concepts in nursing, ed 2, Philadelphia, 1967, JB Lippincott Co.

Holden C: A top priority at NIMH, Science 235(4787):431, 1987.

Holmes MJ: Influences of the new hospital psychiatry on nursing, In The new hospital psychiatry, New York, 1971, Academic Press, Inc.

Holzman D: Baring the brain of a schizophrenic, Insight, July 6:50-51, 1987.

Holzman P: Eye movement dysfuntions and psychosis, Int Rev Neurobiol 27(179):179-205, 1985.

Holzman P et al: Eye-tracking dysfunctions in schizophrenic patients and their relatives, In Cancro R, editor: Annual review of the schizophrenic syndrome, New York, 1974, Brunner/Mazel, Inc.

Howells JG: World history of psychiatry, New York, 1975, Brunner/Mazel, Inc.

Iodice J and Wodarski J: Aftercare treatment for schizophrenics living at home, Soc Work 32(2):122-128, 1987.

Ivker B and Sze W: Social work and the psychiatric nosology of schizophrenia, Soc Casework 68(3):131-139, 1987.

Jackson D: The etiology of schizophrenia, New York, 1960, Basic Books, Inc.

Kallman FJ: The genetics of schizophrenia, New York, 1938, Augustin.

Kanas N: Group therapy with schizophrenics: a review of controlled studies, Int J Group Psychother 36(3):339-349, 1986.

Kasanin JS, editor: Language and thought in schizophrenia, New York, 1944, WW Norton & Co. Inc.

Kendel R et al: Diagnostic criteria of American and British psychiatrists, Arch Gen Psychiatr 25(8):123-130, 1971.

Kendler K and Robinette C: Schizophrenia and the National Academy of Sciences–National Research Council twin registry: a 16-year update, Am J Psychiatr 140(12):1551-1563, 1983.

Kety S: Heredity and environment, In Shershow JC editor: Schizophrenia: science and practice, Cambridge, Mass, 1978, Harvard University Press.

Laing RD: The divided self, London, 1965a, Penguin Books. Mystification, confusion and conflict, In Boszormenyi-Nagy I and Framo JL, editors: Intensive family therapy: theoretical and practical aspects, New York, 1965b, Harper & Row.

Lidz T: The origin and treatment of schizophrenic disorders, New York, 1973, Basic Books.

Mahler M, Pine F, and Bergman A: The psychological birth of the human infant, New York, 1975, Basic Books, Inc.

Matorin S and De Chillo N: Psychopharmacology: guidelines for social workers, Soc Casework 65(10):579-589, 1984.

Maugh T: Biochemical markers identify mental states, Science 214(2):39-41, 1981.

May R: The origins and significance of the existential movement in psychology, In May R et al, editors: Existence: a new dimension in psychiatry and psychology, New York, 1958, Simon & Schuster, Inc.

Mednick S et al: The Copenhagen high risk project, 1962–86, Schizophrenia Bull 13(3):483-495, 1987.

Mellow J: Nursing therapy, Am J Nurs 68(11):2365-2369, 1968.

Mendel W: Schizophrenia: the experience and its treatment, San Francisco, 1976, Jossey-Bass.

Mendel WM and Green GA: The therapeutic management of psychological illness: the theory and practice of supportive care, New York, 1967, Basic Books.

Menninger K: The vital balance, New York, 1963, The Viking Press, Inc.

Mintz L et al: Expressed emotion: a call for partnership among relatives, patients, and professionals, Schizophrenia Bull 13(2):227-235, 1987.

Munich R: Conceptual trends and issues in the psychotherapy of schizophrenia, Am J Psychother 41(1):23-37, 1987.

Neal M: Partial hospitalization: an alternative to inpatient psychiatric hospitalization, Nurs Clin N Am 21(3):461-472, 1986.

New York Times: Newly found drug is said to be of help for severe schizophrenics, NY Times, B12, May 15, 1987.

Newsday: Health watch: handling schizophrenics at home, Newsday, Part II:7, June 21, 1982.

Oden G: There are no mute patients, In Burd S and Marshall M, editors: Some clinical approaches to psychiatric problems, New York, 1963, Macmillan, Inc.

Pao P: Schizophrenic disorders: theory and treatment from a psychodynamic point of view, New York, 1979, International Universities Press.

Pepper B and Ryglewicz H: The stimulus window: stress and stimulation as aspects of everyday experience, Tie-Lines 3(3):1-5, 1986.

Peterson E and Nelson K: How to meet your client's spiritual needs, J Psychosoc Nurs 25(5):34-39, 1987.

Pfeiffer, C: Mental and elemental nutrients: a physician's guide to nutrition and health care, New Canaan, Ct, 1975, Keats Publishing, Inc.

Pittman FS and Flomenhaft K: Treating the doll's house marriage, Fam Proc 9(2):143-155, 1970.

Potkin SG et al: Are paranoid schizophrenics biologically different from other schizophrenics? N Eng J Med 298(2):61-66, 1978.

Rankel H and Rankel L: Carbamazepine in the treatment of catatonia, Am J Psychiat 145(3):361-362, 1988.

Rehab Brief: Fountain House: a club for former mental patients. Rehab Brief 5(2). National Institute of Handicapped Research, Washington, DC, 1982, Office of Special Education and Rehabilitation Services Department of Education.

Roman P and Trice HM: Schizophrenia and the poor, Ithaca, NY, 1967, Cayuga Press.

Rosen J: Direct analysis: selected papers, New York, 1953, Grune & Stratton, Inc.

Rowe CJ: An outline of psychiatry, ed 6, Dubuque, Ia, 1975, William C Brown Co.

Ruesch J: Disturbed communication: the clinical assessment of normal and pathological communicative behavior, New York, 1957, WW Norton & Co.

Sarbin T: Schizophrenia is a myth, born of metaphor, meaningless, Psychol Today 6(June):20-27, 1972.

Schwing G: A way to the soul of the mentally ill, New York, 1954, International Universities Press.

Science News: Schizophrenia: support therapy gets boost, Sci News 126(25/26):388, 1984.

Science News: Schizophrenia: new hope from an old drug, Sci News 131(21):324, 1987a.

Science News: Low-dose caveat for schizophrenia, Sci News 131(24):374, 1987b.

Science News: Low-dose advantage for schizophrenia, Sci News 134(13):196, 1988.

Searles HF: Collected papers on schizophrenia and related subjects, New York, 1965, International Universities Press.

Sechehaye MA: A new psychotherapy in schizophrenia, New York, 1956, Grune & Stratton, Inc.

Seifer R and Sameroff A: A structural equation model analysis of competence in children at risk for mental disorder, Prev Hum Serv I(4), 1982.

Serban G: Stress in schizophrenics and normals, Br J Psychiat 126:397-407, 1975.

Shapiro S: Contemporary theories of schizophrenia: review and synthesis, New York, 1981, McGraw-Hill Book Co.

Shelton R et al: Cerebral structural pathology in schizophrenia: evidence for a selective prefrontal cortical defect, Am J Psychiatr 145(2):154-162, 1988.

Singh M and Kay S: Wheat gluten as a pathogenic factor in schizophrenia, Science 191:401-402, 1976.

Slater E: Psychotic and neurotic illnesses in twins, London, 1953, Her Majesty's Stationery Office.

Snyder K and Liberman R: Family assessment and intervention with schizophrenics at risk for relapse, In New developments in interventions with families of schizophrenics, San Francisco, 1981, Jossey Bass.

Snyder S: Madness and the brain, New York, 1974, McGraw-Hill Book Co.

Spitz R: Innate inhibition of aggressiveness in infancy, Psychoanal Study Child, vol 20, 1965.

Stein L and Wise CD: Possible etiology of schizophrenia: progressive damage to the noradrenergic reward system by 6-hydroxydopamine, Science 171:1032-1036, 1971.

Strackan A: Family intervention for the rehabilitation of schizophrenia: toward protection and coping, Schizophrenia Bull 12(4):678-698, 1986.

Strahl M: Masked schizophrenia: diagnosis and a unified method of treatment, New York, 1980, Springer Publishing Co.

Stroebel CF: Biological rhythm correlates of disturbed behavior in the rhesus monkey, In Rohles FH, editor: Circadian rhythms in nonhuman primates, New York, 1969, S Karger.

Sullivan H: The interpersonal theory of psychiatry, New York, 1953, WW Norton & Co.

Szasz TS: The myth of mental illness, New York, 1961, Dell Publishing Co.

Taft LT and Goldfarb W: Prenatal and perinatal factors in childhood schizophrenia, Develop Med Child Neurol 6:32-34, 1964.

Talbot J and Glick I: The inpatient care of the chronically mentally ill, Schizophrenia Bull 12(1):129-140, 1986.

Taylor E: The biological basis of schizophrenia, Soc Work 32(2):115-121, 1987.

Tienari P et al: Genetic and psychosocial factors in schizophrenia: the Finnish adoptive family study, Schizophrenia Bull 13(3):475-484, 1987.

Torrey E: Surviving schizophrenia, New York, 1983, Harper & Row.

Trotter RJ: Schizophrenia: a cruel chain of events, Sci News, p 394, June 18, 1977.

Von Domarus E: The specific laws of logic in schizophrenia, In Kasanin JS, editor: Language and thought in schizophrenia, collected papers, Los Angeles, 1944, University of California Press.

Winnicott D: The maturational processes and the facilitating environment, New York, 1965, International Universities Press.

Wong D et al: Positron emission tomography reveals elevated D2 dopamine receptors in drug-naive schizophrenics, Science 234:1558, 1986.

Wynne, LC et al: The nature of schizophrenia: new approaches to research and treatment, New York, 1978, John Wiley & Sons, Inc.

Yates W et al: Cerebellar atrophy in schizophrenia and affective disorder, Am J Psychiatr 144(4):465-467, 1987.

ANNOTATED SUGGESTED READINGS

Barnes D: Biological issues in schizophrenia, Science 235(4787):430-433, 1987.

A brief but cogent summary of the current biological issues in the research of schizophrenia. Controversial theories about genetic factors, altered brain dopamine systems, and structural abnormalities of these theories are discussed. Additional readings on these topics are provided.

Goldstein M: Psychosocial issues, Schizophrenia Bull 13(1):157-171, 1987.

This article discusses the psychosocial attributes of individuals and their social environments that play a contributory role in the onset, course, and treatment of the schizophrenia disorder. A vulnerability-stress model is used to examine these factors. The relevance of the EE concept (expressed emotion in families) is reviewed, and a family-based intervention program in combination with appropriate psychopharmacological treatment is viewed as the effective treatment option.

Kasanin J editor: Language and thought in schizophrenia, New York, 1944, WW Norton & Co., Inc.

A compilation of the works of several well-known authors, this classic book describes and analyzes various aspects of the thought and communication processes in schizophrenia. For example, the schizophrenic's tendency to use paralogical thinking is examined.

Pepper B and Ryglewicz H: The stimulus window: stress and stimulation as aspects of everyday experience, Tie-Lines 3(3):1-5, 1986.

Sensory stimulation tolerance levels related to stress/life change units are viewed through a unifying concept called the "stimulus window." Schizophrenics may react to overstimulation such as increased life changes or too many activities by retreating into withdrawal, exhibiting thought disorder or psychotic symptoms such as hallucinations and delusions. The acceptable level of stimulation varies for each individual. The authors postulate that schizophrenic individuals have difficulty interpreting and distinguishing external stimuli and that

they have a narrow functional range. They therefore have a narrow range of comfort in high-stimuli situations. Implications for treatment programs are discussed.

Swearingen L: Transitional day treatment: an individualized goal-oriented approach, Arch Psychiatr Nurs 1(2):104-110, 1987.

This describes one model for the transitional care of chronic psychiatric clients. The model was originally described by Falloon and Talbot (1982) and evolved in response to client needs. It used an individually goal-oriented treatment approach combined with the structure of the more traditional day treatment program. Swearingen conceptualizes transitional day treatment for chronically ill clients as a "bridge" that can facilitate its traveler's movement toward a meaningful place in the community.

Talbott J and Glick I: The inpatient care of the mentally ill, Schizophrenia Bull 12(1):129-140, 1986.

The authors review the history of inpatient care for mentally ill clients, its present-day issues, advantages and disadvantages, its techniques and treatment modalities. How inpatient care may be practiced in the future is also discussed. The reasons for admitting a chronically ill client to the hospital, steps in the hospital treatment, modalities used, and considerations for discharge are reviewed.

Taylor E: The biological base of schizophrenia, Social Work 32(2):115-121, 1987.

A concise overview of the recent findings on the biological basis for schizophrenia. New techniques for investigating the disorder (e.g., CAT scan, PET scan, rCBf techniques, and BEAM) are reviewed. The article also presents a model for working with schizophrenic clients and their families.

FURTHER READINGS

Bower B: Low-dose advantage for schizophrenia, Sci News 134(13):196, 1988.

Nom S and Avison W: Spouses of discharged psychiatric patients: factors associated with their experience of burden, J Marriage Family 50(2):377-389, 1988.

CHAPTER 26

Patterns of impaired brain function

CHAPTER FOCUS

Historically, mental disorders have been attributed to a variety of natural and supernatural forces. In our own era, many people, including prominent research scientists, have come to believe that most, if not all, psychiatric disturbances are related to altered physiological processes within the central nervous system.

Research in neurophysiology during the last quarter century has led to increased knowledge of neuronal functioning and to a better understanding of the complex metabolic processes of the central nervous system. The advancement in knowledge has made improved treatment possible for organic brain dysfunctions, although treatment has not kept pace with the expanding knowledge.

Organic brain dysfunction, in either the acute form or the chronic form, may occur at any point in the life cycle, although it is more common in the later years of life. Alzheimer's disease, the fourth leading cause of death for American adults, may strike as early as the fourth decade for some people, but most of its victims are over 65 years of age (Leroux, 1986).

The organic brain disorders are believed to be among the most prevalent of psychiatric disorders. There is some evidence that the incidence of the acute form of organic brain dysfunction is increasing as more complex medical treatments become possible with advances in medical technology. It may even be endemic in acute health care settings such as intensive care units. Nurses are frequently the health professionals having the most direct and continuous contact with persons experiencing organic brain dysfunction. They are often in the best position to identify early signs and to set in motion

845

the early treatment measures that are essential to a client's health and at times survival. This chapter will focus on the symptoms and explanatory theories and identified factors in organic brain dysfunction and on the modalities that are used to treat these conditions. In addition, attention will be given to primary, secondary, and tertiary prevention in both the acute and the chronic forms of organic brain disorders. Nursing process as it relates to acute and chronic confusional states is included.

CLASSIFICATIONS OF ORGANIC DYSFUNCTIONS

Psychiatric disorders* have been broadly classified as either *functional* or *organic*. The functional disorders included the mood, thought, and personality disorders discussed in previous chapters; they were thought to have their origins in psychogenic or psychological processes. The term *functional* in this context, referred to psychosocial or psychodynamic functioning rather than to biological functioning. The symptoms of functional disorders are usually viewed as defensive responses to stress and anxiety; they differ from symptoms of organic conditions in that disturbances in cognitive functioning either are not present or are secondary to such symptoms as delusions or hallucinations. The term *organic* refers to psychiatric conditions, both chronic and acute, that are known to have their origins in disturbances in neurophysiology or brain tissue functioning. Disturbances in cognitive functioning characterize these disorders.

Current research strongly suggests that there is a neurophysiological contribution to such disorders as schizophrenia (see Chapter 25) and the affective disorders (see Chapter 22). These findings therefore cause some confusion in the use of the terms *organic* and *functional* in the classification of psychiatric disorders.

Organic brain dysfunction is usually classified as either *acute* or *chronic*. Factors underlying altera-

---

*See Appendix A for the many codings for organic mental disorders.

tions in normal brain functioning may produce an acute, temporary dysfunction that responds readily to appropriate therapy and the normal physiological reparative processes, leaving no residual effects. For such conditions the terms *acute* and *reversible* are used. In some instances of organic brain dysfunction, there are residual deficits that result from diffuse alterations of neuron structure or from some continuing interference with neurophysiological processes. The terms *chronic* and *irreversible* are often used to categorize this type of dysfunction. The terms *acute* and *chronic* can be misleading, however, since some brain dysfunctions can progress from acute to chronic, often depending on the underlying basis of the disorder and the effectiveness of treatment. In addition, chronic disorders of unknown origin can appear with a gradual or insidious onset, without an acute phase. Chronic disorders may also be classified as mild, moderate, or severe, depending on the degree of cognitive dysfunction.

The neuropsychiatric disorders associated with impaired brain function may also be classified according to associated factors. Organic brain dysfunction has been associated with systemic disorders; infections; chemical, drug, and alcohol intoxication; nutritional deficiencies; intracranial trauma and neoplasms; neurological disorders; iatrogenic disorders; and genetic factors. Organic syndromes in which the underlying basis is unknown have been termed *primary*, signifying the absence of any known factors. Organic disorders with known underlying factors have been termed *secondary*, to indicate an association with some known pathophysiological process.

CHARACTERISTICS AND UNDERLYING DYNAMICS

The clinical manifestations of organic brain disorders include disturbances in attention, comprehension, memory, orientation, and judgment. Emotional instability, or lability of affect, may also be present. These disturbances in cognitive or intellectual functioning point to brain dysfunction.

Acute brain syndrome

Symptoms of delirium or an acute confusional state generally have an acute onset, associated with some underlying pathophysiology. These symptoms indicate a serious level of brain dysfunction, and they require immediate treatment of the underlying pathology, often as a life-saving measure.

Difficulty in focusing attention and in comprehending incoming stimuli are often the most prominent features in acute brain dysfunction. The difficulty in focusing or maintaining attention will be reflected in an inability to grasp an idea or a simple communication. There will be difficulty in comprehending the facts of a situation and in responding to questions or other verbal communication. Even when grasped or understood, information or ideas will not be retained. There may be a lack of clarity in thinking and an inability to recall or remember pertinent information. Difficulties in focusing attention also lead to an inability to screen out irrelevant stimuli so that anything going on distracts the person's attention. Persons who are experiencing delirium often convey their confusion and lack of comprehension through facial expressions and other forms of nonverbal communication.

In a health care setting, a person with an acute brain dysfunction may have difficulty in comprehending and cooperating with monitoring and treatment activities. People who are regaining consciousness after general anesthesia often display a similar difficulty in sustaining attention and a similar distractibility. They also may experience fluctuations in levels of consciousness. Disturbances in levels of consciousness may vary from a clouding of consciousness, in which the individual is not fully conscious and responsive, to intermittent periods of stupor or coma.

Emotional instability may or may not be present in acute brain dysfunction. Some people respond with sustained fearfulness, apprehension, irritability, and restlessness. In others, such emotions may alternate with periods of calm and lethargy. Other symptoms may appear, often in association with the underlying pathophysiology. Hallucinations and delusions, for example, may appear in a dysfunction that is associated with withdrawal from alcohol or drugs.

Chronic brain syndrome

The onset of symptoms in chronic brain dysfunction is usually insidious. Some chronic dysfunctions may, however, directly follow an acute phase, when the causative agent has resulted in irreversible brain tissue damage, as in some cases of prolonged anoxia or when a disturbance in neurophysiology persists. Although chronic brain syndrome may occur at any age, the majority of cases appear in the geriatric population.

The prominent symptoms of chronic organic brain dysfunction are disturbances in intellectual abilities—particularly memory, orientation, and judgment. Disturbances in attention are reflected in the distractibility that is often present. Fluctuations in emotional tone—that is, lability of affect—are often present. Additional neurological symptoms may also occur, depending on the kind of neurophysiological impairment.

The extent to which chronic organic brain dysfunction disrupts a person's ability to function varies considerably. Some people are able to cope with the deficit and continue to function adequately. Others may be so severely impaired in functions of daily living that they are unable to care for themselves. Disturbances in memory, for example, may be so mild as to be imperceptible to anyone other than the affected person or a close family member. Forgetting where one put down one's eyeglasses or reading material or not remembering the names of people recently met are lapses of memory that most of us experience from time to time. More serious defects in memory, such as a tendency to forget appointments or details of important events, may be compensated for by such special efforts as note taking and association tricks. In severe memory loss, there may be difficulty in recalling what, if anything, one had for breakfast or in the ability to recognize friends and family members. In chronic brain syndrome, memory of recent events is often more impaired than remote memory or memory of earlier phases of life. This is termed *retrograde memory loss.*

Severe memory disturbances are usually accompanied by disturbances in orientation—in the ways in which we relate to and in our environment. Disturbances in orientation may involve time, place, or people. Those which involve time are usually of a gross nature, such as an inability to distinguish night from day or to identify the season, the year, or even the decade. The hour of the day or the day of the month may, however, be unknown to a client who is institutionalized and is shut off from ongoing events. Many of us, when on vacation, may ignore the clock or the calendar. People from cultures that are not highly time oriented may pay little attention to precise times, days, and dates. It is important therefore that an evaluation of time orientation take into account an individual's circumstances.

Disturbances in orientation to place may vary from a recognition of where one is (but an inability to recall how one got there) to an inability to accurately perceive one's present location. The former type is seen in persons who have suffered head injuries followed by a period of coma. A period of amnesia or total loss of memory of events immediately preceding the trauma often occurs. Disorientation in relation to place may also appear spontaneously and for no known reason in persons who suffer from chronic organic dysfunction.

Disorientation in relation to other people is an inability to accurately perceive or comprehend the identity of persons who are in the immediate environment. In a hospital setting, a person may mistake health care providers for family members. In an extreme case of this form of disorientation, there may be a lack of recognition of a close family member.

Disturbances in judgment are manifested by impairment of the ability to perceive, interpret, and respond appropriately or effectively to situations in the environment. Judgment will usually be impaired to the degree or extent to which the other cognitive functions are impaired. Behavioral manifestations may vary from mild peccadilloes that embarrass family and friends to a failure to observe social mores or to use financial and other resources prudently. In some instances, impaired judgment is so extreme that a person can endanger his or her own life or others' lives through imprudent acts.

Certain communication and speech patterns may be found in chronic brain disorders. Among them are circumstantiality, confabulation, and (to some extent) recall and association difficulties.

Circumstantiality is a speech pattern in which a person has difficulty in screening out relevant from irrelevant material in describing an event. There is a tendency to include every detail, often in sequential order. While a raconteur may delightfully embellish a story with interesting details that bring it to life, circumstantiality has the opposite effect, arousing impatience in the listener that may cause him to tune out or lose interest. In a busy health care setting, there may be a tendency on the part of health care providers to complete a story for a person who displays circumstantiality or to intervene in other ways. This tendency may arouse anxiety and anger. If the person is under stress and vulnerable to any additional frustration, pressure to get to the point of the story or omit unnecessary detail may increase confusion or even result in an anxiety reaction.

Circumstantiality may, at times, cause the individual who is affected to lose the point of a story or a question, as one association leads to another and the main thread is forgotten. Often the person, realizing that the main point has been lost, will say so and ask to have a question repeated.

The following vignette illustrates circumstantiality in an older woman who has mild to moderate brain dysfunction. In the situation described here, pain and fear played an important role.

Mrs. M., who lived alone in her own home, phoned a niece and told her that she had hurt her foot and did not know what to do. The niece took her aunt to the emergency room of the local hospital for treatment. Mrs. M. was in pain from the injured foot, and she was very anxious about what would happen if she were unable to walk for any length of time. When asked by a nurse to tell her what had happened, Mrs. M. responded: "I was going to the department store to buy a shower gift for my neighbor's daughter. She's getting married to a very nice boy, and my neighbor across the street is having a shower, and all the people on the block are invited. I am all alone, you know, and have to do everything for myself, and the girl's family has been very good to me. So I wanted to get something nice for the shower. I was reading the paper last night and saw an ad for a coffee pot on sale. I don't have too much money, you know, so I rushed out early this morning to buy it before they were all gone. I don't have anyone to drive me, so I have to do everything for myself. It's awful to be alone." Prodded a bit by the nurse, Mrs. M. continued to explain how, in her rush to get on the bus, she had turned her ankle as she stepped off the curb.

Although Mrs. M. was able to arrive at the appropriate end point in her description of the event, she also included many ramifications that were irrelevant to the immediate situation in the emergency room. The story had been told in the same detail, and almost identical language, earlier, when Mrs. M. told the niece about the accident. The astute observer will also note an underlying theme of dependence, or fear of dependence and helplessness. These emotions and the uncertainty they indicate may have a higher priority of concern for Mrs. M. than the physical injury and pain in this situation.

Another symptom of brain dysfunction that may be demonstrated in speech patterns is difficulty in recalling words, ideas, or events and in making associations with other words, ideas, or events. Difficulties in *recall* and *association* are not uncommon, nor are they limited to persons with brain dysfunction. Who among us has not forgotten words or things that, in retrospect, we should have remembered? When memory is impaired by brain dysfunction, however, the ability to recall or make associations may inhibit communication ability. The symptom may be severe in the more extreme forms of chronic brain syndrome. In Pick's disease, for example, in which cerebral insufficiency is related to damage to the bilateral, frontotemporal areas of the brain having to do with speech and association (Heston et al., 1987), there may be an inability to name such commonly used items as pencils. An affected person may, however, be able to state the purpose for which such an item is used. Even in such a situation, the association loss may be selective; the amount of loss depends on the familiarity and value to the individual of a particular object or idea. For example, Mrs. L. was unable to recall the word for a wristwatch when she was asked to name this commonly used item during an examination, but she could readily identify coins by their monetary value.

Confabulation is a frequently observed phenom-enon in chronic brain syndrome, often seen in residents of nursing homes and psychiatric hospitals. In confabulation, an individual who cannot recall specific aspects of an event will fill in the gaps in memory with relevant but imaginary information. For example, a man whose recent memory was being tested responded to a question about what he had eaten for breakfast by saying a soft-boiled egg and toast, when, in fact, he had been given oatmeal and coffee cake. Confabulation is occasionally viewed by health care providers as a wish-fulfilling fantasy, as a deliberate attempt to deceive, or as evidence of severely impaired memory. It is usually none of these, but represents a face-saving device or defense mechanism in which the person copes by filling in gaps in memory with substitutions. Thus, confabulation can represent a strength: it can be an attempt to cope with an intolerable situation. Recognition of the defensive nature of confabulation can serve a useful purpose in the provision of needed emotional support for such clients.

Factors that influence coping ability

Disturbances in cognitive functioning influence a person's ability to cope with life's experiences. The degree to which the disability is disorganizing to a person is influenced by a variety of factors. Although the extent of neuronal damage or dysfunction may be a factor in some instances, other factors may be of even greater significance as a person attempts to cope with the stress of life. Among these factors are the developmental era in which an organic dysfunction begins and the psychodynamic and sociocultural forces that influence the functioning of everyone.

DEVELOPMENTAL FACTORS
▶ **Acute brain syndrome**

The age of onset of organic dysfunction, particularly when it is early in life, may have a profound influence on the ability to cope with life. A young child who has not yet mastered language and logical thinking will respond to brain dysfunction quite differently from the way an older person, who has mastered these developmental tasks, responds. In a hospitalized child, the failure to focus attention and the irritability or apathy that may be symptomatic of acute organic dysfunction can be confused with the psychological coping process of regression, which often accompanies the stress of illness and separation from home and family. In an older person the symptoms of acute brain dysfunction may mistakenly be attributed to a degenerative process associated with aging (Zisook and Braff, 1986). Conversely, deficits in the sensory apparatus, particularly those involving sight and hearing, may be mistaken for a disturbance in comprehension, especially when such deficits are severe enough to promote a level of isolation that leads to illusions or hallucinatory experiences. Culture shock (see Chapter 4), which many people experience when first admitted to a hospital, may also influence adaptive responses to the hospital setting. This is particularly true when there is a language barrier or when there is a marked cultural difference between the client and the health care providers. Severe pain, apprehension, and anxiety may also distort or be mistaken for symptoms of acute brain dysfunction. The picture is further confused when an organic dysfunction is superimposed upon a functional psychiatric disorder. Because symptoms may be distorted by such factors, a history of an individual's patterns of functioning and ways of coping with stress, prior to the onset of the medical problem underlying the acute brain dysfunction, is an important part of nursing assessment and intervention.

▶ Chronic brain syndrome

The characteristics of chronic brain dysfunction will, of course, be affected by the age of onset. Up to this point we have focused primarily upon the older adult, because the largest number of people with chronic brain syndrome is in this age group. However, since chronic cerebral dysfunction can occur at any age, it is important to mention its effects on the child and the young adult. If organic dysfunction has its onset in the early adult years, the individual has already mastered the language and the learning tasks necessary for adaptation to his or her culture. The person has educational and living experiences to fall back on in coping with the deficit and a variety of coping measures to rely on. The young child, in contrast, must learn language and must negotiate the developmental crises upon which personality and cultural adaptation are founded. A child must also master the knowledge, skills, and other requirements essential to adapting to the people and mores of a complex culture.

Organic brain disease can occur at any point during the developmental process, from conception to the end of life. When the onset is in the prenatal or perinatal period, the child may fail to master language and may be so impaired in the ability to function that severe mental retardation is the result.

Onset later in childhood also may have a profound effect on the child and the family. The memory disturbance makes learning difficult, and the shortened or altered attention span increases the learning difficulties. Such a child has a very low tolerance for frustration and is often restless and hyperactive. The following excerpt illustrates some of the aspects of such brain damage in a child.

Thomas was brought to a mental health clinic by his parents when he was 6 years old. He was of average size for his age and physically well developed and well nourished. He did not respond to any questions or directions and was extremely restless and hyperactive. He had a very pained facial expression, and he exhibited stereotypical movements of the hands: he would hold them in front of him and shake them up and down. He had been excluded from all schools, even those for emotionally disturbed children. The mother reported that he had frequent, severe temper tantrums at home, in which he would break anything in sight. He required constant and direct supervision. The family was very devoted to him and willing to make any sacrifice to get help for him and to care for him at home.

The parents described Thomas' early development as normal. He was a very happy, responsive child whose language development was normal. The father, who was a professional photographer, had taken many movies of the son from birth until the onset of the present symptoms when he was 3 years of age. A review of these movies tended to confirm the parents' assessment of Tommy's early development. Between the ages of 2 and 3, he developed an acute infectious illness, from which he appeared to have an uneventful recovery. But shortly following the illness, language development stopped, and his personality changed from that of the happy, responsive child he had been to the hyperactive, anxious, and unresponsive child he was upon admission to the clinic. Neurological, psychological, and other testing measures confirmed a diagnosis of organic brain dysfunction.

In the young adult, the symptoms closely resemble those in the older adult, although the social and psychological impact may be more devastating in the young adult. Cognitive defects inhibit learning of new material, thus interfering with career plans. Even previously mastered knowledge and skills are affected. For example, a computer programmer may no longer be able to function in that field. In severe cases, the memory defect may be so embarrassing in relationships with peers that it promotes isolation and withdrawal. In instances in which the functional deficit is mild or moderate, a young adult may be more resilient in compensating for and adapting to the cognitive defect than an older person is.

Disturbances in cognitive functioning that result from organic brain dysfunction may, of course, be superimposed upon such functional disorders as the thought and mood disturbances. Depression* and elation frequently accompany organic brain disease. Such mood disorders are functional disturbances secondary to brain dysfunction and may represent a grief and mourning process similar to that which occurs after the loss of a body part. Depression, particularly in the elderly, may be mistaken for brain dysfunction.†

Mrs. S. had been active all her life, participating in running a small store that she and her husband owned. When her husband died, Mrs. S. was in her early 70s. The store was sold, and she moved to a small apartment near her only son, in a community far removed from the one in which she had lived for many years and where she knew many people. Alone much of the time and isolated from old friends and acquaintances, Mrs. S. became severely depressed. She was taken to a mental health center, where she was diagnosed as having chronic brain syndrome. After a few weeks, Mrs. S. was transferred to an adult home,

where she came to the attention of a community mental health nurse. Working with Mrs. S. over a period of time, the nurse became aware that her cognitive abilities were intact but that she was depressed and lonely. Her mental state was exacerbated by a physical infirmity that was not being treated and was somewhat immobilizing. The immobilization increased her feelings of helplessness and abandonment. Working with the son and community agencies, the nurse was instrumental in having Mrs. S. transferred to a health-related facility that was more suitable to her needs. Her medical and psychological problems were treated there. In the new setting, where she felt more safe and secure, Mrs. S. made excellent progress and began to take part in and enjoy social and other activites.

SOCIOCULTURAL FACTORS

Many sociocultural factors influence each of us in our ability to cope with the normal stresses of life. The needs for love, approval, acceptance, status, recognition, and achievement are important to the mental health of everyone. Economic security and the availability of family, friends, and other social support systems are essential to meeting these needs.

For the individual with organic brain dysfunction, many factors combine to limit the ability to satisfy these normal human needs. In an older person, organic brain dysfunction often occurs at a time of sociocultural stress. Loss of family and friends through marriage, death, illness, and change of residence frequently coincides with physical ailments that contribute to organic dysfunction. Forced retirement from productive employment conflicts with one's need to be a useful, constructive member of society. In addition, retirement often leads to economic insecurity and isolation from friends and coworkers.

Although these factors are especially pertinent to older persons, a young person with some cognitive deficits may suffer similar deprivations. Work and earning capacity can be limited by the disability, and isolation from family and peers often occurs.

All these factors influence the ability to cope. The person who can maintain close ties with family and friends and who experiences little disruption in life-style may cope more effectively with the disability.

---

*See Chapter 22.
†See Chapter 18.

PSYCHODYNAMIC FACTORS

Stress and emotional responses to it can be disruptive of anyone's ability to function (see Chapter 8). For an individual with some organic brain dysfunction, such emotional factors as anxiety, anger, hopelessness, and depression may cause greater disorganization of behavior than would be the case for a person with normal brain functioning. This exacerbation of symptoms may be erroneously attributed to cerebral damage. For example, an individual with a mild degree of organic brain dysfunction, when confronted with interpersonal, economic, social, or other crises, frequently experiences increased fear, anxiety, anger, frustration, and feelings of helplessness. These emotions in turn may cause restlessness, inattention, and difficulty in comprehension and memory. All these symptoms, characteristic of organic dysfunction, can become exaggerated under emotional stress. Thus, assessment on the basis of cognitive function alone, without the level of anxiety and coping responses being taken into account, may lead to an inaccurate assessment of the degree of brain dysfunction and to overlooking the strengths of a client.

Clients with organic brain dysfunction may be quite aware of their disability and of their emotional responses to pressure, stress, or assaults upon their self-concept and security. Such individuals may mention that they become very nervous and confused when pressured. They also frequently respond with embarrassment and anger when deficits in memory or other cognitive abilities are pointed out to them.

• • •

Thus, many factors in addition to the cognitive dysfunction influence the coping patterns of people who have organic brain syndrome. The following case summaries illustrate differences in the ways people cope.

Mrs. M., who is in her mid-70s, has lived alone in a single-family dwelling since the death of her husband, which occurred when she was 60. She has no children, but she maintains close family ties with her four siblings and their children. Although she had to drop out of school after the eighth grade to help support her

immigrant family, Mrs. M. is fluent in and able to read and write both English and the language of her ethnic group. She is in good physical health, and she is economically secure. Mrs. M. is able to do her own housework, shopping, and cooking. She also maintains a small yard and flower garden and takes great pride in her home. Always socially active, Mrs. M. continues to entertain family and friends and participates in various social and religious activities with them.

Mrs. M. has several complaints that she associates with aging, which shows a degree of insight. She complains of having trouble remembering things. If one observes her carefully, however, one finds the memory defect to be selective and related to new material or to areas that have little value for her. For example, she cannot remember where her favorite nephew's wedding will be held, although she has heard the plans many times and in detail. But she has no need to remember, since she will be taken there and brought home by a family member. She can, however, remember in detail the previous day's soap opera episode to recount it to a friend who missed the broadcast. In the retelling and in other social interactions, her speech is somewhat stereotypical and circumstantial.

She also complains that she becomes very nervous and upset when she is under any pressure or when she is confronted with a problem in her home that requires maintenance from service people in the community. But she is very effective in using problem-solving techniques and in appealing to appropriate family members or friends for assistance. And she meets the need to feel useful by doing minor alterations and repairs of clothing for family members and close friends.

• • •

Mrs. G., also a widow, is in her late 70s. In many ways, her situation is similar to that of Mrs. M. She is also economically secure and owns her own home. Although she has several married children and a large extended family, her home is at some distance from any of them, so any immediate support or contact with her family is limited. In addition Mrs. G. speaks little English, and since she does not live in a neighborhood where her language is spoken, her community contact is more limited.

She is a strong-willed woman, however, and for several years had been able to manage her affairs and care for herself fairly effectively. Gradually, however, her family began to notice changes in her ability to function. Her memory had become progressively poorer. She would forget where she had put her mon-

ey and other things and whether or not a tenant had given her a check for the rent of an apartment. She also began to make errors in judgment, such as renting the apartment to a second family after she had already rented it and giving to strangers articles of furniture that she needed. When Mrs. G. began to lose weight, a daughter suspected that she had been forgetting to prepare meals or eat an adequate diet. A physical check-up revealed no disease, but the physician convinced the family that Mrs. G's cognitive difficulties were making it impossible for her to continue living alone. At this point, she moved into her daughter's home.

Although immediately following the change she became somewhat disoriented during the night, when she would awaken and think she was still in her own home, Mrs. G's condition has become more stable. She continues to have some defects in memory, but in the protective and supportive environment, with adequate nutrition and the presence of family members, the cognitive defects have become less disabling.

•   •   •

Mrs. A. was also a widow in her late 70s who was economically secure and in good physical health. She lived in a stable ethnic community throughout her lifetime and had many relatives and friends nearby. Within a period of three years Mrs. A. lost both her husband and her only daughter, and her grandsons married and moved away. Much of Mrs. A.'s social activity prior to their deaths had centered around the husband, the daughter, and the daughter's family. The husband had been retired for many years; he did all the shopping for the family and made all of the major decisions. Although he was several years older than Mrs. A., he had, over a period of time, kidded her about her forgetfulness. A few months after the husband's death, Mrs. A.'s neighbors began phoning a son, who lived some distance from his mother, with complaints about Mrs. A.'s behavior. They described her as confused and said she was harassing them about not paying rents, which they had indeed paid. The son and his wife visited Mrs. A. and hired someone to stay with her, but her condition continued to deteriorate. She became increasingly disoriented to time, confusing the night with the day and summer with winter, often appearing outside on very cold days clad only in a sweater. She also began to confuse her neighbor's children with the grandsons, who were grown and married. She began to cook large pots of food for the deceased husband and daughter, which she stored in the refrigerator to await their arrival. She

continued to harass the tenants about the rents and, at times, to confuse them with people from her youth. On one occasion, she left home, saying she was going to visit her mother. She was found some distance from her home, and in a very confused state, by the police. They took her to a psychiatric hospital, where she was admitted with a diagnosis of chronic brain syndrome. In the hospital her general health and cognitive abilities deteriorated until her death about six months later.

EPIDEMIOLOGY AND SOCIOCULTURAL ASPECTS

Organic brain dysfunctions are the most ubiquitous of all mental health problems. Acute forms occur with regularity in many health facilities as complications of physiological and traumatic disorders and their treatment. The chronic forms constitute one of the major mental health problems. Despite, or perhaps because of, this prevalence, definitive data about the incidence of organic brain dysfunction are not currently available. It is estimated, however, that 5% of the population is affected—with most of that number in the older age group (Larue et al, 1985). The multiplicity of underlying factors that may contribute to organic dysfunction, however, suggests a very high and possibly increasing incidence and also is an indication of some of the problems involved in gathering demographic data.

When acute confusional states occur as complications of medical conditions, data are often not compiled on such complications or, when collected, are related to specific underlying diagnoses. In addition, delirium may go undiagnosed by physicians, although nursing staffs are often more aware of the symptoms and record them in their notes.

The incidence of organic dysfunctions of both acute and chronic nature is highest in people over 65 years of age (Leroux, 1986; Zisook and Braff, 1986). Persons in the older age groups are more susceptible to the major health problems (cancer, cardiac and respiratory diseases) with which organic dysfunctions are often associated. Many individuals with some degree of chronic organic impairment are living in the community and do not come into contact with any data collection system. In some instances, a diagnosis of chronic brain syndrome is made purely on the basis of behavioral assessment.

The diagnosis of chronic brain syndrome frequently arouses feelings of hopelessness in physicians, nurses, and other health professionals and leads to a lack of interest in the active treatment of such disorders in the elderly (Karpf, 1982). Such responses may have contributed to the historical paucity of research in this area of psychiatry. There is, however, a growing interest in the neuropsychiatric conditions associated with impaired cerebral functioning, particularly Alzheimer's disease, and there has been an increase in the amount of research into the causes and treatment of such conditions.

Organic brain disturbances occur in all social classes and ethnic groups. Many sociocultural factors contribute, directly or indirectly, to the incidence of organic brain dysfunction. Poverty, with its concomitant poor housing, overcrowding, and malnutrition, may increase the incidence of infectious and other diseases, which can be complicated by organic brain disorders of either an acute or a chronic nature.

Lead poisoning, when untreated, results in chronic brain dysfunction (Whaley and Wong, 1987). Many victims of lead poisoning live in old houses in which lead-based paints had been applied to exterior and interior surfaces. Current legislation has fairly well eliminated the use of lead in paints for most purposes, and many states have directives for preventing inhalation of lead when old paint is removed. In some older dwellings, however, lead paint remains on walls or on furniture (Barry, 1984), where it becomes a source of lead poisoning as a result of flaking, paint removal efforts, and children chewing on painted surfaces.

Social stress and the competitive pressures of highly industrialized society are experienced by people of all classes, ages, and ethnic groups. Pressures on the adolescent to achieve in school, on the adult in many work situations, on the older person forced into retirement and often into isolation, and on minority group members who are excluded from the job market and meaningful participation in other aspects of life are commonplace.

The ways in which people cope with social stress often contribute, directly or indirectly, to organic disease. Social pressures contribute significantly to drug and alcohol abuse, as people increasingly turn to such chemicals in an effort to cope with the pressures of modern life. Suicide attempts may also result in brain damage, depending on the particular method employed and other factors.*

Prejudice, another source of social stress, may contribute indirectly to organic brain dysfunction in a variety of ways, including the failure to provide early or preventive treatment of disorders that can lead to chronic organic dysfunction when they are untreated.

The technological era in which we live may contribute to the incidence of organic dysfunction. Environmental pollution from industry and other sources is an ever-present danger. Advances in medical technology, which have been so effective in prolonging life and functioning ability, have also contributed to the increase in the incidence of organic dysfunction in the elderly (Leroux, 1986). The delirious states associated with cardiac and general surgery, intensive care units, and treatment of renal diseases are also increasing.

High-speed transportation, another aspect of our advanced technology, has increased the incidence of head injury—through automobile and other accidents. While improved treatment has decreased mortality from head trauma, organic dysfunction may be an increasingly common sequela of severe head injury.

EXPLANATORY THEORIES AND IDENTIFIED FACTORS
Acute confusional states

Acute confusional state is a term used to describe the acute brain dysfunction that often accompanies physical illness and injury. Many other diagnostic terms are used, among them *delirium, acute delirious states, acute brain syndrome,* and *toxic psychosis.* The following are some major underlying

---

*Sociocultural aspects of alcohol and drug abuse are discussed in Chapter 20; sociocultural aspects of suicide are discussed in Chapter 22.

factors in an acute confusional state, but it should be remembered that any condition that interferes with complex biochemical or metabolic functions may result in temporary or permanent brain dysfunction.

SYSTEMIC DISORDERS

Among the systemic disorders that may be associated with an acute confusional state are chronic heart and lung diseases, hepatic and renal insufficiencies, acute forms of diabetes, and severe anemias. The specific patterns that such systemic disorders produce vary with the underlying pathological process. Among these patterns are hypoxia, which is particularly prevalent in chronic heart and lung disorders and in severe anemias, and hypoglycemia, which often occurs in severe diabetes. Disturbances in acid-base and electrolyte balances and in the water-sodium balance may be present in any of these physical ailments and in many others. Toxic substances in the blood that accompany renal and hepatic dysfunction can also contribute to brain dysfunction. Uremic toxins may cause such neurological symptoms as seizures and asterixis—a characteristic flapping tremor of the hands—in addition to acute brain dysfunction (Barry, 1984; Seltzer and Frazier, 1978; Zisook and Braff, 1986).

INFECTIOUS DISORDERS

Acute confusional states frequently occur in systemic infectious disorders such as typhoid fever, malaria, pneumonia, and infectious hepatitis. Central nervous system infections such as meningitis and encephalitis may also cause delirium. In the systemic infectious conditions, brain dysfunction is believed to be associated with the high temperature and level of toxicity that are symptomatic of the diseases. The debilitating effects of such an illness may also be a contributory cause. Encephalitis may be followed by a chronic syndrome. Immunization against the communicable diseases of childhood and effective treatment of syphilis with penicillin have nearly eliminated the encephalitis often associated with these diseases. Antibiotic treatment of viral and bacterial encephalitis has also been effective in preventing chronic brain dysfunction as a result of these diseases.

CHEMICAL INTOXICATION

Chemical intoxication is becoming an increasing hazard in industrial societies. The presence of numerous chemical additives in foodstuffs and the chemical pollution of our air, water, and soil have received wide attention because of their potential for the production of cancer and birth defects. There has, however, been far less attention paid to the potential hazard of such chemicals to the normal physiological processes of the central nervous system and the rest of the body.

Two chemicals that have long been associated with brain dysfunction are carbon monoxide and lead. Carbon monoxide poisoning can come about suddenly, from breathing automobile exhaust fumes in a suicide attempt or as a result of a faulty ventilation of a car's interior. In current-model cars in which ventilation depends on a system that brings air into the car when it is in motion and windows are closed, idling a motor when the car is stopped to provide heat or air conditioning is particularly hazardous. In addition, incomplete combustion of fuels, particularly coal, may cause toxic levels of carbon monoxide to be emitted into the air of a home.

Carbon monoxide causes anoxia by combining with blood hemoglobin to form a stable substance, carboxyhemoglobin. This condition prevents the uptake of oxygen by the hemoglobin. When severe or prolonged enough, carbon monoxide poisoning can cause death or permanent brain damage. The symptoms of confusion and a clouding of consciousness may be early indications of carbon monoxide poisoning. Mild cases may appear in persons working in such industries as auto repairing, in which a constant level of carbon monoxide results from motors being run in inadequately ventilated garages.

Several of the heavy metals—lead, mercury, and manganese—may cause brain dysfunction. Lead has received the greatest attention and may be the most commonly found of the heavy metals. The ingestion of lead by children has been greatly reduced as a result of government actions that ban the use of lead in paints, particularly in paints used on toys, children's furniture, and other items that young children may suck or chew on. The habit of pica, or the craving of unnatural foods such as plaster from walls, may still be a hazard to children and occasionally to adults who live in older dwellings in which lead paint remains on the walls.

In adults, lead poisoning is usually caused by inhalation associated with industrial activities. Workers in the construction industry are particularly vulnerable when they are dismantling or removing paint from older structures on which lead paints had been used over a period of time. Removal of lead paint from older houses by homeowners can also result in lead inhalation.

Lead intoxication may produce an acute delirious state, or it may result in chronic brain syndrome—particularly if treatment is delayed or ineffective. Lead produces a fragility of the red blood cell membrane, with subsequent destruction or hemolysis of the cell. Lead may be stored in the bones, which can lead to symptoms recurring as it is later released without further inhalation or ingestion (Billings and Stokes, 1986).

PHARMACOLOGICAL AGENTS

Many pharmaceuticals may cause an acute confusional state in some people. This side effect may occur in susceptible individuals at normal therapeutic dosage levels, as well as in high dosage levels and overdoses. Among the drugs that may cause such a response are anticholinergics, diuretics, digitalis, levodopa, hypnotics, sedatives, and some of the hormonal substances (Zisook and Braff, 1986). Some children and elderly people may develop delirium following application of atropine eye drops (Barry, 1984). The reason why some are so affected is not known. The long-term use of major tranquilizers (such as Mellaril, Thorazine, and Haldol) which has been associated with the physical disorder *tardive dyskinesia** is now being related to a psychological counterpart, a serious mental and emotional disorder that is a side effect and something apart from the functional disorder. The syndrome has been termed *tardive dysmentia* (Herbert, 1983).

Other drugs may produce acute confusional states when taken in overdoses or in combination with other chemicals such as alcohol or other central nervous system depressants. A synergistic or

*See Chapter 25.

potentiating effect takes place when such drugs are taken in combination. The tricyclic antidepressants and lithium salts are drugs that cause delirium and other neurologic symptoms when they are taken in toxic levels. Mild intake of alcohol, in combination with such drugs as phenothiazines, antidepressants, and barbiturates, may produce an acute intoxication and may even lead to coma and death as a result of depression of the respiratory centers.

Many therapeutic procedures may produce an acute confusional state. Diuretic therapy and low-sodium diets, for example, unless carefully monitored, can produce fluid electrolyte imbalances that may lead to symptoms of delirium. Anesthesia and prolonged surgical procedures may also cause an acute brain dysfunction.

ALCOHOL AND DRUG WITHDRAWAL

There are two ways in which alcohol may produce an acute brain syndrome. First, excessive ingestion produces acute alcoholism. Second, for people who habitually consume large quantities of alcohol and who are physiologically addicted, the abrupt withdrawal of the substance may produce the symptom picture known as delirium tremens. This condition is often encountered in persons admitted to a general hospital for treatment of a physical illness or injury. Very often it is not known that the individual is physically addicted to alcohol until the symptoms appear. Withdrawal symptoms, including brain dysfunction, may also occur in individuals addicted to such drugs as opiates, meprobamates, and barbiturates.

NUTRITIONAL DEFICIENCIES

A deficiency in the B vitamins (particularly thiamine) is the most common nutritional deficiency associated with psychiatric and neurological disorders. The condition known as Wernicke's syndrome is caused by a deficiency of thiamine in the diet (Barry, 1984). Pellagra is caused by a nicotinic acid deficiency, and a progressive dementia may accompany severe folic acid deficiency. A lack of B_{12} from pernicious anemia can lead to schizophrenic-like psychosis (Barry, 1984). Because of the addition of the B vitamins to many foods, most people in the United States have an adequate intake of these essential substances. Deficiencies of B vitamins are seen most often in chronic alcoholics, because of the poor nutritional habits and the interference with intestinal absorption that are associated with chronic alcoholism. Thiamine and other B vitamin deficiencies may, however, occur in cases of hyperemesis gravidarum and pernicious anemia and in elderly persons who have inadequate nutritional intake. Delirium may be one of the early symptoms of these deficiencies. Prolonged deficiency of thiamine may also cause permanent neurological damage and chronic dysfunction. The chronic condition is known as Korsakoff's psychosis.

Severe dehydration may also produce delirium. Elderly people living alone may be especially vulnerable in hot summer weather because of inadequate fluid intake or excessive loss of fluids.

HEAD INJURIES

An acute confusional state is often associated with head injuries, particularly in instances involving a concussion and loss of consciousness. The delirium may result from neuronal injury from the concussion, but prolonged or recurring delirium may indicate hemorrhage and intracranial pressure (Barry, 1984; Zisook and Braff, 1986).

Chronic brain syndrome

Like acute brain dysfunction, chronic brain dysfunction may be secondary to many pathological processes. For example, Lehman (1983) states: "Great progress in the prevention of OBS [organic brain syndrome] in the aged would be made with the discovery of an effective prevention or cure for arteriosclerosis." In addition to the toxic, metabolic, and circulatory disorders that may underlie chronic brain dysfunction, examples of which have been noted, intracranial neoplasms, normal-pressure hydrocephalus, and Huntington's disease* (a genetic disorder) are among other factors. Infections include Creutzfeldt-Jakob disease (a slow virus) and general paresis, the neurological complication of third-stage syphilis.

Alzheimer's disease is a disorder that is receiving

---

*Gusella et al. (1983) located the H.D. gene on chromosome 4 of the human genome (Kessler, 1987).

a great deal of attention. Actually, there are two types—Alzheimer's disease (AD) and senile dementia of the Alzheimer's type (SDAT). The two disorders differ in age of onset and rate of progression but are similar in terms of their pathology (Whitehouse et al., 1983). Some believe that these two types of Alzheimer's disease are the most common cause of dementia in middle and late life Leroux, 1986; Whitehouse et al., 1983). Both are characterized by progressive abnormalities of memory, behavior, and cognition. Brain changes include neurofibrillary tangles, neuritic plaques, and loss of specific populations of nerve cells (Coyle et al., 1983). Some work is being done relating brain changes in AD and SDAT to those in Down's syndrome (Delabar et al., 1987; Edwards, 1986; Patterson, 1986). Down's syndrome, or trisomy 21, is a chromosomal abnormality that results in mental retardation and other physical anomalies in the children who are born with it. In the past few decades, autopsy studies have determined that all individuals with Down's syndrome who are over the age of 35 will develop the same sort of abnormal plaques and neurofibrillary tangles in the brain as people who die of Alzheimer's disease (Patterson, 1986). Better medical practice has raised the life expectancy of Down's syndrome individuals to 50 (up from 9 years, in 1910) (Edwards, 1986), and the life expectancy of people in general has also increased so that more people live to the older age at which Alzheimer's disease usually manifests (Leroux, 1986). Deficiencies in the cholinergic neurotransmitter system are thought to be partly responsible in both conditions for the brain plaques (Edwards, 1986). The hippocampus, the section of the brain responsible for memory and that is part of the system that influences motivation and mood states, is affected (Edwards, 1986). Recent work in Paris and at the National Institute of Health (NIH) resulted in reports of an extra gene that is responsible for the production of the protein *amyloid* in the cells of both Down's and Alzheimer's victims. The workers believed that the extra gene may lead to excessive amyloid production and abnormal deposition of the protein in the brain (Delabar et al., 1987; *Science News*, March 21, 1987). However, three later studies in this country and in Europe dispute this—finding no evidence of duplication of the amyloid gene either in familial or nonfamilial Alzheimer's disease. Others remain convinced that gene duplication does play a role in Alzheimer's disease (*New York Times*, October 30, 1987). One of the research experts involved in the later update is James Gusella of Harvard University who identified the Huntington's disease gene that was mentioned earlier in this chapter. His team's findings and those of another team in Belgium suggest that the two genetic defects (Alzheimer's disease and a genetic defect responsible for overproduction of amyloid protein in the brain) are inherited independently (*Science News*, September 19, 1987). Research efforts continue to focus on increasing our understanding of this devastating disease in the hope that prevention and treatment may become a reality. Other areas that are being investigated include head trauma and the possibility of infection by a slow virus (Zinman, 1987).

A light metal, aluminum, is being investigated as a possible causitive agent in Alzheimer's disease (Lerick, 1980; Pajik et al., 1984; Roberts, 1982; Perl and Brody, 1980; Trapp et al., 1978; Wurtman, 1985). Victims of the disorder are found to have high levels of aluminum in their brains on autopsy. Dietary and environmental sources of the metal include many over-the-counter antacids, underarm deodorants (Roberts, 1982), and aluminum cookware (Levick, 1980). "Dialysis dementia," a progressive dementia related to renal dyalisis, was traced to a high concentration of aluminum found in postmortem examination of victims of the syndrome. The large amounts of tap water used to flush out the blood stream were believed to be the source, since many municipalities rely on aluminum to remove impurities from the water supply (Tanne, 1983; Wurtman, 1985). However, current research is focusing more on elevated aluminum in the brain as a symptom rather than a contributory factor (Leroux, 1986). Aluminum appears to interfere with an enzyme, dihydropteridine, which is important for brain activity. This may explain one possible factor in neurological problems such as dementia (*Newsday*, July 14, 1987). At Cornell University, workers found a surprising difference in susceptibility to "aluminum poisoning" between Alzheimer's disease subjects and normal control subjects. The cells of normal subjects were *more* susceptible to aluminum than the cells of Alzheim-

er's disease victims. Citing a need for further study of this phenomenon, they believe that the results support the theory that Alzheimer's disease somehow involves a hereditary change in the body's defenses against the metal (*Alzheimer's Research Review*, Winter 1987-88).

Alzheimer's disease, considered the fourth leading cause of death for American adults, accounts for 150,000 deaths a year. While it can strike as early as the 40s (and very rarely the 20s and 30s), most Alzheimer's disease victims are over the age of 65. It is estimated that of people in this age group, 7 to 9% are suffering from the disease (Leroux, 1986). The estimated cost for Alzheimer's disease is $27 to $31 billion, and this is expected to increase dramatically as the size of our aged population increases (*New York Times*, August 30, 1987). Alzheimer's disease is a major health problem in which the underlying basis remains uncertain (Cooke, 1988).

Systems theory

A systems approach to organic brain dysfunction integrates biopsychosocial processes that are in simultaneous interaction with one another. This means that the various brain syndromes are products of reciprocal interaction among such factors as personal vulnerability to a stressor (e.g., disturbance in neurophysiological processes), the nature and duration of the stressor, the presence and potency of precipitating factors, age of onset, and sociocultural factors governing behavior.

Organic brain syndromes represent complex responses of the central nervous system to disturbances in neurophysiological processes that maintain normal functioning (see Table 26-1). Brain tissue is highly dependent on a constant supply of oxygen, glucose, and certain amino acids to maintain normal functioning. Any systemic or local condition that interferes with these essential elements or that inhibits or alters the normal metabolic processes can produce brain dysfunction of either an acute or a chronic nature. It should be noted that the present state of our knowledge of neurophysiology is not sufficient to explain all of the mechanisms through which systemic disorders affect brain function.

Organic brain disorders may occur at any age along the life span. When chronic dysfunction oc-

TABLE 26-1   Explanatory theories and identified factors of organic brain syndrome

Theoretical and identified factors	Acute	Chronic
Cardiovascular disease	Congestive heart failure Arrhythmias Cardiac infarction Hypovolemia Aortic stenosis Transient ischemic attacks Stroke Subdural hematoma Vasculitis Arteriosclerosis Hypertensive encephalopathy Subarachnoid hemorrhage	Multiple-infarcts dementia Cerebral arteriosclerosis Cerebral vascular accident (stroke) Subarachnoid hemorrhage
Infections	Septicemia Pneumonia Tuberculosis Urinary tract infection Bacteremia Meningitis Encephalitis Septic emboli Neurosyphilis Brain abscess	Encephalitis Meningitis Creutzfeldt-Jakob disease (slow virus) Alzheimer's disease (slow virus?) Third-stage syphilis Chronic brain abscess; aftermath of acute brain abscess
Medications	Analgesics Anticholinergics Antidepressants Antihistamines Antiparkinsonian agents Cimetidine Digitalis glycosides Diuretics Neuroleptics Sedative/hypnotics	Tardive dysmentia from antipsychotic (neuroleptic) drugs
Metabolic disorders	Electrolyte and fluid imbalance Hepatic, renal, or pulmonary failure Diabetes Hyperthyroidism or hypothyroidism Other endocrinopathies	Myxedema (hypothyroid)
Neoplasm	Neoplasm; any site in body Neoplasm, intracranial	Neoplasm, intracranial

Sources: Barry (1984), LaRue et al. (1985), Zisook and Braff (1986).   *Continued.*

TABLE 26-1 Explanatory theories and identified factors of organic brain syndrome—cont'd

Theoretical and identified factors	Acute	Chronic
Toxic conditions	Alcohol: delirium tremens; drunkenness; alcoholic hallucinosis; Wernicke's syndrome Amphetamines Sedative/hypnotics/hallucinogens (LSD) Heavy metals: lead; mercury; manganese; arsenic Solvents: glue Pesticides Carbon monoxide Burns Hip fracture Head injury (subdural, extradural hematomas)	Korsakoff's psychosis—chronic alcoholism Aftermath of poisoning, e.g., retardation from chronic lead poisoning Aluminum—Alzheimer's disease? Alzheimer's disease; head injury? Posttraumatic organic brain syndrome
Genetic diseases		Huntington's disease Alzheimer's disease? Down's syndrome Untreated PKU
Mechanical factor	Head injury	Untreated normal-pressure hydrocephalus Congenital hydrocephalus, microcephalus Minimal brain dysfunction in children?
Nutritional disorders	Protein deficiency Vit. B12 deficiency—postgastrectomy clients at risk Folic acid deficiency Nicotinic acid deficiency (pellagra) Thiamine deficiency (beriberi; Wenicke's and Korsakoff's syndromes)	Untreated folic acid deficiency Untreated pellagra Korsakoff's psychosis Minimal brain dysfunction in children?
Sensory deprivation/ overstimulation	Postoperative syndrome; "bypass psychosis"	
Electrical disorder	Seizure disorders	
Unknown	Multiple sclerosis, sequelae Systemic lupus erythematosus, sequelae	Multiple sclerosis, sequelae Systemic lupus erythematosus, sequelae Parkinson's disease Alzheimer's disease? Pick's disease

curs early in life, the inhibition in learning ability often results in mental retardation. The highest incidence of organic brain disorders, however, is in the older age group (LaRue et al., 1985), in which there are often functional impairments in sensory, motor, and homeostatic mechanisms and in central nervous system integrative efficiency. Persons in this age group are also more susceptible to chronic metabolic or systemic disorders and to psychosocial problems related to changes in role and status that are contributory factors. The emotional responses of grief, anger, and depression may distort the degree of cognitive dysfunction; in older persons, particularly, such symptoms are often mistaken for signs of an organic disorder. Thus, a systems approach emphasizes the interrelationship among an individual, other people, and the environment.

TREATMENT MODALITIES

The treatment of acute brain dysfunction depends on the underlying medical condition with which the dysfunction is associated. Aspects of treatment will be discussed further in the section on nursing intervention.

Many of the chronic brain dysfunctions associated with underlying pathological disorders may be reversed or ameliorated through proper treatment during the early stages. In a few disorders, advances in the treatment of the acute stages have virtually eliminated the appearance of chronic brain disease. For example, early and effective treatment of syphilis with penicillin has prevented the general paresis associated with syphilis, which was at one time a common cause of dementia. Early diagnosis of Wernicke's syndrome and treatment with thiamine cure this acute organic disorder and prevent the development of a chronic dysfunction.

Increased knowledge and better diagnostic procedures have enhanced the possibility of recognition and treatment of underlying pathology. For many years a diagnosis of psychosis with cerebral arteriosclerosis was almost routinely made for persons older than 65 who were admitted to large state mental hospitals. At the present time this diagnosis is being increasingly questioned as a valid cause of chronic brain syndrome (Heston and White, 1983).

Cerebral arteriosclerosis would be more apt to cause an acute condition such as a cerebral vascular accident. There is, however, a possibility of brain damage from multiple cerebral infarcts occurring over a period of time. Such a condition is associated with hypertension; if hypertension is recognized and treated early, such multiple infarctions could be prevented (Heston and White, 1983).

Normal-pressure hydrocephalus is another disorder that has received increased attention during the past decade. Normal-pressure hydrocephalus is characterized by a progressive dementia, accompanied by incontinence and a peculiar gait. As the name indicates, the cerebrospinal fluid pressure is normal in this condition. Diagnosis is made by pneumoencephalogram and other neurological diagnostic measures. A history of head trauma, infection, or another brain disease has been associated with the condition in some cases. A cerebrospinal shunt has been effective in reversing the symptoms in some patients (Heston and White, 1983).

The psychiatric treatment modalities used in therapy for clients with chronic organic brain dysfunction include individual, group, and family psychotherapy; occupational, recreational, and work therapies; activity therapies, including dance and movement therapies; crisis intervention; brief hospitalization; and administration of psychopharmaceuticals. Since most of these forms of treatment have been dealt with in earlier chapters, discussion in this chapter will be limited to aspects that are particularly relevant to clients who have organic insufficiency.

The use of individual and group psychotherapy in the treatment of clients with organic brain syndrome has been increasing since World War II. The extent to which these forms of therapy are available to such clients will depend on a variety of factors. Among those factors are the socioeconomic status of the individual, the availability and interest of psychotherapists, and the willingness of the client to accept these forms of therapy. Perhaps major inhibiting factors are attitudes toward chronic brain dysfunction and toward the elderly population, who make up the largest number of potential clients. Many professionals, including therapists and nurses, experience feelings of hopelessness and helplessness in response to chronic brain dysfunction and to elderly people. Such emotional responses inhibit the ability of the health professional to function or to maintain an interest in working with such clients. Karpf (1982) believes that the presence of chronic organic brain syndrome has been used as a scapegoat for contraindications for psychotherapy. He believes that individual therapy can prevent a rapid decline and that it can help clients to "behave more adaptively to the confines of their limitations." A therapeutic relationship can be of help in an estimated 50% of all cases diagnosed with dementia, according to Karpf. The therapeutic relationship can be made more effective if clients who feel dependent and helpless are offered an opportunity to achieve or to feel that they have achieved mastery and gratification.

Chronic organic brain syndrome (dementia)

In the elderly it is crucial that dementia be differentiated from the pseudodementia that is caused by depression and that is, with treatment, reversible (see Chapter 18 for differences). It is also important that correct diagnosis of other reversible syndromes be made—such as nutritional deficiencies and fluid-electrolyte imbalances. Stress and the emotional responses to it may increase the degree of cognitive dysfunction and the usual ability of an individual to cope with daily living. For this reason assessment in chronic brain disturbances must have a multiple focus in the collection and interpretation of data. That is, in addition to assessment of the cognitive functions of comprehension, memory, and orientation, there is also a need to assess mood or affect and the status of physical health and nutrition, as well as to be alert for the presence of psychosocial factors that may be serving as stressors.

Psychopharmaceuticals are widely employed in the treatment of people with organic dysfunction to control such symptoms as agitation, anxiety, and depression. In addition, many substances have been used and studied in relation to their effect on cognition. Among these are stimulants such as amphetamines, vasodilators, anticoagulants, hormones, vitamins, and procaine. The anticoagulants

continue to be widely used in the geriatric population in the treatment of circulatory and cognitive disorders. The possibility of hemorrhage, from even a minor injury, when anticoagulants are used, requires close monitoring of blood levels and close health supervision. In the case of persons who have organic dysfunctions with memory defects, which may interfere with the ability to follow through prescribed treatment and medication instructions, monitoring by community health nurses is important. Some drugs have been used in an attempt to improve or affect cognitive function, but studies have not supported their effectiveness (Leroux, 1986).

The use of antipsychotic and antidepressant drugs in older people has a higher risk of toxic side effects than it does in younger people.* The absorption, metabolism, and excretion of many of these drugs are altered in the older age group. The side effects that may appear include confusion, disorientation, lethargy or agitation, and aggression. Since confusion and disorientation are common symptoms in organic brain dysfunction in both the acute and the chronic states, antipsychotic or antidepressant drugs may exacerbate these symptoms. Although lower-than-average doses may prevent such side effects, it is important that nursing staff be alert to toxic side effects in assessing client behavior.

Acute organic brain syndrome (delirium)

Treatment of a person in an acute confusional state depends on the underlying process. In view of the fact that such a state may be precipitated by a broad range of medical problems, therapeutic measures may encompass a broad range of treatments. In some conditions, such as drug and alcohol withdrawal, chemical intoxication, head trauma, and intracranial neoplasms or infections, an acute confusional state may be an anticipated complication. In other conditions, an organic dysfunction

---

*For discussion of side effects of antipsychotic drugs, see Chapter 25; for side effects of antidepressant drugs, see Chapter 22.

is far less predictable. Some people may be more vulnerable to organic brain dysfunction than other people are. Older people, for example, may be more vulnerable to the toxic effects of prescribed medications or a fluid electrolyte imbalance. A low-grade fever in an elderly person may not be indicative of the degree of an inflammatory process because the normal physiological responses to inflammation (elevated temperature, elevated white blood count, and so on) may be altered in older people. The temperature, for example, may be only slightly elevated in the presence of a severe inflammatory process. In such a situation, the severity of the disease process may go unrecognized.

EMERGENCY INTERVENTIONS

In the emergency treatment of confusional states, differential diagnosis is extremely important. Acute organic brain syndrome must be differentiated from chronic organic brain syndrome, and the specific underlying factors of acute brain syndrome must be determined. In dementia, it is important to differentiate true dementia from the pseudodementia of depression in the elderly.

Diagnosis and differential diagnosis necessitate an ongoing, current assessment and a carefully constructed history. First observations of the client may include an appraisal of the client's appearance (grooming, body habits, clothing, gait, stance, movements, and speech). If the client was accompanied, the individual who comes to the emergency room (relatives, police) should be interviewed to help construct an accurate history (Phillips and Schwartz, 1982). Level of consciousness should be ascertained. The box on p. 864 describes the levels of consciousness.

Appropriate to the level of consciousness, the mental and neurological state of the client should be determined. The client's orientation to person, place, and time and psychological testing can help to determine the client's mental state. Neurological examination will help to complete the assessment. Table 26-2 summarizes the neurological exam.

TABLE 26-2   The neurological examination

Area examined	Assessments
Mentation	Awareness Orientation (oriented to time, place, and person); level of consciousness (obtunded, stuporous, semicomatose, comatose)
Speech	Normal, dysplasia, dysarthria, dysphonia
General knowledge	Knowledge of current events, vocabulary
Memory	Intact, recent memory impaired, remote memory impaired
Retention and recall	Recall of objects, digits forward and reversed
Reasoning	Judgment, insight, abstraction (interpretation of proverbs, similarities, and differences)
Use of symbols	Calculation, reading, writing
Object recognition	Normal, agnosia
Praxis	Ideational, ideomotor, motor, and constructional apraxias
Perception	Delusions, illusions, hallucinations
Mood	Normal, euphoric, depressed, anxious, agitated
Affect	Normal, flat, inappropriate
Gait, station	Hemiplegic, ataxic, spastic, festinating, hyperkinetic, waddling, apraxia of gait, hysterical gait, step-page gait; Romberg test
Cranial nerves— motor system	Atrophy, fasciculations, tremor, dystonia, involuntary movements, palpation, tone, strength
Coordination	Finger-to-nose and heel-to-shin tests, rapid alternating movements
Reflexes	Superficial reflexes, tendon reflexes
Sensation	Touch, pain, temperature, vibration and position sense, tactile localization, two-point discrimination, bilateral simultaneous stimulation, stereognosis, barognosis, skin writing

From Phillips and Schwartz (1982).   *Continued.*

TABLE 26-2 The neurological examination—cont'd

Area examined	Assessments
Head and neck	Bruises over head and neck, scalp and skull tenderness and deformity, signs of head trauma, cerebrospinal fluid drainage from ears and nose
Spine, skin	Nuchal rigidity, low hairline, shortness of neck, spinal deformity, spinal tenderness, limitation of movement of spine, paravertebral spasm, limitation of straight leg raising, palpation for cervical ribs, pes cavus, peripheral nerve enlargement, adenoma sebaceum, café-au-lait spots, trigeminal hemangioma

Nursing Intervention
PRIMARY PREVENTION

Primary prevention in organic brain dysfunction involves many aspects of our complex social system. The importance of the prevention of a condition that in many instances *is* preventable and that can have a devastating effect upon the individual, the family, and the community cannot be overemphasized. The nurse, as a health professional and as a citizen, has a responsibility to participate in the primary prevention of organic disorders.

Primary prevention in organic disorders focuses on individuals, families, and groups at risk and on factors in the environment that contribute to the disease process. Because organic disorders are associated with a broad range of factors and because they are closely interrelated with other health problems, primary prevention will often be an integral part of general health promotion. The prevention of suicide through "hot lines," for example, or programs that enable nurses to intervene in alcohol and drug abuse may have an impact on the incidence of organic brain disorders.

Social and political action related to such community concerns as environmental pollution, consumer products safety, and highway and transpor-

---

Levels of consciousness

obtundation Client responds to stimuli and obeys commands but usually only for as long as stimulation continues. Confusion during response and arousal may be present.

stupor Painful stimuli produce withdrawal and bodily movement, often with groans; spontaneous movement is present. Some prolonged intervals of responsiveness are brought about by painful stimuli.

semicoma Painful stimuli produce withdrawal response away from stimulus; no spontaneous movement is noted.

coma No response to painful stimuli is evident, and any psychologically understandable response to external stimuli or inner need is absent

coma-vigil (akinetic mutism) Comalike state exists, in which reflex activity (swallowing, sucking, and chewing) may be released by lesions to mesencephalon and in which eye movements may be seen in the absence of other bodily movements and in the presence of unconsciousness.

Adapted from Phillips and Schwartz, 1982.

tation safety may also be part of primary prevention of organic disorders. Although Ralph Nader has demonstrated that one committed individual can have an impact upon public safety, the most effective action has come about through persistent and informed group action.

The degree to which environmental pollution contributes to organic brain disease is not known. It is known, however, that certain chemicals—heavy metals and carbon monoxide, for example—play a very direct role. The ever-increasing number of reports in the news media of severe environmental pollution by industry is alarming. Reports of the long-term pollution of a town in Italy after a single emission of a toxic chemical from a factory and of buried chemicals seeping to the surface in the Love Canal in Niagara Falls, New York, and their destructive impact on the health of residents, are but two examples.

Professional nurses working in industry have

long been involved in occupational health and safety. They have been effective in the early identification of health and safety hazards and in early diagnosis and treatment of health problems. Industrial nurses also have had an opportunity to work with environmental and safety engineers and with the Occupational Safety and Health Administration to identify and eliminate potential hazards to health in industry and to assist in the promotion of safety measures through health teaching and health supervision of workers.

Since brain dysfunction may be a secondary response to underlying metabolic or other systemic disorders, any advances in the prevention of such conditions would automatically have a preventive effect on the incidence of acute brain syndrome. Immunization against communicable diseases and treatment of primary and secondary stages of syphilis are examples of such prevention. Early diagnosis and effective treatment of many systemic disorders—treatment of pneumonia with antibiotics, for example—has also been important. Efforts to prevent alcohol abuse, drug abuse, and toxic substance use have been less than successful despite the expenditure of much effort toward this end. Early identification of people at risk and the availability of community services for effective treatment are important aspects of these efforts. Public education, particularly of the younger population, can play a role. Research into underlying factors may eventually lead to more effective preventive measures.

Primary prevention in chronic brain syndrome is more complex, since the underlying factors are not known in the majority of cases. The increasing interest in such conditions and the awareness that they are disease processes and not normal concomitants of aging are hopeful signs for further research and treatment of these disorders. The greatest advances to date have been in the fields of neuropathology and neurochemistry. A number of people, labeled as having chronic brain syndrome, have symptoms that represent an underlying disorder that in many instances can be alleviated through appropriate treatment. Improved diagnostic measures, including neurological evaluation, could lead to the institution of such treatment. Normal-pressure hydrocephalus, for example, is a neurological condition that is often mistaken for senile dementia

when the diagnosis is based on the symptom picture alone, without an adequate neurological evaluation.

Depression in an older person is also often misdiagnosed as senile dementia. Treatment for the depression alleviates the symptoms in such cases. The prevalence of such conditions in the elderly has become widely enough recognized to have spawned the term *pseudodementia* to describe them. McAllister (1983) suggests that there may be at least two categories of pseudodementia. He believes, based on the available data, that the cognitive impairment that can be associated with depression is more correctly viewed as *depression-induced organic mental disorder*. The prognosis for these individuals tends to be, with adequate psychiatric treatment, very hopeful. The prognosis for those people who have coexisting organic and functional illnesses is less hopeful and is determined by the extent to which the current deficit is being caused by the functional or psychiatric component of their illness (McAllister, 1983).

Professional nurses working in hospitals and communities can be effective in many aspects of primary prevention of chronic brain dysfunction. Early identification and treatment of physical and psychological health problems often rest with the community health nurse, who may be the first health professional to become aware of the existence of such health problems. Differentiating between symptoms of depression and chronic brain dysfunction* may be more possible for a nurse, who frequently has greater contact with a client, than for a physician, who may see the person only briefly. Communication of such observations to other health professionals is important in obtaining appropriate treatment. Case finding among people living alone and somewhat isolated in a community and providing information about resources for recreation, crisis intervention, and social interaction are also appropriate nursing functions that may play a part in prevention.

The frequency with which many health problems coincide with some degree of organic brain dys-

---

*See Chapter 18 for table differentiating depression from dementia.

function, particularly in elderly people, points up the need for and importance of ongoing health supervision and teaching for clients with these health problems. Many such people are receiving medical care and have had drugs prescribed for the treatment of the physical disorders. However, even a mild degree of organic dysfunction, and the memory deficit that accompanies it, often makes it difficult for a person to understand, remember, or carry out prescribed treatment. This situation can be complicated by anxiety, attitudes toward taking drugs, ethnic beliefs about illness, food preferences, and a variety of other factors.

Several aspects of health supervision and teaching are particularly relevant preventive measures in working with such clients. *Counseling* that is oriented toward helping people identify the concerns they may have about medications and other treatments will facilitate nursing intervention and will serve to communicate interest in and concern for clients as individuals.

Frequently, prescribed medical treatment is not followed because a person does not understand or remember the purpose of the therapy or is confused by the variety of pills and capsules ordered by a physician. An understanding of the purpose of each medication and treatment usually overcomes such difficulties. Helping the person to devise an organized system for taking medication can help combat a medication error or omission resulting from a memory deficit. Adapting special diets to accommodate ethnic food preferences may provide a person the incentive necessary to maintain a prescribed dietary regimen. Consultation with family, friends, or people of the same ethnic background as a client can be used for a variety of purposes.

Acting in support of or on behalf of a client—client advocacy—has long been a part of professional nursing practice, and it is currently receiving renewed attention as a part of mental health practice. Client advocacy is particularly important when nurses are working with clients who may be at risk of developing organic brain dysfunction. The objective in both prevention and treatment is to help a person maintain an optimal level of independent functioning. Attempting to cope with the bureaucracies of social agencies, the isolation that confronts older people, and other aspects of our society often requires that a client have the support and assistance of a nurse or other health professionals.

Client advocacy can involve a variety of actions carried out in cooperation with a client or, with permission, on the client's behalf. Maintaining contact and cooperation with a physician, clinic, or health agency can help the nurse to reinforce, clarify, or amplify prescribed medical or other treatment. Assisting a client to contact social, recreational, and other community services and to follow through on appointments are often important aspects of working with people with organic brain disorders. Seeking out social support systems in the community and helping clients to make use of them can help them to overcome isolation and loneliness.

SECONDARY PREVENTION

Secondary prevention in organic brain dysfunction is oriented toward early diagnosis and effective treatment so that a person may be restored to the optimal level of functioning. The professional nurse performs an important function in both aspects of this objective.

For a client in the acute confusional state, early recognition of symptoms of organic dysfunction and prompt treatment of the underlying pathological condition are often essential to preserving the integrity of the brain and, at times, the life of the client. Since the nurse is frequently the health professional in closest contact with the client, he or she may be the first to identify early signs of cognitive dysfunction and thus to take action (including communication of findings to medical and nursing staff) to initiate early treatment. Which treatment is appropriate will depend on the underlying pathology. But it is important to note that symptoms of cognitive dysfunction may, in some instances, be the first indications of systemic and other disorders.

Nursing intervention in acute confusional states is based on the nurse's ability to use the nursing process in assessment and correlation of data and to protect the client and prevent chronicity. Early symptoms include shifting levels of awareness, difficulty in focusing attention, and an inability to screen out irrelevant stimuli. These symptoms may be accompanied by clouding of consciousness or an inability to think clearly or to comprehend what is said. There may be a haziness or vagueness of perception. In later stages there is confusion and disorientation and evidence of memory impairment. In severe stages there may be loss of motor control. Shifts in degrees of awareness and orientation and changes in emotional responses, from calmness to restlessness, fearfulness to apathy, or irritability to placidity, may be suggestive of delirium.

Nursing process

Nursing intervention in an acute confusional state depends on the ability of the nurse to assess and interpret symptoms. The nursing history is an important part of the assessment process in delirious states. An understanding, obtained from the family or the client, of the person's functioning prior to the onset of the illness and of the ways in which the person coped with stress may be important in distinguishing chronic from acute brain syndrome and in identifying early symptoms of organic dysfunctions, particularly in the elderly. Pertinent information about many other factors that can contribute to delirium, such as medication, drug and alcohol use, and diet, are a part of such a history. Correlation of the symptoms with the medical history, the diagnosis, and the laboratory data is also an important aspect of assessment. Communications of findings to other members of the health team, particularly the physician and the nursing staff, is essential to appropriate intervention.

ASSESSMENT

The assessment of a client who is coping with impaired brain function that has led to either an acute or chronic confusional state, should consider the following areas:
1. Presenting symptoms—defects in perception, attention and memory, and so on, that are creating problems for the client
2. Emotional state—such feelings as helplessness, anxiety, or anger that are responses to a stimulus situation

3. Maladaptive coping behaviors—these tend to be regressive patterns (dependency, denial, projection) in attempts to satisfy needs and protect the self-system
4. Origin of maladaptive coping behaviors—identification of stressful experiences in the present that are helping to generate the maladaptive behavior
5. Stimulus situations—stressful life situations that are characterized by a threat to one's security and the frustration of one's attempts to satisfy needs and that can be exacerbated or engendered by losses in cognitive functioning: impaired memory and learning; diminished attention and concentration; distorted perceptions; loss of orientation
6. Holistic health status—physical, intellectual, emotional, sociocultural, and spiritual status of the client, factors that may either facilitate wellness (for example, a concerned and relatively large extended family system may be able to compensate for some of the client's impairment through the care the family members extend to the client) or may impede wellness (for example, the inadequate nutrition of an elderly and poor client may complicate the symptoms of chronic organic brain syndrome)

ANALYSIS OF DATA

As the presenting symptoms, emotional states, maladaptive coping behavior, and stimulus situations are fully assessed, some understanding of the client's (and often of the family's) situation will emerge. Using this understanding, appropriate nursing diagnoses can be made.

PLANNING AND IMPLEMENTATION

The following section is concerned with the nursing diagnoses of *acute confusional state* and *chronic confusional state*. The nursing process as it applies to intervening with children and their families has been discussed in Chapter 17 and will not be repeated here.

NURSING CARE PLAN

Clients with Impaired Brain Function

Long-term Outcomes*	Short-term Outcomes*	Nursing Strategies

Nursing diagnosis: Altered thought processes related to an acute confusional state (NANDA 8.3; DSM-III-R 293.00)

Long-term Outcomes*	Short-term Outcomes*	Nursing Strategies
Prevent any chronicity of impaired brain functioning Restore the client to normal (premorbid) levels of functioning in all areas	Preserve the integrity of the brain Protect the integrity of the organism as a whole (monitoring of nutrition, safety, and skin care; modulation of environment) Help to determine the specific cause of the syndrome Differentiate between chronic and acute syndrome Protect the self-esteem of the client Provide support to family and significant others Communicate any findings, assessment to other members of the health team (physician, nursing staff)	The number of people providing direct care to the client should be limited to the smallest number possible to provide adequate care. Members of the group should function as a team, sharing information and offering guidance and support to each other. A small number of people providing continuity of care will be less demanding of the client's cognitive abilities than a large number and will aid in maintaining orientation to people. Consistency in the staff caring for the client, which is implied in this team concept, will also promote the establishment of supportive relationships. Close supervision of client by team members is important to protect safety. The atmosphere should be as quiet as possible to limit distracting external stimuli. Placing a client in a room near the call box results in distraction, as does a room in which or near which there is a high level of activity. Communication† with clients in acute confusional states should be brief and clear, and abstractions should be avoided. Questioning should be limited to essential information, and it should be terminated if the client becomes more confused or appears frustrated. Staff members should call patients by name and should also identify themselves by name, avoiding asking if clients remember them. Since clients in acute confusional states are often frightened or anxious, reassurance appropriate to the situation can help allay fears. When it is known that a condition is temporary and directly related to a physical condition, a simple explanation of this fact can be reassuring to a client. Often, the presence and understanding of the nurse are the most important factors in helping allay fears. When possible, the presence of a familiar and caring family member can be a stabilizing factor. This is particularly important when ethnic and language differences exist between the client and the health staff. Disorientation is often more severe during the night, when energy levels are lower and darkness increases the possibility of visual distortion. Keeping the room of a client with delirium well lighted at night may prevent the increase in cognitive dysfunction and development of illusions (visual misperceptions). Assume advocacy role for client/family system, as needed.

*When a client is in an acute confusional state, the locus of decision making lies with the nurse.
†Subjective reports are not always reliable in clients who are coping with impaired brain function.

Long-term Outcomes*	Short-term Outcomes*	Nursing Strategies
Nursing diagnosis: Altered thought processes related to a chronic confusional state (NANDA 8.3; DSM-III-R 294.10)		
Restore to highest level of functioning possible in all areas	Undergo ongoing assessment and monitoring of status in all areas	Establish a relationship with the client and family
Family/client system will be sustained throughout the experience of client's disorder	Be protected, as far as integrity of the whole organism is concerned (monitoring of nutrition; safety; skin care; modulation of environment; health teaching and supervision)	Maintain ongoing assessment and monitoring of the client's status in all areas†
		Protect the integrity of the organism as a whole (monitoring of nutrition, safety, skin care; modulation of environment; health teaching and supervision)
	Maintain independent functioning to maximum degree possible	Promote the client's ability for independent functioning to the maximum degree possible
	Build self-esteem in a realistic manner	Protect the self-esteem of the client
		Adequate medical care and health supervision (Treatment and rehabilitation of existing physiological disorders or disabilities are essential. Health supervision and teaching in such areas as nutrition and hygiene are particularly important.)
		Early identification and treatment of emotional disorders, such as depression, which can complicate organic dysfunction should be carried out
		Promote emotional security through use of such resources as family, friends; social, religious, and ethnic groups; and community agencies
		Referral of client/family system, as needed in following:
		• economic assistance
		• crisis intervention and emergency medical and psychiatric care
		• social, recreational, and family respite services
		Assume advocacy role for client/family system, as needed

EVALUATION

Whenever feasible, the client and the client's family or significant others should be included in estimating the client's progress toward attainment of goals. Evaluation should encompass the following areas:

1. Estimation of the degree to which there has been improvement and/or stabilization in coping with impaired brain functioning and associated psychosocial losses. This would include *awareness* of conflicts and problem areas and beginning efforts toward working them through.
2. Estimation of the degree to which goals have been achieved and client functioning has improved or stabilized (demonstrated by decreased anxiety; decreased disorder in interpersonal relationships; increased ability to function in society; decreased tendency to use regressive coping mechanisms; reaching maximum potential for self-care; maintaining an adequate level of safety in functioning through appropriate client-family participation)
3. Identification of goals that need to be modified or revised
4. Referral of the client and the client's family to support systems other than the nurse-client relationship

a. People in the client's and the client's family's social network who are willing to serve as a support system
b. Clinics or individuals for ongoing individual and group psychotherapy for client's family members, when indicated
c. Community agencies that help clients learn to live with disorders that may never be completely eliminated (e.g., day hospital settings structured to meet the needs of organically impaired clients)
d. Centers or organizations that provide support for families of organically impaired clients (e.g., support groups for families of individuals with Alzheimer's disease)

TERTIARY PREVENTION

Some individuals cope with the cognitive impairment of organic brain dysfunction and are able to function adequately except at times of crisis, when supportive services may be needed. In this respect, these individuals differ little from the general population, with the possible exception of a greater vulnerability to stress and a somewhat diminished capacity to cope with stress without assistance.

In other individuals the cognitive dysfunction and associated psychosocial factors may inhibit the ability to care for oneself and may become progressively incapacitating. Perception, memory, orientation, and judgment may be so impaired that an individual cannot be responsible for self-care; these people require a fairly constant level of care and supervision. They may be found living with families who are able to care for them or in mental hospitals or other institutions. Whatever the decision of the family as far as institutionalization is concerned, the nurse can play an important role in providing information during the decision-making process. Support of the family that combats destructive guilt can help maximize a continuing involvement with the client. Organized support groups for the relatives of clients with Alzheimer's disease have been particularly effective. Such groups can help family members deal with the grief that is associated with a loved one's progressive dementia; with the financial and personal burdens of caregiving; with family members' fears about heredity and the disease process (Teusink and Mahler, 1984). *Respite care* was

discussed in Chapter 18 as it applied to the elderly, and it is a valid alternative here, too. The relatives of Alzheimer's disease victims who are caregivers experience a great deal of stress and may be at risk for physical and emotional illness (*Science News*, September 12, 1987). There are also day care facilities that have become available for those who suffer from dementia.

Whether it is given in the home or in a community agency, tertiary care for organic brain syndrome clients has the following major objectives:

1. Promoting and maintaining the optimum level of functioning possible for the individual
2. Promoting a sense of dignity and worth
3. Maintaining physical health and well-being by means of adequate diagnostic measures so that treatment may be instituted for those conditions that may respond to treatment
4. Maintaining and promoting reality orientation
5. Encouraging independent functioning to the degree possible
6. Providing opportunity to meet psychosocial needs, such as recreation, intellectual stimulation, and socialization
7. Providing support when needed

Meeting these treatment objectives necessitates close cooperation between the health team members and, when possible, between the family and the health team. The role of liaison between the client and family and between members of the health team is an important function of the nurse, whether the client resides in an agency or at home.

A therapeutic environment is important for providing protection, support, and rehabilitation for clients. The therapeutic milieu as a treatment that employs all aspects of the environment to promote health has been discussed in Chapter 12. Special emphasis should be placed on providing physical and emotional support, encouraging independent functioning to the extent possible for the individual, and promoting reality orientation.

Maintaining orientation can be encouraged through the placement of large-faced clocks and calendars in prominent places and through individual and group discussions of events of daily living and affairs of interest in the community. Contact between the community and the hospital or agency unit may be used to stimulate interest and interaction between clients and the broader environment. Use of community resources for recreation, health care, and support systems is important in preventing isolation.

Recreational, occupational, and movement therapies promote mental and physical health. Such therapies should be adapted to the interests and physical abilities of clients.

Interpersonal therapies, both individual and group, are helpful in maintaining emotional security. The nurse-client relationship, discussed at length in earlier chapters, provides opportunity for emotional support.

CHAPTER SUMMARY

The organic brain disorders are a group of complex conditions that involve disturbances in cognition related to disruptions in the normal neurophysiological processes that are essential to intellectual functioning. Behavioral manifestations of cognitive impairment include disturbances in levels of awareness, comprehension, memory, association, orientation, and judgment, which interfere with the ability to perceive, interpret, and respond effectively to the environment. The cognitive dysfunction may range from mild to severe, and it is often accompanied by emotional responses of fear, anger, feelings of helplessness, and depression.

Organic brain dysfunction may be acute and temporary, in which case the individual recovers completely in a relatively brief period of time with appropriate treatment and effective restorative processes. In other instances, the brain dysfunction may be chronic and irreversible because of a continuing disturbance in metabolic functioning or a diffuse destruction of brain tissue.

The explanation for organic brain dysfunction may lie in any systemic or central nervous system pathological condition, including metabolic disorders, systemic and central nervous system infections, trauma, and conditions caused by chemicals and drugs. In some chronic forms, the underlying process is unknown, in which case the onset is often slow and insidious, rather than acute.

Treatment of acute organic brain dysfunction includes early diagnosis and treatment of the underlying pathological condition so that cognitive dysfunction may be reversed or contained. In some acute disorders, early diagnosis may be essential to prevent progressive dysfunction, which can lead to coma and death. Which specific treatment is used depends on diagnosis. For the client with acute brain dysfunction, who is most often seen in a general hospital, nursing assessment of cognitive dysfunction may be very important to early diagnosis.

Treatment of chronic brain dysfunction has the objective of promoting independent functioning to the maximum degree possible. It includes adequate medical and nursing care for treatment and rehabilitation of physical and emotional disorders and preventive intervention through health teaching and supervision. Preventive measures to promote emotional security and comfort include client advocacy in the use of community resources to meet psychosocial needs and in the development and strengthening of social networks. In addition, a protective therapeutic environment, all of the forms of psychosocial therapy, and chemotherapy are employed. Treatment settings include general hospitals, private homes, foster homes, nursing homes, and mental hospitals.

Clients with organic brain dysfunction may be found in almost every area in which professional nurses practice. Nursing intervention spans both the preventive and the therapeutic aspects of organic brain disorders, although not every nurse will be involved in every area. Primary prevention encompasses the nurse's role both as a citizen and as a health professional. As a citizen, participation in social, political, and community action groups that seek to reduce environmental pollution, promote occupational safety, or provide community facilities to meet the needs of vulnerable individuals is an important preventive activity. Professional roles include health education, genetic counseling, case finding, and client advocacy in meeting health and psychosocial needs.

Secondary prevention and tertiary prevention include collaboration with the health team, participation in therapeutic modalities, health supervision and promotion, and participation in individual, family, and group activities that promote the emotional comfort and the cognitive functioning of clients.

SELF-DIRECTED LEARNING

Sensitivity-Awareness Exercises

The purposes of the following exercises are:
- Develop awareness about the interrelationship of factors in the underlying basis of organic brain syndromes
- Develop awareness about the subjective experience of clients who are coping with impaired brain functioning
- Develop awareness about the subjective experience of the families of clients who are coping with impaired brain functioning
- Develop awareness about your own feelings and attitudes in working with clients who are coping with impaired brain functioning

1. Try to imagine that you are suffering with either an acute organic brain syndrome or a chronic organic brain syndrome.
2. Describe what you think that experience would entail. Describe some of your symptoms and how you might cope with them.
3. Describe what you think it would be like to be the family member of someone who is suffering from an organic brain syndrome. How would you cope with this situation? What are your thoughts and feelings about institutionalization if a family member of yours was coping with a chronic organic brain syndrome?
4. Develop a plan of care for assisting a family to cope with a client with impaired brain functioning:
   a. When the family has decided that it is necessary to institutionalize the client
   b. When the family has decided to care for the client at home

Questions to Consider

1. Which of the following is an acute organic brain syndrome?
   a. General paresis of the insane
   b. Dementia praecox
   c. Down's syndrome
   d. Delirium tremens
2. Which of the following is a chronic organic brain syndrome?
   a. Pseudodementia
   b. Pick's disease
   c. Second-stage syphilis
   d. Delirium tremens

3. Which of the following statements describes Alzheimer's disease?
   a. It is almost always associated with a chronic vitamin B deficiency
   b. The incidence is declining in most communities because of the increased research efforts
   c. An individual with the same genetic structure as a victim of Down's syndrome is somehow protected from it
   d. Structural brain changes are found on autopsy

Match the following columns:

4. Huntington's disease   a. Viral
5. Korsakoff's psychosis   b. Syphilis
6. General paresis   c. Genetic
7. Creutzfeldt-Jakob disease d. Vitamin B deficiency

8. Tertiary prevention for Alzheimer's disease includes:
   a. Brain imaging methods such as the CAT scan and the PET scan
   b. Organized support groups for the families of victims
   c. Health teaching in the elderly about the avoidance of aluminum-containing antacids
   d. Genetic counseling
9. Memory of recent events is often more impaired than remote memory in individuals who are suffering from chronic organic brain syndrome. This is termed:
   a. Confabulation
   b. Retrograde memory loss
   c. Current memory loss
   d. Benign senescent memory loss
10. In caring for a client who is experiencing an acute confusional state, it is important to:
    a. Limit the number of personnel providing direct care
    b. Initiate an active program of sensory stimulation to prevent regression
    c. Keep the room somewhat darkened to cut down on stimuli
    d. Allow the client to make decisions

Answer key

1. d	5. d	8. b
2. b	6. b	9. b
3. d	7. a	10. a
4. c		

REFERENCES

Alzheimers Research Review: Cornell researchers investigate the systemic nature of Alzheimer's disease, Alzheimer's Res Rev (Winter):3, 1987-88.

Barry P: Organic brain syndrome, In Barry P: Psychosocial nursing assessment and intervention, Philadelphia, 1984, JB Lippincott Co.

Billings D and Stokes L: Medical surgical nursing, ed 2, St. Louis, 1986, The CV Mosby Co.

Cooke R: The Alzheimer's puzzle, Newsday, May 10, Section 2: pp 1 and 3, 1988.

Coyle J, Price D, and DeLong M: Alzheimer's disease: a disorder of cortical cholinergic innervation. Science 219:1184-1189, 1983.

Delabar J et al: Beta amyloid gene duplication in Alzheimer's disease and karotypically normal Down syndrome, Science 235(4794):1390-1392, 1987.

Edwards D: A common medical denominator, Sci News 129(4): 60-62, 1986.

Gusella J et al: A polymorphic DNA marker genetically linked to Huntington's disease, Nature 306:234-238, 1983.

Herbert W: Mental illness from psychiatric drugs? Sci News 124(14):214, 1983.

Heston L and White J: Dementia: a practical guide to Alzheimer's disease and related illnesses, New York, 1983, WH Freeman & Co.

Heston L et al: Pick's disease, Arch Gen Psychiatr 44:409-411, 1987.

Karpf R: Individual psychotherapy with the elderly, In Horton A, editor: Mental health interventions for the aging, New York, 1982, Praeger Publishers.

Kessler S: Psychiatric implications of presymptomatic testing for Huntington's disease, Am J Orthopsychiatr 57(2):212-219, 1987.

La Rue A et al: Aging and mental disorders, In Birren J and Schaie K, editors: The Handbook of the psychology of aging, New York, 1985, Van Nostrand Reinhold Company, Inc.

Lehman, H: Psychopharmacological approaches to the organic brain syndrome, Comp Psychiatr 24(5):412-430, 1983.

Leroux C: Coping and caring: living with Alzheimer's disease, Washington, DC, 1986, American Association of Retired Persons in cooperation with the Alzheimer's Disease and Related Disorders Association.

Levick S: Dementia from aluminum pots? N Engl J Med 303(3):164, 1980.

McAllister T: Overview: pseudodementia, Am J Psychiatr 140(5):528-532, 1983.

Newsday: Alzheimer's study, Newsday June 2, Section 3:10, 1987.

Newsday: Aluminum finding, Newsday July 14, Section 4:10, 1987.

New York Times: Alzheimer's costs, NY Times, August 30, Section 3:1, 1987.

New York Times: Gene's causative link to Alzheimer's is disputed, NY Times October 30, Section D:24, 1987.

Pajik M et al: Continuing education: Alzheimer's disease, Am J Nurs 84(2):215-232, 1984.

Patterson D: The causes of Down syndrome, Sci Am 257(2):52-60, 1986.

Perl D and Brody A: Alzheimer's disease: x-ray spectrometric evidence of aluminum accumulation in neurofibrillary tangle-bearing neurons, Science 208:297-299, 1980.

Phillips F and Schwartz J: The client with an organic disorder, In Gorton J and Partridge R, editors: Practice and management of psychiatric emergency care, St. Louis, 1982, The CV Mosby Co.

Roberts E: Potential therapies in aging and senile dementias, In Alzheimer's disease, Down's syndrome, and aging, Ann NY Acad Sci 396:175, 1982.

Science News: Alzheimer/Down syndrome bond tightens, Sci News 131(12):188, 1987.

Science News: Taking care of immunity, Sci News 132(12):181, 1987.

Seltzer B and Frazier SH: Organic mental disorders, In Nicholi AM Jr, editor: The Harvard modern guide to psychiatry, Cambridge, Mass, 1978, Belknap Press of Harvard University Press.

Tanne J: Alzheimer's and aluminum: an element of suspicion, Am Health 2(5):48-54, 1983.

Teusink J and Mahler S: Helping families cope with Alzheimer's disease, Hosp Commun Psychiatr 35(2):152-156, 1984.

Trapp G et al: Aluminum levels in brain in Alzheimer's disease, Biolog Psychiatr 13:709-718, 1978.

US Department of Health and Human Services: The dementias: hope through research, Washington, DC, 1983, Office of Scientific and Health Reports, National Institute of Neurological and Communicative Disorders and Stroke.

Whaley L and Wong D: Nursing care of infants and children, ed 3, St Louis, 1987, The CV Mosby Co.

Whitehouse P et al: Alzheimer's disease and senile dementia: loss of neurons in the basal forebrain, Science 215:1237-1239, 1982.

Wurtman R: Alzheimer's disease, Sci Am 252(1):62-74, 1985.

Zinman D: Losing minds: more Alzheimer's, no new treatments, Newsday April 14, Section 5: pp 1 and 3, 1987.

Zisook S and Braff D: Delirium: recognition and management in the older patient, Geriatrics 41(6): 66-78, 1987.

ANNOTATED SUGGESTED READINGS

Edwards D: A common medical denominator, Sci News 129(4):60-62, 1986.

A very good overview of the specific neuropathological changes that can be found in Alzheimer's disease and in Down syndrome and how these similarities are helping research scientists to increase their understanding of both disorders. The examinations and comparisons are carried out with the hope of finding improved methods of treatment. Several research efforts in this area are described.

Hughes D: Alzheimer's disease and psychiatric nursing: treating the depression, Persp in Psychiatr Care 24(1):5-8, 1987.

This describes some of the problems of clients and staff as a research psychiatric unit, set up to treat depression, was converted to a unit for the treatment of Alzheimer's disease. The symptoms and behavior associated with depression were evi-

dent in many clients. One of the clinical staff's tasks was to differentiate pathological depression from a grief reaction to the losses encountered with Alzheimer's disease. A therapeutic, structured atmosphere and adaptations of treatment are discussed. The importance of family support groups and individual family sessions with the patient are noted. The author concludes that Alzheimer's disease victims can respond to therapy for their depressions and that an improved quality of life for client and family results from active intervention.

Leroux C: Coping and caring: living with Alzheimer's disease, Washington, DC, 1986, The American Association of Retired Persons in association with the Alzheimer's Disease and Related Disorders Association.

This helpful publication explains the nature and history of Alzheimer's disease, tells "what it is not," provides socioeconomic facts such as statistics of incidence and prevalence and costs to the nation. Treatment and caregiving and legal issues are also covered. There are sections on how to obtain financial help and how to choose a nursing home. Research into the disorder is briefly reviewed.

Pajik M, Reisberg B, and Beam I: Continuing education: Alzheimer's disease, Am J Nurs 84(2):215-232, 1984.

Three separate articles comprise this continuing education presentation for credit units: "Inpatient care" by M. Pajik; "Stages of cognitive decline" by B. Reisberg; and "Helping families survive" by I. Beam. These articles represent a comprehensive approach to understanding some of the underlying factors, course, and treatment of Alzheimer's disease. Appropriate interventions for each level of cognitive impairment and for supportive care for the family are included.

Wurlman R: Alzheimer's disease, Sci Am 252(1):62-74, 1985.

Six conceptual models for understanding Alzheimer's disease are discussed in some detail: genetic model, abnormal protein model, infectious-agent model, toxin model, blood-flow model, acetylcholine model. The author points out that the integration of all of these models—a multifactorial model—may be closer to the truth. He terms this the elephant model *after the parable of six blind men describing an elephant, each from a different vantage point.*

Zisook S and Braff D: Delirium: recognition and management in the older patient, Geriatrics 41(6):66-78, 1986.

The article describes signs and symptoms (core symptoms and associated symptoms) of delirium. The underlying factors of an acute confusional state are discussed, and a listing of the systemic and CNS correlates for delirium is provided. The authors also make suggestions for the management of this acute disorder.

FURTHER READINGS

Grady D: The ticking of a time bomb in the genes, Discover 8(6):26-37, 1987.

Heslon L et al: Pick's disease, Arch Gen Psychiatr 44:409-411, 1987.

Jess L: Investigating impaired mental states, Nursing 88 18(6):42-50, 1988.

Kessler S: Psychiatric implications of presymptomatic testing for Huntington's disease, Am J Orthopsychiatr 57(2):212-219, 1987.

GLOSSARY

acculturation Process of reciprocal retentions, losses, and/or adaptations of culture patterns that results when members of two or more cultural groups interact

acquired immunodeficiency syndrome (AIDS) Disease caused by the human immunodeficiency virus (HIV), which reduces the body's ability to resist other diseases. It is transmitted primarily by sharing drug needles and syringes with an infected person and by having sex with an infected person

activity theory Theory of aging that supports the belief that the greatest satisfaction comes from continuing activities and social roles into late life

acute confusional state Acute brain dysfunction caused by any interference with the complex biochemical or metabolic processes essential to brain functioning. Symptoms include disturbances in cognition, levels of awareness, memory, and orientation, accompanied by restlessness, apprehension, irritability, and apathy. SYNONYMS: delirium, acute delirious state, acute brain syndrome, toxic psychosis

adaptation Adjusting one's responses to cope with internal or external stress

ageism Systematic stereotyping and discrimination against people because they are old

agoraphobia Irrational fear of open spaces or of entering public places alone, because of a psychic phenomenon in which internal fears or anxiety are projected onto an aspect of the environment

alienation Failure in reciprocal connectedness between a person and significant others; estrangement of self from others

ambivalence Simultaneous existence of strong feelings of both love and hate toward a person, an object, or a situation

amnesia Emergency response to stress and anxiety in which a part or all of a person's past life is forgotten or forced out of awareness through repression

anal phase In psychosexual development, the stage that encompasses ages 15 months to 3 years. Libidinal energy is shifted from the mouth as a source of gratification to the anus

andropause Return to the nonreproductive state of function of the male genitalia. Andropause occurs later than menopause, usually beginning in the middle to late 50s

anger Sense of intense tension or discomfort that arises when a goal is thwarted

anhedonia Inability to find pleasure in situations that would normally be pleasurable

anomie State of alienation and disassociation from social values and beliefs; normlessness

anorexia nervosa Condition characterized by excessive dieting, which is often carried to the point of severe malnutrition and emaciation and which, in some instances, leads to death through starvation

anticipatory planning Identification of possible stressors in one's life—for example, pregnancy or change in job—and the initiation of the problem-solving process to reduce or eliminate a crisis situation before it occurs

antisocial personality Characterized by impulsive and asocial behavior, poor judgment, irresponsibility, and lack of insight into the consequences of one's behavior

anxiety Diffuse feeling of apprehension and dread of being threatened or alienated. The threat may be real or perceived. Anxiety can maintain one's alertness, or it can immobilize an individual

anxiety disorders Conditions characterized by overt physiological and psychological manifestations of anxiety in which there are no stable defense mechanisms to enable the person to cope with the anxiety. This form of neurosis may be chronic, or it may occur in acute attacks. Generalized anxiety disorder, panic disorder, phobic disorders, and obsessive-compulsive disorders are types of anxiety disorders

apathy Blunting of affect; an absence of feeling from a psychological point of view

associative looseness Thinking disorder in which relationships among ideas are autistically determined

asthenic personality Characterized by constant and extreme fatigue, listlessness, and indecisiveness. Asthenic personality is believed to be a precursor of neurasthenia

attention deficit disorders Disorders characterized by short attention span, clumsiness, lack of symmetry of hand movements, intellectual and memory faults, restlessness, and quarrelousness. Hyperactivity may or may not be present

attitudes Major integrative forces in the development of personality that give consistency to an individual's behavior. Attitudes are cognitive in nature, formed through interactions with the environment. Attitudes serve to direct an individual's commitments and responsibilities; they reflect innermost convictions about what is good or bad, right or wrong, desirable or undesirable

authority Right to use power to command behavior, enforce rules, and make decisions. Authority is often based on rank or position in a social hierarchy, and it may be either of two types: line authority or staff authority

autism Exclusive focus is on the self. Subjective, introspective thinking and a good deal of fantasy are prominent aspects of autism

autistic phase In Mahler's system of preoedipal development, the stage from birth to 1 month. This is termed *normal autism*, and it gradually changes as children become aware that they cannot satisfy their needs by themselves

aversion therapy Type of negative conditioning that uses learning theory to change behavior from maladaptive to adaptive

basic group identity Shared social characteristics such as world view, language, and value and ideological systems. Basic group identity evolves from membership in an ethnic group

beneficence Right to health care that maximizes benefits to the client while minimizing harm and suffering. Benefits and harm are calculated in physiological, social, cultural, emotional, financial, and spiritual terms

benign senescent forgetfulness This implies a normal change in most people as they age—forgetfulness tends to increase. It is not to be confused with the massive memory loss associated with the various types of dementia

biogenic Motivated by physiological states

biological aging Refers to changes that occur in the body over time, ending with the death of the individual

bipolar depressive response Affective disorder that is characterized by symptoms of both depression and mania

bisexuality Preference for a sexual partner may be either of the same sex or the opposite sex. In most cases, there is a preference for one gender

blame placing Process of placing responsibility for one's behavior, and especially misbehavior, on others

body image Individual's conscious and unconscious perceptions of his or her body. Body image is an integral component of self-concept

boundary maintenance mechanisms Behavior and practices that exclude members of some groups from the customs and values of a particular group

bulimia Eating disorder characterized by binge eating (often done in secret) and by self-induced purging

castration Removal of the testes in a male or the ovaries in a female

catatonic schizophrenia Type of schizophrenia. In the *catatonic stupor* form, prominent symptoms may include stupor, stereotypical behavior, cerea flexibilitas (waxy flexibility), and negativism. In the *catatonic excitement* form, there may be hyperkinesia, stereotypical behavior, bizarre mannerisms, and impulsivity

catharsis Therapeutic outpouring of repressed ideas or conflicts through verbalization and working through of conscious material. An appropriate emotional reaction accompanies catharsis

cerea flexibilitas Waxy flexibility—a symptom seen in catatonic schizophrenia. The individual's muscular system is in a condition that permits the molding of arms and legs into any position where they will remain indefinitely

change agent Person who tries to influence the making and implementing of decisions in the direction of change

character neuroses Personality organizations characterized by excessive anxiety and unconscious conflict in which the compromise solutions needed to maintain adjustment or adaptation result in rigidity of personality and inhibit interpersonal relations, although there are no overt clinical symptoms

childhood-onset pervasive developmental disorders Disturbances in thought, affect, social relatedness, and behavior that emerge between the ages of 30 months and 12 years

childhood triad Three types of behavior (firesetting, bedwetting, and cruelty to animals) that when used in combination and consistently may predict emerging sociopathy

chronic, undifferentiated schizophrenia Symptoms of more than one of the classic types of schizophrenia (simple, paranoid, catatonic, hebrephrenic) are demonstrated in this category

circum-speech Behavior characteristic of conversation. Instrumentals, markers, interactional behavior, demonstratives, and stress kinesics are types of circum-speech

circumstantiality Speech pattern in which there is difficulty in screening out irrelevant material in describing an event. The inclusion of many irrelevant details results in a lengthy and rambling account before the end point is reached. This speech pattern may be found in chronic brain dysfunction

clarification seeking Attempting to make clear ambiguous or global statements

coalition across generational boundaries Conspiracy or alliance between a parent and a child. Such a conspiracy is usually against the other parent

cognitive dissonance Refers to a state of inconsistent cognitions that generates discomfit (an aversive state of arousal)

cognitive restructuring Focusing on positive aspects of life; reframing events so that they contribute to self-esteem

cohesiveness, group Quality of unity that characterizes a group. It results from all the factors, evident and subtle, that interact to encourage close bonds among group members so that the group tends to stay together

command hallucination Hallucinated voice that an individual experiences as commanding him or her to perform a certain act. Command hallucinations may influence a person to engage in behavior that is dangerous to himself, herself, or others

complementarity Ongoing mutual interaction between human and environmental fields

communication theme Recurrent idea or concept that underlies and ties together communication. There are three types of communication themes: content theme (the idea that underlies or links together seemingly varied topics of discussion), mood theme (the affect or emotion an individual communicates), interaction theme (the idea or concept that best describes the dynamics between communicating participants)

community mental health Prevention, early diagnosis, effective treatment, and rehabilitation of people with mental disorders and disabilities in geographically defined communities through a network of collaborative health and social welfare systems, community organizations, and consumers

compulsion Persistent, irrational need or urge to perform a particular act or acts. A compulsion, which often has the quality of a ritual, serves a defensive purpose by controlling anxiety, guilt, and other noxious feelings

concrete thinking Part of the thought disorder characteristic of schizophrenia. Concrete thinking is a primitive way of thinking in which an individual tends to take the literal meanings of ideas. It is indicative of a difficulty in abstracting

conduct disorders Disorders of childhood characterized by either socialized or unsocialized aggressive behaviors, such as stealing, lying, truancy, promiscuity, and cheating. The purpose of such behavior is to enhance self-esteem and provide courage in anxiety-producing situations.

conductor Family therapist who uses his or her own dynamic personality to give direction to a family in therapy

confabulation Adaptive or defensive phenomenon in which a person with memory deficits fills in gaps in memory with relevant but imaginary information

confrontation Pointing out ambivalent or discrepant statements

conscience Part of the superego system that monitors thoughts, feelings, and actions and measures them against internalized values and standards

conscious Conscious level of experience includes those aspects of experience that are in awareness at any given time. Consciousness is a psychodynamic concept that embraces three levels of awareness, each of which influences behavior. These levels are the conscious, the preconscious, and the unconscious

consensual validation Comparing one's evaluations of experience with those of another person

consolidation of individuality and emotional object constancy Fourth and final subphase of the separation-individuation phase of preoedipal development (in Mahler's system). It begins toward the end of the second year, and it is seen as open ended. A degree of object constancy is accomplished, and separation of self and object representations is established

consumer Individual, group, or community that utilizes a product or service. In the area of mental health, consumerism refers to the utilization of all levels of mental health services (services designed for primary, secondary, and tertiary prevention of mental illness)

continuity theory Theory of aging that takes into account the continuing influence of early personality patterns, patterns of coping, and family situations

conversion Transformation of unacceptable, anxiety-provoking impulses into sensorimotor symptoms such as paralysis or blindness. There is no organic basis for such impairment. Conversion is an emergency response to stress

coping mechanisms Measures utilized to reduce tension. These measures are often learned through early interactions with significant others in the environment

coprolalia Excessive use of profane language

countersociety Society that runs counter to or against the established society in which it exists

countertransference Emotional and often unconscious process in the helping person that is related to the client and that has an effect on the therapeutic interaction between therapist and client

crystallized intelligence Intelligence based on learned ability, experience, and stored information. It reflects cultural assimilation and is highly influenced by formal and informal education. Growth of crystallized intelligence *is* limited by neurophysiology, and increments do become smaller as we age, but crystallized intelligence continues to increase throughout life (see **fluid intelligence**)

crisis Situation that cannot be readily resolved by an individual's normal repertoire of coping strategies. A crisis is precipitated by an actual or perceived threat to self-esteem or physical integrity

crisis intervention Provision of immediate treatment for individuals undergoing acute psychological distress

culturally specific Unique to a particular culture and a function of that cultural context

culture Ordered system of shared and socially transmitted symbols and meanings that structures world view and guides behavior

culture shock Drastic change in the cultural environment that is both precipitated by and a response to cognitive dissonance

cyclothymic personality Characterized by vacillation between depression and elation. Differentiation between cyclothymic personality and manic depressive psychosis is a matter of degree of symptomatology

day hospital Psychiatric facility where formerly hospitalized clients participate in a therapeutic program during the normal working hours

deinstitutionalization Practice of discharging chronically mentally ill clients into the community

delirium See **acute confusional state**

delusion False belief (other than a commonly believed myth or superstition of a culture)

dementia praecox Outdated term used to describe schizophrenia. Dementia (insanity) praecox (youthful) was used to distinguish schizophrenia from the dementias of later life, such as senility

demonstrative Type of circum-speech that accompanies and illustrates speech

denial Unconsciously motivated behavior that manifests itself as evasion or negation of objective reality

dependence Reliance on others in the environment to meet needs for nurturance, security, love, shelter, and sustenance

depersonalization State in which an individual feels a loss of personal identity. The feeling that the environment is also changed and unreal may also be present. This latter feeling is termed **derealization**

depression Extension of the grieving process that is considered abnormal. Depression is described by DSM-III-R as a disturbance in mood which may be accompanied by some form of manic or depressive syndrome

developmental crisis Period of vulnerability encountered as one progresses from one developmental stage to the next

differentiation First subphase of the separation-individuation phase in Mahler's system of preoedipal development. It occurs from approximately 5 months to 9 months of age. This phase coincides with maturation of partial locomotor functioning and the differentiation of a primitive but distinct body image. At this time, the child begins tentative moves away from the mother and begins to view her as a separate being

disability Condition that results in a partial or total limitation of the normal life activities of a person (see **impairment**)

discreditable people Refers to people who, if their socially deviant behavior were visible or known, would be devalued and condemned by society. For instance, "secret" alcoholics and prostitutes are discreditable people

discredited people Refers to people who, because their socially deviant behavior is visible or known, are devalued and condemned by society. For instance, known alcoholics and prostitutes are discredited people

disengagement theory Theory of aging that contends that there is a natural and mutual agreement between an aging person and society that interactions with others will gradually decrease. Earlier social roles of the person will become less important

displacement Unconscious transferal of strivings or feelings from the original object to a different object, activity, or situation

dissociative disorders Characterized by psychiatric symptoms that represent a form of psychological flight from the self. A part or all of the personality is denied or dissociated from present reality. Psychogenic amnesia, psychogenic fugue, and multiple personality are types of dissociative disorders

domestic violence Emotional and/or physical abuse or

neglect perpetrated by one family member against another family member(s). Domestic violence includes consort abuse, child abuse, and elder abuse and is a symptom of family dysfunction

double-bind communication Communication pattern that involves the giving of two conflicting messages at the same time. One message may be verbal and the other nonverbal, or both messages may be verbal. The conflicting nature of the messages serves to immobilize and confuse the listener

dyad Combination of two—for example, husband and wife, parent and child

dyspareunia Abnormal condition in women, in which pain is experienced during sexual intercourse. The condition may be caused by inadequate lubrication of the vagina

dysthymia Chronic nonpsychotic disorder characterized by depressed mood accompanied by loss of interest in activities or persons in the environment. Must be of 2 years duration or longer with continuous or intermittent mood disturbance

echolalia Imitating and repeating the speech of another person. Echolalia is a pathological form of speech that is demonstrated by some schizophrenic individuals

echopraxia Imitating and repeating the body movements of another person. Echopraxia is a symptom demonstrated by some schizophrenic individuals

educational therapy Educational and vocational training programs designed to develop self-esteem, group identification, and school and occupational adjustment

ego Part of the personality that is in interaction with the external environment and with somatic and psychic aspects of the internal environment. Ego functions, which encompass intellectual and social abilities, maintain an equilibrium between id and superego, as well as the integrity of the personality in coping with stress

egocentricity Tendency to view one's own thoughts and ideas as the best possible, without considering the views of others

ego-dystonic Adjective used to describe ideas, defenses, or behaviors that are unacceptable to a person and inconsistent with his or her total personality. SYNONYM: ego-alien

ego-syntonic Adjective used to describe ideas, defenses, or behaviors that are acceptable to a person and consistent with his or her total personality

eldercare Concept of employer support for caregivers of the elderly. It includes information and referral; flexible work hours; company-sponsored day-care centers; financial support and insurance coverage for long-term care

eldering Process of moving into age-appropriate roles. The process occurs as people retire, become empty-nesters and grandparents

electroconvulsive therapy (ECT) Somatic therapy in which electric current is applied to the brain through electrodes placed on the temporal areas of the skull. The desired generalized convulsion is precipitated by applying 70 to 130 volts for 0.1 to 0.5 seconds. The treatment is used in mania, depression, and certain cases of schizophrenia. SYNONYM: electrostimulation therapy (EST), electric shock therapy

emotional divorce Schism that occurs when emotional investment between spouses is withdrawn

empathy Ability to understand and share the emotions and thoughts of another person without losing one's objectivity

enculturation Process of learning the conceptual and behavioral systems of one's culture

environmental manipulation Modifying the physical and/or social environment

erectile dysfunction (impotence) Recurrent or persistent inhibition of sexual excitement manifested by the inability to maintain an erection

eros According to Freud, the instinct for life

ethnic culture Attitudinal, value, and behavioral patterns associated with an ethnic group

ethnic enclave Area in a city, town, or village that is populated by a minority ethnic group

ethnic group Collectivity of people organized around an assumption of common origin

ethnocentrism Attitude that one ethnic group's folkways are superior and right and those of other ethnic groups are inferior and wrong. Each ethnic group uses its culture as a standard for judging all other cultures

euthymism Normal mood responses

explosive personality Characterized by episodes of uncontrollable rage and physical abusiveness in response to relatively minor pressures

experience Person's reaction, consisting of perception, interpretation and response, to a situation or event

extended family Family unit consisting of three or more generations

family Group of people who are united by bonds of kinship, at least two of whom are conjugally related

family disorganization Breakdown of the family system; associated with parental overburdening and/or loss of significant others who served as role models for children or support systems for family members. Such a breakdown of the family may contribute to the loss of social controls that families usually impose on their members

family myths Communication pattern involving the construction of myths that serve to deny the reality of family situations

family therapy Simultaneous treatment of more than one family member in the same session. The family's communication patterns and their patterns of relating are considered the focus of the treatment

feedback Regulatory function of a system. It serves to monitor, reinforce, and/or correct the structure and conditions of a system. Positive feedback facilitates change within a system, while negative feedback promotes system stability

feminization of poverty Refers to a multiplicity of factors that keep women in a more economically vulnerable position than men while at the same time increasing their economic responsibilities

fictive kin Refers to people who are not related by consanguinal or affinal bonds but who are regarded as "just like family." Fictive kinship binds people together in ties of affection, concern, obligation, and responsibility

fixation Concentration of libidinal energies in one psychosexual stage of development, because of over gratification or under gratification in that stage

flight of ideas Communication that is characterized by rapid movement from one idea to another. There is a connection between the ideas, but it is tenuous and often influenced by the immediate environment. This phenomenon is sometimes demonstrated in manic-depressive psychosis

fluid intelligence Processing of information that reflects the functioning of neurological structures. These are at their peaks of efficiency in adolescence and in young adulthood. (See Crystallized intelligence)

forensic psychiatry Subspecialty in psychiatry that deals with the legal facets of mental illness

formation Cluster of people that occupies, and thereby defines, a quantum of space

frame of reference Individual's personal guidelines, taken as a whole. A person's frame of reference reflects his or her social situation, cultural norms, and ideas

fugue Dreamlike or trance state, during which a person may travel distances from home, act out impulsively, or engage in childish behavior. Fugue is an emergency response to stress and anxiety, and it may precede amnesia

genogram Diagram that depicts family relationships over at least three successive generations. It is useful as a tool for tapping into the process of a family system over time

geronting Process of coping with the interaction of *senescing* and *eldering* (see these). The organism repatterns in response to inner, biological forces and to outer, societal forces and, simultaneously, to how these forces interact with each other

grief Series of subjective responses that follow a significant loss—for example, loss of body function, a body part, status, or a relative

group boundary Physical or psychological factor that separates relevant regions within the group. For example, an internal boundary distinguishes the leader from the group members. An external boundary separates the group from the external environment

group cohesiveness All the forces that act on group members to encourage them to remain as a group

group norms Rule or standard to which group members are expected to adhere. Norms define the behavior that will be tolerated within the group

group process *Everything* that happens within a group—who talks to whom; who "pairs"; who sits where; the tone and atmosphere of the group; the norms; the conflicts

guilt Tension between ego and superego that occurs when one falls short of standards set for oneself

hallucination False sensory perception; a perception for which there is no apparent external stimulus. Any of the senses may be involved; individuals have experienced hallucinations that are auditory, visual, tactile, olfactory, gustatory, or kinesthetic

hebephrenic schizophrenia Type of schizophrenia that is characterized by severe thought and emotional disorders. Behavior is bizarre, silly, and inappropriate. *Regression* is the main defense mechanism that is used in an exaggerated form. Hallucinations and delusions are present. This form of schizophrenia is generally believed to have the poorest prognosis. The age of onset tends to be young—before the 20s. This term is no longer included in DSM-III-R

helicy Refers to the nature of human and environmental change, which is a continuous developmental process that is evolutionary, creatively complex, diverse, differentiated, probablistic, and goal-directed

helplessness State characterized by the existence of an unfulfilled need and the inability to meet that need. Helplessness can be a learned response

holistic health Refers to the view that people are organic wholes. Well-being evolves from the development and integration of the component dimensions of this organic whole: the physical, the intellectual, the psychological, the sociocultural, and the spiritual

homeodynamics Refers to a state of relative balance and flux in a system

homeostasis Refers to the maintenance of equilibrium or to a steady state of balance in a system

homosexuality Preference for a sexual partner of one's own sex

hopelessness Situation characterized by the belief that all efforts to alter one's life situation will be fruitless

hospice Alternative care model whose goals are to provide supportive care for the dying client and his/her family and to facilitate the aging process to ensure a dignified death when medical treatment regimens are no longer appropriate

hostility Tendency of an organism to do something harmful to another organism or to itself. Hostility may be passively rather than actively expressed

household Group of people bound together by common residence, economic cooperation, and the task of child rearing. Members of a household may or may not be united by bonds of kinship. A household is not concerned with the function of procreation

human ecosystem Refers to the interaction between human beings and their environment, specifically their physical and social environment

humor Culturally influenced concept of what is funny, whimsical, capricious, and/or ludicrous

hydrotherapy Form of treatment for mental illness that involved the use of water at various temperatures. Hydrotherapy is mostly of historical interest; it included such measures as continuous tub baths, application of wet sheet packs, and use of shower sprays

hypochondriasis Morbid preoccupation with the state of one's health, usually accompanied by physical symptoms or the conviction that some disease process is present that cannot be substantiated by medical evidence

hypomania State of elation. A hypomanic individual has boundless energy; is witty and outgoing, and is considered the life of the party. Hypomanic behavior is purposeful and goal-directed

hysterical neurosis Emergency psychological response to overwhelming anxiety. Hysterical neurosis includes a variety of symptom formations, such as amnesia and fugue state

hysterical personality Characterized by extremely excitable, emotionally labile, and overly dramatic behavior

id In psychoanalytical theory, one of three interacting systems of the personality. The id represents the early or archaic parts of the personality. Id functioning occurs on an unconscious level, the existence of which can only be inferred through dreams, impulsive acts, and such psychiatric symptoms as primitive or unacculturated drives, needs, and so forth

idealized image Person who has a compulsive craving for perfection and admiration may come to view himself or herself as unreal and to create instead a self-concept based on high and often unattainable goals. Such a person then tries to live up to this ideal conceptualization and to receive affirmation from others that the self and the ideal conceptualization are one and the same

ideas of reference Pathological belief system that the actions and speech of others have reference to oneself. For example, an individual who is experiencing ideas of reference may believe that what a television announcer is saying is actually a coded reference to him or her. Since ideas of reference can occur in degrees, this example might be termed a *delusion of reference*

identification Process whereby an individual imitates the desired qualities of a significant person in the environment

impaired female excitement Recurrent or persistent inhibition of sexual excitement during sexual activity manifested by partial or complete failure to maintain the lubrication phase of sexual excitement

impaired female orgasm Recurrent or persistent inhibition of female orgasm manifested by delay or absence of orgasm following normal sexual excitement

impairment Physiological or psychological abnormality that does not interfere with normal life activities in the individual (see Disability)

impotence Inability of the male to achieve or maintain an erection

inadequate personality Characterized by faulty judgment and poor physical and emotional endurance

incest Form of sexual abuse where generational boundaries are crossed. Sexual relations occur between people who ignore cultural prohibitions, such as mother and son, father and daughter, or between close family members

infantile autism Disorder characterized by profound disturbances of speech, perception, and neurological functioning in children under the age of 30 months

inhibited sexual desire Low interest in sexual activity and lack of responsiveness to initiatives made by partner

instrumental Type of circum-speech that is task oriented. Walking, smoking, and eating, when carried on while a person is speaking, are examples of instrumentals

insulin coma therapy Production of a coma, with or without convulsions, through intramuscular administration of insulin. The treatment, introduced by Sakel, was once used with schizophrenic persons. It is now of historical interest only

integrated drinking Refers to the incorporation of drinking alcoholic beverages into the life-style of a cultural group

intellectualization Defense mechanism in which reasoning is used as a defense against the conscious realization of an unconscious conflict

interaction coaching Attempt to modify disturbed mother-infant interactions. The goal is to improve the interactional "fit" between mother and child

interactional behavior Type of circum-speech that includes body shifts or movements that increase, decrease, or maintain space between interacting individuals

interactional model Model of family therapy that views the family as a communication system comprised of interlocking subsystems (the individual family members). Family dysfunction is seen as occurring when the rules that govern family interaction become vague and ambiguous. The goal of family therapy is to help the family clarify the rules that govern family relationships

intrapsychic Taking place *within* the mind

introject Mental image of someone or something that becomes incorporated into one's ego system. The process of introjection is opposite to that of projection. An introject becomes emotionally invested for the individual and is involved in the process of identification and superego development

introjection Incorporation of qualities of a loved or hated object or individual into one's own ego structure. Introjection is an unconscious mechanism

involutional melancholia Form of depression that occurs during the middle to later periods of life. One of its primary characteristics is agitation

isolation State in which the linkage between facts and emotions has been broken. Facts are allowed into the individual's experience, yet the emotional component is excluded from awareness

kinesics Use of body movements to communicate meaning

latency Stage of development, according to Freud and Erikson, that encompasses ages 6 to 12

liaison nursing Provision, by clinical specialists in psychiatric nursing, of consultation services for nursing colleagues and members of other disciplines working in medical-surgical, parent-child, and geriatric settings

libido According to Freud, one's sexual drive

life review, the Universal mental process that occurs naturally in individuals. It is characterized by:

1. a progressive return to consciousness of past experiences
2. the resurgence of unresolved conflicts

3. a simultaneous review and integration of these reviewed experiences and conflicts.

The life review is sometimes encouraged by clinicians working with the elderly to foster healthy coping and accomplishment of the developmental tasks of aging

loss Relinquishing of supportive objects, persons, functions, or status

mania Extreme state of elation characterized by rapid motor activity, inappropriate dress, and illogical thought processes

manic-depressive response Cluster of behaviors characterized by mood swings, ranging from profound depression to euphoria, with periods of normalcy in between

manipulation Habitual use of others to gratify one's own needs and desires

markers Type of body movement that aids in communication. Markers act as punctuation points and indicators

menopause Return to the nonreproductive state of function of the female genitalia; usually begins in the early to late 40s

metacommunication Communication that indicates how verbal communication should be interpreted. Metacommunication may support or contradict verbal communication

milieu therapy Treatment of a hospitalized person that makes use of the entire hospital environment: workers, scheduled and unscheduled activities, the physical plant, and so on (see Therapeutic community)

mirroring Observing a person's behavior and giving the person that feedback

monopolization Domination of the discussion within a group by one member of the group

morpheme Group of minimal meaningful sounds that cannot be broken down into smaller meaningful sounds. Morphemes are a basic unit of the expressive system (sound system) of spoken language

motivation Reasons for one's actions, for what one experiences, and for the way one experiences one's actions. These reasons can be on a conscious, preconscious, or unconscious level

mourning Psychological processes or reactions activated by an individual to assist him or her in overcoming a loss. The process is finally resolved when reinvestment in a new object relationship has occurred

multifactorial Having a variety of causes

multigenerational model Model of family therapy that focuses on reciprocal role relationships over time and thus takes a longitudinal approach to family therapy. The family is viewed as an emotional system where patterns of interacting and coping, as well as unresolved issues, can be passed down from generation to generation and can cause stress to the family members on whom they are projected. Family dysfunction is viewed as the transmission of undifferentiation across generational lines. The goal of family therapy is to help family members attain a higher level of differentiation

multiple personality Disorder characterized by a primary personality that is usually shy and introverted and two or more alter or secondary personalities, each exhibiting values and behaviors and sometimes ages and sexual orientations that differ from each other and from the primary personality. Multiple personality usually develops as a means of coping with severe physical and/or sexual abuse in one's childhood

mutism Inability or unwillingness to speak

mutual cuing Circular interaction process between mother and infant by which they empathically read one another's signs and signals and react to each other

mystification Habitual communication process that may include vagueness, tangentiality, double-bind communication, and family myths. Mystification serves to maintain the equilibrium of a family system even while it confuses family members

narcissism Self-love or self-admiration. Depending upon degree and consequential behavior, narcissism can be healthy or pathological

neologism Invented word that has an obscure and purely subjective meaning. Neologisms are very often symbolic for a person; they are sometimes demonstrated in the speech of schizophrenic individuals

networking Mechanism for providing support and sharing information among members of a group (e.g., a professional group such as one of the specialty area groups within the American Nurses' Association)

neuroses Group of disorders characterized by excessive anxiety and unconscious conflict. Although there is no gross distortion of the personality, the compromise solutions and defense mechanisms needed to cope with anxiety and conflict can inhibit personality functioning and may result in pathological symptoms. The terms *neuroses* and *psychoneuroses* are used synonymously

non-with spaces Spaces in which interacting persons use body parts and regions to show that they have different spatial orientations and thus are unaffiliated with one another

nuclear family Family unit composed of a man, a woman, and their children

nursing process Method of scientific inquiry used to explore and intervene in a client's experience. The steps in the nursing process are assessment, analysis of data, formulation of a plan of care, implementation of the care plan, and evaluation. The nursing process forms the cognitive framework for nursing practice

object constancy This occurs in the development of a child when the child is able to maintain mental and emotional representations of mother (as first object). This is an indication that the child has been able to synthesize "good" and "bad" object representations to be able to relate to a whole object (person)

obsession State in which a repetitive thought or thought pattern keeps recurring despite the individual's efforts to banish it or prevent it from recurring

obsessive-compulsive personality Characterized by orderly, methodical, ritualistic, inhibited, and frugal behavior

obsessive-compulsive disorder Psychiatric disorder characterized by repetitious performance of ritualistic behavior and the presence of obsessive thoughts that cannot be banished

Oedipus complex Direction of a child's erotic attachment toward the parent of the opposite sex, during the phallic stage of development. Concurrently, there is jealousy toward the parent of the same sex

omigenous family Family unit consisting of the family that is formed when parents divorce and remarry. A complex kinship system of relatives and steprelatives may develop. The omigenous family is also referred to as a blended family

open charting Charting system in which a client has access to his or her chart. The more progressive mental health facilities have open charting in varying degrees

oral phase Freudian developmental phase that encompasses approximately the first 15 months of life. This period is characterized by a concentration of libidinal energies in the oral zone, particularly the mouth and lips

organic brain dysfunctions Neuropsychiatric conditions caused by any disturbance in brain tissue functions and characterized by the following syndrome: disturbances in comprehension, memory, orientation, and judgment and lability of emotional responses. Brain dysfunctions may be either acute or chronic. SYNONYM: Organic brain syndromes

orgasmic dysfunction Inability of the female to achieve orgasm. Women may be "preorgasmic," referring to those who have never achieved an orgasm

orientation phase First stage of the nurse-client relationship. During this stage, the framework of the relationship is established, the client maps out areas of concern, and the nurse begins the process of assessment

outcome criteria Criteria identified by the American Nurses' Association Division on Psychiatric and Mental Health Nursing Practice that focus on observable or measurable results of nursing activities and mental health services

overinclusiveness Association disturbance seen in the thought disorder of schizophrenia. The individual is unable to think in a precise manner because of an inability to keep irrelevant elements outside of perceptual boundaries

paranoid personality Characterized by extremely sensitive, rigid, suspicious, and jealous behavior. An individual makes exaggerated use of projection in an attempt to cope with insecure and negative feelings

paranoid schizophrenia Form of schizophrenia in which the paramount symptoms include suspicion, hallucinations, and delusions. The delusions are often grandiose or persecutory

passive-aggressive personality Characterized by both independent and hostile behavior. Aggressiveness is usually covertly expressed through obstinateness, procrastination, vacillation, and helplessness

patient (client) government Organization, composed of clients, through which clients have some influence in the running of a unit

perceptual deprivation/restriction Absence of or decrease in the meaningful grouping of stimuli, caused, for example, by an ever-present hum or constant dim lighting

perceptual monotony State characterized by a lack of variety in the normal pattern of everyday stimuli. Perceptual monotony can result, for example, from having the television on all day

pervasive developmental disorders Those disorders of infancy and childhood characterized by severe impairment of relatedness and behavioral aberrations previously known as childhood psychoses. Infantile autism, childhood schizophrenia, and symbiotic psychosis are included in this category

pet therapy Pairing people and companion animals for mutual benefit. Pet therapy can help to combat the problems of loneliness in the elderly. Pets provide companionship, physical contact, affection, and meaning to life through the responsibility required in caring for an "other"

phobia Irrational or illogical fear of some object or aspect of the environment, because of the externalization of inner fears or anxiety

phobic disorder Psychiatric condition in which internal anxiety and conflict are displaced or externalized onto some object in the environment, which can then be avoided

phoneme Minimal unit of sound that distinguishes one utterance from another. Phonemes are a basic unit of the expressive system (sound system) of spoken language

physical dependence Addiction; marked by a physiological need for a substance and by physical withdrawal symptoms when a substance is abruptly terminated

planned change Altering the status quo by means of a carefully formulated program. Planned change is characterized by four phases: motivation, establishing a change relationship, changing, and assimilating and stabilizing

point behavior Orienting body parts in some direction within a quantum of space

polarization Within a group, the concentration of members' interests, beliefs, and allegiances around two conflicting positions

political nursing Use of knowledge about power processes and strategies to influence the nature and direction of health care and professional nursing. The constituency of political nursing is clients: communities, groups, and individuals, both diagnosed and potential

politics Process of achieving and using power for the purpose of influencing decisions and resolving disputes between factions

positional behavior Orienting body regions in order to claim a quantum of space. Positional behavior involves four body regions: head and neck, upper torso, pelvis and thighs, and lower legs and feet

posttraumatic stress disorder Disorder characterized by the development of symptoms following a psychological event that is outside the range of human experiences. Major characteristics include a reexperiencing of the traumatic event, avoidance of stimuli related to the event, and blunted responsiveness to external stimuli

power Ability to act, to do, and/or to control others. Power may be wielded in three predominant ways. These ways are referred to as instruments of power and include condign power, compensatory power, and conditioned power

powerlessness Inability to effect change in one's environment

practicing Second subphase of the separation-individuation phase in Mahler's system of preoedipal development. In this subphase, the child is able to move away from mother and return to her. The child feels elation in response to this investigation of the environment and through practicing locomotor skills

preconscious Those areas of mental functioning in which information is not in immediate awareness but is subject to recall

prefrontal lobotomy Psychosurgical procedure in which some of the connections between the prefrontal lobes of the brain and the thalamus are severed. The procedure was used as a treatment for long-standing schizophrenia involving uncontrollable, destructive behavior. After surgery, individuals were often apathetic, docile, and lacking in social graces. The procedure is rarely used today, and it is frowned upon by many mental health professionals. The operation is called a lobotomy if tissue is removed; if only white fibers are severed, the procedure is called prefrontal leucotomy

premature ejaculation Sexual dysfunction which is characterized by the ejaculation of semen before partners reach a state of mutual enjoyment

premenstrual syndrome (PMS) Group of symptoms both psychological and physiological that occur prior to the onset of menstruation each cycle

preoperational thought phase According to Piaget, the phase of development during which the child focuses on the development of language as the tool to meet his or her needs. This period encompasses ages 2 to 7

preschizophrenic state Period before psychosis is evident. The individual deviates from normality but does not demonstrate grossly psychotic symptoms such as delusions, hallucinations, or stupor

primary prevention Health promotion with individuals, families, groups, and communities through the identification and alleviation of stress-producing factors

primary processes Unconscious processes, originating in the id, that obey different laws from those of the ego (reality, logic, and the environment influence the ego). These processes are seen in the least disguised forms in infancy and in the dreams of the adult. Much of the distorted thinking of an acutely psychotic person is based on primary process thinking

primary triad In Beck's theory of depression, the three major cognitive patterns that force the individual to view self, environment, and future in a negativistic manner

primitive idealization Primitive defense mechanism in which the individual tends to see another person as *all good* and powerful and a necessary help against *all bad* objects (including one's own bad parts)

privacy Culturally specific concept defining the degree of one's personal responsibility to others and behaviors that are regarded as interpersonally intrusive

process criteria Criteria identified by the American Nurses' Association Division on Psychiatric and Mental Health Nursing Practice that focus on nursing activities

process schizophrenia In contrast to reactive schizophrenia, organic, inborn factors are seen as paramount. The premorbid adjustment is usually poor, and onset is early in life. The process develops gradually and progresses to irreversibility

projection Unconscious mechanism that involves the attributing of one's own unacceptable thoughts, wishes, fears, and actions to another person or object

projective drawing Family therapy technique that spatially depicts relational patterns among family members

projective identification More primitive level of the defense mechanism of projection. It is characterized by a tendency to experience impulses that are simultaneously projected onto another person. The individual using projective identification then fears the recipient of this projection and feels the need to control this now "dangerous" person

proxemics Use of space to communicate meaning

pseudodementia Cognitive impairment associated with depression, particularly in the elderly. It may occur as (1) depression-induced organic mental disorder or (2) coexisting organic and functional disorder

pseudomutuality Term used in family therapy theory and practice. It denotes an atmosphere, maintained by family members, in which there is surface harmony and a high degree of agreement with one another. The atmosphere of agreement covers deep and destructive intrapsychic and interpersonal conflicts

psychodrama Type of group treatment in which an individual is encouraged to act out his or her conflicts and problems in a supervised setting. Other people in the group take on the roles of significant others in the person's life. Insight and/or catharsis may develop through the use of psychodrama as a therapy

psychological dependence Habituation; marked by a craving for drug-induced effects or mood changes and by emotional withdrawal symptoms when the substance is abruptly terminated

psychoneuroses See Neuroses

psychosomatogenic Causing or leading to the development of psychophysiological coping measures that are learned as responses to stressful situations. Minuchin describes the "psychosomatogenic family" as one in which a child receives positive reinforcement for symptoms

psychotic insight Stage in the development of psychosis that follows the initial experience of confusion, bizarreness, and apprehension. When the individual reaches the point of psychotic insight, everything begins to fit together and to become understandable. He or she then understands the external world in terms of this new system of thinking: the delusional system explains all of the things he or she had been confused by. The individual experiences this development as the attainment of exceptionally lucid thinking. The defensive nature of this phenomenon is obvious

quality assurance Activities designed to indicate the quality of health care or to improve the quality of health care

rape Sexual intercourse without the partner's consent. It is an act of violence, not an act of passion

rapprochement Third subphase of the separation-individuation phase of Mahler's system of preoedipal development. This subphase occurs from approximately 14 months to 2 years or more. This stage is characterized by a rediscovery of mother after the initial separation of the practicing subphase. The narcissistic inflation of the practicing subphase is replaced by a realization of separation and vulnerability. The subphase of rapprochement is seen as extremely significant in the subsequent development of borderline personality pathology

rationalization Process of constructing plausible reasons to explain and justify one's behavior

reaction formation Unconscious assumption of behavior patterns that are in direct opposition to what a person really feels or believes

reactive schizophrenia In contrast to process schizophrenia, reactive schizophrenia is attributed more to environmental factors than to inborn factors. There is usually a fairly good premorbid adjustment, onset is rapid, and the psychotic episode is usually brief

reality Culturally constructed world of preception, meaning, and behavior that members of any given culture regard as an absolute

reality orientation Correcting a person's distorted perceptions of reality

reciprocal Type of body movement that aids in communication. A reciprocal indicates affiliation between people

reductionism Approach that tries to explain a form of behavior or an event in terms of a particular category of phenomena (for example, biological, psychological, or cultural), negating the possibility of an interrelation of causal phenomena

reframing Involves paradoxical intent and symptom prescription; a person is directed to take a new, exaggerated approach to a situation

regression Return to an earlier stage of behavior, where modes of gratification had been more satisfying and needs had been met and where the ego had been acted upon rather than initiating the action

relationship therapy Therapy that emerges out of the totality of a client-therapist relationship. The therapist *begins where the client is* and encourages the growth of self in the client. Relationship therapy is an experience in living that takes place within a relationship with another person

relativism Attitude or belief that all cultures are logically consistent and viable and can only be understood and examined in terms of their own standards, attitudes, values, and beliefs. Relativism is the opposite of ethnocentrism

religiosity Psychiatric symptom characterized by the demonstration of excessive or affected piety

remotivation group Type of treatment group that is often used to stimulate the interest, awareness, and communication of withdrawn and institutionalized clients

repression Defense mechanism through which unpleasant thoughts, memories, and actions are pushed out of conscious awareness involuntarily. Repression is the cornerstone of defense mechanisms

resistance Conscious or unconscious reluctance to bring repressed ideas, thoughts, desires, or memories into awareness

resonancy Tendency of human and environmental fields to function according to patterns that can be identified and studied

respite care Care provided on an intermittent basis to the family or care giver of an elderly or disabled person. Temporary relief from continuous and stressful involvement with a chronically ill person is provided

retarded ejaculation Inability of the male to ejaculate after having achieved an erection. This often accompanies the aging process

retention procedure Method established by state statute or mental health code for committing a person to a psychiatric institution. Most states recognize four types of retention: informal, voluntary, emergency, and involuntary

role blurring Tendency for professional roles to overlap and become indistinct

scapegoating Process of consciously or unconsciously projecting blame, hostility, suspicion, etc., onto another person

schizoaffective schizophrenia Schizophrenic illness in which affective symptoms (depression, elation, and excitement) are prominent

schizoid personality Characterized by eccentric, introverted, withdrawn, and aloof behavior. The differentiation between schizoid personality and schizophrenia is a matter of degree of symptomatology

schizophrenogenic Adjective used to describe behavior that is believed by some family therapy theorists to cause schizophrenia

school phobia Disorder in children that is characterized by increased anxiety secondary to separation from parenting figure in relation to school. Parental fears of separation and uncertainty are transferred to the child

scripting Technique of family therapy involving the development of new family transactional patterns

sculpting Technique of family therapy involving the construction of a live family portrait that depicts family alliances and conflicts

secondary prevention Early diagnosis and treatment through the provision of referral services, the facilitation of the use of these services, and the rapid initiation of treatment

self-concept Mental picture that includes an individual's identity—strengths, weaknesses, and self-perception—based on reflected appraisals from the environment

self-esteem Amount of worth and competence an individual attributes to himself or herself, which acts as a protective mechanism against anxiety

self-fulfilling prophecy Distortion of an event or situation that eventually leads an individual to behave as he or she is expected to behave by others in the social setting

senescing Term used to describe biological processes that render a person vulnerable to physical deterioration over a period of time. It culminates in the death of the person

sensorimotor phase According to Piagetian theory, the developmental phase encompassing the period from birth to 2 years

sensory deprivation/restriction Reduction of environmental stimuli to a minimum

sensory-perceptual overload State characterized by an increase in the intensity and amount of stimuli to the point that a person loses the ability to discriminate among varying incoming stimuli

separation-individuation phase In Mahler's system of preoedipal development, this phase begins when the infant begins to "hatch" from the "symbiotic orbit" with the mother and to see itself as separate. This occurs in the period from approximately five months to two and one half years and it evolves through four distinct subphases (see Differentiation, Practicing, Rapprochement, and Consolidation of individuality and Emotional object constancy)

sexism Attitude or belief that one sex is inferior or superior to the other

sex role Expectations held by society about what constitutes appropriate or inappropriate behavior for each sex

sexual dysfunction Psychophysiological disorder in which the experiencing of sexual pleasure is inhibited because of psychosocial factors and in some cases physical factors

sexuality Integral part of the human condition. Sexuality integrates the physical, emotional, intellectual, sociocultural and spiritual dimensions of human beings. Sexuality continues throughout the life cycle and does not disappear as one ages

sexually deviant personality Characterized by sexual behavior that significantly differs from society's norms. Either the quality of sexual drives or the object of sexual drives is at variance with cultural norms for adults. While these forms of sexual behavior are considered deviant for adults, most of them are part of normal psychosexual growth and development

significant other Person in the environment who is considered by another as being special and as having an impact on that individual

simple schizophrenia Form of schizophrenia in which impoverishment of emotions, intellect, and will is evident but in which secondary symptoms such as hallucinations and delusions are absent. The person is often viewed as eccentric, isolated, and dull

single-parent family Family unit consisting of a man or a woman and his or her children

site Quantum of space occupied and defined by a cluster of people

situational crisis Crisis that occurs when a person is confronted with a stressful event of such unusual or extreme intensity or duration that the habitual methods of coping are no longer effective. SYNONYM: Incidental crisis

social class Grouping of persons who have similar values, interests, income, education, and occupations

social deviance Behavior that violates social standards, engendering anger, resentment, and/or the desire for punishment in a significant segment of society

social mobility Process of moving upward or downward in the social hierarchy

social network An interconnected group of cooperating significant others, both relatives and non relatives, with whom a person interacts

sociogenic Motivated by social values and constraints

sociolinguistics Study of the relationship between language and the social context in which it occurs

somatoform disorders Characterized by physical symptoms without organic basis. Somatoform disorders are a response to overwhelming anxiety. Such disorders as hypochondriasis and conversion disorder are types of somatoform disorders

sorting Family therapy technique that asks a client to use a different pattern for selecting information (e.g., focusing on strengths rather than weaknesses)

spatial zones Spatioperceptual fields in which people interact. There are four spatial zones: intimate zone (distance of 18 or fewer inches), personal zone (1½ to 4 feet), social zone (4 to 12 feet), and public zone (12 to 25 feet or more)

splitting Primitive defense mechanism that when overused, represents a developmental arrest. There is a failure to synthesize the positive and negative experiences and ideas one has of oneself, other people, situations or institutions

spot Small quantum of space that becomes the territorial object and extension of point behavior

stereotype Assignment of a set of characteristics by one group of people to themselves (autostereotype) or to others (heterostereotype)

stereotypical behavior Pattern of body movements that has autistic and symbolic meaning for an individual

stress kinesic Type of circum-speech that serves to mark the flow of speech and that generally coincides with linguistic stress patterns

stress management Series of techniques utilized by individuals to identify stressors and to implement strategies to reduce or alleviate potential and/or actual stressors. Such strategies include: progressive relaxation, guided imagery, biofeedback and active problem solving

structural model Model of family therapy that views the family as an open system and identifies subsystems within the family that carry out specific family functions. When faced with demands for change, individual family members, family subsystems or the family as a whole may respond with growth behaviors or with maladaptive behaviors. Family dysfunction is seen as occurring because these maladaptive behaviors are dysfunctional transactional patterns (scripts) for organizing family life and family relationships. The goal of family therapy is to help the family learn new scripts or transactional patterns

stupor Condition in which an individual's senses are blunted and in which the person is, to some degree, unaware of his or her environment

sublimation Directing of unacceptable libidinal energies into socially acceptable channels

substance intoxication State that results when a person ingests toxic amounts of a substance—for example, alcohol or another drug

suicide Infliction of bodily harm on self that results in death

summarizing Expressing in one statement several ideas or feelings and/or their relationship

superego In psychoanalytical theory, the system of the personality that represents the internalized ethical precepts and taboos of parents and others who are responsible for the enculturation of the child. The ego ideal and the conscience are aspects of the superego system

symbiotic phase In Mahler's system of preoedipal development, the stage from 1 month to approximately 5 months of age. The child participates in a "symbiotic orbit" with the mother. All parts of mother (including voice, gestures, clothing, and space in which she moves) are joined with the infant

symptom neuroses Psychological disorders in which dysfunctional coping mechanisms appear as clinical symptoms that represent direct manifestations of anxiety or the unconscious defenses utilized to cope with anxiety

syntax Property of language. Syntax refers to structural cues for the arrangement of words into phrases and sentences. In English, the usual order of a sentence is subject-verb-object

system Set of component parts that are in dynamic interaction. A system is characterized by interrelatedness, flow of information, feedback, and boundaries. Feedback, boundary-maintenance mechanisms, and self-corrective mechanisms serve a regulatory function in maintaining order within a system

tangentiality Association disturbance characterized by the tendency to digress from one's original topic of conversation. Tangentiality can destroy or seriously hamper a person's ability to communicate effectively with other people

tardive dysmentia Syndrome of emotional disturbance associated with tardive dyskinesia. Both are believed to be related to the long-term use of phenothiazines. The syndrome is sometimes termed *iatrogenic schizophrenia*

termination phase Last stage of the nurse-client relationship. During this stage, nurses and clients evaluate goals attained and outcomes achieved. During this stage, nurses may also help clients establish networks of support, other than the nurse-client relationship, that may be of assistance in coping with problems that might arise in the future

territorial Type of body movement that aids in communication. A territorial frames an interaction and defines a territory

territory Area or space over which an animal or human being maintains some degree of control. Both the claiming of space and acknowledgment of the claim are necessary for the establishment of a territory

tertiary prevention Rehabilitative process. Its goals are the reduction of the severity of a disability or dysfunction and the prevention of further disability

thanatos According to Freud, the instinct for death

therapeutic community Concept that every aspect of

hospitalization should be used as treatment for a client. In a therapeutic community all staff members work together as a team, and the environment is structured to be of maximum benefit to clients. (see Milieu therapy)

token economy   Therapeutic program that uses reward procedures (or positive reinforcement) in order to effect desirable behavioral change in individuals. This therapy is sometimes used in day hospitals, halfway houses, and wards for chronically ill persons in psychiatric hospitals

tolerance   Larger and larger amounts of a substance are required to produce the desired effect

touch   Tactile means of communicating such emotions as love, sympathy, hostility and fear. One's use of and response to touch is culturally influenced

toxic psychosis   See Acute confusional state

transference   Displacement of feelings and attitudes originally experienced toward significant others in the past onto persons in the present

transitional object   Object used by a child to provide comfort and security while he or she is moving away from a secure base (such as mother or home)

transsexual behavior   Transsexual is an individual who feels trapped in the body of the wrong sex. It is believed to relate to ineffective development of core gender identity. May eventually result in sex-reassignment surgery

triad   Combination of three—for example, two parents and a child

trust   Risk-taking process whereby an individual's situation depends upon the future behavior of another individual

unconscious   Psychodynamic concept that refers to mental functioning that is out of awareness and cannot be recalled. Drives, wishes, ideas, and so forth that are in conflict with internalized standards and ideals are maintained in the unconscious level through repression and other mental mechanisms

undoing   Performing a specific action that is intended to negate, in part, a previous action or communication. Undoing is related to the magical thinking of childhood

unipolar depressive response   Affective disorder that is characterized by symptoms of depression only

vaginismus   Development of spasticity in the pelvic muscles surrounding the vagina, which results in decreased probability of penetration

vagueness   Communication pattern involving the use of global pronouns and loose associations that lead to ambiguity and confusion in communication

verbal language   Culturally organized system of vocal sounds that communicate meaning

verbalizing the implied   Stating directly what a person has inferred

violence   Refers to behavior that has the physical intent of inflicting harm on people or property. For violence to be considered criminal, the behavior must conform to the definition of violent behavior delineated by the society in which it occurs

wellness   Dynamic condition of well-being that evolves from the development and integration of the five dimensions of a person: physical, intellectual, psychological, sociocultural and spiritual. Wellness is a process of ongoing growth toward self-actualization

with spaces   Spaces in which interacting persons use body parts and regions to show that they share a similar spatial orientation and thus are affiliated

word salad   Type of speech characterized by phrases that are confusing and apparently meaningless. A word salad may contain neologisms. Only the client can provide the meaning of such highly personal, coded communication

working phase   Second stage of the nurse-client relationship. During this stage, clients explore their experiences. Nurses assist clients in this process of exploration by helping them to describe and clarify their experiences, to plan courses of action and try out the plans, and to begin to evaluate the effectiveness of their new behavior. Should new behavior prove ineffective, nurses may assist clients to revise their courses of action

worthlessness   Component of low self-esteem; a feeling of uselessness and inability to contribute meaningfully to the well-being of others or to one's environment

APPENDIX A

DSM-III-R classification: axes I and II categories and codes

The *Diagnostic and Statistical Manual of Mental Disorders* is published by the American Psychiatric Association and is periodically revised. The revised third edition (DSM-III-R) appeared in 1987.

The *Manual* categorizes and codifies psychiatric diagnoses. A description of diagnostic criteria accompanies each diagnosis. Categories and codes are used by physicians when they make diagnoses and by institutional personnel when they compile statistics and complete insurance forms. The uses of DSM-III-R are discussed in Chapter 1.

All official DSM-III-R codes are included in ICD-9-CM. Codes followed by * are used for more than one DSM-III-R diagnosis or subtype to maintain compatibility with ICD-9-CM.

A long dash following a diagnostic term indicates the need for a fifth digit subtype or other qualifying term. The term *specify* following the name of some diagnostic categories indicates qualifying terms that clinicians may wish to add in parentheses after the name of the disorder.

DISORDERS USUALLY FIRST EVIDENT IN INFANCY, CHILDHOOD, OR ADOLESCENCE

NOS = Not Otherwise Specified
The current severity of a disorder may be specified after the diagnosis as:

mild
moderate
severe

} currently meets diagnostic criteria

in partial remission (or residual state)
in complete remission

DEVELOPMENTAL DISORDERS
Note: These are coded on Axis II.
Mental retardation

317.00	Mild mental retardation
318.00	Moderate mental retardation
318.10	Severe mental retardation
318.20	Profound mental retardation
319.00	Unspecified mental retardation

Pervasive development disorders

299.00	Autistic Disorder *Specify* if childhood onset
299.80	Pervasive developmental disorder NOS

Specific developmental disorders
Academic skills disorders

315.10	Developmental arithmetic disorder
315.80	Developmental expressive writing disorder
315.00	Developmental reading disorder

Language and speech disorders

315.39	Developmental articulation disorder
315.31*	Developmental expressive language disorder

Motor skills disorder

315.40	Developmental coordination disorder
315.90*	Specific developmental disorder NOS

Other developmental disorders

315.90*	Developmental disorder NOS

Reprinted with permission from the *Diagnostic and Statistical Manual of Mental Disorders, Third Edition, Revised.* Copyright 1987 American Psychiatric Association.

Disruptive behavior disorders

314.01	Attention deficit hyperactivity disorder
	Conduct disorder
312.20	group type
312.00	solitary aggressive type
312.90	undifferentiated type
313.81	Oppositional defiant disorder

Anxiety disorders of childhood or adolescence

309.21	Separation anxiety disorder
313.21	Avoidant disorder of childhood or adolescence
313.00	Overanxious disorder

Eating disorders

307.10	Anorexia nervosa
307.51	Bulimia nervosa
307.52	Pica
307.53	Rumination disorder of infancy
307.50	Eating disorder NOS

Gender identity disorders

302.60	Gender identity disorder of childhood
302.50	Transsexualism
	Specify sexual history: asexual, homosexual, heterosexual, unspecified
302.85*	Gender identity disorder of adolescence or adulthood, nontranssexual type
	Specify sexual history: asexual, homosexual, heterosexual, unspecified
302.85*	Gender identity disorder NOS

Tic disorders

307.23	Tourette's disorder
307.22	Chronic motor or vocal tic disorder
307.21	Transient tic disorder
	Specify: single episode or recurrent
307.20	Tic disorder NOS

Elimination disorders

307.70	Functional encopresis
	Specify: primary or secondary type
307.60	Functional enuresis
	Specify: primary or secondary type
	Specify: nocturnal only, diurnal only, nocturnal and diurnal

Speech disorders not elsewhere classified

307.00*	Cluttering
307.00*	Stuttering

Other disorders of infancy, childhood or adolescence

313.23	Elective mutism
313.82	Identity disorder
313.89	Reactive attachment disorder of infancy or early childhood
307.30	Stereotypy/habit disorder
314.00	Undifferentiated attention-deficit disorder

ORGANIC MENTAL DISORDERS
Dementias arising in the senium and presenium

	Primary degenerative dementia of the Alzheimer type, senile onset
290.30	with delirium
290.20	with delusions
290.21	with depression
290.00*	uncomplicated
	(Note: code 331.00 Alzheimer's disease on Axis III)

Code in fifth digit:
1 = with delirium, 2 = with delusions,
3 = with depression, 0* = uncomplicated.

290.1x	Primary degenerative dementia of the Alzheimer type, presenile onset, _____ (Note: code 331.00 Alzheimer's disease on Axis III)
290.4x	Multi-infarct dementia, _____
290.00*	Senile dementia NOS
	Specify etiology on Axis III if known
290.10*	Presenile dementia NOS
	Specify etiology on Axis III if known (e.g., Pick's disease, Jakob-Creutzfeldt disease)

Psychoactive substance-induced organic mental disorders

	Alcohol
303.00	intoxication
291.40	idiosyncratic intoxication
291.80	uncomplicated alcohol withdrawal
291.00	withdrawal delirium
291.30	hallucinosis
291.10	amnestic disorder
291.20	Dementia associated with alcoholism
	Amphetamine or similarly acting sympathomimetic
305.70*	intoxication
292.00*	withdrawal

292.81*	delirium
292.11*	delusional disorder

Caffeine
305.90*	intoxication

Cannabis
305.20*	intoxication
292.11*	delusional disorder

Cocaine
305.60*	intoxication
292.00*	withdrawal
292.81*	delirium
292.11*	delusional disorder

Hallucinogen
305.30*	hallucinosis
292.11*	delusional disorder
292.84*	mood disorder
292.89*	posthallucinogen perception disorder

Inhalant
305.90*	intoxication

Nicotine
292.00*	withdrawal

Opioid
305.50*	intoxication
292.00*	withdrawal

Phencyclidine (PCP) or similarly acting arylcyclohexylamine
305.90*	intoxication
292.81*	delirium
292.11*	delusional disorder
292.84*	mood disorder
292.90*	organic mental disorder NOS

Sedative, hypnotic, or anxiolytic
305.40*	intoxication
292.00*	Uncomplicated sedative, hypnotic, or anxiolytic withdrawal
292.00*	withdrawal delirium
292.83*	amnestic disorder

Other or unspecified psychoactive substance
305.90*	intoxication
292.00*	withdrawal
292.81*	delirium
292.82*	dementia
292.83*	amnestic disorder
292.11*	delusional disorder

292.12	hallucinosis
292.84*	mood disorder
292.89*	anxiety disorder
292.89*	personality disorder
292.90*	organic mental disorder NOS

Organic mental disorders associated with Axis III physical disorders or conditions, or whose etiology is unknown.
293.00	Delirium
294.10	Dementia
294.00	Amnestic disorder
293.81	Organic delusional disorder
293.82	Organic hallucinosis
293.83	Organic mood disorder
	Specify: manic, depressed, mixed
294.80*	Organic anxiety disorder
310.10	Organic personality disorder
	Specify: if explosive type
294.80*	Organic mental disorder NOS

PSYCHOACTIVE SUBSTANCE USE DISORDERS

Alcohol
303.90	dependence
305.00	abuse

Amphetamine or similarly acting sympathomimetic
304.40	dependence
305.70*	abuse

Cannabis
304.30	dependence
305.20*	abuse

Cocaine
304.20	dependence
305.60*	abuse

Hallucinogen
304.50*	dependence
305.30*	abuse

Inhalant
304.60	dependence
305.90*	abuse

Nicotine
305.10	dependence

Opioid
304.00	dependence
305.50*	abuse

Phencyclidine (PCP) or similarly acting arylcyclohexylamine
304.50*	dependence
305.90*	abuse

Sedative, hypnotic, or anxiolytic
304.10	dependence

305.40*   abuse
304.90*   Polysubstance dependence
304.90*   Psychoactive substance dependence NOS
305.90*   Psychoactive substance abuse NOS

SCHIZOPHRENIA

Code in fifth digit: 1 = subchronic, 2 = chronic, 3 = subchronic with acute exacerbation, 4 = chronic with acute exacerbation, 5 = in remission, 0 = unspecified.

Schizophrenia,
295.2x   catatonic, _____
295.1x   disorganized, _____
295.3x   paranoid, _____
    Specify if stable type
295.9x   undifferentiated, _____
295.6x   residual, _____
    Specify: if late onset

DELUSIONAL (PARANOID) DISORDER

297.10   Delusional (Paranoid) disorder
    Specify: type: erotomanic
        grandiose
        jealous
        persecutory
        somatic
        unspecified

PSYCHOTIC DISORDERS NOT ELSEWHERE CLASSIFIED

298.80   Brief reactive psychosis
295.40   Schizophreniform disorder
    Specify: without good prognostic features or with good prognostic features
295.70   Schizoaffective disorder
    Specify: bipolar type or depressive type
297.30   Induced psychotic disorder
298.90   Psychotic disorder NOS (Atypical psychosis)

MOOD DISORDERS

Code current state of Major Depression and Bipolar Disorder in fifth digit:
1 = mild
2 = moderate
3 = severe, without psychotic features
4 = with psychotic features (*specify* mood-congruent or mood-incongruent)
5 = in partial remission
6 = in full remission
0 = unspecified

For major depressive episodes, *specify* if chronic and *specify* if melancholic type.

For Bipolar Disorder, Bipolar Disorder NOS, Recurrent Major Depression, and Depressive Disorder NOS, *specify* if seasonal pattern.

Bipolar disorders

Bipolar disorder,
296.6x   mixed, _____
296.4x   manic, _____
296.5x   depressed, _____
301.13   Cyclothymia
296.70   Bipolar disorder NOS

Depressive disorders

Major Depression,
296.2x   single episode, _____
296.3x   recurrent, _____
300.40   Dysthymia (or Depressive neurosis)
    Specify: primary or secondary type
    Specify: early or late onset
311.00   Depressive disorder NOS

ANXIETY DISORDERS (or anxiety and phobic neuroses)

Panic disorder
300.21   with agoraphobia
    Specify current severity of agoraphobic avoidance
    Specify current severity of panic attacks
300.01   without agoraphobia
    Specify current severity of panic attacks
300.22   Agoraphobia without history of panic disorder
    Specify with or without limited symptom attacks
300.23   Social phobia
    Specify if generalized type
300.29   Simple phobia
300.30   Obsessive compulsive disorder (or Obsessive compulsive neurosis)
309.89   Post-traumatic stress disorder
    Specify if delayed onset
300.02   Generalized anxiety disorder
300.00   Anxiety disorder NOS

SOMATOFORM DISORDERS

300.70*   Body dysmorphic disorder
300.11   Conversion disorder (or Hysterical neurosis, conversion type)
    Specify: single episode or recurrent

300.70*	Hypochondriasis (or Hypochondriacal neurosis)
300.81	Somatization disorder
307.80	Somatoform pain disorder
300.70*	Undifferentiated somatoform disorder
300.70*	Somatoform disorder NOS

DISSOCIATIVE DISORDERS (or hysterical neuroses, dissociative type)

300.14	Multiple personality disorder
300.13	Psychogenic fugue
300.12	Psychogenic amnesia
300.60	Depersonalization disorder (or Depersonalization neurosis)
300.15	Dissociative disorder NOS

SEXUAL DISORDERS
Paraphilias

302.40	Exhibitionism
302.81	Fetishism
302.89	Frotteurism
302.20	Pedophilia
	Specify: same sex, opposite sex, same and opposite sex
	Specify if limited to incest
	Specify: exclusive type or nonexclusive type
302.83	Sexual masochism
302.84	Sexual sadism
302.30	Transvestic fetishism
302.82	Voyeurism
302.90*	Paraphilia NOS

Sexual dysfunctions

Specify: psychogenic only, or psychogenic and biogenic (Note: If biogenic only, code on Axis III)
Specify: lifelong or acquired
Specify: generalized or situational

	Sexual desire disorders
302.71	Hypoactive sexual desire disorder
302.79	Sexual aversion disorder
	Sexual arousal disorders
302.72*	Female sexual arousal disorder
302.72*	Male erectile disorder
	Orgasm disorders
302.73	Inhibited female orgasm
302.74	Inhibited male orgasm
302.75	Premature ejaculation
	Sexual pain disorders
302.76	Dyspareunia

360.51	Vaginismus
302.70	Sexual dysfunction NOS

Other sexual disorders

302.90*	Sexual disorder NOS

SLEEP DISORDERS
Dyssomnias

	Insomnia disorder
307.42*	related to another mental disorder (nonorganic)
780.50*	related to known organic factor
307.42*	Primary insomnia
	Hypersomnia disorder
307.44	related to another mental disorder (nonorganic)
780.50*	related to a known organic factor
780.54	Primary hypersomnia
307.45	Sleep-wake schedule disorder
	Specify: advanced or delayed phase type, disorganized type, frequently changing type
	Other dyssomnias
307.40*	Dyssomnia NOS

Parasomnias

307.47	Dream anxiety disorder (Nightmare disorder)
307.46*	Sleep terror disorder
307.46*	Sleepwalking disorder
307.40*	Parasomnia NOS

FACTITIOUS DISORDERS

	Factitious disorder
301.51	with physical symptoms
300.16	with psychological symptoms
300.19	Factitious disorder NOS

IMPULSE CONTROL DISORDERS NOT ELSEWHERE CLASSIFIED

312.34	Intermittent explosive disorder
312.32	Kleptomania
312.31	Pathological gambling
312.33	Pyromania
312.39*	Trichotillomania
312.39*	Impulse control disorder NOS

ADJUSTMENT DISORDER

	Adjustment disorder
309.24	with anxious mood
309.00	with depressed mood
309.30	with disturbance of conduct

309.40	with mixed disturbance of emotions and conduct
309.28	with mixed emotional features
309.82	with physical complaints
309.83	with withdrawal
309.23	with work (or academic) inhibition
309.90	Adjustment disorder NOS

PSYCHOLOGICAL FACTORS AFFECTING CONDITION

| 316.00 | Psychological factors affecting physical condition |

Specify physical condition on Axis III

PERSONALITY DISORDERS
Note: These are coded on Axis II.

Cluster A

301.00	Paranoid
301.20	Schizoid
301.22	Schizotypal

Cluster B

301.70	Antisocial
301.83	Borderline
301.50	Histrionic
301.81	Narcissistic

Cluster C

301.82	Avoidant
301.60	Dependent
301.40	Obsessive compulsive
301.84	Passive aggressive
301.90	Personality disorder NOS

V CODES FOR CONDITIONS NOT ATTRIBUTABLE TO A MENTAL DISORDER THAT ARE A FOCUS OF ATTENTION OR TREATMENT

| V62.30 | Academic problem |
| V71.01 | Adult antisocial behavior |

| V40.00 | Borderline intellectual functioning (Note: This is coded on Axis II.) |

V71.02	Childhood or adolescent antisocial behavior
V65.20	Malingering
V61.10	Marital problem
V15.81	Noncompliance with medical treatment
V62.20	Occupational problem
V61.20	Parent-child problem
V62.81	Other interpersonal problem
V61.80	Other specified family circumstances
V62.89	Phase of life problem or other life circumstance problem
V62.82	Uncomplicated bereavement

ADDITIONAL CODES

300.90	Unspecified mental disorder (nonpsychotic)
V71.09*	No diagnosis or condition on Axis I
799.90*	Diagnosis or condition deferred on Axis I

| V71.09* | No diagnosis or condition on Axis II |
| 799.90* | Diagnosis or condition deferred on Axis II |

MULTIAXIAL SYSTEM

Axis I	Clinical Syndromes V Codes
Axis II	Developmental Disorders Personality Disorders
Axis III	Physical Disorders and Conditions
Axis IV	Severity of Psychosocial Stressors
Axis V	Global Assessment of Functioning

APPENDIX B

Selected psychotropic drugs

Psychopharmacology figures prominently in the treatment of mental illness. Nursing activities range from administration of psychopharmaceuticals to teaching clients about the medications they are receiving. To safely and effectively carry out these nursing activities, nurses need to be knowledgeable about the characteristics of psychotropic drugs (e.g., actions, dosages, untoward side effects). The following tables use selected psychotropic drugs to exemplify the characteristics and nursing implications of psychotropic medications frequently prescribed for clients with psychiatric disorders.

Cerebral stimulating agents*

Generic name	Trade name	Major indications	Usual adult dosages
AMPHETAMINES			
Amphetamine sulfate	Benzedrine	Narcolepsy	5 to 60 mg P.O. daily in divided doses
Dextroamphetamine sulfate	Dexampex Dexedrine	Adjunct treatment of exogenous obesity	5 to 30 mg P.O. daily in divided doses before meals

Nursing implications

- Instruct client about CNS and cardiovascular side effects (e.g., overstimulation, headache, insomnia, hypertension, tachycardia, palpitations). Monitor client's pulse and blood pressure.
- Do not use concurrently with general anesthetics, tricyclic antidepressants, or MAO inhibitors or within 14 days of administration of MAO inhibitor.
- Contraindicated in such conditions as glaucoma, cardiovascular disease, hypertension, hyperthyroidism, anxiety states, and excessive restlessness. Alters diabetic drug requirements and dietary restrictions.
- Educate client about the habit-forming potential of amphetamines.
- Instruct client that physical coordination and/or mental alertness may be impaired.
- Administer the last dose at least 6 hours before bedtime to prevent insomnia; sustained-release capsules should be administered 10-14 hours before bedtime; administer other doses 30-60 minutes before mealtime to suppress appetite.
- Instruct client not to chew sustained-release capsules.
- Gradually decrease dosage before discontinuing the drug to avoid withdrawal symptoms.
- Administer with caution to elderly and/or debilitated clients or to clients with histories of suicidal, homicidal, or addictive tendencies.
- Gradually decrease dosage to avoid psychotic symptoms and lethargy, which are associated with abrupt withdrawal.

*Nursing implications modified from McKenry L and Salerno E: Pharmacology in nursing, ed 17, St. Louis, 1989, The CV Mosby Co.

896

Generic name	Trade name	Major indications	Usual adult dosages
NONAMPHETAMINE ANOREXIGENIC AGENTS			
Mazindol	Mazanor Sanorex	Adjunct treatment for exogenous obesity	1 mg P.O. before meals or 2 mg 1 hour before lunch
Phendimetrazine tartrate	Bontril Phenazine Plagine		35 mg P.O. b.i.d. or t.i.d. 1 hour before meals
Phenmetrazine hydrochloride	Preludin		25 mg P.O. b.i.d. or t.i.d. not to exceed 75 mg daily
Phenylpropanolamine hydrochloride	Acutrim Dexatrim Prolamine		25 mg P.O. t.i.d. 1 hour before meals or 75 mg P.O. of a sustained-release form once daily
Fenfluramine hydrochloride	Pondimin		20 mg P.O. t.i.d. to a maximum of 120 mg/day in divided doses before meals

Nursing implications

- Pharmacologically resemble amphetamines, demonstrating amphetamine actions and side effects. See amphet-Amines.
- Fenfluramine increases serotonin levels and long-term use depletes catecholamines. It may produce paranoia, depression, and psychosis. Its interaction with anesthesia may result in cardiac arrest.
- Educate client about the habit-forming potential of the drug.
- Instruct client that physical coordination and/or mental alertness may be impaired.

Generic name	Trade name	Major indications	Usual adult dosages
PSYCHOTHERAPEUTIC CNS STIMULANTS			
Methylphenidate hydrochloride	Ritalin	Narcolepsy (adults)	10 to 60 mg P.O. daily in divided doses
		ADHD (children)	Initially 5 mg before breakfast and lunch with 5 to 10 mg increments weekly not to exceed 60 mg/day
Nikethamide	Coramine	Treatment of CNS depression in acute alcoholism	1.25 to 5 g I.V. p.r.n.
Cocaine hydrochloride		Included in Brompton's cocktail (oral analgesic)	

Nursing implications

- Methylphenidate is contraindicated in clients with known sensitivity to the drug and in those with glaucoma.
- Methylphenidate may lower the seizure threshold. Use with caution for clients with epilepsy.
- Methylphenidate should be used with caution for clients with hypertension, anxiety states, emotional instability, or a history of substance abuse.
- Do not give methylphenidate concurrently with MAO inhibitors or within 14 days of administration of MAO inhibitors.
- Educate client about the habit-forming potential of methylphenidate.
- Monitor client for weight loss from appetite suppression effects of methylphenidate.
- Methylphenidate is not recommended for pregnant or lactating women.
- Administer last dose of methylphenidate at least 6 hours before bedtime to prevent insomnia.
- Monitor client when discontinuing methylphenidate since depression may occur.

Sedative and hypnotic agents*

GENERAL INFORMATION ON SEDATIVE-HYPNOTICS

- Individual responses vary. Discuss with the client the quality and quantity of sleep to assess whether adjustments in dosage and/or medication are indicated.
- Irritation to the gastric mucosa and aftertaste may be minimized by administration with fruit juice, milk, or a bedtime snack if dietary requirements allow this.
- Safety measures, such as siderails and assistance with ambulation, should be implemented shortly after ingestion. Hypnotic doses often have a rapid onset of action, resulting in transient dizziness and excitation. This occurs most frequently when administered on an empty stomach or to an ambulating client.
- Clients may complain of "morning hangover," drowsiness, blurred vision, and transient hypotension on arising. Explain to the client the need for arising first to a sitting position, equilibrating, and then standing. Again, assistance with ambulation may be required. If "hangover" becomes troublesome, there should be a reduction in dosage and/or change in medication.
- These drugs are psychologically and/or physiologically habit-forming. Withdrawal after long-term use may produce symptoms of anxiety, insommnia, tremors, vivid dreams, agitation, and confusion. Use as many natural aids as possible (for example, a relaxing backrub, a warm cup of milk, a quiet and soothing environment, a clean body and bed) to help produce relaxation and sleep.
- Therapeutic, toxic, and fatal blood levels are much lower when more than one CNS depressant (for example, alcohol, tranquilizers, antihistamines, anesthetics, narcotics) have been ingested.

Generic name	Trade name	Major indications	Usual adult dosages
BARBITURATES			
Amobarbital			
Amobarbital sodium	Amytal	Sedative for anxiety and tension	30 to 50 mg P.O. or I.M. b.i.d. or t.i.d.
		Hypnotic for insomnia, acute convulsive disorders, manic disorders	65 to 200 mg P.O. or I.M. h.s.
		Sedative prior to anesthesia	200 mg P.O. or I.M. 1 to 2 hours before operative procedure
Mephobarbital	Mebaral	Daytime sedative to relieve anxiety, tension, and apprehension; adjunct treatment of grand mal and petit mal epilepsy	32 to 100 mg P.O. t.i.d. or q.i.d.
Pentobarbital	Nembutal	Daytime sedative for relief of nervous tension	20 to 40 mg P.O. b.i.d. to q.i.d.
		Sedative before surgery	150 to 200 mg P.O. or I.M.
Butabarbital sodium	Butisol Buticaps	Daytime sedative for anxiety disorders and anxiety	15 to 30 mg P.O. t.i.d. or q.i.d.
		Hypnotic for insomnia, emergency control of convulsions; may be given I.V. for status epilepticus	100 mg P.O., 120 to 200 mg rectal, 100 to 200 mg I.M.
Phenobarbital Phenobarbital sodium	Luminal	Daytime sedative to relieve mild to moderate anxiety	15 to 30 mg P.O. b.i.d. to q.i.d.
		Sedative before surgery	100 to 200 mg I.M. 60 to 90 minutes before surgery

*Nursing implications are from Clayton B: Mosby's handbook of pharmacology, ed 4, St. Louis, 1987, The CV Mosby Co.

Generic name	Trade name	Major indications	Usual adult dosages
		Hypnotic for insomnia, anticonvulsant	100 to 320 mg P.O. or I.M. h.s.

Nursing implications

- General adverse effects of barbiturates include drowsiness, lethargy, headache, muscle or joint pain, and mental depression. Barbiturate "hangover" frequently occurs after administration of hypnotic doses or with long-term anticonvulsant therapy. Clients may display dulled affect, subtle distortion of mood, and impaired coordination.
- Elderly clients and those in severe pain may respond paradoxically to barbiturates with excitement, euphoria, restlessness, and confusion.
- Hypersensitivity reactions to barbiturates are infrequent, but the sequelae are quite serious and potentially fatal. Barbiturate therapy should be discontinued immediately if the client develops symptoms of hypersensitivity, including high fever, inflammation of mucous membrane, or any type of dermatitis.
- Blood dyscrasias have been attributed to barbiturate administration. Blood counts should be repeated periodically during long-term therapy. The client should be reminded to report symptoms, including sore throat, easy bruisability, fever, or petechiae.
- Barbiturates readily cross the placental barrier, appearing in fetal circulation. They are also present in breast milk. Neonates and nursing infants whose mothers receive barbiturates must be observed for signs of toxicity.
- See general information on sedative-hypnotics.

BENZODIAZEPINES

Generic name	Trade name	Major indications	Usual adult dosages
Lorazepam	Ativan	Hypnotic for insomnia from anxiety or transient situational stress, the management of anxiety disorders, and short-term relief of anxiety, or anxiety associated with depressive symptoms	2 to 4 mg P.O. h.s.
		Sedative before surgery	0.5 mg/kg up to 4 mg I.M. 2 hours before operative procedure
		Drug of choice for symptoms of alcohol withdrawal	
Triazolam	Halcion	Hypnotic for insomnia from physical or psychological states	0.5 mg P.O. h.s.

Nursing implications

- The most common side effects observed are extensions of pharmacologic activity and include drowsiness (14%), dizziness (7%), and light-headedness (5%). Other side effects include nausea, headache, confusion, euphoria, tachycardia, and brief memory impairment. Rare adverse effects include nightmares, taste alterations, insomnia, tinnitus, and paresthesias.
- Overdosage may be manifested by somnolence, confusion, impaired coordination, slurred speech and ultimately coma. Treatment consists of general physiologic and supportive measures, including the use of levarterenol, dopamine, or metaraminol for hypotension, maintenance of an airway, and administration of oxygen.
- Benzodiazepines are contraindicated for use in pregnant women. Clients should be warned to discontinue use before becoming pregnant or discontinue use immediately if pregnancy is suspected.
- See General information on sedative-hypnotics

Continued.

Sedative and hypnotic agents—cont'd

Generic name	Trade name	Major indications	Usual adult dosages
NONBENZODIAZEPINES-NONBARBITURATES			
Chloral hydrate	Noctec SK-Chloral Hydrate	Daytime sedative	250 mg P.O. or 325 mg rectal t.i.d. after meals
		Hypnotic for insomnia	0.5 to 1 g P.O. or rectal 15 to 30 minutes before bedtime

Nursing implications

- The habitual use of chloral hydrate may result in physical dependence and addiction similar to that of alcohol. Sudden withdrawal may result in delirium.
- Allergic reactions, although rare, include erythema, urticaria, and dermatitis. The eruption usually begins on the face or back and spreads to the neck, chest, and arms. The dermatitis may occur soon after administration or for as long as 10 days after administration.
- Large doses may produce false-positive results with Clinitest tablets.
- Chloral hydrate passes the placental barrier and is excreted in breast milk.
- See General information on sedative-hypnotics.

Paraldehyde	Paral	Sedative	5 to 10 ml P.O. or rectal
		Hypnotic for insomnia	10 to 30 ml P.O. or rectal
		Treatment of alcohol withdrawal symptoms	5 to 10 ml P.O. or 5 ml I.M. every 4 to 6 hours to a maximum of 40 to 60 ml P.O. or 30 ml I.M. daily
		Seizures	5 to 10 ml I.M.; divide 10 ml into 2 injections. I.V. 0.2 to 0.4 ml/Kg in N.S. injections

Nursing implications

- Paraldehyde must be used with caution in clients with hepatic disease. The drug is metabolized more slowly, and the hypnotic effects may be prolonged.
- Paraldehyde by-products are excreted through the lungs, giving the breath a characteristic odor.
- The most frequent adverse effects associated with normal doses are gastric irritation and erythematous skin rash.
- Acetaldehyde, a metabolic by-product, may produce false-positive serum and urine ketone values when Acetest tablets are used.
- Paraldehyde readily diffuses across the placenta and appears in fetal circulation in quantities sufficient to induce respiratory depression in newborn infants.
- See General information on sedative-hypnotics

Antidepressant and antimanic agents*

Generic name	Trade name	Major indications	Usual adult dosages
MAO INHIBITORS			
Trancylcypromine sulfate	Parnate	Depression not respondent to tricyclic antidepressants	10 mg P.O. b.i.d., increased to a maximum of 30 mg/day after 2 to 3 weeks, if necessary
Isocarboxazid	Marplan	Depression not respondent to tricyclic antidepressants	30 mg P.O. daily in a single dose or divided doses, reduced to 10 to 20 mg/day when condition improves

Nursing implications

- Do not administer to any client with confirmed or suspected cardiovascular disease or hypertension or a history of severe headaches.
- Do not administer to clients over 60 years of age, because of the possibility of cerebral sclerosis with damaged vessels.
- Do not administer to clients with a known or suspected pheochromocytoma. These tumors secrete catecholamines that produce severe hypertension.
- *Dietary restrictions:* MAO inhibitors act throughout the body, inhibiting monoamine oxidase. Foods and other drugs are not metabolized as rapidly and may accumulate to toxic levels. Foods with a high tyramine content must be avoided to prevent these serious interactions. Clients must be instructed not to ingest cheese (particularly strong or aged varieties), sour cream, Chianti wine, sherry, beer, pickled herring, liver, canned figs, raisins, bananas, or avocados (particularly if overripe), chocolate, soy sauce, the pods of broad beans (fava beans), yeast extracts, or meat prepared with tenderizers.
- Manifestations of depression may improve within a few days (that is, increase in appetite, sleep, and psychomotor activity). However, the depression still exists and usually takes several weeks of therapeutic doses of antidepressants and psychotherapy before improvement is noted. Suicide precautions should be maintained during this time.
- Postural hypotension and dizziness are observed more frequently as dosages exceed 30 mg/day. They may be relieved by having the client lie down until blood pressure returns to normal. Clients should be taught to rise slowly from a horizontal position to a sitting position and then flex the arms and legs several times before standing. The client should be forewarned to sit or lie down with the onset of weakness and dizziness.
- Other side effects reported with MAO inhibitors include dizziness, tachycardia, drowsiness, dryness of mouth, nausea, anorexia, diarrhea, abdominal pain, and constipation.
- Administer MAO inhibitors with caution to clients with hyperthyroidism. Clients with this disease are quite sensitive to increased levels of norepinephrine and serotonin.
- Administer with caution in clients with diabetes mellitus. MAO inhibitors have been reported to contribute to hypoglycemic episodes in diabetic clients being treated with insulin or oral hypoglycemic agents.
- Use with caution in clients at risk for angina pectoris. MAO inhibitors may suppress anginal pain that would otherwise serve as a warning of myocardial ischemia.
- It is recommended that MAO inhibitors be discontinued 7 days before elective surgery to allow time for recovery of monoamine oxidase levels before anesthetic agents are administered.
- Use MAO inhibitors with extreme caution in pregnancy and only when the benefits of therapy significantly outweigh the risk of exposure to MAO inhibitors to the fetus. Laboratory tests indicate that MAO inhibitors cross the placental barrier and are secreted into breast milk.
- When switching from MAO inhibitors to tricyclics, wait 1 to 2 weeks for synthesis to occur.

*Nursing implications are from Clayton B: Mosby's handbook of pharmacology, ed 4, St. Louis, 1987, The CV Mosby Co.

Continued.

Antidepressant and antimanic agents—cont'd

Generic name	Trade name	Major indications	Usual adult dosages
TRICYCLIC ANTIDEPRESSANTS			
Amitriptyline hydrochloride	Elavil Emitrip Endep	Depression	50 to 75 mg P.O. h.s. increased to 200 mg/day, then to a maximum of 300 mg daily, if needed; or 20 to 30 mg I.M. q.i.d. or as a single dose h.s.
Imipramine hydrochloride	Presamine Tofranil	Depression Phobia	50 to 75 mg P.O. increased to a maximum of 300 mg/day
Doxepin hydrochloride	Adapin Sinequam	Depression	25 to 50 mg P.O. daily initially, increased to a maximum of 300 mg daily, if necessary

Nursing implications

• The most common side effects are those associated with anticholinergic activity. These include dry mucous membranes, metallic taste, constipation, mydriasis, and cycloplegia resulting in blurred vision, epigastric distress, and urinary retention. Sugarless hard candy or chewing gum may help the dry mouth. The use of stool softeners such as docusate (Colace) or the occasional use of a potent laxative such as bisacodyl (Dulcolax) may be required for constipation. Reduction in dosage of the antidepressant may relieve symptoms of urinary retention. Tolerance to these side effects tends to develop with continued therapy.

• Extrapyramidal side effects are rare, but a fine rapid tremor of the hands may occur in about 10% of the clients receiving tricyclic therapy. Occasionally, clients have reported numbness and tingling of arms and legs. The tremor may be controlled with small doses of propranolol. If parkinsonian symptoms develop, the tricyclic antidepressant dosage must be reduced or discontinued. Antiparkinsonian medications will not control tricyclic antidepressant-induced symptoms.

• Clients with cardiovascular disorders must be observed for development or aggravation of existing arrhythmias, congestive heart failure, sinus tachycardia, and hypotension. The tricyclic antidepressants inhibit the reuptake of norepinephrine in cardiac tissue and have direct, quinidine-like depressant effects on the myocardium. Orthostatic hypotension is commonly seen with therapeutic dosages. Tricyclic antidepressants may cause flattening or inversion of the T wave of an electrocardiogram in about 20% of clients without previous history of cardiovascular disease. Deaths from coronary occlusion, cardiac arrest, and ventricular fibrillation have been reported, as well as cases of severe arrhythmias.

• High doses of tricyclic antidepressants lower the seizure threshold. Seizures may occur in those with and without a history of seizure activity. Adjustment of anticonvulsant therapy may be required, especially in those seizure-prone clients.

• Safe use in pregnancy has not been established. Fetal malformation, urinary retention, lethargy, and withdrawal symptoms have been reported in neonates whose mothers ingested tricyclic antidepressants during pregnancy.

SECOND-GENERATION ANTIDEPRESSANTS

Trazodone hydrochloride	Desyrel	Depression	150 mg P.O. daily in divided doses, increased by 50 mg/day every 3 to 4 days up to a maximum of 400 mg/day; (600 mg/day for severely ill)

Nursing implications

• Manifestations of depression may improve within a few days (that is, increase in appetite, sleep, and psychomotor activity). However, the depression still exists, and it usually takes several weeks of therapeutic doses of antidepressants and psychotherapy before improvement is noted. Suicide precautions should be maintained during this time.

• After an optimal response has been obtained, dosage should be reduced to the minimum necessary to maintain relief of depression.

Generic name	Trade name	Major indications	Usual adult dosages

- Drowsiness and decreased energy are the most commonly reported adverse effects. Other CNS effects reported are fatigue, lightheadedness, dizziness, ataxia, mild confusion, and inability to think clearly.
- Cardiovascular side effects reported are orthostatic hypotension, tachycardia, and palpitations. Syncope, arrhythmias, angina, and bradycardia have rarely occurred.
- Fetotoxicity and teratogenic effects have been reported in laboratory animals. Trazodone should not be administered to pregnant clients unless therapeutic benefits significantly outweigh possible adverse effects to the fetus.

LITHIUM

Generic name	Trade name	Major indications	Usual adult dosages
Lithium carbonate	Eskalith Lithane Lithobid	Mania and bipolar disorder prophylaxis	300 mg P.O. t.i.d. to q.i.d., adjusted to achieve lithium blood level of 1 to 1.5 mEq/liter for acute mania; 300 mg t.i.d. or q.i.d. to achieve maintenance blood levels of 0.6 to 1.2 mEq/liter for bipolar disorder prophylaxis; blood levels should not exceed 2 mEq/liter; administer with food
Lithium citrate			

Nursing implications

- Side effects frequently reported early in the course of therapy are nausea, anorexia, stomach irritation, and diarrhea. These effects are frequently minimized by administration with meals. Polyuria and excessive thirst are common in the first week of therapy because of sodium diuresis. Fine hand tremor and mild, transient ataxia are also occasionally observed.
- Persistent vomiting, profuse diarrhea, hyperreflexia, lethargy, and weakness are all signs of impending serious toxicity. Dosages should be reduced or discontinued.
- Rarely, long-term lithium therapy (greater than 6 months) produces hypothyroidism. The mechanism of action is unknown. The hypothyroid state should be treated with thyroid replacement.
- Chronic lithium therapy rarely initiates a diabetes insipidus-like syndrome characterized by polyuria and polydipsia. Temporarily discontinuing therapy for a few days corrects the problem. Reinitiation of therapy at lower doses rarely reactivates the syndrome. Monitor clients closely for fluid and electrolyte balance.
- Other adverse effects that have been reported with lithium therapy include albuminuria, oliguria, renal tubular damage, transient hyperglycemia, leukocytosis, worsening of organic brain syndrome, generalized pruritis with and without rash, edematous swelling of the ankles and wrists, and metallic taste.
- Lithium should be avoided in pregnancy, especially in the first trimester, if at all possible. The use of lithium early in pregnancy may be associated with an increased incidence of cardiovascular abnormalities in the neonate. Breast-feeding during lithium therapy is also not recommended. Significant amounts of lithium are excreted in breast milk, and toxicities have been reported.
- Advise client to monitor his/her degree of alertness and coordination, especially when beginning lithium therapy.

Antianxiety agents*

Generic name	Trade name	Major indications	Usual adult dosages
BENZODIAZEPINES			
Chlorazepate dipotassium	Tranxene	Anxiety	15 to 60 mg daily in divided doses
		Alcohol withdrawal	Day 1—30 mg P.O. followed by 30 to 60 mg P.O. in divided doses; Day 2—45 to 90 mg P.O. in divided doses; Day 3—22.5 to 45 mg P.O. in divided doses; Day 4—15 to 30 mg P.O. in divided doses; gradually reduced to 7.5 to 15 mg P.O. daily
Diazepam	Valium Valrelease	Anxiety	2 to 10 mg P.O. b.i.d. to q.i.d.
		Alcohol withdrawal	10 mg P.O. t.i.d. or q.i.d. for 24 hours, decreased to 5 mg t.i.d. or q.i.d.
		Skeletal muscle spasms	2 to 10 mg P.O. t.i.d. or q.i.d.
		Status epilepticus	5 to 10 mg slow I.V. push repeated every 10 to 15 minutes to a maximum of 30 mg
Alprazolam	Xanax	Anxiety disorders, short-term anxiety, and anxiety with depression	0.25 to 0.5 mg P.O. t.i.d.

Nursing implications

- The more common side effects of benzodiazepines are extensions of their pharmacologic properties. Drowsiness, fatigue, lethargy, and ataxia are relatively common, dose-related, adverse effects of this class of agents.
- Paradoxic reactions occasionally occur within the first few weeks of therapy. These reactions are manifested by increased anxiety, hyperexcitation, hallucinations, acute rage, and insomnia.
- Physical and psychologic dependence are relatively rare but may occur on discontinuance after prolonged therapy with high dosages. Abrupt withdrawal may result in seizure activity and symptoms similar to barbiturate withdrawal. The symptoms may not appear for more than a week after discontinuance as a result of the long half-lives and conversion to active metabolites.
- Benzodiazepines should be administered with caution to clients with a history of blood dycrasias or hepatic or renal damage. Cases of agranulocytosis, jaundice, and elevated AST, ALT, bilirubin, and alkaline-phosphatase levels have been reported.
- Benzodiazepines should not be administered during the first trimester of pregnancy. Congenital malformations have been reported.
- Chronic administration during pregnancy may cause physical dependence with withdrawal symptoms in the infant after delivery.
- Benzodiazepines and their metabolites are secreted in breast milk in sufficient quantities to produce drowsiness and feeding difficulties in infants.

Generic name	Trade name	Major indications	Usual adult dosages
MISCELLANEOUS			
Buspirone hydrochloride	Buspar	Anxiety	5 mg P.O. t.i.d., increased by 5 mg q 2 to 3 days, as needed, to a maximum of 60 mg/day

Nursing implication

- Monitor the client closely, because expected reactions to this relatively new drug are unknown.

*Nursing implications are from Clayton B: Mosby's handbook of pharmacology, ed 4, St. Louis, 1987, The CV Mosby Co.

Antipsychotic agents*

Generic name	Trade name	Major indications	Usual adult dosages
PHENOTHIAZINES			
Chlorpromazine hydrochloride	Thorazine	Relief of psychotic symptoms	150 to 600 mg P.O. initially, increased to a maintenance dose of 500 to 1,000 mg P.O. daily in divided doses
Fluphenazine decanoate	Prolixin decanoate	Relief of psychotic symptoms	Initially 12.5 to 25 mg I.M. or S.C. every 1 to 4 weeks, then 25 to 50 mg p.r.n. for maintenance
Fluphenazine hydrochloride	Permitil hydrochloride Prolixin		

Nursing implications

- Some of the most troublesome side effects noted with antipsychotic agents are extrapyramidal effects. These include the parkinsonian symptoms of tremor, muscular rigidity, masklike facies, shuffling gait, and loss or weakness of motor function; dystonias and dyskinesias, which are spasmodic movements of the body and limbs (dystonias) and coordinated, involuntary rhythmic movements (dyskinesias); and akathisias, which consist of involuntary motor restlessness, constant pacing, inability to sit still, and are often accompanied by fidgeting, with lip and limb movements.
- Tardive dyskinesia is a drug-induced neurologic disorder manifested by facial grimaces and involuntary movement of the lips, tongue, and jaw, producing smacking and frequent, recurrent protrusions of the tongue. This adverse drug effect is usually irreversible and appears after several years of antipsychotic therapy. The incidence appears to be higher in clients taking both antiparkinsonian and antipsychotic agents concomitantly. It has been reported that fine movements of the tongue may be an early sign of tardive dyskinesia. If the medication is stopped with gradual reduction of dosage, the syndrome may not develop.
- Dry mouth and constipation are other frequent side effects that may cause decreased compliance. Sugarless hard candy or gum may help the dry mouth. The use of stool softeners such as docusate (Colace) and occasionally a potent laxative such a bisacodyl (Dulcolax) may be required for constipation.
- Chronic drowsiness and fatigue may occur during initiation or adjustment in therapy. Tolerance will usually develop, but a single daily dose at bedtime may also be effective.
- Phenothiazines lower the seizure threshold. Seizures may occur in those with and without a history of seizure activity. Adjustment of anticonvulsant therapy may be required, especially in those seizure-prone clients.
- Hypersensitivity reactions include cholestatic jaundice (upper abdominal pain, yellow skin, rash, fever, eosinophilia, elevated liver function tests), blood dyscrasias, dermatoses, and photosensitivity. Most hypersensitivity reactions occur within the first few months of therapy.
- Adverse effects, listed according to organ systems involved, include:
  a. Hematologic: blood dyscrasias are rare, but the mortality rate can be high. Agranulocytosis occurs most frequently in women and after 4 to 10 weeks of therapy. Leukopenia frequently occurs after prolonged therapy with high dosages of phenothiazines and is usually an indication to stop therapy. Other blood dyscrasias include eosinophilia, hemolytic anemia, thrombocytopenia, and aplastic anemia. If signs of blood dyscrasias (sore throat, fever, weakness) occur, phenothiazine therapy should be discontinued until a complete blood count has eliminated the possibility of a blood dyscrasia.
  b. Hepatic: a cholestatic jaundice may appear in 0.5% to 4% of those clients ingesting phenothiazines. It usually appears within 2 to 4 weeks after initiating therapy. Clients may complain of upper abdominal pain, yellow skin, rash, and fever, and display elevated levels in liver function tests (AST, ALT, bilirubin, alkaline phosphatase).

*Nursing implications are from Clayton B: Mosby's handbook of pharmacology, ed 4, St. Louis, 1987, The CV Mosby Co.

Continued.

Antipsychotic agents—cont'd

Generic name	Trade name	Major indications	Usual adult dosages

   c. Skin: photosensitivity may develop while a client is on phenothiazine therapy. Clients should be warned to wear protective clothing and avoid direct sunlight. A contact dermatitis may develop in those clients who have contact with solutions of phenothiazine derivatives. These clients should avoid physical contact with these solutions. Skin pigmentation, usually yellowish brown but possibly changing to grayish purple, may result from long-term (3 years or more) administration of large doses of phenothiazines. The pigmentation is more frequent in women, is usually restricted to exposed areas of the body, and may fade on discontinuance of therapy.

   d. Ophthalmic: long-term administration may lead to deposition of fine particulate matter in the lens and cornea. These eye lesions appear to be reversible on discontinuance of phenothiazine therapy.

   e. Cardiovascular: hypotension, tachycardia, fainting, and dizziness may occur, especially after parenteral administration. ECG changes similar to those caused by hypokalemia or quinidine may also occur.

   f. Endocrine: menstrual irregularities, delayed ovulation, galactorrhea, alterations in libido, glycosuria, hypoglycemia, weight gain, and high or prolonged glucose tolerance curves may occur.

   g. Other: phenothiazines may produce a myriad of side effects other than those already listed. These include gastrointestinal effects, alterations in body temperature regulation, particularly hypothermia, and respiratory depression, especially in those with impaired pulmonary function.

- Phenothiazines cross the placental barrier and may appear in the milk of nursing mothers. The effects of phenothiazine therapy on the human fetus is unknown. Therefore, these derivatives should be used on a risk versus benefit basis in pregnant women or those women planning to become pregnant while on phenothiazine therapy.

NONPHENOTHIAZINES

Haloperidol	Haldol	Relief of psychotic symptoms; relief of dyskinesia in Gilles de la Tourette's syndrome	0.5 to 5 mg P.O. b.i.d. or t.i.d. increased up to 100 mg/day if necessary

Nursing implications

- Extrapyramidal symptoms (akathisia or parkinsonian manifestations of marked drowsiness and lethargy, drooling and hypersalivation, fixed stare, and muscular rigidity) are the most common side effects of haloperidol. These symptoms often occur during the first few days of therapy and may require reduction in dosage, initiation of antiparkinsonian drug therapy (benztropine [Cogentin] 2 to 4 mg) or complete discontinuance of haloperidol therapy. Antiparkinsonian drugs should be continued after haloperidol has been discontinued because the slow elimination of haloperidol may cause a recurrence of the extrapyramidal symptoms.
- Tardive dyskinesia, manifested by recurrent protrusion of the tongue, puffing of the cheeks, puckering of the mouth, and chewing movements, may develop with long-term treatment with haloperidol. There appears to be a higher incidence in elderly female clients on high-dose therapy. This syndrome is irreversible in some clients, but may be prevented if the drug is discontinued at the first sign of fine tremorlike movements of the tongue.
- Haloperidol should be administered with caution in clients prone to seizures, since haloperidol may lower the convulsive threshold. Dosages of anticonvulsant therapy may require readjustment.
- Hypotension occurs infrequently but may be observed on IM injection or overdosage. It may be treated with IV fluids, plasma, albumin, or vasopressors such as norepinephrine or phenylephrine. *Do not use epinephrine*, since haloperidol blocks its vasopressor effects, resulting in further lowering of blood pressure.
- Other general adverse effects of haloperiodol include mild and transient leukopenia and leukocytosis, impaired liver function and/or jaundice, skin rashes and alopecia, anorexia, dry mouth, constipation, nausea and vomiting, blurred vision, urinary retention, bronchospasm, drowsiness, euphoria, and agitation.
- Haloperidol therapy is not recommended in pregnant women. Teratogenic effects have been reported; however, a causal relationship has not been established. Haloperidol also appears in the milk of lactating mothers.

ANA standards of psychiatric and mental health nursing practice

Standard I. Theory   The nurse applies appropriate theory that is scientifically sound as a basis for decisions regarding nursing practice.

Standard II. Data collection   The nurse continuously collects data that are comprehensive, accurate, and systematic.

Standard III. Diagnosis   The nurse utilizes *nursing diagnoses* and standard classification of mental disorders to express conclusions supported by recorded assessment data and current scientific premises.

Standard IV. Planning   The nurse develops a nursing care plan with specific goals and interventions delineating nursing actions unique to each client's needs.

Standard V. Intervention   The nurse intervenes as guided by the nursing care plan to implement nursing actions that promote, maintain, or restore physical and mental health, prevent illness, and effect rehabilitation.

Standard V-A. Psychotherapeutic interventions   The nurse (generalist) uses *psychotherapeutic interventions* to assist clients to regain or improve their previous coping abilities and to prevent further disability.

Standard V-B. Health teaching   The nurse assists clients, families, and groups to achieve satisfying and productive patterns of living through health teaching.

Standard V-C. Self-care activities   The nurse uses the activities of daily living in a goal-directed way to foster adequate self-care and physical and mental well-being of clients.

Standard V-D. Somatic therapies   The nurse uses knowledge of somatic therapies and applies related clinical skills in working with clients.

Standard V-E. Therapeutic environment   The nurse provides, structures, and maintains a therapeutic environment in collaboration with the client and other health care providers.

Standard V-F. Psychotherapy   The nurse (specialist) utilizes advanced clinical expertise in individual, group, and family psychotherapy, child psychotherapy, and other treatment modalities to function as a psychotherapist and recognizes professional accountability for nursing practice.

Standard VI. Evaluation   The nurse evaluates client responses to nursing actions in order to revise the data base, nursing diagnoses, and nursing care plan.

Standard VII. Peer review   The nurse participates in peer review and other means of evaluation to assure quality of nursing care provided for clients.

Standard VIII. Continuing education   The nurse assumes responsibility for continuing education and professional development and contributes to the professional growth of others.

Standard IX. Interdisciplinary collaboration   The nurse collaborates with interdisciplinary teams in assessing, planning, implementing, and evaluating programs and other mental health activities.

Standard X. Utilization of community health systems The nurse (specialist) participates with other members of the community in assessing, planning, implementing, and evaluating mental health services and community systems that include the promotion of the broad continuum of primary, secondary, and tertiary prevention of mental illness.

Standard XI. Research The nurse contributes to nursing and the mental health field through innovations in theory and practice and participation in research.

ANA standards of child and adolescent psychiatric and mental health nursing practice

PROFESSIONAL PRACTICE STANDARDS

Standard I. Theory   The nurse applies appropriate, scientifically sound theory as a basis for nursing practice decisions.

Standard II. Assessment   The nurse systematically collects, records, and analyzes data that are comprehensive and accurate.

Standard III. Diagnosis   The nurse, in expressing conclusions supported by recorded assessment and current scientific premises, uses nursing diagnoses and/or standard classifications of mental disorders for childhood and adolescence.

Standard IV. Planning   The nurse develops a nursing care plan with specific goals and interventions delineating nursing actions unique to the needs of each child or adolescent, as well as those of the family and other relevant interactive social systems.

Standard V. Intervention   The nurse intervenes as guided by the nursing care plan to implement nursing actions that promote, maintain, or restore physical and mental health, prevent illness, effect rehabilitation in childhood and adolescence, and restore developmental progression.

Standard V-A. Intervention: Therapeutic environment   The nurse provides, structures, and maintains a therapeutic environment in collaboration with the child or adolescent, the family, and other health care providers.

Standard V-B. Intervention: Activities of daily living   The nurse uses the activities of daily living in a goal-directed way to foster the physical and mental well-being of the child or adolescent and family.

Standard V-C. Intervention: Psychotherapeutic interventions   The nurse uses psychotherapeutic interventions to assist children or adolescents and families to develop, improve, or regain their adaptive functioning, to promote health, prevent illness, and facilitate rehabilitation.

Standard V-D. Intervention: Psychotherapy*   The child and adolescent psychiatric and mental health specialist uses advanced clinical expertise to function as a psychotherapist for the child or adolescent and family and accepts professional accountability for nursing practice.

Standard V-E. Intervention: Health teaching and anticipatory guidance   The nurse assists the child or adolescent and family to achieve more satisfying and productive patterns of living through health teaching and anticipatory guidance.

Standard V-F. Intervention: Somatic therapies   The nurse uses knowledge of somatic therapies with the child or adolescent and family to enhance therapeutic interventions.

Standard VI. Evaluation   The nurse evaluates the response of the child or adolescent and family to nursing actions in order to revise the data base, nursing diagnoses, and nursing care plan.

---

*Standards V-D and X apply only to the clinical specialist in child and adolescent psychiatric and mental health nursing. Reprinted with permission of the American Nurses' Association, 2420 Pershing Road, Kansas City, MO 64108. Copyright 1985.

PROFESSIONAL PERFORMANCE STANDARDS

Standard VII. Quality assurance The nurse participates in peer review and other means of evaluation to assure quality of nursing care provided for children and adolescents and their families.

Standard VIII. Continuing education The nurse assumes responsibility for continuing education and professional development and contributes to the professional growth of others studying children's and adolescents' mental health.

Standard IX. Interdisciplinary collaboration The nurse collaborates with other health care providers in assessing, planning, implementing, and evaluating programs and other activities related to child and adolescent psychiatric and mental health nursing.

Standard X. Use of community health systems* The nurse participates with other members of the community in assessing, planning, implementing, and evaluating mental health services and community systems that attend to primary, secondary, and tertiary prevention of mental disorders in children and adolescents.

Standard XI. Research The nurse contributes to nursing and the child and adolescent psychiatric and mental health field through innovations in theory and practice and participation in research, and communicates these contributions.

ANA standards of gerontological nursing practice

Standard I. Organization of gerontological nursing services All gerontological nursing services are planned, organized, and directed by a nurse executive. The nurse executive has baccalaureate or master's preparation and has experience in gerontological nursing and administration of long-term care services or acute care services for older clients.

Standard II. Theory The nurse participates in the generation and testing of theory as a basis for clinical decisions. The nurse uses theoretical concepts to guide the effective practice of gerontological nursing.

Standard III. Data collection The health status of the older person is regularly assessed in a comprehensive, accurate, and systematic manner. The information obtained during the health assessment is accessible to and shared with appropriate members of the interdisciplinary health care team, including the older person and the family.

Standard IV. Nursing diagnosis The nurse uses health assessment data to determine nursing diagnoses.

Standard V. Planning and continuity of care The nurse develops the plan of care in conjunction with the older person and appropriate others. Mutual goals, priorities, nursing approaches, and measures in the care plan address the therapeutic, preventive, restorative, and rehabilitative needs of the older person. The care plan helps the older person attain and maintain the highest level of health, well-being, and quality of life achievable,

as well as a peaceful death. The plan of care facilitates continuity of care over time as the client moves to various care settings and is revised as necessary.

Standard VI. Intervention The nurse, guided by the plan of care, intervenes to provide care to restore the older person's functional capabilities and to prevent complications and excess disability. Nursing interventions are derived from nursing diagnoses and are based on gerontological nursing theory.

Standard VII. Evaluation The nurse continually evaluates the client's and family's responses to interventions to determine progress toward goal attainment and to revise the data base, nursing diagnoses, and plan of care.

Standard VIII. Interdisciplinary collaboration The nurse collaborates with other members of the health care team in the various settings in which care is given to the older person. The team meets regularly to evaluate the effectiveness of the care plan for the client and family and to adjust the plan of care to accommodate changing needs.

Standard IX. Research The nurse participates in research designed to generate an organized body of gerontological nursing knowledge, disseminates research findings, and uses them in practice.

Standard X. Ethics The nurse uses the code for nurses established by the American Nurses' Association as a guide for ethical decision making in practice.

Standard XI. Professional development The nurse assumes responsibility for professional development and contributes to the professional growth of interdisciplinary team members. The nurse participates in peer review and other means of evaluation to assure the quality of nursing practice.

Reprinted with permission of the American Nurses' Association, 2420 Pershing Road, Kansas City, MO 64108. Copyright 1987.

ANA standards of addictions nursing practice

Standard I. Theory The nurse uses appropriate knowledge from nursing theory and related disciplines in the practice of addictions nursing.

Standard II. Data collection Data collection is continual and systemic and is communicated effectively to the treatment team throughout each phase of the nursing process.

Standard III. Diagnosis The nurse uses nursing diagnoses congruent with accepted nursing and interprofessional classification systems of addictions and associated physiological and psychological disorders to express conclusions supported by data obtained through the nursing process.

Standard IV. Planning The nurse establishes a plan of care for the client that is based upon nursing diagnoses, addresses specific goals, defines expected outcomes, and delineates nursing actions unique to each client's needs.

Standard V. Intervention The nurse implements actions independently and/or in collaboration with peers, members of other disciplines, and clients in prevention, intervention, and rehabilitation phases of the care of clients with health problems related to patterns of abuse and addiction.

Standard V-A. Intervention: Therapeutic alliance The nurse uses the "therapeutic self" to establish a relationship with clients and to structure nursing interventions to help clients develop the awareness, coping skills, and behavior changes that promote health.

Standard V-B. Intervention: Education The nurse educates clients and communities to help them prevent and/or correct actual or potential health problems related to patterns of abuse and addiction.

Standard V-C. Intervention: Self-help groups The nurse uses the knowledge and philosophy of self-help groups to assist clients in learning new ways to address stress, maintain self-control or sobriety, and integrate healthy coping behaviors into their life-style.

Standard V-D. Intervention: Pharmacological therapies The nurse applies knowledge of pharmacological principles in the nursing process.

Standard V-E. Intervention: Therapeutic environment The nurse provides, structures, and maintains a therapeutic environment in collaboration with the individual, family, and other professionals.

Standard V-F. Intervention: Counseling The nurse uses therapeutic communication in interactions with the client to address issues related to patterns of abuse and addiction.

Standard VI. Evaluation The nurse evaluates the responses of the client and revises nursing diagnoses, interventions, and the treatment plan accordingly.

Standard VII. Ethical care The nurse's decisions and activities on behalf of clients are in keeping with personal and professional codes of ethics and in accord with legal statutes.

Standard VIII. Quality assurance The nurse participates in peer review and other staff evaluation and quality assurance processes to ensure that clients with abuse and addiction problems receive quality care.

Standard IX. Continuing education The nurse assumes responsibility for his or her continuing education and professional development and contributes to the professional growth of others who work with or are learning about persons with abuse and addiction problems.

Standard X. Interdisciplinary collaboration The nurse collaborates with the interdisciplinary treatment team and consults with other health care providers in assessing, planning, implementing, and evaluating programs and other activities related to addictions nursing.

Standard XI. Use of community health systems The nurse participates with other members of the community in assessing, planning, implementing, and evaluating community health services that attend to primary, secondary, and tertiary prevention of addictions.

Standard XII. Research The nurse contributes to the nursing care of clients with addictions and to the addictions area of practice through innovations in theory and practice and participation in research and communicates these contributions.

Index

A

Psychiatric nursing—cont'd
  definition of, 45
  future directions for, 45-46
  levels of preparation for, 5
  and liability insurance coverage, 45
  modern, development of, 41-46
  principles of, 327-330
  relevance of, to professional nursing, 5-6
  supervisory process in, 330
Psychiatric nursing generalist, 5
Psychiatric nursing specialist, 5
Psychiatrist on mental health team, 7, 8
Psychiatry
  community, crisis theory and, 419-420
  forensic, 76
  orthomolecular, 795
  preventive, 30, 32
Psychodrama in therapeutic milieu, 349-350
Psychodynamic theory, 17-20
Psychoeducation of families of schizophrenic clients, 813-815
Psychologist, clinical, on mental health team, 6-7, 8
Psychoneuroimmunology, 570
Psychopharmaceuticals; *see also* Drugs, antipsychotic
  characteristics and nursing implications of, 896-906
  for chronic brain syndrome, 862
  for neuroses, 734
  for schizophrenia, 808-812
Psychopharmacology for depression, 694-695
Psychophysiologic dysfunction, 555-556, 573-574, 578
  and accident-prone behavior, 567-568
  biochemical theory of, 570-571, 572t
  classification of, 557-572
  and conditioned or learned response, 569-570
  development of, 567-568
  early identification of, 575
  emergency intervention for, 572
  explanatory theories of, 568-572, 572t
  and family, 571
  family and, nursing implications of, 572t
  family therapy for, 573
  high-risk groups for, identifying, 574
  historical perspectives of, 556
  individual and group therapy for, 573
  intervention in, focus of, 575
  learned response and, 572t
  nursing assessment of, 576
  nursing intervention for, 573-578
  pharmacology for, 572-573
  psychoanalytic theory of, 568, 572t
  psychodynamic theory of, 568, 572t
  stress and change and, 568-569, 572t
  systems theory and, 571-572
  systems theory of, nursing implications of, 572t
  treatment modalities for, 572-573
  underlying dynamics of, 556-557

Psychosis
  amphetamine, 798
  mescaline, and schizophrenia, 801
Psychotherapy
  for borderline personality disorder, 764-766
  group, for neuroses, 732-733
  for organic brain dysfunction, 861-862
  psychoanalytic, for neuroses, 732
  research in, nursing's involvement in, 79
  for schizophrenia, 812-813
Pyroluria, 795

Q

Quality assurance, definition of, 72

R

Rape, 638-640
  two-phase response to, 639t
Rape-trauma syndrome, 322, 639
Rapist, types of, 638t
Rationalization
  personality development and, 156t
  by substance and practice abusers, 584
Rauwolfia serpentina for schizophrenia, 808
rCBF; *see* Regional cerebral blood flow
Reactive disorders in children, 475-476
Reality
  codification of, 105-106
  perception of, without distortion, 165, 174
Reassurance in nurse-client relationship, 329
Recall, difficulty in, in chronic brain syndrome, 849
Reciprocals, in nonverbal communication, 284, 286t
Recreational therapist, on mental health team, 7, 8
Regional cerebral blood flow, 800
Rehabilitation following human abuse, professional services for, 664
Reinterpretation, in group therapy, 649
Relationship(s)
  abusive, mourning loss of, 635, 636t
  inter-ethnic, 103-104
Religion
  enculturation and, 95-97
  and personality development, 148-149
  and sexuality, 204-205
Religiosity
  in schizophrenia, 791
  sexual behavior and, 204-205
Relocation, assistance with, for homeless mentally ill, 447t
Remembering, steps in, 534
Repoise; *see* Butaperazine
Report of the Joint Commission on Mental Health of Children, 469, 470
Report of the Joint Commission on Mental Health and Mental Illness, 419
Repression, 17-18
Reproductive system, effects of alcohol on, 592t
Research, vulnerability of, in schizophrenia, 816
Reserpine, 808

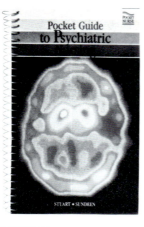

POCKET NURSE GUIDE TO PSYCHIATRIC NURSING
by Gail Wiscarz Stuart, Ph.D., R.N., M.S.; Sandra J. Sundeen, R.N., M.S. (5270-7)

POCKET NURSE GUIDE TO PSYCHIATRIC NURSING, by Gail Stewart and Sandra Sundeen is an easy to use reference that puts psychiatric nursing interventions at the reader's fingertips. This practical guide uses tables, charts, and lists to succinctly, but thoroughly, present interventions.

- Organizes material in two units — Foundations of Psychiatric Nursing Practice and Psychiatric Nursing Interventions.
- Includes NANDA-approved nursing diagnoses, and the revised DSM-III classifications.
- Features the latest information on psychotropic drugs.

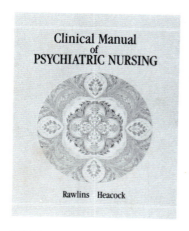

CLINICAL MANUAL OF PSYCHIATRIC NURSING
by Ruth Parmelee Rawlins, R.N., M.S.E., C.S.; Patricia Heacock, R.N., Ph.D. (4096-2)

CLINICAL MANUAL OF PSYCHIATRIC NURSING is a practical, A-to-Z clinical reference that takes a holistic approach to over 30 maladaptive behaviors within a nursing process framework.

- Gives a conceptual framework for holistic care that consistently addresses the five dimensions of health: physical, emotional, intellectual, social, and spiritual.
- Includes for each disorder: definitions theoretical principles, assessment, diagnosis, planning, implementation and evaluation, case studies, and references.
- Provides a handy assessment tool that thoroughly, yet succinctly familiarizes you with all assessment areas.
- Enumerates interventions step by step and explains the rationale for each action.
- Offers case studies for applying knowledge to clinical examples.

Both of these handy references are a must for your reference library, as you prepare for your clinical rotation. To order, ask your bookstore manager or call toll-free 800-221-7700, ext. 15A. We look forward to hearing from you.